Urinalysis in the
Dog and Cat

Urinalysis in the Dog and Cat

Dennis J. Chew

DVM Diplomate ACVIM (Internal Medicine)
Professor Emeritus
Veterinary Medical Center
The Ohio State University, Columbus, OH, USA

Patricia A. Schenck

DVM, PhD
Veterinary Consulting
DeWitt, MI, USA

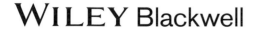

Registered Offices
John Wiley & Sons, Inc., 111 River Street, Hoboken, NJ 07030, USA

Editorial Office
111 River Street, Hoboken, NJ 07030, USA

For details of our global editorial offices, customer services, and more information about Wiley products visit us at www.wiley.com.

Wiley also publishes its books in a variety of electronic formats and by print-on-demand. Some content that appears in standard print versions of this book may not be available in other formats.

Library of Congress Cataloging-in-Publication Data applied for
[PB ISBN: 9781119226345]

Cover Design: Wiley
Cover Images: Dennis Chew, Michael L. Horton
Cover Illustration: Tom Vojt

Set in 9.5/12pts of STIXTwoText by Straive, Pondicherry, India

Printed in Singapore
M063699_260123

This book is dedicated TO Dr. Richard C. Scott and Dr. Carl A. Osborne for their untiring efforts to promote the value of the complete urinalysis, encouraging all veterinarians to both perform and interpret the urinalysis with accuracy.

Dr. Scott ("Scotty") emphasized the need to perform urine microscopy within 15 minutes of urine collection. That was the practice of the day at the Animal Medical Center, New York, NY during the evaluation of sick dogs and cats being seen by the Medicine Service and on all consults for other hospital services. The so-called rare urinary elements were found with surprising frequency (e.g. WBC casts, RBC casts, and renal tubular epithelium) when fresh warm urine was examined. Dr. Scott's influence in this arena cannot be overstated, due to the large numbers of interns and residents that were engaged in the routine viewing of urine microscopy and integration of those findings into the two other components of the complete urinalysis (physical properties and urine chemistry) as part of daily rounds. Dr. Scott routinely acquired photomicrographs of urine sediment to assist in his teaching, some of which are in this book. I continue to admire Scotty for all of his contributions to nephrology, but I believe his biggest contribution was sharing his expertise and philosophy regarding the value of urine microscopy.

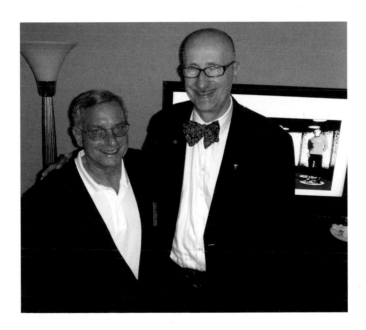

Dr. Osborne's influence in urology and nephrology was extensive and also pioneering in so many instances. Dr. Osborne believed in the need for the profession to reconfigure its thinking, to understand that it was ESSENTIAL to get a urine sample on all patients and then integrate the results of the complete urinalysis with the blood work from those patients. He detailed how to interpret results from urinalysis during his many extensive continuing education lectures, which influenced generations of graduate veterinarians and students. His mantra that using the results of a partial urinalysis was analogous to doing a CBC without a differential cell count is legendary. Dr. Osborne enthusiastically promoted the use of routine urinalysis and emphasized that a medical workup was incomplete without it. His numerous publications usually referenced the value that results of a complete urinalysis brought to case management and to understanding the pathophysiology of a particular disease. "Just get the urine sample and submit the urinalysis, you will be glad that you did."

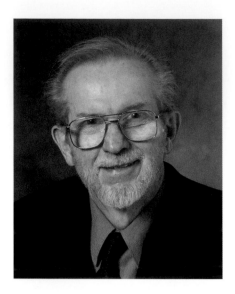

A shout-out to the fathers of modern veterinary nephrology in addition to Dr. Carl Osborne; Drs. Del Finco, Don Low, Ken Bovee, and Jerry Ling. It is necessary to acknowledge the foundation laid for all of the advances in veterinary urology and nephrology that were to follow. There were many veterinarians, too numerous to list, trained or heavily influenced by these pioneers, that contributed to the growth and advancement of the field of urology and nephrology.

Further thanks to the many students, interns, residents, and graduate veterinarians who asked those basic and clinically relevant questions, that were at times difficult to answer with certainty, for spurring me on to try to find answers. And I must especially thank my patients, the animals for which we were privileged to study their urine and their diseases in our attempts to help them and to the many cats and dogs in my home that taught me way more than I thought possible about urinary diseases and life in general.

To the performance of a complete urinalysis along with every CBC and biochemistry submitted.

To the collection of fresh warm urine for immediate urinalysis – make it so!

Brief Contents

Table of Contents

5 | Chemical Properties of Urine

7   Proteinuria   236

8 Atlas 317

9 Frequently Asked Questions (FAQ) 383

10 Case Studies 406

Glossary 500

Index 514

How to Read and Use this Book

This book largely reflects how I think findings from the components of the complete urinalysis (urine physical properties, urine chemistry, and urine microscopy) can best be clinically integrated and interpreted. My clinical experience combined with an extensive review of the literature informs much of this interpretation, but high-quality evidence may not be available to support some of my opinions, conclusions, and recommendations. I have tried to be clear where my experience and opinion are the primary support for a conclusion. Basic to advanced information is provided in most chapters. References are extensive by design, as many of the references are old and difficult to find. This book has been written largely from a urine-centric view, meaning that findings from urine are featured first and then other data from cytology or histopathology, hematology, serum biochemistry, and imaging are integrated afterward.

As with any scientific book, some information in this book may already be outdated due to current research. But core concepts for performing and interpreting the urinalysis have remained stable and are not expected to quickly or radically change over time. The chapter on proteinuria (Chapter 7) is the chapter most likely to be affected by current and ongoing research, yielding new information of clinical consequence for the diagnosis and management of renal proteinuria. It is also likely that new information will be published regarding the use of automated urinary sediment readers, as this is a recent technological advancement. Readers of this book should be aware that Internet Websites listed in this work may have changed or disappeared between when this work was published and when you read it.

The information in this book is accurate to the best of my abilities, but nearly all books have inadvertent errors or insufficient coverage of some topics. I believe that the content in this book is complete to the extent that a clinical book of this nature should be. Always question anything in this book that does not make sense to you. You should always double-check and verify drug dosages. Ultimately, it is your obligation to decide what you believe to be accurate and useful in your clinical practice. I would appreciate hearing from you (dennischew@me.com) about any specific places in the book that you find to be unclear, suspect to be in error, that contains discrepancies with other places in the book, or is missing some important part of urinalysis which you expected to find.

This book is not likely to be read in its entirety from start to finish, except by the most interested readers. It is a reference – not a novel. It is expected that you will pick and choose selected sections that have information relevant to a current need for understanding or a clinical question. There is some overlap in content and concepts between the chapters that is by design, as repetition can reinforce learning of important or complicated material. The outline at the beginning of each chapter should help you find relevant subheadings quickly and the detailed index should also help you get to the specific information you are seeking.

Each chapter has the basic information in the beginning and progresses to more advanced and detailed/technical information later. Where relevant, clinically applied sections follow discussions of diagnostics and pathophysiology. This book was primarily written to be useful to students, veterinarians in general practices, and veterinary technicians. However, residents and specialists in internal medicine, nephrology and urology, clinical pathologists, and anyone seeking more will find advanced concepts in most chapters which should be of use to them, both in teaching and in practice.

This book is visually rich with hundreds of high-quality photomicrographs, medical illustrations, tables, and algorithms. Most of the images for urinary sediment were collected during my time at The Ohio State University College of Veterinary Medicine – initially using a film photomicroscope system and later with digital capture. Other images were given to me to use by permission as noted in the legends. The legends for many of the urine microscopy images are often detailed and contain history or outcome when available.

Legends for some of the medical illustrations (those drawn by Tim Vojt) are quite detailed. The language in the legends generally parallels that in the main text but may be modified to tell the story in a slightly different way. It is best to read both the figure legend and the main text that aligns with that illustration in order to best understand the illustration. Tables that summarize important concepts are included in most chapters.

There are numerous algorithms in this book designed to capture a plausible decision-making flow after you identify a particular abnormality. Some of these algorithms are simple and some are complex. In general, readers usually either like or hate the concept of algorithms in decision-making. As almost no algorithm is perfect in all clinical situations, do not blindly follow any one of the algorithms; rather, use them for general guidance in your particular situation.

If you are perplexed about a particular finding from a urinalysis result on one of your patients and cannot find an adequate answer after searching in this book or others, consultation with a clinical pathologist or specialist in urology and nephrology is recommended. Sending pictures from urine microscopy that contain mysterious or unidentified elements to specialists is recommended in order to gain more definitive information. These pictures can be taken using your smartphone camera during manual microscopy, or from digital images acquired during automated microscopy.

If you are weak in renal physiology, Renal Anatomy and Applied Renal Physiology (Chapter 1) offers a review of basic renal functions with extensive review of how urine is concentrated. A general understanding of this chapter is needed as background for content that follows in most of the other chapters.

If you are intimidated by the scope and depth of this book, I suggest that you start by reading Frequently Asked Questions (Chapter 9) and Urinalysis Case Examples (Chapter 10) that are not so heavy on pathophysiology. These two chapters are filled with clinically relevant scenarios that have the potential to whet your appetite to read the more formal detailed chapters and will get you excited about going back to the earlier chapters to better understand what you are seeing in the case examples (and your own patient's urinalyses). Reading the Glossary is also likely to be helpful. I recommend that you read the detailed chapter on Proteinuria (Chapter 7) last, since this is the most complex chapter in this book.

If you do not want to read the formal text in each chapter right now:

1. Review the figures and read their legends, realizing that the legends are a supplement to the text.

2. Review the tables and their legends in order to get a feel for the chapter detail to follow, again realizing that you will be getting an incomplete picture without referring to the text.

3. Review the algorithms and their legends as a supplement to the text.

4. For serious students of urology and nephrology, READ EVERYTHING.

Foreword

It is my honor to introduce the first edition of *Urinalysis in the Dog and Cat*. Dr. Dennis Chew is a giant among those of us who have dedicated our careers to veterinary nephrology and urology. Dr. Chew possesses a wealth of knowledge and experiences that comes only after decades of consulting with veterinarians about, and having primary case responsibility for, dogs and cats with diseases of the urinary tract. He has been able to give back so much of this expertise to our profession in the pages of this book.

The book is designed to be a comprehensive yet useful guide to understanding all aspects of urine and the urinalysis. It is rich in algorithms, tables, images, and beautiful artwork that enhance the contents of the book but also provide for quick reference as needed. The FAQ and case examples serve to consolidate the information. Although meant as a reference rather than a book to be read from cover to cover, I had trouble putting the book down because the content is so interesting and I was able to discover relevant information that could be applied to several of my current patients. *Urinalysis in the Dog and Cat* should soon find its place in the hands of anyone who wants to "go for the gold" and practice high-quality small animal medicine.

Shelly L. Vaden, DVM, PhD, DACVIM
Founder ACVNU
Professor of Nephrology and Urology
College of Veterinary Medicine
North Carolina State University

Many years ago when I was a third-year veterinary student at The Ohio State University, a young newly minted bowtie-wearing assistant professor walked <u>into</u> our urinary system course and began teaching us about how the kidneys function and how urine is produced. This was our introduction to the inimitable Dr. Dennis Chew.

Dr. Chew is the consummate professor and has had a long and distinguished career teaching veterinary students, interns and residents, veterinary technicians, and legions of veterinarians all around the world. One of the things that struck me during those early lectures has remained true throughout Dr. Chew's tenure as a veterinary educator of the highest level. Dennis is as passionate today as he was then about the importance of urinalysis and doing things right, and this is clearly evidenced through the excellence of this new book, *Urinalysis of the Dog and Cat*.

Throughout my career as a specialist and while serving as chief medical officer for VCA for many years, I have had the opportunity to work closely with over a thousand small animal hospitals of all sizes in primary care as well as specialty. Veterinary medicine has advanced leaps and bounds over the last four decades, and we have witnessed many technological advances. Today we routinely perform ultrasonography, echocardiography, endoscopy, advanced imaging using CT and MRI, and we rely on many types of antigen and PCR tests to help us diagnose our patients' illnesses with ever greater accuracy and understanding. Despite all of the high-tech options, however, urinalysis remains a critical component of the minimum database and is a must as we evaluate our patients not only when they are ill, but also every time we perform wellness screening/early detection tests. We still underutilize this important test and it is essential for us to be more thorough. We must also know how to interpret the results accurately!

Urinalysis of the Dog and Cat is a *must have* for all small animal hospital libraries. I am excited about this book because we now have an all-encompassing practical new reference work to not only instruct us on how to accurately interpret results but also correctly obtain and manage urine samples. But there is so much more at the fingertips of the reader. I enjoyed reviewing the chapters, and it was hard to stop reading as there are so many updates on patient management tips, i.e. what do we do with the results once we have them. Small animal veterinarians all see patients with some type of urinary tract disorder every month. What do we do about subtle early changes in laboratory tests? Early detection and intervention is always our goal, and it all starts with the minimum database. Chapter 1 sets the stage through a review of renal physiology and evaluation of function, Chapter 7 delves deeply into proteinuria (timely update!), and Chapter 9 presents 127 Frequently Asked Questions (FAQ) that can serve as entire "short course" on urinary tract issues. It is written in trademark Dennis Chew style: thorough, clear, and conversational. Common misconceptions and errors in interpretation are explained (e.g. overemphasis on crystals, potential for misinterpretation of "cocci" in urine sediment, and what SDMA is and isn't, among many others).

Chapter 10 includes 47 cases for which the complete urinalysis is presented and then detailed interpretation, recommendations for further diagnostics, and final diagnosis are given. No doubt readers will recognize similar cases from their own practices and be able to compare notes on interpretation and diagnostic pathways as well as how to get the most out of basic testing when everything on the diagnostic menu just can't be done due to financial constraints. Test yourself!

Dr. Chew is famous for his "isms" which he has interjected in his teaching over the years, and readers will see these interspersed throughout the book. I have always enjoyed these "isms" because they continually remind us about the importance of doing things right! Among my favorites from Dr. Chew are, "JUST DO IT! (urinalysis), FAKE NEWS: USG and urine chemistry dipstrip results are good enough without urine sediment microscopy," and "When blood test results return without results of urinalysis at the same time, you are driving partly blind-folded." Readers will find great value throughout this text, as I did on my first review, and their patients will be the beneficiaries of their veterinarians always striving to stay up to date and practice evidence-based medicine. The ability to help animals in need is what makes veterinary medicine such a great profession to be a part of.

It is an honor for me to write this Foreword.

Todd R. Tams, DVM, DACVIM
Vice President for External Affairs
Mars Veterinary Health
VCA Chief Medical Officer (Emeritus)
Los Angeles, California

Preface

"Superficially it might be said that the function of the kidneys is to make urine, but in a more considered view one can say that the kidneys make the stuff of philosophy itself." Homer William Smith: A Memoir, New York University Press 1965; Homer Smith: The Evolution of the Kidney, Lectures on the Kidney 1943.

The initial impetus for writing this book was the desire to share my extensive collection of urinary sediment images, originally captured as Kodachrome slides and then with digitally acquired photomicrographs, collected over a period of nearly 40 years. These images provide multiple examples of common abnormal urinary elements, which show the many slight variations in appearance that are possible. Many of the urine microscopy images are designed to show routine abnormalities, whereas other images feature uncommonly described or rarely recognized elements. Though these images, with their legends can often stand alone, I believe there is more value when the images are combined with the fuller explanations provided in the various chapters.

Thus, the scope of this book grew and became an effort to provide a comprehensive look into the complete urinalysis, emphasizing integration of findings from physical properties (e.g. USG), urine chemistry by dipstrip, and urine microscopy (evaluation of urinary sediment). The Renal Anatomy and Applied Renal Physiology (Chapter 1) provides the backdrop showing how urine is formed by a combination of glomerular filtration and then extensive modification of that initial fluid by tubular secretion and/or reabsorption of water and small molecules. Proteinuria (Chapter 7) provides a more detailed look into the world of proteinuria than that provided in the Chemical Properties of Urine (Chapter 5) that emphasized measurement by dipstrip.

The primary intent for this book "Urinalysis in the Dog and Cat" is for it to be a useful reference which will allow practicing veterinarians to more fully recognize abnormal findings, and to understand, integrate, and interpret the results from a urinalysis to improve their understanding of their patient's illnesses. Except for guidelines on how to mitigate renal proteinuria (Chapter 7), the treatment of specific conditions is not the goal of this book. Rather, the numerous images of urinary sediment in Urinary Microscopy (Chapter 6) and Atlas (Chapter 8) along with their detailed legends are presented to help veterinary technicians and attending veterinarians more accurately identify abnormal elements, from both manual and automated in-house urinalysis. Similarly, veterinary students should find these images useful, allowing them to more confidently identify elements during urine microscopy. There is additional value to this book when it is read by clinicians wanting a greater understanding of their patients by revealing how findings from urinalysis could help improve the diagnosis and management of cases in primary care and specialty practices. This book should also prove useful during clinical training of residents in internal medicine and in clinical pathology.

In addition to detailed pathophysiology, I provide nuggets of clinically useable information throughout the chapters. When appropriate, nuts and bolts technical information has been provided (e.g. how to set up for urine microscopy). Pitfalls are also identified, explaining what can go wrong when performing or evaluating the results of a urinalysis, whether considering physical, chemical, and/or microscopic properties.

Extensive referencing has been provided for those wanting to know where this content arose and for those in academia wanting to dive deeper. The Frequently Asked Questions (Chapter 9) and Urinalysis Case Examples (Chapter 10) provide clinical details appropriate for veterinary students as well as for graduate veterinarians who want a hook that will encourage them to read the more formal chapters. See "How to Read/Use This Book" (front matter below) for suggestions on how those with different learning styles might gain the information they are seeking more readily.

Ultimately, I hope this book sparks some excitement that shows the ultimate value of routinely performing urinalysis on patients that allows that component of the diagnostic testing profile to achieve the respect it deserves. If that happens, I believe our canine and feline patients, and you – my colleagues – will benefit from more accurate diagnoses and

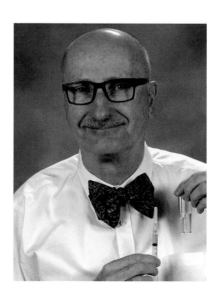

treatment plans. You can expect to gain increasingly nuanced interpretation of urinalysis results after reading and processing the information in this book. I am also hopeful that the ability of our technicians to generate increased accuracy of their results when performing in-house urinalyses will result from the lessons presented in this book. Performing automated (microscopy, urine chemistry dipstrip) or manual urinalysis in-house provides increased value to your practice, your patients, and your clients when the highest standards for urine handling and technical performance are in place.

"Go for THE GOLD" (Dr. Craig Greene).
"Learn to Love the Secret Language of Urine." (Dr. Jonathan Reisman Opinions, Washington Post November 23, 2016)

Acknowledgements

Dr. Stephen DiBartola (DVM, DACVIM) and I spent over 30 years working together at the Ohio State University (OSU) College of Veterinary Medicine. We pushed each other to be the best urinary specialists we could be, as we provided each other frequent feedback in clinics, classroom teaching, research, and publications. Our combined clinical experiences, case management philosophies, and publications are reflected in the contents of this book. Thanks to Steve for some of the early editing in this project.

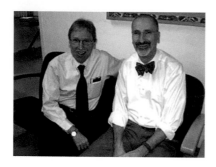

Dr. Arthur Lage (DVM, DACVIM) showed me that it was possible to both develop special expertise in urology and nephrology in private practice and also still be productive in an academic research program. His mentoring as I performed my first 24-hour quantitative urinalysis during the first week of my internship helped to enforce the value of the quantitative urinalysis in addition to that of the more routine complete urinalysis in my early training.

Dr. Dennis DeNicola (DVM, PhD, DACVP) critiqued an early version of the urine microscopy chapter in this book that helped me gain greater focus. He also convinced me that a comprehensive book on urinalysis was really needed and encouraged me to keep writing. He was kind enough to provide me access to the IDEXX SediVue® digital images that are provided in the Urine Microscopy and Atlas chapters.

Dr. Michelle Larsen (DVM) for providing digital images acquired by Zoetis SA® in the Urine Microscopy and Atlas chapters.

Dr. Heather Wamsley (DVM, PhD, DACVP) provided many of the urine sediment abnormal element images found in the Urine Microscopy and Atlas chapters. Her expertise regarding and enthusiasm for urine evaluation, especially the examination of urinary sediment, energized me at important steps during this project. It was fun and empowering to have a colleague with this level of skill sharing with me, in text messages and emails, the interesting things she discovered during her daily clinical pathology work evaluating urine samples.

I am thankful for the willingness of Dr. **Jessica Hokamp** (DVM, PhD, DACVP), **Dr. Mary Nabity** (DVM, PhD DACVP), **Dr. Rachel Cianciolo** (DVM, PhD DACVP), **Dr. Kendal Harr** (DVM, MS, DACVP), and **Dr. Meryl Littman** (VMD, DACVIM) to share their expertise about urine chemistry, renal proteinuria, glomerular diseases, and urine microscopy while answering quite a few of my questions along the way. They are acknowledged as personal communications in the chapters. A shoutout to **Dr. Valerie Parker** for evaluating concepts regarding dietary treatment of glomerular proteinuria.

Dr. Patricia Schenck (DVM, PhD) was pivotal for the role she provided in organizing and editing content within all the chapters. I am not a linear writer – so this was a big challenge. She tried to teach me to use an outline to no avail. She spent many tedious hours organizing my writing so that it appeared in a logical sequence. She was a stickler for detail in use of language, punctuation, and clarity. She provided me valuable and continuing feedback regarding better strategies on how to approach topics in several places throughout the book. She reviewed the algorithms in detail to ensure that they made sense. As we had worked together on several prior projects, she often knew what I was really trying to say more clearly than what was written on the pages. Dr. Schenck provided me great energy as she used her editing skills to improve these chapters. Perhaps most importantly, she would not let me give up during the past two years of intense writing and editing.

Thanks to **Erica Judisch** – Executive Editor, Veterinary Medicine and Dentistry at Wiley-Blackwell who appreciated the need for and had a vision for this book at the start of this project. In its original conception, the content level appropriate for this book was a moving target but over time evolved into the design and writing of this comprehensive work. She always was on board to help us as the writing and figure developments matured.

Rosie Hayden was the Senior Managing Editor with Wiley-Blackwell when the manuscript was first submitted in full. I appreciate her availability and efforts to see this project through to completion.

Special thanks to the talented medical photographers and medical illustrators over the years at **The OSU College of Veterinary Medicine's Department of Biomedical Media**. **Dr. Phil Murdick** deserves tremendous credit for his vision that a biomedical media section within the veterinary school would enrich the teaching, research, and publication lives of OSU faculty. **Dan Patton** was the original head of biomedical media, and he hired and mentored the talent in this group. He manned an amazing photomicrography station with top-of-the-line quality of photomicroscopic equipment and cameras. He soon realized that it was very important to immediately take pictures of elements in the urine sediment; otherwise, cellular degeneration or breakup of fragile elements like casts and renal tubular epithelium could easily happen quickly. He was usually able to accommodate my request for a photomicrograph within 10 minutes of a urine sediment being created for which I remain grateful.

Tim Vojt is the medical illustrator at The Ohio State College of Veterinary Medicine who contributed numerous figures and drawings to this book. He is the sole survivor of that section of the biomedical media department, due to relentless budget cuts over the years. I am thankful that recent administrations have chosen to support his work. We had several traditional medical illustrators in the past who did great work by hand. Tim took medical illustration to a whole new level with his digital drawing abilities, which I think you will appreciate throughout this book. I am amazed at Tim's ability to understand how his drawings will fit into whatever concepts I am trying to develop for a project. After each meeting with me to try to understand how best the drawing could come into being, Tim became one with his art. Tim researched just about everything related to the drawings, especially anatomy and physiology. Tim was always gentle and willing to deal with me despite my scattershot approach to ideas that were frequently emerging while he was constructing the first drafts of his images. I come close to weeping when I review the stunning quality of many of the illustrations that he developed for use in this book.

To **Ron Sacks** for steadfast love and support during a much longer time to finish this project than could possibly have been imagined at the start: Thanks for putting up with me and my endless babbling of things related to urine.

Abbreviations

1,25(OH)$_2$-vitamin D	1,25-dihydroxyvitamin D, calcitriol	Cr	creatinine
25D	25-hydroxyvitamin D	CRF	chronic renal failure
ACE2	angiotensin II converting enzyme 2	CRGV	cutaneous and renal glomerular vasculopathy
ACE-I	angiotensin-converting enzyme inhibitor	CT	collecting tubule
ACTH	adrenocorticotrophic hormone	CT	computed tomography
ACVIM	American College of Veterinary Internal Medicine	CV	coefficient of variation
		d	diameter
ADH	antidiuretic hormone	dDAVP	l-deamino-8-D-arginine vasopressin, desmopressin
AG	aminoglycoside		
AG	angiotensin	DHA	docosahexaenoic acid
AI/ML	artificial intelligence/ machine learning	DIC	disseminated intravascular coagulation
AIHA	autoimmune hemolytic anemia	DM	diabetes mellitus
AKI	acute kidney injury	DNA	deoxyribonucleic acid
ALP	alkaline phosphatase	DOCA	desoxycorticosterone acetate
ALT	alanine transaminase	DT	distal tubule
ANA	antinuclear antibodies	ECC	endogenous creatinine clearance
ANOVA	analysis of variance	ECF	extracellular fluid
APPD	apparent psychogenic polydipsia	ECFV	extracellular fluid volume
AQP	aquaporin	EDTA	ethylenediaminetetraacetic acid
ARB	angiotensin-II receptor blockers	EG	ethylene glycol
AST	aspartate aminotransferase	ELISA	enzyme-linked immunoassay
ATN	acute tubular necrosis	EM	electron microscopy
ATP	adenosine triphosphate	EMT	renal epithelial to mesenchymal cell transitioning
AVP	arginine vasopressin		
BHA	beta-hydroxybutyric acid	EPA	eicosapentaenoic acid
BP	blood pressure	epi	epithelial cell
BRAF	serine/threonine-protein kinase B-Raf, proto-oncogene B-Raf	FC	fractional clearance
		FDA	Food and Drug Administration
BUN	blood urea nitrogen	FeLV	feline leukemia virus
Ca:P	calcium:phosphorus ratio	FeMV	feline morbillivirus
CAH	copper-associated hepatopathy	FGF-23	fibroblast growth factor-23
cAMP	cyclic adenosine monophosphate	FIC	feline idiopathic/interstitial cystitis
CaR	calcium receptor	FIP	feline infectious peritonitis
CAV-1	canine adenovirus	FIV	feline immunodeficiency virus
CBB	Coomassie brilliant blue	FN	field number
CBC	complete blood count	FNA	fine needle aspirate
CCB	calcium channel blockers	FOV	field of view
CDI	central diabetes insipidus	Fr	French
CFU (cfu)	colony forming unit	FSGS	focal segmental glomerulosclerosis
CHF	congestive heart failure	GAG	glycosaminoglycan
CK	creatine kinase	GBM	glomerular basement membrane
CKD	chronic kidney disease	GDI	gestational diabetes insipidus
CNN	convolutional neural network	GFR	glomerular filtration rate
CNS	central nervous system	GI	gastrointestinal

GN	glomerulonephritis	PDH	pituitary-dependent hyperadrenocorticism
HAC	hyperadrenocorticism		
HMW	high molecular weight	PGE2	prostaglandin E2 (also listed as PgE$_2$)
HN	hereditary nephropathy	PgI$_2$	prostaglandin I$_2$
HPF	high-power field	PKD	polycystic kidney disease
HPLC	high-performance liquid chromatography	PLE	protein-losing enteropathy
		PLN	protein-losing nephropathy
HTG	hypertriglyceridemia	POC	point of care
HUS	hemolytic uremic syndrome	P$_{osm}$	plasma osmolality
HW	heartworm	PPD	psychogenic polydipsia, primary polydipsia
ICGN	immune-complex glomerulonephritis		
		PRM	pyrogallol red molybdate
ICU	intensive care unit	PSS	portosystemic shunt
IFA	Immunofluorescent antibody	PTH	parathyroid hormone
Ig	immunoglobulin	PTHrP	parathyroid hormone related protein
IHC	idiopathic hypercalcemia	PU/PD	polyuria/polydipsia
IRIS	International Renal Interest Society	PUBS	purple urine bag syndrome
ISCAID	International Society for Companion Animal Infectious Diseases	PUFA	polyunsaturated fatty acids
		RAAS	renin–angiotensin–aldosterone system
IV	intravenous		
IVRPS	International Veterinary Renal Pathology Service	RAAS-I	Renin–angiotensin–aldosterone system inhibition
kD (kDa)	kiloDalton	RBC	red blood cell
LC/MS	liquid chromatography/mass spectrometry	RBF	renal blood flow
		RBP	retinol binding protein
L-DOPA	levodopa, L-3,4-dihydroxyphenylalanine	RCF	relative centrifugal force
		RPGN	rapidly progressive glomerulonephritis
LE	leukocyte esterase		
LMW	low molecular weight	RI	refractive index
LPF	low-power field	RIA	radioimmunoassay
LUT	lower urinary tract	RPF	renal plasma flow
MA	microalbumin	rpm	revolutions per minute
MA	microalbuminuria	RTE	renal tubular epithelium
MMB	3-mercapto-3-methylbutanol; mercaptan	S3	straight part of the distal proximal tubule
MR	mineralocorticoid receptor	SAA	serum amyloid A
MRA	mineralocorticoid antagonists	SCWT	Soft-coated Wheaten Terrier
MRB	mineralocorticoid receptor blocker	SDMA	symmetric dimethylarginine
MRI	magnetic resonance imaging	SDS-PAGE	sodium dodecyl sulphate-polyacrylamide gel electrophoresis
mTAL	medullary thick ascending limb		
MW	molecular weight	SEM	standard error of the mean
MWO	medullary washout	SGLT2	sodium-glucose cotransporter 2
NDI	nephrogenic diabetes insipidus	SGOT	serum glutamic-oxaloacetic transaminase (also known as AST)
NEW	nutrient-enriched water		
NIST	National Institute of Standards and Technology	SIAD	syndrome of inappropriate antidiuresis
NKCC2 transporter	sodium potassium chloride 2 cotransporter	SIADH	syndrome of inappropriate antidiuretic hormone
NRC	National Research Council	SIRS	severe (systemic) inflammatory response syndrome
NS	nephrotic syndrome		
NSAID	nonsteroidal anti-inflammatory drug	SLE	systemic lupus erythematosus
OHE	ovariohysterectomy	SNGFR	single-nephron glomerular filtration rate
PAS	Periodic-acid Schiff stain		
P$_{Cr}$	plasma concentration of creatinine	S$_{osm}$	serum osmolality
PCR	polymerase chain reaction	SQ	subcutaneous

SSA	sulfosalicylic acid	UG	urogenital
SUN	serum urea nitrogen	UGGT/U_{Cr}	urinary GGT to urinary creatinine ratio
T4	thyroxine		
TCC	transitional cell carcinoma	ULS	ultrasound
Tc-DTPA	technetium-labeled diethylenetri-aminepentaacetic acid	UO	urethral obstruction
		U_{osm}	urine osmolality
TEM	Transmission electron microscopy	UPC	urinary protein-to-creatinine ratio
TGF-B	transforming growth factor beta	UPC	urine protein-to-creatinine ratio
THG	Tamm–Horsfall glycoprotein		
THP	Tamm–Horsfall protein, uromodulin	USG	urine specific gravity
T_{max}	maximal ability of proximal tubular cells to reabsorb filtered glucose	UT-A1	urea transporter-A1
		UT-A2	urea transporter-A2
TMB	3,3′,5,5′-tetramethylbenzidine	UT-A3	urea transporter-A3
TNTC	too numerous to count	UT-A4	urea transporter-A4
TRPC6	transient receptor potential cation channel 6	UT-B	urea transporter-B
		UTI	urinary tract infection
UA	urinalysis	UV	ultraviolet
UAC	urine albumin to creatinine ratio	V2R	vasopressin type-2 receptor
UC	urothelial carcinoma	VDBP	vitamin D binding protein
U_{Ca}	urinary calcium concentration	VDR	vitamin D receptor
UCC	urothelial cell carcinoma (TCC)	VEGF	vascular endothelial growth factor
UCCR	urinary cortisol to creatinine ratio	WBC	white blood cell
U_{Cr}	urinary concentration of creatinine	WDT	water deprivation testing
U_{creat}	urinary creatinine concentration	XLHN	X-linked hereditary nephropathy

Renal Anatomy, Physiology, and Evaluation of Function

GENERAL FUNCTIONS OF THE KIDNEY

The kidneys perform many important functions, including excretion of solute and water, conservation of solute and water, and biosynthesis of hormones. Normal kidney function is vital to the maintenance of a constant internal milieu. The most widely recognized kidney function is to excrete waste products (urea nitrogen, creatinine, nitrogen waste products, phosphorus, symmetric dimethylarginine (SDMA), hemoglobin breakdown products, and hormone metabolites) that are not needed and are potentially dangerous, as they would otherwise accumulate in the body. Waste products are eliminated into urine by various combinations of glomerular filtration and tubular reabsorption and tubular secretion.

Proper kidney function is important for the regulation of water and balance of electrolytes. To maintain homeostasis, the kidneys are able to vary the volume of water excreted into urine, depending on the physiological need of the body. Urine volume can be very small when water is needed to minimize change in the plasma osmolality during times of limited water intake. The combination of glomerular filtration and tubular activity on renal tubular fluid ultimately determines what is excreted and what is conserved from the initial filtrate delivered into Bowman's space.

The kidneys are also responsible for the regulation of arterial pressure, the regulation of acid–base balance, gluconeogenesis, and biosynthesis of erythropoietin, calcitriol, and renin, but discussion of these processes is beyond the scope of this book. The interested reader is referred to detailed reports of renal anatomy and functions elsewhere [1–7].

ANATOMY OF THE KIDNEY

The kidneys are located outside the peritoneal cavity on the dorsal wall of the abdomen. The hilus of the kidney (the indentation on the medial side) is the area in which the renal artery and vein, lymphatics, nerve supply, and ureter enter the kidney. The two major regions of the kidney are the cortex more superficially and more deeply the medulla (Figure 1.1). The cortex contains superficial and juxtamedullary nephrons (glomeruli and tubules) that undergo filtration and tubular processing of filtrate. The medulla contains the long loops of Henle from juxtaglomerular nephrons as well as parts of some loops of Henle from more cortical nephrons, the straight part of the proximal tubule (PT) (S_3) of juxtaglomerular nephrons, connecting tubules, collecting ducts, and vasa rectae. The border of the renal pelvis contains diverticulae that radiate into the deeper medulla. The collecting ducts terminate in the renal pelvis and diverticulae which continues into the upper end of the ureter. Contractile elements in the diverticulae, renal pelvis, and ureters propel urine into the urinary bladder where urine is stored until voided [1, 8].

RENAL BLOOD SUPPLY

An elaborate network of renal blood vessels allows for normal glomerular filtration and tubular processing of filtrate that results in urine formation. Once the renal artery enters the kidney, it progressively branches into the interlobar arteries, arcuate arteries, interlobular arteries (radial arteries), afferent arterioles, and finally, glomerular capillaries where fluid is filtered (Figure 1.1). The distal ends of the glomerular capillaries coalesce into the efferent arterioles, which lead to the peritubular capillaries that surround the renal tubules. The peritubular capillaries empty progressively into the interlobular veins, arcuate veins, interlobar veins, and, finally, the renal vein [1, 8].

The glomerular capillaries are unique in that they lie between two arterioles (afferent and efferent arteriole). The hydrostatic pressure of these capillary beds can be altered by changing the resistance of the afferent and efferent arterioles, resulting in a change in the rate of glomerular filtration and tubular reabsorption [2, 7].

ANATOMY OF THE NEPHRON

The nephron is the functional unit of the kidney. Each feline kidney contains approximately 200000 nephrons, and each canine kidney contains about 400000 [2, 9–12]. The nephron

contains the blood vessels and tubular cellular structures for glomerular ultrafiltration of blood into tubular fluid for further processing. At the core of the nephron is the glomerulus containing the glomerular capillaries, which are covered by visceral epithelial cells. The glomerulus is encased by Bowman's capsule, which includes visceral and parietal epithelial cells (Figure 1.2). Fluid filtered from the glomerulus first passes into Bowman's space and then flows into the PT (Figure 1.3). The PT includes the proximal convoluted tubule and the straight portion distally (also known as S3 or pars recta). The PT starts at the junction with Bowman's space and ends at the junction with Henle's loop. S3 extends into the outer medulla when parent nephrons are juxtaglomerular. The filtered fluid continues to flow into the loop of Henle, which extends into the renal medulla. The loop of Henle consists of three anatomically and functionally different parts. The loop starts from the end of the PT (S3) and ends as it joins the distal tubule. The thin descending limb ends at the hair pin turn, and the thin ascending limb starts at the hair pin turn of the

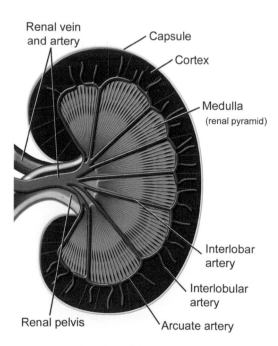

FIGURE 1.1 Sagittal section of the canine kidney. Note vascular architecture from renal artery, to interlobar, arcuate, and interlobular arteries. The afferent arteriole then extends to the glomerular vessels (not shown). Source: Illustration by Tim Vojt, reproduced with permission of The Ohio State University.

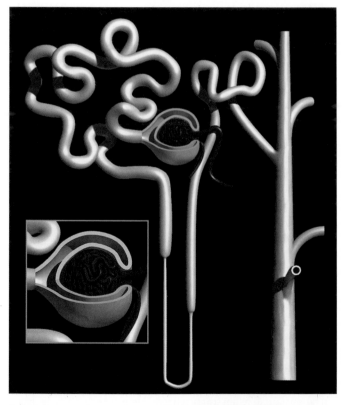

FIGURE 1.2 The renal corpuscle consists of the glomerulus and its covering with visceral and parietal epithelium shown in blue. Bowman's space is the area in between those two layers of epithelium and is where plasma is filtered across the glomerulus to form tubular fluid as it enters the proximal tubule. The insert shows an enlarged view of the renal corpuscle. Note that the afferent arteriole is shown to be larger than the efferent arteriole, since about 30% of the blood volume is filtered across the glomerulus to form the initial tubular fluid. Source: Illustration by Tim Vojt, reproduced with permission of The Ohio State University.

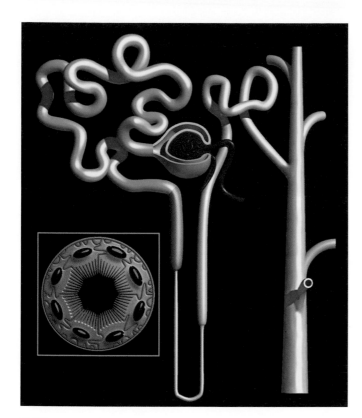

FIGURE 1.3 The proximal tubule (PT) includes the proximal convoluted tubule (blue) and the straight portion distally (pink) (also known as S3 or pars recta). The PT starts at the junction with Bowman's space and ends at the junction with Henle's loop. S3 extends into the outer medulla when parent nephrons are juxtaglomerular. The insert shows the histology of the PT featuring its brush border. Source: Illustration by Tim Vojt, reproduced with permission of The Ohio State University.

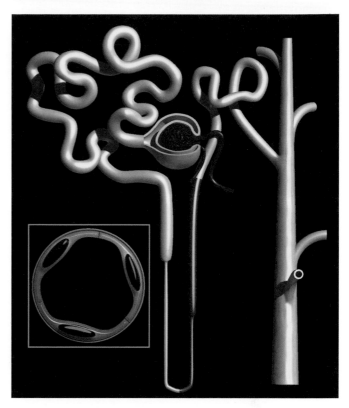

FIGURE 1.4 The loop of Henle has three anatomically and functionally different parts. The loop starts from the end of the proximal tubule (S3) and ends as it joins the distal tubule. The thin descending limb (shown in blue) ends at the hair pin turn and the thin ascending limb (shown in pink) starts at the hair pin turn of the loop. The medullary thick ascending limb (mTAL) (purple) contains considerable metabolic apparatus for energy consuming activities that occur in this region. The insert shows the histology of the thin limbs. Source: Illustration by Tim Vojt, reproduced with permission of The Ohio State University.

loop. The descending limb and beginning portion of the ascending limb are very thin, and as the ascending limb passes through the medulla and back into the cortex, the walls become much thicker (medullary thick ascending limb [mTAL]) (Figure 1.4). At the end of the ascending limb, there is a short segment of the initial distal tubule known as the macula densa, containing specialized epithelial cells (Figures 1.5 and 1.6). There is close apposition of the specialized macula densa cells of the distal tubule with the juxtaglomerular cells of the afferent arteriole. Cells of the macula densa are important in sensing solute flowing by this region and then sending signals to the afferent arteriole that control vascular tone of the afferent arteriole, which changes glomerular filtration rate (GFR). Past the macula densa, fluid flows progressively into the later distal tubule (Figure 1.7), connecting tubule, cortical collecting tubule (Figure 1.8), and cortical collecting duct. Collecting ducts merge to form the medullary collecting duct; these collecting ducts merge and empty into the renal pelvis.

Nephron structure and function differs depending on the location within the renal cortex. Nephrons that have glomeruli located in the outer portion of the cortex are called cortical nephrons, and these nephrons only penetrate a short distance into the medulla (Figure 1.9). Some nephrons have short loops of Henle [8, 13, 14]. Glomeruli that are located deeper in the cortex are termed juxtamedullary nephrons. Tubules from these nephrons extend much deeper into the renal medulla from some combination of having longer loops of Henle and closer proximity of parent glomeruli to the medulla. One source notes that all nephrons in both the dog and cat have long loops of Henle and vary by how much of the loop extends into the medulla [2]. The blood supply to the juxtamedullary nephrons is slightly different in that the efferent arterioles are much longer and extend into the outer medulla where they divide into specialized peritubular capillaries (vasa recta). The vasa recta extend into the medulla parallel with the loop of Henle and then return to the cortex to empty into cortical veins. The vasa recta are important in the concentration of urine (described in detail below).

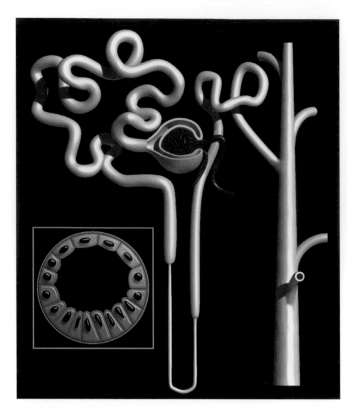

FIGURE 1.5 The first part of the distal tubule is shown in blue to be in close anatomical proximity to the afferent arteriole. This region of the distal tubule contains specialized cells of the distal tubule called the macula densa (shown as the thin long cells in the cut out). Source: Illustration by Tim Vojt, reproduced with permission of The Ohio State University.

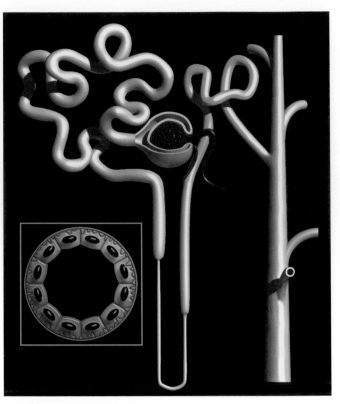

FIGURE 1.7 The distal tubule (DT shown in blue) consists of early (proximal) and late (more distal) portions that have different functions. Some of the DT is convoluted. The DT starts at the end of the mTAL and ends at the junction with the connecting tubule. Source: Illustration by Tim Vojt, reproduced with permission of The Ohio State University.

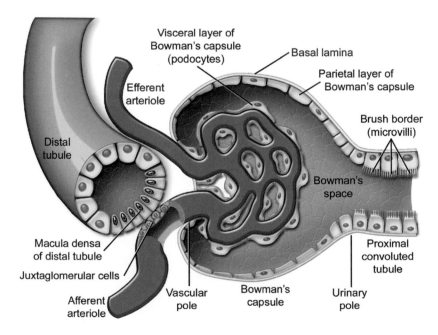

FIGURE 1.6 Juxtaglomerular apparatus. Notice the close apposition of the specialized macula densa cells of the distal tubule with the juxtaglomerular cells of the afferent arteriole. Cells of the macula densa are important in sensing solute flowing by this region and then sending signals to the afferent arteriole that control vascular tone and GFR. Source: Illustration by Tim Vojt, reproduced with permission of The Ohio State University.

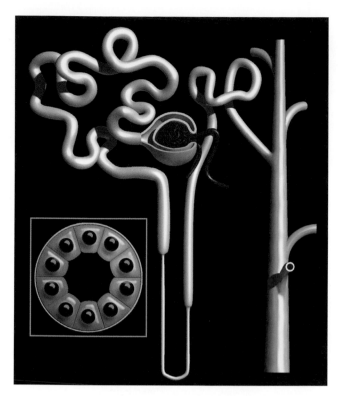

FIGURE 1.8 Collecting tubule (CT). The CT has very different functions depending on whether it is the cortical CT, outer medullary CT, or inner medullary CT. The CT is where most of the final adjustments are made as to how concentrated the urine will be based on water reabsorption under the influence of ADH. Source: Illustration by Tim Vojt, reproduced with permission of The Ohio State University.

Extensive details describing renal vascular tubular organization and relationships in dogs have been reported. It appears that some postglomerular efferent arterioles provide blood supply to tubules from different nephrons than from the original parent nephron [13–15]. This heterogeneity of vascular tubular relationship is not usually mentioned in traditional renal physiology courses, but it could be important in understanding patchy tubular necrosis that develops in some cases with ischemic acute kidney injury (AKI).

URINE

URINE FORMATION

Ultrafiltration of plasma across the glomerulus into Bowman's space is the first step in the formation of urine. Fluid that enters Bowman's space is quite similar to that of plasma with the exception of protein content. Only small-molecular-weight substances are easily filtered across the glomerulus. Large-molecular-weight proteins in plasma, such as albumin, are excluded from this ultrafiltrate; thus, this fluid is nearly devoid of plasma proteins in healthy individuals (Figure 1.10). The glomerular and tubular handling of filtered proteins is

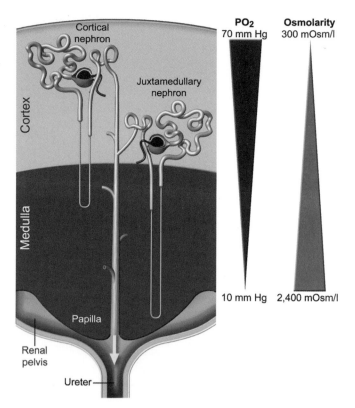

FIGURE 1.9 Cortical and juxtamedullary nephrons. Not all nephrons are identical anatomically. Juxtamedullary nephrons are those that have long loops of Henle that are vital in the generation of medullary hyperosmolality and the ability to maximally concentrate and dilute urine. There are many more cortical nephrons, which explains why renal blood flow is much greater in the cortex than in the medulla. Note that there is a progressive decrease in oxygen saturation from the outer cortex to the inner medulla. This oxygen gradient helps explain the development of certain types of acute kidney injury that happen in regions of relatively low oxygen delivery and high metabolic demand (such as occurs in S3 and the mTAL in juxtamedullary nephrons). Note also the gradient from low to high osmolality in the renal interstitium from outer cortex to inner medulla. Initial interstitial osmolality in the cortex parallels that of plasma (300 mOsm/L) that becomes many times increased over that of plasma in the medulla due to the process of countercurrent multiplication. The maximal osmolality achieved at the turn of Henle's loop parallels the maximal urine concentration that can be elaborated. Source: Illustration by Tim Vojt, reproduced with permission of The Ohio State University.

discussed in greater detail in Chapter 7. Tubular fluid is extensively modified in volume and quantity of solute and water as it traverses the tubular lumens along the PT, the loop of Henle, distal tubule, connecting tubule, and the collecting tubules. Isosmotic reabsorption of tubular fluid occurs until the end of the PT [2, 7]. The majority of filtered solutes and water are reabsorbed in the PT. The PT is inherently permeable to water due to the presence of constitutively expressed aquaporins (AQPs) [16] that facilitate transcellular movement of water, as well as some paracellular movement

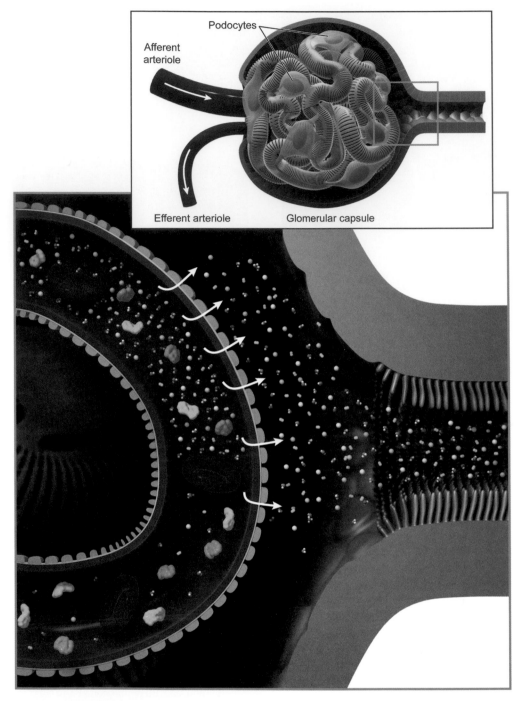

FIGURE 1.10 Glomerular tuft (insert) and view of glomerular filtration process are illustrated. The afferent arteriole, glomerular capillary, efferent arteriole, Bowman's Space and junction with proximal tubule are shown in the insert; podocytes (visceral epithelium) are shown as an outer cover of the glomerular vessel. About 30% of the plasma volume coming in from the afferent delivery is filtered across the glomerulus into Bowman's space. Approximately 2–4 mL/min/kg of fluid traverses the glomerulus into Bowman's space in normal dogs and cats, and this volume is referred to as the glomerular filtration rate (GFR). GFR is largely a function of the algebraic sum of Starling's forces that include glomerular capillary pressure, oncotic pressure within the glomerulus, and tubular pressure in Bowman's space. Glomerular capillary pressure develops as a function of plasma flow into the glomerulus and the resistance to flow of fluid out of the glomerulus. In addition to Starling forces, GFR also depends on the surface area of the glomerular capillaries and their inherent permeability characteristics (Kf). The larger image below shows that only the smaller molecular weight and size molecules are filtered into Bowman's space. Proteins with higher molecular weight and size (shown as larger blue and orange elements within the glomerular capillary) do not cross the glomerulus. This figure also shows that cells (RBC shown) stay within the glomerular capillary and do not cross the glomerulus. Source: Illustration by Tim Vojt, reproduced with permission of The Ohio State University.

due to the absence of tight junctions in this region [17]. From 60% to 80% of the glomerular ultrafiltrate undergoes isosmotic reabsorption by the end of the PT, which is important in reduction of fluid volume delivered to more distal nephron segments for further processing. The thin descending limb of Henle's loop is permeable to water due to the presence of AQPs [17], and fluid undergoes reabsorption due to the hyperosmolality of the interstitium that surrounds them. Tubular fluid becomes progressively more concentrated as it travels along the descending loop of Henle (water and solute permeable) and then becomes progressively less concentrated as it travels along the ascending loop of Henle (water impermeable due to the absence of AQPs and presence of extensive tight junctions) [17]. The thin and thick segments of the ascending limb of Henle's loop are often referred to as the "diluting segments" as solute is reabsorbed but water is not, which reduces tubular fluid osmolality. The thick ascending limb is responsible for reabsorption of 20–25% of the filtered load of sodium and chloride, a process that is facilitated by the Na-K-2Cl cotransporter (NKCC2) [18]. Progressive tubular fluid hypotonicity develops in this region, while the degree of interstitial hypertonicity increases at the same time, a development that is important to allow elaboration of urine with maximal concentration. NKCC2 activity in the cells of the macula densa allows a signaling process that controls preglomerular afferent arteriolar tone through tubuloglomerular feedback [18, 19]. Hypotonic fluid (100 mOsm/kg) is presented from Henle's loop to the distal convoluted tubule. The osmolality of tubular fluid within the medullary and cortical thick ascending limb of Henle's loop is low as it joins the distal tubule, regardless of high or low circulating antidiuretic hormone (ADH) status.

Tubular fluid that is delivered from the collecting tubules to the renal pelvis can be either more dilute or more concentrated than the initial (approximately 300 mOsm/kg) glomerular ultrafiltrate, depending on the needs of the animal. The degree of urine concentration is largely determined by the response to ADH, which is discussed in more detail below. Normal urine is markedly different from plasma that was initially filtered across the glomerulus into Bowman's space (waste products, pH, urine concentration). No further modification of fluid occurs after it enters the renal pelvis on its way to the urinary bladder for storage. The interested reader is referred to an excellent veterinary review of basic applied renal physiology and disorders of sodium metabolism for more detail [2, 20, 21]. Failure to conserve water, potassium, glucose, and plasma proteins are processes that can be detected in urine and will be discussed in specific sections of this book that follow. An overview of the functions and physiological processes that occur in each nephron segment is presented in Figure 1.11.

URINARY CONCENTRATION AND DILUTION

See Chapter 4 for clinical details about urine concentration based on urinary specific gravity (USG) and urine osmolality.

The ability to concentrate or dilute urine is critical to maintain a healthy plasma osmolality (285–310 mOsm/L population-based reference range for dogs and cats). Normal plasma osmolality is maintained within a very narrow range for an individual animal but can vary according to the volume of fluid intake and solute consumed in the diet, as well as by losses of fluid and electrolytes that alter plasma osmolality. Dehydration from loss of mostly water increases plasma osmolality, which stimulates the release of ADH and elaboration of concentrated urine. More rarely, a decrease in plasma osmolality happens when loss of fluid is replaced by mostly water, and the ability to excrete dilute urine is essential to restore normal plasma osmolality when the serum osmolality was reduced. The kidneys can excrete dilute urine with an osmolality of about one-sixth the osmolality (50 mOsm/L) of normal. The kidneys are also able to regulate solute excretion independently of water excretion, which is important when there is limited fluid intake [22].

Glomerular ultrafiltrate is modified in order to conserve needed solute and water or to excrete excess solutes and wastes and water when needed to maintain the constancy of the internal milieu. Urine volume, in general, is related to the degree of urine concentration in health. A larger urine volume is associated with a lower urine concentration, and a smaller urine volume is associated with a higher urine concentration. Small volumes of highly concentrated urine allow conservation of body water when needed, whereas high volumes of minimally concentrated urine allow excretion of excess water in normal individuals. There is a divergence in this general pattern in patients with severe oligo-anuric AKI, as a small urine volume is associated with minimally concentrated urine.

Urine Concentration

The degree of urine concentration in health is largely determined by plasma osmolality and its association with ADH release. Juxtamedullary nephrons contribute more to urinary concentration than cortical nephrons. There are three main mechanisms within the kidney that control urine concentration. First, the transport of sodium chloride without water from the ascending limb of the loop of Henle creates and maintains interstitial hypertonicity and tubular fluid hypotonicity in this region that is essential to allow the option for the elaboration of either concentrated or diluted urine. Second, the secretion and action of ADH (vasopressin) increases water permeability of the collecting duct to allow concentrated urine to form. Third, urea reabsorption from the medullary collecting tubule under the influence of ADH and urea entry into the descending limb of Henle's loop importantly contribute to interstitial hypertonicity to allow urine that is maximally concentrated to be formed.

The fluid that is filtered by the glomerulus has approximately the same osmolality of plasma (about 300 mOsm/kg). Most of the water and solute that has been filtered by the glomerulus is reabsorbed in the proximal convoluted tubule; yet, the osmolality remains unchanged due to isosmotic reabsorption of

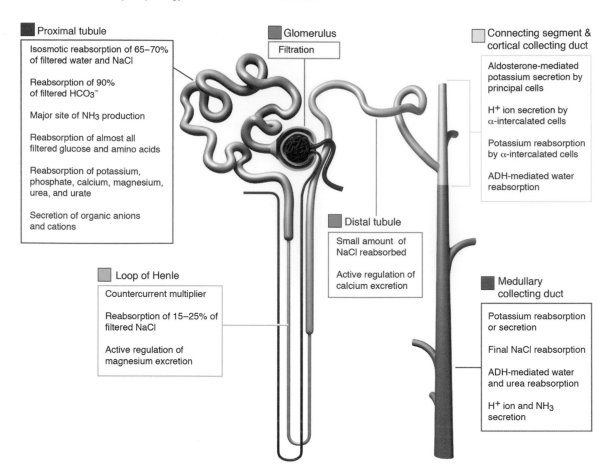

Proximal tubule

Isosmotic reabsorption of 65–70% of filtered water and NaCl

Reabsorption of 90% of filtered HCO₃⁻

Major site of NH₃ production

Reabsorption of almost all filtered glucose and amino acids

Reabsorption of potassium, phosphate, calcium, magnesium, urea, and urate

Secretion of organic anions and cations

Glomerulus

Filtration

Connecting segment & cortical collecting duct

Aldosterone-mediated potassium secretion by principal cells

H⁺ ion secretion by α-intercalated cells

Potassium reabsorption by α-intercalated cells

ADH-mediated water reabsorption

Distal tubule

Small amount of NaCl reabsorbed

Active regulation of calcium excretion

Loop of Henle

Countercurrent multiplier

Reabsorption of 15–25% of filtered NaCl

Active regulation of magnesium excretion

Medullary collecting duct

Potassium reabsorption or secretion

Final NaCl reabsorption

ADH-mediated water and urea reabsorption

H⁺ ion and NH₃ secretion

FIGURE 1.11 General overview of functions and physiological processes that occur by nephron segment. See text for more details about GFR, tubular secretion, tubular reabsorption, and urine concentration or dilution. Source: Illustrated by Tim Vojt. Illustration by Tim Vojt, reproduced with permission of The Ohio State University.

water and solute. Approximately 60–80% of filtered fluid is reabsorbed in the proximal convoluted tubule, along with sodium, amino acids, glucose, phosphate, chloride, potassium, and bicarbonate.

Fluid with an osmolality of about 300 mOsm/kg continually enters the descending limb of the loop of Henle from the PT. The descending and ascending loops of Henle have a hairpin turn configuration, which is the basis for countercurrent multiplication, which allows for the multiplication of a single osmotic effect (Figure 1.12). The descending limb of the loop of Henle is permeable to water, but relatively impermeable to electrolytes. The interstitium of the renal medulla, which surrounds the loop of Henle, is maintained at a higher osmolality due to high concentrations of sodium and urea. As fluid travels down the descending limb of the loop of Henle, water exits the descending limb in an effort to equilibrate with the surrounding interstitium. By the time the fluid within the loop reaches the bottom of the descending limb, the osmolality is greatly increased as compared to the original filtrate.

From the descending limb, fluid passes into the ascending limb of the loop of Henle. The ascending limb is impermeable to water, but is permeable to electrolytes, which is opposite to the descending limb. There is active transport of sodium in the thick portion of the ascending limb, which generates an

osmotic gradient of approximately 200 mOsm/kg. The activity of the basal membrane Na⁺-K⁺-ATPase pump of these cells maintains an electrochemical gradient that drives entry of sodium from the tubular fluid into the cell by facilitated diffusion (Figure 1.13). The carrier Na⁺-K⁺-2Cl⁻ (NKCC2) binds one sodium ion, one potassium ion, and two chloride ions in the lumen, which then transports these electrolytes into the cell and then into the interstitium [18]. Adequate chloride binding to the carrier is the rate-limiting step in transport. Loop diuretics, such as furosemide, bind to the chloride-binding site within the pocket of the NKCC2 carrier molecule of the mTAL, thereby impairing its function resulting in increased excretion of sodium, chloride, and potassium [18, 24].

The osmotic gradient generated between the tubular fluid and the interstitium is multiplied over the length of the loop of Henle. The magnitude of the gradient from the beginning of the descending limb to the bottommost part where the ascending limb begins is a function of the length of the loop, which is an important component of the countercurrent multiplier concept. The vasa recta are also an important part of the countercurrent system through what is called countercurrent exchange (Figure 1.14). Vasa recta are parallel vessels of the renal medulla that provide much lower blood flow than that in the cortex [17]. The descending vasa recta

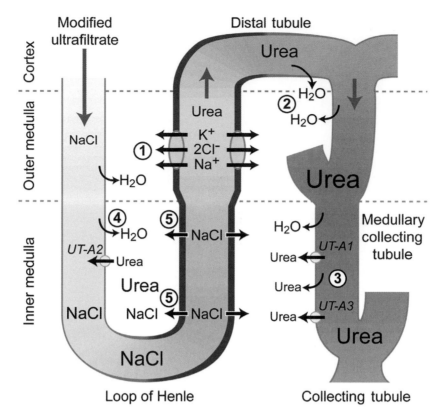

FIGURE 1.12 Factors involved in the elaboration of concentrated or dilute urine. The major factors needed to elaborate maximally concentrated urine are shown in this illustration (excluding the isosmotic reabsorption of solute and water that transpired along the proximal tubule). A critical minimal number of healthy nephrons are needed to make concentrated urine, and the body must be capable of synthesizing and releasing ADH in adequate quantity. The integrity of the collecting tubule V-2 receptor to bind to ADH and initiate intracellular signals for the phosphorylation of aquaporin-2 is essential. The major stimulus for the release of ADH is an increase in plasma osmolality perfusing the hypothalamus; most domestic animals have evolved to produce concentrated urine for much of the day. The ability to concentrate or dilute the urine centers on the ability of the medullary thick ascending limb of the loop of Henle's ability to actively reabsorb sodium and chloride without water. The ascending limb of the loop of Henle is impermeable to water so that the osmolality of tubular fluid progressively decreases during ascent of the loop. At the same time, the osmolality of the interstitium increases as solute is added to this region. ADH increases the permeability of the cortical collecting duct to water but not urea, so the concentration of urea progressively increases as it descends the cortical collecting duct. The increased concentration of urea is represented by the size of the font. The medullary collecting duct is inherently permeable to urea, contributing importantly to the hyperosmolality of this region as urea diffuses into the interstitium. The permeability of the inner medullary collecting duct to urea is enhanced by ADH interaction with specific urea transporters (UT A-1 and UT A-3), which are variably located along the apex, within the tubule cell, and along the basolateral membranes [23] that further movement of urea into the interstitium. The thin descending limb of Henle's loop has a specific urea transporter (UT A-2) that facilitates recycling of urea from the interstitium into the tubular lumen. Step 1: the Na-K-2Cl cotransporter provides the energy that initially generates interstitial hyperosmolality. This process also generates tubular fluid hypoosmolality since this segment of the nephron is not permeable to water. Step 2: in the late distal tubule and cortical collecting tubule, ADH increases water but not urea permeability. Water leaves the tubules from these segments due to the hyperosmolality of the interstitium generated by step 1. Since water but not urea leaves these segments, note that the tubular fluid concentration of urea increases. Step 3: as tubular fluid reaches the medullary collecting tubule, the concentration of urea is quite high. The high concentrations of urea at this location favor diffusion in this region that is permeable to urea. Urea transporters here favor diffusion from tubular fluid into the interstitium, increasing the osmolality of this region. Urea contributes substantially to the solute concentration of this region. Urea transporters also favor the uptake of urea from the interstitium into the thin descending limb of Henle's loop. Step 4: the high concentration of urea and NaCl in the interstitium favors the movement of water out of the descending thin limb of Henle's loop. The thin descending limb is highly permeable to water and not so soluble for sodium and chloride. As a consequence, the concentration of sodium and chloride progressively increases until the point of the hair pin turn of Henle's loop is reached. Step 5: sodium and chloride are shown leaving the thin ascending limb of Henle's loop down their concentration gradient. This occurs because sodium and chloride are relatively permeable in this region and have achieved a high concentration from processes that happened previously in the descending loop (Step 4). The thin ascending limb is impermeant to water, which contributes to the progressive development of hypoosmolality as solute, but not water, is removed from the ascending limb. The sodium and chloride that leave the ascending thin limb contribute to the interstitial hyperosmolality of that region, which further facilitates water movement from the collecting tubule in the presence of ADH activity. Source: Illustration by Tim Vojt, reproduced with permission of The Ohio State University.

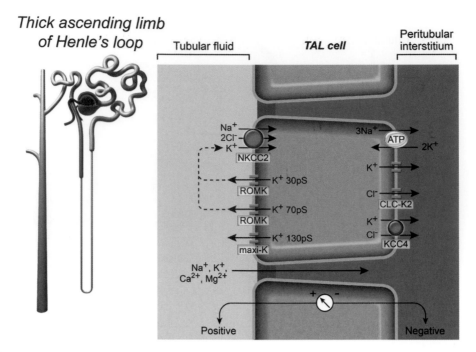

FIGURE 1.13 Medullary thick ascending limb (mTAL) reabsorption of sodium, potassium, and chloride. The apical surface of the mTAL epithelium contains the Na-K-2Cl cotransporter (NKCC2) that is important in the reclamation of 20–25% of the filtered load of sodium and chloride. All four molecules must occupy this cotransporter at the same time in order to allow facilitated uptake of sodium, chloride, and potassium inside the cell. The active sodium–potassium ATPase pump on the basolateral membrane maintains low intracellular sodium concentration, which favors sodium entry into the cell from the apical side. The diuretic furosemide is secreted into tubular fluid and then binds to this transporter in place of chloride, which renders the transporter inoperative. Source: Illustration by Tim Vojt, reproduced with permission of The Ohio State University.

originate from the efferent arterioles of juxtamedullary nephrons, supplying blood to capillary plexuses at multiple levels within the medulla. Ascending vasa recta arise from the capillary plexuses and travel parallel to the descending vessels. This unique anatomical arrangement allows countercurrent flow of water and solutes to occur at local levels without dissipating the hypertonicity of the medulla. Sodium, chloride, and urea enter while water leaves descending vessels; the process is reversed in ascending vessels in that sodium, chloride, and urea leave and water enters. This process of countercurrent exchange is facilitated by the presence of AQP-1 water channels and by urea transporter-B urea transporters in the endothelial cells of the descending vasa recta. Without the vasa recta, the hyperosmotic gradient of the interstitium would quickly dissipate. Hypertonicity of the medulla can be disrupted by disorders or conditions that increase blood flow in the vasa recta.

By the time fluid enters the distal convoluted tubule, it is hypoosmotic to plasma (approximately 100 mOsm/kg). The distal convoluted tubule is minimally permeable to water, but sodium and chloride can be reabsorbed from the tubular fluid into the interstitium further lowering tubular fluid osmolality. From the distal tubule, hypoosmotic tubular fluid enters the collecting duct. Even though most water and solute reabsorption occurs in the proximal convoluted tubule and the loop of Henle, the final urine volume is ultimately determined by the collecting ducts. The collecting duct is divided into three

segments: the cortical collecting duct, outer medullary collecting duct, and inner medullary collecting duct. In the presence of ADH, the hypoosmotic tubular fluid equilibrates osmotically with the cortical interstitium, and about two-third of the tubular water is removed before delivery to the outer medullary collecting duct. The cortical collecting duct is also permeable to sodium and chloride, and more water can be reabsorbed depending on how much sodium reabsorption occurs in response to aldosterone. The cortical collecting duct is not permeable to urea; thus, fluid with a very high urea concentration is delivered to the medullary collecting duct as water but not urea is reabsorbed from the tubular lumen. The fluid that is delivered to the medullary collecting duct is isosmotic with plasma and greatly reduced in volume.

The action of ADH controls the water permeability of the collecting duct and, therefore, the final concentration of urine. An adequate number of functioning nephrons are necessary for this system to conserve or excrete water. ADH is synthesized by the hypothalamus and secreted by the posterior pituitary [25, 26]. Humans and most mammals secrete arginine-ADH as the predominant form, but pigs and marsupials secrete lysine-ADH as the predominant form [27–29]. The antidiuretic activity of arginine-ADH was greater and lasted longer than that from lysine-ADH in dogs [30]. Increasing plasma osmolality is sensed by osmoreceptors in the hypothalamus that trigger the release of ADH, resulting in water conservation by the kidney. Decreases in plasma osmolality inhibit the release of ADH, which facilitates

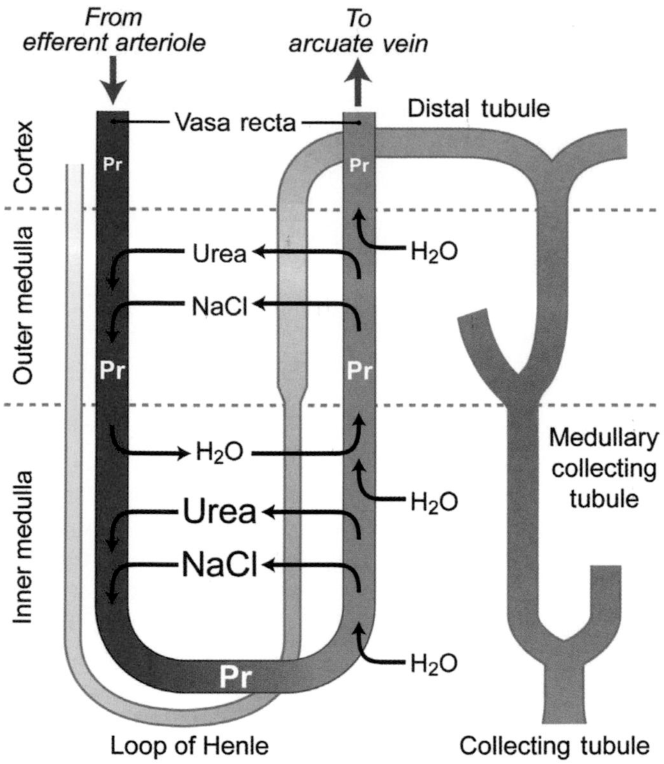

FIGURE 1.14   Vasa recta countercurrent exchanger system. The vasa recta consist of postglomerular efferent arterioles from juxtaglomerular nephrons. This system of vessels (interconnections not shown) runs parallel to the loops of Henle. Solute (NaCl, urea) enters the descending limb and leaves the ascending limb of the vasa recta. Water leaves the descending limb and enters the ascending limb of the vasa recta. The function of this vascular array allows preservation of medullary solute at local levels within the medulla, while still returning extra water to the systemic circulation as needed. Note that the concentration of protein increases within the descending vessel as water leaves and then decreases during ascent as water enters. The size of the font is proportional to the quantity of the compound. This process is sometimes called the Countercurrent Exchanger, and it works in concert with countercurrent multiplication as generated by the loop of Henle. The rate of blood flow through the vasa recta is normally very slow to allow this system to work properly. It is possible for some diseases to increase blood flow through the vasa recta, which dissipates interstitial hyperosmolality, thus reducing the ability to elaborate highly concentrated urine. This process creates one form of medullary washout. Source: Illustration by Tim Vojt, reproduced with permission of The Ohio State University.

excretion of excess water by the kidney [17, 31]. An increased concentration of circulating ADH increases the water permeability of principal cells of the late distal tubules, connecting tubules, and collecting ducts via AQPs, which allows water reabsorption and excretion of a more concentrated urine. Increased ADH activity also increases the activity of the Na-K-2Cl pump in the mTAL. This increases sodium, chloride, and potassium absorption across the medullary thick ascending loop of Henle that further increases interstitial solute concentration (osmolality) while lowering tubular fluid osmolality [16].

In the presence of ADH, water is removed from the collecting duct, and the tubular fluid equilibrates with the hyperosmotic medullary interstitium. The maximal urine osmolality can approach 2800 mOsm/kg in dogs and 3000 mOsm/kg in cats. Less than 1% of the fluid filtered across the glomerulus is excreted as the final urine volume under these circumstances.

The role of prostaglandin E2 (PGE2) in urinary concentration is not fully understood and most likely depends on which receptor is activated under varying physiologic conditions. PGE2 has been thought to have negative effects on urine concentration until recently. Water reabsorption and water excretion by the kidney can be facilitated by PGE2, and increased prostaglandin effects have been implicated in some polyuric conditions, especially in hypercalcemia. In some studies, polyuria was decreased by administering anti-prostaglandin medications [32].

Urine Dilution

When there is excess water in the extracellular fluid (ECF), the plasma osmolality decreases. To remove excess water from the body, the glomerular filtrate needs to be diluted as it passes through the nephron. This is accomplished by the reabsorption of solutes to a greater extent than water. The tubular fluid remains isosmotic to plasma as it passes through the proximal convoluted tubule, and fluid is reabsorbed as it passes through the descending limb of the loop of Henle, becoming more concentrated. In the ascending limb of the loop of Henle, sodium, potassium, and chloride are reabsorbed, and the tubular fluid becomes more dilute as it flows to the distal convoluted tubule.

As a result of the decreased plasma osmolality, there is a decrease in the secretion of ADH by the posterior pituitary. In the absence of ADH effect, the collecting duct remains impermeable to water. As the tubular fluid enters the collecting duct, it has an osmolality of approximately 100 mOsm/kg. Sodium chloride continues to be reabsorbed in the cortical and inner medullary collecting duct, without the reabsorption of water. The hypoosmolar fluid becomes even more dilute and can be as low as 50 mOsm/kg (maximally dilute urine) in the absence of ADH.

The Role of Urea

Along with the active transport of sodium and chloride from the thick ascending limb of the loop of Henle and passive transport in the thin ascending limb, urea is also important in establishing and maintaining high interstitial osmolality that is important in the function of the urinary concentrating mechanism [2]. There is a low permeability to urea in most segments of the thin descending limb of the loop of Henle, but there is high permeability to water in this segment. The high concentration of urea in the medullary interstitium causes water to be removed osmotically from the thin descending limb of the loop of Henle, as well as from the medullary collecting tubule in the presence of ADH. Urea increases medullary interstitial osmolality without changing the sodium concentration in this region. In the descending limb, the concentration of sodium of the tubular fluid eventually exceeds medullary interstitial sodium concentration due to the low permeability for sodium. There are select segments of the descending limb that are permeable to urea; these are segments that express the urea transporter UT-A2. This urea transporter is likely important to reclaim urea that entered the medullary interstitium from the medullary collecting duct [16]. The excretion or reabsorption of urea along the tubules is in part dependent on the rate of urine flow. Faster tubular flow rates result in less time for reabsorption of urea along the tubules resulting in more urea excretion. The opposite happens when tubular flow rates are slow (as in dehydration) and there is increased reabsorption of urea.

As the tubular fluid enters the thin ascending limb of the loop of Henle, the sodium in the tubular fluid is reabsorbed passively into the medullary interstitium down a concentration gradient. The entire ascending limb of Henle is impermeable to water, which promotes dilution of tubular fluid as solute is removed but water is not. In the inner medullary collecting duct, the permeability to urea is increased by ADH via urea transporters UT-A1, UT-A3, and possibly UT-A4, which are variably located along the apex, within the tubule cell, and along the basolateral membranes [16, 23]. ADH additionally upregulates the number of urea channels [16]. There is limited permeability to urea in the distal convoluted tubule, cortical collecting duct, and outer medullary collecting duct; thus, the urea concentration of tubular fluid markedly increases in these portions of the nephron.

When the concentration of plasma ADH increases (in times of water conservation), water permeability of the cortical collecting duct increases without an increase in urea permeability, so the concentration of urea progressively increases as it descends the cortical collecting duct. With increased ADH, urea permeability of the inner medullary collecting duct increases via urea transporters, so more urea diffuses into the medullary interstitium. With the entry of urea into the interstitium, maximally concentrated urine can be produced by osmotic equilibration of tubular fluid with the hyperosmotic interstitium in the presence of ADH. In times of water conservation (antidiuresis), urea constitutes more than 40% of the total medullary solute in dogs, but only accounts for about 10% during water diuresis [33].

The Role of Aquaporins

Aquaporins (AQPs) are small membrane proteins that act as semipermeable channels that facilitate water transport. AQPs consist of six alpha helices that span the membrane, containing a central water-transporting pore. Four AQP monomers combine to form a tetramer, which is the functional unit. Water can cross a lipid membrane by diffusion, but the presence of AQP channels greatly increases the water permeability of the membrane [34].

Thirteen AQPs have been identified in mammals (AQP0-12), which are expressed in various tissues. AQPs are highly expressed in renal epithelial cells where they are important in water movement [35]. Eight different AQPs are expressed in the kidney, and five are important in water homeostasis (AQP-1, AQP-2, AQP-3, AQP-4, and AQP-7). AQP-2 is most important, as it is regulated by ADH [34, 36, 37]. AQP-1 is located in the membranes of proximal convoluted tubules, descending

limb of the loop of Henle (of long-looped nephrons), and descending vasa recta. AQP-2, AQP-3, and AQP-4 are present in the connecting tubule and collecting duct. AQP-7 is present in PTs. Defects in the expression of any of the AQPs can result in significant impairment of urine concentration.

AQP-2 plays the biggest role in urinary concentration. It is expressed in principal cells of the connecting tubule and collecting ducts and is modulated by the presence of ADH (Figure 1.15) ADH upregulates the expression and half-life of AQP-2 and also promotes phosphorylation of AQP-2, facilitating its migration and insertion into the luminal membrane via exocytosis and inhibition of endocytosis. AQP-2 is endocytosed and degraded in the absence of ADH [16, 17, 40, 41].

ADH binds to the vasopressin type-2 receptor inducing a cascade of events, including G-protein-mediated activation of adenylate cyclase, an increase in intracellular cAMP, activation of protein kinase, and a redistribution of AQP-2 to the apical membranes. Thus, luminal water can enter the cells via AQP-2 and leaves the cells via AQP-3 and AQP-4 in the basolateral membrane. This process results in a concentration of urine. Once ADH levels decrease, AQP-2 is internalized, and the water permeability of the apical membranes return to basal levels. AQP-2 can either be degraded or stored for future use. Without functioning AQP-2, urinary concentrating ability is severely decreased.

A number of conditions characterized by a lack of urinary concentration have been shown to be related to altered function or expression of AQP-2 in humans. In humans, about 10% of congenital nephrogenic diabetes insipidus (NDI) cases are due to mutations in AQP-2 [35]. Acquired causes of NDI that are related in part to altered AQP-2 include hypokalemia, hypercalcemia, urinary tract obstruction, AKI, and lithium treatment [16, 36, 41].

RENAL FUNCTION ASSESSMENT

FRACTIONAL CLEARANCE OF ELECTROLYTES

Evaluation of the concentration of any urinary electrolyte has little meaning by itself. For example, a urinary sodium concentration of 20 or 200 mEq/L could be appropriate depending on the status of the extracellular fluid volume (ECFV), signals for sodium reabsorption, and how much water is excreted or reabsorbed in tubular fluid. A general rule that a urinary sodium of <15 mEq/L indicates prerenal azotemia as used in human medicine appears to be misleading in veterinary medicine.

The fractional clearance of electrolytes is more useful in the evaluation of renal function than the concentration of the electrolyte in urine by itself. The fractional clearance of electrolytes is defined as the ratio of the clearance of the electrolyte in question to that of creatinine [42, 43]. The fractional clearance is calculated by dividing the ratio of the urinary concentration of the electrolyte (U_x) to the plasma concentration of the electrolyte (P_x) by the ratio of urinary

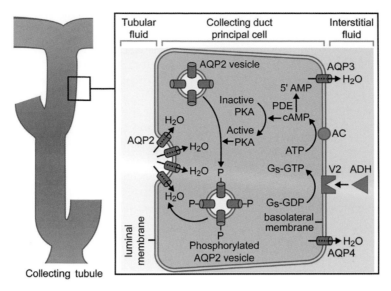

FIGURE 1.15 ADH actions in the principal cells of the collecting tubule. Callout to right is taken from the collecting tubule; the urine side of the collecting tubule (luminal) is on the left and the blood side (basolateral) on the right of this image. Aquaporin-2 (AQ-2) is phosphorylated under the influence of ADH, and then, this vesicle is inserted along the luminal membrane serving as a water channel that facilitates water crossing the collecting tubular lumen into the interstitium [38], [39]. The development and maintenance of a hypertonic interstitium is an overarching requirement to allow water to move out of the descending loop of Henle and out of the collecting duct under the influence of ADH. Circulating ADH binds to a specific receptor (V-2) on the basal side of the collecting duct, which then activates cyclic adenosine monophosphate (cAMP) and a series of intracellular events that lead to phosphorylation of AQ-2. AQ-2 then migrates to the luminal membrane of the collecting duct, where it is inserted allowing it to act as water channel that facilitates water transport across these cells. Under the influence of ADH, urine of low volume and high osmolality is excreted. AC, adenyl cyclase; AQP, aquaporin; Gs, stimulatory guanine nucleotide regulatory protein; GDP, guanosine diphosphate; GTP, guanosine triphosphate; PDE, phosphodiesterase; PKA, protein kinase A; V2, vasopressin receptor. Source: Illustration by Tim Vojt, reproduced with permission of The Ohio State University.

concentration of creatinine (U_{Cr}) to the plasma concentration of creatinine (P_{Cr}) × 100. $FC_x = (U_x/P_x)/(U_{Cr}/P_{Cr}) \times 100$. The fractional clearance is expressed as a percentage. Normal values for urinary fractional clearance of electrolytes in dogs and cats are summarized in Table 1.1. However, normal values may be lower in greyhounds for potassium, chloride, calcium, and phosphorus [47]. The advantage of this measurement is that a timed urine collection is not necessary. In normal animals, the fractional clearances of all electrolytes are much less than 100% implying net conservation. Higher values for fractional excretion of potassium and phosphorus exist than

for sodium and chloride and can exceed 100% for potassium during some forms of chronic kidney disease (CKD).

The fractional clearance of sodium may be useful in the differentiation of prerenal and primary renal azotemia. In animals with prerenal azotemia and volume depletion, sodium conservation should be avid and the fractional clearance of sodium very low (<1%). Higher numbers suggest the presence of primary kidney disease in this setting. A significantly increased urinary fractional excretion of electrolytes (sodium, chloride, potassium, calcium, magnesium, and phosphorus) allowed early identification of dogs with intrinsic AKI compared to volume responsive AKI. Increased urinary fractional excretion of electrolytes was also associated with nonsurvival in this study [49].

The fractional clearance of potassium may be useful in the evaluation of hypokalemic patients to determine if the kidneys are contributing to the hypokalemia. The fractional excretion of potassium should be low during states of hypokalemia if the kidneys are functioning normally; a high value incriminates the kidneys as contributing to the hypokalemia. The fractional excretion of phosphorus is often high in CKD due to the effects of increased parathyroid hormone and fibroblast growth factor-23 that decrease proximal tubular reabsorption of phosphate. An increased fractional excretion of phosphorus may delay the onset of hyperphosphatemia in early CKD as a compensatory mechanism [44]. A decrease in the fractional excretion of phosphorus can sometimes be used

Table 1.1 General reference values for fractional electrolyte clearance (%). Values will vary by fasting, dietary intake, and particular study. Several studies provide further details [42–46].

Analyte	Dog	Cat
Sodium	<1	<1
Potassium	<20	<24
Chloride	<1	<1.3
Phosphorus	<39	<73
		<45
Calcium (total calcium)	<1	<1

Source: Adapted from Lefebvre et al. [42], DiBartola et al. [43], Parker et al. [46], Bennett et al. [47], Carr et al. [48].

to document the effectiveness of dietary and intestinal phosphate binding treatment during CKD [45].

The fractional clearance of calcium based on serum total or ionized calcium and the use of urinary-calcium-to-urinary-creatine ratio may be useful for investigation of risk factors or diagnostic indices in dogs with calcium containing urinary stones [48, 50, 51], dogs with CKD [46], in cats with idiopathic hypercalcemia [52], and in obscure cases of hypercalcemia.

GLOMERULAR FILTRATION

Glomerular filtration is a passive process within the kidneys that largely depends on systemic blood pressure and blood volume that perfuse the kidneys. GFR represents the sum of all the single-nephron glomerular filtration rates (SNGFRs) of all nephrons in both kidneys. The SNGFR varies among nephron populations; thus, an average SNGFR value is typically evaluated. Glomerular capillaries are impermeable to large-molecular-weight plasma proteins and cells, so the normal glomerular filtrate is almost protein-free and devoid of cellular elements.

The kidneys receive about 25% of the cardiac output [3]. GFR is about 20–30% of the renal plasma flow (RPF) (GFR/RPF or filtration fraction) [2]. This high rate of glomerular filtration depends on a high blood flow to the kidney and on properties of the glomerular capillary membranes. Glomerular capillaries are thicker than most other capillaries, but are more porous to water and small molecules, enabling a high fluid filtration rate (mL/minute). GFR is determined by the hydrostatic and colloid osmotic forces across the glomerular membrane and the glomerular capillary filtration coefficient, which is the product of the permeability and filtering surface area of the capillaries. Forces favoring filtration include glomerular hydrostatic pressure and Bowman's capsule colloid osmotic pressure, and forces opposing filtration include Bowman's capsule hydrostatic pressure and glomerular capillary colloid osmotic pressure. Changes in these forces impact GFR [53].

Since the glomerulus does not normally filter protein, the colloid osmotic pressure of fluid within Bowman's capsule is essentially zero and does not contribute to GFR. Alterations in the glomerular capillary filtration coefficient can increase or decrease GFR, but this is not a primary mechanism for day-to-day regulation of GFR. Chronic hypertension, diabetes mellitus, and progressive CKD can increase the thickness of the glomerular capillary basement membrane, thereby decreasing the capillary filtration coefficient. Changes in the hydrostatic pressure of Bowman's capsule can increase or decrease GFR in disease, but this is also not a primary mechanism for day-to-day regulation. Increased hydrostatic pressure of Bowman's capsule occurs with urinary tract obstruction or with renal edema that develops during AKI, which decreases GFR.

Glomerular capillary colloid osmotic pressure importantly impacts GFR. As blood passes from the afferent arteriole to the efferent arteriole, the plasma protein concentration progressively increases since water is being filtered by the glomerulus, but protein is not. Thus, there is loss of fluid, increasing the concentration of protein as the plasma flows through the glomerulus. This increase in protein increases the capillary colloid osmotic pressure, progressively decreasing GFR from the highest near the afferent arteriole to the lowest near the efferent arteriole. The increased oncotic pressure in blood leaving the glomerulus is important in regulating reabsorption of tubular fluid and solutes into the peritubular capillaries.

A change in capillary hydrostatic pressure is the primary mechanism for the regulation of GFR. An increase in this pressure will increase GFR, and GFR is decreased with a decrease in capillary hydrostatic pressure. The glomerular capillary hydrostatic pressure is controlled by arterial pressure and the resistance of both the afferent and efferent arterioles. Increased systemic blood pressure will raise the glomerular hydrostatic pressure, which can increase GFR. However, there are autoregulation mechanisms in place to maintain a relatively constant glomerular pressure as arterial pressure fluctuates. Autoregulation in healthy individuals ensures that GFR and RBF remain relatively constant over a wide range of systemic arterial blood pressures from 80 to 180 mmHg [2, 7].

A decrease in afferent arteriole (preglomerular) resistance leads to an increase in both renal blood flow (RBF) and GFR. An increase in afferent arteriole resistance leads to a decrease in both RBF and GFR. When the resistance decreases in the efferent arterioles (postglomerular), RBF increases, but GFR decreases. Conversely, when the resistance increases in efferent arterioles, RBF decreases and GFR increases. These changes in arteriolar resistance allow for rapid alterations in glomerular blood flow, minimizing changes in GFR [2, 7].

The resistance of the afferent and efferent arterioles is regulated by the autonomic nervous system and vasoactive mediators. Vasoconstrictors of both afferent and efferent arterioles include norepinephrine, angiotensin II, endothelin, and thromboxane. ADH (vasopressin) also causes constriction of the efferent arteriole but not the afferent arteriole. Norepinephrine is released by stimulation of the sympathetic nervous system, causing constriction of both the afferent and efferent arterioles; however, constriction of efferent arterioles predominates, decreasing RBF while minimizing changes in GFR. Angiotensin II also causes more vasoconstriction in the efferent arterioles than in the afferent vessels. Vasodilators of both afferent and efferent arterioles include acetylcholine, nitric oxide, dopamine, bradykinin, prostacyclin, and prostaglandin I_2 (PgI_2). PGE2 causes relaxation in afferent arterioles, but not efferent arterioles. The release of norepinephrine, angiotensin II, and ADH causes vasoconstriction and, at the same time, promotes the production of prostaglandins that promote vasodilation. The production of PGE2 and PgI_2 is important in maintaining RBF when norepinephrine and angiotensin II concentrations are increased (hypovolemic states). The balance between afferent and efferent arteriolar tone (vasodilation or vasoconstriction) determines the effective transglomerular hydrostatic pressure available to drive glomerular filtration [2, 7].

Approximation of Glomerular Filtration Rate

GFR is directly related to functional renal mass in health and in those with acute loss of renal mass (AKI). Measurement of GFR (mL/min, mL/min/kg, mL/min/m²) is the gold standard for the assessment of renal function and the detection of renal disease progression. It is important to recognize that there is discordance between the percentage of renal mass that is initially lost and the percentage of decrease in measured GFR, due to renal hypertrophy and increases in SNGFR that occur as adaptations over time in chronic disease [54]. Consequently, the percentage loss of renal mass is greater than the percent decrease in GFR during CKD. Determination of RBF also can be useful in detecting progression of renal disease but is less commonly evaluated than GFR.

Sedatives and anesthetics have little effect on GFR. In one study, GFR was similar in dogs sedated with butorphanol and diazepam, acepromazine and butorphanol, and diazepam and ketamine. GFR in sedated dogs was not significantly different from that of awake dogs [55]. Ketamine and acepromazine have minimal effects on GFR in cats [56]. A combination of medetomidine, butorphanol, and atropine has been evaluated in dogs using technetium-labeled diethylenetriamine-pentaacetic acid (99 m) renal scintigraphy as an estimate of GFR and was found to have effects on GFR, similar to those observed after saline alone [57].

GFR is not routinely measured in the evaluation of renal function due to technical difficulties and costs. Instead, surrogates for GFR such as blood urea nitrogen (BUN), serum creatinine, and SDMA concentrations, are used because they are more easily determined than is GFR. The simultaneous evaluation of various combinations of circulating surrogates for GFR (including creatinine, cystatin C, galectin-3, and SDMA) improves the accuracy for the calculation of estimated GFR in humans [58, 59]. This is likely to also be true for veterinary medicine, though equations that accurately predict GFR have yet to be successfully developed. An attempt to increase the accuracy for prediction of measured GFR based on serum creatinine and an estimation of muscle mass failed to adequately perform in one study of cats [60].

An ideal substance for estimation of GFR should be excreted from the body entirely by the kidneys, produced at a constant rate in the body, have little binding to plasma proteins, be freely filtered by the glomerulus, and undergo no tubular reabsorption or secretion. It also should not alter renal function if injected, should be well distributed and restricted to the ECF, and should not be metabolized by the kidney.

GFR and serum analytes used to estimate GFR often have wide reference ranges for the general population, which limits their usefulness to detect early changes in renal function in individuals. General reference ranges for clinical tests related to glomerular function are provided in Table 1.2. Individual animals have far less variability in these measurements. Due to large variation in veterinary patient size, GFR is usually normalized to body weight or surface area. The use of age- and breed-specific reference ranges can increase the utility

Table 1.2 General reference ranges for clinical tests related to glomerular function. The reference range provided by a specific laboratory should be used.

Test (Units)	Dog	Cat
Blood urea nitrogen (mg/dL)	8–25	15–35
Serum creatinine (mg/dL)	0.3–1.3	0.8–1.8
Serum cystatin C (mg/dL)	0.5–1.5	0.6–2.0 [61]
SDMA (µg/dL)	<14	<14
	<18 IRIS	<18 IRIS
Endogenous creatinine clearance (mL/min/kg)	2–5	2–5
Exogenous creatinine clearance (mL/min/kg)	3–5	2–4
Iohexol clearance (mL/min/kg)	1.7–4.1	1.3–4.2
24-hour urine protein excretion (mg/kg/day)	<30	<20
U_{Pr}/U_{Cr}	<0.5	<0.4
	<0.2 for most	<0.2 for most
Microalbuminuria (mg/dL)	<1	<1
	<2.5	<2.5

of these measurements to detect early renal disease. Trending for increases in the concentration of molecules used to estimate GFR can also provide meaningful evidence for progressive renal disease, even when their concentrations are still within the reference range. Analytic variability of a particular analyte should also be considered during the evaluation of changes in reported values from serial samples [54].

GFR was measured by scintigraphy in one study of client-owned dogs with either a diagnosis of CKD or those likely to have CKD. GFR was compared to serum creatinine, SDMA, and cystatin C. The sensitivity for the finding of a serum creatinine >1.3 mg/dL or SDMA >14 µg/dL to predict a low GFR was 90%, whereas the specificity was 90% for creatinine and 87% for SDMA. Overall performance of SDMA or serum creatinine to predict a low GFR was similar in this study, but cystatin C was inferior to both creatinine and SDMA [62].

The relationship between GFR measured by iohexol, SDMA, and serum creatinine was reported in one study of client-owned nonazotemic dogs. Serum creatinine and SDMA were only moderately correlated to GFR and to each other. An SDMA cutoff of >14 µg/dL was sensitive at 90% for the detection of dogs with a ≥40% decreased in GFR, but specificity was low at 50%. More than half of the dogs with an increased SDMA >14 µg/dL had GFR values that were either increased or decreased by <20% of the expected normal GFR. Sensitivity was maintained at 90%, but specificity increased to 83% when the SDMA cutoff was increased to >18 µg/dL for the detection of those with ≥40% decreased GFR [63].

RENAL CLEARANCE

The renal clearance of a substance is that volume of plasma that would have to be filtered by the glomeruli each minute to account for the amount of that substance appearing in the urine each minute. The renal clearance of a substance (x) that is neither reabsorbed nor secreted by the tubules is equal to the GFR. Thus, GFR equals the concentration of the substance in the urine (U_x mg/dL) times the volume of urine per total minutes (V^o mL/min), divided by the concentration of the substance in the serum or plasma (P_x mg/dL) times the weight of the animal (W kg) ($GFR = U_x V^o / P_x W$). This method for precise GFR is mostly restricted to the research environment. Nuclear scintigraphy can also be used to determine GFR at tertiary referral centers [64].

GFR is classically measured by physiologists and researchers using serum/plasma along with urine samples that have been accurately collected by volume over time. Inulin clearance is the gold standard, but it is not easily measured and not available at commercial laboratories. Bolus and continuous infusion of inulin or exogenous creatinine are usually the molecules employed for the most precise results. Endogenous creatinine clearance can be used to calculate GFR as a less accurate alternative than exogenous creatinine clearance [65–67]. Single-injection plasma clearance methods using inulin, iohexol, or creatinine have been used to estimate GFR. Plasma clearance of the substance is calculated using the area under the plasma concentration-versus-time curve. These methods do not require urine collection, but accuracy depends on the number of plasma samples and the timing of their collection [64, 68, 69].

Iohexol is readily available for clinical use to estimate GFR [70, 71], but a laboratory with special equipment must be available to measure it. Very few veterinary commercial laboratories offer iohexol determination. Iohexol is given IV and plasma samples collected after administration. It was recommended in one report to collect samples at 5 and 120 minutes following injection for dogs and at 20 and 180 minutes for cats when using the two-sample method. For the single-sample method, sampling at 120 minutes in dogs and 80 minutes in cats was recommended [72, 73]. Iohexol clearance may be useful in further investigation of renal function to determine if occult renal disease is present or not when routine serum surrogates for GFR (BUN, creatinine, SDMA) are normal. Although not specifically reported in dogs and cats, hypersensitivity to iohexol is possible. Because 1 mL/kg of iohexol is given IV relatively rapidly, caution should be used in those with marginal cardiac function and should not be used if the patient is overhydrated.

GFR determined by iohexol clearance (mL/min and mL/per/kg) was significantly higher for normal dogs in the lowest quartile of body weight (1.9-12.4 kg) of one study [74] similar to that found in another study of healthy dogs [72]. Age did not exert a significant effect on GFR in this study when all dogs were considered. A weak trend for increasing age associated with a decrease in GFR was found only in dogs of the lowest quartile body weight. It was suggested that a separate reference range for GFR of dogs with low body weight should be used [74].

Creatinine is produced endogenously from muscles (see details below) and excreted by glomerular filtration. Thus, its clearance can be used to estimate GFR. For endogenous creatinine clearance determination in clinical cases, collect all urine for 12 or 24 hours and record the volume [43]. Failure to collect all urine produced will decrease the calculated clearance value. The animal's body weight should be recorded, and the serum and urine creatinine concentrations should be determined. Normal endogenous creatinine clearance is approximately 2–5 mL/min/kg in the dog and cat [2]. However, endogenous creatinine clearance measurements are higher than adult reference ranges in puppies from 9 to 21 weeks of age [75]. The main indication for determination of endogenous creatinine clearance in clinical practice is the suspicion of renal disease in a patient with polyuria and polydipsia that has a normal BUN and serum creatinine concentrations.

For exogenous creatinine clearance, administer creatinine (100 mg/kg) SQ or IV to increase the serum creatinine concentration approximately 10-fold. Approximately 40 minutes later, collect at least one timed urine sample using an indwelling urinary catheter (e.g. all urine produced in 20 minutes). The average of three 20-minute collection periods is recommended to minimize collection errors. Determine the animal's body weight and serum and urine creatinine concentrations. Exogenous creatinine clearance exceeds endogenous creatinine clearance and approximates inulin clearance (the gold standard for determination of GFR) in the dog [64, 66]. In cats, exogenous creatinine clearance may be slightly lower than inulin clearance [64].

Renal excretion of urea occurs by glomerular filtration, and BUN concentrations are inversely proportional to GFR. However, urea clearance is not a consistently reliable estimate of GFR, and in the face of volume depletion, decreased urea clearance may occur without a decrease in GFR due to increased tubular reabsorption of urea.

BLOOD UREA NITROGEN/SERUM UREA NITROGEN

More than 90% of urea is excreted by the kidney, with minor excretion in the gastrointestinal (GI) tract and skin [76]. The production and excretion of urea are not constant depending on dietary protein intake, degree of tissue catabolism, liver function, and renal tubular fluid flow rate. Urea is produced primarily from ammonia in the liver via the urea cycle (also known as the ornithine cycle or Krebs–Henseleit cycle), which effectively removes excess ammonia from the circulation. A small amount of urea is also generated in brain tissue [77]. The urea cycle disposes of approximately 90% of circulating nitrogen [78]. The rate of urea production depends on the amount of ammonia produced from protein catabolism from dietary sources and endogenous protein, primarily derived from muscle [76]. Ammonia enters the urea cycle either directly from the blood or from the breakdown of glutamine. Ammonia and bicarbonate form carbamoyl phosphate, which combines with ornithine to form citrulline. Citrulline and aspartate combine to form arginosuccinate, resulting in the release of fumarate and the production of arginine. With the action of arginase, urea is released and ornithine forms, completing the cycle [79]. Carnivores are unique in that they are unable to synthesize ornithine from proline and glutamine; thus, ornithine is produced exclusively from arginine, which is required in the diet [79]. After urea is produced, urea distributes evenly in the total body water since it is able to diffuse through cell membranes.

Circulating levels of urea nitrogen have long been used to assess renal function and still have value today when close attention is paid to nonrenal factors involved in its interpretation. The term "blood urea nitrogen" is often used, but since the measurement is rarely performed on whole blood, the term "serum urea nitrogen" (SUN) should be used to reflect the measurement utilizing serum.

Urea is measured primarily by enzymatic methods. Urea in the sample is hydrolyzed with urease to generate ammonia, and the ammonia is then quantified. The analysis actually measures urea and is converted to a urea nitrogen measurement for reporting as BUN or SUN. In the USA, BUN/SUN in mg/dL is the typical reported value and is NOT equivalent to the true measurement of urea. In most parts of the world, the reporting of urea concentration in mmol/L is preferable. Urea contains two nitrogen atoms (each with a mass of 14), and the mass of urea is 60. Thus, the concentration of urea in mg/dL is 60/28 (2.14) times the urea nitrogen concentration in mg/dL. To convert to molar units, 1 mg/dL BUN (or SUN) = $10 \times 2.14/60 = 0.357$ mmol/L urea. Multiply the BUN concentration in mg/dL by 0.357 to get the urea concentration in mmol/L. [76]

Reagent test strips have also been used for rapidly estimating BUN concentration. These strips group results into 4 categories: category 1, 5-15 mg/dL, category 2, 15-26 mg/dL, category 3, 30-40 mg/dL, and category 4, 50-80 mg/dL. For dogs in one study, category 1 and 2 results were considered nonazotemic and categories 3 and 4 were considered azotemic. In cats, category 1-3 results were considered nonazotemic and category 4 results were azotemic. Results from the test strips were compared to an automated analyzer measurement of SUN and were found to have high sensitivity and specificity in both dogs and cats. Since the test strips only give a semiquantitative measurement, BUN/SUN should be verified by quantitative measurement [80].

The age of the patient can have a significant impact on the urea nitrogen concentration [81]. In a study of 68 puppies, BUN was higher in puppies as compared to adults until 28 days of age. From days 28 through 84 (end of study), BUN levels were lower in the puppies than in adult dogs [82]. In Borzoi and beagle puppies, plasma urea concentrations were higher than that for the adult reference range from birth to one week old [83]. Reference intervals based on adult dogs should not be used for puppies. A mechanism for the higher BUN in puppies was not obvious. Gender did not appear to significantly affect BUN concentration in 896 dogs less than one year of age [81]. Yorkshire terriers have been anecdotally noted to have an increased BUN independent of increased serum creatinine as a breed predisposition, and some have also been noted with renal proteinuria. Most are not clinically ill for long periods of time [84, 85].

Both postprandial and diurnal effects were found for urea concentrations in one study from cats. Mean plasma concentrations of urea were 15% higher when measured at 8 p.m. compared to 8 a.m. [86]. The circulating urea concentration can be increased in any condition characterized by increased (endogenous tissue or exogenous dietary intake) protein catabolism [87]. The effect of some drugs (e.g. long-term glucocorticosteroids, azathioprine, or tetracyclines) on BUN has not been well studied, but it appears to be minimal. The feeding of higher protein diets to dogs with CKD preferentially increases BUN over creatinine. BUN will decrease during the feeding of lower protein content diets due to less generation of BUN despite decreased GFR during CKD. Lower protein dietary intake may be associated with a slight increase in serum creatinine concentration due to the decreased GFR during CKD. During the feeding of higher protein diets, serum creatinine may decrease some due to increased GFR.

Comparing preprandial and four-hour postprandial BUN concentrations in dogs, BUN increased from 13.7 to 16.0 mg/dL in dogs receiving a 5% protein (as-fed) diet, and increased from 16.0 to 26.8 mg/dL in dogs receiving an 8.5% protein (as-fed) diet [88]. In general, the BUN concentration increased significantly within three hours of a meal and peaked at about six to nine hours. This elevation lasted up to 18 hours [89]. Therefore, an 18-hour fast has been recommended prior to the measurement of BUN [90]. The feeding of small amounts of diet tends to decrease the magnitude of the increase in BUN [89, 91]; thus, feeding multiple small meals during the day may be better to maintain BUN at a lower level. It is likely that increases in BUN following feeding will be more pronounced in those that have underlying renal disease and decreased GFR.

Low BUN is detected less frequently than increased BUN. Polyuria is often considered as a potential cause for a low BUN since tubular reabsorption of urea is heavily influenced by the tubular fluid flow rate. Higher tubular flow rates are associated with lower BUN due to less reabsorption of urea, an effect that does not occur with creatinine [92].

When protein is limited in the diet in the presence of adequate nonprotein calories, the BUN decreases because most of the ingested protein is used for protein synthesis with little waste left over for excretion [90]. However, in a study of 152 very underweight or emaciated dogs with chronic disease (starvation), BUN was increased. BUN was increased more frequently than serum creatinine, and the BUN/Cr ratio was elevated due to some combination of accelerated catabolism and loss of muscle mass [93].

SERUM CREATININE

For a more detailed veterinary review of creatinine, refer to the articles by Braun [94], Kovarikova [95], and Finco [96]. Measurement of serum creatinine concentration is the most commonly used surrogate to estimate GFR in clinics. Serum creatinine is generally preferred over BUN for evaluation of renal function since creatinine has fewer nonrenal variables [94, 97, 98]. Creatine is taken up by muscle from the circulation after its synthesis by kidney, liver, and pancreas. Creatine is enzymatically phosphorylated to phosphocreatine inside muscle cells. Both creatine and phosphocreatine undergo spontaneous conversion to creatinine, which is released into the circulation at a relatively steady rate for each individual animal [76]. The daily rate for creatinine production is determined by age, sex, and muscle mass of the individual. The small-molecular-weight nonprotein-bound creatinine undergoes glomerular filtration but negligible tubular secretion or reabsorption in the dog and cat [94]. Increased concentration of circulating creatinine can lead to less creatinine generation by several postulated mechanisms including negative feedback for creatine synthesis [76].

Since creatinine arises from muscles, serum creatinine concentration is lower than it would otherwise be in patients that have lost substantial amounts of lean muscle mass regardless of the cause. In these instances, serum creatinine overestimates the degree of excretory renal function in that animal. During the progression of CKD, loss of lean muscle mass can parallel loss of renal function, which results in little or no change in serum creatinine concentration. This phenomenon reduces the ability for serum creatinine to detect ongoing CKD progression early, even when tracking serial changes in serum creatinine.

An increased serum creatinine is not associated with a decreased GFR, however, in some instances [99]. Healthy dogs and cats with large lean muscle mass can have higher serum creatinine concentrations than those with less muscle mass [98, 100, 101]. Increased production of creatinine by heavily muscled normal dogs can increase serum creatinine concentration to some degree, as can release of preformed creatinine from muscle into the circulation during rhabdomyolysis.

Greyhounds have higher reference range serum creatinine than the general reference range for all breed dogs [102–104], despite also having higher GFR than average for other breeds [105]. Whippet, Afghan hound, and Saluki dogs have also been described with a higher reference range for serum creatinine [106]. Birman cats had higher serum creatinine compared to Abyssinian, Norwegian Forest, and Siberian cats of one study [107], a finding that was confirmed in another study using mostly domestic short-hair cats as the control group [108]. Physiologically higher serum creatinine concentrations may also occur in Siberian, Siamese, and Somali cats [108, 109].

Serum creatinine concentrations are often lower in puppies and kittens than those encountered in adults [100, 101, 110, 111]. Serum creatinine concentrations slowly rise as they age [75]. Normal client-owned puppies at 8 and 16 weeks of age from two different large-breed litters had either a 0.4 or 0.5 mg/dL serum creatinine (Chew and Meuten 1982 unpublished observations). Five-month-old Beagle puppies had a mean serum creatinine of 0.5 mg/dL [112], and mean serum creatinine was 0.46–0.54 mg/dL in healthy mongrel puppies at 10, 20, and 30 days of age in another study [113]. In normal beagles, mean creatinine was 0.4 mg/dL at four and six weeks, which increased and stabilized to 0.9 mg/dL at six months of age [114]. Creatinine concentrations in Borzoi and beagle puppies up to eight weeks of age were lower than the adult reference range, varying from 24 to 51 μmol/L (0.27–0.58 mg/dL) [83]. Compared to the adult reference range, lower creatinine values were also found in puppies from a variety of breeds between 16 and 60 days old. Median creatinine concentration in these puppies was from 41 to 50 μmol/L (0.46–0.57 mg/dL) [115]. In a study of healthy dogs of various breeds, sex, body size, and age, median circulating creatinine and urea concentrations were lower in puppies than in adults. Median creatinine was 0.45 mg/dL in four-to-eight-week-old puppies and the creatinine values progressively increased in older puppies until a median creatinine of 1.05 mg/dL was reached in dogs >52 weeks of age. Similarly, urea was a median of 20 mg/dL in four-to-eight-week-old puppies and progressively increased to a median urea of 34 mg/dL in dogs >52 weeks of age. Sex and body size did not impact creatinine or urea values in this study [116]. An increase in serum creatinine may not be readily recognized in this population when using an adult reference range. The same concerns exist during the measurement of serum creatinine in small-breed and geriatric dogs. A reference interval for serum creatinine was suggested to be used for specific breeds that differed from those used for mixed breeds. Serum creatinine was significantly lower in all dogs <1 year of age and serum creatinine values were lower in small breed than that found in larger breeds of this study [117].

In contrast, mean serum creatinine progressively declined in normal beagles from 10 to 14 years of age in one study, possibly attributed to loss of lean muscle mass in this age group. The mean serum creatinine was 0.57 mg/dL at 14 years old compared to 0.88 mg/dL at one year of age [118]. In another study of normal beagles, the median creatinine decreased from 0.9 mg/dL at three years old to 0.6 mg/dL at nine years old [119].

Creatinine concentrations are not constant throughout the day, with higher concentrations observed in the afternoon or in the evening [86, 95]. In one study of normal cats, plasma creatinine concentrations were lower during feeding than following fasting, possibly an effect of feeding that increases GFR. This finding was different than that encountered in the dog in which increased circulating creatinine occurred after feeding. The composition of the diet and the amount eaten also factor into these effects [86]. A circadian rhythm has been shown for creatinine in both the dog [120] and cat [86]. Mean serum creatinine was 18% higher when measured at 8 p.m. compared to 8 a.m. in one study of normal cats [86]. The magnitude of disparity in serum creatinine concentrations from these different methods of collection (preanalytical) is not likely to be of clinical importance unless the serum creatinine values are slightly above or below the upper reference range or near levels used by the International Renal Interest Society (IRIS) for staging.

Creatinine can be measured in plasma or serum, but creatinine was 5–10 μmol/L (0.06–0.1 mg/dL) higher in serum compared to plasma from dogs [121]. Plasma creatinine values were higher in most samples when blood was collected from the jugular vein compared to the cephalic vein in dogs, with a maximal difference of 15 μmol/L (0.17 mg/dL) [122].

The concentration of serum creatinine concentration is generally considered to change little over weeks, months, and years in individual healthy dogs and cats [54]. However, in 20 normal dogs studied at nine time points, even though all values were within the normal reference range for serum creatinine, there was a high interindividual variability [123]. Analytic variability in the measurement of serum creatinine in the same sample is minimal in some labs, but differences in serum creatinine have been reported to be as high as 0.45 mg/dL when measured by the same laboratory and up to 0.57 mg/dL when measured by different laboratories. The variability in measurement of serum creatinine was greater in the same laboratory and between laboratories in the face of moderate-to-severe azotemia. It appears that an increase in serum creatinine of ≥0.3 mg/dL is a clinically relevant indicator of decreased renal function even when the creatinine value is still within the reference range if measurements are made with the same analyzer and laboratory [54].

The median upper reference limit for creatinine and BUN varied by breed of cats in one study between Holy Birman, Chartreaux, Maine Coon, and Persian cats, with Birman having the highest median values [109]. The median and range reference values for creatinine and BUN were significantly different, but the degree of difference was small in four large-breed dogs [124]. The reference interval for circulating creatinine concentrations in various breeds of small dogs (<12 kg) was lower than for the general population, 45–90 μmol/L (0.51–1.0 mg/dL) in comparison to 54–144 μmol/L (0.61–1.63 mg/dL) in one study. It has been suggested that the use of breed-specific reference intervals is important in order to allow early diagnosis of renal impairment in small-breed dogs based on creatinine [125, 126]. A narrower reference range for serum creatinine was established for the dog breed Dogue de Bordeaux compared to the general population [127].

The type and volume of meat consumed as well as the timing of the blood sample have the potential to influence serum creatinine [76]. Cooking of meat favors the conversion of creatine to creatinine, which increased serum creatinine by as much as 20% in one study of dogs consuming a pelleted food [128]. No change in serum creatinine occurred after the feeding of dry, semimoist, or canned food to dogs in another study; BUN increased after the feeding of these diets in all dogs with the greatest increases observed in dogs consuming canned food [129]. Fasting prior to collection of blood is recommended to limit the degree of dietary impact on the measurement of serum creatinine [128].

Most laboratories use automated methods to measure serum and urine creatinine by the Jaffe colorimetric method, which employs alkaline picrate to bind with creatinine to form a reddish complex [130, 131]. The basic Jaffe picric acid reaction overestimates the amount of true creatinine since some noncreatinine molecules contribute to the color that develops. The original Jaffe method was subject to measurement of noncreatinine chromogens in addition to true creatinine that can slightly increase the creatinine value reported [65, 128, 131, 132]. In a study of multiple domestic species, the kinetic Jaffe reaction was positively influenced by acetone and glucose, whereas there was negative bias from acetoacetic acid, bilirubin, and lipid. The enzymatic method to measure creatinine was not affected by acetoacetic acid, acetone, or glucose, but was negatively affected by bilirubin and lipid [131]. The overestimation of true circulating creatinine is most noticeable in healthy animals with low total creatinine values. Total creatinine chromogens measured by the original Jaffe method were compared to that following extraction with Lloyd's reagent to determine true creatinine. True creatinine accounted up to 55% and pseudocreatinine up to 45% of the total circulating creatinine in normal dogs of this study [133]. A pseudocreatinine chromogen correction of −0.3 mg/dL is arbitrarily applied by some automated analyzers to generate the reported circulating value [134].

A concern is that measurement of noncreatinine chromogens in addition to true creatinine could falsely increase total creatinine to a higher value within or above the reference range [128]. An increase in creatinine from noncreatinine chromogens becomes less clinically relevant in animals with azotemic kidney disease since most of the increase in creatinine is now from true creatinine [94, 133]. Interfering noncreatinine chromogens in urine do not occur as frequently as those in serum [76], so the use of the Jaffe method on urine does not overestimate urine creatinine. The kinetic method currently used is an improvement as this decreases the detection of interfering pseudocreatinine compounds [131]. Some interfering molecules in the circulation can also lower the amount of creatinine that is detected [131].

Deproteination of the sample before creatinine measurement improves the accuracy but does not remove all interfering substances. Methods to modify the sample to an alkaline pH allow only true creatinine to combine with picric acid, allowing a more accurate measurement of creatinine. Many different modifications of the basic Jaffe method are used by commercial laboratories that are designed to remove or account for interfering substances. Consequently, it is difficult to accurately compare serum creatinine results generated between different commercial laboratories or results from different in-house analyzers on the same patient. It has been recommended that all methods to measure creatinine be standardized to that using the method of stable isotope dilution tandem mass spectrometry in order to allow comparison of results between laboratories [135].

Standardization in the measurement of serum creatinine is common in human medicine laboratories, but there is no such standardization in veterinary laboratories. Repeatability for the measurement of serum creatinine (intralaboratory precision) among 10 veterinary laboratories was high using the same analyzer in the same laboratory, but there was quite a bit of variation between results reported by some laboratories (interlaboratory imprecision) [136, 137].

Enzymatic methods to measure creatinine result in lower values than those generated using the Jaffe method [94, 131]. Use of enzymatic methods to measure serum creatinine allowed endogenous creatinine clearance to approximate that of inulin clearance in one study of dogs [65]. Automated enzymatic methods to measure creatinine are more costly, and these reagents have a shorter shelf life than that needed for Jaffe measurements. Some authors have advocated to measure creatinine only by enzymatic methods in order to improve the quality of data for clinical decision-making, especially at low levels of circulating creatinine [130].

In a study of over 300 healthy dogs from 32 breeds, the mean fasting plasma creatinine determined with an enzymatic method was 0.93 ± 0.24 mg/dL with a range of 0.45–1.40 mg/dL for the general population. Mean serum creatinine varied by body weight category in this study. Serum creatinine magnitude was the lowest in dogs with a body weight of 0–10 kg (0.70 ± 0.12, range 0.48–1.02) and progressively increased in dogs 11–25 kg (0.85 ± 0.16, range: 0.55–1.24), 26–45 kg (1.01 ± 0.26, range: 0.60–2.01), and dogs >45 kg (1.19 ± 0.24, range: 0.88–1.82). Males had a higher creatinine (1.00 ± 0.25 mg/dL) compared to females (0.90 ± 0.24 mg/dL) in this study [126]. Dogs with a body weight of 1–10 kg had a mean serum creatinine of 0.79 mg/dL, 0.91 mg/dL when 11–25 kg, and 1.08 mg/dL when >25 kg in another study using the Jaffe methodology [138]. Creatinine was lower in adult small-sized dogs of seven breeds at 45–90 μmol/L (0.51–1.0 mg/dL) compared to the population-based reference range of 54–144 μmol/L (0.61–1.62 mg/dL) [125]. The median creatinine for Greyhound puppies was 0.8 mg/dL, similar to that for other breeds but lower than that for adult Greyhounds [139].

Population-based reference ranges are broader than the reference range for an individual animal. For this reason, population-based reference ranges are less sensitive than an individual's reference range [140] for the diagnosis of CKD using surrogates of GFR such as creatinine or SDMA. An individual's reference range includes inherent random biological variation for the concentration of an analyte around its homeostatic set point [140].

The utility of serum creatinine to accurately detect renal disease can be increased when population-based reference intervals for creatinine are adjusted to account for small-, medium-, and large-breed dogs (based on body weight) to interpret results. Interpretation of serum creatinine should also take into account different reference ranges for animals that are very young and old. When available, specific breed reference ranges should be used instead of population-based reference ranges [95]. Small changes in serum creatinine can indicate clinically relevant changes in GFR as long as the conditions of blood collection and specific analyzer used are kept the same.

For a discussion of urinary creatinine measurement, refer to Chapter 7.

SYMMETRIC DIMETHYLARGININE

Although SDMA was discovered decades ago, there is renewed interest in this molecule as a surrogate to improve estimated GFR in humans [59] and as another surrogate for GFR in veterinary medicine. SDMA is largely eliminated by the kidneys [54, 141] and changes in circulating SMDA parallel that for GFR in the dog [142] and the cat [143]. SDMA results from methylation of arginine that occurs in all nucleated cells and then enters the circulation. Dietary intake does not appear to affect SDMA concentrations regardless of amino acid intake [54]. SDMA is excreted almost entirely into urine by glomerular filtration without further tubular processing and, consequently, increases in blood as GFR decreases. Urinary concentration of SDMA has not been used to study renal function in clinical practice to date. The measurement of SMDA offers an advantage over the measurement of serum creatinine in some patients, as SDMA is not influenced by lean muscle mass in cats [144] or dogs [100]. Consequently, SDMA concentration can be increased when serum creatinine concentration is still within the reference range in those with low lean muscle mass and reduced kidney function.

Liquid chromatography tandem mass spectrometry (LC/MS/MS) methodology has been validated as precise and accurate to measure SDMA concentration in dogs and cats [142, 144]. An automated proprietary clinical immunoassay that correlates with the LC/MS/MS method [145] is offered by one commercial veterinary laboratory (IDEXX); an in-house test for veterinarians to measure circulating SMDA concentration is also available from the same laboratory [146]. A competing veterinary laboratory (Antech) now measures SDMA by a different methodology as of late 2019, but comparisons of measured SDMA between these two methods have not yet been published. For IDEXX, SDMA in the dog and cat ≤14 μg/dL is normal, 15–19 μg/dL is mildly increased, 20–24 μg/dL is moderately increased, and ≥25 μg/dL is severely increased [147]. For Antech, normal SDMA is <14 μg/dL for the dog and <15 μg/dL for the cat. A mild increase is 14–16 μg/dL for the dog and 15–20 μg/dL for the cat. A high increase is >16 μg/dL for the dog and >20 μg/dL for the cat [148].

There was wide dispersion of SDMA results measured by a commercial immunoassay method in cats of one study. Dispersion includes variability in a measured analyte based on both analytical imprecision and biological variability. Biological and analyzer variability were considered important factors to consider for proper clinical interpretation, especially values that are at the edges of the reference range or medical decision threshold (such as IRIS CKD staging). Without this nuanced interpretation, it is possible for clinicians to ascribe too much clinical relevance to small changes in SDMA [149].

There was wide dispersion in SDMA results when analyzed by both a proprietary commercial laboratory method using high-throughput immunoassay and a proprietary point-of-care analyzer method in another study of cats. Results were not comparable in 20–50% of SDMA values generated by these two methods. A measured SDMA of 14 μg/dL could represent values from 8 to 20 μg/dL based on results from this study. Interpretation of SDMA values near the reference limit or threshold for medical decisions (slightly above or below) is difficult to make with certainty due to analytical and biological variability. Consequently, reference intervals based on specific analyzers were recommended [150].

SDMA measured with IDEXX SDMA using high-throughput competitive immunoassay, SDMA measured with the DLD SDMA ELISA on microtiter plates, and the gold standard of SDMA measured by liquid chromatography–mass spectrometry were compared. IDEXX SDMA exhibited less bias and less variation in the measurement of low and high concentrations of SDMA than when measured by the DLD SDMA ELISA method and was considered more suitable for veterinary patients in one study [151].

In general, the upper limit reference range for SDMA is <14 μg/dL for both adult dogs and cats, though the concentration of SDMA occasionally reaches or exceeds the 14 μg/dL reference limit in juvenile dogs [54]. The IDEXX reference range for puppies is currently 0–16 μg/dL; the reference range for kittens is the same as for adults. The average SDMA concentration was higher in nonracing Greyhounds than for the general population; the upper reference range was near 20 μg/dL [152]. SDMA and serum creatinine concentrations were evaluated in pretraining Greyhound puppies (three to eight months old) in one study. The median SDMA of 14 μg/dL (11–19 μg/dL) for puppies was similar to that for previously reported adults (median 14 μg/dL; 9–20 μg/dL). It was suggested that a reference range of ≤20 μg/dL for SDMA could be used for both age populations of Greyhounds. SDMA concentration also was higher in normal Birman cats than in cats of other breeds, though it was less commonly increased than serum creatinine concentration [108]. An SDMA <18 μg/dL is used as one criterion in the assignment of IRIS CKD stage 1, and an SDMA persistently >14 μg/dL can be used to diagnose CKD based on IRIS 2019 recommendations [153]. An SDMA >18 μg/dL was considered optimal for detection of ≥40% decrease in GFR in dogs of one study [63].

It is important to consider total variability in the interpretation of serum creatinine and SDMA when comparing multiple measurements over time. Total variability includes biological and analytical variability. It appears that total variability for serum creatinine is about ±0.2 mg/dL with the analytical variability at ±0.1 mg/dL. Similarly, for SDMA, total variability is about ±2 μg/dL and analytic variability is about ±1 μg/dL. More analytic variability is expected during repeated measurements of the same sample at the extreme upper limits of measurement, but variability in those measurements is not usually important since it is unlikely to result in a level that would substantially change clinical decision-making. For a hypothetical example, it is possible that the serum creatinine was 20 mg/dL on the first run through the analyzer and 15 mg/dL on a second run immediately thereafter on the same sample. In this instance, the interpretation of high-magnitude azotemia will not change. If the creatinine was first measured as 20 mg/dL and the creatinine repeated on the same sample was 5 mg/dL, there is an error in the measurement of one or both samples. Analytical variability can be much higher when comparing results of the same samples on different analyzers, as often occurs for measurements determined in-house compared to those sent to a referral laboratory (Mack-Gertig personal communication October 2020). Excellent analytic performance for SDMA measurement was shown in one study of dogs; SDMA was highly stable in serum and plasma [142]. The interested reader is referred to an extensive recent review of SDMA and circulating creatinine for the evaluation of excretory renal function in the dog and cat [136].

The biological variability for serum creatinine and SDMA was determined over nine time points of varying intervals in 20 normal dogs [123]. There was considerable variability in the values for these analytes so that values exceeded the upper reference range at times in some dogs. In order to be considered different values on sequential measurement, SDMA had to change by 1.34 μg/dL [123]. In a study of week-to-week variability in dogs with hereditary nephritis, serum creatinine and SDMA had to change by 21–24% in order to be confident for a true increase or decrease from baseline values [154]. SDMA and serum creatinine were measured once weekly for six weeks to determine biological variability in a study of healthy cats. The degree of variability in the magnitude of these analytes was higher than generally appreciated, but similar to findings in dogs [155]. Findings from these studies support the recommendation to evaluate SDMA and serum creatinine on sequential samples and not a single sample, especially for values that are near the reference range limits or near values used in IRIS staging.

It appears that, on average, SDMA concentration increases when there has been about a 40% decrease in GFR. The concentration of SDMA can increase in CKD patients when there is as little as 25% loss of renal mass and GFR at times [142, 156]. Concentrations of SDMA have been shown to increase above the reference range before serum creatinine increased in multiple studies of dogs and cats eventually diagnosed with azotemic CKD [101, 141, 142, 144, 157–159]. The concentration of SDMA increased many months before serum creatinine concentration when relatively high values for the upper limit of creatinine reference (above 2.0 mg/dL) ranges were used to diagnose the onset of CKD. When lower creatinine values were used for the upper limit as the comparator, SDMA concentration still increased before creatinine but by a shorter time. The concentration of SDMA was increased much more frequently than serum creatinine concentration in both dogs and cats when measured on the same sample (diagnostic discordance) [160], but it is not clear how many of these patients will develop progressive azotemic CKD.

A creatinine at >1.9 mg/dL and SDMA >18 μg/dL were used as surrogates for decreased GFR in a study of dogs. Decreased GFR using this definition was common in older dogs of most breeds, especially dogs >10 years of age. Using both creatinine and SDMA identified more dogs with decreased GFR than with either test alone. Fourteen breeds were identified to be at increased risk to discover an increased creatinine or SDMA. Geriatric and senior Shetland sheepdogs, Yorkshire terriers, and Pomeranians were significantly overrepresented with increased creatinine or SDMA. Boxers were also identified with significant increases in creatinine or SDMA up to 10 years of age [161].

CKD was diagnosed by a variety of criteria in 51.2% of initially healthy senior dogs when followed for over the next four years. Increased serum SDMA ≥14 μg/dL occurred in 8 of the 22 dogs diagnosed with CKD, compared with only 2 of 22 dogs with increased serum creatinine >1.8 mg/dL. A persistent increase in SDMA was documented in all dogs diagnosed with CKD. Based on these results, it was recommended to include SDMA as part of routine screening of elderly dogs [159].

A first-time mild increase in SDMA (15–19 μg/dL) was found to persist (>14 μg/dL) in the subsequent measurement in many dogs and cats of one study. This was observed in 33% of cats that had an initial SDMA of 15 μg/dL and in 62% of cats with an initial SDMA of 19 μg/dL. Increased SDMA persisted similarly in dogs, in 44% with an initial SDMA of 15 μg/dL and in 68% of dogs with an SDMA of 19 μg/dL [162].

The concordance between increased SDMA and serum creatinine was assessed in one large study in dogs and cats. When SDMA was increased, serum creatinine was increased in 30% of cats and in 28% of dogs, a finding that increased to 57% in cats and 54% of dogs one year later. When serum creatinine was increased, SDMA was increased in 75% of cats and in 69% of dogs, a finding that increased to 93% of cats and 87% of dogs one year later [163].

SDMA and serum creatinine were significantly correlated to each other and to GFR measured with iohexol clearance in one study of azotemic and nonazotemic cats. Plasma SDMA and serum creatinine were similar in sensitivity for the detection of reduced excretory renal function, but creatinine had higher specificity. Increased SDMA identified cats with decreased GFR in this study, but the superiority of SDMA over serum creatinine as a value-added test for early detection, as highly touted for detection of decreased GFR in other reports, was not demonstrated in this study. Thirty-nine of 49 cats had concordant results between serum creatinine and plasma SDMA. Discordant results were observed in 10 of 49 cats. SDMA was increased in eight cats, while serum creatinine was within the reference range; six of these eight cats, however, had normal GFR indicating a false positive test result for SDMA. SDMA was within the reference range in two cats, in which the serum creatinine was increased and GFR was reduced, indicating a false negative result for SDMA. Using a cutoff of 14 μg/dL was associated with many false positives for SDMA; increasing the cutoff to 18 μg/dL resulted in a more optimal sensitivity and specificity for SDMA [164].

Elevated SDMA with normal renal function has been identified on occasion in some reports [165, 166], a finding that has also been anecdotally noted by others [136] and also observed by this author. SDMA was reported to be lower in cats with diabetes mellitus than in control cats of one study [165]. An increased SDMA was considered to be falsely positive in 32% of dogs evaluated for the presence of kidney disease in dogs, whereas there were no false positives for increased serum creatinine at the same time; the gold standard of reduced GFR measured by iohexol clearance was used to define the presence of kidney disease [166].

There is sometimes discordance between the finding of a very high IDEXX SDMA value compared to a minimal or no increase in serum creatinine at the same time in animals with cancer [167]. Reductions in GFR to account for this magnitude of increase in SDMA were considered unlikely, as these patients had minimal clinical signs that would typically be expected in those with CKD. One proposed theory is that cancer cells infiltrating the kidney change the filtration barrier in some way that inhibits filtration of cationic SDMA but does not inhibit the filtration of nonpolar creatinine, allowing SDMA to increase, sometimes greatly, without an accompanying increase, or minimal increase, in serum creatinine [167]. Neoplastic infiltration of the kidney was shown to occur in all animals studied with a variety of cancers that had an increased SDMA with normal serum creatinine in one study [168]. Some dogs with lymphoma of another report had a disproportionate increase in SDMA at a time of reference range serum creatinine; SDMA declined when the lymphoma went into remission. Whether the increased SDMA reflected a reduced GFR was not determined. A large burden of tumor cells that were synthesizing SDMA was also considered as an alternative explanation for the preferential increase in SDMA [169].

CYSTATIN C

Serum cystatin C concentration appears to be a useful marker of GFR though its use has not entered routine clinical practice because measurement of this molecule is not yet available from veterinary referral laboratories, and a clear superiority for use of cystatin C has not been demonstrated. Measurement of serum and urine concentrations of cystatin C has been validated for use in the dog and cat using methods employed in human medicine [170].

Cystatin C is a protease inhibitor freely filtered by the glomeruli, does not undergo tubular secretion, and is almost completely reabsorbed by the proximal tubular cells [95]. Cystatin C is produced at a constant rate in all nucleated cells, and its excretion is not dependent on age, sex, or diet. Cystatin C has been extensively reviewed for its possible use in dogs and cats [61, 95, 170–172]. Normal cystatin C concentration is approximately 1 mg/L in dogs and 0.6–2.0 mg/L in cats [95, 171, 173]. Serum cystatin C concentration may also be increased by the presence of inflammation [174] or some types of neoplasia [175]. There are many reports with no consensus for the use of serum cystatin C in dogs and cats to evaluate renal function. Cystatin C appears to be less useful as a surrogate for GFR in cats than in dogs. There is no convincing evidence that cystatin C is superior to the use of serum creatinine in the evaluation of renal disease in the dog or cat [95].

INTERPRETATION OF RENAL FUNCTION TESTS

INTERPRETATION OF RENAL FUNCTION TESTS IN RENAL DISEASE

Serum creatinine concentration is the most commonly used serum biochemical indicator of renal function in the clinical setting. The relationship between GFR and serum creatinine is described as curvilinear, exponential, or hyperbolic [94, 96]. There is an exponential relationship between decreasing GFR and increasing serum creatinine (Figure 1.16). Notice that despite a substantial decrease in GFR, there is a minimal increase in serum creatinine concentration until a pivot point is reached at the exponential rise part of the curve. At that point, each subsequent further decrease in GFR is associated with a much larger increase in serum creatinine concentration. The slope of the curve is small when GFR is mildly or moderately decreased but large when GFR is severely reduced. Thus, large changes in GFR early in the course of renal disease cause small increases in BUN or serum creatinine concentration. Small changes in GFR in advanced renal disease cause large changes in BUN or serum creatinine concentration.

Neither BUN nor serum creatinine concentrations are specific enough for an early diagnosis of renal disease or clear identification of patients with normal renal function. BUN and serum creatinine are reported to increase at nearly the same time during the diagnosis of CKD in dogs and cats, neither being more sensitive than the other, but BUN concentrations are impacted by many more nonrenal factors [90, 176].

In a patient with primary renal disease, a serum creatinine concentration above the population reference range (>2.0 mg/dL) is often interpreted to be associated with a loss of greater than 75% of functional renal mass and GFR [54, 94, 177, 178]. When a lower value for the upper limit of serum creatinine such as 1.4, 1.5, or 1.6 mg/dL is used, an increased serum creatinine concentration is associated with a loss of about 50% renal mass and GFR [54]. Thus, the diagnostic utility of serum creatinine to detect decreased renal function as a surrogate for GFR can be enhanced when the upper limit of the reference range is lowered (<1.4 in dogs and <1.6 mg/dL in cats), when seemingly small increases in serum creatine ≥0.3 mg/dL are interpreted to be important, when breed- and age-specific dynamics for serum creatinine are brought into consideration, and when the same analyzer and conditions are used during the measurement of serum creatinine. An individual patient's serum creatinine concentration will increase over time with progression of renal disease, and trending patterns of increasing serum creatinine concentrations should not be ignored even if the results are still within the reference range. This is due to a high interindividual variation in serum creatinine values. Trends for increasing serum creatinine and BUN concentrations in individual animals are helpful for earlier detection of CKD [54, 179].

It has been recommended to adjust reference ranges for an individual animal's serum creatinine results to improve the

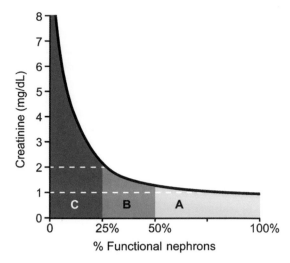

FIGURE 1.16 Serum creatinine concentration compared to the percent of functional nephrons (GFR). Note that the relationship of serum creatinine concentrations to GFR is exponential and described as a rectangular hyperbola. The slope of the curve is relatively flat when GFR is mildly or moderately decreased, but steep when GFR is severely reduced. Thus, decreases in GFR early in the course of renal disease cause only small increases in serum creatinine. With further decrease in GFR, a larger magnitude of increased serum creatinine occurs while on the exponential rise part of the curve (to the left). Small increases or decreases in GFR along the exponential steep rise part of the curve can create large numerical change in serum creatinine. Classically, a 75% decrease in GFR must occur before serum creatinine increases above the reference range, but this depends on what value for the upper end of the reference range for creatinine is used. When lower values for the upper reference range of serum creatinine are used, a decrease in GFR of about 50% can be detected when serum creatinine is found to be increased. In CKD, the area up to 50% decrease in GFR is referred to as that of decreased renal reserve, from 50% to 75% loss is referred to renal insufficiency, and 75% loss is renal failure associated with azotemia. Area A represents diminished renal reserve with advancing chronic renal disease (International Renal Interest Society [IRIS] Stage 1). Area B represents renal insufficiency (late IRIS Stage 1 and early IRIS Stage 2); submaximally concentrated urine is often documented in dogs but less commonly in cats in this stage. Area C represents overt azotemic renal failure (IRIS Stages 3 and 4). The percent of nephron mass loss and the decrease in GFR are parallel when there is an acute loss of nephron mass. In those with CKD, adaptive hypertrophy of the surviving remnant nephrons (anatomically and physiologically) over weeks to months limits the decrease in GFR, so that the percentage loss of GFR is less than compared to the loss of nephron mass. Illustration by Tim Vojt, reproduced with permission of The Ohio State University.

interpretation. The animal's breed, body weight, and muscle/body condition scores can be factored into the assessment as one way to increase the utility of serum creatinine to diagnosis CKD. Similarly, trends for an increasing serum creatinine within the general population reference range can increase the sensitivity for the diagnosis of CKD over a period of months or over days for the diagnosis of AKI. The use of a previously established baseline creatinine for individual patients allows values that escalate within the reference range to be detected early [54, 95].

The loss of renal mass is proportional to the decrease in GFR during an acute insult, but there is discordance between the percentage loss of renal mass and decrease in GFR in chronic disease. In CKD, GFR gradually increases over weeks to months following an initial loss of renal mass due to adaptive mechanisms of renal hypertrophy and increases in SNGFR [54, 180, 181].

The magnitude of a single high BUN, serum creatinine, or SDMA concentration cannot be used to predict whether azotemia is prerenal, primary renal, or postrenal in origin and cannot be used to distinguish between acute and chronic, reversible and irreversible, or progressive and nonprogressive processes. In addition, the finding of a reference range BUN, serum creatinine, or SDMA concentration does not exclude the possibility of renal disease. A reference range BUN, serum creatinine, or SDMA concentration implies that at least 25–40% of renal mass is functional, but how much more renal mass is functional cannot be determined by these tests. In some situations, either the BUN or serum creatinine is increased, but not both at the same time (discussed previously). It is not always possible to explain discordant results between BUN and serum creatinine concentrations (Table 1.3).

Table 1.3 Discordant results between blood urea nitrogen (BUN) and serum creatinine (SCr) concentrations.

↑ BUN-to-SCr ratio	↓ BUN-to-SCr ratio
(high BUN, low creatinine, combinations)	(low BUN, high creatinine, combinations)
Dehydration and volume depletion-early oliguria	Polyuria
High-protein-content meal	Low-protein-content meal
Gastrointestinal hemorrhage	Anorexia/hyporexia
Loss of lean muscle mass	Highly muscled individual
Emaciated animal – chronic disease	Sighthounds
	Acute muscle injury
Hyperthyroidism	Anabolic steroids
Physiological low muscle mass – young animal	Liver disease
Geriatric – normal aging low muscle mass	
Uroabdomen (early)	
Congestive heart failure	

Discordance between serum creatinine and SDMA is common, with increases in SDMA being reported more commonly than increases in creatinine in both dogs and cats [160]. SDMA is reported to increase earlier than serum creatinine in both dogs and cats, and in dogs that are eventually diagnosed with azotemic CKD. SDMA and creatinine concentrations both varied within the same normal dog when blood was sampled at multiple time points in one study. Both of these analytes are limited as individual screening tests because of this individual variation. Serial monitoring and trend detection were recommended to detect early renal dysfunction before concentrations escalate above the population reference range. SDMA had less biological and analytical variability than serum creatinine in this study suggesting SDMA to be a superior early biomarker for detection of kidney dysfunction [123]. In another study, median SDMA concentrations were increased to the same magnitude in dogs with CKD or AKI, but serum creatinine concentrations were significantly higher in dogs with AKI compared to dogs with CKD. The ratio of SDMA (μg/dL) to serum creatinine (mg/dL) was significantly higher in dogs with CKD (median 10.0) than in dogs with AKI (median 6.5). Unfortunately, substantial overlap in this ratio limits its usefulness to distinguish CKD from AKI [182]. An SDMA-to-creatinine ratio >10 was associated with a higher risk of death in dogs and cats with CKD in one report. Most dogs and cats with CKD have an SDMA-to-creatinine ratio of <10. The use of this ratio for prognosis should not be used for dogs and cats with values within the reference range as they can have ratios >10 that would be very misleading [183]. The prognostic value for this ratio in dogs with CKD was not confirmed in another study [182].

Serum creatinine and/or SDMA are used to assign an IRIS CKD stage [153]. Serum creatinine and urine output are the mainstays for assigning an IRIS AKI grade, though SDMA can be used to provide evidence for Grade 1 AKI [184]. Staging is performed AFTER CKD has been diagnosed in patients that have stable CKD. The CKD staging system uses an upper reference range for creatinine of <1.6 mg/dL for cats and <1.4 mg/dL for dogs and an SDMA <18 μg/dL for both dogs and cats. CKD stages from 1 to 4 are assigned based on escalating magnitude of serum creatinine concentration and/or SDMA. Substages for CKD are assigned based on blood pressure and magnitude of proteinuria measured by urinary-protein-to-urinary-creatinine ratio (UPC) (discussed later in Chapter 7). An acute increase of ≥0.3 mg/dL serum creatinine is used to help assign IRIS AKI stage 1.

SDMA concentration was added to the IRIS CKD staging and treatment recommendations in 2019 (Table 1.4). Adding SDMA is helpful to further characterize CKD and the degree of renal dysfunction in patients in which serum creatinine concentration underestimates the decline in GFR. The finding of a serum creatinine concentration <1.6 mg/dL for the cat and <1.4 mg/dL for the dog, and an SDMA concentration that is

Table 1.4 IRIS CKD staging guidelines (updated 2019).

		Dog	Cat	Units	Comments
Stage 1	Creatinine	<1.4	<1.6	mg/dL	Other abnormalities are found that support primary kidney disease (USG, renal imaging, UPC, others)
		<125	<140	μmol/L	
	SDMA	<18	<18	μg/dL	SDMA persistently >14 μg/dL may be used to diagnose CKD
Stage 2	Creatinine	1.4–2.8	1.6–2.8	mg/dL	Clinical signs minimal or absent
		125–250	140–250	μmol/L	
	SDMA	18–35	18–25	μg/dL	
Stage 3	Creatinine	2.9–5.0	2.9–5.0	mg/dL	Early and late-stage 3 based on severity of clinical signs
		251–440	251–440	μmol/L	
	SDMA	36–54	26–38	μg/dL	
Stage 4	Creatinine	>5.0	>5.0	mg/dL	Increasing risk for systemic signs and uremic crisis
		>440	>440	μmol/L	
	SDMA	>54	>38	μg/dL	

<18 μg/dL, provides one entry point into IRIS Stage 1 CKD in the presence of other abnormalities that suggest primary kidney disease (urinalysis with low USG, high systemic blood pressure, increased UPC, renal imaging changes) [153].

The same IRIS CKD stage will be assigned in most patients based on both SDMA and serum creatinine concentrations. Guidelines for the use of SDMA concentration in combination with serum creatinine concentration continue to be evaluated due to concerns that serum creatinine may underperform in its estimation of declining GFR, especially in patients with low lean muscle mass. During times of discordant staging between creatinine and SDMA, the higher stage is chosen based on the highest value of either of these analytes [153]. Most discordant results will be associated with a creatinine suggesting a lower stage and SDMA suggesting a higher stage, likely due to loss of lean muscle mass that generates a lower serum creatinine concentration. An SDMA >18 μg/dL in a dog with a serum creatinine <1.4 mg/dL, or <1.6 mg/dL in a cat, is upstaged to Stage 2 rather than Stage 1 when based on creatinine alone. Patients designated as Stage 2 by serum creatinine should be restaged to Stage 3 if the SDMA is >35 μg/dL in dogs or if the SDMA is >25 μg/dL in cats. Similarly, an SDMA >54 μg/dL in the dog or >38 μg/dL in the cat would result in an assignment of Stage 4 in those originally assigned to stage 3 based on creatinine [153].

The BUN/serum creatinine ratio has also been used to evaluate renal disease. The BUN/creatinine ratio often is 15:1 to 30:1 in mature healthy dogs and cats. In one study, the median BUN/serum creatinine ratio in healthy dogs was 14.4 [185]. This ratio may be increased in prerenal and postrenal azotemia as a result of increased tubular reabsorption of urea at lower tubular flow rates or easier absorption of urea than creatinine across peritoneal membranes in animals with uroabdomen. Hyperthyroid cats may also have an increased ratio due to increased GFR and loss of lean muscle mass. It may be increased during cachexia as a result of lower serum creatinine concentration due to loss of lean muscle mass. The BUN/serum creatinine ratio may be decreased after fluid therapy as a result of increased tubular flow and decreased tubular reabsorption of urea, rather than as a result of a change in GFR.

It is important to remember that any analyte serving as a surrogate for GFR will be influenced by prerenal, primary renal, and postrenal factors. In addition, the finding of normal serum creatinine, BUN, and/or SDMA concentrations does NOT exclude the presence of primary renal disease, as loss of substantial renal mass and renal function must occur before the concentrations of these molecules increase above the reference range. Discordant test results between serum creatinine, SDMA, and BUN occur at times, so it is important to not rely solely on the results of just one test of renal function. Close attention to results of urinalysis (especially USG and proteinuria, as well as cylindruria and renal epithelial cyturia) can suggest the presence of ongoing renal disease when renal parameters on routine blood testing are normal.

Thyroid Status and Renal Function Evaluation

Functional thyroid hormone status should be considered during evaluation of renal function parameters since thyroid status influences GFR and creatinine synthesis. High levels of circulating thyroid hormones increase RBF and GFR [186, 187], whereas low levels decrease them [188, 189]. Extremes of thyroid functional status (hypothyroid or hyperthyroid) can be of clinical significance for an effect on GFR especially for evaluation of patients with underlying CKD. Dogs with naturally occurring hypothyroidism were reported with slightly higher serum creatinine concentrations than euthyroid dogs in one study, but they were rarely above the reference range [190]. In dogs with experimental hypothyroidism, decreased GFR was documented, but no change was observed in serum creatinine. Decreased synthesis of creatinine accounted for the failure of serum creatinine to increase in the face of decreased GFR in these hypothyroid dogs [189]. Reduced GFR was documented in dogs with clinical hypothyroidism, and GFR was restored to higher levels following thyroxine supplementation [188].

Hyperthyroidism is associated with increased RPF and GFR following some combination of increased cardiac output, increased blood volume, renal vasodilatation, and activation of the renin–angiotensin–aldosterone system [187, 191–193]. Around 11–41% of cats with hyperthyroidism have been reported with azotemia prior to treatment [187, 194–198]. There was discordance in the frequency of increased BUN (11%) compared to increased creatinine (6%) in hyperthyroid cats prior to treatment in one report [191]. An increased BUN-to-creatinine ratio in hyperthyroidism can occur due to some combination of increased BUN and decreased creatinine. Increased production of urea from increased body protein turnover can increase the BUN, and decreased muscle mass can result in less creatinine synthesis and lower circulating creatinine concentrations [191, 192]. SDMA was more frequently increased in a large series of hyperthyroid cats (20%) than was creatinine (3.5%) in one report [199]. Higher total thyroxine (T4) concentrations were associated with lower serum creatinine concentrations in cats diagnosed with hyperthyroidism, but SDMA was not affected by the level of T4 in one study [200].

In patients with underlying CKD, increased GFR associated with hyperthyroidism can "mask" its detection based on BUN, serum creatinine, and SDMA that are lower than they would otherwise be during euthyroidism [186, 192, 198, 201–204]. Some of the lowering of serum creatinine concentrations can also be associated with the loss of muscle mass associated with hyperthyroidism [201].

Azotemia emerges as a new finding or increases in magnitude from baseline in some cats following treatment for hyperthyroidism. Around 10–51% of cats have been reported to develop "overt" renal failure following various treatments for hyperthyroidism that resulted in euthyroidism or hypothyroidism [191, 194, 197, 201, 203–207] [187]. The process of conversion from nonazotemia to a diagnosis of azotemic CKD is often referred to as "unmasking" of subclinical CKD that was not apparent during the "masked" hyperthyroid state associated with increased GFR [201, 206]. Post-treatment increases in circulating creatinine are attributed to decreases in GFR associated with a return to euthyroidism or iatrogenic hypothyroidism. GFR was significantly higher in cats with hyperthyroidism compared to control cats and significantly decreased when euthyroidism was achieved during methimazole treatment in one study. Mean BUN and serum creatinine did not significantly increase after treatment, but overt azotemia developed in 2 of 12 cats [203].

Cats with hyperthyroidism were studied after treatment with bilateral thyroidectomy, I-131, or methimazole treatment. Mean values for T4, BUN, and serum creatinine were not different between treatment groups at baseline, 30, or 90 days after treatment. Mean serum creatinine and BUN at 30 and 90 days were significantly higher and T4 significantly lower than before treatment in all treatment groups. Mean increases of up to 1.0 mg/dL for serum creatinine and up to 9 mg/dL for BUN over baseline developed following treatment for hyperthyroidism in these cats. Though mean BUN and serum creatinine were within the reference range before treatment, up to 27% of these cats had BUN or serum creatinine above the reference range [198].

In another study, the mean GFR decreased by 44% at 30 days following bilateral thyroidectomy in 13 cats with hyperthyroidism [204]. At the same time, mean serum creatinine (1.26 versus 2.05 mg/dL) and BUN (26.6 versus 34.9 mg/dL) were significantly increased over baseline and T4 was significantly decreased. Seven of 13 cats had post-treatment T4 levels below the reference range, but none developed azotemia. Two of 13 cats in this study developed overt renal failure following treatment and both had normal reference range T4 [204].

Following I-131 treatment of hyperthyroid cats, T4 declined at six days, but there were no significant changes in GFR, BUN, or creatinine at this time in one study. Significant increases in BUN and serum creatinine were observed at 30 days along with further decreases in T4. Nine of 22 cats were in renal failure (serum creatinine >1.8 mg/dL) prior to treatment and 13 cats were in renal failure 30 days following treatment [194].

The decrease in GFR following restoration of euthyroidism stabilizes within one month of treatment [208] and is of the same magnitude following thyroidectomy, methimazole or carbimazole, or I-131 treatments [187]. Some increase in BUN, creatinine, and SDMA is expected at this time, but creatinine can continue to increase for up to six months [187] from a combination of decreased GFR and increased muscle mass [187, 191, 197, 201, 205, 206]. GFR was above the reference range before treatment of hyperthyroid cats in another study of hyperthyroid cats and decreased significantly following treatment with I-131 at one month without further significant decrease by six months. BUN and serum creatinine were significantly increased at one month. Creatinine continued to increase at three and six months likely the result of increased muscle mass, but BUN did not increase further [209].

SDMA was increased more frequently than serum creatinine at baseline, one, three, and six months following treatment of hyperthyroidism in cats of one study [210]. Body weight, creatinine, and SDMA increased up to 30 days following treatment for hyperthyroidism. Creatinine but not SDMA continued to increase during weight gain in these cats [200].

Though SDMA and serum creatinine were positively correlated in another study of hyperthyroid cats, SDMA was increased in 30% of samples at a time that serum creatinine was within the reference range. In 5% of samples, serum creatinine was increased when SDMA was normal. SDMA was relatively higher than creatinine in hyperthyroid compared to euthyroid or hypothyroid cats. The assignment of renal status was often discordant between SDMA and serum creatinine in this study [202].

Overt azotemia following treatment of hyperthyroidism is more likely to occur in cats during iatrogenic hypothyroidism. It can take up to six months for hypothyroidism to develop in some cats after radioiodine treatment [207]. Significantly more cats with hypothyroidism had azotemia (16 of 28) compared to euthyroid cats (14 of 47) following treatment in one study [207]. It has been estimated that about 10% of cats are expected to develop iatrogenic hypothyroidism following I-131 treatment for hyperthyroidism [206], but this was encountered in nearly half of cats following bilateral thyroidectomy [202]. Hypothyroidism was documented in 45–67% of cats with "unmasked" azotemic CKD following I-131 or bilateral thyroidectomy treatment [201, 206]. In hyperthyroid cats that were nonazotemic before treatment, a >2.1 mg/dL serum creatinine developed at a median of six months in 16% of these cats.

Overmedication with antithyroid medications in cats with hyperthyroidism can cause iatrogenic hypothyroidism (low T4, high TSH) and an increase in serum creatinine concentrations. Restoration of euthyroidism following dose reduction of antithyroid medications was associated with a significant reduction in plasma creatinine (median 2.61 versus 2.07 mg/dL) in one study [211]. Serum creatinine decreased in all hypothyroid cats following supplementation with thyroxine in another study, but most creatinine concentrations were still above the reference range [206].

An increased SDMA concentration above the reference interval prior to treatment had a high specificity but poor sensitivity for the prediction of post-treatment azotemia [210] similar to results from a previous study [201]. SDMA concentration showed few false positives for the prediction of azotemia, but failed to predict the emergence of azotemia in most cats [201].

INTERPRETATION OF RENAL FUNCTION TESTS IN NONRENAL DISEASES

Gastrointestinal Disorders

GI bleeding can increase BUN concentration more so than serum creatinine because digested blood provides an endogenous protein load that preferentially increases BUN over serum creatinine. The elevation in BUN is largely related to the amount of hemorrhage [90] but can also be influenced by the degree of ECFV contraction associated with the hemorrhage (prerenal azotemia) that can increase both BUN and serum creatinine as a form of prerenal azotemia. In a very early study of normovolemic dogs, the maximal increase in BUN was proportional to the amount of protein fed in the form of whole blood, plasma, packed red blood cells (RBCs), lean round steak, or casein. The globin component of hemoglobin from RBCs was demonstrated to be readily digested in this study [212]. An increase in BUN by two to threefold over baseline was commonly observed in dogs fed blood [87, 212]. Greater increases in BUN were seen in dogs fed blood when they were dehydrated or hypotensive [87]. Dogs with upper GI hemorrhage in one clinical study had significant increases in both serum creatinine and BUN. There was a larger increase in BUN that was obvious, while the increase in creatinine was still within the reference range, resulting in a nearly doubling of the BUN-to-serum-creatinine ratio [185]. In one study of dogs with protein-losing enteropathy, mean serum creatinine was 0.4–0.7 mg/dL and mean BUN was 12–16 mg/dL [213], suggesting loss of lean muscle mass affecting creatinine without an increase in BUN from bleeding. Anecdotally, chronic bleeding from bad teeth and periodontal disease can cause an increase in the BUN/creatinine ratio in addition to classic GI bleeding.

In one study of dogs with chronic enteropathy, serum creatinine was low in 75% and within the reference range in 25%, while the urea nitrogen was above the reference range in 14% and normal in 85%. Consequently, the urea-to-creatinine ratio will be increased most of the time since creatinine is low most of the time regardless of whether the urea is increased or not [214]. Occult fecal bleeding was common in one study of CKD, even in IRIS CKD Stage 2. The urea-nitrogen-to-creatinine ratio was increased in dogs of this study from stage 2 to stage 4 [215].

Cardiac Conditions

BUN may be increased in cardiac conditions. This can be attributed to prerenal factors that result in reduced delivery of blood to the kidneys and or to high-level activation of the renal tubular urea transporters during the body's perception of reduced cardiac output and increased ADH release [76, 216]. There is discordance between BUN and serum creatinine in this setting as BUN is increased more so than would be predicted by decreased GFR alone. The BUN-to-creatinine ratio is increased in part due to the effects of increased circulating ADH on renal tubular urea transporters that increase the reabsorption of urea into the blood stream. Additionally, the BUN could be preferentially increased due to catabolism or intake of higher protein intake diets, whereas the creatinine could be decreased due to loss of lean muscle mass due to cardiac cachexia [217].

It appears that BUN can be used as a biomarker for the prognosis of heart failure in humans by serving as a surrogate for the degree of neurohormonal activation [76, 216]. A high

BUN/creatinine ratio was an independent predictor of death in humans with acute heart failure [218]. Discordance of BUN and serum creatinine has been noted in some dogs or cats with congestive heart failure (CHF). Both BUN and serum concentrations were significantly increased in a review of 31 dogs with aortic thrombosis, but the BUN was above the reference range more frequently than creatinine [219]. In a study of 145 dogs and cats with acute CHF, 52% exhibited elevated BUN at the time of admission, but creatinine was increased in only 17% at the same time [220]. Cats with CHF and cachexia had higher BUN and BUN/serum creatinine ratios than those cats with CHF but without cachexia; serum creatinine concentrations were not different between these groups. Maximal values for BUN were 112 mg/dL, 4.6 mg/dL for serum creatinine, and BUN/creatinine ratio of 77 in cats of this study [217]. There was no difference in BUN or serum creatinine concentrations in dogs with or without cardiac cachexia, but dogs with cardiac cachexia had a significantly higher BUN-to-creatinine ratio. BUN was as high as 107 mg/dL and serum creatinine as high as 2.7 mg/dL in this study [221].

Portosystemic Shunt

In animals with portosystemic shunts (PSS), ammonia metabolism is disrupted, and hyperammonemia develops as a result of shunting of portal blood into the systemic circulation [79]. Both dogs and cats with PSS typically have low BUN concentrations, most likely due to decreased urea cycle function to synthesize urea with decreased hepatic perfusion [222–224]. Impaired creatine synthesis in the liver can contribute to lower serum creatinine concentrations [225, 226]. GFR is higher than normal in dogs with shunts, which can in part additionally account for the finding of low serum creatinine and BUN that occurs in this population. After correction of the shunt, BUN and serum creatinine raise to a normal level as GFR declines and as more normal liver metabolism returns [226].

Periodontal Disease

In a study of 38 healthy dogs with periodontal disease, BUN concentration significantly increased after treatment of the periodontal disease from a median of 13–17 mg/dL but remained within the reference range (5–30 mg/dL); the creatinine did not change before or after treatment [227]. The reasons for the discordance between the change in BUN and serum creatinine in this study were not apparent.

Primary Hyperparathyroidism

Sixty-three percent of dogs with primary hyperparathyroidism in one study had a BUN below the reference compared to only 4% of dogs with a low serum creatinine. The reason for this discordance was not identified but might be explained by polyuria preferentially affecting BUN [228].

Exercise

With vigorous exercise, muscle produces increasing amounts of ammonia, which potentially could increase BUN generation in the liver. An increased release of creatinine from muscle is also possible depending on the degree of muscle insult. The effect of vigorous exercise on BUN and creatinine in dogs is highly variable. No change in BUN or creatinine was seen following agility competition in one study [229]. A decrease in BUN was observed in Labrador Retrievers following field trial competition; creatinine was not measured [230]. An increase in BUN occurred after exercise in sled dogs without a change in creatinine in another study [231].

Creatinine variably increased, was not changed, or decreased in dogs undergoing heavy exercise in four other studies. Creatinine significantly increased by about 20 μmol/L (0.23 mg/dL) after sprinting in Greyhounds at a time of no change in BUN [232]. Creatinine increased by 50% over baseline following sled dog performance in one study; BUN was not measured [233]. Increases in serum creatinine could result from increased muscle release of creatinine or decreased creatinine clearance following decreased GFR associated with exercise. Creatinine decreased and BUN increased at some time points following sled dog racing of another study, but the magnitude of these changes was small [234]. Creatinine decreased by about 10% from baseline in untrained Beagles after running for reasons that were not apparent; BUN was not measured [235].

Immune-mediated Thrombocytopenia

In a study of 73 dogs with immune-mediated thrombocytopenia, a high BUN at the time of admission was significantly associated with failure to survive compared to dogs without increased BUN. BUN exceeded the reference range more often than serum creatinine (22% versus 5%); serum creatinine was not associated with survival in this study. The disparity between the number of dogs with BUN and serum creatinine increases is likely due to those that had melena, which was also associated with failure to survive [236].

Infectious and Parasitic Diseases

Infectious and parasitic diseases can decrease renal function through mechanisms that promote an inflammatory process to the organism in the kidneys, creative oxidative stress and renal injury, or damage the kidneys through immune complex injury in response to the infecting organism [237–243]. Animals that are sick from a systemic infection can have reduced ECFV and reduced GFR to account for some of the increases in BUN and creatinine (prerenal azotemia). These processes are likely to affect BUN and serum creatinine to the same degree, unless there is GI bleeding that will preferentially increase BUN or if there is chronic catabolism with loss of muscle mass in which the creatinine will be preferentially decreased. There was discordance in the frequency of increased creatinine compared to increased BUN in one study of dogs with babesiosis. BUN was increased about twice as often as was the finding of an increased serum creatinine (62.4% versus 30.7%) and the degree of azotemia was mild in most cases. A reason for this discordance was not apparent. A decreased BUN happened rarely that was attributed to hepatic dysfunction and decreased synthesis of urea [244]. In 51 dogs with vena caval syndrome due to heartworm infection, BUN and serum creatinine were elevated presurgically and decreased significantly after surgical removal of the heartworms in dogs that survived. Ten days post worm removal, the mean BUN/serum creatinine ratio was 18 in survivor dogs and 33 in nonsurvival dogs [245].

Uroperitoneum (Uroabdomen)

BUN and serum creatinine both progressively increase following the accumulation of urine in the peritoneal cavity as one form of postrenal azotemia. Ruptured bladder is the most common cause for uroperitoneum, but urine leakage can also occur following major trauma to the kidneys, ureter, and urethra. The concentrations of creatinine and urea in urine initially entering the peritoneal cavity are much higher than that in the circulation, which favors concentration-dependent movement of these molecules from the abdominal fluid into the circulation. Urine that enters the peritoneal cavity is modified by reabsorption of solutes from the abdominal fluid and entry of water into the abdominal fluid by osmotic and concentration-dependent dynamics. An increase in BUN is the first biochemical abnormality to be detected in uroabdomen. Urea is more readily absorbed across the peritoneal membranes than is creatinine due to its lower molecular weight resulting in an increase in BUN before serum creatinine in the early hours following urine accumulation in the abdominal cavity. The greatest discordance between BUN and serum creatinine is observed early when azotemia is minimal. In an experimental model of uroabdomen in the dog, an increased BUN above the reference range was the first significant biochemical change observed by 5 hours and an increased serum creatinine above the reference range was documented by 21 hours after urine entered the abdominal cavity. There was a concordant increase in both BUN and serum creatinine from 21 to 69 hours following the development of uroabdomen when moderate to severe

azotemia had developed. In the clinical condition, the magnitude and rate of increase in BUN and serum creatinine concentrations may be magnified by concomitant prerenal factors that commonly accompany trauma such as shock and hypotension [246]. The higher molecular weight of creatinine in the abdominal fluid urine causes it to be reabsorbed across the peritoneal membranes more slowly than urea. This allows the ratio of abdominal fluid creatinine to serum creatinine to definitively identify the abdominal fluid as urine when a large gradient is detected, even before serum creatinine is increased. The concentration of urea nitrogen in the abdominal fluid is often nearly the same as in the blood after 24 hours or more making this ratio of little value later on. A large gradient of abdominal fluid potassium to serum potassium is also useful to confirm the diagnosis of uroabdomen [246–250]. The combination of metabolic acidosis, hyperkalemia, hyponatremia, and azotemia that often are discovered in patients with uroperitoneum can be confused with similar findings in hypoadrenocorticism, especially when there is no clear history of trauma.

In summary, the kidneys are integral in maintaining the constancy of the internal milieu, largely through the excretion of metabolic waste products, conservation or excretion of water and electrolytes, and acid–base balance. In addition, the kidneys are integral in the regulation of arterial blood pressure and the secretion, metabolism, and excretion of hormones. The kidneys are endocrine organs that secrete erythropoietin to stimulate RBC production from the bone marrow, as well in the synthesis and secretion of the most active metabolite of vitamin D ($1,25(OH)_2$-vitamin D or calcitriol) vital in the regulation of calcium metabolism and in general cellular health. Pathology in any part of the kidney can have vast consequences on a variety of physiological processes resulting in serious disease. Failure to conserve water, glucose, amino acids, and plasma proteins are processes that can be detected in urine as well as additions of cells (RBC, white blood cells, epithelial cells) from the kidneys or lower urinary tract that can be detected in urine sediment. Many severe or advancing kidney diseases are associated with the loss of ability to elaborate concentrated urine and renal origin proteinuria. The specifics of these alterations in urinalysis will be discussed in sections of this book that follow.

REFERENCES

1 Clarkson, C.E. and Fletcher, T.F. (2011). Anatomy of the kidney and proximal ureter. In: *Nephrology and Urology of Small Animals* (ed. J. Bartges and D. Polzin), 3–22. Chichester: Wiley.

2 DiBartola, S.P. (2012). Applied renal physiology. In: *Fluid, Electrolyte, and Acid-Base Disorders in Small Animal Practice* (ed. D.B. SP), 26–43. St. Louis, Missouri: Elsevier Saunders.

3 Verlander, J.W. (2013). Glomerular filtration. In: *Cunningham's Textbook of Veterinary Physiology*, 5e (ed. B.G. Klein), 460–468. St. Louis, Missouri: Elsevier Saunders.

4 Verlander, J.W. (2013). Solute reabsorption. In: *Cunningham's Textbook of Veterinary Physiology*, 5e (ed. B.G. Klein), 460–479. St. Louis, Missouri: Elsevier Saunders.

5 Verlander, J.W. (2013). Water balance. In: *Cunningham's Textbook of Veterinary Physiology*, 5e (ed. B.G. Klein), 481–487. St. Louis, Missouri: Elsevier Saunders.

6 Verlander, J.W. (2013). Acid-base balance. In: *Cunningham's Textbook of Veterinary Physiology*, 5e (ed. B.G. Klein), 481–487. St. Louis, Missouri: Elsevier Saunders.

7 Costanzo, L.S. (2018). Renal physiology. In: *Physiology*, 6e (ed. L.S. Costanzo), 245–310. Philadelphia, PA: Elsevier.

8 Hall, J.E. (2016). The urinary system. In: *Guyton and Hall Textbook of Medical Physiology*, 13e (ed. J.E. Hall), 323–333. Philadelphia, PA: Elsevier.

9 Osborne, C.A., Low, D.G., and Finco, D.R. (1972). Applied anatomy of the urinary system. In: *Canine and Feline Urology* (ed. C.A. Osborne, D.G. Low and D.R. Finco), 3–10. Philadephia, PA: W.B. Saunders Co.

10 Horster, M., Kemler, B.J., and Valtin, H. (1971). Intracortical distribution of number and volume of glomeruli during postnatal maturation in the dog. *J. Clin. Invest.* 50: 796–800.

11 Kunkel, P.A. (1930). The number and size of of the glomeruli of several mammals. *Bull. Johns Hopkins Hosp.* 47: 285–291.

12 Rytand, D.A. (1938). The number and size of mammalian glomeruli as related to kidney and to body weight with methods for their enumeration and measurement. *Am. J. Anat.* 62: 507–520.

13 Beeuwkes, R. 3rd. (1971). Efferent vascular patterns and early vascular-tubular relations in the dog kidney. *Am. J. Physiol.* 221: 1361–1374.

14 Beeuwkes, R. 3rd and Bonventre, J.V. (1975). Tubular organization and vascular-tubular relations in the dog kidney. *Am. J. Physiol.* 229: 695–713.

15 Beeuwkes, R. 3rd. (1980). The vascular organization of the kidney. *Annu. Rev. Physiol.* 42: 531–542.

16 Knepper, M.A., Kwon, T.H., and Nielsen, S. (2015). Molecular physiology of water balance. *N. Engl. J. Med.* 373: 1349–1358.

17 Danziger, J. and Zeidel, M.L. (2015). Osmotic homeostasis. *Clin. J. Am. Soc. Nephrol.* 10: 852–862.

18 Castrop, H. and Schiessl, I.M. (2014). Physiology and pathophysiology of the renal Na-K-2Cl cotransporter (NKCC2). *Am. J. Physiol. Renal Physiol.* 307: F991–F1002.

19 Huang, X., Dorhout Mees, E., Vos, P. et al. (2016). Everything we always wanted to know about furosemide but were afraid to ask. *Am. J. Physiol. Renal Physiol.* 310: F958–F971.

20 DiBartola, S.P. (2012). Disorders of sodium and water: hypernatremia and hyponatremia. In: *Fluid, Electrolyte, and Acid-Base Disorders in Small Animal Practice St* (ed. S.P. DiBartola), 51–85. Louis, MO: Elsevier Saunders.

21 DiBartola, S.P. (2012). Applied physiology of body fluids in dogs and cats. In: *Fluid, Electrolyte, and Acid-Base Disorders in Small Animal Practice* (ed. D.B. SP), 26–43. St. Louis, MO: Elsevier Saunders.

22 Hall, J.E. (2016). Urine concentration and dilution; regulation of extracellular fluid osmolarity and sodium concentration. In: *Guyton and Hall Textbook of Medical Physiology*, 13e (ed. J.E. Hall), 371–387. Philadelphia, PA: Elsevier.

23 Fenton, R.A. (2009). Essential role of vasopressin-regulated urea transport processes in the mammalian kidney. *Pflugers Archiv: Eur. J. Physiol.* 458: 169–177.

24 Ellison, D.H. (2019). Clinical pharmacology in diuretic use. *Clin. J. Am. Soc. Nephrol.: CJASN* 14: 1248–1257.

25 Robertson, G.L., Shelton, R.L., and Athar, S. (1976). The osmoregulation of vasopressin. *Kidney Int.* 10: 25–37.

26 Shiel, R.E. (2012). Disorders of vasopressin production. In: *BSAVA Manual of Canine and Feline Endocrinology* (ed. C.T. Mooney and M.E. Peterson), 15–27. Quedgeley, Gloucester, England: British Small Animal Veterinary Association.

27 Braileanu, G.T., Simasko, S.M., Hu, J. et al. (2001). Effects of arginine- and lysine-vasopressin on phospholipase C activity, intracellular calcium concentration and prostaglandin F2alpha secretion in pig endometrial cells. *Reproduction* 121: 605–612.

28 Acher, R. and Chauvet, J. (1988). Structure, processing and evolution of the neurohypophysial hormone-neurophysin precursors. *Biochimie* 70: 1197–1207.

29 Wallis, M. (2012). Molecular evolution of the neurohypophysial hormone precursors in mammals: comparative genomics reveals novel mammalian oxytocin and vasopressin analogues. *Gen. Comp. Endocrinol.* 179: 313–318.

30 Ali, M.N. (1958). A comparison of some activities of arginine vasopressin and lysine vasopressin on kidney function in conscious dogs. *Br. J. Pharmacol. Chemother.* 13: 131–137.

31 van Vonderen, I.K., Kooistra, H.S., and Rijnberk, A. (1997). Intra- and interindividual variation in urine osmolality and urine specific gravity in healthy pet dogs of various ages. *J. Vet. Intern. Med.* 11: 30–35.

32 Olesen, E.T. and Fenton, R.A. (2013). Is there a role for PGE2 in urinary concentration? *J. Am. Soc. Nephrol.* 24: 169–178.

33 Levitin, H., Goodman, A., Pigeon, G. et al. (1962). Composition of the renal medulla during water diuresis. *J. Clin. Invest.* 41: 1145–1151.

34 Kortenoeven, M.L. and Fenton, R.A. (2014). Renal aquaporins and water balance disorders. *Biochim. Biophys. Acta* 1840: 1533–1549.

35 Moeller, H.B., Fuglsang, C.H., and Fenton, R.A. (2016). Renal aquaporins and water balance disorders. *Best Pract. Res. Clin. Endocrinol. Metab.* 30: 277–288.

36 Nielsen, S., Kwon, T.H., Frokiaer, J. et al. (2007). Regulation and dysregulation of aquaporins in water balance disorders. *J. Intern. Med.* 261: 53–64.

37 Agre, P. and Homer, W. (2000). Smith award lecture. Aquaporin water channels in kidney. *J. Am. Soc. Nephrol.* 11: 764–777.

38 Li, Y., Wang, W., Jiang, T., and Yang, B. (2017). Aquaporins in urinary system. *Adv. Exp. Med. Biol.* 969: 131–148.

39 Brown, D. (2017). The discovery of water channels (aquaporins). *Ann. Nutr. Metab.* 70 (1): 37–42.

40 Li, C. and Wang, W. (2017). Molecular biology of Aquaporins. *Adv. Exp. Med. Biol.* 969: 1–34.

41 Kwon, T.H., Frokiaer, J., and Nielsen, S. (2013). Regulation of aquaporin-2 in the kidney: a molecular mechanism of body-water homeostasis. *Kidney Res. Clin. Pract.* 32: 96–102.

42 Lefebvre, H.P., Dossin, O., Trumel, C. et al. (2008). Fractional excretion tests: a critical review of methods and applications in domestic animals. *Vet. Clin. Pathol.* 37: 4–20.

43 DiBartola, S.P., Chew, D.J., and Jacobs, G. (1980). Quantitative urinalysis including 24-hour protein excretion in the dog. *J. Am. Anim. Hosp. Assoc.* 16: 537–546.

44 Martorelli, C.R., Kogika, M.M., Chacar, F.C. et al. (2017). Urinary fractional excretion of phosphorus in dogs with spontaneous chronic kidney disease. *Vet. Sci.* 4: 67–76.

45 Hansen, B., DiBartola, S.P., Chew, D.J. et al. (1992). Clinical and metabolic findings in dogs with chronic renal failure fed two diets. *Am. J. Vet. Res.* 53: 326–334.

46 Parker, V.J., Rudinsky, A.J., Benedict, J.A. et al. (2020). Effects of calcifediol supplementation on markers of chronic kidney disease-

mineral and bone disorder in dogs with chronic kidney disease. *J. Vet. Intern. Med.* 34: 2497–2506.

47 Bennett, S.L., Abraham, L.A., Anderson, G.A. et al. (2006). Reference limits for urinary fractional excretion of electrolytes in adult non-racing greyhound dogs. *Aust. Vet. J.* 84: 393–397.

48 Carr, S.V., Grant, D.C., DeMonaco, S.M. et al. (2020). Measurement of preprandial and postprandial urine calcium to creatinine ratios in male miniature schnauzers with and without urolithiasis. *J. Vet. Intern. Med.* 34: 754–760.

49 Troia, R., Gruarin, M., Grisetti, C. et al. (2018). Fractional excretion of electrolytes in volume-responsive and intrinsic acute kidney injury in dogs: diagnostic and prognostic implications. *J. Vet. Intern. Med.* 32: 1372–1382.

50 Furrow, E., Patterson, E.E., Armstrong, P.J. et al. (2015). Fasting urinary calcium-to-creatinine and oxalate-to-creatinine ratios in dogs with calcium oxalate urolithiasis and breed-matched controls. *J. Vet. Intern. Med.* 29: 113–119.

51 Groth, E.M., Lulich, J.P., Chew, D.J. et al. (2019). Vitamin D metabolism in dogs with and without hypercalciuric calcium oxalate urolithiasis. *J. Vet. Intern. Med.* 33: 758–763.

52 Midkiff, A.M., Chew, D.J., Randolph, J.F. et al. (2000). Idiopathic hypercalcemia in cats. *J. Vet. Intern. Med.* 14: 619–626.

53 Benzing, T. and Salant, D. (2021). Insights into glomerular filtration and albuminuria. *N. Engl. J. Med.* 384: 1437–1446.

54 Hokamp, J.A. and Nabity, M.B. (2016). Renal biomarkers in domestic species. *Vet. Clin. Pathol.* 45: 28–56.

55 Newell, S.M., Ko, J.C., Ginn, P.E. et al. (1997). Effects of three sedative protocols on glomerular filtration rate in clinically normal dogs. *Am. J. Vet. Res.* 58: 446–450.

56 Winter, M.D., Miles, K.G., and Riedesel, D.H. (2011). Effect of sedation protocol on glomerular filtration rate in cats as determined by use of quantitative renal scintigraphy. *Am. J. Vet. Res.* 72: 1222–1225.

57 Grimm, J.B., Grimm, K.A., Kneller, S.K. et al. (2001). The effect of a combination of medetomidine-butorphanol and medetomidine, butorphanol, atropine on glomerular filtration rate in dogs. *Vet. Radiol. Ultrasound* 42: 458–462.

58 Ji, F., Zhang, S., Jiang, X. et al. (2017). Diagnostic and prognostic value of galectin-3, serum creatinine, and cystatin C in chronic kidney diseases. *J. Clin. Lab. Anal.* 31: e22074.

59 El-Khoury, J.M., Bunch, D.R., Hu, B. et al. (2016). Comparison of symmetric dimethylarginine with creatinine, cystatin C and their eGFR equations as markers of kidney function. *Clin. Biochem.* 49: 1140–1143.

60 Finch, N.C., Syme, H.M., and Elliott, J. (2018). Development of an estimated glomerular filtration rate formula in cats. *J. Vet. Intern. Med.* 32: 1970–1976.

61 Ghys, L.F., Meyer, E., Paepe, D. et al. (2014). Analytical validation of a human particle-enhanced nephelometric assay for cystatin C measurement in feline serum and urine. *Vet. Clin. Pathol.* 43: 226–234.

62 Pelander, L., Haggstrom, J., Larsson, A. et al. (2019). Comparison of the diagnostic value of symmetric dimethylarginine, cystatin C, and creatinine for detection of decreased glomerular filtration rate in dogs. *J. Vet. Intern. Med.* 33: 630–639.

63 McKenna, M., Pelligand, L., Elliott, J. et al. (2020). Relationship between serum iohexol clearance, serum SDMA concentration, and serum creatinine concentration in non-azotemic dogs. *J. Vet. Intern. Med.* 34: 186–194.

64 Von Hendy-Willson, V.E. and Pressler, B.M. (2011). An overview of glomerular filtration rate testing in dogs and cats. *Vet. J.* 188: 156–165.

65 Finco, D.R., Tabaru, H., Brown, S.A. et al. (1993). Endogenous creatinine clearance measurement of glomerular filtration rate in dogs. *Am. J. Vet. Res.* 54: 1575–1578.

66 Finco, D.R., Brown, S.A., Crowell, W.A. et al. (1991). Exogenous creatinine clearance as a measure of glomerular filtration rate in dogs with reduced renal mass. *Am. J. Vet. Res.* 52: 1029–1032.

67 Finco, D.R., Coulter, D.B., and Barsanti, J.A. (1981). Simple, accurate method for clinical estimation of glomerular filtration rate in the dog. *Am. J. Vet. Res.* 42: 1874–1877.

68 Barthez, P.Y., Chew, D.J., and DiBartola, S.P. (2000). Effect of sample number and time on determination of plasma clearance of technetium Tc 99m pentetate and orthoiodohippurate sodium I 131 in dogs and cats. *Am. J. Vet. Res.* 61: 280–285.

69 Barthez, P.Y., Chew, D.J., and DiBartola, S.P. (2001). Simplified methods for estimation of 99mTc-pentetate and 131I-orthoiodohippurate plasma clearance in dogs and cats. *J. Vet. Intern. Med.* 15: 200–208.

70 Brown, S.A., Finco, D.R., Boudinot, F.D. et al. (1996). Evaluation of a single injection method, using iohexol, for estimating glomerular filtration rate in cats and dogs. *Am. J. Vet. Res.* 57: 105–110.

71 Finco, D.R., Braselton, W.E., and Cooper, T.A. (2001). Relationship between plasma iohexol clearance and urinary exogenous creatinine clearance in dogs. *J. Vet. Intern. Med.* 15: 368–373.

72 Goy-Thollot, I., Chafotte, C., Besse, S. et al. (2006). Iohexol plasma clearance in healthy dogs and cats. *Vet. Radiol. Ultrasound* 47: 168–173.

73 Goy-Thollot, I., Besse, S., Garnier, F. et al. (2006). Simplified methods for estimation of plasma clearance of iohexol in dogs and cats. *J. Vet. Intern. Med.* 20: 52–56.

74 Bexfield, N.H., Heiene, R., Gerritsen, R.J. et al. (2008). Glomerular filtration rate estimated by 3-sample plasma clearance of iohexol in 118 healthy dogs. *J. Vet. Intern. Med.* 22: 66–73.

75 Lane, I.F., Shaw, D.H., Burton, S.A. et al. (2000). Quantitative urinalysis in healthy Beagle puppies from 9 to 27 weeks of age. *Am. J. Vet. Res.* 61: 577–581.

76 Lamb, E.J. and Jones, G.R.D. (2018). Kidney function tests. In: *Tietz Textbook of Clinical Chemistry and Molecular Diagnostics*, 6e (ed. N. Rifai, A.R. Horvath and C.T. Witter), 479–516. St. Louis, MO: Elsevier.

77 Lyman, J.L. (1986). Blood urea nitrogen and creatinine. *Emerg. Med. Clin. North Am.* 4: 223–233.

78 van Straten, G., van Steenbeek, F.G., Grinwis, G.C. et al. (2014). Aberrant expression and distribution of enzymes of the urea cycle and other ammonia metabolizing pathways in dogs with congenital portosystemic shunts. *PLoS One* 9: e100077.

79 Dimski, D.S. (1994). Ammonia metabolism and the urea cycle: function and clinical implications. *J. Vet. Intern. Med.* 8: 73–78.

80 Berent, A.C., Murakami, T., Scroggin, R.D. et al. (2005). Reliability of using reagent test strips to estimate blood urea nitrogen concentration in dogs and cats. *J. Am. Vet. Med. Assoc.* 227: 1253–1256.

81 Sako, T., Mori, A., Lee, P. et al. (2011). Age-specific plasma biochemistry reference ranges in <1 year old dogs in Japan. *Vet. Res. Commun.* 35: 201–209.

82 O'Brien, M.A., McMichael, M.A., Le Boedec, K. et al. (2014). Reference intervals and age-related changes for venous biochemical, hematological, electrolytic, and blood gas variables using a point of care analyzer in 68 puppies. *J. Vet. Emerg. Crit. Care (San Antonio)* 24: 291–301.

83 Rosset, E., Rannou, B., Casseleux, G. et al. (2012). Age-related changes in biochemical and hematologic variables in Borzoi and Beagle puppies from birth to 8 weeks. *Vet. Clin. Pathol.* 41: 272–282.

84 Allen, J. (2019). Increased & decreased blood urea nitrogen. *Clin. Brief* July: 31.

85 Allen J. (2021). Top 5 Breed-Associated Biochemical Abnormalities. *Clinicians Brief.* 21–25. http://cliniciansbrief.com.

86 Reynolds, B.S., Brosse, C., Jeunesse, E. et al. (2015). Routine plasma biochemistry analytes in clinically healthy cats: within-day variations and effects of a standard meal. *J. Feline Med. Surg.* 17: 468–475.

87 Gregory, R., Ewing, P.L., and Levine, H. (1945). Azotemia associated with gastrointestinal hemorrhage. *Arch. Intern. Med.* 75: 381–394.

88 Anderson, R.S. and Edney, A.T. (1969). Protein intake and blood urea in the dog. *Vet. Rec.* 84: 348–349.

89 Street, A.E., Chesterman, H., Smith, G.K. et al. (1968). Prolonged blood urea elevation observed in the beagle after feeding. *Toxicol. Appl. Pharmacol.* 13: 363–371.

90 Finco, D.R. and Duncan, J.R. (1976). Evaluation of blood urea nitrogen and serum creatinine concentrations as indicators of renal dysfunction: a study of 111 cases and a review of related literature. *J. Am. Vet. Med. Assoc.* 168: 593–601.

91 Street, A.E., Chesterman, H., Smith, G.K. et al. (1968). The effect of diet on blood urea levels in the beagle. *J. Pharm. Pharmacol.* 20: 325–326.

92 Tripathi, N.K., Gregory, C.R., and Latimer, K.S. (2011). Urinary system. In: *Duncan and Prasse's Veterinary Laboratory Medicine: Clinical Pathology* (ed. K.S. Latimer), 253–282. West Sussex, UK: Wiley.

93 Pointer, E., Reisman, R., Windham, R. et al. (2013). Starvation and the clinicopathologic abnormalities associated with starved dogs: a review of 152 cases. *J. Am. Anim. Hosp. Assoc.* 49: 101–107.

94 Braun, J.P., Lefebvre, H.P., and Watson, A.D. (2003). Creatinine in the dog: a review. *Vet. Clin. Pathol.* 32: 162–179.

95 Kovarikova, S. (2018). Indirect markers of glomerular filtration rate in dogs and cats: a review. *Vet. Med.* 63: 395–412.

96 Finco, D.R., Brown, S.A., Vaden, S.L. et al. (1995). Relationship between plasma creatinine concentration and glomerular filtration rate in dogs. *J. Vet. Pharmacol. Ther.* 18: 418–421.

97 Concordet, D., Vergez, F., Trumel, C. et al. (2008). A multicentric retrospective study of serum/plasma urea and creatinine concentrations in dogs using univariate and multivariate decision rules to evaluate diagnostic efficiency. *Vet. Clin. Pathol.* 37: 96–103.

98 Medaille, C., Trumel, C., Concordet, D. et al. (2004). Comparison of plasma/serum urea and creatinine concentrations in the dog: a 5-year retrospective study in a commercial veterinary clinical pathology laboratory. *J. Vet. Med. A Physiol. Pathol. Clin. Med.* 51: 119–123.

99 Samra, M. and Abcar, A.C. (2012). False estimates of elevated creatinine. *Perm. J.* 16: 51–52.

100 Hall, J.A., Yerramilli, M., Obare, E. et al. (2015). Relationship between lean body mass and serum renal biomarkers in healthy dogs. *J. Vet. Intern. Med.* 29: 808–814.

101 Hall, J.A., Yerramilli, M., Obare, E. et al. (2014). Comparison of serum concentrations of symmetric dimethylarginine and creatinine as kidney function biomarkers in healthy geriatric cats fed reduced protein foods enriched with fish oil, L-carnitine, and medium-chain triglycerides. *Vet. J.* 202: 588–596.

102 Feeman, W.E. 3rd, Couto, C.G., and Gray, T.L. (2003). Serum creatinine concentrations in retired racing greyhounds. *Vet. Clin. Pathol.* 32: 40–42.

103 Zaldivar-Lopez, S., Marin, L.M., Iazbik, M.C. et al. (2011). Clinical pathology of greyhounds and other sighthounds. *Vet. Clin. Pathol.* 40: 414–425.

104 Dunlop, M.M., Sanchez-Vazquez, M.J., Freeman, K.P. et al. (2011). Determination of serum biochemistry reference intervals in a large sample of adult greyhounds. *J. Small Anim. Pract.* 52: 4–10.

105 Drost, W.T., Couto, C.G., Fischetti, A.J. et al. (2006). Comparison of glomerular filtration rate between greyhounds and non-greyhound dogs. *J. Vet. Intern. Med.* 20: 544–546.

106 Hilppo, M. (1986). Some haematological and clinical-chemical parameters of sight hounds (Afghan hound, saluki and whippet). *Nord. Vet. Med.* 38: 148–155.

107 Paltrinieri, S., Ibba, F., and Rossi, G. (2014). Haematological and biochemical reference intervals of four feline breeds. *J. Feline Med. Surg.* 16: 125–136.

108 Paltrinieri, S., Giraldi, M., Prolo, A. et al. (2017). Serum symmetric dimethylarginine and creatinine in Birman cats compared with cats of other breeds. *J. Feline Med. Surg.* 10: 905–912.

109 Reynolds, B.S., Concordet, D., Germain, C.A. et al. (2010). Breed dependency of reference intervals for plasma biochemical values in cats. *J. Vet. Intern. Med.* 24: 809–818.

110 Grundy, S.A. (2006). Clinically relevant physiology of the neonate. *Vet. Clin. North Am. Small Anim. Pract.* 36: 443–459, v.

111 von Dehn, B. (2014). Pediatric clinical pathology. *Vet. Clin. North Am. Small Anim. Pract.* 44: 205–219.

112 Riviere, J.E. and Coppoc, G.L. (1981). Pharmacokinetics of gentamicin in the juvenile dog. *Am. J. Vet. Res.* 42: 1621–1623.

113 Cowan, R.H., Jukkola, A.F., and Arant, B.S. Jr. (1980). Pathophysiologic evidence of gentamicin nephrotoxicity in neonatal puppies. *Pediatr. Res.* 14: 1204–1211.

114 Wolford, S.T., Schroer, R.A., Gohs, F.X. et al. (1988). Effect of age on serum chemistry profile, electrophoresis and thyroid hormones in beagle dogs two weeks to one year of age. *Vet. Clin. Pathol.* 17: 35–42.

115 Rortveit, R., Saevik, B.K., Eggertsdottir, A.V. et al. (2015). Age-related changes in hematologic and serum biochemical variables in dogs aged 16–60 days. *Vet. Clin. Pathol.* 44: 47–57.

116 Montoya Navarrete, A.L., Quezada Tristan, T., Lozano Santillan, S. et al. (2021). Effect of age, sex, and body size on the blood biochemistry and physiological constants of dogs from 4 wk. to > 52 wk. of age. *BMC Vet. Res.* 17: 265.

117 Chang, Y.M., Hadox, E., Szladovits, B. et al. (2016). Serum biochemical phenotypes in the domestic dog. *PLoS One* 11: e0149650.

118 Fukuda, S., Kawashima, N., Iida, H. et al. (1989). Age dependency of hematological values and concentrations of serum biochemical constituents in normal beagles from 1 to 14 years of age. *Nihon Juigaku Zasshi* 51: 636–641.

119 Lowseth, L.A., Gillett, N.A., Gerlach, R.F. et al. (1990). The effects of aging on hematology and serum chemistry values in the beagle dog. *Vet. Clin. Pathol.* 19: 13–19.

120 Singer, U. and Kraft, H. (1989). Biological rhythms in the dog. *Kleintierpraxis* 36: 167–174.

121 Thoresen, S.I., Tverdal, A., Havre, G. et al. (1995). Effects of storage time and freezing temperature on clinical chemical parameters from canine serum and heparinized plasma. *Vet. Clin. Pathol.* 24: 129–133.

122 Jensen, A.L., Wenck, A., Koch, J. et al. (1994). Comparison of results of haematological and clinical chemical analyses of blood samples obtained from the cephalic and external jugular veins in dogs. *Res. Vet. Sci.* 56: 24–29.

123 Kopke, M.A., Burchell, R.K., Ruaux, C.G. et al. (2018). Variability of symmetric dimethylarginine in apparently healthy dogs. *J. Vet. Intern. Med.* 32: 736–742.

124 Sharkey, L., Gjevre, K., Hegstad-Davies, R. et al. (2009). Breed-associated variability in serum biochemical analytes in four large-breed dogs. *Vet. Clin. Pathol.* 38: 375–380.

125 Misbach, C., Chetboul, V., Concordet, D. et al. (2014). Basal plasma concentrations of routine variables and packed cell volume in clinically healthy adult small-sized dogs: effect of breed, body weight, age, and gender, and establishment of reference intervals. *Vet. Clin. Pathol.* 43: 371–380.

126 Craig, A.J., Seguela, J., Queau, Y. et al. (2006). Redefining the reference interval for plasma creatinine in dogs: effect of age, gender, body weight, and breed; abstract 107. *J. Vet. Intern. Med.* 20: 740.

127 Lavoue, R., Geffre, A., Braun, J.P. et al. (2013). Breed-specific biochemical reference intervals for the adult Dogue de Bordeaux. *Vet. Clin. Pathol.* 42: 346–359.

128 Evans, G.O. (1987). Post-prandial changes in canine plasma creatinine. *J. Small Anim. Pract.* 28: 311–315.

129 Epstein, M.E., Barsanti, J.A. et al. (1984). Postprandial changes in plasma urea nitrogen and plasma creatinine concentrations in dogs fed commercial diets. *J. Am. Anim. Hosp. Assoc.* 20: 779–782.

130 Schmidt, R.L., Straseski, J.A., Raphael, K.L. et al. (2015). A risk assessment of the Jaffe vs enzymatic method for creatinine measurement in an outpatient population. *PLoS One* 10: e0143205.

131 Jacobs, R.M., Lumsden, J.H., Taylor, J.A. et al. (1991). Effects of interferents on the kinetic Jaffe reaction and an enzymatic colorimetric test for serum creatinine concentration determination in cats, cows, dogs and horses. *Can. J. Vet. Res.* 55: 150–154.

132 Goren, M.P., Osborne, S., and Wright, R.K. (1986). A peroxidase-coupled kinetic enzymatic procedure evaluated for measuring serum and urinary creatinine. *Clin. Chem.* 32: 548–551.

133 Balint, P. and Visy, M. (1965). True creatinine and pseudocreatinine in blood plasma of the dog. *Acta Physiol. Acad. Sci. Hung.* 28: 265–272.

134 Cobas (2010). CREJ2 Creatinine Jaffé 04810716190V10. *Cobas C Systems*. Indianapolis, Indiana Roche Diagnostics. 1–5.

135 Moore, J.F. and Sharer, J.D. (2017). Methods for quantitative creatinine determination. *Curr. Protoc. Hum. Genet.* 93: A 3O 1–A 3O 7.

136 Sargent, H.J., Elliott, J., and Jepson, R.E. (2020). The new age of renal biomarkers: does SDMA solve all of our problems? *J. Small Anim. Pract.* 62: 71–81.

137 Ulleberg, T., Robben, J., Nordahl, K.M. et al. (2011). Plasma creatinine in dogs: intra- and inter-laboratory variation in 10 European veterinary laboratories. *Acta Vet. Scand.* 53: 25.

138 Suárez, P.C.B., Martínez, C.A.C., and Ruiz, I.C. (2014). Standardization of serum creatinine levels in healthy dogs related to body weight at the South Valley of Aburra, Colombia. *Rev. Med. Vet.* 27: 33–40.

139 Couto, G.C., Murphy, R., Coyne, M. et al. (2019). Serum symmetric dimethylarginine concentrations in greyhound puppies – evidence for breed specific physiologic differences NU07. *J. Vet. Intern. Med.* 33: 2522.

140 Walton, R.M. (2012). Subject-based reference values: biological variation, individuality, and reference change values. *Vet. Clin. Pathol.* 41: 175–181.

141 Relford, R., Robertson, J., and Clements, C. (2016). Symmetric dimethylarginine: improving the diagnosis and staging of chronic kidney disease in small animals. *Vet. Clin. North Am. Small Anim. Pract.* 46: 941–960.

142 Nabity, M.B., Lees, G.E., Boggess, M.M. et al. (2015). Symmetric dimethylarginine assay validation, stability, and evaluation as a marker for the early detection of chronic kidney disease in dogs. *J. Vet. Intern. Med.* 29: 1036–1044.

143 Braff, J., Obare, E., Yerramilli, M. et al. (2014). Relationship between serum symmetric dimethylarginine concentration and glomerular filtration rate in cats. *J. Vet. Intern. Med.* 28: 1699–1701.

144 Hall, J.A., Yerramilli, M., Obare, E. et al. (2014). Comparison of serum concentrations of symmetric dimethylarginine and creatinine as kidney function biomarkers in cats with chronic kidney disease. *J. Vet. Intern. Med.* 28: 1676–1683.

145 Patch, D., Obare, E., and Xie, H. (2015). High throughput immunoassay that correlates to gold standard liquid chromatography mass spectrometry (LC-MS) assay for the chronic kidney disease (CKD) marker symmetric dimethylarginine (SDMA) [abstract]. *J. Vet. Intern. Med.* 29: 1216.

146 Bilbrough, G, Evert, B, Hathaway, K, et al. (2018). IDEXX Catalyst SDMA Test for in-house measurement of SDMA concentration in serum from dogs and cats. White Paper. IDEXX Laboratories, Inc.

147 IDEXX (2019). IDEXX SDMA Algorithm. https://www.idexx.com/files/idexx-sdma-test algorithm.pdf: IDEXX.

148 Ogeer, J, Aucoin, D, Andrews, J. (2020). Antech SDMA ELISA Performs Well in Comparison Study with IDEXX SDMA and Liquid Chromatography Mass Spectrometry (LCMS): Antech.

149 Baral, R.M., Freeman, K.P., and Flatland, B. (2021). Analytical quality performance goals for symmetric dimethylarginine in cats. *Vet. Clin. Pathol.* 50: 57–61.

150 Baral, R.M., Freeman, K.P., and Flatland, B. (2021). Comparison of serum and plasma SDMA measured with point-of-care and reference laboratory analysers: implications for interpretation of SDMA in cats. *J. Feline Med. Surg.* 10: 906–920.

151 Ernst, R., Ogeer, J., McCrann, D. et al. (2018). Comparative performance of IDEXX SDMA test and the DLD SDMA ELISA for the measurement of SDMA in canine and feline serum. *PLoS One* 13: e0205030.

152 Liffman, R., Johnstone, T., Tennent-Brown, B. et al. (2018). Establishment of reference intervals for serum symmetric dimethylarginine in adult nonracing greyhounds. *Vet. Clin. Pathol.* 47: 458–463.

153 IRIS (2020). IRIS Staging of CKD (Modified 2019) http://iris-kidneycom/2019; http://iris-kidney.com/pdf/IRIS_Staging_of_CKD_modified_2019.pdf (ACCESSED March 10, 2020)

154 Nabity, M.B., Lees, G.E., Boggess, M. et al. (2013). Week-to-week variability of iohexol clearance, serum creatinine, and symmetric dimethylarginine in dogs with stable chronic renal disease NU-14. *J. Vet. Intern. Med.* 27: 734.

155 Prieto, J.M., Carney, P.C., Miller, M.L. et al. (2020). Biologic variation of symmetric dimethylarginine and creatinine in clinically healthy cats. *Vet. Clin. Pathol.* 49: 401–406.

156 Nabity, M.B., Lees, G.E., Cianciolo, R. et al. (2012). Urinary biomarkers of renal disease in dogs with X-linked hereditary nephropathy. *J. Vet. Intern. Med.* 26: 282–293.

157 Grauer, G.F. (2015). Feline friendly article: feline chronic kidney disease. *Today's Vet. Pract.* 5: 36–41.

158 Yerramilli, M., Farace, G., Quinn, J. et al. (2016). Kidney disease and the nexus of chronic kidney disease and acute kidney injury: the role of novel biomarkers as early and accurate diagnostics. *Vet. Clin. North Am. Small Anim. Pract.* 46: 961–963.

159 Guess, S.C., Yerramilli, M., Obare, E.F. et al. (2018). Longitudinal evaluation of serum symmetric dimethylarginine (SDMA) and serum creatinine in dogs developing chronic kidney disease. *Intern. J. Appl. Res. Vet. Med.* 16: 122–130.

160 IDEXX (2016). White Paper SDMA Creatinine Azotemia Cats Dogs

161 Coyne, M., Szlosek, D., Clements, C. et al. (2020). Association between breed and renal biomarkers of glomerular filtration rate in dogs. *Vet. Rec.* 187: e82.

162 Mack-Gertig, R, Hegarty, E, McCrann, D. (2020). The probability of persistence of an increased SDMA in Cats and Dogs. Paper presented at American College of Veterinary Internal Medicine Forum

163 Mack-Gertig, R., Hegarty, E., and McCrann, D. (2020). Agreement of renal biomarkers: longitudinal evaluations of increased SDMA and creatinine in cats and dogs. *Paper presented at American College of Veterinary Internal Medicine Forum.*

164 Brans, M., Daminet, S., Mortier, F. et al. (2020). Plasma symmetric dimethylarginine and creatinine concentrations and glomerular filtration rate in cats with normal and decreased renal function. *J. Vet. Intern. Med.* 35: 303–311.

165 Langhorn, R., Kieler, I.N., Koch, J. et al. (2018). Symmetric dimethylarginine in cats with hypertrophic cardiomyopathy and diabetes mellitus. *J. Vet. Intern. Med.* 32: 57–63.

166 Pelligand, L, Cotter, D, Williams, S, et al. (2017). Early detection of kidney disease in dogs: a comparison of serum SDMA and creatinine versus GFR measured by iohexol clearance. *Proceedings of British Small Animal Veterinary Association*

167 IDEXX (2021). How does cancer affect IDEXX SDMA?. https://www.idexx.com/en/veterinary/reference-laboratories/sdma/sdma-faqs/#:~:text=Cancer%20patients%20with%20increased%20SDMA,disease%20and%2For%20its%20treatment: IDEXX

168 Yerramilli, M., Farace, G., Robertson, J. et al. (2017). Symmetric Dimethylarginine (SDMA) as kidney biomarker in canine and feline cancer – ESVNU-P-4. *J. Vet. Intern. Med.* 31: 251.

169 Abrams-Ogg, A., Rutland, B., Phillipe, L. et al. (2017). Lymphoma and symmetric dimethylarginine concentrations in dogs a preliminary study. *J. Vet. Intern. Med.* 31: 1584–1585.

170 Ghys, L., Paepe, D., Smets, P. et al. (2014). Cystatin C: a new renal marker and its potential use in small animal medicine. *J. Vet. Intern. Med.* 28: 1152–1164.

171 Ghys, L.F., Paepe, D., Duchateau, L. et al. (2015). Biological validation of feline serum cystatin C: the effect of breed, age and sex and establishment of a reference interval. *Vet. J.* 204: 168–173.

172 Paepe, D., Ghys, L.F., Smets, P. et al. (2015). Routine kidney variables, glomerular filtration rate and urinary cystatin C in cats with diabetes mellitus, cats with chronic kidney disease and healthy cats. *J. Feline Med. Surg.* 17: 880–888.

173 Miyagawa, Y., Takemura, N., and Hirose, H. (2009). Evaluation of the measurement of serum cystatin C by an enzyme-linked immunosorbent assay for humans as a marker of the glomerular filtration rate in dogs. *J. Vet. Med. Sci.* 71: 1169–1176.

174 Muslimovic, A., Tulumovic, D., Hasanspahic, S. et al. (2015). Serum cystatin C – marker of inflammation and cardiovascular morbidity in chronic kidney disease stages 1–4. *Mater. Sociomed.* 27: 75–78.

175 Guo, S., Xue, Y., He, Q. et al. (2017). Preoperative serum cystatin-C as a potential biomarker for prognosis of renal cell carcinoma. *PLoS One* 12: e0178823.

176 Braun, J.-P. and Lefebvre, H.P. (2008). Kidney function and damage. In: *Clinical Biochemistry of Domestic Animals*, 6e (ed. J.J. Kaneko, J.W. Harvey and M.L. Bruss), 485–528. Burlington, MA: Elsevier.

177 Pressler, B.M. (2015). Clinical approach to advanced renal function testing in dogs and cats. *Clin. Lab. Med.* 35: 487–502.

178 De Loor, J., Daminet, S., Smets, P. et al. (2013). Urinary biomarkers for acute kidney injury in dogs. *J. Vet. Intern. Med.* 27: 998–1010.

179 Bradley, R., Tagkopoulos, I., Kim, M. et al. (2019). Predicting early risk of chronic kidney disease in cats using routine clinical laboratory tests and machine learning. *J. Vet. Intern. Med.* 33(6): 2644–2656.

180 Bricker, N.S., Klahr, S., and Rieselbach, R.E. (1964). The functional adaptation of the diseased kidney. I. Glomerular filtration rate. *J. Clin. Invest.* 43: 1915–1921.

181 Brown, S.A., Finco, D.R., Crowell, W.A. et al. (1990). Single-nephron adaptations to partial renal ablation in the dog. *Am. J. Physiol.* 258: F495–F503.

182 Dahlem, D.P., Neiger, R., Schweighauser, A. et al. (2017). Plasma symmetric dimethylarginine concentration in dogs with acute kidney injury and chronic kidney disease. *J. Vet. Intern. Med.* 31: 799–804.

183 Yerramilli, M., Murthy Yerramilli, M., Obare, E. et al. (2015). Prognostic value of symmetric dimethylarginine (SDMA) to creatinine ratio in dogs and cats with chronic kidney disease (CKD). *J. Vet. Intern. Med.* 29: 1274.

184 IRIS (2020). IRIS Grading of Acute Kidney Injury (Modified 2016) http://iris-kidneycom/2016; http://iris-kidney.com/pdf/IRIS_Staging_of_CKD_modified_2019.pdf (accessed March 10, 2020).

185 Prause, L.C. and Grauer, G.F. (1998). Association of gastrointestinal hemorrhage with increased blood urea nitrogen and BUN/creatinine ratio in dogs: a literature review and retrospective study. *Vet. Clin. Pathol.* 27: 107–111.

186 Adams, W.H., Daniel, G.B., and Legendre, A.M. (1997). Investigation of the effects of hyperthyroidism on renal function in the cat. *Can. J. Vet. Res.* 61: 53–56.

187 Vaske, H.H., Schermerhorn, T., and Grauer, G.F. (2016). Effects of feline hyperthyroidism on kidney function: a review. *J. Feline Med. Surg.* 18: 55–59.

188 Gommeren, K., van Hoek, I., Lefebvre, H.P. et al. (2009). Effect of thyroxine supplementation on glomerular filtration rate in hypothyroid dogs. *J. Vet. Intern. Med.* 23: 844–849.

189 Panciera, D.L. and Lefebvre, H.P. (2009). Effect of experimental hypothyroidism on glomerular filtration rate and plasma creatinine concentration in dogs. *J. Vet. Intern. Med.* 23: 1045–1050.

190 Dixon, R.M., Reid, S.W., and Mooney, C.T. (1999). Epidemiological, clinical, haematological and biochemical characteristics of canine hypothyroidism. *Vet. Rec.* 145: 481–487.

191 Langston, C.E. and Reine, N.J. (2006). Hyperthyroidism and the kidney. *Clin. Tech. Small Anim. Pract.* 21: 17–21.

192 DiBartola, S.P. and Brown, S.A. (2000). The kidney and hyperthyroidism. In: *Kirk's Current Veterinary Therapy XIII* (ed. J.D. Bonagura), 337–339. Philadelphia: WB Saunders.

193 Williams, T.L., Elliott, J., and Syme, H.M. (2013). Renin-angiotensin-aldosterone system activity in hyperthyroid cats with and without concurrent hypertension. *J. Vet. Intern. Med.* 27: 522–529.

194 Adams, W.H., Daniel, G.B., Legendre, A.M. et al. (1997). Changes in renal function in cats following treatment of hyperthyroidism using 131I. *Vet. Radiol. Ultrasound* 38: 231–238.

195 Broussard, J.D., Peterson, M.E., and Fox, P.R. (1995). Changes in clinical and laboratory findings in cats with hyperthyroidism from 1983 to 1993. *J. Am. Vet. Med. Assoc.* 206: 302–305.

196 Peterson, M.E., Kintzer, P.P., Cavanagh, P.G. et al. (1983). Feline hyperthyroidism: pretreatment clinical and laboratory evaluation of 131 cases. *J. Am. Vet. Med. Assoc.* 183: 103–110.

197 Williams, T.L., Peak, K.J., Brodbelt, D. et al. (2010). Survival and the development of azotemia after treatment of hyperthyroid cats. *J. Vet. Intern. Med.* 24: 863–869.

198 DiBartola, S.P., Broome, M.R., Stein, B.S. et al. (1996). Effect of treatment of hyperthyroidism on renal function in cats. *J. Am. Vet. Med. Assoc.* 208: 875–878.

199 Relford, R. (2017). Hyperthyroid cats: the IDEXX SDMA test is a more reliable indicator of kidney function than creatinine. *Todays Vet. Pract.* 7: 112–113.

200 Szlosek, D., Robertson, J., Quimby, J. et al. (2020). A retrospective evaluation of the relationship between symmetric dimethylarginine, creatinine and body weight in hyperthyroid cats. *PLoS One* 15: e0227964.

201 Peterson, M.E., Varela, F.V., Rishniw, M. et al. (2018). Evaluation of serum symmetric dimethylarginine concentration as a marker for masked chronic kidney disease in cats with hyperthyroidism. *J. Vet. Intern. Med.* 32: 295–304.

202 Covey, H.L., Chang, Y.M., Elliott, J. et al. (2019). Changes in thyroid and renal function after bilateral thyroidectomy in cats. *J. Vet. Intern. Med.* 33: 508–515.

203 Becker, T.J., Graves, T.K., Kruger, J.M. et al. (2000). Effects of methimazole on renal function in cats with hyperthyroidism. *J. Am. Anim. Hosp. Assoc.* 36: 215–223.

204 Graves, T.K., Olivier, N.B., Nachreiner, R.F. et al. (1994). Changes in renal function associated with treatment of hyperthyroidism in cats. *Am. J. Vet. Res.* 55: 1745–1749.

205 Riensche, M.R., Graves, T.K., and Schaeffer, D.J. (2008). An investigation of predictors of renal insufficiency following treatment of hyperthyroidism in cats. *J. Feline Med. Surg.* 10: 160–166.

206 Peterson, M.E., Nichols, R., and Rishniw, M. (2017). Serum thyroxine and thyroid-stimulating hormone concentration in hyperthyroid cats that develop azotaemia after radioiodine therapy. *J. Small Anim. Pract.* 58: 519–530.

207 Williams, T.L., Elliott, J., and Syme, H.M. (2010). Association of iatrogenic hypothyroidism with azotemia and reduced survival time in cats treated for hyperthyroidism. *J. Vet. Intern. Med.* 24: 1086–1092.

208 van Hoek, I., Lefebvre, H.P., Peremans, K. et al. (2009). Short- and long-term follow-up of glomerular and tubular renal markers of kidney function in hyperthyroid cats after treatment with radioiodine. *Domest. Anim. Endocrinol.* 36: 45–56.

209 Boag, A.K., Neiger, R., Slater, L. et al. (2007). Changes in the glomerular filtration rate of 27 cats with hyperthyroidism after treatment with radioactive iodine. *Vet. Rec.* 161: 711–715.

210 DeMonaco, S.M., Panciera, D.L., Morre, W.A. et al. (2020). Symmetric dimethylarginine in hyperthyroid cats before and after treatment with radioactive iodine. *J. Feline Med. Surg.* 6: 531–538.

211 Williams, T.L., Elliott, J., and Syme, H.M. (2014). Effect on renal function of restoration of euthyroidism in hyperthyroid cats with iatrogenic hypothyroidism. *J. Vet. Intern. Med.* 28: 1251–1255.

212 Yuile, C.L. and Hawkins, W.B. (1941). Azotemia due to ingestion of blood proteins. *Am. J. Med. Sci.* 201: 162–167.

213 Nakashima, K., Hiyoshi, S., Ohno, K. et al. (2015). Prognostic factors in dogs with protein-losing enteropathy. *Vet. J.* 205: 28–32.

214 Kathrani, A., Sanchez-Vizcaino, F., and Hall, E.J. (2019). Association of chronic enteropathy activity index, blood urea concentration, and risk of death in dogs with protein-losing enteropathy. *J. Vet. Intern. Med.* 33: 536–543.

215 Crivellenti, L.Z., Borin-Crivellenti, S., Fertal, K.L. et al. (2017). Occult gastrointestinal bleeding is a common finding in dogs with chronic kidney disease. *Vet. Clin. Pathol.* 46: 132–137.

216 Kazory, A. (2010). Emergence of blood urea nitrogen as a biomarker of neurohormonal activation in heart failure. *Am. J. Cardiol.* 106: 694–700.

217 Santiago, S.L., Freeman, L.M., and Rush, J.E. (2020). Cardiac cachexia in cats with congestive heart failure: prevalence and clinical, laboratory, and survival findings. *J. Vet. Intern. Med.* 34: 35–44.

218 Matsue, Y., van der Meer, P., Damman, K. et al. (2017). Blood urea nitrogen-to-creatinine ratio in the general population and in patients with acute heart failure. *Heart* 103: 407–413.

219 Lake-Bakaar, G.A., Johnson, E.G., and Griffiths, L.G. (2012). Aortic thrombosis in dogs: 31 cases (2000–2010). *J. Am. Vet. Med. Assoc.* 241: 910–915.

220 Goutal, C.M., Keir, I., Kenney, S. et al. (2010). Evaluation of acute congestive heart failure in dogs and cats: 145 cases (2007–2008). *J. Vet. Emerg. Crit. Care (San Antonio)* 20: 330–337.

221 Ineson, D.L., Freeman, L.M., and Rush, J.E. (2019). Clinical and laboratory findings and survival time associated with cardiac cachexia in dogs with congestive heart failure. *J. Vet. Intern. Med.* 33: 1902–1908.

222 Johnson, C.A., Armstrong, P.J., and Hauptman, J.G. (1987). Congenital portosystemic shunts in dogs: 46 cases (1979–1986). *J. Am. Vet. Med. Assoc.* 191: 1478–1483.

223 Blaxter, A.C., Holt, P.E., Pearson, G.R. et al. (1988). Congenital portosystemic shunts in the cat: a report of nine cases. *J. Small Anim. Pract.* 29: 631–645.

224 Berger, B., Whiting, P.G., Breznock, E.M. et al. (1986). Congenital feline portosystemic shunts. *J. Am. Vet. Med. Assoc.* 188: 517–521.

225 Allen, L., Stobie, D., Mauldin, G.N. et al. (1999). Clinicopathologic features of dogs with hepatic microvascular dysplasia with and

without portosystemic shunts: 42 cases (1991–1996). *J. Am. Vet. Med. Assoc.* 214: 218–220.

226 Deppe, T.A., Center, S.A., Simpson, K.W. et al. (1999). Glomerular filtration rate and renal volume in dogs with congenital portosystemic vascular anomalies before and after surgical ligation. *J. Vet. Intern. Med.* 13: 465–471.

227 Rawlinson, J.E., Goldstein, R.E., Reiter, A.M. et al. (2011). Association of periodontal disease with systemic health indices in dogs and the systemic response to treatment of periodontal disease. *J. Am. Vet. Med. Assoc.* 238: 601–609.

228 Feldman, E.C., Hoar, B., Pollard, R. et al. (2005). Pretreatment clinical and laboratory findings in dogs with primary hyperparathyroidism: 210 cases (1987–2004). *J. Am. Vet. Med. Assoc.* 227: 756–761.

229 Rovira, S., Munoz, A., and Benito, M. (2007). Fluid and electrolyte shifts during and after agility competitions in dogs. *J. Vet. Med. Sci.* 69: 31–35.

230 Steiss, J., Ahmad, H.A., Cooper, P. et al. (2004). Physiologic responses in healthy Labrador retrievers during field trial training and competition. *J. Vet. Intern. Med.* 18: 147–151.

231 Burr, J.R., Reinhart, G.A., Swenson, R.A. et al. (1997). Serum biochemical values in sled dogs before and after competing in long-distance races. *J. Am. Vet. Med. Assoc.* 211: 175–179.

232 Rose, R.J. and Bloomberg, M.S. (1989). Responses to sprint exercise in the greyhound: effects on haematology, serum biochemistry and muscle metabolites. *Res. Vet. Sci.* 47: 212–218.

233 Hammel, E.P., Kronfeld, D.S., Ganjam, V.K. et al. (1977). Metabolic responses to exhaustive exercise in racing sled dogs fed diets containing medium, low, or zero carbohydrate. *Am. J. Clin. Nutr.* 30: 409–418.

234 Hinchcliff, K.W., Olson, J., Crusberg, C. et al. (1993). Serum biochemical changes in dogs competing in a long-distance sled race. *J. Am. Vet. Med. Assoc.* 202: 401–405.

235 Chanoit, G.P., Concordet, D., Lefebvre, H.P. et al. (2002). Exercise does not induce major changes in plasma muscle enzymes, creatinine, glucose and total proteins concentrations in untrained beagle dogs. *J. Vet. Med. A Physiol. Pathol. Clin. Med.* 49: 222–224.

236 O'Marra, S.K., Delaforcade, A.M., and Shaw, S.P. (2011). Treatment and predictors of outcome in dogs with immune-mediated thrombocytopenia. *J. Am. Vet. Med. Assoc.* 238: 346–352.

237 Ezeokonkwo, R.C., Ezeh, I.O., Onunkwo, J.I. et al. (2012). Comparative serum biochemical changes in mongrel dogs following single and mixed infections of *Trypanosoma congolense* and *Trypanosoma brucei brucei*. *Vet. Parasitol.* 190: 56–61.

238 Heidarpour, M., Soltani, S., Mohri, M. et al. (2012). Canine visceral leishmaniasis: relationships between oxidative stress, liver and kidney variables, trace elements, and clinical status. *Parasitol. Res.* 111: 1491–1496.

239 Ybanez, A.P., Ybanez, R.H., Villavelez, R.R. et al. (2016). Retrospective analyses of dogs found serologically positive for *Ehrlichia canis* in Cebu, Philippines from 2003 to 2014. *Vet. World* 9: 43–47.

240 Grauer, G.F., Culham, C.A., Bowman, D.D. et al. (1988). Parasite excretory-secretory antigen and antibody to excretory-secretory antigen in body fluids and kidney tissue of Dirofilaria immitis infected dogs. *Am. J. Trop. Med. Hyg.* 39: 380–387.

241 Grauer, G.F., Culham, C.A., Cooley, A.J. et al. (1987). Clinicopathologic and histologic evaluation of *Dirofilaria immitis*-induced nephropathy in dogs. *Am. J. Trop. Med. Hyg.* 37: 588–596.

242 Grauer, G.F., Culham, C.A., Dubielzig, R.R. et al. (1989). Experimental *Dirofilaria immitis*-associated glomerulonephritis induced in part by in situ formation of immune complexes in the glomerular capillary wall. *J. Parasitol.* 75: 585–593.

243 Grauer, G.F., Culham, C.A., Dubielzig, R.R. et al. (1988). Effects of a specific thromboxane synthetase inhibitor on development of experimental *Dirofilaria immitis* immune complex glomerulonephritis in the dog. *J. Vet. Intern. Med.* 2: 192–200.

244 Zygner, W., Rapacka, G., Gojska-Zygner, O. et al. (2007). Biochemical abnormalities observed in serum of dogs infected with large Babesia in Warsaw (Poland). *Pol. J. Vet. Sci.* 10: 245–253.

245 Kitagawa, H., Kitoh, K., Ohba, Y. et al. (1998). Comparison of laboratory test results before and after surgical removal of heartworms in dogs with vena caval syndrome. *J. Am. Vet. Med. Assoc.* 213: 1134–1136.

246 Burrows, C.F. and Bovee, K.C. (1974). Metabolic changes due to experimentally induced rupture of the canine urinary bladder. *Am. J. Vet. Res.* 35: 1083–1088.

247 Schmiedt, C., Tobias, K.M., and Otto, C.M. (2001). Evaluation of abdominal fluid: peripheral blood creatinine and potassium ratios for diagnosis of uroperitoneum in dogs. *J. Vet. Emerg. Crit. Care* 11: 275–280.

248 Richardson, D.W. and Kohn, C.W. (1983). Uroperitoneum in the foal. *J. Am. Vet. Med. Assoc.* 182: 267–271.

249 Grimes, J.A., Fletcher, J.M., and Schmiedt, C.W. (2018). Outcomes in dogs with uroabdomen: 43 cases (2006–2015). *J. Am. Vet. Med. Assoc.* 252: 92–97.

250 Aumann, M., Worth, L.T., and Drobatz, K.J. (1998). Uroperitoneum in cats: 26 cases (1986–1995). *J. Am. Anim. Hosp. Assoc.* 34: 315–324.

Introduction to Urinalysis

"When the patient dies the kidneys may go to the pathologist, but while he lives the urine is ours. It can provide us day by day, month by month, and year by year with a serial story of the major events within the kidney. Dr. Thomas Addis (1881–1949)"

INTRODUCTION

Urine has been examined for over 6000 years [1]. The use of microscopy to examine urine sediment was initiated in the nineteenth century, making the analysis of urine an important clinical diagnostic tool. Routine urinalysis is an extremely valuable and relatively inexpensive diagnostic tool that sometimes is overlooked in veterinary practice [2, 3]. Complete urinalysis includes the evaluation of physical and chemical properties as well as a thorough examination of the urinary sediment. Unfortunately, either for convenience or extremely small sample size, the dipstick chemical analysis of urine is sometimes the only component of urinalysis that is performed in private practice. Dipstrip urine chemistry provides an incomplete total picture for the interpretation of results in the absence of urinary physical and sediment findings. Findings from urinalysis should not be interpreted in isolation. Unfortunately, only 57% of survey participants that performed in-house urinalyses always performed a sediment examination in one report [4]. Proper assessment of urinalysis requires the integration of findings from history, physical examination, hematology, routine serum biochemistry, abdominal imaging with radiographs or ultrasound, urine culture, and/or histopathology results from renal or lower urinary tract tissue. Quality assurance for three components of the urinalysis (physical properties, dry reagent pad [dipstrip] urine chemistry, and urine sediment microscopy) is less well established than for hematology and cytology. Guidelines detailing quality control assurance in general and for urinalysis in specific are available for the interested reader [5–8].

WHEN TO PERFORM URINALYSIS

Routine urinalysis (along with hemogram and serum biochemical profile) is a useful starting point for the evaluation of any animal with nonspecific signs of illness, such as anorexia, lethargy, or weight loss (Table 2.1). A complete urinalysis should be performed anytime that a complete blood count and routine serum biochemistry are submitted in order to be able to integrate and maximize the interpretation of findings.

The minimum database for any animal with suspected or known urinary tract disease should include a urinalysis. This includes dogs or cats with clinical signs of lower urinary tract disease, such as those with pollakiuria, stranguria, dysuria, hematuria, inappropriate urinations, or urinary incontinence. Animals with a history of urolithiasis or urinary tract infection (UTI) can also benefit from urinalysis for diagnosis and surveillance. Changes in the character of a pet's urine as observed by an owner (e.g., darker, bloody, paler, sticky) should also prompt the clinician to perform a urinalysis.

A urinalysis should be performed in any animal with known or suspected renal disease to evaluate the possibility for ongoing changes in urine concentration, proteinuria, or development of an active sediment (increases in WBC, RBC, urothelial cells, bacteria, or casts). All patients with a history of polyuria and polydipsia should undergo urinalysis to determine the degree of urine concentration achieved and also if there is an increased level of urinary sediment activity. This is an important first step in determining if the cause of the polyuria and polydipsia is related to abnormal kidney function or an endocrine disorder. Sequentially collected urine samples may be of special value in an animal whose condition is changing over time. All animals with systemic hypertension, most often associated with renal disease, should undergo urinalysis to assess for proteinuria and damaging effects on renal function that can include minimal ability to concentrate urine.

Urinalysis in the Dog and Cat, First Edition. Dennis J. Chew and Patricia A. Schenck.
© 2023 John Wiley & Sons, Inc. Published 2023 by John Wiley & Sons, Inc.

Table 2.1 When should urine be submitted for analysis?

Upper urinary tract disease

    Chronic kidney disease (CKD)

    Acute kidney injury (AKI)

    Neoplasia

Lower urinary tract disease

    Cystitis

    Urinary tract infection (UTI)

    Urolithiasis

    Incontinence

    Neoplasia

Systemic medical diseases

    Inflammatory or immune-mediated

    Infectious

    Neoplasia

Surgical diseases – pre-operative

Endocrine diseases

    Diabetes mellitus

    Diabetes insipidus

    Hyperadrenocorticism

    Hyperthyroidism

Systemic hypertension

    Any cause

Polyuria & polydipsia (PU/PD)

Febrile conditions

Dehydration

Proteinuria already known

Preanesthetic screening

Wellness and geriatric exams

When nonrenal systemic diseases are present, urinalysis can be a helpful evaluation tool. For example, animals with hepatic disease or portosystemic shunts may have bilirubinuria or ammonium biurate crystals. Patients with hypercalcemia may have minimally concentrated urine caused by ionized hypercalcemia. Proteinuria due to glomerular disease may complicate several chronic infectious diseases. All animals with endocrine diseases, such as hyperadrenocorticism, hyperthyroidism, diabetes insipidus, and diabetes mellitus, should have a complete urinalysis performed to assess urine-concentrating ability and to determine if proteinuria or UTI is present.

Urinalysis should be performed in febrile animals, because UTI can be a source of sepsis without obvious urinary tract clinical signs. Completion of urinalysis in dehydrated animals before beginning fluid therapy is crucial for the preliminary evaluation of renal function. A high urine specific gravity (USG) in a dehydrated animal may be reassuring with respect to renal function, whereas low USG in a dehydrated animal is cause for concern for possible underlying renal disease.

As part of a wellness examination, routine urinalysis can serve as a useful reference point during future evaluations. The ability to appropriately concentrate urine and the absence of proteinuria are hallmarks of healthy dogs and cats that can change over time. Preoperative and preanesthetic evaluation should also include a complete urinalysis to fully evaluate renal function, especially urinary concentrating ability and proteinuria.

Many diagnoses and possibilities for treatment interventions are missed when urinalysis is not performed [2]. Abnormalities in urinalysis can be detected despite the absence of obvious clinical signs, especially during early stages of chronic kidney disease (CKD), endocrine disorders, and some chronic infectious and neoplastic diseases. Pathological changes in urine often occur BEFORE changes occur in blood, especially in those with early CKD. Urinalysis is uniquely able to provide information about kidney function and disease that cannot be determined with blood testing, as with the finding of minimally concentrated urine, proteinuria, casts (cylindruria), and the presence of infectious organisms (bacteria, fungi, yeast). Additionally, crystals in urine can provide information that is useful in the evaluation of dogs and cats forming calculi or urethral plugs. The presence of some crystals in urine can indicate toxicity from ethylene glycol ingestion (calcium oxalates) or from food contamination (melamine-cyanuric acid from tainted food).

PERFORMING A URINALYSIS

The method of urine collection and handling of the sample influence interpretation, and will be discussed in Chapter 3. Once urine is collected, the decision is made as to where and how the urinalysis will be performed (Table 2.2). The author estimates that about two-third of veterinarians run some form of urine analysis in-house, and the other one-third send samples to commercial laboratories for analysis. A hybrid of in-house urinalysis and those sent out to referral laboratories are used by some practices [9].

For urine samples being analyzed in-house, about two-third are run as complete urinalyses and one-third only undergo dipstrip chemical analysis. Some practices have established a protocol to examine fresh urinary sediment in-house in addition to sending a urine sample to a commercial lab. Most in-house analyses use standard manual methods of dipstrip reading and sediment microscopy along with the determination of USG using an optical refractometer. Many private practices have adopted automated methods to read the urinary chemistry dipstrip. Digital refractometry to measure USG is ever increasing in availability as an option, instead of optical refractometry. Manual methods of urinalysis take an estimated 18–25 minutes to perform and generate a report. In-house automated methods of urinalysis (chemistry and urine microscopy) allow the

Table 2.2 Advantages and disadvantages of manual or automated in-house urine analysis (UA) and reference lab.

In-House UA: Manual		In-House UA: Automated dipstrip and microscopy	
Advantages	Disadvantages	Advantages	Disadvantages
Convenience to client	18–25 minutes to perform complete UA	Increased laboratory efficiency	Initial cost of equipment – expensive
Quick turnaround time	Technicians	Use of technician time	Initial training in use of automated methods
Allows in-hospital consultation	Interrupted workflow – not linear	More linear work flow	Technician or DVM review of urine sediment
Convenience to DVM	Different skill levels	Five minutes estimated time to generate report for complete UA	Should be done as quality control in general
No need to pack and ship	Multiple technicians performing UA	Standardized time when machine reads dipstrip	Not all sediment is accurately identified automatically
No need to call back owner	Nonstandardized techniques	Standardization of technique for microscopy	Some sediment is not assigned any identification
Less delay in starting therapy	Supravital stain versus no stain	Volume examined	Nonhyaline casts must be further examined and identified
• Not waiting on results	Urine volume and sediment volume	Centrifugation time and force	Some crystals need manual identification
Better owner compliance	Centrifugation time and force	Terminology generated for identified elements	Nonsquamous cells need manual identification
• Immediate consultation	Microscope quality	Digital pictures of urine sediment generated	Clumps of cells – need further identification
Improved quality of results	Lacking in microscope skills & settings	Permanent storage	WBC clumps
Greater preservation of urinary elements	Condenser	Inclusion in medical record	Epithelial clumps
Fragile casts	Lighting	Technician can override automated enumeration and identification of elements	
Less lysis of RBC and WBC	Fine-focus "rocking"		
Greater cellular detail in general	Repeatability of findings varies on same sample, even with same examiner		
Less postcollection artifacts	Vague terminology – "few" or "many"		
Minimizes ex vivo crystal formation			
Minimizes bacterial multiplication			
Income generation to practice			

Reference laboratory UA

Some UA results are better than no results	Results available in 5–24 hours
	Degradation of urine sample
Improved accuracy of results when only nontrained or nonskilled in-house personnel	Fragile elements no longer available to be identified and enumerated
	Lysis of WBC, RBC
	Casts, especially cellular
	Increased number of bacteria
	Loss of cellular detail
	Development of crystals not originally there

complete urinalysis to be performed, and a report generated within five minutes. This includes the time to visually confirm that the abnormalities reported in urine sediment accurately match up the acquired digital pictures. An increasing number of private practices have transitioned to automated methods of urine microscopy for reasons of increased efficiency and accuracy of analysis (described further in Chapter 6).

In-house analysis of urine is preferred as evaluation of fresh warm urine always provides more accurate results for the enumeration and identification of elements in urinary sediment. Many fragile elements, especially cellular casts, are identified when fresh urine is examined within 15 minutes, and these elements are frequently no longer seen during analysis hours later.

Complete urinalysis form - sample

Owner's name _____   Pet Name   _____

Date _____   Working Diagnosis _____

Volume submitted   _____mL
Time Sample Collected   _____Time Sample Analyzed _____
Refrigeration   Yes No
Preservatives   Yes No
Sediment Stain   Yes No

Source of Sample:

Void: From Owner	Mid-Stream	End-Stream	Begin-Stream	Expression
Postvoid:	Table/Floor	Cage Paper/Pads	Nonabsorbent Litter	
Catheter:	Single	Indwelling		
Cystocentesis:	Palpate/Blind	ULS-Guided		

Drugs: Steroids   Antibiotics   Chemotherapy   Other

Reason for submission: Lower urinary signs   Abnormal urine color/clarity
                             Pre-Op   Wellness screening
                             Systemic illness   Endocrine disease
                             Other

Automated strip reader: Yes No   Automated microscopy: Yes No

Color   _____

Appearance   _____

Specific Gravity_____

pH   _____

Protein   _____

Occult blood   _____
      Intact RBC
      Hemolyzed

Glucose   _____

Ketones   _____

Bilirubin   _____

Comments: _____

Casts   / LPF
   Hyaline   _____
   Granular   _____
   Waxy   _____
   Cellular   _____

WBC   _____   /HPF
      Free
      Clumped

RBC   _____   /HPF

Epithelial cells   /HPF
   Squamous_____
   Transitional_____
   Free
   Clumped
   Renal   _____

Crystals 0   Few   Mod   Many
Crystal type _____

Bacteria 0   Few   Mod   Many
           Rods   Coccci Mixed

Miscellaneous:

FIGURE 2.1   Complete Urinalysis Form. LFP – low powered field; HPF – high powered field; RBC – red blood cells; WBC – white blood cells.

There appears to be an increasing trend for veterinary hospitals to send out urine specimens for analysis instead of performing them on site. Some veterinary practices feel that performing in-house urinalysis is too time consuming, and they lack the confidence in their level of skill to report findings accurately. One of the purposes of this book is to expose and train in-house technicians and veterinarians in standard methods of urine microscopy to build confidence for accurate identification of common urinary elements and bacteria. Performing in-house complete urinalysis generates income that is justifiable with the practice of good medicine. It is important to routinely use a standard form to record the results of urinalysis as part of the patient's medical record (Figure 2.1).

REFERENCES

1   Magiorkinis, E. and Diamantis, A. (2015). The fascinating story of urine examination: from uroscopy to the era of microscopy and beyond. *Diagn. Cytopathol.* 43: 1020–1036.

2   Parrah, J.D., Moulvi, B.A., Gazi, M.A. et al. (2013). Importance of urinalysis in veterinary practice – a review. *Vet. World* 640–646.

3   Piech, T.L. and Wycislo, K.L. (2019). Importance of urinalysis. *Vet. Clin. North Am. Small Anim. Pract.* 49: 233–245.

4   Gibbs, N.H., Heseltine, J., Rishniw, M., and Nabity, M. (2020). Survey of the practice of canine and feline urinalyses in the United States and Canada:Abstract NU30. *J Vet Intern Med* 34: 2936.

5   Arnold, J.E., Camus, M.S., Freeman, K.P. et al. (2019). ASVCP guidelines: principles of quality assurance and standards for veterinary clinical pathology (version 3.0): developed by the American Society for Veterinary Clinical Pathology's (ASVCP) Quality Assurance and Laboratory Standards (QALS) committee. *Vet. Clin. Pathol.* 48: 542–618.

6   Camus, M.S., Flatland, B., Freeman, K.P. et al. (2015). ASVCP quality assurance guidelines: external quality assessment and comparative testing for reference and in-clinic laboratories. *Vet. Clin. Pathol.* 44: 477–492.

7   Gunn-Christie, R.G., Flatland, B., Friedrichs, K.R. et al. (2012). ASVCP quality assurance guidelines: control of preanalytical, analytical, and postanalytical factors for urinalysis, cytology, and clinical chemistry in veterinary laboratories. *Vet. Clin. Pathol.* 41: 18–26.

8   Monti, P. and Archer, J. (2016). Quality assurance and interpretation of laboratory data. In: *BSAVA Manual of Canine and Feline Clinical Pathology*, 3e (ed. E. Villiers and J. Ristic), 11–26. Gloucester England British Small Animal Veterinary Association.

9   Bilbrough, G. (2016). In-house versus external testing. In: *BSAVA Manual of Canine and Feline Clinical Pathology*, 3e (ed. E. Villiers and J. Ristic), 1–10. Gloucester England British Small Animal Veterinary Association.

CHAPTER 3

Urine Sample Collection and Handling

INTRODUCTION

Urine samples can be collected during voiding, following voiding (post-voiding), by urinary catheterization, and by cystocentesis. The advantages and disadvantages of the urine collection method are outlined in Table 3.1. The appropriate method of urine collection is chosen after the consideration of the likelihood of obtaining a diagnostic urine sample using the particular method, the risk of traumatizing or infecting the urinary tract, the expense of collection equipment and procedure time, animal restraint required, and the level of technical expertise required or available to collect the urine sample. It is important to always note on the laboratory record how the urine sample was obtained, since the technique of urine collection influences the interpretation of findings in urinalysis.

The overarching goal for the collection of urine is to obtain and analyze urine samples that reflect what was in the urine immediately prior to collection in order to gain the most accurate information for clinical interpretation. Consequently, great care should be taken to eliminate or minimize artifacts that can occur from the method of urine collection (discussed later in this chapter) and also those that can develop following collection and storage of urine prior to analysis (see Chapter 6). It is important to remember that settling of formed elements and crystals can occur within the bladder. In these instances, urine samples collected by midstream void, catheter, or cystocentesis will not accurately represent the number of cells and crystals in the total bladder urine, so efforts to resuspend gravitated sediment should be made prior to urine collection. Though a single urinalysis can reveal important findings, there can also be increased clinical value for the serial collection and analysis of urine from patients over time. Serial urinalyses may be especially helpful in the evaluation of patients whose conditions are changing over time, before and after treatment, and before and after invasive urinary procedures.

It historically has been recommended to submit 10–12 mL of urine for urinalysis, but this volume of urine often is not available to be collected from dogs and cats, especially if they have signs of lower urinary tract urgency and frequently void. We recommend that a minimum of 3 mL should be submitted, though a complete urinalysis can be done on 1–2 mL of urine (see Chapters 4–6). The container used to transport the urine sample to the laboratory must be clean and free of contamination with detergents, other cleaning agents, and disinfectants that could lead to spurious results. An airtight container is preferred to avoid pH changes in the sample. Labels noting the method of sample collection, patient identification, and the date and time of collection should be written or affixed to the container (not the lid) or tube to be submitted to the laboratory.

Disposable unpowdered latex gloves should be worn during collection and handling of urine as a safety measure [1].

Urinalysis in the Dog and Cat, First Edition. Dennis J. Chew and Patricia A. Schenck.
© 2023 John Wiley & Sons, Inc. Published 2023 by John Wiley & Sons, Inc.

Table 3.1 Urine collection methods: advantages and disadvantages.

	Advantage	Disadvantage
Voided	No risk to patient for urinary trauma or to acquire urinary infection	Contamination by urethra and genital tract
	Client can collect sample	Contamination from environment (especially when collected by owners)
	Suitable for initial screening	
	Method of choice to evaluate hematuria (no RBC added by trauma of collection)	Less useful for urine culture, unless no growth
	Comparison of initial, mid, and final stream useful to localize process	
Manual expression	Easy to acquire under anesthesia	In awake animals, method easily adds RBC, protein to sample-trauma
		Bladder rupture possible
		Same others as listed for voided
Post-void	Some urine available for analysis	Small volume harvested to submit
		Contamination likely
		Absorption or adsorption of elements or urine fluid possible into surfaces
		Same others as listed for voided
Catheterized	Limits contamination from genital tract compared to voided sample	Trauma from method can introduce RBC, epithelial cells, and protein to sample
	Sample acquisition when urine volume in bladder is small	Iatrogenic UTI possible
	Useful for urine culture when use critical cutoff cfu/mL	Distal urethral flora can be introduced into bladder
		Urethral or bladder trauma – inflammation to rupture
Cystocentesis	Bypass urethral and genital contamination	Iatrogenic RBC and protein added to urine
	Ideal for urine culture	Possible TCC seeding
	No risk for UTI in immunosuppressed animals	Urine leakage when bladder atony or obstruction is present
		Caudal vena cava or aortic entry possible – poor technique
		Enterocentesis – poor technique

Urine can harbor infectious bacteria that cause leptospirosis infection or urinary tract infection (UTI) (e.g. *Escherichia coli*) in animals that could be a threat to human health. Protective eye wear is also recommended to prevent splashes of urine into the eyes. Human exposure to urine is more likely to occur with samples collected by voiding and catheterization, though it could occur with cystocentesis when samples are transferred to transport tubes. Hands should not touch the face until gloves are removed after the sample has been collected.

Urine samples collected at random times of the day usually are sufficient for routine diagnostic evaluation. Samples from dogs that are collected first thing in the morning before the animal has eaten or consumed water are most likely to have the highest urine specific gravity (USG) and be most useful in evaluation of urinary concentrating ability (described in detail in Chapter 4). Timing for urine collection is not as important in cats, as they vary their degree of urine concentration less over the day. A first morning urine sample includes the possibility of increased numbers of cellular elements and bacteria in these samples, but this must be balanced against the possibility of more fragile elements (e.g. casts and cells) degenerating overnight in the bladder. In some conditions, it can be informative to compare the first morning sample to another sample collected a few hours later. It is best to collect urine before drugs or parenteral fluids have been administered. Glucocorticoids and diuretics are examples of drugs that interfere with renal concentrating ability. Erroneous conclusions are potentially drawn from the USG about renal function during the use of these drugs and fluid therapy because of the elaboration of less concentrated urine. Antimicrobial drugs may affect the numbers of leukocytes and bacteria observed in the urine sediment, and some antimicrobials may precipitate in the urine leading to unfamiliar crystals in the urine sediment.

Ideally, urinalysis should be performed on samples right after collection in order to limit artifacts that develop following storage at room temperature or in the refrigerator (detailed in subsequent chapters) [2–6]. If urinalysis cannot be performed within 10 minutes of collection, the sample should be refrigerated until analysis can occur. Delay in examination may allow growth of contaminating bacterial organisms, change in urinary pH, loss of cellular detail, and disruption of fragile elements (especially casts). Unrefrigerated urine can cause relatively rapid lysis of erythrocytes and leukocytes [7]. Delay can also result in ex vivo precipitation of crystals in the urine sample. Refrigeration should be limited to four hours but one hour or less is better. Samples that are analyzed after overnight refrigeration provide suboptimal results. It is best to collect and ship samples performed in a timely manner. It is best to not add preservatives to urine before analysis as these can alter chemical analysis at times. Recently, a boric acid sponge preservative system was shown to be effective for reliable bacterial culture for 24 hours in nonrefrigerated urine samples [8]. When sending to a reference laboratory, ensure that urinalysis is selected on the work order and not fluid analysis.

Gram-negative organisms can double their concentration every 30 minutes in urine kept at room temperature [9]. This can allow bacteria to be visualized in urine sediment that were not originally there in sufficient quantity to be seen. When gram-negative and gram-positive organisms exist in the same urine sample submitted for bacterial culture, gram-negative organisms with a shorter doubling time can overgrow other organisms that have a longer doubling time in samples that are not properly refrigerated. Urine samples kept under refrigeration for too long yield false-negative bacterial culture results [10].

COLLECTION OF VOIDED AND POST-VOID URINE SAMPLES

URINE COLLECTED BY VOIDING

Collection of voided urine requires no special equipment, no need for animal restraint, and does not subject the animal to urinary tract trauma or introduction of bacterial infection from instrumentation. Depending on the timing of collection, a voided urine sample can reflect urine from the initial stream, midstream, endstream, combined all stream, or collected from surfaces post-voiding. Voided midstream urine specimens are acceptable for initial routine evaluation of suspected urinary disorders and for medical screening purposes, though the other timings of voided sample collection may also reveal valuable information.

Urine samples collected by voiding can add cells and protein from the passage of urine through the distal urethra, vagina, or prepuce and may contact perineal or preputial hair as additional sources for contamination of the sample. In male dogs, urine that passes through preputial exudate commonly adds inflammatory cells, protein, and bacteria to the sample (Figure 3.1). Urine voided by normal female dogs is less contaminated than urine from male dogs, but if the female is in estrus, the degree of contamination with red blood cells

(RBC) and epithelial cells added to the urine sample can be substantial (Figure 3.2). Minimal contamination of voided urine specimens occurs in cats of either sex [10]. Cleansing the vulva or tip of the prepuce with soap and water followed by sponge gauze application of benzalkonium or alcohol may lessen sample contamination when a voided sample is collected by veterinary personnel, especially when these areas are obviously soiled or have exudate.

Urinalysis on voided urine collected by owners at home can provide meaningful information, but these samples are more likely to be contaminated with elements in urine sediment that come from the environment (soil, plant material, spores, fungal elements, fibers, hair) and chemicals like soap or bleach from make-shift urine containers. It is usually unclear if initial, mid, or endstream portions of the urine stream were sampled during collection by the owner. If the

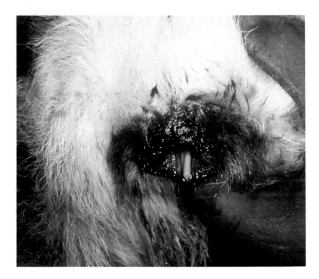

FIGURE 3.2 Bloody vulvar discharge in a female dog in heat. Voided urine will easily pick up RBC and protein from this type of discharge that must be considered during evaluation of urinalysis results.

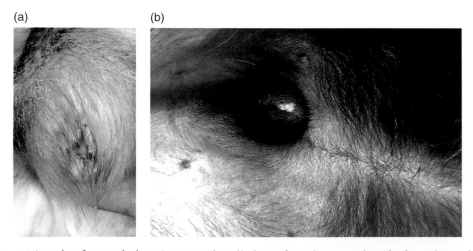

FIGURE 3.1 (a, b) Preputial exudate from male dogs. Some purulent discharge from the external urethral opening and prepuce is common in normal male dogs. This exudate easily contaminates voided urine samples and so can add WBC and protein to the urinalysis results.

urinalysis results could possibly be due to contamination, urine collection by another method may be needed.

In general, a voided midstream urine sample is the best portion to collect to assess disease processes occurring in the bladder, ureters, or kidneys. A voided urine sample is the method of choice to evaluate (confirm or exclude) the presence of excess RBC in the urine. No trauma to the urinary tract is involved with this method of urine collection, in contrast to that incurred during collection with urinary catheters or cystocentesis. The initial urine stream mechanically flushes out cells, bacteria, and debris that enter the sample from the urethra, vagina, prepuce, or perineum. Initial urine stream samples may be more diagnostic for evaluation of disease processes that are distal to the bladder (e.g., urethra, vagina, prepuce, prostate). Comparison of urinalysis results from initial stream, midstream, and endstream voided urine specimens is sometimes helpful to more precisely determine the anatomic origin of cells and protein in the urine sample. If initial stream urine contains numerous RBC and white blood cells (WBC) but the midstream and endstream urine samples have very few cells, the lesion is likely to be in the distal urethra or genitalia. If cellular elements are numerous in the endstream urine sample and absent in initial stream samples, the lesion is more likely to be in the urinary bladder. If substantial settling of elements within the bladder has occurred, end of urination samples can reveal cells, crystals, and bacteria that are only observed when the bladder is more completely evacuated. Sometimes, end-urination samples exacerbate bleeding and the detection of RBC and protein in the urine sample as the bladder contracts over a lesion (e.g. bladder calculi, bladder tumor). It is the impression of some oncologists that the end-urination voided samples, particularly after straining, are the most likely to provide a high yield of abnormal transitional epithelial cells in those with urothelial cell carcinoma (UCC) (transitional cell carcinoma [TCC]).

Successful collection of voided samples from dogs often requires ingenuity and quickness of hand. It can be difficult to collect an adequate volume of voided samples from male dogs due to their tendency to have multiple discontinuous small volume urinations, some of which are related to marking behaviors. The low squatting posture of female dogs makes it difficult to collect a voided specimen at times. The gradual placement of a clean pie plate or similar container can be helpful in these cases (Figure 3.3). Some dogs are startled by the abrupt placement of the urine collection container and stop urinating. Devices that have a handle attached to a collection container or a ladle (Figures 3.4 and 3.5a,b) can allow capture of urine from a distance without frightening the dog. A simple handle made from an unwrapped wire coat hanger can be attached to a cup for urine collection (Figure 3.6). After urine has been obtained using a bowl, pie plate, ladle, cup, etc. the bowl should be removed quickly to avoid spillage. Voided urine should be immediately aspirated into a syringe and transferred to a plain sterile tube using a needle to avoid contamination from the environment (Figure 3.7a–c).

Collection of midstream urine samples from cats during voiding is rarely successful unless the cat has severe polyuria.

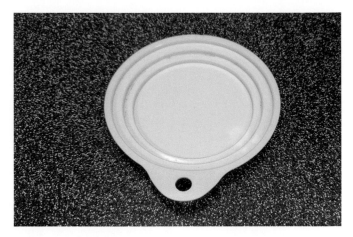

FIGURE 3.3 Silicone canned food lid cover/cap used to collect voided urine. The inverted lid cover provides a shallow collection chamber with a small diameter that fits more readily under female dogs. This method may be more successful than with the use of larger collection containers that are more likely to touch the back legs, which causes urination to immediately cease. The lid cover can be slid into position by hand or extended into position with a grabber.

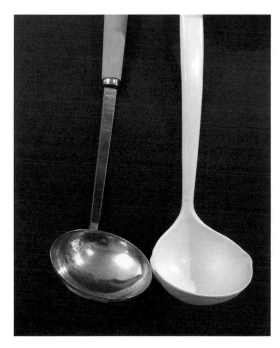

FIGURE 3.4 Kitchen ladles can be used to help catch voided urine samples from dogs.

It is sometimes possible to collect a voided sample from cats that have not had access to the litter box overnight. After this restriction, some cats will immediately void when a litter box is provided and a post-voided sample can be collected [1]. Removal of the litter pan may also inadvertently provide stress to certain cats, which can change some of the findings in the urinalysis such as pH. Some cats like to use the cat box immediately after cleaning and/or adding fresh litter, so this can be a good time to try to collect a post-voided sample.

(a)

(b)

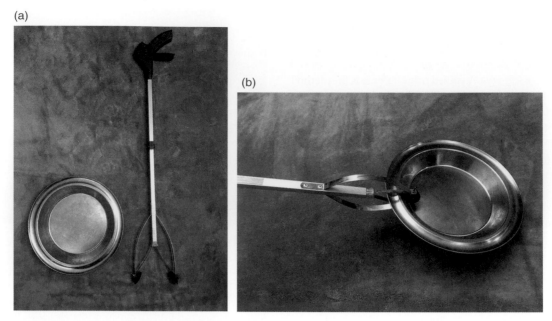

FIGURE 3.5 (a) Grabber-reacher tool next to pie pan. (b) Pie pan attached to grabber-reacher tool allows urine collection from more distance which is less likely to startle the dog, especially females.

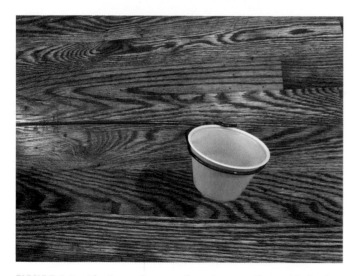

FIGURE 3.6 Plastic cup homemade system to collect voided urine. A wire coat hanger is taken apart, straightened out, and then the end is custom wrapped around the chosen container.

Voiding of urine is often stimulated from neonatal puppies or kittens after the prepuce or vulva is licked by the dam or queen. This urinating behavior can also be stimulated following gentle massage of these areas with a warm moist cotton ball. Once urination starts, the puppy or kitten can be held up so that urine drips into a container [11].

In some instances, comparison of urinalysis results obtained from a voided urine specimen to those obtained from urine collected by catheterization or cystocentesis may be helpful in anatomical localization of the disease process. For example, if urine microscopic abnormalities are readily observed in urine obtained by voiding, yet inapparent on samples obtained by cystocentesis or urethral catheterization,

the lesion is located distal to the bladder sphincter. If the abnormalities are apparent on cystocentesis or catheterization but absent in a voided sample, trauma from the collection method should be considered a source of the abnormalities.

MANUAL EXPRESSION OF URINE BY DIGITAL PALPATION AND COMPRESSION OF THE BLADDER

Gentle palpation of the urinary bladder with gradually increasing pressure may stimulate reflex voiding or can expel urine directly as intravesical pressure exceeds urethral resistance. It is usually more difficult to express urine from unanesthetized male dogs and cats due to greater urethral resistance than in females. It is common for an animal that failed to expel urine during attempts at manual compression to void urine shortly thereafter. Consequently, the clinician should be prepared to collect a post-voided sample from a clean surface.

Though this method of urine collection has commonly been employed in veterinary medicine, it is no longer recommended for the collection of routine urine samples for several reasons. Manual expression of urine often introduces red cells and protein into the sample from trauma to the bladder. It is likely that the diseased bladder will more readily add RBC to the urine sample during bladder trauma from this method of urine collection. As with spontaneously voided urine samples, specimens collected by manual expression are subject to contamination as urine passes through the distal urogenital tract. It is also possible that increased bladder hydrostatic pressure that develops during this procedure may force infected urine from the bladder retrograde into the ureters and extend a bacterial urinary infection into the kidneys. Rupture of the normal

(a)

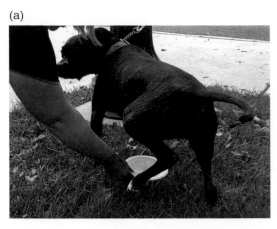

(b)

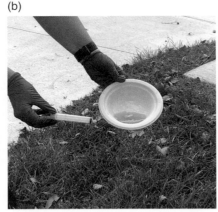

(c)

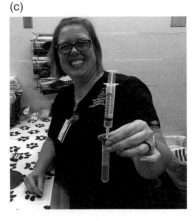

FIGURE 3.7   (a) Male dog voiding into disposable bowl. The bowl is placed into the urine stream just after the dog starts to evacuate urine. (b) It is important to remove the bowl as quickly as possible so that the dog does not knock it over. Immediately aspirate the voided urine into a syringe to eliminate contamination from the environment and to further limit chances for spillage. (c) Urine that was aspirated from the bowl into the syringe is transferred to a plain sterile tube using a needle facilitating transport to the laboratory. Source: Used with permission of Amanda Waln, RVT, The Ohio State University College of Veterinary Medicine.

urinary bladder can occur if excessive pressure is applied, and rupture of a diseased bladder may occur more readily. Expression of urine samples should not be attempted when urethral obstruction exists, severe bladder tissue devitalization has occurred, major bladder trauma has been sustained, or if recent cystotomy has been performed. Expression of urine from animals under anesthesia is acceptable since urethral resistance is usually far lower than that encountered in awake animals.

COLLECTION OF POST-VOIDING URINE SAMPLES

Urine that is collected from surfaces after the animal has spontaneously voided is referred to as a post-voided urine specimen. Urine samples collected from the cage floor, metabolism cages, hallways, litter pans, and examination tables are the least desirable samples for urinalysis, but some animals with pollakiuria may not accumulate sufficient urine in their bladders to allow collection by other methods. The analysis of post-voided samples still may be useful if environmental contamination (e.g. hair, fibers, chemicals, bacteria, particulate debris) is taken into consideration. It is important to clearly mark the laboratory requisition form as post-voided urine collected off the exam table, floor, cage papers or pads, or from a litter box.

Urine is occasionally collected from animals on the surgery table at various times before, during, and after the procedure (post-void sample or manual expression). Extremely high USG has been observed in some of these samples that is likely from contamination of the urine sample with surgical scrub (personal communication Heather Wamsley 2020).

Voiding shortly after failed attempts to collect urine by cystocentesis or manual expression sometimes occurs [1]. Consequently, it is best to perform these procedures in a place that has clean dry nonabsorbent surfaces, such as a metal examination table, that readily allows collection of post-voided urine. Collection of post-voided urine samples from soaked cage pads is not recommended. Collection from the surface of cage papers may be acceptable if urine has not yet soaked in. Syringes with or without needles can be used to aspirate urine from these surfaces [12], preferably from the top of the urine bubble if present. Alternatively, a pipette, eyedropper, or vacuum tube can be used to aspirate the sample. Consolidation methods to retrieve very small volumes of urine from surfaces have been described. A glass microscope slide that it tilted can be advanced over the urine layer to lift a volume of urine that can then be aspirated [12]. In a variation of this method, two glass microscope slides are moved toward each other using a V-shaped angle over the surface with the voided urine. This allows very small volumes of urine to be scraped or scooped into a narrow space, rather than being spread out. This provides more volume in a small space allowing urine to be aspirated by needle between the slides [1, 13].

House cats accustomed to using a litter pan may void in the pan even after the litter has been removed and the box cleaned. Soap and bleach should be thoroughly rinsed from the litter pan after cleaning to avoid artifacts in the chemical analysis of urine using chemical dipstrips. Placing plastic cellophane wrap loosely over the litter is another technique that occasionally is helpful. The use of a nonabsorbable cat litter (Nosorb®) allows voided urine specimens from cats to be aspirated or poured into a container (Figure 3.8a,b). Other nonabsorbable materials such as aquarium gravel or plastic packing materials may also be used. Aquarium gravel made of limestone may not be ideal since it consists of calcium carbonate, which can raise the pH of urine collected in this manner.

A commercial form of hydrophobic sand used as cat litter is also available (Kit4Cat®; Coastline Global) to collect spontaneously voided urine from cats. Urine accumulates in droplets either on top of the sand or under the sand after the cat has covered voided urine with this litter. Urine is aspirated from droplets on the surface of the sand or from droplets that appear after moving the sand aside, until a suitable volume for urinalysis has been acquired (Figure 3.9a,b). Urinalysis results were similar in samples collected by cystocentesis or from hydrophobic sand in a small number of cats [14].

(a)

(b)

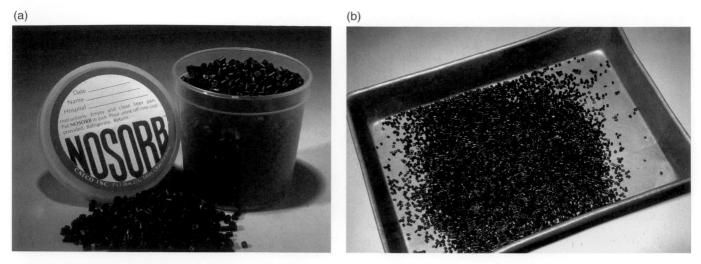

FIGURE 3.8 (a, b) Plastic beads used as nonresorbable litter. It is important to ensure that the litter pan is clean and free of disinfectants and soaps before the litter is placed in the pan. Urine can be easily poured out of the pan into the original plastic container.

(a)

(b)

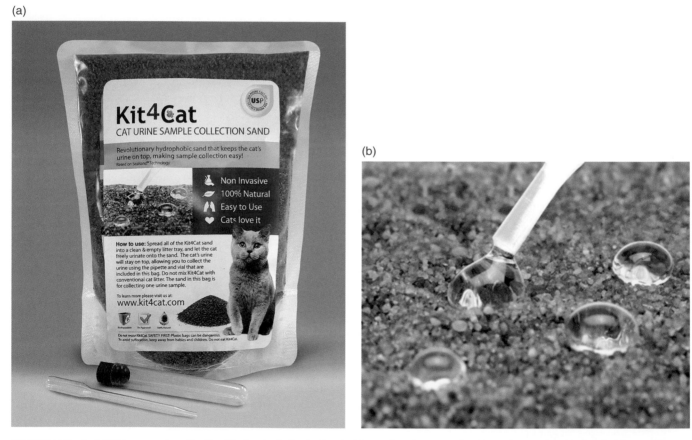

FIGURE 3.9 (a, b) Urine sample collection kit that includes hydrophobic sand, a pipette, and vial to submit urine. Hydrophobic sand litter allows voided urine to form spheres on top that can be aspirated with the pipette. Also, urine under the litter can be collected after parting the sand over the urine to reveal the spheres. Source: Used with permission of Alon Rosenberg, Kit4Cat®, Coastline Global Inc, West Chester PA

There was good agreement between the UPC determined in cats from urine samples collected from a proprietary nonabsorbent hydrophobic sand litter after 24 hours in a covered petri dish compared to UPC at baseline in samples collected by cystocentesis. UPC measured using this litter was considered acceptable for IRIS substaging [15].

Comparable results for urine chemistry were found between the use of hydrophobic sand and metabolic cages in rats, though evaporation over time reduced the total urine volume that was able to be collected [16, 17]. "Dust" from hydrophobic sand residue is identified by its characteristic appearance during urine microscopy and is readily distinguished from urinary crystals (see Chapter 6). Bags of unopened hydrophobic sand are sterile, but bacteria could be introduced into the litter and urine sample by cats as they walk around and cover their excrement. It appears that cats often willingly accept hydrophobic sand as cat litter.

Litter box systems utilizing nonabsorbent cat litters are available. These systems allow drainage of urine into a collection device or pad below the litter. One such system uses litter consisting of mineral-based pellets with liquid repellant coating (Purina Tidy Cats Breeze`, Figure 3.10), which results in minimal absorption or adsorption to the pellets. Voided urine can be collected in these litter boxes when the refillable adsorbent pads are not placed in the container below the nonabsorbent litter. This allows owners to submit voided urine specimens collected from their cats at home or by veterinary personnel in hospitalized cats using a convenient system. Studies comparing the effects of pre- and post-litter pellet exposure on urinalysis results have yet to be published for this proprietary system, but preliminary experience suggests minimal difference.

A recent study compared results of urinalysis from urine retrieved from cats by cystocentesis to that from the residual urine sample added to a nonabsorbent litter and then retrieved from the tray. Most dipstrip results and urine protein-to-creatinine ratio were comparable for up to 12 hours in this litter system. Ketone measurement was unreliable at all time points, and clinically relevant discordance in USG results was seen by three hours [18]. Urine

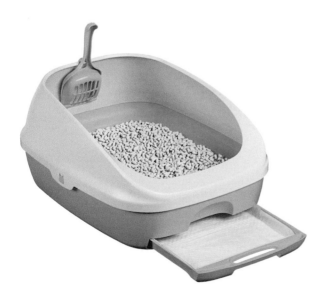

FIGURE 3.10 Urine collection litter box system (Purina Tidy Cats Breeze). Voided urine from the cat drains through nonabsorbent pellets into a drain space below. When an absorbent pad is not placed in the pan, freshly voided urine can be collected from this tray.

was collected from 6 cats using a proprietary nonabsorbent plastic granule litter and compared to urine that did not enter this litter. Urinary phosphate increased by a mean of 7.65 mmol/L after sitting in this litter for 2 hours. Urine samples collected by this method were considered suitable for determination of urinary phosphate as an alternative to collecting urine by urinary catheterization [19]. In another study, cat urine was collected from a proprietary plastic nonabsorbent spherical pellet litter after one hour at room temperature. UPC did not differ in this urine when compared to fresh urine collected by cystocentesis [20]. We recommend that urine be harvested from nonabsorbent or hydrophobic sand litter within three hours after voiding to minimize the effects of evaporation on the urine sample.

URINE COLLECTED BY URINARY CATHETERIZATION

We do not recommend that urine samples be collected by urethral catheterization for routine urinalysis. Urethral catheterization is associated with trauma to the urinary tract and an increased risk of iatrogenic bacterial UTI. Catheterization should not be used for routine urine collection from male cats due to increased risk to acquire a urethral obstruction. This method should not be used if the urethra or urinary bladder is friable. Urethral catheterization is acceptable for urine culture in male dogs and both male and female cats when quantitative culture guidelines for diagnosis of UTI using cfu/mL are used. Urethral catheterization for urine culture is not acceptable in female dogs because of considerable bacterial contamination from the vestibule and distal urethra. If the urinary bladder is too small for cystocentesis, then urethral catheterization can be considered when collection of urine is immediately necessary. Urethral catheterization is an acceptable method of urine collection in severely ill animals both as a single procedure or through an indwelling urethral catheter. A fee separate from the urinalysis is warranted to cover the cost of materials needed for this method of urine collection. A step-by-step approach to urethral catheterization in dogs has been reviewed [21].

The first few milliliters of urine collected during urethral catheterization should be discarded since this portion is more likely to be contaminated with bacteria or cells that entered the catheter during initial insertion [10]. Urine collected through a urinary catheter may display quite different urinalysis findings depending on whether the sample is collected from the initial urine aspirated, midway through bladder emptying, or as the bladder is nearly empty, mostly due to effects of settling of cells and crystals. (Figure 3.11). Palpation and agitation of the bladder prior to collection of a catheterized urine sample may yield a more representative sample of a disease process in these instances as elements are resuspended.

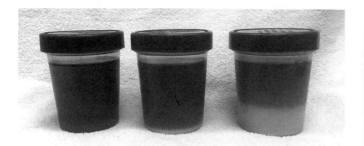

FIGURE 3.11 Three equine urine samples collected by a urethral catheter. From left to right, an initial sample, a middle sample, and an end sample are shown as the bladder was emptied. This illustrates how different the urinalysis results could be if settling of urinary elements has occurred. In this instance, the settling in the dependent bladder was accounted for by numerous calcium oxalate crystals. Source: Courtesy of Dr. Harold Schott, Michigan State University.

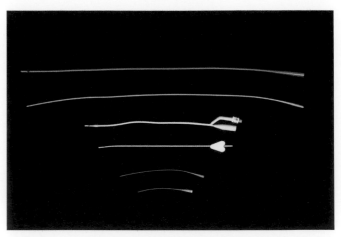

FIGURE 3.12 Various sizes (width and length) and chemical composition of urinary catheters are available for use in male and female dogs and cats. From top to bottom: red rubber, polypropylene, Foley, metal bitch catheter, and Tom-Cat catheters of two sizes (polyurethane, silicone, or polypropylene).

Urine specimens collected by careful catheterization of the urinary bladder bypass much of the contamination from the distal urogenital tract, but urethral trauma and contamination may still occur. Urethral catheterization may increase the number of RBC, transitional epithelial cells, squamous cells [1] and protein to the urine sample because of trauma. The amount of difficulty encountered during catheterization should be considered when evaluating the presence of cellular elements in the urine sediment. Bladder or urethral epithelium may be inadvertently dislodged by advancement of the catheter or aspirated by suction on the catheter. In these instances, clumps of transitional epithelial cells may be identified during urine microscopy. When urine samples are obtained from patients with indwelling catheters, catheter-induced elements are more likely (urothelial cells, RBC, WBC) to be identified during urine microscopy.

CATHETER TYPES

We encourage the use of single-use disposable urethral catheters instead of urinary catheters that undergo cold sterilization prior to reuse, since chemicals from the reused catheter can enter the urine sample and influence urine chemistry dip-strip reactions [1]. Gas sterilization of reused urinary catheters is an acceptable alternative. Aseptic technique should be used for urethral catheterization, and all equipment should be sterilized. For specula, cold sterilization is acceptable; sterile, aqueous lubricant should be used; individual sterile packets of lubricating jelly are preferred over a large multiple-use tube to limit the possibility of bacterial contamination.

Flexible-to-semiflexible urinary catheters are available that vary in their chemical composition that includes polypropylene, polyvinyl, red rubber, silicone, and medical grade silastic (Figure 3.12). A rigid metal catheter (the bitch catheter) with a bent end is available in varying lengths for use in female dogs that can facilitate catheterization in some instances. This type of catheter may also be used in female cats. Softer catheters are chosen for indwelling purposes. The diameter of the catheter is generally from 3.5 French (Fr) to 12 Fr for use in dogs, depending upon the size of the dog and specific anatomy (Note: one French unit equals 1/3 mm). Side-hole and end-hole rigid plastic catheters are available for use in male cats at 3.5 or 5.0 Fr diameter in most instances. The same diameter catheters are often used for catheterization of female cats using longer and softer polyvinyl catheters. The appropriate length of catheter is chosen after estimating the length from the external urethral orifice to the approximate area of neck of the bladder by laying the catheter over the anatomy on the animal's body. A metal or hard-plastic stylet inserted into the lumen of soft urethral catheters is often needed in order to provide stability that then allows insertion and advancement of the catheter within the urethra. The same types of urethral catheters used for male dogs can be used in female dogs.

SPECULA TYPES

To facilitate the passage of a urethral catheter in females, the use of a sterile speculum is recommended that allows direct visualization of the external urethral orifice. A variety of types and sizes of specula exist; the best have self-retaining light systems. Anoscopes designed for humans adapt well for use in most female dogs and are available in small, medium, and large sizes (Figures 3.13a,b). The obturator of the anoscope facilitates entry through the vulva into the vestibule while also preventing contamination of the lumen of the anoscope. The tip of the anoscope is positioned just caudal to or over the urethral orifice after the obturator has been removed. Sterile otoscopic heads can also be used for this purpose. Vaginal specula in a variety of sizes can also be used, but a light source is additionally needed.

(a)

(b)

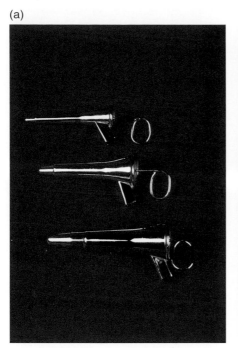

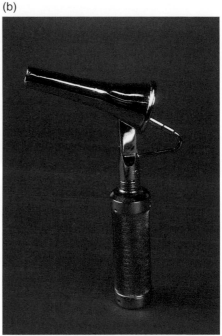

FIGURE 3.13 (a) Three different sizes of human anoscope heads that fit into the vestibule of most female dogs. The smallest head also can fit into larger female cats. Notice that the obturator is in place to facilitate advancement of the device through the vulva. The obturator is then removed and the position of the tip of the scope confirmed to be near the external urethral orifice. (b) Anoscope head attached to self-retaining light source and battery pack. The obturator has been removed allowing the operator to easily view the vestibule and position of the external urethral orifice.

The smallest size of anoscope head performs well for the placement of a urethral catheter in larger female cats. A small sterile otoscope also can work well for direct visualization of the external urethral orifice in both large and small female cats. A blind technique can be used after inserting the otoscope speculum into the vestibule and then allowing the urinary catheter to follow the ventral floor of the vestibule and possibly enter the urethral orifice.

CHEMICAL RESTRAINT

Chemical restraint or anesthesia is needed for atraumatic urethral catheterization in cats. Animals that have urethral obstruction will require heavier sedation or general anesthesia for urethral catheterization. Full anesthesia in dogs is not usually necessary, but catheterization is greatly facilitated by some degree of sedation. There are numerous protocols of sedation or anesthesia using varying combinations of butorphanol, acepromazine, medetomidine, oxymorphone, propofol, ketamine, diazepam, and midazolam that can be chosen based on the clinician's knowledge and level of comfort with these agents.

PREPARATION AND POSITIONING

Male Dogs

To prepare for catheterization, keep the hair away from the tip of the penis (hair may need to be clipped) and cleanse the

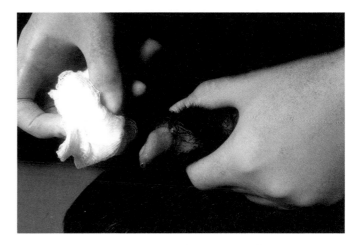

FIGURE 3.14 Prolapsed penis in dog. The gloved operator has prolapsed the penis, which is then cleansed with a disinfectant wipe prior to the passage of a urethral catheter to collect urine.

external genitalia with a gentle disinfectant (benzalkonium chloride). Gently cleanse exudate from the tip of the penis and external urethral orifice by flushing with sterile saline if needed. Gently wash the prolapsed penis with mild disinfectant and rinse with sterile saline (Figure 3.14).

We prefer to catheterize male dogs positioned in lateral recumbency, though the standing position can also be used [10]. The penis is prolapsed by an assistant, and then, the external urethral orifice is cleansed and rinsed as described above.

Female Dogs

For females, clip the hair surrounding the vulva and cleanse the external genitalia with benzalkonium chloride. We prefer to catheterize female dogs in sternal recumbency, though the standing position can be used [10]. Lateral or dorsal recumbency changes the effect of gravity on the anatomy that may facilitate passage in some circumstances. Clipping or combing long hair out of the way may be needed beforehand. Follow with cleansing as outlined under preparation above. Speculum techniques, especially those that are closed such as the anoscope, allow placement of the catheter directly on the external urethral orifice, minimizing vaginal or vestibular contamination. The urinary catheter is then advanced under direct visualization into the external urethral orifice and further along the lumen of the urethra until urine is obtained as the bladder is entered. Stylets are usually necessary in order to advance Foley catheters and most catheters of small caliber.

Cats

The area surrounding the penis or vulva is prepped as above for dogs. For catheterization of male cats, the patient is placed in lateral recumbency or in dorsal recumbency with legs pulled back, depending on personal preference. It is important to fully extend the penis caudally so as to straighten out the natural bend in the urethra (Figure 3.15) [10].

After sedation or anesthesia, female cats are often placed in ventral recumbency with the legs hanging over the edge of the table, and the tail pulled dorsally. Some operators prefer dorsal recumbency.

CATHETERIZATION

Prior to catheterization, all materials needed should be assembled. To handle the catheter in both dogs and cats, the packaging surrounding the sterile catheter can be clipped to create a

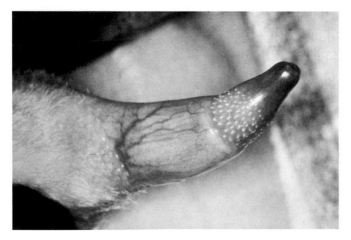

FIGURE 3.15   Penis of intact male cat (note barbs on penis). The penis has been prolapsed out of the prepuce and extended caudally. This positioning allows a urethral catheter to more easily be advanced.

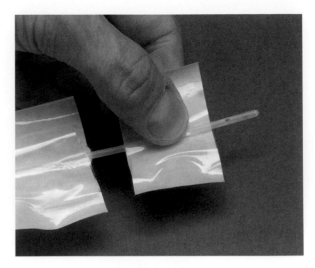

FIGURE 3.16   Cut sterile bag technique for male dog urethral catheterization. A sterile bag containing the urethral catheter can be cut to allow sterility to be maintained as the catheter is advanced without need for sterile towels and gloves.

sterile "handle" so that the catheter can be passed without touching the sterile catheter (Figure 3.16). Alternatively, the catheter wrap can be used as a handle to advance the urinary catheter as the catheter emerges from the sterile bag. This method minimizes exposure of the sterile catheter to air and environmental contamination, since it remains in the bag until the catheter is passed. Alternatively, sterile gloves can be used to remove the catheter from the packaging, and the catheter can be placed on a sterile towel. Liberally lubricate the end of the catheter with sterile lubricating jelly and insert the urinary catheter through the external urethral orifice. Force on the urinary catheter should stay parallel to the abdominal wall to facilitate catheter passage. It is essential to use feather-touch technique to minimize undue trauma to the urinary tract. Never force advancement of the urinary catheter since rupture of the urethra or bladder and traumatic urethritis can be consequences of poor technique. Detailed protocols for placement and maintenance of indwelling urethral catheters in critical care dogs have been developed that minimize the development of UTI [22, 23].

Male Dogs

In male dogs, resistance to advancement of the urethral catheter may be encountered at the junction of the turn from the penile to the perineal urethra behind the os penis, and also at the level of the ischial arch as it becomes the pelvic urethra (Figure 3.17). If resistance is excessive, external perineal palpation is used to redirect the catheter tip at the perineal point, or rectal palpation is used if at the ischial arch point. This kind of obstruction occurs mostly with rigid polypropylene catheters. More flexible catheters often require a stylet to provide needed rigidity to allow passage. The catheter is usually passed just to the first level of urine drainage, so as to not traumatize

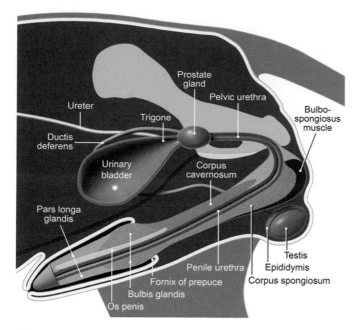

FIGURE 3.17   Lower urinary tract anatomy – intact male dog. Source: Illustration by Tim Vojt, reproduced with permission of The Ohio State University.

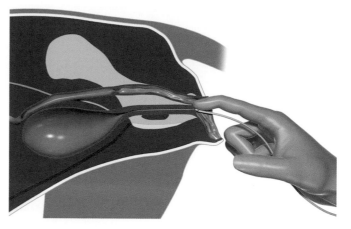

FIGURE 3.18   Blind placement of urinary catheter in female dog. Placing the tip of the finger just cranial to the urethral opening helps guide the urinary catheter into the external urethral orifice. Source: Illustration by Tim Vojt, reproduced with permission of The Ohio State University.

the bladder. In cases of obstruction, the catheter may be advanced further to allow better drainage of urine from the overdistended bladder.

Female Dogs

We do not recommend blind urethral catheterization techniques in female dogs unless direct visualization techniques have failed, as this technique increases the chances to inoculate the urethra and bladder with bacteria, especially from the vestibule. Blind techniques entail placement of a sterile gloved finger cranial to the urethral orifice and then sliding the urinary catheter along the floor of the vestibule into the external urethral orifice (Figure 3.18). The external urethral meatus is located on the ventral midline in the vestibule just before the opening into the vagina (Figure 3.19). The protrusion of the urethral meatus can sometimes be palpated during digital palpation within the vestibule. If the meatus cannot be palpated, the digit is inserted as far craniad as possible to obstruct entry into the vagina. Experienced personnel using this technique often perform atraumatic urethral catheterization, but contamination from perivulvar hair, vulva, the vestibule, and the vagina is greater than with speculum techniques that limit this type of contamination.

A technique has been described to facilitate urethral catheterization of neonatal and adult female dogs. A Foley catheter is first advanced through the vestibule into the vagina, and then, the balloon is inflated. The urethral catheter is fed along the ventral wall of the vestibule until it enters the urethral orifice. Since the inflated balloon is in the vagina, there

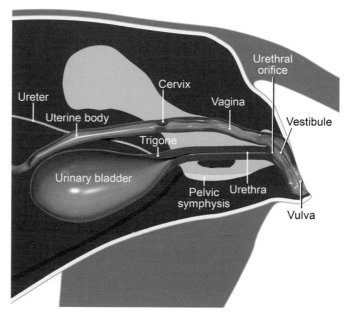

FIGURE 3.19   Lower urinary tract anatomy – female dog. Source: Illustration by Tim Vojt, reproduced with permission of The Ohio State University.

is only one orifice remaining for the catheter to advance. During the use of a vaginal speculum with light, the urethral orifice can be more readily seen when the inflated Foley catheter is gently pulled caudally [24].

A cystoscope can be used to visualize the anatomy of the vestibule, external urethral meatus, and vagina when other methods of catheter placement have failed, and it is considered imperative to place an indwelling urinary catheter (Figure 3.20). This allows the catheter to be directed under visualization into the urethral meatus and confirmation of the catheter advancement.

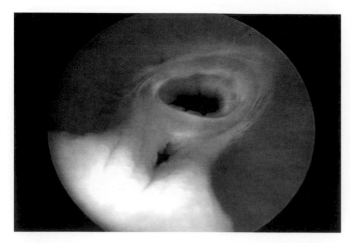

FIGURE 3.20 Cystoscopic view of the vestibule, urethral meatus, and vagina of the female dog. The cingulum is the junction of the vestibule with the vagina (larger opening at the top). The urethral opening is the slit like opening at the bottom of this image.

Male Cats

Collection of catheterized urine samples from male cats is generally avoided for routine purposes, since this trauma may predispose to urethral obstruction. Catheters placed as a therapeutic procedure to reestablish urethral patency for cats under anesthesia are justifiable for urine collection at the time of the procedure, but these urine samples are often altered by flush solution. If the penis is not fully extended caudally so as to straighten out the natural bend in the urethra, there may be resistance to the passage of the urinary catheter at this point [10] (Figure 3.21) and an erroneous assumption of an obstruction at this location. Stay sutures in the reflection of penis and prepuce (or mosquito hemostats) may facilitate adequate exposure of the penis.

Female Cats

A small sterile otoscopic speculum works well for direct visualization of the external urethral orifice (Figure 3.22), and the catheter is advanced by direct visualization or using the blind technique through the scope as described earlier. The blind technique is facilitated in some cats when performed with the cat in dorsal recumbency.

COMPLICATIONS OF URETHRAL CATHETERIZATION

Complications resulting from urethral catheterization include UTI and trauma. The development of an acquired UTI is a possibility even with the best sterile technique. Introduction of organisms into the urinary tract can occur due to poor aseptic technique during placement of the catheter or may result from the introduction of resident bacteria from the distal urethra, vestibule, vagina, or prepuce. The risk of iatrogenic UTI from a single urethral catheterization is low in male dogs, but was as high as 20% in previously healthy female

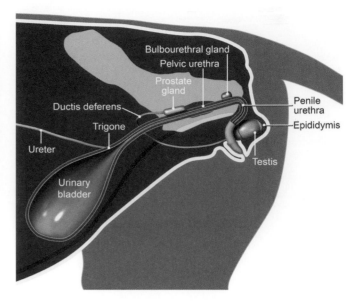

FIGURE 3.21 Lower urinary tract anatomy of the intact male cat. Source: Illustration by Tim Vojt, reproduced with permission of The Ohio State University.

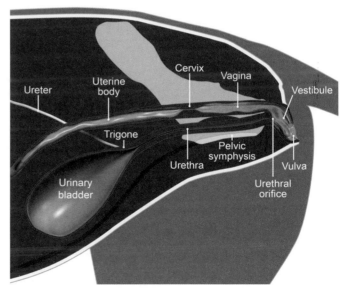

FIGURE 3.22 Lower urinary tract anatomy of the female cat. Source: Illustration by Tim Vojt, reproduced with permission of The Ohio State University.

dogs [25]. Immunosuppressed animals and those with abnormal urinary tract anatomy or function may be at greater risk to develop UTI following catheterization [10]. We recommend that urine collected by cystocentesis be examined one to two weeks following urethral catheterization to exclude the presence of an acquired UTI, though this is not recommended by the International Society for Companion Animal Infectious Diseases (ISCAID) if there are no clinical signs at that time. Although it is common in some practices to administer prophylactic antibiotics for three to five days following a single urethral catheterization, there is no published evidence that this is effective in prevention of post catheter acquired UTI and is not recommended by ISCAID [26].

TRAUMATIC URINARY CATHETERIZATION

Sometimes, it is desirable to use a traumatic urinary catheterization technique to obtain diagnostic tissue for histopathology or cells for cytology from masses within the urethra or the bladder. Either soft red rubber or semirigid plastic urinary catheters can be used for this purpose. Extra caution must be used when using semirigid urinary catheters as it is easier to damage and possibly perforate the urethra with this type of catheter. During this procedure, the urinary catheter side holes are directed next to the suspected lesion, and then, suction is provided from an attached syringe to create a vacuum against the mass. The goal of the vacuum is to aspirate tissue into the lumen of the catheter that is then collected as the catheter is moved quickly back and forth about 1–2 inches. A sharp pull on the catheter while the vacuum is maintained is another variation on this technique that can successfully shear tissue into the catheter. If aspiration on the syringe easily retrieves urine, the side holes of the catheter are not aligned with the mass, and the catheter should be rotated until a vacuum can be established [27, 28]. This technique is easily performed on masses within the urethra. Rectal palpation (males and female dogs) or perineal palpation (male dogs) can be used to further ensure that the urethral catheter is passed into the region of the urethral mass. It is more difficult to accurately direct the catheter tip to the lesion in the bladder using only bladder palpation unless the mass is large. Ultrasound guidance increases the chance that the tip of the urinary catheter will be placed accurately against the mass in the bladder. When the bladder is large, some fluid may need to be drained to allow proper catheter placement against the mass. Fluid may need to be infused into the bladder to improve ultrasonographic visualization of the mass when the bladder is inadequately distended. It is also possible to bring the bladder lesion to the catheter tip using external palpation documented during real-time ultrasonography when it is otherwise difficult to direct the catheter tip to the mass [28]. An adequate volume of sheared tissue for histopathology is usually obtained during this procedure, especially when the lesion is from TCC (UCC) that is often friable and easily aspirated into the catheter lumen. Cytologic evaluation often provides a tentative diagnosis until the tissue biopsy report provides the definitive diagnosis.

URINE COLLECTED BY CYSTOCENTESIS

Antepubic cystocentesis (vesicopuncture) refers to needle puncture and aspiration of urine from the bladder to acquire a urine sample. The value of cystocentesis for diagnosis and treatment has been recognized for over 100 years [29] and has been safely performed as a routine procedure in veterinary medicine for over four decades. The procedure is relatively simple to perform, does not require specialized equipment, usually provides samples of superior diagnostic value due to less contamination, poses no risk for acquiring an iatrogenic UTI, and is well tolerated by most dogs and cats with minimal restraint [30, 31]. Cystocentesis can be performed during bladder palpation and immobilization, using blind technique (dogs only), or with ultrasonographic guidance.

Urine samples collected by cystocentesis usually are the most diagnostically useful since they are not subject to contamination from the distal urogenital tract, skin, or perineal hair. Elements arising from the proximal urethra and prostate gland still may be found in specimens collected by cystocentesis due to retrograde movement into urine. In general, collection of urine by cystocentesis results in the lowest numbers of cellular elements (e.g. RBC and WBC) in the sediment of urine from normal animals [10, 30].

In cases of bladder inflammation, cystocentesis may be considered a provocative procedure that exposes the underlying inflammatory process as RBC are more readily introduced into the sample instead of occurring as an artifact as would occur from a normal bladder. Cystocentesis is considered the best method for the collection of urine to submit for bacterial culture.

Prevention of voiding before attempting cystocentesis is helpful to ensure sufficient bladder urine volume for the procedure to be successful. Carrying small dogs into the hospital and exam room and keeping cats in their carrying case or a hospital cage without a litter pan will decrease opportunities for voiding. Some patients have great urgency and increased frequency of voiding that makes it difficult for the bladder to contain enough urine to collect via cystocentesis. Administration of drugs to provide analgesia and tranquilization (e.g. buprenorphine and acepromazine or midazolam) one to two hours before cystocentesis can be successful in alleviating urgency to urinate and allow an adequate volume of urine to accumulate in the bladder [32].

Reluctance to perform cystocentesis in animals that have a distended bladder from urethral obstruction is pervasive despite decades of experience demonstrating the safety of this procedure. In this setting, it is important to perform decompressive (therapeutic) cystocentesis that removes as much of the bladder urine volume as possible. Less complete urine evacuation from the bladder (diagnostic cystocentesis) can result in leakage of urine along the cystocentesis path into the abdomen if the intravesical pressure remains high. More complete evacuation of bladder urine is facilitated when the cystocentesis needle is attached to an extension tube, three-way stopcock, and large syringe. Urinalysis results in these instances are unaltered by flush solution that otherwise is added to urine during advancement of urethral catheters. As an additional benefit, decompressive cystocentesis facilitates the passage of urethral catheters into the bladder with less resistance and less danger for bladder rupture during infusion of fluid into the urethra under high pressure. No rupture of the bladder occurred in 47 male cats with urethral obstruction initially managed by cystocentesis followed by the placement of an indwelling urinary catheter [33]. There is concern that cystocentesis will lead to urine leakage into the abdomen, but this is not likely when bladder pressure remains low after placement of an indwelling urethral catheter. Abdominal effusion has commonly been detected in male cats with urethral obstruction before cystocentesis was performed [33–36]. Abdominal ultrasonography revealed as many as 60% of cats with abdominal effusion before cystocentesis in one study [34]. Abdominal radiography is less sensitive for detection of abdominal effusion in this population. In another study, one-third of male cats with urethral obstruction had abdominal effusion identified by ultrasonography at initial presentation that was considered scant in most and mild in a few cats. An additional 15% of cats in this same study developed scant abdominal effusion 15 minutes following cystocentesis. No clinically relevant complications secondary to cystocentesis were identified [36].

A small volume of urine leakage into the abdomen following cystocentesis is not likely to be problematic in cats since urine at the time of initial urethral obstruction is almost always sterile [37]. Male cats with urethral obstruction that underwent initial decompressive cystocentesis followed by urethral catheterization were compared to those that only underwent urethral catheterization in a prospective and randomized study. Similar to other studies, those cats undergoing decompressive cystocentesis did not have an increased risk for abdominal effusion or development of uroabdomen. Decompressive cystocentesis did not have a significant effect on the time or ease of catheterization compared to the urethral catheterization only group, nor was there an observed benefit on biochemical parameters and clinical outcome [38].

PREPARATION OF THE CYSTOCENTESIS SITE

Full surgical preparation of the skin at the site of cystocentesis is not necessary [13]. Soap and water should be used to first cleanse the site if it is soiled, and obvious areas of dermatitis and pyoderma should be avoided. Clipping of hair and disinfection of the skin with solutions of benzalkonium chloride or alcohol at the puncture site prior to cystocentesis is advocated by some [10, 13, 32, 39], but many practices do not routinely employ skin preparation prior to cystocentesis. We do not recommend clipping hair and disinfecting the skin prior to routine cystocentesis. If disinfectant is used, we recommend waiting for the skin to dry before cystocentesis is performed. Omission of skin preparation increases the efficiency of cystocentesis and removes potential owner concerns regarding the cosmetic appearance of altered hair and skin.

There is concern that a small amount of disinfectant may contaminate the urine specimen potentially inhibiting bacterial growth in samples submitted for bacterial urine culture. Disinfectant contamination also has the potential to alter chemical reactions on dipstrip analysis. There is little data comparing the effects of skin preparation on urine culture, urinalysis results, or the possibility for acquiring a bacterial UTI from the procedure. The effect of clipping hair and disinfection of skin at the puncture site for cystocentesis was studied in cats from an animal shelter immediately following euthanasia. Each cat had cystocentesis performed first using lateral bladder puncture after clipping hair and disinfecting the skin at the puncture site with chlorhexidine and alcohol. Cystocentesis was then performed using lateral bladder puncture on the other side without any clipping or disinfecting. No difference in urinalysis or quantitative urine culture results was detected between the two methods of preparation for urine collection [40]. Based on this study, it is unlikely that there would be a large enough degree of bacterial contamination that would clinically increase bacterial growth or alter chemical reagent pad reactions using a cystocentesis sample collected with no clipping of hair and skin disinfection. The impact on the health of the animal or bladder status following cystocentesis performed without skin preparation has not been specifically investigated. Samples collected by cystocentesis pose less risk of acquiring a UTI and are better tolerated by the patient as compared to samples collected by catheterization in most instances [13].

BLADDER PALPATION AND IMMOBILIZATION FOR CYSTOCENTESIS

Routine cystocentesis (manual palpation with bladder immobilization) is easier to perform, and trauma is less likely if the urinary bladder is readily palpable. Aggressive or unmanageable animals should be sedated if necessary, but this is not commonly needed for this procedure alone. The position of the animal during cystocentesis is chosen so that the bladder can be immobilized prior to puncture. The chosen position depends on patient size, degree of animal cooperation, and operator preference. Large dogs are often more easily sampled from a lateral approach while standing on all four limbs, or occasionally while an assistant raises the forelimbs forcing the dog to stand on its rear limbs. Smaller dogs may be sampled while in lateral or dorsal recumbency. The relatively hairless ventral midline is targeted for puncture when the patient is in dorsal recumbency. For male dogs in dorsal recumbency, the puncture is made on the midline after pushing the penis and prepuce to the side. Alternatively in male dogs, the puncture can be made 2–4 cm lateral to the sheath and posterior to the umbilicus [10]. Cystocentesis is performed on cats either in dorsal (Figure 3.23) or lateral recumbency. For cats, a single assistant is usually able to adequately restrain and stretch the cat in lateral recumbency so that the abdomen becomes thinner and the bladder more easily palpated. Compressing the bladder from the opposite side of the abdomen from the operator when the animal is standing or in lateral position often facilitates its identification on palpation when the bladder is pushed toward the operator (Figure 3.24).

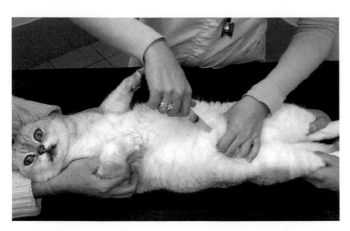

FIGURE 3.23 Cystocentesis in the cat. In this example, the cat is restrained in dorsal recumbency and the bladder is palpated and immobilized during aspiration of urine. Notice the optimal 45° angle of needle penetration that is aiming toward the pelvic inlet. Notice also that hair has not been clipped or wet with disinfectant. Source: Paepe, D., et al. (2013). "Routine health screening: findings in apparently healthy middle-aged and old cats." J Feline Med Surg 15(1): 8-19.

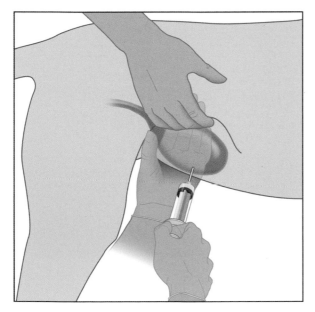

FIGURE 3.24 Cystocentesis in a large standing dog. The operator stabilizes the bladder just cranial to the hind limb with the left hand while an assistant elevates the skin of the flank dorsally and caudally. With the right hand, the operator punctures the near lateral wall of the bladder. Source: Illustration by Tim Vojt, reproduced with permission of The Ohio State University.

CYSTOCENTESIS TECHNIQUE

We have observed dramatic differences in urinalysis results from urine samples collected before and after agitating the bladder in some cases. Consequently, we recommend agitation of the bladder immediately prior to bladder puncture to

increase chances that settled sediment will now be available for microscopic evaluation following its suspension in urine. Alternatively, consider elevating the rear legs to a wheel barrow position to accomplish dispersal of sediment throughout the urine to be sampled [13]. Urine settling of elements and crystals is most likely to occur in dogs in which urine is collected via cystocentesis while standing (lateral bladder wall is penetrated) and in cats in dorsal recumbency (ventral bladder wall is penetrated). When ultrasonography demonstrates gravity-dependent mobile sediment, agitation of the bladder should be performed just prior to the ultrasound-guided cystocentesis as settling can occur quickly. Alternatively, just after the needle enters the bladder, the syringe can be aspirated and flushed back into the bladder to resuspend elements that have settled in order to acquire a more representative urine sample.

To perform cystocentesis, the bladder's position is first stabilized by palpation. Then, either the ventral or lateral regions of the bladder are targeted for needle entry depending on body position, though the ventral midline of the bladder is relatively less vascular. A 22 or 23 gauge, 1–1.5-inch hypodermic needle is usually selected for cystocentesis in adult dogs and cats of average body condition [10]. To lessen the chance for accidental entry of the needle into viscera, we recommend the use of shorter needle lengths in conjunction with palpation that compresses the distance between the abdominal wall and bladder, rather than using longer needles. Longer hypodermic needles or spinal needles may be needed for cystocentesis in very large or obese dogs. Needles as small as 26–29 gauge are appropriate for use in neonates. Needles are usually attached to a 3–6-mL syringe for urine aspiration. No local anesthetic agent is required prior to puncture since this procedure using small gauge needles does not appear to be painful.

A "dart-like" one-hand technique allows the collection of urine without the need to change hands or finger position on the syringe following bladder puncture. Two fingers are arranged to steady the barrel end as the needle advances for bladder puncture. The barrel end then provides a platform for the third finger to pull the plunger back [32]. This method of cystocentesis is likely to create less iatrogenic hematuria as needle movement is minimized during insertion and aspiration of urine.

Ideally, the needle should be introduced through the skin, abdominal musculature, bladder wall, and into the bladder lumen at an oblique angle of about 45° (Figure 3.25). This angle allows the needle tract to seal as the needle is removed and the muscle of the bladder wall collapses over the tract. Additionally, the needle tract lumen is forced closed as pressure increases during bladder filling providing another mechanism that can reduce urine leakage following this procedure [13]. Even though we advocate trying to achieve this angle, we have not identified urine leakage as a problem following cystocentesis technique in which the oblique angle was not achieved. The needle should be directed toward the

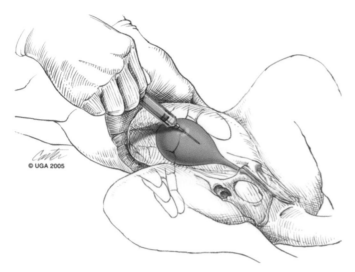

FIGURE 3.25   Cystocentesis with animal in dorsal recumbency. The palpating hand is positioned to hold the bladder back against the pelvic brim. Note that the needle entry through the bladder is angled and pointed toward the pelvic inlet. Source: Used with permission of Elsevier, from Infectious diseases of the Dog and Cat 3rd edition 2006, Craig Green Editor, Figure 91-1, page 941.

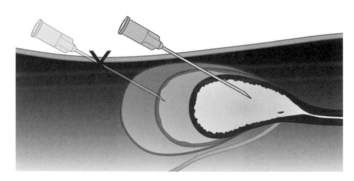

FIGURE 3.26   Cystocentesis showing optimal placement of the puncture needle; animal is in dorsal recumbency. The needle is shown penetrating at a 45° angle away from the apex of the bladder. The bladder can retract substantially as urine is removed when the needle punctures near the apex requiring reinsertion of the needle, shown with an X here. The needle tip should avoid touching the far bladder wall especially near the trigone and ureteral openings as the bladder empties. Source: Illustration by Tim Vojt, reproduced with permission of The Ohio State University.

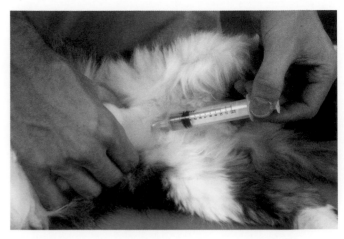

FIGURE 3.27   Cystocentesis in a cat. Notice that the needle is aimed at the apex of the bladder (toward the cat's head) instead of the optimal direction toward the pelvic canal (toward the cat's tail). This increases the chances for the needle tip to traumatize the bladder wall as urine is withdrawn and the bladder contracts in size.

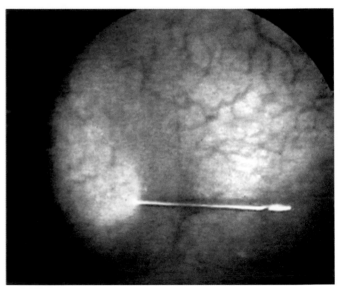

FIGURE 3.28   Cystoscopic view of needle puncture during cystoscopy. Note that the needle has been fully inserted into the bladder lumen, avoiding the potential for aspiration of blood from local trauma at the puncture site. Notice urine layer to the right.

pelvic canal (Figure 3.26) so that the needle tip does not contact and traumatize the mucosa of the bladder as the bladder contracts caudally as urine is removed (Figure 3.27). Gentle suction on the syringe allows the operator to immediately know when the lumen of the bladder has been accessed as urine enters the syringe. It is preferred to aspirate urine into the syringe once the needle tip is seated well within the lumen of the bladder rather than just next to the mucosa, as this minimizes contamination from iatrogenically introduced RBC (Figure 3.28). Excessive suction through the syringe can traumatize the mucosa when bladder volume is small and the mucosa is adjacent to the needle tip resulting in iatrogenic RBC contamination of the urine sample. Suction through the syringe should be stopped before removing the needle from the bladder in order to avoid aspirating elements from muscle, subcutaneous tissue, skin, and contaminants from the environment. To minimize urine leakage around the needle, avoid excessive bladder palpation and the attending increased bladder pressure while the cystocentesis needle is in place.

A new needle and syringe should be used during each attempt at cystocentesis to lessen chances for contamination of the urine sample [41]. Also, a new needle should be placed on the syringe before injecting or squirting urine into a urine culture container to minimize bacterial contamination from the original needle that could have occurred during needle entry or withdrawal [10, 41].

Failure to gain a urine specimen from attempted cystocentesis may be due to inadequate bladder distension from low urine volume, improper bladder immobilization, or the inability to identify the bladder by palpation, often due to obesity of the patient or inexperience of the operator. If the failure to retrieve urine was due to low urine volume in the bladder, another attempt can be made after the animal has been allowed time to make more urine. Alternatively, furosemide at 2 mg/kg given subcutaneously can be given and cystocentesis attempted again after 20–30 minutes when the bladder has partially filled with urine. This technique makes evaluation of urine concentration based on USG impossible, but abnormal elements in urine often can still be identified. Urine culture can still be submitted following administration of furosemide, but one log lower of growth based on cfu/mL can be expected at times.

BLIND CYSTOCENTESIS

When initial efforts to obtain urine using manual palpation and bladder stabilization for cystocentesis have failed, the so-called blind technique can be considered for use in dogs. Blind techniques are not appropriate for use in cats since the cat's bladder is much more mobile than that in the dog, and its anatomical location is much less predictable when the bladder cannot be palpated. To perform a blind cystocentesis, the dog is first placed in dorsal recumbency and the anterior rim of the pubis is identified. The penis and prepuce in male dogs are first deflected to one side in order to expose the midline prior to needle puncture. In one method, the needle is inserted perpendicular to the abdominal wall approximately 1 inch cranial to pubis on the ventral midline. Gentle suction is maintained on the syringe during needle insertion in order to know when the bladder lumen has been penetrated. Another method for blind cystocentesis is to make an X connecting teats 4 and 5 on contralateral sides. At the intersection of these lines on the midline, attempt a needle stick to aspirate urine. If this fails to retrieve urine and the bladder is very small, choose a more caudal insertion site on the midline between both fifth teats (closer to the pubis). If the bladder is very large, choose a more cranial insertion point for the needle on the midline between the fourth teats. If blind techniques for cystocentesis fail to obtain urine from these three locations, further attempts at blind cystocentesis should be abandoned. Cystocentesis can be tried again after enough time has passed to allow the bladder to achieve a larger fill volume. Sometimes, when the bladder cannot be palpated, the bladder can be visualized as a slight bulge along the midline when the abdominal viscera are pushed caudally with one hand in dorsal recumbency. The needle puncture is then aimed into the area that the bulge developed. We estimate that about 60% of attempts using blind cystocentesis successfully obtain urine.

ULTRASOUND GUIDANCE FOR CYSTOCENTESIS

Ultrasound guidance to perform cystocentesis can be considered when manual palpation with bladder immobilization or blind techniques has failed to obtain a urine sample. Ultrasound guidance for cystocentesis is particularly helpful when the bladder cannot be identified by palpation, if the bladder is small, or if the animal is obese. In some private primary care practices, the standard of care is to obtain urine by cystocentesis with ultrasound guidance as the first option to increase patient safety and to ensure an adequate sample size (Figure 3.29a–c) [42]. Ultrasound guidance techniques for cystocentesis offer an opportunity to determine the presence or absence of bladder masses or urolithiasis at the same time of the urine collection. This knowledge allows increased clinical interpretation of urinalysis findings for cases in which more extensive abdominal imaging has not yet been performed. Business professionals recommend charging clients for urine collection by cystocentesis as a separate fee rather than including the fee in the urinalysis cost [42].

CONTRAINDICATIONS/COMPLICATIONS OF CYSTOCENTESIS

Cystocentesis should not be performed if the urinary bladder is known to be severely devitalized, if the bladder has sustained recent major trauma, if a cystotomy has recently been performed, or bladder atony exists. We recommend abandoning any attempt to perform cystocentesis in patients with platelet counts less than 25 000/μL due to the increased chance for local bleeding at the puncture site (Figure 3.30). Cystocentesis should be avoided if the patient is known to have emphysematous cystitis, as this likely increases the chance for urine leakage following the procedure. It is controversial as to whether cystocentesis can be performed safely in animals with known bladder masses (discussed further below). Bladder palpation should be avoided for several hours after cystocentesis to prevent potential leakage of urine into the peritoneal space [13].

It is generally safe to perform cystocentesis as a routine procedure in animals with bacterial UTI when there is no urethral obstruction. In these instances, infected urine does not leak or contaminate the needle track into the peritoneal cavity or soft tissues when proper technique is employed [13]. Septic peritonitis was reported following decompressive cystocentesis in a dog with infected urine and urethral obstruction [43].

Complications from cystocentesis are rare with the most common being transient microscopic or macroscopic

(a)

(b)

(c)

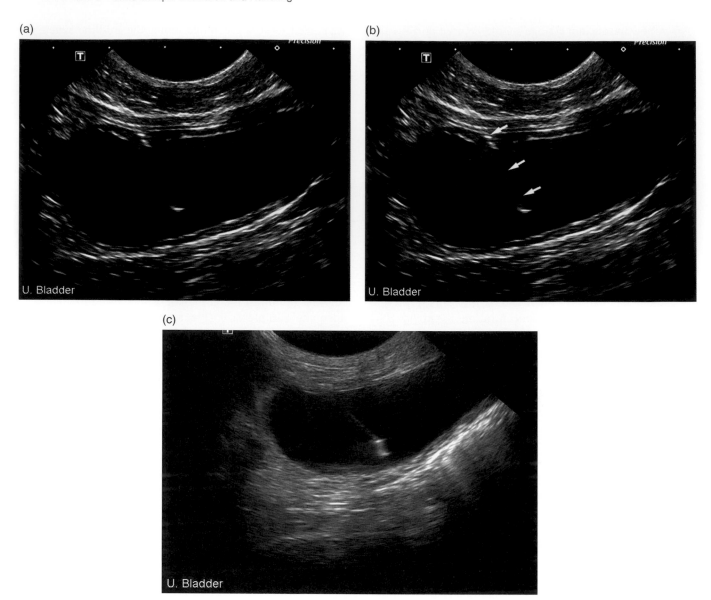

FIGURE 3.29 (a–c) Ultrasound guided cystocentesis. Needle is seen entering through the ventral bladder on the ventral midline. (a, b) are from the same image – arrows align with the needle. (c) Needle is very close to the dorsal bladder wall as bladder distension decreases as urine is aspirated. This could allow trauma of the mucosa and iatrogenic entry of RBC. The needle position should be adjusted away from the bladder wall as urine is removed.

hematuria. Needle tip laceration or excessive syringe suction can cause iatrogenic hematuria, especially if the bladder is minimally distended. Even with good technique, up to 50 red cells per high-power field occasionally may be found as a result of inadvertent trauma from the needle puncture during cystocentesis. It is likely that cystocentesis adds RBC to the urine sample when the bladder is inflamed due to the needle penetration of congested or engorged blood vessels associated with the inflammation [13].

It is controversial as to whether cystocentesis can be safely performed in patients with TCC regarding the risk for tumor seeding along the needle passage path. The occurrence of tumor implantation following cystocentesis is con-

sidered rare, but does occur. Localized tumor invasion of the bladder wall was reported to occur at the site of fine needle aspiration biopsy in three dogs (two bladder and one prostate) in one study [44], and in one dog undergoing cystocentesis in another study [45]. The frequency for implantation may increase with larger bore needles, multiple needle passages, and the particular type of tumor (Figure 3.31) [44]. To reduce these possibilities, at some institutions, the collection of urine via urinary catheterization is recommended when there is a known bladder mass [44, 45]. Cystocentesis is still performed in those with known TCC by other investigators, but the needle is directed under ultrasound guidance as far away from the known mass as possible [46]. Directing

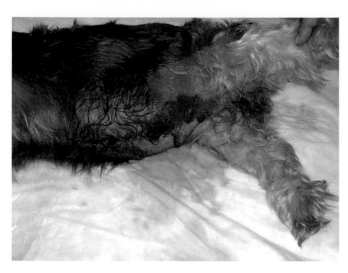

FIGURE 3.30 Subcutaneous bleeding immediately following cystocentesis in a Yorkshire dog. At the time of the procedure, it was unknown that this dog had only 10 000 platelets/μL. We do not recommend attempting cystocentesis when the platelet count is less than 25 000/μL.

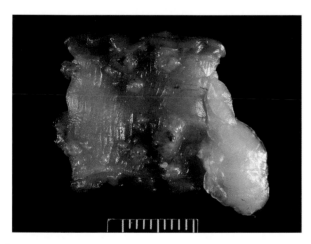

FIGURE 3.31 Carcinomatosis of cat's abdominal wall. This cat had TCC of the bladder and had undergone multiple cystocentesis to install local drug treatment within the bladder.

the needle away from an obvious mass does not guarantee that contact will not be made with other smaller masses not previously identified. Cystocentesis performed without ultrasound guidance increases the risk for tumor seeding in those with TCC. Cystotomy resulted in considerably more implantation of TCC into the abdominal wall of dogs (10.2%) than for those that did not have surgery (1.6%) [45]. The frequency for detection of metastasis along the needle tract site may be under diagnosed as patients could succumb to their disease before the metastatic process becomes apparent [44]. No episodes of TCC implantation were identified in dogs that had cystocentesis performed a median of two times in the same dog as part of surveillance to detect bacterial UTI.

Most of the samples in this study were collected using ultrasound guidance [46].

A rare complication of cystocentesis is penetration of other viscera, but this is usually of no clinical consequence in well-restrained patients due to the small gauge needles used in this procedure. Inadvertent penetration of the small intestine or colon (enterocentesis) may confuse interpretation of urinalysis and bacterial culture results because enteric bacteria contaminate the sample (Figure 3.32) [13, 47]. Severe abdominal hemorrhage following aortic laceration occurred during an unsuccessful attempt at blind cystocentesis in an unsedated struggling dog; the dog survived following surgical repair [48]. Though aortic or caudal vena cava penetration is possible, it should not happen under conditions of adequate animal restraint and cautious advancement of the cystocentesis needle with proper technique. Attempts at cystocentesis should immediately be abandoned at any point that bright or dark red blood or intestinal contents appear in the syringe.

We have observed that some cats salivate excessively or vomit right after cystocentesis, a finding that we have attributed to a vagovagal response. Rarely a cat will collapse after cystocentesis, possibly due to catecholamine release; this effect may be more severe in cats with underlying cardiovascular disease. It is our impression that rapid removal of a large volume of urine during cystocentesis can also amplify these responses. A role for stress during restraint and needle puncture during the procedure is also likely. Two cats with feline interstitial cystitis were reported to have dramatic episodes of collapse with combinations of vocalization, open mouth breathing, tachypnea, bradycardia, voiding of bloody urine, vomiting, and defection immediately following blind cystocentesis. Recovery from these signs occurred within 30–45 minutes [49]. It is unknown if another cystocentesis in the same cat will result in the same adverse effect again or not.

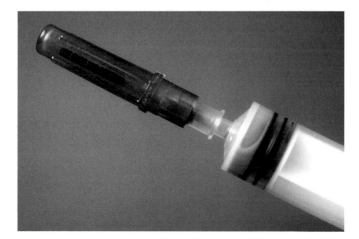

FIGURE 3.32 Inadvertent penetration of colon (enterocentesis) during attempted cystocentesis in a cat. This is a rare complication during cystocentesis. This cat developed mild fever for 24 hours and recovered uneventfully.

REFERENCES

1 Rizzi, T.E., Valenciano, A., Bowles, M. et al. (2017). Sample collection and handling. In: *Atlas of Canine and Feline Urinalysis*, 3–46. Hoboken, N.J.: John Wiley and Sons, Inc.

2 Duderstadt, J.M. and Weingand, K.W. (1990). Effects of overnight refrigeration on routine dog urinalysis (abstr). *25th Annu Meet Am Soc Vet Clin Pathol.* 20.

3 Culhane, J.K. (1990). Delayed analysis of urine. *J. Fam. Pract.* 30: 473–474.

4 Padilla, J., Osborne, C.A., and Ward, G.E. (1981). Effects of storage time and temperature on quantitative culture of canine urine. *J. Am. Vet. Med. Assoc.* 178: 1077–1081.

5 Acierno, M.J., Partyka, M., Waite, K. et al. (2018). Effect of refrigeration of clinical canine urine samples on quantitative bacterial culture. *J. Am. Vet. Med. Assoc.* 253: 177–180.

6 Albasan, H., Lulich, J.P., Osborne, C.A. et al. (2003). Effects of storage time and temperature on pH, specific gravity, and crystal formation in urine samples from dogs and cats. *J. Am. Vet. Med. Assoc.* 222: 176–179.

7 McIntyre, M. and Mou, T.W. (1965). Persistence of leukocytes and erythrocytes in refrigerated acid and alkaline urine. *Am. J. Clin. Pathol.* 43: 53–57.

8 Hedstrom, M., Moller, M., Patsekhina, H. et al. (2021). The effect of urine storage temperature and boric acid preservation on quantitative bacterial culture for diagnosing canine urinary tract infection. *BMC Vet. Res.* 17: 379.

9 Chew, D.J. and Kowalski, J. (1981). Urinary tract infections. In: *Pathophysiology of Surgery in Small Animals* (ed. M.J. Bojrab), 255–270. Lea & Febiger.

10 Ling, G.V. (1995). Techniques of Urine Collection and Handling. In: *Lower Urinary Tract Diseases of Dogs and Cats* (ed. G.V. Ling), 23–27. St. Louis: Mosby-Year Book, Inc.

11 Johnston, S.D., Root Kustritz, M.V., and Olson, P.N. (2001). The neonate- from birth to weaning. In: *Canine and Feline Theriogenology*, 1e (ed. R. Kersing), 146–167. Philadelphia: WB Saunders.

12 Osborne, C.A. and Stevens, J.B. (1999). Collection of urine. In: *Urinalysis: A Clinical Guide to Compassionate Patient Care* (ed. C.A. Osborne and J.B. Stevens), 45–50. Shawnee Mission, KS: Bayer.

13 Osborne, C.A., Lulich, J., and Albasan, H. (2011). The ins and outs of urine collection. In: *Nephrology and Urology of Small Animals* (ed. J. Bartges and D. Polzin), 28–42. Wiley-Blackwell.

14 Rosenberg, A. (2019). Hydrophobic sand: Uses and techniques. *J. Feline Med. Surg.* 21: 51.

15 Kennils, J.M., Maunder, C.L., and Costa, M.T. (2022). The effect of non-absorbent hydrophobic sand litter on the urine protein-to-creatinine ratio in feline urine. *Vet Clin Pathol.* 51: 85–390.

16 Hoffman, J.F., Fan, A.X., Neuendorf, E.H. et al. (2018). Hydrophobic sand versus metabolic cages: a comparison of urine collection methods for rats (*Rattus norvegicus*). *J. Am. Assoc. Lab Anim. Sci.* 57: 51–57.

17 Hoffman, J.F., Vergara, V.B., Mog, S.R. et al. (2017). Hydrophobic sand is a non-toxic method of urine collection, appropriate for urinary metal analysis in the rat. *Toxics* 5: 25–40.

18 Pebre, J.G., Lefebvre, H.P., and Reynolds, B.S. (2018). ESVNU – O – 13 Effects of a non-absorbent litter on urinalysis results in cats. *J. Vet. Intern. Med.* 32: 565.

19 Delporta, P.C. and Fourie, L.J. (2005). Katkor® cat litter, a non-invasive method of collecting cat urine for phosphate determination. *J. S. Afr. Vet. Assoc.* 76 (4): 233–234.

20 Giraldi, M., Paltrinieri, S., Rossi, G. et al. (2021). Influence of preanalytical factors on feline proteinuria. *Vet Clin Pathol* 50 (3): 369–375.

21 Powell, L.L. (2019). Urinary catheter placement in dogs. *Clinician's Brief.* https://www.cliniciansbrief.com/article/urinary-catheter-placement-dogs 62–67.

22 Smarick, S.D., Haskins, S.C., Aldrich, J. et al. (2004). Incidence of catheter-associated urinary tract infection among dogs in a small animal intensive care unit. *J. Am. Vet. Med. Assoc.* 224: 1936–1940.

23 Sullivan, L.A., Campbell, V.L., and Onuma, S.C. (2010). Evaluation of open versus closed urine collection systems and development of nosocomial bacteriuria in dogs. *J. Am. Vet. Med. Assoc.* 237: 187–190.

24 Moore, E.S., Fine, B.P., and Edelmann, C.M. Jr. (1970). Catheterization of the urinary bladder in young female animals. *Biol. Neonate* 16: 256–259.

25 Biertuempfel, P.H., Ling, G.V., and Ling, G.A. (1981). Urinary tract infection resulting from catheterization in healthy adult dogs. *J. Am. Vet. Med. Assoc.* 178: 989–991.

26 Weese, J.S., Blondeau, J., Boothe, D. et al. (2019). International Society for Companion Animal Infectious Diseases (ISCAID) guidelines for the diagnosis and management of bacterial urinary tract infections in dogs and cats. *Vet. J.* 247: 8–25.

27 Holt, P.E., Lucke, V.M., and Brown, P.J. (1986). Evaluation of a catheter biopsy technique as a diagnostic aid in lower urinary tract disease. *Vet. Rec.* 118: 681–684.

28 Lamb, C.R., Trower, N.D., and Gregory, S.P. (1996). Ultrasound-guided catheter biopsy of the lower urinary tract: technique and results in 12 dogs. *J. Small Anim. Pract.* 37: 413–416.

29 Kruger, J.M., Osborne, C.A., and Ulrich, L.K. (1996). Cystocentesis. Diagnostic and therapeutic considerations. *Vet. Clin. North Am. Small Anim. Pract.* 26: 353–361.

30 Ling, G.V. (1976). Antepubic cvstocentesis in the dog: an aseptic technique for routine collecton of urine. *Calif. Vet.* 30: 50–52.

31 Krawec, P. and Odunayo, A. (2020). Cystocentesis. *Clin. Brief* May: 61–68.

32 Lulich, J.P. and Osborne, C.A. (2004). Cystocentesis: lessons from thirty years of clinical experience. *Clin. Brief* 2: 11–14.

33 Hall, J., Hall, K., Powell, L.L. et al. (2015). Outcome of male cats managed for urethral obstruction with decompressive cystocentesis and urinary catheterization: 47 cats (2009-2012). *J. Vet. Emerg. Crit. Care (San Antonio)* 25: 256–262.

34 Nevins, J.R., Mai, W., and Thomas, E. (2015). Associations between ultrasound and clinical findings in 87 cats with urethral obstruction. *Vet. Radiol. Ultrasound* 56: 439–447.

35 Eisenberg, B.W., Waldrop, J.E., Allen, S.E. et al. (2013). Evaluation of risk factors associated with recurrent obstruction in cats treated medically for urethral obstruction. *J. Am. Vet. Med. Assoc.* 243: 1140–1146.

36 Gerken, K.K., Cooper, E.S., Butler, A.L. et al. (2020). Association of abdominal effusion with a single decompressive cystocentesis prior to catheterization in male cats with urethral obstruction. *J. Vet. Emerg. Crit. Care (San Antonio)* 30: 11–17.

37 Cooper, E.S., Lasley, E., Daniels, J.B. et al. (2019). Incidence of bacteriuria at presentation and resulting from urinary catheterization in feline urethral obstruction. *J. Vet. Emerg. Crit. Care (San Antonio)* 29: 472–477.

38 Reineke, E.L., Cooper, E.S., Takacs, J.D. et al. (2021). Multicenter evaluation of decompressive cystocentesis in the treatment of cats with urethral obstruction. *J. Am. Vet. Med. Assoc.* 258: 483–492.

39 Alleman, R. and Wamsley, H.L. (2017). Complete urinalysis. In: *BSAVA Manual of Canine and Feline Nephrology and Urology* (ed. J. Elliott, G.F. Grauer and J.L. Westropp), 60–83. Gloucester, UK: BSAVA.

40 Fry, D.R. and Holloway, S.A. (2004). Comparison of normal urine samples collected by cystocentesis with and without prior skin disinfection. *Austral. Vet. Pract.* 34: 2–5.

41 Poulin, R.V. (2017). Using cystocentesis to obtain sterile urine samples. *Vet. Team Brief.* https://www.veterinaryteambrief.com/article/using-cystocentesis-obtain-sterile-urine-samples?utm_medium=email&utm_source=Clinician%27s+Brief+Newsletter&utm_campaign=Online+171129&ajs_uid=1017F7693790G6V: http://veterinaryteambrief.com 51–55.

42 Tassava, B. (2017). Fees for cystocentesis. *Vet. Team Brief* https://www.veterinaryteambrief.com/article/setting-fees-cystocentesis 57–59.

43 Specht, A., Chan, D., O'Toole, T. et al. (2002). Acute staphylococcal peritonitis following cystocentesis in a dog. *J. Vet. Emerg. Crit. Care* 12: 183–187.

44 Nyland, T.G., Wallack, S.T., and Wisner, E.R. (2002). Needle-tract implantation following us-guided fine-needle aspiration biopsy of transitional cell carcinoma of the bladder, urethra, and prostate. *Vet. Radiol. Ultrasound* 43: 50–53.

45 Higuchi, T., Burcham, G.N., Childress, M.O. et al. (2013). Characterization and treatment of transitional cell carcinoma of the abdominal wall in dogs: 24 cases (1985-2010). *J. Am. Vet. Med. Assoc.* 242: 499–506.

46 Budreckis, D.M., Byrne, B.A., Pollard, R.E. et al. (2015). Bacterial urinary tract infections associated with transitional cell carcinoma in dogs. *J. Vet. Intern. Med.* 29: 828–833.

47 Vap, L.M. and Shropshire, S.B. (2017). Urine cytology: collection, film preparation, and evaluation. *Vet. Clin. North Am. Small Anim. Pract.* 47: 135–149.

48 Buckley, G.J., Aktay, S.A., and Rozanski, E.A. (2009). Massive transfusion and surgical management of iatrogenic aortic laceration associated with cystocentesis in a dog. *J. Am. Vet. Med. Assoc.* 235: 288–291.

49 Odunayo, A., Ng, Z.Y., and Holford, A.L. (2015). Probable vasovagal reaction following cystocentesis in two cats. *J. Feline Med. Surg. Open Rep.* 1: 1–4.

CHAPTER 4

Physical Properties of Urine

INTRODUCTION

The physical properties of urine have been studied for over 6000 years [1]. Descriptions of color, clarity (turbidity), odor, volume, viscosity, and taste were included in these observations. Modern urinalysis still includes the subjective assessment of physical properties in addition to urine chemistry and urinary microscopy [2]. Odor, volume, viscosity, and taste, however, are not routinely reported today. Urine concentration usually estimated by urine specific gravity (USG) is another important physical property of urine (Table 4.1). Shaking or agitating urine and observing foam formation, along with its persistence and color, have been used to indicate the presence of protein or bilirubin. Agitation of normal urine results in the formation of scant white foam that dissipates rapidly after shaking. Stable white foam suggests moderate-to-severe proteinuria (Figure 4.1). Yellow or green foam suggests the presence of bilirubin [3, 4]. The verification of the presence of protein or bilirubin requires further evaluation by urine chemistry (e.g. dipstrip measurements). Quantitative urinalysis using timed urine volume collection (12 or 24 hour) is not commonly performed in veterinary medicine.

URINE COLOR

Urine color should be evaluated by looking through or down into a clear container against a white background with good lighting. Urine color varies considerably in normal animals and in those with disease processes and is affected by the patient's hydration status. Also, color changes can develop in urine over time during storage as a consequence of oxidative processes and, thus, is best to record color using fresh urine. Ideally, terms to describe normal and abnormal color should be standardized for use by all laboratory personnel to minimize subjectivity. An objective method for reporting urine color in cats using comparison to a printed color scale has been reported [5]. This eight-degree scale originally was developed for use in human athletes in an effort to determine hydration status [6]. This scale would not be appropriate for use in animals with abnormal urine color associated with other conditions (e.g. bilirubinuria).

Normal urine is light (pale) yellow, yellow, or dark yellow (amber) (Figure 4.2a,b). This color is due primarily to the presence of the pigment urochrome, which forms after oxidation of urochromagen, with minor contributions from urobilin and uroerythrin [2]. Bilirubin and urobilin may

Urinalysis in the Dog and Cat, First Edition. Dennis J. Chew and Patricia A. Schenck.
© 2023 John Wiley & Sons, Inc. Published 2023 by John Wiley & Sons, Inc.

Table 4.1 Physical properties typically reported in urinalysis from normal dogs and cats.

Color	Straw, yellow or light amber
Appearance	Clear
Specific gravity	
Dogs	1.015–1.050 (random time of day)
	>1.040 a.m. sample before eat/drink – most dogs
	>1.030 a.m. sample before eat/drink – nearly all dogs
	>1.040 if dehydrated
Cats	1.035–1.070 (dry food)
	1.025–1.050 (canned food)
	Time of day – not as important as in dogs
	> 1.040 if dehydrated

(a)   (b)

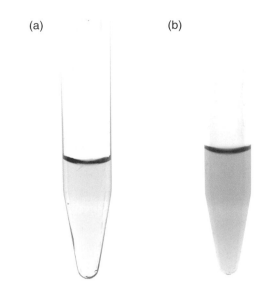

FIGURE 4.2   (a) Yellow clear urine (Normal). (b) Darker yellow urine is sometimes reported as amber. Amber urine is normal and darker amber colors are often described in urine that is highly concentrated.

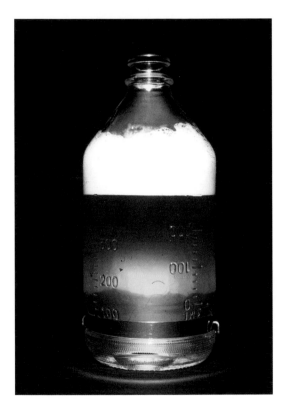

FIGURE 4.1   Urine was from a dog with heavy renal proteinuria. Note large foam head that stays at the top of this urine sample following shaking.

contribute to the color of urine in some dogs with highly concentrated urine. Increased excretion of urochrome may occur during fever and starvation as a result of increased catabolism. Urochrome excretion is relatively constant over a 24-hour period in normal subjects [7, 8]. Thus, the color may be dark amber if the urine is highly concentrated, or light yellow to colorless if the urine is more dilute.

A color chart was developed in an effort to standardize how urine color is assigned in human urine. Color categories

were yellow, pale yellow-clear, milky, pink, red, tea-colored, orange, blue–green, purple, and gray–black [9]. In a study of normal human athletes utilizing a standardized color reference chart, urine color was strongly correlated with urine concentration (USG and osmolality) when differentiating between various hydration states [10], but such a correlation has not been established in veterinary patients. Although urine color may indicate the urine concentration, disparity may occur, and urine concentration should be verified by refractometry (USG) or determination of urine osmolality. Colorless or pale-yellow urine often is dilute, but deeply colored urine may be concentrated or instead may contain increased amounts of specific pigments (e.g. bilirubin).

Abnormal urine color sometimes is the primary complaint of the animal's owner, and this concern is confirmed or refuted by observation of urine color in the laboratory, as well as by assessment of microscopic findings during urinalysis. Another reason to note urine color is that urine color can interfere with interpretation of the color changes on chemical reagent dipstrip pads [11]. In one study, approximately 6% of urine samples from dogs and 20% of samples from cats had abnormal color. Over 90% of urine samples with abnormal color from dogs and cats in this study had microscopic abnormalities that supported the observed color [12]. Normal urine color does not ensure that the urine is normal, because abnormalities still may be discovered during chemical analysis and sediment examination.

Abnormal urine color can be described along a spectrum that includes dark yellow (dark amber), pink, red, port-wine, reddish-brown, dark brown, orange–brown, black, yellow–brown, yellow–green, green, greenish-blue, white (chalky, milky), and colorless (Table 4.2). Whether or not an abnormal color clears upon centrifugation or upon standing provides clues about the cause of the color initially observed. If the color clears,

Table 4.2 Causes of abnormally colored urine.

Color of urine	Possible cause
Pink/Red/Brown	Hematuria
	Hemoglobinuria
	Myoglobinuria
	Porphyrins
	Dietary dyes
Very dark brown/black	Methemoglobin
Deep amber (yellow–brown/green–brown)	Concentrated urine
	Bile pigments
Yellow–orange	Urobilin
	Phenazopyridine
	Nitrofurantoin
Yellow–green	Bilirubin
Blue/blue–green/green	*Pseudomonas spp.*
	Methylene blue
	Amitryptilline
	Metoclopramide
	Propofol
	Herbicides
Bright yellow	Riboflavin
	Sodium fluorescein (ethylene glycol)
Pale/colorless	Dilution – low USG, any cause
White	Pyuria
	Lipiduria
	Chyluria
	Crystalluria
Purple	Some bacteria UTI
	Purple urine bag syndrome (PUBS)

then elements not dissolved in urine and subject to gravity were responsible for the color. The patient's history should be reviewed because many therapeutic or diagnostic agents can result in abnormal urine color. Unusual colors may be due to drugs or their metabolites and diagnostic agents excreted into urine [2, 3, 13]. Urine pH can influence the color of some substances in urine, because pH may affect their state of ionization [3].

PINK, RED, OR BROWN URINE

The most common abnormal urine color is pink, red, or reddish brown and can be attributed to intact red blood cells (RBC), hemolyzed RBC, muscle pigments, food pigments, or porphyrins (Figure 4.3). The most common cause of pink to red urine is the presence of intact RBC (hematuria) (Figure 4.4a–e). Intact RBC in urine impart a pink to brown color to urine, depending on the number of RBC, urine pH, and length of time the RBC have been in the urine [2]. A substantial number of RBC must be present in urine before a pink or red color is observed (Figure 4.5). Light pink color was observed in urine from dogs when approximately 600 RBC/hpf were present in

the urine sediment and dark pink color was observed when 800–950 RBC/hpf were present [14]. Red color from intact RBC in urine clears with centrifugation or settling (Figure 4.6). Hemoglobinuria from intravascular hemolysis or lysis of previously intact red cells in the urine specimen (*in vivo* or *in vitro*) also may cause reddish color that persists in the supernatant after settling or centrifugation (Figure 4.7a,b). Uncommonly, the presence of myoglobinuria, or rarely porphyrinuria, may cause a reddish color (see also Chapter 5, occult blood). Rarely, dyes used in the manufacture of some dry dog foods or ingestion of an unusual food item will impart a pink color to the urine. Discoloration caused by free hemoglobin, myoglobin, porphyrin, or dyes will persist in the urine supernatant after centrifugation, because they are dissolved in the urine.

The term "beeturia" has been used to describe pink to deep red discolored urine from human patients after eating beets or foods that have been colored with beet pigments. Betacyanuria is the preferred scientific term that describes these red pigments in urine. Betanin and its epimer isobetanin contribute most of this red color. Urine can become progressively pinker when beetroot pigments are exposed to sunlight. High performance liquid chromatography (HPLC) can be used to definitively identify beetroot pigments in urine, but this is not clinically necessary since beeturia is a benign condition. A main concern in human medicine is that beeturia can be misdiagnosed as painless hematuria [15]. The occurrence of beeturia in urine of dogs and cats is not known.

Myoglobin and free hemoglobin impart a reddish color to the urine that does not clear with settling or centrifugation (Figure 4.8a,b). Both pigments can turn darker over time, while the sample awaits analysis, but myoglobin more consistently turns reddish-brown to brown in color [2]. In this situation, the reagent pad will be positive for occult blood (see Chapter 5), but intact erythrocytes are not seen in the urinary sediment. In patients with hemoglobinuria, the serum will be pink owing to hemoglobin binding to haptoglobin. Myoglobin has no carrier protein, and its presence does not result in discoloration of serum because it is rapidly cleared from the circulation. A simple screening test using ammonium sulfate can discriminate between myoglobin and hemoglobin in urine. Myoglobin in urine largely stays in solution when exposed to 80% saturation of urine with ammonium sulfate, whereas hemoglobin is completely precipitated [16]. Although evaluation of serum color and use of ammonium sulfate precipitation testing can presumptively distinguish between hemoglobinuria and myoglobinuria, definitive differentiation requires urinary protein electrophoresis. Myoglobinuria probably occurs more commonly than diagnosed because it is easily confused with hemoglobinuria. Myoglobinuria sometimes is observed with exertional rhabdomyolysis in horses and dogs, and during postanesthetic rhabdomyolysis in horses [17–19].

Porphyrins in urine turn red after oxidation of porphobilinogen. This color intensifies upon standing and often is described as red or port wine [3]. The color of the urine supernatant does not change after centrifugation. In cats, porphyrinuria has been described as imparting an orange–brown color to urine that becomes orange–pink during fluorescence. Teeth of affected

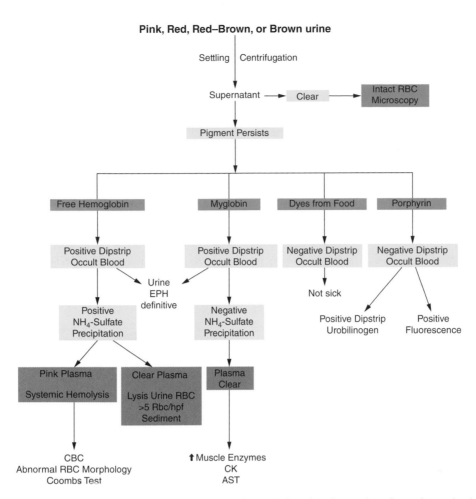

FIGURE 4.3 An algorithm for further evaluation of pigmented urine that is pink, red, or brown in order to determine its likelihood to be from intact RBC, hemolyzed RBC, muscle pigment, food pigments, or porphyrins. Porphyrin in urine contains no iron, so the reaction for occult blood should be negative. Intense pigmenturia can cause the reagent pad to appear colored despite lack of reaction with iron (false positive). RBC = red blood cells; EPH = electrophoresis; CBC = complete blood count; CK = creatine kinase; AST = aspartate aminotransferase.

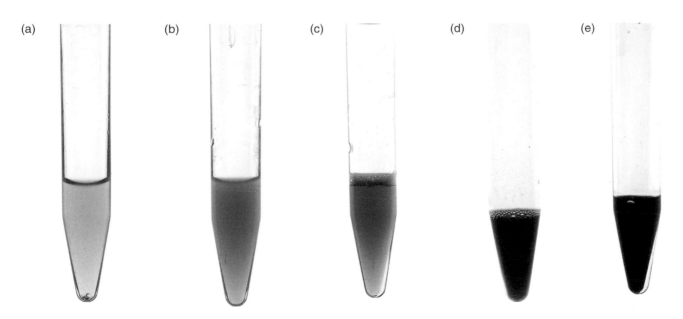

FIGURE 4.4 (a) Slightly pink, clear. Note settling of RBC in small clump at bottom of tube. (b) Cloudy orange–red urine due to numerous RBC. (c) Slightly cloudy red urine due to mostly intact RBC; some contribution from lysed RBC within urine. Supernatant color cleared upon centrifugation but not completely. (d) Dark red cloudy urine. TNTC RBC. TNTC = too numerous to count. (e) Dark red to black opaque urine. The color was so intense as to make it impossible to read the dipstrip chemistry reactions. 40–60 RBC/HPF were reported. Some of the dark color is likely imparted by oxidation of hemoglobin.

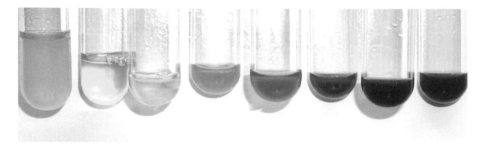

FIGURE 4.5 Increasing number of RBC per HPF in representative tubes from left to right (approximate numbers per HPF). Tube 1 < 5, tube 2 and 3 (light yellow) have between 100 and 200, tube 4 (dark yellow) 250–400, tube 5 (light pink) 600, tube 6 (dark pink) 800–950, tube 7 (red) 900–1500, and tube 8 (red) 1000–2000[1]. HPF = high powered microscopic field. Source: Vientós-Plotts et al. [14]. Used with permission of Am J Vet Research.

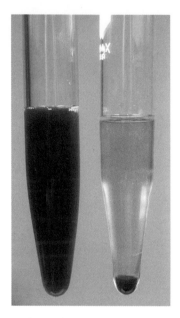

FIGURE 4.6 Note obviously red urine in the tube on the left. After centrifugation, the supernatant in the tube on the right is clear indicating the presence of formed elements mostly comprised of RBC that have settled on the bottom. Note also a thin layer at the top of the pedicel that is lighter consisting of WBC as identified later during urine microscopy.

cats are also discolored with an orange–brown shade and undergo red fluorescence [20–23]. Intermittent porphyria and congenital erythropoietic porphyria have been described in cats [23]. Rabbits often can have red urine as a result of ingesting porphyrins in cabbage, carrots, dandelions, parsley or broccoli, and this red color can be a normal finding [24]. King George III of England (1738–1820) reportedly had urine that was blue as a consequence of hereditary intermittent porphyria [25].

VERY DARK BROWN OR BLACK URINE

This coloration most often is the result of oxidation of hemoglobin to methemoglobin in acidic urine [2], a process that can occur while urine is stored in the bladder or in the laboratory while awaiting analysis [3]. The color varies from pink to black depending on how much heme pigment is present, its contact time in urine, and urine pH [3].

(a) (b)

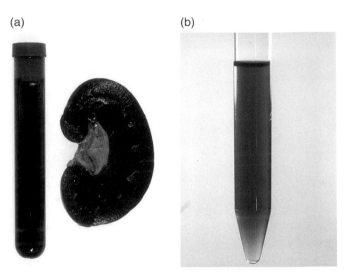

FIGURE 4.7 (a) Hemoglobinuric nephrosis. This young Great Dane suffered acute hemolysis following ingestion of chlorinated naphthalene (moth balls). Red top tube contains dark brown urine that did not change color of supernatant after centrifugation. (b) Hemoglobinuria in a dog with heartworms and caval syndrome. Note that the red color did not clear after settling or centifugation.

(a) (b)

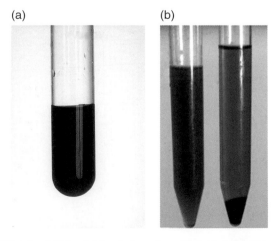

FIGURE 4.8 (a) Myoglobinuria from dog with heat stroke. Urinary electrophoresis was used to confirm this pigment as myoglobin. (b) Cloudy red urine before settling on left. Large pedicel of RBC in tube on the right after centrifugation. Supernatant is still moderately colored likely due to hemoglobin from ruptured RBC.

Melaninuria is suspected in human patients with melanoma when urine turns black in color while standing, but the chemical reagent dipstrip is negative for blood. Melanogen, which is colorless, must first be oxidized to melanin, which is black in color. Similarly, urine containing homogentisic acid can turn black at alkaline pH in human patients with inborn errors of metabolism for phenylalanine (alkaptonuria) [2]. Neither condition has been reported in domestic animals, to our knowledge.

DEEP AMBER (YELLOW–BROWN OR GREEN–BROWN) URINE

Yellow–brown or green–brown discoloration could be the result of highly concentrated urine in normal or dehydrated patients, or increased amounts of bile pigments in the urine. Normal concentrated urine will produce transient white foam upon shaking, whereas dark urine caused by bilirubin will produce yellow foam upon shaking. Urine containing bilirubin may turn green or yellow–green upon standing as bilirubin is photo-oxidized to biliverdin [2].

YELLOW–ORANGE URINE

Photo-oxidation of urobilinogen to urobilin can impart a yellow–orange or yellow–brown color to urine (Figure 4.9). This change is most likely to occur when urine has been allowed to stand [2]. Phenazopyridine (alone or in combination with sulfonamides) is a dye that provides local analgesia for human patients with urinary tract infections (UTIs). It commonly causes yellow–orange urine and may cause fever, yellow discoloration of the skin and eyes, methemoglobinemia, vomiting, hematuria, serious allergic reactions, hepatitis, acute interstitial nephritis, or pyelonephritis [26–28]. This compound

FIGURE 4.9 Orange urine; slightly cloudy.

should not be prescribed for use in dogs or cats because of the potential for serious adverse effects. Nitrofurantoin used to treat UTI can also impart an orange color to urine [2].

YELLOW–GREEN URINE

Bilirubin contributes to the yellow–green to yellow–brown coloration of urine. A green shade of urine color is caused by biliverdin, which is an oxidation product of bilirubin. This green color intensifies over time [3].

BLUE, BLUE–GREEN, AND GREEN URINE

Pigments imparted by *Pseudomonas spp.* UTIs occasionally result in bluish-green urine. Methylene blue is a urinary antiseptic that should not be used in dogs or cats because of the risk of Heinz body hemolytic anemia, but if inadvertently used, it can result in green urine [29]. Amitriptyline [2], metoclopramide [30, 31], and propofol [32] are drugs that have the potential to cause greenish discoloration of urine. "Grass" green discoloration of urine has been noted with propofol administration in humans [33] and has recently been described after the infusion of propofol in a dog (Figure 4.10 a–c) [34]. Green-colored urine has also been reported after the ingestion of some herbicides [35].

BRIGHT YELLOW URINE

Several ingested compounds can cause bright yellow discoloration of urine. Large doses of riboflavin (vitamin B2) may turn urine bright yellow [3, 36]. Sodium fluorescein is added to some commercial antifreeze preparations to aid in the detection of radiator fluid leaks. Animals that have consumed antifreeze containing this compound may have urine that has a bright yellow–green color if examined soon after ingestion. Ultraviolet light examination of urine facilitates detection of this fluorescent compound and potentially aids in the early diagnosis of ethylene glycol poisoning. Negative fluorescence does not exclude a diagnosis of ethylene glycol intoxication, because not all ethylene-glycol-based antifreeze solutions have fluorescein added [37–39]. Negative fluorescence is also expected if the time between the ingestion of antifreeze and examination of urine is more than 6–12 hours. False-positive fluorescence can arise from many substances, and this situation has been especially problematic in human pediatrics. Fluorescence detection varies among readers and with the type of container in which the urine is being examined [40, 41]. This potential problem has not been critically evaluated in veterinary medicine.

PALE TO COLORLESS URINE

Lack of urine color usually indicates high urine volume and associated urine dilution that occurs in a variety of diseases (e.g. chronic kidney disease [CKD], diabetes mellitus,

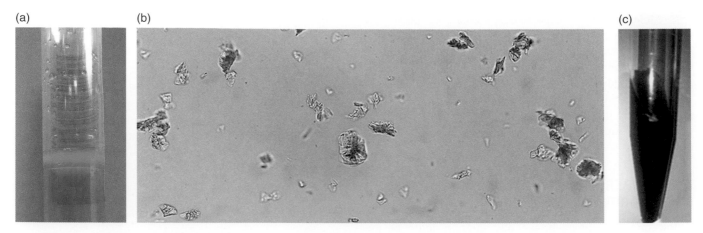

(a) (b) (c)

FIGURE 4.10 (a, b) Green urine from a dog. Large number of unidentified crystals in urine sediment. Green urine most often occurs following exposure to certain drugs or injectable anesthetic like propofol. Source: Reproduced with permission of Dr. Heather L. Wamsley, Bradenton, FL. (c) Green urine possibly related to propofol. Source: Reproduced with permission of Dr. Heidi Ward, Sarasaota FL.

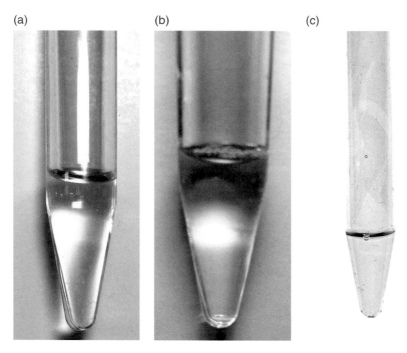

(a) (b) (c)

FIGURE 4.11 (a) Pale to colorless and clear urine sample. The USG was 1.019 in the absence of minimal color illustrating that guessing the urine concentration from color of urine is misleading at times. (b) Colorless urine with a 1.013 USG. The urine is more concentrated based on USG that its color would suggest. (c) Colorless urine. There is so little color in this sample causing one to question whether the sample is really urine or urine that has been adulterated. It could be that the sample is actually water, urine contaminated with water, or extremely dilute urine from the patient. The USG on this sample was 1.001.

hyperadrenocorticism (HAC), diabetes insipidus, psychogenic polydipsia [PPD]). This lack of color is expected in normal patients with high fluid intake, those on intravenous (IV) fluids, or those treated with diuretics (Figure 4.11a–c). Some dogs are extremely sensitive to glucocorticoids (by injection, orally administered, or in topical products for use in the ears and eyes) and produce very dilute pale urine [42]. It is also important to determine that the urine sample has not been contaminated with water or dilute fluids from other sources [3].

WHITE URINE

White urine rarely is observed in dogs and cats. Pyuria can cause the urine to appear white in some instances before the cells settle out (Figure 4.12a,b). Lipiduria can contribute to a white color, but this situation is uncommon. Chyluria may manifest itself as chalky white urine, which has been observed occasionally in humans [3]. We have only rarely observed this situation in animals. Given the extensive network of

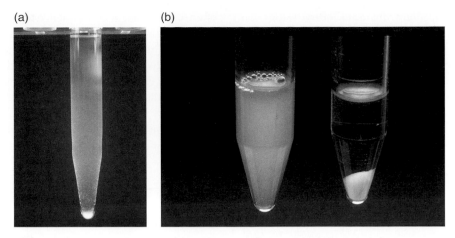

FIGURE 4.12   Whitish color to urine due to pyuria. (a) White color is settling out by gravity. (b) Before and after centrifugation. Note supernatant is clear and lacking in color after centrifugation; large pedicel at bottom right.

lymphatic venous anastomoses that are present in the abdomen, chyluria is a possible finding in patients with chylothorax, but this occurrence has not been systematically evaluated in veterinary medicine. When crystals are numerous, a white color can be imparted to the urine, but this color will not persist in the supernatant after settling. Although this phenomenon occasionally is observed in small animals, it often is an artifact observed after storage and refrigeration of urine that allows *ex vivo* precipitation of crystals that alter the color of the sample after mixing before analysis. Macroscopic alteration of urine color or clarity as a result of calcium carbonate crystalluria occasionally is observed in fresh urine samples from horses [19]. Large quantities of struvite and calcium carbonate crystals in normal rabbit urine can also result in opaque urine of light white color. Clear urine in rabbits actually may be pathological as a result of low calcium excretion during renal failure, or it may be physiological during lactation [24].

PURPLE URINE

Purple urine bag syndrome (PUBS) occurs at times in geriatric humans with indwelling urinary catheters and underlying bacterial UTIs. The purple color is described in urine [43], but this color may only develop after reaction of the urine with plastic in the collection bag and lines [44]. Tryptophan in food is metabolized to indole by intestinal bacteria, and then, indole is converted to indoxyl sulfate in the liver and excreted in urine. UTI by bacteria with indoxyl phosphatase/sulfatase activity can result in conversion of indoxyl sulfate to indigo or indirubin, which can react with the catheter bag, producing a purple color [45, 46]. The most common bacteria with indoxyl phosphatase/sulfatase activity are *Providencia stuartii*, *Klebsiella pneumoniae*, and *Enterobacter agglomerans* [47]. Whether or not this situation occurs in veterinary emergency critical care patients has not been critically evaluated.

CLARITY (TRANSPARENCY AND TURBIDITY)

Color and clarity are determined at the same time. The clarity of urine is described as a continuum from complete transparency to nearly complete opacity (complete turbidity). As with the assessment of color, it is best to determine clarity using fresh warm (i.e. body or room temperature) urine after the sample has been well mixed. Clarity should be assessed in a clear container while holding the sample in front of a light source and against a white background. Terms used to describe clarity should be standardized among laboratory personnel to allow more certainty and reproducibility of reported results. The terms clear, hazy, cloudy, turbid, and milky are used to describe progressively increasing amounts of particulates in the urine sample. It is helpful to describe clarity in relation to how easy it is to see print through the sample. Print can be easily read through a clear urine sample; it will appear blurred through cloudy urine and cannot be seen through a turbid urine sample [2]. Some laboratories restrict the description of clarity to clear, hazy, or cloudy [3]. It is helpful to evaluate clarity before and after centrifugation or after time has been allowed for elements to settle by gravity (cells and crystals) or rise (lipids).

Turbid urine is classified by causes that are either nonpathological or pathological. Mucus, sperm, prostatic secretions, squamous epithelial cells, crystals that have formed during refrigeration or after prolonged standing of the sample, fecal contamination, bacterial growth at room temperature, glove powder, lubricant, and environmental contaminants are categorized as nonpathological causes of urine turbidity. Turbidity arising from lipids usually is classified as nonpathological, especially in cats. Excessive numbers of white blood cells (WBC), RBC, transitional epithelial cells, bacteria, fungi, casts, and crystals are classified as pathological causes of turbidity (Figures 4.13, 4.14a–c, 4.15a–c, and 4.16). In urine that has stood over time, lipids will rise to the top of the tube, whereas crystals or cells causing turbidity will fall by gravity

(Figure 4.17) [11]. Flocculent material often settles on standing and usually consists of aggregates of WBC or occasionally clumps of epithelial cells (Figure 4.18a,b). Small calculi (i.e. "sand" or "gravel") also may contribute to turbidity.

Urine from normal dogs and cats usually is clear [48], especially urine that is fresh and at body temperature. Cloudy urine often is a result of crystalluria, most often in refrigerated samples in which cooling has favored crystal precipitation. Fresh urine from horses, rabbits, goats, and guinea pigs is often cloudy as a consequence of mucus and abundant calcium carbonate crystals. Cloudiness was found in 68.5% of urine specimens from dogs with various urinary and nonurinary tract diseases; 73.4% of urine specimens from cats in this study were cloudy. Of the cloudy urine samples, 55% of dog samples and 63% of cat samples subsequently were found to have microscopic abnormalities [12]. Cloudy urine from dogs and cats may be normal in the absence of other abnormal macroscopic or microscopic findings [12].

ODOR

The assessment of odor is not reported as part of the routine urinalysis, but unusual odors can be recorded under comments. Normal urine has a slight odor that has been attributed to volatile aliphatic amines [49]. The intensity of this odor varies greatly among individual dogs and cats and is in part related to the degree of urine concentration and dietary intake. Ingestion of onions, garlic, and asparagus imparts characteristic urine odors in some humans, but these foods are not commonly ingested by dogs and cats. The urine of intact male cats has a characteristic strong odor related to metabolism of the sulfur-containing amino acid felinine (2-amino-7-hydroxy-5,5-dimethyl-4-thiaheptanoic acid). Large amounts of felinine are excreted into urine of domestic cats [50], with higher concentrations found in intact male cats than in castrated males and females. Plasma testosterone concentration is highly correlated

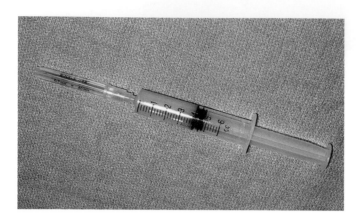

FIGURE 4.13 Cloudy urine from urine sample collected by cystocentesis. Severe increases in WBC and bacteria account for the cloudy appearance.

(a)   (b)   (c)

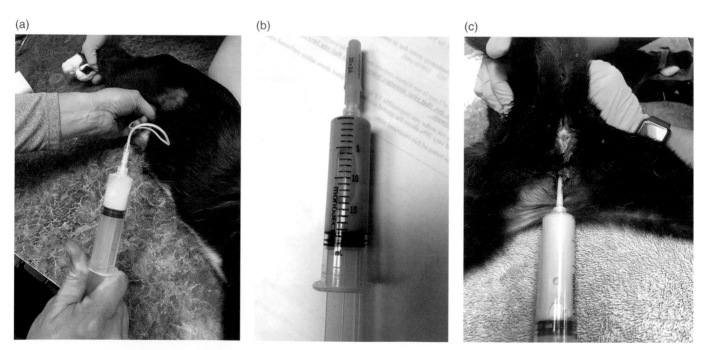

FIGURE 4.14 (a) Green urine aspirated by cystocentesis from female cat with urethral obstruction. (b) Darker green urine sample after the bladder was more fully evacuated. (c) Cream colored urine retrieved following urethral catheterization. Urinalysis showed many WBC and rod bacteria but urine culture was not performed. Following urethral catheterization and a 10-day course of enrofloxacin, the cat was clinically normal. An underlying cause for the presumed bacterial UTI was not found. The greenish color could be imparted by certain bacteria growing in the urine, as is known to happen with *Pseudomonas spp.* Reproduced with permission of Dr. Heidi Ward, Sarasota FL. Source: Courtesy of Dr. Heidi Ward.

(a)

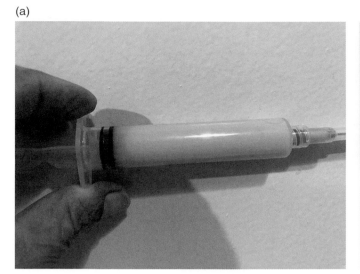

(b)

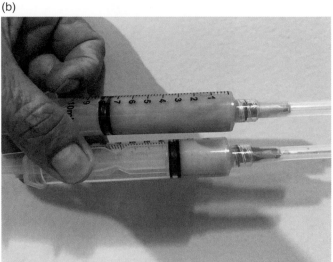

(c)

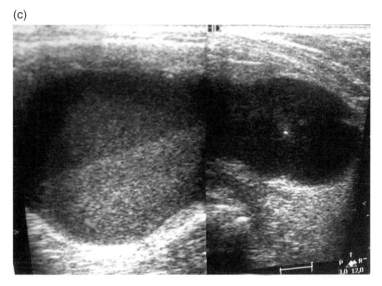

FIGURE 4.15   Dog with bacterial cystitis and prostatitis with abscess. (a) Opaque urine sample obtained by cystocentesis from a nine-year-old intact male dog. (b) Prostatic aspirate (top tube) compared to cystocentesis sample. (c) Highly echogenic material in the dog's bladder (left) and an enlarged prostate (right) with cavity lesions during ULS. This dog presented with dysuria, stranguria, pollakiuria, and progressive inappetence for two weeks. The owners noted "thick" urine. Abdominal palpation was painful – rectal palpation was not performed due to pain. There was no response to prior treatment with amoxicillin and with cephalexin. WBC count was 25 000 with normal serum biochemistry. Urinalysis showed many abnormalities. Turbid cloudy thick urine was noted with a USG 1.040, pH 8, 4+ protein, >50 WBC/HPF, and a large amount of rod bacteria on urine microscopy. No bacterial cultures were performed. Treatment consisted of castration, ULS guided drainage of cavitary prostatic lesions (abscess), lavage of the bladder via urinary catheter, and oral enrofloxacin at 5 mg/kg BID for 60 days. ULS guided drainage of prostatic lesions was repeated 10 days after the first drainage. CBC, biochemical profile and UA were normal at 60 days and the dog had no clinical signs. The dog did well in long term follow-up. Source: Reproduced with permission of Dr. Janis Gonzalez – Londrina State University; Universidade Estadual de Londrina.

with urinary felinine concentration in male cats [51, 52]. Felinine production is controlled by urinary cauxin, a carboxylesterase excreted in feline urine, a metabolic pathway unique to cats [53]. Felinine production can be altered by dietary ingredients. For example, dietary cystine can increase felinine production, whereas dietary arginine can decrease felinine production [54]. Felinine is odorless, but its metabolite, mercaptan

(3-mercapto-3-methylbutanol [MMB]), is the major source of urine odor in cats [53, 55].

Abnormal urine odor most often is ammoniacal [48] after release of ammonia from urea metabolism by urease-producing bacteria that cause urinary infections or bacterial contamination of the specimen. Ammonia can also be released in urine samples that have not been properly stored before

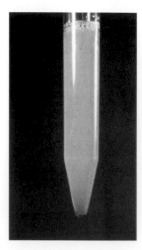

FIGURE 4.16 Markedly opaque or milky appearance to uncentrifuged urine before settling by gravity has had a chance to occur. This appearance could be created by an abundance of WBC, epithelial cells, crystals, or sperm. Mucus could also contribute to this opacity.

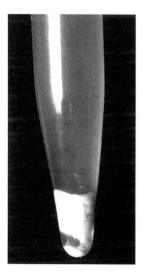

FIGURE 4.17 Cloudy urine settling by gravity. Purulent urine sample – cow.

analysis. Bacterial degradation of proteins in urine (i.e. putrefaction) or sloughing of necrotic tissue may result in a foul urine odor. Occasionally, some clinicians can detect the sweet smell of ketonuria in the urine of a diabetic animal. Some drugs excreted into urine can also impart an unusual odor.

URINE CONCENTRATION

GENERAL CONCEPTS

Urine concentration is the most important physical property reported on the urinalysis, because it provides quantitative information about renal tubular function. In most patients, urine concentration progressively decreases with loss of renal

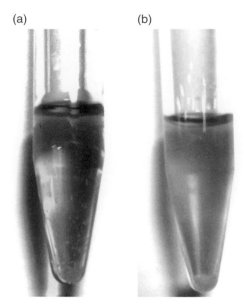

(a)   (b)

FIGURE 4.18 (a) Amber to dark yellow sample. Note flocculent material floating within urine tube and especially as it accumulates at the tip of the tube by gravity. (b) Same tube as above with more time elapsed for standing and settling of flocculent particles to bottom of tube. Supernatant cleared after settling.

mass. However, the ability to concentrate urine to a USG >1.035 was preserved in 13 of 14 cats with 5/6 experimental reduction in renal mass that was associated with reduced glomerular filtration rate (GFR) and azotemia. The ability of the cat to continue to make urine with a high USG at times despite the presence of substantial nephron loss makes the detection or suspicion of primary renal disease more challenging. The diagnosis of CKD has traditionally included the presence of a USG <1.035 in cats often in the presence of azotemia [56]. Dogs characteristically lose the ability to elaborate concentrated urine much earlier during progressive CKD compared to cats.

Nonrenal conditions can also alter the kidney's ability to produce highly concentrated urine (e.g. central diabetes insipidus (CDI), nephrogenic diabetes insipidus [NDI], hypercalcemia, hypokalemia, PPD). The proper interpretation of urine concentration requires the integration of findings from the patient's hydration status, presence or absence of azotemia, and timing of eating and drinking in relation to when the urine sample was collected. Semiquantitative urine chemistry dipstrip reactions should be evaluated in light of USG findings. For example, a +1-protein reaction in association with a USG of 1.015 usually represents more protein excretion than does a 1+ protein reaction in a urine sample with a USG of 1.045. The degree of urine concentration is also used in the evaluation of the number of formed elements seen during microscopic evaluation of the urine sediment. For example, the finding of 5 RBC/hpf in urine with a USG of 1.010 is more likely to be clinically relevant than the same result in a sample with a USG of 1.055 [57].

Total urine solute concentration is an important tool for the clinical evaluation of renal function. The most precise method to determine urine concentration is to measure the weight of the solutes in a precise volume of urine, but this is cumbersome and only done in research settings using a pycnometer [2, 58]. Instead, in a clinical setting, urine concentration is estimated by urinometry, refractometry, or osmometry. Harmonic oscillation densitometry determines how the frequency of sound waves entering a solution is altered in proportion to the density of the solution, but this method is rarely used today. Urinometry (hydrometry gravitometry) uses a weighted float attached to a scale that displaces a volume of liquid equal to its own weight. The level to which the float sinks is read from the scale and represents the USG, but this method requires a larger urine volume than often is available from dogs and cats (Figure 4.19). Urinometry is less accurate than refractometry in the estimation of USG [59], but it is still used in some countries to report USG. USG as determined by urinometry is highly correlated to refractometry in dogs, but varies by 0.004–0.008 USG in concentrated urine [60]. When using a urinometer, it is important to observe the reference temperature printed on the urinometer, along with measuring the temperature of the urine sample during testing. A temperature correction then can be calculated based on the temperature difference.

The measurement of urine osmolality (U_{osm}) is the definitive method by which to assess the degree of urine concentration [61–63] because the kidneys function in units of osmoles for excretion and not excretion by weight. USG as determined by refractometry, however, is most commonly used to assess the degree of urine concentration in routine clinical practice. USG as determined by refractometry approximates total solute concentration but does not yield a precise concentration of solute.

Estimates of USG measured by chemistry reagent dipstrips are used as a screening test in people but are not accurate in domestic animals (see Chapter 5). The reagent strip changes color in proportion to the number of ions in solution depending on changes in the dissociation constant (pK_a) of multiple electrolytes in an alkaline environment. USG is reported in increments of 0.005 depending on the color that develops from blue at very low USG to green for moderate USG and yellow at a USG of ≥1.030. Samples with urinary pH >6.5 can cause falsely low USG readings by interference with the color indicator pad. Large amounts of protein increase the USG reading [64]. In dogs, the test strip is considered unreliable because of its poor correlation with USG as determined by refractometry or urine osmolality [65–67]. USG measured by dipstrip differed by >0.005 compared to refractometry in 77.5% of all samples, a difference that decreased to 60% when correction was made for samples with pH >6.5 [65]. USG determined by test strip was lower than that determined by refractometry in both of these studies, often by large amounts [65, 66].

Excellent correlation between USG determined by refractometry and urine osmolality has been reported in four studies of dogs [60, 65, 66, 68] and two studies of cats [5, 69]. In one study of dogs with a variety of diseases, USG was correlated to urine osmolality, but a relatively wide range of osmolalities was predicted from USG [62]. In another study, three dogs with a USG of 1.048 had osmolalities of 1734, 1820, and 1978 mOsm/L [70]. The discordance between USG and urine osmolality is not high enough to affect the clinical assessment of renal tubular functions in most cases. Urine osmolality and USG by refractometry were highly correlated in dogs with medical conditions, but osmolality predicted from USG was wide. For example, a USG of 1.020 predicted an osmolality of 300–1000 mOsm/kg using 95% confidence intervals. Ketonuria had a small negative effect on urine osmolality [71].

In one study of dogs, predicted U_{osm} was calculated from USG by the formula $y = 3.60 \times 10^4 (x-1)$, where y is U_{osm} in mOsm/kg and x is USG. For example, U_{osm} of a urine sample with a specific gravity of 1.030 is estimated to be $3.60 \times 10000 \times (0.030) = 3.60 \times 300 = 1080$ mOsm/kg [60]. A simpler way to arrive at the same result is to multiply the last two digits to the right of the decimal point of the USG by 36 (in this example, $30 \times 36 = 1080$ mOsm/kg). This rule may be misleading if the urine sample contains a large amount of high-molecular-weight solute, because substances with high molecular weights have a greater effect on specific gravity than on osmolality.

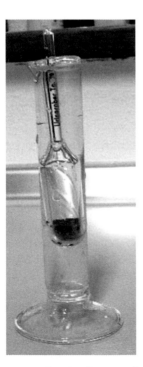

FIGURE 4.19 Urinometer showing flotation device in urine sample. The degree of flotation is proportional to the USG. This method is uncommonly used to estimate USG today.

URINE SPECIFIC GRAVITY

General Principles of Measurement of USG by Refractometry

The interested reader is referred to an excellent review of refractometry in veterinary medicine [72]. USG is the ratio of the mass (density) of urine compared to the mass of an equal volume of pure water at the same temperature. USG represents the average mass of all solutes, based on the mass contributed by each of the individual solutes present in the urine [73]. In recent years, the term specific gravity has fallen out of favor in scientific literature and is being replaced with the term "relative density." However, in some industries like urine testing, salinity, and beer brewing (regionally), the term specific gravity is still customarily used for its historical significance.

Despite the fact that refractometry does not measure USG directly, it provides an approximation of urine solute concentration, which is important in the evaluation of renal excretory and tubular functions. USG can be calculated by formulas that use simple additive functions for the individual concentration of the various molecules that are dissolved in urine, but not all of these particles are easily identified or measured. Urine concentration based on USG is determined by the urinary excretion of both organic and inorganic molecules [74].

Refractometry is the recommended and most commonly used method for approximating specific gravity during routine urinalysis. Refractometers provide an affordable method to quickly estimate and report urine concentration by USG in in the laboratory, examination room, or cage-side. A refractometer costs less than $500 in North America, and no further cost is incurred because no reagents are needed. The use of the refractometer is easy, and special training or expertise is not required. Reference laboratories have the ability to automate the measurement of USG and clarity, as the urine sample is dispensed onto a fiber optic through which light is transmitted. In these instances, USG is measured by the light refractive fiber-optic method and clarity is objectively assigned following both transmission and scattering of light that is detected [75].

USG or relative density measurement is dimensionless (no units) because it is a ratio (density of urine divided by density of water). However, USG has recently been reported in g/mL in the veterinary and human literature, despite the definition of USG as a unitless number [5, 76]. This usage is in error because g/mL refers to a concentration or urine density (mass per volume) and not USG [58]. An effort has been made in the scientific community to move away from specific gravity or relative density measurement in favor of measuring density directly. Because density is a mass/volume calculation, it can be expressed as an absolute value, as opposed to a dimensionless ratio.

The veterinary refractometer (Figure 4.20) does not directly measure USG, but instead measures the refractive index (RI) of urine and then reports a specific gravity reading to the user based on the mathematical relationship between

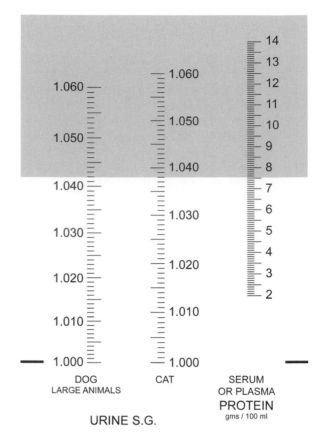

FIGURE 4.20 Dog and cat specific scales are used to read the USG as estimated by refractometry. Note the gray line intersects at a USG of 1.042 for the dog scale, and 1.038 for the cat scale. Cat urine measured using the dog scale will read higher USG values than those determined on refractometers that have separate scales. For example, if cat urine reads out on the dog scale at 1.035 it will read at 1.031 or 1.032 on the cat scale. Source: Illustration by Tim Vojt, reproduced with permission of The Ohio State University.

RI and USG. RI is the ratio of the velocity of light through air, compared to the velocity of light through a solution (urine), and is reported as a dimensionless number together with a reference wavelength and temperature. RI varies with the specific gravity, but it is not identical to the specific gravity. An approximate relationship exists between the specific gravity determined by refractometry and the total solute concentration in urine. Specific gravity is dependent on molecular size and weight as well as the total number of solute molecules, whereas osmolality depends only on the number of molecules [62]. The measured RI is read from a scale that usually is calibrated in terms of specific gravity or total solids, but it can also be reported as RI, which is the most accurate measurement. Handheld analog and digital refractometers operate on the same general principles, but internal software converts RI to USG that is displayed digitally on digital devices.

A traditional analog refractometer consists of a series of lenses and prisms, which image a shadow line, created by the critical angle of urine (a property directly related to its RI), onto a tiny scale etched onto a glass reticle [77]. The reading is taken at the point the shadow line intersects the reticle scale. In this device, RI is correlated with specific gravity based on the design of the reticle. Temperature and the wavelength of light during the measurement markedly influence RI. Therefore, some traditional analog refractometers contain a bimetallic strip capable of moving lenses and prisms to perform rudimentary compensation to a reference temperature. Temperature compensation is not available on all traditional analog refractometers, but it is an essential feature when selecting a refractometer for USG testing.

Digital refractometers assess fluids in a similar fashion, but instead of projecting the shadow line on a tiny glass reticle, it is projected onto a linear array of photosensitive detector elements. The RI of the solution is determined by the relative position of the shadow line on the detector array, and a microcontroller applies an algorithm to convert the reading to specific gravity. Digital refractometers remove the subjectivity present in traditional analog refractometers, are more capable of controlling wavelength, and usually can apply more accurate temperature correction. An added benefit of a digital refractometer is that urine samples do not need to be brought close to the operator's face and eyes, and this decreases the likelihood that the operator will be exposed to urine and, thus, increases safety in the laboratory.

A difference in RI exists between the urine of dogs and cats, and thus, it has been considered necessary to employ a refractometer with species-specific scales in order to report accurate USG results [72, 78]. This difference in RI for cats was demonstrated in cats that were consuming an all fish diet in the late 1950s and has not been evaluated in cats consuming commercial cat foods in recent years [72]. The RI of cat urine was shown to be higher than that of dogs or humans [78]. Therefore, the USG reported for cats using a scale designed for humans or dogs will be falsely increased, an error that increases as urine becomes more concentrated. In these instances, USG is overestimated by 0.002 using samples with USG of 1.010 and by 0.006 using samples with USG of 1.040 [72]. As an alternative, USG in cats can be calculated from the value measured on a USG scale designed for dogs or humans by use of the correction formula: $0.846 \times USG$ (from a scale designed for dogs or humans) $+ 0.154$ [72]. The need for a different scale to measure USG in cats has recently been challenged by one group [58].

Veterinarians expect USG results to be the same when measured by different refractometers, but variation in reported results among various instruments seems to be greater than generally appreciated. Some of the variability in USG results may be accounted for by design differences in analyzers from different manufacturers [72]. Lack of temperature compensation, failure to properly calibrate, or poor-quality devices could be responsible for much of the variability among refractometers. We recommend only using refractometers equipped with automatic temperature compensation or

correction. Excellent correlation of USG was found between measurements made with an analog (Schmidt & Hensch Goldberg; 1.040 maximal USG) and digital refractometer (Atago PAL-USG; 1.080 maximal USG) in dogs and cats. However, clinically relevant decreases in USG were observed with the digital device. The discordance was particularly disturbing in 10 samples with USG >1.030 reported on the analog device that were associated with digital measurements of 1.023–1.028 [79]. Investigation of five refractometers by the same group identified significantly different USG results, and imprecision of USG measurements was both increased and decreased in comparison to gold-standard USG determinations made using dried total solids or pycnometry [58]. A mean USG of 1.031 was obtained from cats when measured by optical analog refractometry, compared to 1.027 obtained by digital refractometry using a cat-specific USG scale. The mean difference in USG between these analyzers was approximately 0.003, a difference not likely to impact clinical decision-making in most instances. Excellent correlation was found between both methods of measuring USG when compared to urine osmolality [69]. In another study, USG and U_{osm} also were highly correlated in normal cats [5]. In a similar study of dogs, USG by optical refractometry was significantly higher than that determined using a digital refractometer, but this difference was very small and unlikely to be clinically relevant. USG differed by <0.002 in over 90% of the cases [68]. Analytical validity for this analyzer was confirmed in humans [80].

Analyzer Types Used for Refractometry in Animals

Refractometers used in veterinary practices are mostly handheld optical devices (Figure 4.21a,b). Certain traditional analog refractometers can be connected to a stand that provides consistent lighting (Figure 4.22). There is widespread belief that all the refractometers are similar in quality, but substantial differences can exist among analyzers in the results generated. We recommend the use of a refractometer engineered to provide separate RI scales for urine from dogs and cats. When making a decision for purchase of a refractometer to measure both USG and total protein concentration, it should be noted that refractometers manufactured in Asia often use a different formula to calculate total protein concentration than the formula used in other parts of the world. This difference impacts the estimates of total protein concentration generated, but does not impact USG results [81]. Based on research studies and general observation, the use of digital refractometers is increasing in veterinary medicine. Measurements acquired using digital handheld refractometers (Figure 4.23a,b) appear to be more precise (closeness of agreement of repeated measurements on the same sample) than those obtained from traditional handheld refractometers. A digital refractometer was considered easier to read and eliminated the subjective variability in visual determination of USG in one study of cats [69].

The use of a refractometer designed to evaluate human urine is not recommended for use in domestic species, because

(a)

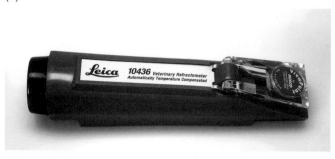

(b)

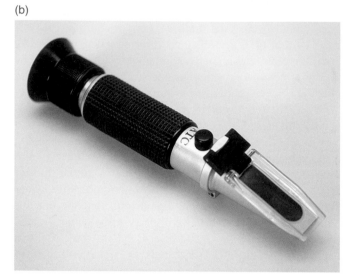

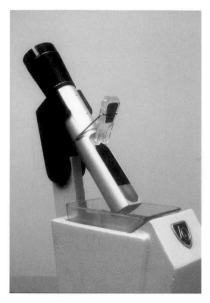

FIGURE 4.22 Optical refractometer, stand, and light source. Using a stand ensures that the refractometer is always in the same place and ready to use with good lighting.

the maximal upper limit of measurement that is reported is usually 1.035. It is not acceptable to report USG as >1.035, because it is clinically important to know the precise urine concentration in some urinary tract diseases (e.g. urolithiasis, feline idiopathic cystitis). Because dogs, cats, and horses can elaborate urine of much higher USG than that of humans, the use of a specifically designed veterinary refractometer that can measure USG of at least 1.060 is recommended. The RI of

FIGURE 4.21 (a) Veterinary optical refractometer. Source: Leica 10 436; Misco Products Division. (b) Veterinary optical refractometer. Source: ATC Model FG-311.

(a) (b)

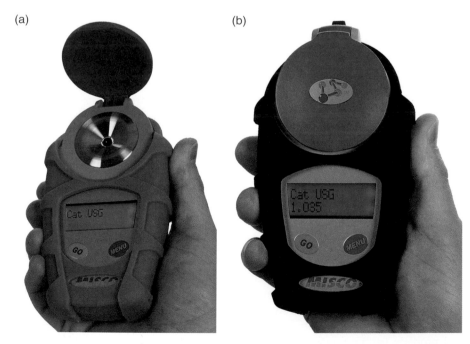

FIGURE 4.23 (a, b) Handheld digital refractometer (Misco®). In the first panel (orange shell), the urine chamber is open, the species selected (between dog, cat, horse, other), and the USG selected to be measured. In the second panel (black shell), a drop of urine has been added to the well, the lid on the urine chamber has been closed and USG measured and digitally displayed. The nD (principal refractive index) value can also be reported as the original parameter that is used to calculate the USG. Note that the scale for reporting has been set to the cat.

canine urine was determined in early studies to a maximum USG of 1.045 [82, 83], but because the scale is linear, it has been extrapolated to higher USG values.

How to Measure USG by Refractometry

First, the refractometer should be calibrated each day using known fluids that are minimally, moderately, and highly concentrated [2]. The refractometer should also be calibrated daily using distilled water to be sure that, before, a value of 1.000 is obtained [3]. Reference solutions with documented National Institute of Standards and Technology concentrations should be used for calibration when highly accurate results are needed. Calibration with 5% NaCl should result in a USG reading of 1.022 ± 0.001, or calibration with 9% sucrose should give a USG of 1.034 ± 0.001 [2]. On the canine USG scale at 20 °C, a 5% m/m (mass/mass; mass of solute/total mass of solution) NaCl solution should read 1.024 and 9% m/m sucrose solution should read 1.035. These values will be different using the feline USG scale [84, 85]. Measurement of NaCl or sucrose solutions should be performed as close to 68 °F (20 °C) as possible to avoid temperature compensation errors. Instrument readings may drift over time, and thus, ongoing surveillance is important. Some veterinary refractometers maintain their calibration for years, and thus, the need for daily calibration has been questioned [72].

Stored refrigerated urine samples should be mixed well before USG testing to force any condensed water droplets on the inside of the container back into solution. It is not necessary to analyze urine at room temperature because the thermal mass of the urine sample is quite small compared with the thermal mass of the refractometer, and temperature equilibration should occur quickly. Ideally, one should wait approximately 30 seconds for every 10 °F difference between the sample temperature and room temperature (68 °F or 20 °C) to ensure temperature equilibration. For the most accurate USG readings, the temperature of the sample, the device, and the room should be in equilibrium and within the range of the temperature compensation of the refractometer.

The measuring surface on the refractometer should be clean and dry before USG measurement. For analog refractometers, add one or two drops of urine to the measuring surface, ensuring that the entire glass surface is covered with urine (Figure 4.24). The refractometer is then pointed toward a suitable light source, and the USG is read looking through the eyepiece to determine the point that the shadow line intersects with the USG scale. Be sure no air bubbles are trapped between the sample cover and the measuring surface, because they may cause a reading failure or inaccuracy in determining where the shadow line intersects the USG scale. Similarly, a highly turbid sample may cause the shadow line to appear blurred and make it difficult to report an accurate value. For a digital refractometer with an internal light source, one to three drops of urine are added to the measuring surface and the USG is displayed digitally. A slightly larger amount of

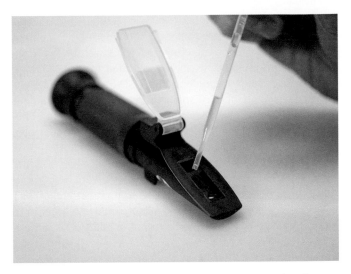

FIGURE 4.24 Handheld optical refractometer – open chamber (Heska; HSK-VET). A drop of urine is placed on the chamber glass and the lid closed. It is important to make sure that enough urine covers the glass in order to avoid artifacts of reading the USG intersection line. The eyepiece is placed near the eye after pointing the analyzer to a lighted area to allow optimal light transmission through the chamber.

urine may be needed for digital refractometers because the urine is not spread evenly against a prism by the sample cover, as with analog refractometers. After each measurement, rinse urine from the measuring surface and cover with distilled water, and then, dry the instrument.

If the measured USG is higher than the upper end of the scale (i.e. refractometers for use in humans have a maximal USG of 1.035 on their scale), the measurement can be repeated after diluting the urine sample with an equal volume of distilled water. After dilution, multiply the last two digits of the value to the right of the decimal point by two to obtain the USG [11, 70, 79]. For example, if the diluted sample reads 1.034, the calculated USG value for the undiluted urine sample would be 1.068. This method is less desirable than a direct reading of USG using an extended scale, because this technique can introduce dilution errors that are magnified by the multiplication factor.

Veterinarians usually expect the USG measured by different refractometers to generate the same results, but variability in these results can be greater than generally appreciated at times. The reproducibility of USG measurement by refractometry is very high when evaluating replicates using the same urine sample and analyzer. Discordance of USG determined on the same urine sample using different analyzers is of minimal clinical relevance in urine samples with low or very high USG. USG values that are close to a cutoff threshold of 1.030 (dog) or 1.035 (cat) could be difficult to interpret, because the reported value could be falsely above or below that threshold, resulting in inaccurate assessment about adequate urine concentration.

Results of USG from urine of 100 dogs presenting to a veterinary teaching hospital were compared following measurement by three optical (Reichert, Heska, and AO) and one digital (Misco) refractometers. Agreement between analyzers for USG was evaluated for all USG and for five USG ranges (from most to least concentrated urine). Though statistical differences were found for USG between refractometer pairs evaluated, very small differences were found for USG as determined between three (Reichert, Heska, and Misco) of the four refractometers. Results using these analyzers were thought to be interchangeable as the differences in USG were consistently <0.002. Differences in USG between the Heska, Reichert, and Misco refractometers were > 0.001 in only 5% of the measurements. The AO refractometer had much greater differences in USG results than the other analyzers. Based on these findings, a recommendation for the use of rigid cutoff points to assess whether the USG is "adequate" or "not adequate" is problematic when the reported USG is within ±0.002 of the prescribed cutoff USG value. For example, if the dog's USG is 1.028 and a USG of 1.030 is used to be considered "adequate" as a cutoff, a rigid interpretation would be that the USG is inadequate when, in reality, the USG might be 1.030 when measured by another refractometer. USG results close to any cutoff point should be repeated later to see if they are still in the same category or not. USG from all the four refractometers was strongly correlated with urinary osmolality, but it was not possible to accurately predict USG from urine osmolality or to predict urine osmolality from USG. A wide range of urine osmolality was predicted from any one USG in this [86] and another study [62].

USG in urine from dogs and cats was determined with a single-scale refractometer and compared to results using a refractometer with separate scales for dogs and cats. The single-scale refractometer generated higher mean USG values that varied by <0.001 USG in dogs and 0.003 in cats. Based on this minimal discordance, the authors of this study concluded that it was not necessary to measure USG on a refractometer with different scales for dogs and cats [87].

Analytical Errors in USG Determination

Several factors can cause errors in the determination of USG. The method of urine collection does not affect the measurement of urine concentration, except in rare instance when the urine sample has been contaminated by other fluids (e.g. water) that could dilute the urine, a situation most likely to occur with voided samples collected by pet owners. The change in USG determined after dilution of urine with water has been reported to be an inverse linear function related to the magnitude of dilution in human urine [74]. However, in one study of dog and cat urine employing dilution with water for urine samples with USG >1.035 measured by one refractometer, USG was neither linear nor accurate compared to pycnometry. In this study, USG by refractometer was falsely increased following dilution [58].

Errors can occur related to laboratory methodology. As mentioned above, air bubbles between the measuring surface and the sample cover of an analog refractometer can affect the

USG reading or lead to misinterpretation of the intersection of the shadow line with the USG scale. Also, a falsely low reading could occur if water remains in the chamber after cleaning its surface. Likewise, reusing disposable pipettes to apply urine to the measurement surface could cause errors as a result of mixing of the new urine sample with residual fluid in the pipette. Failure to verify or calibrate the refractometer before the determination of USG can also lead to erroneous USG results. Some solutes, such as acetone, may cause false increases in specific gravity determined by refractometry as compared to osmolality measurements [71], because ketones increase refraction but are less dense than water [72].

Urine concentration is stable over a few days if the sample is stored in an airtight container to prevent evaporation. Storage time under refrigeration or at room temperature did not significantly alter USG at 6 and 24 hours in 31 dogs and 8 cats in one study, when compared to analysis within 60 minutes of collection [88]. USG did not change up to 72 hours when urine from dogs was stored in refrigerated plain glass tubes in one study. USG significantly increased when urine samples were stored at room temperature in preservative-containing tubes, but the magnitude of increase was not considered clinically relevant [89]. Loss of volatile fatty acids and CO_2 from bicarbonate in the urine contributes to a lower USG after 24 hours of exposure to air [74], which is why it is recommended to store urine in containers preventing these losses before USG is measured. Storage of whole urine or supernatant at either 4 °C or −20 °C for up to six months had no significant effect on USG in urine from dogs and cats in one study [87]. However, urine samples that are not kept tightly sealed during storage are subject to evaporation of water from the sample, which will falsely increase USG. Also, during refrigeration, water vapor from the urine sample may condense on the inside of the container, which will increase USG, emphasizing the need to fully mix the condensate with the rest of the urine sample. Thus, all stored urine samples should be mixed gently before USG measurement.

Solutes can precipitate from solution during storage and refrigeration, which will decrease USG. Visible crystalline precipitates do not readily go back into solution. Suspended elements that do not settle out have the potential to falsely increase USG. An increase in USG of up to 0.005 can occur in urine that is very turbid due to crystals or the presence of numerous WBC and bacteria. USG should be determined on the supernatant to avoid concern about the possibility of turbidity falsely increasing USG [68, 69], (Dr. Hokamp personal communication). Theoretically, urine turbidity that is the result of suspended particles (cells, crystals, mucus) should not affect USG measured by refractometry [90], since USG depends on refraction of light by dissolved molecules. In one study, USG determined from both well-mixed fresh urine and fresh urine from supernatant in dogs and cats was not significantly different [87].

Large amounts of protein or glucose in the urine will increase the USG approximately 0.004 for each g/dL of glucose and 0.003 for each g/dL of protein [2, 48, 91]. A corrected USG in these instances will be more accurate for the purpose of renal function evaluation. Using the guidelines above, the amount of glucose or protein in the urine as measured by a chemical reagent dipstrip can be converted to USG units and subtracted from the original USG to obtain the corrected USG. However, proteinuria up to 100 mg/dL exerted an insignificant effect on measurement of USG in one study [87]. The urinary content of chloride, urea, sulfate, phosphate, creatinine, and bicarbonate accounted for 70–90% of the USG in normal humans with varying intake of dietary protein. On higher protein diets, urea, sulfate, and phosphate contributed more to the USG. Uncommonly measured organic molecules in urine contributed to the remaining 10–30% of the USG (urea and creatinine comprise 50–70% of the organic molecules in urine) [74].

Voided midstream urine was collected from 15 dogs into polystyrene cups and then aspirated into syringes. Urine was applied from the syringe to diapers or mixed into a cup with a standard amount of nonresorbable litter. Urine was aspirated from the diaper and litter at 30 minutes and then hourly up to five hours and USG recorded. Urine stored in the closed syringe had USG measured by refractometry at the same time points. Mean USG from urine in the closed syringe did not change from baseline over these time points, but there was a significant increase in USG beyond the 30-minute time in samples (hours 1–5) compared to baseline from the diaper and litter. Seven samples in the closed syringe stayed the same, seven increased the USG by 0.001, and in one sample, the USG increased by 0.003. Mean USG increased from the litter sample by 0.004 (0.0–0.010), whereas the USG from the diaper sample increased by 0.008 (0.002–0.019 range). The increase in USG occurred more quickly in samples retrieved from the diaper compared to the litter, and an increased USG over time occurred more frequently in samples that had more concentrated urine at baseline. Based on these findings, urine should be retrieved from diapers or nonresorbable litter by 30 minutes after voiding in order to record the most clinically useful results. USG results from urine in a closed syringe were nearly identical for up to five hours [92].

Normal dogs that received saline intravenously at 20 mL/kg for 60 minutes experienced a parallel decrease in USG and urine osmolality, as expected. Urine osmolality decreased, but USG increased in the same dogs after they received hetastarch IV at 20 mL/kg over the same time period. The peak increase in USG occurred at 60 minutes, with a mean USG of 1.070 ± 0.021 (range, 1.036–1.104). The appearance of the large hetastarch molecules (670 kDa) in urine increases USG but not urine osmolality, resulting in the overestimation of renal concentrating ability based on USG [93].

Client-owned healthy cats had USG determined before and during infusion of IV Lactated Ringer's solution or normal saline for 24 hours at 4 mL/kg/hr. Median USG significantly decreased at 12 and 24 hours of fluid infusion, but not at the two- and six-hour time points. Based on these results, obtaining a urine sample up to six hours after starting low-volume IV fluid therapy may allow valuable information about urinary concentration to be gained before it becomes more diluted from the fluid therapy at least in healthy cats [94].

Glucose was added to pooled urine samples of varying USG from dogs and cats, and then, the difference in USG was calculated. Glucose concentration in the urine varied from 50 to 2400 mg/dL. The addition of glucose increased USG, but this change was surprisingly small and not considered clinically important by the authors, even in the presence of high-magnitude glucosuria. USG increased ≤0.005 in most instances but could approach an increase in USG up to 0.010 in some instances especially in the face of higher urinary glucose concentrations. The addition of glucose to urine samples had the greatest increase in USG from samples that were less concentrated, an effect that was greater in urine from dogs than in cats. The authors concluded that it is unlikely that increases in USG in the presence of glucosuria would change a decision as to adequate versus inadequate urine concentration [95], but a change in USG up to 0.005 or up to 0.010 at times could change a clinical interpretation if the USG initially was near accepted cutoff for expected USG. It should also be noted that the mechanical addition of glucose to urine ex vivo does not simulate the decrease in USG that develops following osmotic diuresis when glucose is not reabsorbed by the proximal tubules, as in diabetes mellitus.

IV injection of radiocontrast material makes assessment of USG difficult, because of variable effects on measured USG in dogs. By 15 minutes postinjection, USG increased by as much as 0.034 in some dogs and decreased by as much as 0.037 in other dogs. USG increased in 22 of 30 dogs that received three different doses of radiocontrast material, an effect that appeared to be more marked when baseline USG was <1.040. A positive linear relationship between USG measured by refractometry and amount of radiocontrast material introduced into the bladder (as might occur during urethrocystography) has also been observed [96].

Preservatives in urine (as added tablets or lyophilized in tubes) variably increase USG measured by refractometry from 0.002 to 0.007 units when added to 20–40 mL of human urine. Increases of up to 0.025 units can occur in 5 mL of urine [57].

USG was significantly higher in dark pink and red samples following addition of RBC than in undiluted urine for both dogs and cats in one study. The median USG did not change for dogs following the addition of RBC, but the lower range increased by 0.008 in urine samples graded as red. The median USG for cats increased by 0.005–0.008 in urine graded as dark pink or red following addition of RBC [14].

Expected Urine Concentration: USG by Refractometry

USG in Dogs and Puppies

The USG of healthy dogs varies widely among individual dogs and in the same dog, depending on the time of day. Healthy, hydrated dogs have somewhat concentrated urine when USG is averaged over the course of a day. USG values of

1.018–1.025 were common in urine samples collected randomly throughout the day in healthy dogs in one report [62], and USG values from 1.015 to 1.045 were observed in another report [97]. USG values in dogs are likely to be highest in urine samples obtained in the morning, before the consumption of food and water. Male and female dogs have similar urine concentration.

Most studies of USG in dogs have been carried out using dogs that either were housed in or presented to a veterinary hospital. A mean USG of 1.038 (range, 1.023–1.064) was reported in one study of 20 normal laboratory dogs having free access to water [70]. The mean USG of 60 young dogs on the day of presentation for routine neutering was 1.035 (range, 1.032–1.039) [98]. Mean USG was 1.044 ± 0.009 (range, 1.024–1.059) in 17 mature healthy dogs of both sexes, using samples collected in a veterinary hospital [99].

A mean USG of 1.031 ± 0.012 was reported for 99 apparently healthy senior and geriatric dogs in one study. There was no difference between the combined group data for mean USG and that by senior or geriatric dogs. For the combined group, USG ≥1.030 was found in 58%, USG >1.013–1.030 in 36%, and a USG of 1.007–1.013 in 6% of dogs. Urine samples were collected by ultrasound-guided cystocentesis, but a specific time of the day or protocol for fasting was not reported. An increased serum creatinine was noted in 31 of these dogs, which challenges the notion that they were healthy dogs [100].

In a large study of healthy client-owned dogs, considerable intra- and interindividual variation was observed for USG. Owners of 89 healthy dogs collected voided urine samples in the morning during the first walk of the day and in the afternoon during the last walk for two consecutive days. Details about feeding practices before the walks were not provided, but presumably food and water were consumed before the morning walk. USG varied widely throughout the day in these client-owned dogs. A maximal USG of 1.050 was obtained, but this result may have been a limitation of the refractometer used in the study. USG was lower in the evening (mean, 1.031) than in the morning (mean, 1.035). USG at both times excluded data from 27 young dogs with USG >1.050. USG did not vary by sex but decreased with increasing age in both the morning and evening samples. USG ranged from 1.006 to >1.050 when data from the morning and afternoon samples were combined [97]. The coefficient of variation for USG in individual dogs was approximately 33%, but it was high as 42%. The authors suggested that providing a reference range for USG is not appropriate, given the wide range of USG values in these apparently healthy dogs. Based on these results, normal dogs appear to vary widely in their water drinking behavior, unrelated to physiological needs, which results in considerable variability in USG throughout the day.

USG was measured with the same digital refractometer in 103 apparently healthy dogs using owner-collected, voided urine samples in one study (Figure 4.25) [101]. Urine was collected from each dog in the morning before eating or drinking,

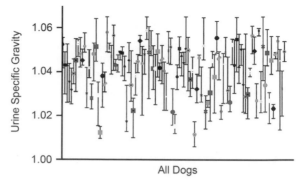

FIGURE 4.25 Variability in median and range for USG in voided first morning urine samples from 103 apparently healthy dogs. This degree of variation in day to day and week to week USG values is considerable and could impact clinical decisions based on rigid cutoff points for expected USG in health. For example, 33% of the dogs in this study had a USG both above and below 1.030 as the frequently used cutoff considered for adequate urinary concentration in the dog. USG was 1.031–1.060 in 83% of dogs in this study. Source: Rudinsky et al. [101] / John Wiley & Sons.

and before any exercise for three consecutive days during two consecutive weeks. The mean USG for the 618 urine samples was 1.040 ± 0.011 with a range of 1.011–1.060. The mean difference between the minimum and maximum USG for each dog was 0.015 ± 0.007. The mean difference in USG for each dog was much smaller when weeks 1 and 2 were evaluated separately. The mean variability in USG in all time points was 15.6%. Over 80% of first morning USG were >1.030, and >1.040 in over 60% in these dogs. USG was 1.051–1.060 in 20.4%, 1.041–1.050 in 40.8%, 1.031–1.040 in 21.4%, 1.021–1.030 in 13.6%, and 1.010–1.020 in 3.4% of these dogs; there were no dogs with hyposthenuria. A total of 42.7% of individual dogs were above and below the cutoff point for USG of 1.050, 47.6% were above and below the cutoff point of 1.040, 33% were above and below the cutoff point of 1.030, 13.6% were above and below the cutoff point of 1.020, and 1.9% were above and below the cutoff of 1.010. The mean difference in USG during the six time points of 0.015 for dogs in this study was large enough that it could change what would be interpreted to be appropriate or inappropriate urinary concentration from day to day or week to week depending on what USG cutoffs are used. The only variable that correlated to decreased USG was increased age in this study [101] as was also found in another study [97]. Decreased maximal urine concentration during "normal" aging could be the result of decreased expression of aquaporins, urea transporters, and vasopressin V-2 receptors that are pivotal in urine concentration [102, 103]. It is also possible that reduced urinary concentrating capacity in the aged is from renal disease that has not been detected [101]. Variation in urine concentration in this study was less than occurred in the van Vonderen study. It seems that careful attention to timing for urine sample collection (i.e. before eating, drinking or exercise) decreases the variability in USG that has been reported in other studies. First morning urine samples before eating, drinking, or exercise are likely to be the most concentrated samples of the day, because healthy pet dogs do not often drink water at night and, thus, are likely to elaborate more concentrated urine as the morning approaches. Clinicians should be aware of the apparently normal fluctuations in USG that can occur in first morning urine samples from normal dogs, both between day to day and week to week that could affect clinical decision-making [101].

The impact of different laboratory personnel reading USG by analog or digital refractometry (variability) was reported from dogs presenting to a veterinary teaching hospital. Urine samples that were positive for glucose, blood, protein, or ketones on urinary dipstrip or those that had crystalluria or bacteriuria on urine microscopy were excluded from this study. Strong agreement in the USG results recorded by three registered veterinary technicians was shown, with a maximal disagreement in USG of 0.002 in either direction between pairs of observers in over 95% of the samples. A USG that differed between observers by 0.005 and 0.006 occurred on two occasions when measured by the analog refractometer. Greater agreement and repeatability of results were reported for USG measured by the digital refractometer. The variability in USG measurement by these highly trained individuals was considered trivial, but it could affect decision-making when the USG is close to a chosen cutoff point (e.g. 1.030 in dogs and 1.035 in cats). Similar studies examining variability for the reporting of USG by different laboratory personnel have not been conducted in dogs with abnormalities on the urinary dipstrip and urinary sediment [104]. In one study of urine from dogs, USG did not significantly differ between samples with an active compared to an inactive urinary sediment [105]. Variability in the measurement of USG as recorded between and within observers was also minimal in another study of dogs and cats [87].

There was no difference in the measurement of USG between observers with various levels of laboratory experience in another study of dogs' urine using four different optical refractometers [90]. There was high agreement in categorization for the degree of urine concentration as highly concentrated (>1.030 USG), moderately concentrated (1.013–1.029 USG), isosthenuric (1.008–1.012 USG), or hyposthenuric (<1.009 USG) for the four refractometers used in this study of dogs. Discordance in categorization for the degree of urine concentration existed in 18 of 59 samples between refractometers when USG values were near the upper and lower limits of the defined USG range. All refractometers measured USG at <1.030 in those with renal azotemia [90].

At a time of slight dehydration after water deprivation of 30–96 hours, maximal USG was 1.062±0.007 (range, 1.050–1.076 USG) in one study of laboratory dogs. The mean duration of water deprivation required to obtain maximal USG was 42 hours, but the duration of time required was highly variable among dogs (range, 0–78 hours). Based on this study, 95% of young dogs that are slightly dehydrated should elaborate urine with USG of at least a 1.048. Interestingly, urine concentration did not maintain maximal USG and most dogs achieved maximal urine concentration mid-way through the water deprivation test (WDT) [70].

After exogenous antidiuretic hormone (ADH) administration to laboratory dogs, maximal USG was lower than that achieved after water deprivation [70, 106–108]. In water-loaded dogs, a mean maximal USG of 1.042±0.009 (range, 1.028–1.057) was achieved after repositol ADH administration. A linear increase in USG was seen starting one hour after the administration of ADH and continued for up to 11 hours in some dogs (mean, 8.38 hours to achieve maximal USG). Water loading in these experimental dogs potentially mimicked polyuria (PU) and renal medullary washout (MWO), resulting in diminished urinary concentration [108]. The mean maximal USG gravity was 1.021±0.0058 (range, 1.012–1.033) after IV administration of aqueous ADH and was achieved after 60 minutes in all but one dog in which USG peaked at 90 minutes. USG rapidly decreased over the next 60 minutes [107].

Urinary concentrating ability in very young puppies is less than that of adult dogs [109–111], but varies considerably. The kidney is functionally and structurally immature at birth and nephrogenesis continues for at least the first two weeks of life [111]. USG was significantly lower in puppies from 0 to 3 weeks of age (mean USG 1.018) compared to puppies 4–24 weeks of age (mean USG >1.032). The highest USG recorded was 1.038 in the zero-to-three-week age group and 1.055 in the 4–24-week age group. The mean USG of puppies >4 weeks of age was comparable to that of adult dogs [112]. USG was higher when two-month-old Beagles (mean, 1.042) were compared to six-to-nine-year-old Beagles (mean, 1.035) [113]. In one study of Great Dane puppies, USG was less concentrated for the first 14 days of life (mean USG <1.020) and then USG increased to become similar to values expected in adults by four weeks of age (mean USG 1.027). USG in these puppies did not vary by litter or sex. The mean USG was 1.014±0.005 when one day old [114].

USG in Cats and Kittens

The widely held clinical impression that healthy cats usually elaborate urine of specific gravity >1.035 as evaluated from random urine samples was supported by one large study of apparently healthy cats examined at first opinion practices. Most cats had USG of 1.040–1.065. The USG was >1.030 in 91% and >1.035 in 88% of these cats. In 121 of 976 adult cats with USG <1.035, no cause was identified in 43, no diagnosis was pursued in 51, and a pathological cause was found in 27 (CKD or hyperthyroidism). USG <1.035 was found in 5 of 64 cats <6 months of age, without identifiable cause. Older cats with USG <1.035 were more likely to have a pathological cause identified [115].

Clinical experience suggests that cats eating mostly dry foods as compared to those eating mostly canned foods have higher USG. This effect may not be as great as generally thought, because the effect of dietary water intake had minimal impact on USG in two studies of client-owned cats [115, 116]. Increasing dietary moisture was associated with lower USG in female but not in male cats, and most cats still had USG >1.040 regardless of dietary moisture [115]. Cats consuming a high moisture diet (73.3%) had USG 1.036 ± 0.002 (standard error of the mean, SEM) compared to a USG of 1.052 ± 0.002 SEM and 1.054 ± 0.002 SEM for cats consuming foods with lower moisture content. No difference in USG was found in cats consuming 6.3%, 25.4%, or 53.2% moisture [117].

A proprietary mix of organic osmolytes, glycerol, amino acids, gum, whey protein, poultry digest, and flavorings (HydraCare® Purina) is now marketed to increase water intake and more optimally maintain hydration in cats. The dry ingredients are added to water to create a nutrient-enriched water (NEW) that is usually served alongside a bowl of tap water to allow the cat a choice of which water source to consume. The gum increases the viscosity of the water. Drinking of NEW increased water intake and urine volume and decreased urine concentration (USG, Uosm) in cats [5, 118] and dogs [119]. A substantial drop in USG occurred from a mean USG of 1.054 at the start to a mean USG of 1.037 over time in association with an increase in water consumed and urine output when NEW without flavoring was consumed by cats. This effect was greater when poultry flavors were added as the mean USG of 1.055 at the start decreased to a mean USG of 1.021 over time [118]. In another study of cats by the same group, mean USG decreased from 1.053 at baseline to a mean USG of 1.031–1.041 depending on time during the consumption of NEW without flavoring. Control cats consuming tap water consistently maintained mean USG from 1.052 to 1.058 over time in this study. The mean USG for cats consuming tap water was 1.054 ± 0.001 (SEM) with most values varying <0.006 over time. Mean USG was lower (1.040 ± 0.002) in cats consuming NEW in this study [120]. Dogs that drank NEW also experienced a substantial decrease in USG from a mean USG at baseline of 1.026 to a mean USG of 1.014–1.018 over time [119]. Consequently, the usual guidelines for the expected USG in healthy cats and dogs may not be operative for use in animals consuming NEW.

The time of day that urine was collected did not influence USG in one study [115]. In an earlier study of colony cats, the time of day also did not affect USG, and no effect of meal versus continuous feeding on USG was found [121]. In 62 healthy cats, mean USG was 1.049 ± 0.013, with a median of 1.052 and range of 1.012–1.075. Thirteen percent of these cats had USG <1.035 [122]. Ninety-nine middle-aged and older apparently healthy cats had a mean USG of 1.046 ± 0.010 in another study by the same group. Fifteen of these cats had a USG < 1.035 [123]. USG of cats evaluated at a teaching hospital ranged from 1.005 to 1.042 (mean, 1.042; median, 1.044) [124].

USG for colony cats eating dry food ranged from 1.041 to 1.072 (mean, 1.056), and from 1.034 to 1.060 (mean, 1.050) when the cats were eating all meat or canned food [125]. In another study, normal adult male colony cats had USG of 1.023–1.084 (mean, 1.057; median, 1.058). Water loading (4–10 mL/kg one to four hours before sampling) in a subset of these male cats resulted in USG of 1.013–1.064 (mean, 1.037; median, 1.040) [124]. USG was determined several times over nine months in nine healthy young colony cats consuming a dry renal diet. The median USG for individual cats ranged from 1.041 to 1.060. Considerable variability in USG was observed in the same cat over time (Figure 4.26). USG was <1.035 in 7.5% of the urine samples and occurred occasionally in five of the nine cats. Time of day did not affect USG in these cats [126] as noted in a study of dogs [97].

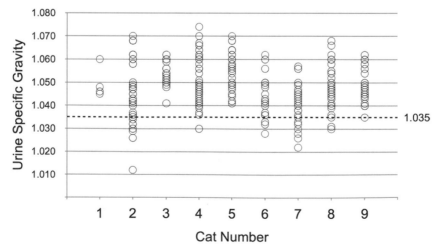

FIGURE 4.26 Individual urine specific gravity variation within nine laboratory cats under normal physiological conditions. Samples were obtained over nine months. The dotted line represents the usual cutoff point at 1.035 used for clinical decision-making in cats. Notice that in five cats, the USG vacillates above and below the 1.035 marker. Source: Adapted from Pelligand et al. [126].

USG was evaluated in 99 apparently healthy cats from 6 to 10 years old (middle-aged), ≥10 years (old), and combined groups. The combined group USG was 1.046 ± 0.010, 1.047 ± 0.010 in cats 6–10 years of age, and 1.044 ± 0.012 in cats >10 years old. Overall, 15% of cats of this study had a USG <1.035, with a frequency of 10.7% in middle aged and 20.9% in old cats. USG from 1.035 to 1.040 occurred in 8% overall, and in 12.5% of middle aged and in 2.3% of old cats. USG >1.040 occurred in 77%, which did not differ from that in middle aged or old cats. The presence of subclinical renal disease could not be excluded in this study [123].

Cats with surgical reduction in nephron mass and azotemia retained considerable ability to concentrate urine, much more so than observed in dogs [127]. Cats became azotemic, and maximal USG decreased, but most cats still had USG >1.040. In another study, despite 5/6 reduction in renal mass and azotemia, 13 of 14 cats with induced chronic renal failure (CRF) retained the ability to concentrate urine to USG >1.035 in at least one of several samples. Cats with induced azotemic CKD eating higher protein diets elaborated less concentrated urine (mean USG, 1.038) than did cats eating a lower protein diet (mean USG, 1.050). Mean USG for individual control cats was 1.050–1.061, a finding that was not significantly different when cats were eating a high or low protein diets [56]. In yet another study, mean USG for 28 normal colony cats was approximately 1.050 before surgical reduction and approximately 1.033 after 11/12 surgical reduction of nephron mass [128].

Less information about urine concentration after water deprivation is available for cats as opposed to dogs. Mean maximum USG was 1.067 ± 0.015 (range, 1.047–1.087) in laboratory cats that achieved 5% body weight loss during water deprivation in one study [127].

USG in apparently healthy kittens was 1.020–1.038 at four weeks of age, 1.024–1.026 at six weeks of age, and 1.047–1.080 at eight weeks of age [129]. In a study of urine from 106 kittens up to 32 weeks of age, the median USG by optical refractometry was 1.060 (range: 1.012–1.070) for all cats. Kittens of this study were able to highly concentrate their urine in most samples in all age groups up to 32 weeks, though 13 kittens had <1.035 USG. Burmese kittens had a significantly lower USG when compared to random-bred kittens. Urine glucose was absent in all but one kitten. Urine protein was commonly detected on dipstrip at trace, 1+ or 2+. Dipstrip reactions to blood were very uncommon in spite of the potentially traumatic method of urine collection by cystocentesis using a 29-gauge needle. Urine pH was most often neutral (Kendall 2021, personal communication).

URINE OSMOLALITY

When available, measurement of urine osmolality by osmometry is a more precise way to determine urine concentration as opposed to USG estimated by refractometry. A higher solute concentration in urine lowers the freezing point, increases the boiling point, increases osmotic pressure, and decreases vapor point pressure. Osmometers employ either vapor point or freezing point methods to measure osmolality, but freezing point depression methods are used much more commonly [2]. It is best to measure both urine and serum (or plasma) osmolality at the same time. Doing so gives better insight into the appropriateness of the urine osmolality as compared to serum or plasma osmolality. For example, in patients with increased plasma osmolality and normal ADH release, urine osmolality should be high in response. The kidney in healthy domestic animals functions as an osmole generator, allowing water conservation over much of a given 24-hour period. Consequently, the ratio of urine osmolality to serum (or plasma) osmolality (U_{osm}/P_{osm}) usually is high (>3) in most dogs and cats over a 24-hour time period.

Simultaneous measurement of urine and serum (or plasma) osmolality is an underutilized method to more critically evaluate urinary concentrating ability and is recommended in challenging cases in which urine does not seem to be adequately concentrated. The U_{osm}/P_{osm} ratio can be very informative in cases for which the cause for PU and polydipsia (PD) is not readily apparent. The basal U_{osm}/P_{osm} ratio and the ratio after water deprivation and ADH administration provide the basis for establishing a definitive diagnosis in these difficult cases of CDI, PPD, and NDI.

Expected Urine Concentration (U_{osm}) in Dogs and Puppies

As with USG, U_{osm} varies widely in order to maintain P_{osm} within narrow limits. Urine osmolality measured on randomly collected urine samples from normally hydrated dogs ranges from 500 to 1200 mOsm/kg [62, 97]. Urine osmolality ranged from approximately 1000 to 2500 mOsm/kg in well-hydrated experimental dogs [70]. Excellent correlation was found between USG by refractometry and U_{osm} in urine from dogs and cats in some studies [5, 87].

Urine osmolality varied greatly throughout the day in 89 apparently healthy dogs using samples collected at home, ranging from 161 to 2830 mOsm/kg. As with USG, U_{osm} was higher in the morning (mean, 1541 ± 527 mOsm/kg; range, 273–2620 mOsm/kg) than in the evening (mean, 1400 ± 586 mOsm/kg; range, 161–2830 mOsm/kg). No effect of sex on U_{osm} was observed. Urine osmolality decreased significantly with age in both morning and later day samples [97].

Urine osmolality ranged from 1400 to 2425 mOsm/kg after 18 hours of water deprivation in one study of dogs [106]. During water gavage in this study, U_{osm} of 400–800 mOsm/kg was observed. In another study, mean maximal U_{osm} was 2289 ± 251 mOsm/kg (range, 1768–2564 mOsm/kg) at a time of mild dehydration. Based on the 95% confidence interval reported in this study, U_{osm} should be at least 1787 mOsm/kg by the time dehydration is detected [70]. Mean maximal urine osmolality was achieved after 39 hours of water deprivation (range, 0–72 hours). As with USG, U_{osm} did not plateau after maximal U_{osm} was achieved [70].

As with USG, the administration of ADH to laboratory dogs results in mean maximal U_{osm} that is lower than that observed after water deprivation. Mean maximal U_{osm} of 1518 ± 242 mOsm/kg (range, 1052–1850 mOsm/kg) was measured after repositol ADH administration in water-loaded laboratory dogs, most often between 9 and 12 hours after injection [108]. Mean maximal U_{osm} was 933 ± 252 mOsm/kg (range, 525–1428 mOsm/kg) after IV administration of aqueous ADH to water-loaded dogs. This U_{osm} was achieved by 60 minutes in most dogs (range, 30–90 minutes), an effect that rapidly dissipated by 120 minutes [107]. Signs of water intoxication were observed in the dogs that were water-loaded and treated with repositol ADH. These signs occurred at the time of maximal urine concentration and lowest serum osmolality as a consequence of concurrent water loading and ADH administration. These signs included pulmonary edema and death in one dog. ADH testing in dogs that are not water-loaded and without opportunity to drink would be unlikely to create signs of water intoxication [108].

A minimal increase in USG or U_{osm} is expected when exogenous ADH is given to normal dogs that have already undergone a WDT. In four dogs that achieved approximately 4.5% body weight loss after 24-hour water deprivation, U_{osm} increased a mean 25 mOsm/kg (range, 10–90 mOsm/kg). Mean U_{osm} increased approximately 2% (range, 0.7–7.3%) over baseline one hour after subcutaneous administration of two units of lysine vasopressin. In this modified WDT, exogenous ADH was administered after hourly measurements of U_{osm} increased <5% between consecutive hourly urine collections [130].

Mean U_{osm} in puppies at 10, 20, and 30 days of age varied from 706 to 743 mOsm/kg in one study [131]. Mean U_{osm} osmolality was higher in puppies (1572 ± 400 mOsm/kg) than in mature dogs six to nine years of age (1241 ± 338 mOsm/kg) in another report [113]. In a study of Beagle puppies, the U_{osm}/P_{osm} ratio increased progressively from 2.0 at two days of age to 7.0 at 77 days of age. The progressive increase was attributed to continued growth in the length of the Loops of Henle that occur during this time [132].

U_{osm}/P_{osm} Ratio in Dogs

Although evaluation of U_{osm} by itself usually is adequate to evaluate urine concentration, the comparison of U_{osm} to P_{osm} can be useful in the evaluation of polyuric conditions (see Section 4.5.6). The U_{osm}/P_{osm} ratio indicates the number of times the kidney concentrates urine over plasma osmolality. This ratio allows the clinician to assess whether U_{osm} is appropriate for the prevailing P_{osm}. The U_{osm}/P_{osm} ratio always is >1.0 when determined from pooled urine samples from healthy animals with free access to water and is usually ≥ 3.0 [62]. In one study of healthy client-owned dogs, the mean U_{osm}/P_{osm} ratio was 6.13 ± 1.37 (range, 2.71–8.1) [99]. In a study of experimental dogs with free access to water, the U_{osm}/P_{osm} ratio was 3.3–8.3 [70].

The U_{osm}/P_{osm} ratio was 4.2–7.5 after 18 hours of water deprivation in one study of dogs [106]. In another study, during water deprivation, the mean maximal urine-to-serum-osmolality (S_{osm}) ratio was 7.3 ± 0.8 (range, 5.7–8.5). Based on these results, 95% of young normal dogs subjected to water deprivation sufficient to produce a slight degree of dehydration should have a U_{osm}/S_{osm} ratio of at least 5.7–1. Serum osmolality increased in 16–20 dogs in this study after dehydration. A significant mean increase in S_{osm} of 13.3 mOsm/kg occurred during water deprivation between initial (mean, 303 mOsm/kg; range, 292–308 mOsm/kg) and final (mean, 315 mOsm/kg; range, 296–328 mOsm/kg) measurements [70].

The mean maximal U_{osm}/S_{osm} ratio for water-loaded dogs after treatment with repositol ADH was 5.6 ± 0.9 (range, 3.8–6.7) [108]. The mean maximal U_{osm}/S_{osm} ratio observed after IV infusion of aqueous ADH to water-loaded dogs was 3.29 ± 0.88 (range, 1.83–5.10) [107].

Expected Urine Concentration (U_{osm}) in Cats and Kittens

A maximal U_{osm} of 3200 mOsm/kg was observed in cats of one early study [133], but other studies have identified even higher maximal U_{osm}. Urine osmolality for laboratory cats eating dry food ranged from 1997 to 4890 mOsm/kg (mean, 2781 mOsm/kg) and from 1147 to 3420 mOsm/kg (mean, 2311 mOsm/kg) when the cats were eating all meat or canned food [125]. In normal laboratory cats that achieved 5% dehydration during water deprivation, mean maximal U_{osm} was 2270 ± 407 mOsm/kg (range, 1581–2984 mOsm/kg). Excellent correlation was found between USG and U_{osm} in this study [127]. In cats of another study, mean baseline U_{osm} was 2612 ± 861 mOsm/kg, and it increased to 3983 ± 1108 mOsm/kg after 5% weight loss induced by water deprivation [134].

In healthy kittens, U_{osm} was 748–1374 mOsm/kg at four weeks of age, 896–2238 mOsm/kg at six weeks of age, and 1697–2903 mOsm/kg at eight weeks of age [129]. The U_{osm}/P_{osm} ratio in kittens increased from 4.6 at 4–6 weeks of age to 8.9 at 13–19 weeks of age in another report [135].

Calculated U_{osm} was highly correlated to the measured U_{osm} in a report from young healthy cats. The employed formula to calculate U_{osm} was $1.25 \times$ urea $+ 1.1 \times$ sodium $+ 67 \times$ glucose (with all units in mmol/L); alternatively, $20.87 \times$ urea (g/L) $+ 1.1 \times$ sodium (mmol/L) $+ 3.72 \times$ glucose (mg/dL). The calculated U_{osm} was an average of 7.30 mOsm/L lower than the measured U_{osm}. This formula has yet to be verified in sick cats [136]. The expense for measurement of these urinary analytes to calculate U_{osm} is likely to exceed that for a measured U_{osm}.

POLYURIA/POLYDIPSIA

Dogs and cats frequently undergo clinical evaluation for excessive consumption of water and increased volume of urine production, sometimes associated with an increased number of urinations and urine house soiling. Table 4.3 details the numerous causes of PU/PD and the likely mechanisms involved. The most common causes of PU/PD in dogs are CKD, diabetes mellitus, or HAC. In cats, the most

Table 4.3 Differential diagnoses and mechanisms for polyuria and polydipsia, or minimally concentrated urine in dogs and cats.

Disease	Diuresis type	Mechanism(s)	Comments
Renal:			
CKD	Solute	Osmotic diuresis in decreased number of remnant nephrons Disruption of renal medulla by renal lesions	Azotemic and non-azotemic CKD when enough nephrons have been lost
AKI	Solute	ATN – ischemia or nephrotoxins Acute interstitial nephritis (allergic or leptospirosis) Impaired sodium reabsorption CT insensitivity to ADH – water diuresis Redistribute blood flow from cortex to medulla (MSW) Eliminate retained solute during conversion from azotemic oliguria to non-oliguria Acquired renal glucosuria in some	Oligo-anuria, non-oliguria, and polyuria are possible depending on cause and extent of acute renal damage
Pyelonephritis	Water	*Escherichia coli* endotoxin ADH antagonism MSW from Increased RBF Acquired renal parenchymal lesions	
Nephrogenic DI	Water	Congenital or familial lack of ADH response (rare) – Huskies Acquired insensitivity to ADH: Idiopathic See hypokalemia, hypercalcemia, endotoxemia, MSW, drugs Autophagic degradation AQP2 Decreased generation cAMP or ATP Decreased expression/activity of Na-K-2Cl cotransporter in mTAL Structural renal mecullary disease – medullary interstitial amyloidosis, PKD, chronic pyelonephritis Drugs – glucocorticosteroids (injection, pill, topical drops), lithium, demeclocycline, inhalational anesthesia, vinblastine, colchicine	Normal or high ADH
Postobstructive diuresis	Solute	Excretion of previously retained solutes Impaired ADH action in CT Impaired tubular sodium reabsorption	
Partial urinary obstruction, chronic	Solute	RBF redistribution Impaired sodium reabsorption CKD – hydronephrosis, renal atrophy	

(Continued)

Table 4.3 (Continued)

Disease	Diuresis type	Mechanism(s)	Comments
Endocrine:			
Diabetes mellitus	Solute	Osmotic diuresis from glucosuria that follows hyperglycemia	
Hyperadrenocorticism	Water	Impaired ADH release (CDI)	
		Impaired ADH action in kidneys (NDI)	
		Psychogenic	
Hyperthyroidism	Mixed	Psychogenic	
		MSW from increased RBF	
		Hypercalciuria	
		Concurrent CKD	
Central DI	Water	Complete or partial loss of ADH synthesis, transport, or secretion	Low ADH
		Reduced circulating ADH available to exert effect in CT;	
		Aquaporin downregulation	
		MSW	
		Congenital: Rare	
		Pituitary and hypothalamic malformations	
		Acquired:	
		Idiopathic	
		Neoplasia (primary or metastatic) pituitary or hypothalamic; other intracranial	
		Brain trauma	
		Encephalitis	
		Post hypophysectomy	
		Parasitic migration	
		Drugs – ethanol, phenytoin, glucocorticoids	
Gestational DI (Transient DI of pregnancy)	Water	Increased vasopressinase activity from placental trophoblasts enhances ADH degradation; related to placental weight during pregnancy	Low ADH
			Suspected but not reported in dogs
		Liver dysfunction leads to less clearance of vasopressinase	Resolves postpartum
			Evaluate liver function
Hypoadrenocorticism	Solute	Decreased renal sodium reabsorption and MSW	
		Ionized hypercalcemia	

Table 4.3 (Continued)

Disease	Diuresis type	Mechanism(s)	Comments
Hyperparathyroidism – primary	Water	Ionized hypercalcemia CKD late – solute diuresis	
Hypoparathyroidism – primary	Water	Psychogenic from low ionized calcium? Hypercalciuria from low PTH effect to reclaim tubular fluid calcium – NDI	
Primary hyperaldosteronism	Solute	ECF volume expansion Systemic hypertension Pressure diuresis CKD develops later	
Acromegaly or hypersomatotropism (Growth hormone excess)	Solute	Anterior pituitary adenoma Insulin antagonism from GH leading to hyperglycemia and glucosuria – diabetes mellitus in cats Renomegaly and CKD CDI when expanding mass invades posterior pituitary or hypothalamus – late advanced disease – water diuresis component then	
Miscellaneous			
Psychogenic polydipsia (primary polydipsia, apparent psychogenic polydipsia)	Water	ECF volume expansion, increased RBF, MSW Thirst center/osmoreceptor hypothalamic dysfunction Neurobehavioral – anxiety?	USG can vary widely over the day (dogs) Exclude hyperadrenocorticism and liver disease Transient phenomenon in some puppies Low ADH
Liver disease (hepatopathy)	Water	Decreased urea synthesis – less medullary solute hypertonicity Decreased clearance/metabolism of endogenous hormones (cortisol, aldosterone, vasopressinase) Psychogenic during hepatic encephalopathy	
Ethylene glycol ingestion (EG)	Solute	EG is low MW and freely filtered at the glomerulus leading to osmotic diuresis	Early before AKI and oligo-anuria are apparent
Renal glucosuria	Solute	Primary renal glucosuria Congenital Fanconi syndrome (Basenji dog) Acquired: Fanconi syndrome (drugs), Jerky treats, tubular phosphatopathy from diets too high in phosphorus (cats)	

(Continued)

Table 4.3 (Continued)

Disease	Diuresis type	Mechanism(s)	Comments
Hypercalcemia	Water	Interference with ADH binding in CT Impaired generation of cAMP in CT Impaired aquaporin expression and action in CT Increased AQP2 degradation by autophagy Increased medullary blood flow – MSW Impaired mTAL Na and Cl reabsorption – (solute diuresis) Psychogenic Development of CKD	
Hypokalemia Potassium depletion (kaliopenia) with or without hypokalemia	Water	Impaired ADH effects in CT – NDI Enhanced AQP2 degradation by autophagy Increased RBF and MSW (solute diuresis) Decreased mTAL sodium reabsorption Psychogenic Development of CKD – (solute diuresis)	GI Losses Hyperaldosteronism Renal wasting Dietary deficiency Marginal dietary potassium repletion in acidifying diet (cats)
Hyponatremia with dehydration – any cause	Solute	MWO	GI hemorrhage common
Pyometra	Water Solute	E. coli endotoxin effect on CT Pyelonephritis Immune complex GN and CKD	
Systemic hypertension	Solute	Pressure induced diuresis	Not well studied
Medullary solute washout	Water	Medullary solute depletion (urea, sodium, chloride, potassium) Polyuric conditions High renal blood flow conditions Low urea nitrogen generation – low protein diet or liver disease	
Hypothermia	Water	Decreased secretion of ADH Decreased tubular responsiveness to ADH Glucosuria in some instances – solute diuresis component	

Table 4.3 (Continued)

Disease	Diuresis type	Mechanism(s)	Comments
Drugs		See NDI and CDI list – water diuresis Furosemide – solute diuresis Mannitol – solute diuresis Dopamine – solute diuresis Desoxycorticosterone – with or without hypokalemia IV iodinated contrast agents – solute diuresis Alpha-adrenergic agents – inhibit AC in CT – water diuresis Potassium bromide – solute diuresis Phenobarbital – uncertain; hepatopathy Glucocorticosteroids – NDI, CDI, PPD, hepatopathy Catecholamines – CDI, NDI, pressure natriuresis	
IV or SQ fluids	Water or solute	Excess water excreted in salt poor fluids Excess solute excreted in salt rich fluids	
High salt intake: diet and some treats	Solute diuresis	Excess salt excreted	
Rare			
Endotoxemia	Water	Impaired ADH effects in CT	
Polycythemia	Water	Unknown; plasma viscosity?	
Multiple myeloma	Water	Unknown; plasma viscosity?	
Splenomegaly	Water	Dipsinogens from splenic tumor – PPD	Not studied; anecdotal
SIAD or SIADH	Solute	ADH released despite low plasma osmolality Increased V2 receptor binding by ADH in CT – USG higher than expected Mild ECF volume expansion Pressure diuresis and natriuresis	Dirofilariasis, encephalitis, hydrocephalus, brain neoplasia, malignant neoplasia, aspiration pneumonia, vinblastine

CKD – chronic kidney disease; AKI – acute kidney injury; ATN – acute tubular necrosis; MSW – medullary solute washout; ADH – antidiuretic hormone, or vasopressin; PKD – polycystic kidney disease; CT – collecting tubule; RBC – renal blood flow; CDI – central diabetes insipidus; NDI – nephrogenic diabetes insipidus; ECF – extracellular fluid; cAMP – cyclic adenosine monophosphate; mTAL – medullary thick ascending limb of Henle's loop; GN – glomerulonephritis; IV – intravenous; SQ – subcutaneous; AC – adenylate cyclase; SIAD – syndrome of inappropriate diuresis; SIADH – syndrome of inappropriate ADH.
Source: Adapted from Bruyette and Nelson [137] and DiBartola [138].

common causes of PU/PD are CKD, diabetes mellitus, or hyperthyroidism.

PD is defined as a larger than normal consumption of water per day. Normal water intake in the dog is approximately 30 mL/lb/day (60 mL/kg/day) or 1 oz of water per pound body weight per day. A small number of normal dogs drink up to 100 mL/kg/day. Cats typically drink less water than dogs, with a maximal water intake of 20 mL/lb/day (45 mL/kg/day). PU is defined as the excretion of a larger than normal quantity of urine per day. Normal urine production in dogs and cats is approximately 12–24 mL/lb BW/day, or 0.5–1.0 mL/lb BW/hour.

PU and PD usually occur together in the animal, and in most instances, obligatory PU occurs first followed by compensatory PD. Occasionally, PD will be the primary problem with compensatory PU, as occurs in PPD. Any alterations in the production of urine (hypothalamic–pituitary–adrenal–kidney axis) or the thirst mechanism can cause PU/PD. Inaccuracy of the client-reported history is likely in most cases in which there appears to be isolated PU or PD. PD may be present without PU, but this is rare. This may occur when there are high ambient temperatures with increased respiratory loss, excessive exercise, a large atonic bladder with increased residual capacity, correction of previous dehydration, and during lactation. This may also occur when there is third space distribution of consumed water into the gastrointestinal (GI) tract, peritoneal space, or pleural space. True PD must be distinguished from pseudo-PD in which the animal appears to be drinking excessively, but in reality, the water does not enter the mouth properly for swallowing, as can happen in those with neurological conditions such as trigeminal palsy with jaw drop. It is essential to distinguish between PU/PD and causes of lower urinary tract distress, in which urine volume is normal to small as discussed further in the next section.

History and Physical Examination

A patient may be presented for the primary problem of PU/PD, or it may only be uncovered after further questioning of the owner. Usually, PU and PD occur together, and it can be difficult to determine which started first. Owners sometimes only recognize PD, and this tends to be more reliable than the recognition of PU. It is helpful to have the owner estimate how much water the animal is drinking in terms of bowls, cups, quarts, etc. Owners typically do not observe cats drinking more water, and it may be necessary to measure the actual amount of water consumed. The fact that a cat is observed drinking water at all may be an important new finding in support of possible PD. It can be difficult to determine the amount of water consumed by an individual when multiple animals are present in the household. The suspected patient may need to be isolated with its own water source for a few days to identify PD. In the history, it is important to make sure that drugs, such as glucocorticoids or diuretics, are not being given. These drugs impair the urinary

concentrating mechanisms resulting in PU/PD. Glucocorticoids administered either systemically or topically (skin, eye, ear) can cause marked PU/PD in dogs. This effect is less pronounced in cats.

Owners may not be able to recognize that PU is present or assess the volume of urine their pet is producing. A negative history of PU/PD does not exclude the possibility that it is present. Dog owners will usually recognize PU/PD more often than cat owners. Increased amounts of saturated litter or larger clumps of clumpable litter in the litter box or an increased urine odor suggest PU/PD in a cat.

The actual volume of water being consumed is not often helpful in determining the cause; however, PU/PD tends to be more severe with PPD and CDI, and more variable in those with NDI. USG in these conditions is typically in the hyposthenuric range (1.001–1.007) at least some of the time. Owners often will confuse pollakiuria (i.e. increased frequency of urination) with PU. Pollakiuria indicates inflammation in the lower urinary tract (i.e. bladder, urethra) regardless of any change in urine volume. Causes of pollakiuria are very different from the causes of PU and must be clearly differentiated from PU when the history is obtained. Animals with PU may have a history of increased frequency of urination because of their need to eliminate a larger volume of urine, whereas animals with pollakiuria void small volumes of urine, often with straining and sometimes hematuria. Nocturia (i.e. urinating during sleeping hours) often accompanies PU and may be the first sign detected by the owner of dogs. Nocturia may be the presenting complaint because PU/PD during the day is not always appreciated.

Physical examination findings may provide some indication as to the cause of PU/PD. Identification of small irregular kidneys on abdominal palpation suggests underlying chronic renal disease; a neck mass in a cat suggests hyperthyroidism. Palpation of abdominal masses can be associated with paraneoplastic hypercalcemia, or PPD sometimes observed in those with various types of splenic masses possibly due to the production of dipsinogens by the mass (unpublished observations by Dr. Couto and Dr. Chew).

Diagnostic Testing

A minimum database, including CBC, serum biochemistry profile, routine urinalysis, and assessment of thyroid function (particularly in cats), should be performed in all animals in which PU/PD is strongly suspected. Diagnostic evaluation in patients with PU/PD is aimed at the identification of the underlying disease, rather than focusing on the urinary concentrating defect. If the USG is minimally concentrated (<1.030 in the dog or <1.035 in the cat), the minimum database is immediately warranted in those with a history of PU/PD, whereas if the USG is higher than expected (>1.030 in the dog or >1.035 in the cat), the owner may be asked to quantitate the patient's water consumption at home for several days before proceeding with an extensive evaluation.

Results from routine serum biochemistry can reveal obvious kidney, liver, or adrenal gland dysfunction that readily account for PU/PD from NDI. A biased review of serum or plasma electrolytes is indicated to exclude those with overt hypercalcemia, hypocalcemia, or hypokalemia that could account for PU/PD from NDI. Increased serum ionized calcium concentration sometimes is discovered when the serum total calcium concentration is normal, so this test should be considered in cases with uncertain origin or PU/PD in those in which total calcium is near the upper range cutoff. Those with a low sodium-to-potassium ratio should be further evaluated for hypoadrenocorticism with post adrenocorticotrophic hormone (ACTH) stimulation cortisol or aldosterone measurement, though some with this diagnosis do not have a low ratio especially when the defect is mostly in the production of glucocorticosteroids. Plasma cortisol or aldosterone concentrations post ACTH stimulation testing should be considered in those with an obscure origin of PU/PD to exclude a diagnosis of hypoadrenocorticism. Suppression testing to measure cortisol post dexamethasone is needed to secure a diagnosis of HAC, often in combination with adrenal imaging especially in dogs. WDT and ADH challenge testing and measurement of urine and plasma osmolality are not indicated when a likely cause for the PU/PD has been discovered from a minimal or extended data base.

A number of underlying disorders may be identified by evaluation of the minimum database, such as renal failure, liver disease, hypercalcemia, hypokalemia, hyperthyroidism, and diabetes mellitus. If the diagnosis is not clear after evaluation of the history, physical examination, and minimum database, further diagnostic evaluation is indicated, including diagnostic tests to exclude HAC in the dog (post dexamethasone cortisol suppression testing). WDT and ADH challenge testing may also be indicated in more obscure cases.

The clinical approach to the evaluation of PU/PD in dogs and cats is presented in Figure 4.27a,b. Submaximal concentration of urine is expected in patients with PU/PD. The USG of normal dogs that are water-deprived should be 1.050–1.076, and 1.047–1.087 in normal cats. A USG of 1.040 is considered the minimum expected value in dehydrated sick dogs or cats. In dogs with PU/PD, WDT is the next step after HAC, CKD, hyperthyroidism, or other metabolic conditions have been ruled out, and only if the dog or cat is not currently dehydrated.

Water Deprivation Testing

A WDT and exogenous ADH administration are sometimes necessary to establish the cause of persistently dilute urine (Figure 4.28). Water deprivation testing assesses the physiologic response of the patient to the hypertonicity of plasma perfusing the hypothalamus. Water deprivation testing is designed to stimulate the release of endogenous ADH into the circulation as P_{osm} increases. Mild dehydration causes release of ADH into the peripheral circulation, where it can exert its effects on the collecting ducts of the kidney to concentrate urine following

water reabsorption that increases the USG. Circulating ADH will increase if the hypothalamic sensing system (i.e. osmoreceptors) and the ability of the pituitary gland to synthesize and release ADH are intact. All water is withheld during the WDT, and food should also be withheld during this time to avoid confusion from the effects of dietary water and solute intake.

WDT results can facilitate definitive diagnosis, but care must be taken to ensure that the patient is not harmed by the test. Water deprivation testing should not be performed in dehydrated animals, and animals with severe PU that does not abate during a WDT are at greatest risk to develop dehydration and marked increases in P_{osm}. The patient's bladder should be emptied and an accurate body weight obtained at the beginning of the study. The patient should be weighed hourly during the initial evaluation period to ensure that no more than 5% loss of body weight occurs. The use of an indwelling urinary catheter will allow frequent evaluation of USG and U_{osm} during the WDT, and after ADH administration if needed.

The WDT must be tailored to the individual patient in terms of what constitutes failure or success. A predefined 12-hour or 24-hour WDT is not appropriate because some animals rapidly become dehydrated and lose sufficient weight (5% of initial body weight) that the test must be stopped, whereas others require a very long time to achieve maximal urine concentration, with only mild weight loss and without clinical signs of dehydration. When the USG fails to increase appropriately after loss of 3–5% of body weight, the test is stopped. When USG (>1.030 in dogs and >1.035 in cats) or U_{osm} increases substantially during the WDT and reaches a plateau (i.e. minimal change between hourly urine samples) with some body weight loss, the test is also concluded.

The exogenous ADH response test is usually performed after a failed WDT (i.e. after USG or U_{osm} has reached a subnormal plateau), but, sometimes, it is used instead of a WDT in fragile patients in order to avoid dehydration (i.e. patients with nonazotemic CKD). Urinary concentrating ability is assessed by administration of exogenous ADH and observation of its effect on USG or U_{osm} [139]. Administration of exogenous ADH ensures that the circulating concentration of ADH is sufficient to allow a positive effect on urine concentration to occur, provided that the countercurrent multiplier and exchanger systems are intact and functional after ADH binding to the V2 receptors of the collecting duct tubular cells. An alternative to such diagnostic testing is to prescribe a therapeutic trial with 1-deamino-8-D-arginine vasopressin (dDAVP, desmopressin) and determine its clinical success as assessed by a reduction in the patient's urine volume and increase in USG or U_{osm} [140].

In the modified WDT, food (but not water) is withheld 12 hours before testing. Urine osmolality and P_{osm} are measured at time zero, and then, all water is withheld. After emptying the bladder, urine osmolality is measured hourly using an indwelling urinary catheter. The modified WDT is continued until <5% change in U_{osm} is observed between hourly measurements, at which time exogenous ADH is injected. In this protocol, two units of lysine vasopressin are injected subcutaneously and U_{osm} and P_{osm} are measured one hour later. Use of the modified WDT allows differentiation of severe CDI, partial CDI, and PPD [130]. In another study of dogs, aqueous ADH (5 mU/0.45 kg) was administered IV over 60 minutes to evaluate urine concentration. Dilution of one unit of vasopressin in 1 L of lactated Ringer's was used to achieve a vasopressin concentration of 1 mU/mL [107].

Pitressin® Tannate in Oil was an extract from the bovine posterior pituitary gland designed for the management of CDI by subcutaneous or intramuscular injection. It was the formulation of ADH originally studied for its effect on

urine concentration in dogs. With the availability of dDAVP, Pitressin Tannate in Oil was withdrawn from the market in 1998.

Synthetic arginine vasopressin (AVP) designed for intramuscular or subcutaneous administration (20 USP units/mL) is manufactured as an aqueous solution (Pitressin vasopressin injection USP) and is approved for use in humans with CDI. The effects of this synthetic form of arginine ADH on urine concentration in dogs have not been reported.

Desmopressin (dDAVP®) is a synthetic analog of the naturally occurring 8-arginine vasopressin. Desmopressin

(a)

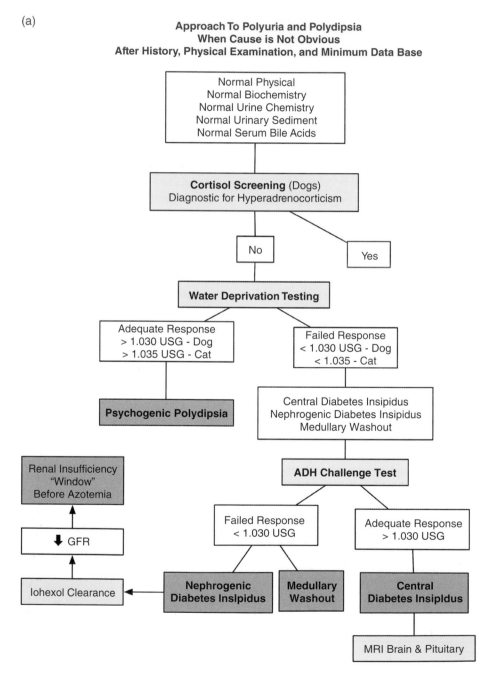

Approach To Polyuria and Polydipsia
When Cause is Not Obvious
After History, Physical Examination, and Minimum Data Base

FIGURE 4.27 (Continued)

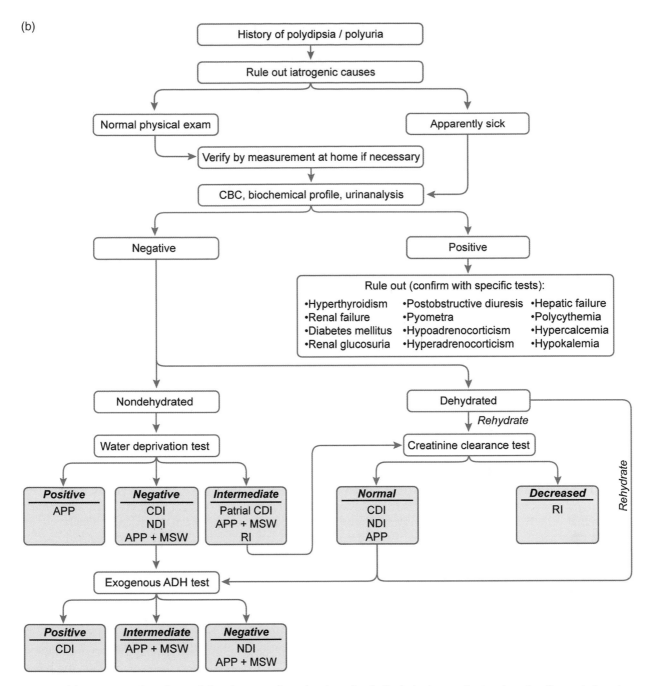

FIGURE 4.27 (a) An approach to determining the cause for polyuria and polydipsia in dogs and cats when the diagnosis is not apparent after evaluation of history, physical examination, and a minimal data base (CBC, serum biochemistry, urinalysis, and imaging). General categories of diagnoses are usually achieved after careful analysis of water deprivation testing (WDT) and exogenous ADH testing. Caution should be exerted to ensure that patients do not become clinically dehydrated during WDT. Clinically fragile patients should not undergo WDT; consider ADH testing instead. (b) This algorithm presents a possible clinical approach to achieve a diagnosis for the patient with polydipsia and polyuria and persistent minimally concentrated to dilute urine. APP, Apparent psychogenic polydipsia; CBC, complete blood count; CDI, central diabetes insipidus; MSW, medullary solute washout; NDI, nephrogenic diabetes insipidus; RI, renal insufficiency with solute diuresis. Source: Illustration by Tim Vojt, reproduced with permission of The Ohio State University.

possesses increased antidiuretic activity and markedly decreased pressor activity compared to the naturally occurring hormone. The antidiuretic-to-pressor ratio is 1:1 for the natural compound and from 2000:1 to 4000:1 for dDAVP. The antidiuretic action is longer lasting than that of the natural hormone, which is attributed in part to a longer half-life [141, 142]. The most common indication for the use of dDAVP is treatment of PU associated with CDI in humans.

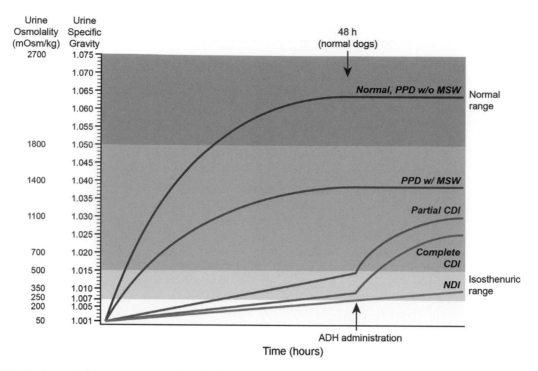

FIGURE 4.28   Idealized expected response to water deprivation testing and exogenous ADH testing in patients with various disorders of water balance. CDI, Central diabetes insipidus; NDI, nephrogenic diabetes insipidus; MSW, medullary solute washout; ADH, antidiuretic hormone. Source: Illustration by Tim Vojt, reproduced with permission of The Ohio State University.

dDAVP challenge testing is often chosen in place of WDT for fragile patients in which dehydration may push them into a crisis (hypotension, AKI). This approach also seems logical for patients that have persistent hyposthenuria and serum sodium that is high or at the high end of the reference range. It is likely that the underlying diagnosis in this scenario is CDI or NDI, both of which will fail the WDT.

There are no reports on the physiological effects of dDAVP on urine concentration in normal dogs or cats, but there are case reports of its use as treatment for CDI. Preparations of dDAVP approved by the FDA, including generics, are available as intranasal aqueous spray (100 μg/mL), sterile IV injection (4 μg/mL), and tablets for oral use (0.1, 0.2 mg). All three formulations appear to effectively decrease urine diuresis in both dogs and cats. Occasionally subcutaneous administration of dDAVP will decrease urine output and increase urine concentration when oral or conjunctival administration does not. During the diagnostic evaluation of patients with PD, PU, and hyposthenuria, subcutaneous injection of dDAVP appears to be more effective than oral or conjunctival administration. According to one protocol, 2–10 μg dDAVP (depending on the animal's body weight) are given IV, and then, USG or U_{osm} is measured every 30 minutes for two hours and then every hour until eight hours after dDAVP was administered. Maximal response to dDAVP   usually occurs within 4–8 hours and rarely after 12–24 hours [143].

Oral administration of dDAVP in conscious dogs led to a dose-dependent increase in peak plasma concentrations of dDAVP as well as the area under the curve [144]. Orally administered dDAVP at a dose of 25–50 μg every 8–12 hours effectively increased USG in five cats with complete CDI. USG in these cats ranged from 1.015 to 1.032 at variable time points after the oral administration of dDAVP [145]. Orally administered dDAVP is also effective in treatment of dogs with CDI [146]. An oral dose of 50–100 μg every 8–12 hours has been recommended for both dogs and cats [145]. GI absorption of dDAVP varies considerably among individuals, which consequently affects the urinary concentrating response. The oral route of administration of dDAVP is not effective in some patients because of inadequate GI absorption, and in some patients, the effect is short-lived despite adequate absorption [143].

The recommended dose of dDAVP for conjunctival administration is 1.5–16 μg (one to four drops of the product designed for intranasal administration in humans) every 12–24 hours; each drop of intranasal solution delivers approximately 1.5–4.0 μg. The response to one to two drops per eye, once or twice daily, was considered excellent in 17 dogs with CDI [147]. Sterile injectable dDAVP (4 μg/mL) is dosed at 0.5–5 μg subcutaneously every 12–24 hours for the treatment of CDI. Preparations designed for intranasal use can be given subcutaneously by injection as this approach is less costly than using the product designed for injection, but the intranasal formulation is not guaranteed to be sterile [143, 146]. Compounded dDAVP (0.01% solution; 100 μg/mL) can be administered using a 100 U/mL insulin syringe (1 μg per U marked on the syringe is delivered).

Hyponatremia rarely develops as a serious adverse effect during dDAVP testing or treatment in clinical patients. It can occur in those that continue to drink excessively when ADH receptors in the kidney are activated by dDAVP to effectively reabsorb water. This scenario is most likely to occur in dogs that have PPD. Water intoxication associated with hyponatremia was observed in all experimental dogs that were water loaded at the time of repositol ADH administration [108].

Urine osmolality is expected to increase by at least 50% over baseline (USG >1.020 or U_{osm} >650 mOsm/kg) after administration of dDAVP to patients with complete CDI. Urine osmolality increases by at least 10–15% in patients with partial CDI. Little to no increase in U_{osm} (<10%) after administration of dDAVP suggests a diagnosis of NDI or PPD [146, 148].

Measurement of Endogenous ADH

The ability to accurately and easily measure basal concentrations of circulating ADH as well as concentrations during dehydration potentially could eliminate the need for WDT and exogenous ADH testing of hyposthenuric patients [149]. Knowing the plasma concentration of ADH could help distinguish among partial and complete CDI. Radioimmunoassay (RIA) methods have been developed to measure extremely low plasma concentrations of ADH (i.e. 10^{-13} mol/L), but it is challenging to develop accurate testing methods because antibodies against ADH are especially susceptible to large molecular substance interference [149]. Measurement of circulating ADH is also difficult under clinical conditions, because ADH undergoes rapid proteolysis after blood collection. To minimize proteolysis, it is necessary to use chilled collection tubes, cold centrifugation, rapid separation of plasma from cellular elements and platelets, and immediate freezing of plasma [143]. The use of protease inhibitors (e.g. aprotinin A) in collection tubes may help stabilize ADH after blood collection. Concurrent measurement of P_{osm} and ADH facilitated the diagnosis of polyuric conditions in dogs in one study and was considered essential to conclusively establish the diagnosis in some instances [139, 148]. Normal cats responded to water restriction with a significant increase in plasma ADH concentration; low ADH concentrations before and after water deprivation were useful in establishing a definitive diagnosis of complete CDI in one cat [134]. Unfortunately, the measurement of plasma ADH concentration is not currently available from commercial veterinary clinical pathology laboratories. Assessment of basal plasma ADH concentration does not always allow a definitive diagnosis because of pulsatile ADH secretion in dogs [150] and the effects of chronic changes in hydration status that alter sensitivity for ADH release [151]. Urinary aquaporin excretion can serve as a surrogate for collecting tubule (CT) exposure to ADH, and its measurement has some technical advantages over measurement of ADH. Urinary aquaporin-2 excretion is upregulated or downregulated after the interaction of ADH with V2 receptors in the principal cells of the CT in healthy dogs after hypertonic or hypotonic saline infusion, respectively [152]. The clinical utility of measuring urinary aquaporins has not been evaluated in dogs or cats with hyposthenuria.

Copeptin is the C-terminal portion of the AVP precursor protein and its secretion mirrors that of AVP secretion. Copeptin is more stable that AVP and is more easily measured, overcoming preanalytic and analytic errors encountered in the measurement of AVP in humans. The use of copeptin to differentiate the causes of hypotonic PU in humans has become more commonplace in recent times either alone or in combination with WDT [153–157]. Studies of copeptin concentrations in dogs and cats that are normal and with a variety of disorders associated with loss of maximal concentrating ability appear warranted. A validated copeptin assay for use in dogs and cats has the potential to more readily allow the differentiation of CDI from NDI.

Mechanisms of PU/PD

Patients with PU/PD can be categorized into those caused by CDI, NDI (including MWO), PPD, or combinations of these disorders. Patients with CDI and NDI often have increased plasma osmolality due to obligatory PU, whereas those with PPD often have normal to low plasma osmolality following primary water intake. High plasma osmolality is associated with increased circulating ADH in health, and low plasma osmolality is generally associated with decreased circulating ADH. Measurement of urine and plasma osmolality along with evaluation of the U_{osm}-to-P_{osm} ratio can be quite helpful in the assessment of difficult or obscure cases with PU/PD. A U_{osm}-to-P_{osm} ratio of >3 is often encountered during adequate urine concentration in dogs and cats. A ratio >1.0 indicates some degree of urinary concentration, a ratio of close to 1.0 defines isosthenuria, and a ratio <1.0 defines hyposthenuria.

The level of plasma osmolality can be used to predict circulating ADH when the hypothalamic–pituitary axis is intact. CDI (partial or complete) is associated with normal to low levels of circulating ADH during times of increased plasma osmolality, whereas PPD is associated with low circulating ADH in association with normal to low plasma osmolality. Treatment with exogenous ADH (desmopressin) restores the ability to elaborate highly concentrated urine in those with CDI but not NDI. NDI accounts for many causes of PU, including MWO from any long-standing cause of PU/PD in association with high but ineffective levels of ADH. As of yet, we do not have clinically available accurate assays for circulating ADH, nor do we have easy access to surrogates for ADH such as the measurement of urinary aquaporins or plasma copeptin. Based on results of WDT and ADH challenge testing along with measurement of plasma and urine osmolality, we often can accurately determine the likely status of endogenous circulating ADH and its activity within the kidneys.

There are four organ systems that must be considered in the pathogenesis of PU/PD: nervous, endocrine, renal, and hepatic systems. The nervous system includes the cerebral cortex and hypothalamus, and the endocrine system includes the pituitary gland, adrenal glands, pancreas, thyroid gland, and paraneoplastic systems. Renal causes could be due to primary renal disease or secondary influences on renal function from systemic disease or another organ dysfunction.

Conditions Associated with Low Circulating ADH

Any disorder that decreases circulating ADH concentrations (CDI, PPD) reduces the ability of the kidneys to elaborate highly concentrated urine. Increased plasma osmolality is the normal stimulus for the release of ADH; thus, low plasma osmolality inhibits the release of ADH into the circulation. PPD leading to PU/PD is often associated with decreased plasma osmolality that then inhibits the secretion of ADH into the circulation. Volume repletion and expansion with IV hypotonic fluids can also lead to decreased plasma osmolality and inhibited release of ADH. Volume expansion with isotonic fluids can also lead to PU/PD from renal mechanisms that do not depend on actions of ADH. In CDI, there is an inability to synthesize, transport, or secrete ADH regardless of plasma osmolality [158]. More rarely, an accelerated degradation of ADH can account for low circulating ADH (described later). Less ADH interaction with its receptor along the CT results in less expression and activation of aquaporins [158], decreased water reabsorption, and the development of hypotonic tubular fluid. Also, less ADH interaction with urea transporters lessens urea reabsorption by the medullary CTs into the interstitium. Less action of ADH on the cortical CT to increase water reabsorption without urea reabsorption also importantly lessens the concentration of tubular fluid urea presented to the medullary CTs. Less ADH action in the mTAL (Na-2Cl-K transporter) results in decreased tubular reabsorption of sodium, potassium, and chloride into the renal interstitium as another mechanism for MWO; high interstitial osmolality is needed to maximally concentrate urine. See Chapter 1 to review the normal physiology of urine concentration.

Central Diabetes Insipidus

Lesions within the hypothalamus or pituitary gland (neoplasia, inflammation, trauma) can result in lower circulating ADH. CDI may be caused by disruption of synthesis or transport of ADH from the paraventricular and supraoptic nuclei in the hypothalamus to the posterior pituitary. Additionally, pituitary lesions can interfere with the release of ADH from the posterior pituitary in CDI. Hypophysectomy always results in CDI, and deficits of hormones secreted by the anterior pituitary are also expected [158]. The release of ADH from the posterior pituitary may be impaired by drugs such as ethanol (alcohol consumption in humans or in treatment of ethylene glycol intoxication in animals), phenytoin (an anticonvulsant not commonly used today), and glucocorticosteroids. Rarely, the osmoreceptor sensitivity may be reset so that a higher plasma osmolality is required before ADH is released into the circulation in some diseases.

The low concentrations of circulating ADH that occur in patients with CDI and with long-standing PPD result in downregulation of aquaporin-2 channel synthesis in principal cells of the CT. This creates a form of NDI that is reversible (see NDI below) [158]. One goal of treatment is to upregulate the synthesis of aquaporin channels after ADH levels have been increased by exogenous ADH supplementation, or by the reduction of excessive water drinking that allows endogenous generation of ADH to increase in those with primary PD. This process may take several days and accounts for why there is often a lag time for the patient to regain the ability to elaborate maximally concentrated urine after treatment has been started despite high concentrations of ADH in the circulation [158, 159]. MWO has been the mechanism most commonly considered in veterinary patients to account for failure to elaborate maximally concentrated urine despite adequate treatment, but these other mechanisms just described are likely to also be important.

The expected decrease in USG will vary by the magnitude of reduction in circulating ADH in CDI and PPD at the time urine was collected. Patients with a maximal absence of circulating ADH will display hyposthenuria (1.001–1.007 USG). Those with minimal to moderate absence of circulating ADH will have higher USG ranging from isosthenuria (1.008–1.017 USG) to minimally concentrated urine (<1.035 USG in cats and <1.030 USG in dogs).

Patients with CDI fail to adequately concentrate urine during WDT, but an increase in their USG, at least in part, is expected following ADH supplementation. Less than maximal urine concentration is expected in some with CDI due to concurrent MWO and decreased aquaporin expression during early treatment with ADH (desmopressin) as a form of reversible NDI. Progressive increases in USG are expected during chronic treatment as AQP expression increases and medullary hypertonicity is restored [158].

Hypothermia

Hypothermia can result in a water diuresis and low USG secondary to decreased release of ADH and decreased tubular responsiveness to ADH. Glucosuria due to reduced proximal tubular reabsorption of glucose can also be observed in human patients [160]. Urine flow has been noted to increase as body temperatures decline, sometimes called cold diuresis [161] that can be associated with reduction in urinary concentration [162]. A marked increase in urine volume and reduction in USG occurred in dogs undergoing experimental hypothermia. Urine volume and GFR returned to normal after rewarming usually by 24 hours [163–165].

Gestational Diabetes Insipidus (GDI)

GDI, or transient diabetes of pregnancy, has not been reported in pregnant dogs or cats, but its presence has been suspected in some pregnant dogs that developed PU and PD. GDI is a rare phenomenon that usually occurs in the third trimester of human pregnancy and resolves postpartum. Lower circulating levels of ADH (AVP) develop mostly as a consequence of increasing activity of vasopressinase by placental trophoblasts resulting in a higher rate for the degradation of ADH, oxytocin, and other small molecules. Vasopressinase activity can increase by as much as 1000-fold in later pregnancy as the placental weight increases, and in those with multiple fetuses. Vasopressinase clearance is decreased in those with liver dysfunction, which is why liver function should be evaluated when GDI is the working diagnosis. Total body water and plasma volume increase substantially during pregnancy, which could increase ADH clearance through increased blood flow to the liver and kidneys. Antagonism to the effect of ADH (NDI) by prostaglandins in pregnancy is another consideration for the development of hypotonic urine. GDI can exacerbate or expose previously unrecognized CDI or NDI [166, 167].

The diagnosis of GDI is strengthened by the finding of hypotonic urine and a low ratio for urine to plasma osmolality; plasma osmolality is normal to increased. Increased urine concentration following treatment with desmopressin secures the diagnosis further. Water deprivation testing could be dangerous to the mother and fetus and is not recommended.

Desmopressin is more resistant to degradation by vasopressinase than AVP and effectively treats this condition in humans [166, 167]. In pregnant dogs with this suspected diagnosis, bacterial UTI (endotoxin effects) and systemic hypertension (pressure diuresis) should be ruled out as other potential causes of PU and PD.

Psychogenic Polydipsia or Apparent Psychogenic Polydipsia (APPD)

Primary PD (PPD) includes two types in humans: dipsogenic and psychogenic. In those with dipsogenic origin, the patient is thirsty despite lack of a physiological need for water intake, due to a lowering of the threshold or setpoint (osmolality, pharyngeal receptors) to initiate thirst. In psychogenic origin, the patient drinks water compulsively without thirst sensation [159]. We are not able to distinguish between these two forms in veterinary medicine.

Primary PD or PPD occurs when excessive water intake occurs beyond that needed for normal physiological needs to maintain hydration, extracellular fluid volume (ECFV), and plasma osmolality [168]. APPD has been suggested as a preferred term by one author, since the ability to diagnose psychoses or neurosis is limited in veterinary medicine and the diagnosis is largely one of exclusion of other known causes of PU/PD [169]. Excess water intake in PPD is the primary driver of the PU that develops as a secondary compensatory response. Several possible mechanisms for PPD were extensively reviewed in an early study of rats [170].

Consumption of water during or just after meals has been commonly observed in animals, but the signals for increased water drinking during these times are not known. The mechanisms involved in this increased intake of water following meals extend beyond that of the dry mouth theory. Dogs are often observed to drink more water soon after eating compared to other times. This is considered to be a normal transient physiological event in most instances. Urine samples after this surge in water drinking can exhibit submaximal urine concentration depending on the time of urine collection after water drinking. Increased water intake can also be observed in experimental animals when there are long pauses without activity or between meals [170]. Excess water drinking during PPD in puppies could occur as a means to feel full when they are not getting enough food, or when there are large gaps in time between feedings. Increasing the volume of food or reducing the time between feedings is sometimes helpful to mitigate PPD in these instances.

In the hypothalamus, there are osmoreceptors that stimulate or inhibit thirst in the so-called drinking center. Plasma hypertonicity stimulates thirst and hypotonicity inhibits thirst in normal animals. Increased temperature of blood perfusing the hypothalamus, dryness of the mucous membranes of the mouth and pharynx, hypotension, and decreased ECFV all stimulate thirst necessary to maintain the constancy of circulating plasma osmolality in health [168, 169, 171–174]. Hypothalamic lesions may adversely affect thirst centers. The stimulation of dipsic or drinking neurons or inhibition of satiety neurons may result in primary PD. Psychogenic factors may be present that cause primary PD with secondary PU. Low plasma osmolality from primary water drinking decreases ADH secretion and action within the kidneys. This can be from an acquired habit that may represent a form of neurosis with no recognizable organic brain lesions in some dogs. PPD can also occur as a result of stimulation of thirst centers by various metabolites (e.g. hepatic encephalopathy), electrolytes disorders (hypokalemia and hypercalcemia), or hormones produced in nonneurologic diseases.

The USG in dogs with psychogenic or primary PD (PPD) will usually be hyposthenuric (≤1.007) at some time points, depending on access to water and the time the urine sample is collected. Complete CDI becomes more likely when all the USG measurements remain in the hyposthenuric range. Water intake is quite variable in those with PPD; thus, more concentrated urine will be seen at other times depending on how much water is ingested. PPD is the only condition in which wide swings in USG from hyposthenuria to highly concentrated urine can be demonstrated on sequential urine samples over a short span. The notion that PPD is uncommon in dogs is not correct in my experience. It is likely that this condition is under diagnosed by academic institutions since primary care veterinarians often handle PPD successfully. Anxiety of some form or psychological disturbances appear to be comorbidities in some with PPD.

Water deprivation testing usually results in a substantial increase in USG over baseline in patients with PPD. The response to increased endogenous ADH during WDT may initially be submaximal due to concurrent MWO or to down-regulation of aquaporin 2 expression that occurs during the suppression of ADH activity in the CTs [172]. Treatment with exogenous ADH to restore medullary hypertonicity and increase aquaporin-2 expression is rarely necessary. WDT can be both diagnostic and therapeutic for PPD. Some dogs with PPD dramatically reduce their water intake as a result of the stress of hospitalization, and this can be a useful diagnostic observation.

Though not specifically studied, PPD appears to be common in some puppies up to six months of age as a transient phenomenon. Why some puppies overdrink water beyond their physiological needs is not known, but they usually outgrow this. It is conceivable that osmoreceptor function in the hypothalamus could continue to mature as some puppies grow.

It appears that adult onset PPD occurs more commonly in large breed dogs and that German Shepherds are an overrepresented breed. PPD was not diagnosed in toy breeds or cats in this series. PU/PD existed for one week to six months before the diagnosis of PPD was made. PPD was more likely to be diagnosed in those with large volume PD in this report. Low-volume PD (1.5 to 2× normal water intake) also occurs in dogs with PPD, usually when evaluated for something else, possibly indicating an early or mild form of PPD [169]. PPD occurs rarely, if at all, in cats. In some instances, the owner may report that the dog has a nervous disposition or that PD developed after some stressful event. Some hyperactive dogs placed in an exercise restricted environment have developed PPD, and some dogs seem to have developed it as a learned behavior to get attention from the owner. Rarely, PPD will be encountered in dogs with primary brain lesions.

In one study, dogs with PPD had daily water consumption of 150–250 mL/kg, USG of 1.001–1.003, urine osmolality of 102–112 mOsm/kg, plasma osmolality of 285–295 mOsm/kg, and serum sodium concentration of 131–140 mEq/L. Although not consistently present, slightly low serum sodium concentration in a dog with PU/PD and marked hyposthenuria supports a diagnosis of PPD. In the same study, approximately 67% of dogs with PPD had a normal response to water deprivation, whereas the others had some degree of renal MWO of solute, but responded to gradual water deprivation or the Hickey–Hare test (response to infusion of hypertonic saline) [169].

Three dogs with primary GI disease of one report had concurrent PU/PD that was associated with PPD, as each was able to highly concentrate urine following water deprivation and no other organ dysfunctions were identified. PU/PD resolved when the GI disease was successfully treated and the clinical signs resolved, but the mediators of primary thirst stimulation were not determined [175].

PPD often can be successfully treated by gradual water restriction into the normal physiological range over several days. This approach usually corrects any renal MWO of solute that is present and allows increased expression of aquaporins as endogenous circulating ADH increases. Lower levels of plasma osmolality and sodium increase to within the normal range during water deprivation and the USG increases. The owner must be careful to eliminate other less obvious sources of water such as toilet bowls or dripping faucets. Water restriction at times during the day or at night may be needed to decrease bouts of excessive water drinking. The shock of hospitalization in a veterinary clinic sometimes corrects PPD at least transiently in some dogs. Treatment of PPD with ADH (desmopressin) is usually not indicated unless MWO is not responsive to gradual water deprivation. Treatment with desmopressin in PPD is potentially dangerous for the development of water intoxication (hyponatremia and brain edema) if excess water drinking persists during the elaboration of concentrated urine. Behavioral modification may be needed in those in which PU/PD returns shortly after water deprivation.

Conditions Associated with Normal to High Circulating ADH
Nephrogenic Diabetes Insipidus

By definition, the urinary concentrating defect associated with PU in NDI is the resistance to the action of vasopressin, despite normal to high concentrations of circulating ADH. Interference with the action of normal or increased concentrations of circulating ADH on the CTs defines both congenital and acquired NDI. Congenital or familial NDI is associated with V-2 receptor mutations in 85–90% of humans, whereas mutations in the aquaporin 2 water channel gene account for the other 10–15% [172, 176, 177]. Congenital NDI is very rare in dogs and cats [178–181]. Hereditary diabetes insipidus was reported in a family of Huskies, in which there were normal numbers of V2-receptors but the affinity for AVP was reduced 10-fold [178, 182].

NDI contains the most expansive number of possible causes and mechanisms for PU/PD. Drug-induced NDI is a common phenomenon [183]. Circulating ADH concentrations in NDI are often high but are not effective within the kidneys. NDI often occurs in association with an increased plasma osmolality that follows obligatory PU from water diuresis when more water than solute loss occurs.

ADH binding to the V-2 receptor increases AQP2 expression, phosphorylation, and trafficking to the apical membrane of the CT principal cell in health is required to generate maximally concentrated urine [184–186]. AQP2 expression in the normal dog kidney determined by immunohistochemistry was located mainly in the apical and subapical region of the collecting duct epithelial cells [187]. Downregulation of AQP2 expression is an important mechanism that accounts at least in part for the PU that develops during the development of NDI in experimental animals with lithium toxicity, hypokalemia, hypercalcemia, ureteral obstruction, ischemic AKI, and CKD [172, 188]. Downregulation of the Na-K-2Cl cotransporter in the mTAL leads to decreased renal interstitial hypertonicity as another mechanism that contributes to ADH resistance.

Interference with the action of ADH occurs when there are not enough V-2 receptors on the CT (as in decreased renal mass), binding to the V-2 receptor on the CT is impaired, or with deficient generation of cyclic adenosine monophosphate (cAMP) and decreased expression or activation of aquaporins after ADH binding to its receptor. The extent of interference with the action of ADH will determine the USG that is elaborated. Obligatory PU occurs in the form of at least a partial water diuresis, such that a USG <1.035 in the cat and <1.030 in the dog will be elaborated. When interference with ADH action is extensive, much lower USG can be expected from minimally concentrated (USG 1.018–1.029 in the dog or USG 1.018–1.034 in the cat), to isosthenuric (USG 1.008–1.017), to hyposthenuria (USG 1.001–1.007).

Medullary Washout

A special form of NDI exists when MWO of solute exists that can develop during long-standing PU of diverse causes. When medullary hypertonicity is reduced for any reason, the osmotic gradient necessary for the movement of water from the collecting ducts into the interstitium and back into the bloodstream is disrupted. The normal hypertonicity of the renal medulla is crucial for the elaboration of highly concentrated urine. MWO is the term used to describe the mechanisms for some polyuric conditions that arise, at least in part, from this lack of interstitial hypertonicity. Depending on the degree of MWO, urine concentration can range from minimally impaired (USG <1.035 in cats and <1.030 in dogs) through a spectrum of further decline to hyposthenuria (1.001–1.007 USG). MWO of solute can occur with long-standing PU/PD of any cause as an accelerated rate of tubular fluid flow diminishes the tubular reabsorption of urea and sodium into the interstitium. Loss of medullary solutes (e.g. sodium, chloride, and urea) reduces interstitial osmolality that is necessary for the elaboration of highly concentrated urine.

Structural lesions do not need to be present for the impairment of concentration to occur during MWO. Increased medullary blood flow in some instances is associated with long-standing PU/PD that can accelerate the removal of solutes by the vasa recta into the systemic circulation. The amount of urea available to enter the renal interstitium is ultimately determined by the amount or urea entering tubular fluid (GFR × the concentration of plasma urea). Reduced urea synthesis that occurs in severe liver disease or PSS decreases the circulating concentration of urea, as does the consumption of very low protein diets, or starvation. Less urea is available in these instances to populate the interstitium with enough solute to maintain the high degree of medullary hypertonicity required to elaborate highly concentrated urine. Urea normally accounts for approximately half of the osmolality of the medullary interstitium. The possibility of MWO as a complicating factor in any disorder associated with PU/PD must be considered in patients that initially fail WDT and ADH challenge testing. Correction of MWO through gradual water deprivation, provision of extra salt in the diet, and treatment with exogenous ADH (desmopressin) is needed at times to replete medullary hypertonicity that then allows the underlying diagnosis to be made with more certainty.

Primary Renal Disease

A critical mass of normally functioning nephrons is required in order to elaborate highly concentrated urine. Both CKD and AKI can result in the elaboration of submaximally concentrated urine and PU as functioning nephrons are lost [188]. PU is commonly encountered in those with CKD, but this can also happen in those with polyuric forms of AKI (e.g. aminoglycoside toxicity sepsis). Isosthenuria occurs in those with azotemic and nonazotemic CKD, classically after the loss of at least two-third of the original nephron mass in that individual animal. Dogs with nonazotemic CKD often develop less concentrated or minimally concentrated urine after the loss of >50% of the original nephron mass, before the loss of enough nephrons to cause azotemia. It appears that a surprising number of experimental cats with more than two-third loss of the original nephron mass continue to be able to elaborate highly concentrated urine; many clinical cats with overt azotemia will be found with minimally concentrated urine. Hyposthenuria (USG 1.001–1.007) is uncommon in CKD, whereas isosthenuria (1.008–1.017 USG) is common in CKD patients with overt azotemia. Some patients will maintain the ability to elaborate urine with minimal concentration (1.018–1.034 in cats or 1.018–1.029 in dogs) especially if the patient is nonazotemic or minimally azotemic. WDT and ADH testing are not indicated in those with CKD. WDT can be dangerous in those with CKD to potentially add an element of renal ischemia and development of AKI on top of CKD.

The major cause of impaired concentrating ability in CKD is the necessity to excrete the daily solute load with a decreased number of functional nephrons resulting in a solute diuresis [189]. Increased fractional urinary excretion of sodium and other electrolytes supports this mechanism. There are several chronic renal diseases that are associated with structural (i.e. histopathologic) abnormalities that preferentially affect the renal medulla that can also contribute to impaired concentrating ability following disruption of the hypertonic medullary interstitium (e.g., pyelonephritis, medullary amyloidosis, polycystic kidney disease [PKD]). Reduced nephron mass in CKD translates to less opportunity for ADH to interact with the CT to allow highly concentrated urine to be elaborated. Additionally, CKD is often associated with renal fibrosis that disrupts the hypertonic renal medulla that disallows maximal urinary concentration. Circulating ADH is expected to be high along with an increased plasma osmolality in CKD patients that often border on dehydration due to increased urinary fluid losses. Despite high circulating ADH, there is renal resistance to effects of ADH to increase tubular fluid water reabsorption [189]. Isosthenuria is common in dogs and cats evaluated with azotemic AKI. Minimally concentrated urine can be encountered when AKI is detected in early phases. Defects in urine concentration occur in AKI due to solute diuresis that follows damaged renal tubules that have a reduced ability to reabsorb sodium from tubular fluid. ADH insensitivity from damaged CT can also be a factor in failure to concentrate urine during AKI.

Usually, in CKD, there is a balanced loss of function in the glomeruli and tubules, so that concentrating capacity is lost after substantial loss of GFR (so-called glomerulotubular balance). Glomerulotubular balance occurs because renal anatomical structure (renal blood vessels, glomeruli, tubules, and interstitium) and renal function are to a large extent interdependent. In some instances, glomerulotubular imbalance can occur. In this situation, the ability to concentrate urine is conserved despite decreased GFR and increased serum creatinine concentration. Glomerulotubular imbalance may occur in dogs when glomerular disease occurs before substantial reduction in postglomerular blood supply and consequent tubular atrophy develop.

A USG of >1.030 in dogs and >1.035 in cats does not exclude the possibility of CKD. A USG >1.035 in cats with experimental and clinical CKD occurs with some frequency, especially during earlier stages of CKD. As CKD advances, reduction in urinary concentrating ability occurs. Why so many cats with both experimental and early clinical CKD are often able to concentrate their urine despite substantial loss of renal mass remains unclear.

Reduced urinary concentration (<1.030 USG) sometimes develops following increased systemic blood pressure by the process of so-called pressure diuresis [190]. This phenomenon has not been well studied in dogs or cats in those with and without underlying CKD. Presumably, the USG would increase to a higher level when normal systemic blood pressure was achieved during treatment.

In patients with CKD, there is nothing that can be done to restore a higher degree of urinary concentrating capacity. However, the magnitude of excess urine volume can be reduced during the feeding of renal diets that are lower in protein and salt intake that reduce the degree of obligatory renal solute excreted.

ENDOCRINE DISORDERS

Adrenal Gland Dysfunction

Hypoadrenocorticism

Dogs with hypoadrenocorticism often have impaired urinary concentrating ability at presentation despite having structurally normal kidneys and ECFV contraction. The combination of low USG and azotemia often results in the erroneous diagnosis of primary renal disease, as the azotemia is prerenal and usually highly responsive to ECFV replacement [191].

Hypoadrenocorticism associated with hyponatremia and hypoosmolality is expected to decrease ADH secretion early on as a form of CDI. As dehydration and ECFV contraction advance, the low extracellular volume and blood pressure signals for the release of ADH predominate over inhibitory signals to release ADH from the low osmolality, but urine is still not maximally concentrated. Aldosterone deficiency in hypoadrenocorticism impairs NaCl reabsorption in the collecting ducts and contributes to MWO of solute and less ability to elaborate concentrated urine as a form of NDI. Ionized hypercalcemia that develops in some dogs with hypoadrenocorticism can contribute to lower USG as another form of NDI; this hypercalcemia is transient and rapidly abates during IV fluid treatment [192, 193].

The USG in dogs with hypoadrenocorticism at presentation has been reported at <1.030 despite dehydration in 58–88% of dogs [191, 194, 195]. Instead of maximally concentrated urine in volume depleted dogs with hypoadrenocorticism, greater than half (99 of 172) of the dogs in one report had a USG <1.030 at initial presentation. USG overall was 1.004–1.055 with a median USG of 1.021 (1.015–1.029 25th to 75th percentile). MWO as a consequence of inability to adequately reclaim filtered sodium needed to replete the hypertonic renal interstitium was considered an important factor in the impaired urine concentration [191]. In another study, USG of 1.010–1.016 was documented during times of hyponatremia, dehydration, and azotemia from different underlying diseases in 11 dogs, two of which had hypoadrenocorticism. Nine of the 11 dogs had evidence for GI blood loss. USG increased to 1.035–1.055 following the correction of hyponatremia in eight of eight dogs with follow-up. It was concluded that hyponatremia could be caused by hemorrhage and that urinary concentrating ability was impaired by hyponatremia irrespective of its cause [196].

Experimental studies in glucocorticoid deficient rats attributed submaximal urinary concentration to reduced interstitial osmolality associated with decreased Na-K-2Cl cotransporter activity in the mTAL. Decreased expression of aquaporins (AQP2) and urea transporters (UT-A1) additionally contributed to elaboration of more dilute urine [172, 197]. Normal urinary concentrating capacity is restored during treatment with physiological doses of mineralocorticoids and glucocorticosteroids in those with hypoadrenocorticism [191, 198].

Hyperadrenocorticism and Glucocorticoid Administration

HAC is most commonly caused by adrenal gland hyperplasia secondary to increased ACTH secretion from a small pituitary tumor, and less commonly by an adrenal gland adenoma or adenocarcinoma. Hypercortisolism characterizes this disorder which can create PU/PD by some combination of CDI, NDI, or PPD. So, depending on the predominant mechanism in a particular patient, the USG can range from hyposthenuric through minimally concentrated. HAC is diagnosed by a combination of cortisol stimulatory (post ACTH) and inhibitory testing (post dexamethasone), measurement of the urinary cortisol to creatinine ratio, and/or adrenal gland imaging. Mechanisms for PU/PD following treatment with exogenous glucocorticosteroids are the same as for excess endogenous cortisol. Some dogs are extremely sensitive to the effects of excess cortisol commonly resulting in PU/PD, and sometimes with polyphagia and or panting.

Minimally concentrated or dilute urine is common in dogs with HAC (canine Cushing's disease) or following exogenous administration of glucocorticosteroids in dogs.

The suspicion for the diagnosis HAC in dogs should be high in those without obvious other causes of PU/PD (e.g. CKD, diabetes mellitus, hypercalcemia) after evaluation of the minimum data base. A varying degree of submaximally concentrated urine will be documented (from hyposthenuria to isosthenuria, and less commonly with minimally concentrated urine). The presence of submaximally concentrated urine, systemic hypertension, and proteinuria is common in dogs with HAC. Cortisol suppression testing should be evaluated in these instances to exclude or confirm HAC as the diagnosis before considering WDT and ADH testing. Dogs with HAC usually fail WDT and ADH testing. Rarely, some cases with psychogenic effects from excess cortisol respond with highly concentrated urine following WDT. Cortisol suppression testing should be analyzed before WDT or ADH testing is employed. The effect of glucocorticosteroids to lessen the degree of urinary concentration in cats is less known.

Glucocorticosteroids are likely to cause PU by inhibiting the release of ADH from the pituitary gland (CDI) by decreasing the reactivity of the osmoreceptor system [42, 199–201] or by interfering with the action of circulating ADH at the level of the CT (NDI) [202]. The expected level of circulating ADH will vary depending on how much effect the excess hormone exerts to create CDI, PPD, and or NDI. Vasopressin-resistant massive PU was acquired following a routine dose of IV dexamethasone in one report in humans [203]. PPD has been encountered by the author in some dogs with excess glucocorticoid activity that produced highly concentrated urine after accidental WDT, though this mechanism has not been reported.

The treatment of HAC with mitotane or trilostane is highly successful in constraining excess circulating cortisol in dogs. A return to lower levels of circulating cortisol usually results in a return to much lower amounts of water consumed, urine volume produced, and an increase in the USG to higher levels. Though not specifically reported, there are anecdotes of dogs with well-controlled HAC based on cortisol levels that still have PU/PD that subsequently respond to exogenous ADH supplementation (desmopressin).

Cortisol administration at 16 mg/kg/day to normal dogs decreased median U_{osm} from 1600 (500–2270 mOsm/kg) to 225 mOsm/kg (70–730 mOsm/kg) and median U/P osmolality ratio from 5.35 (1.70–7.40) to 0.85 (0.23–2.40). Median urine volume increased from 26 (4–93 mL/kg/day) to 300 mL/kg/day (100–750) [202].

Intramuscular injections of cortisone (50–300 mg daily) resulted in a high magnitude of PU/PD in dogs of an early study [204]. The USG decreased substantially in all these dogs during treatment. USG ranged from 1.027 to 1.050 at baseline and from 1.007 to 1.037 during treatment; USG was 1.007 or 1.008 in three of five dogs, 1.018 in one dog, and 1.037 in one dog. Administration of posterior pituitary hormone extract corrected the PU/PD and increased the magnitude of urine concentration [204].

Oral prednisone was given to seven laboratory dogs at anti-inflammatory doses (0.5 mg/kg BID), followed one week later by the addition of desmopressin (5 mcg SQ BID) for five days in an attempt to ameliorate the PU that follows the administration of glucocorticoids to most dogs. Baseline mean USG was 1.034, 1.020 during prednisone alone, 1.047 during prednisone and desmopressin, and 1.015 on prednisone alone after desmopressin had been discontinued. Mean serum sodium was 143.4 mEq/L at baseline, 142.9 mEq/L while on prednisone, 136.2 mEq/L during prednisone and desmopressin, and then 145.2 mEq/L on prednisone after desmopressin had been discontinued. During treatment with desmopressin and prednisone, water intake decreased to levels consumed by control dogs. Though dogs of this study tolerated the combination of prednisone and desmopressin well as they decreased their water intake and increased the USG, the magnitude of hyponatremia that developed was clinically relevant. Hyponatremia developed as a consequence of retention of free water from the activation of ADH receptors on the CTs (higher USG during desmopressin than during any other condition studied). Acute decreases in circulating sodium affect brain function and can result in cerebral edema and seizures. The effect of desmopressin was not studied beyond five days, so close surveillance of serum electrolytes should be undertaken if this protocol is used in clinical patients. The total dose or frequency of the administration of desmopressin could then be adjusted to blunt the development of hyponatremia, if needed, based on the trend in the decline of circulating sodium [205].

Glucosuria: Hyperglycemia, Diabetes Mellitus, and Proximal Tubular Dysfunction

Obligatory solute diuresis in the kidneys occurs in diabetic patients with hyperglycemia above the renal threshold. The filtered load of glucose in hyperglycemic diabetic patients exceeds the reabsorptive capacity of the renal tubules and results in an osmotic diuresis and glucosuria. During euhydration, the USG will be isosthenuric during high levels of tubular fluid glucose excretion. Many diabetic patients with hyperglycemia and glucosuria can concentrate their urine normally at times of dehydration and when the tubular fluid glucose load is minimal. Infusion of 5% or 10% dextrose in water can result in hyperglycemia and glucosuria from the same mechanism. Rarely, a defect in renal tubular reabsorption of glucose (i.e. renal glucosuria; Fanconi syndrome) can be the cause of glucosuria and osmotic diuresis. Solute diuresis is expected to result in the elaboration of isosthenuric urine, though dogs and cats with diabetes mellitus and glucosuria often elaborate urine that is moderately to highly concentrated.

Thyroid Disorders
Hyperthyroidism

Hyperthyroidism is commonly listed in textbooks as a differential for PU/PD and submaximally to minimally concentrated urine in cats. Though there are many potential mechanisms that could account for reduced urinary concentration, impaired ability to concentrate urine solely from hyperthyroidism in cats appears to be uncommon. Reports of PU/PD in cats diagnosed with hyperthyroidism do not easily distinguish between those with and without underlying concomitant CKD. Detection of CKD in cats with hyperthyroidism can be especially challenging since the hyperthyroid state increases GFR. An increased GFR decreases the level of commonly measured GFR surrogates such as serum creatinine, which can mask the diagnosis of CKD. Normal cats that were injected daily with thyroxine for 30 days that induced hyperthyroidism experienced no significant change in USG after treatment (1.041±0.011) compared to before treatment (1.043±0.018) in one study despite increased renal blood flow (RBF) and GFR [206].

Primary PD was proposed as the main mechanism to account for PU/PD in some human thyrotoxic patients, possibly from effects in the hypothalamus [207]. Another study revealed resetting of the osmostat as the threshold of plasma osmolality needed to stimulate thirst and for release of ADH was reduced during the thyrotoxic state. Molecular mechanisms for altered function in the hypothalamus and increased thirst during hyperthyroidism are not currently understood. Another consideration that could account for thirst as a primary mechanism (PPD) is the effect of excess thyroid hormones on higher brain centers, possibly associated with anxiety before treatment [208]. Cats with hyperthyroidism have not been investigated specifically for the possibility of PPD as the main mechanism for increased thirst or submaximally concentrated urine.

Impairment of urine concentration during hyperthyroidism could develop secondary to increased RBF (as reviewed in Chapter 1) and associated MWO. Other considerations for impaired urine concentration include pressure diuresis in those with systemic hypertension and following rare instances of ionized hypercalcemia. Mild hypercalcemia and hypercalciuria occur rarely in humans with thyrotoxicosis due to accelerated bone turnover, sometimes with the development of nephrocalcinosis and renal insufficiency [209, 210]. Impaired urine concentration could be a consequence of underlying CKD and loss of nephron mass that is not related to hyperthyroidism, or alternatively due to CKD that is occurring secondary to glomerular hyperfiltration from the hyperthyroidism.

In a model of hyperthyroidism in rats, increased cardiac output, mean arterial pressure, renal artery pressure, and RBF occurred compared to controls. PD and PU along with increased food intake and increased solute excretion were observed in the hyperthyroid rats. It appeared that the impaired urine concentration occurred in part as a consequence of decreased AQP1 and AQP2 expression in the CT despite adequate ADH. Increased solute excretion occurred despite an increased expression of the Na-K-2Cl cotransporters during hyperthyroidism. It appeared that the decreased filtration fraction and pressure diuresis contributed to solute diuresis in addition to the water diuresis that developed from less aquaporin expression [211].

Mean USG was 1.031 (1.009–1.050) in 57 hyperthyroid cats of an early study [212]. Ten years later, the same group reported another series of 106 hyperthyroid cats in which mean USG was 1.036 (1.010 to >1.050); USG was >1.035 in 52% of the cats in this report [213]. Mean USG in hyperthyroid cats was significantly lower (1.038±0.014) compared to normal cats (1.058±0.008) in another study [214]. Mean USG was 1.046±0.014 in hyperthyroid cats before treatment with radioactive iodine, 1.042±0.015 in cats before methimazole treatment, and 1.033±0.017 in cats treated with surgery. USG at 30 and 90 days following treatment to restore euthyroidism did not change [215]. Prior to methimazole treatment, the mean USG of hyperthyroid cats was 1.041±0.016; four to six weeks after treatment, mean USG declined to 1.033±0.016 [216]. In another series of cats with hyperthyroidism, the mean USG was 1.042±0.016 (1.018–1.070) in cats that did not develop post-treatment azotemia. Mean USG was 1.035±0.014 (1.015–1.058) in cats that developed azotemia post-treatment. Half of the cats that developed post-treatment azotemia had a pretreatment USG of ≥1.035 [217]. In 13 hyperthyroid cats without CKD prior to treatment, the USG was 1.043±0.013, which significantly declined to 1.032±0.013 following conversion to euthyroidism after I-131 treatment [206]. Median USG was 1.035 (1.008–1.084) in 220 hyperthyroid cats prior to treatment of another study. USG <1.024 was found in 28%, 1.024–1.036 in 26%, 1.036–1.046 in 23%, and >1.046 in 23% of cats in this study. Mean USG at initial diagnosis was 1.030 (1.020 25th percentile, 1.049 75th percentile) in those that developed azotemia within 240 days of treatment for hyperthyroidism, whereas the initial mean USG was 1.040 (1.028 25th percentile and 1.060 75th percentile) that did not develop azotemia. USG was significantly associated with survival in this study [218]. In a study of 600 cats with hyperthyroidism before treatment, 51.5% had a USG ≥1.035 and 48.5% had a USG <1.035. Post-treatment with radioiodine, the USG was ≥1.035 in 46% and <1.035 in 54% of the cats. The USG remained concentrated in 78% (241/309) and became dilute in 22% (68/309) post-treatment. Urine that was originally dilute stayed dilute in 88% (256/291) and converted to concentrated in 12% (35/291) post-treatment. Hyperthyroid cats with dilute urine prior to treatment were significantly older and had significantly higher serum creatinine values. Cats with more dilute urine had significantly higher median total serum calcium values that were still within the reference range, and the only three cats with hypercalcemia were in this group. There was no difference in median potassium concentration between groups with more and less concentrated urine, making it unlikely for potassium depletion to adversely affect urine concentration. Following treatment, median serum creatinine increased from 0.9 (0.7–1.1 mg/dL 25th to 75th percentile) to 1.5 mg/dL (1.2–1.7 mg/dL 25th to 75th percentile) in cats with initially concentrated urine. In cats with initially less concentrated urine, the median serum creatinine increased from 1.2 (1.0–1.5 mg/dL 25th to 75th percentile) to 1.9 mg/dL (1.5–2.4 mg/dL 25th to 75th percentile) following treatment. Azotemia (>2.0 mg/dL serum creatinine) developed following treatment in some cats with an initial USG ≥1.035, but this finding was much more common in cats with USG <1.035 prior to treatment [219].

Hypothyroidism

Though hypothyroidism is a common diagnosis in dogs, detailed attention to renal function and urinary concentrating capacity has not been a focus of most clinical reports. PU/PD is not a likely clinical sign in dogs with hypothyroidism. Maximal urine concentration following water deprivation was impaired in a rat model of hypothyroidism. A decreased expression of the Na-K-2Cl cotransporter in the mTAL and resulting decreased medullary hypertonicity and downregulation of AQP2 and AQP3 accounted for the impaired urine concentration; ADH was also not decreased [172]. The GFR was decreased by about 30% during induced hypothyroidism in dogs of one study, but CKD has not been reported in association with hypothyroidism [220]. Hypothyroid dogs had a mean USG of 1.028 ± 0.015 (1.007–1.050) that did not significantly change following treatment with thyroxine, but maximal urine concentrating capacity was not evaluated in this report [221].

Hypercalcemia

Characteristics

Ionized hypercalcemia is frequently associated with urine that has submaximal concentration (lower than expected USG, U_{osm}), especially in dogs. Unlike dogs, many cats appear to retain a high degree of urinary concentrating ability in the face of ionized hypercalcemia, unless they have concomitant CKD [222, 223]. The USG was <1.020 in over 90% of dogs affected with hypercalcemia in one report of 72 cases [224]. Some dogs appear to be exquisitely sensitive in the development of PU/PD after minimal increases in serum ionized calcium concentration. The most common causes for chronic ionized hypercalcemia include malignancy, CKD, primary hyperparathyroidism, and idiopathic (cats); hypervitaminosis D occurs sporadically. CKD in dogs that is associated with increased serum total calcium often is associated with normal ionized calcium [225, 226]. In contrast, cats with CKD and a total calcium above the reference range very frequently had congruent increases in circulating ionized calcium [227].

Both hypercalcemia and hypokalemia are associated with decreased urinary concentrating ability that is out of proportion to other measurements of renal dysfunction early in the process [228], such as GFR and surrogates of GFR including creatinine and SDMA. During more severe and prolonged hypercalcemia, excretory renal function can be decreased by both functional and structural lesions that develop within the kidneys.

Mechanisms of PU/PD in Hypercalcemia

The mechanisms underlying NDI associated with hypercalcemia and or hypercalciuria have been extensively studied in rats and humans, and to some extent in dogs but not in cats. An extensive review for the causes of hypercalcemia is beyond the scope of this chapter; the interested reader is referred elsewhere for reviews [229–237].

The mechanism(s) for impaired urinary concentration during ionized hypercalcemia involve PPD and NDI. Initially, PU/PD appears to follow the functional effects of ionized hypercalcemia on the drinking centers and within the kidneys. Structural kidney lesions that develop during chronic hypercalcemia account for PU/PD in later stages. Hyposthenuria (USG 1.001–1.006) is documented frequently in dogs with ionized hypercalcemia, though isosthenuria (USG 1.007–1.017) or minimally concentrated urine (USG 1.018–1.029) is elaborated at times in some dogs.

In humans, hypercalcemia can directly stimulate thirst centers as the cause for PD, independent of calcium effects on the kidneys [183, 238]. This mechanism has not been confirmed in dogs or cats. In other instances, obligatory PU occurs as a form of NDI when the osmotic gradient in the renal medulla is reduced as a consequence of impaired sodium chloride transport into the interstitium [183]. Hypercalcemia can also interfere with the binding of ADH to its V-2 receptor and disturb post-receptor-binding actions within the CT as another form of NDI. Restoration of normocalcemia following acute or subacute hypercalcemia is typically associated with a rapid return in the ability to elaborate more concentrated urine [238] if there has not been chronic structural damage to the kidneys. Renal concentrating defects may not be reversible with chronic hypercalcemia due to structural renal tubular and interstitial lesions acquired from the hypercalcemia [239].

Decreased GFR and RBF have been demonstrated in humans and experimental animals in both the acute and chronic forms of hypercalcemia. Excess calcium ions alone or in concert with AG-II can mediate renal vasoconstriction that results in this decreased GFR and RBF. The synthesis of renal vasodilatory prostaglandins is stimulated by the excess calcium ions, which then counteracts the vasoconstrictor response to excess calcium. There was a marked increase in the urinary excretion of prostaglandins in one study of rats with chronic hypercalcemia. The role for excess calcium ions in renal vasoconstriction was independent of the effects from AG-II or renal prostaglandins, indicating its primary role in this process. Vasoconstriction from hypercalcemia resulted in greater reduction in GFR than RBF in this study [239].

In one model of chronic hypercalcemia in rats, the maximal mean urinary osmolality was reduced (1669 mOsm/kg) compared to normocalcemic controls (2609 mOsm/kg). Exogenous ADH administration did not increase the degree of urinary concentration, and circulating ADH levels were similar in hypercalcemic and nonhypercalcemic rats supporting NDI as the underlying mechanism. Water restriction in the hypercalcemic rats resulted in a decrease in urine volume and an increase in the mean maximal urinary osmolality compared to hypercalcemic rats consuming ad lib water. Despite water restriction, mean maximal urine osmolality was less and urine volume higher than in the normocalcemic controls. Urinary prostaglandin excretion was markedly increased in hypercalcemic rats (both ad libitum and restricted water intake), but the urinary concentration defects were found to be prostaglandin independent [240]. In contrast, the PU associated with hypercalcemia in rats of another study was found to be prostaglandin dependent [241]. Decreased medullary hypertonicity has been consistently demonstrated during hypercalcemia in most studies. The inner medullary solute concentration correlated with the mean maximal urinary concentration in the rat study by Levi. The lowest tissue solute concentration occurred in hypercalcemic rats with ad libitum water, intermediate solute concentration in water restricted hypercalcemic rats, and the highest medullary solute concentration was encountered in normocalcemic control rats. It was not possible to determine if PD occurred before obligatory PU developed in this study, but the authors concluded that primary PD was unlikely and that the PU was likely to be from a primary renal defect in urine concentration. A marked increase in inner medullary RBF was documented in hypercalcemic rats that could account for decreased interstitial osmolality in this region due to MWO in this study [240].

One author concluded that the most important mechanism contributing to the PU of hypercalcemia was from the decreased renal medullary solute concentration generated as a result of the increased medullary blood flow created by the hypercalcemia. Suppressed secretion of ADH did not appear to play a role in the PU associated with hypercalcemia [242]. Acute and chronic hypercalcemia were associated with marked increases in medullary blood flow in experimental dogs. Redistribution of blood flow from the renal cortex to the deeper regions of the medulla was demonstrated. Dilated vasa recta were demonstrated using vascular casts in dogs with hypercalcemia of this study. This increase in local RBF could largely account for the hyposthenuria of hypercalcemia commonly encountered, due to the washout of medullary interstitial solute that decreased the corticomedullary interstitial osmotic gradient. Another explanation that could account for the hyposthenuria of hypercalcemia, at least in part, is the failure of adequate circulating ADH to increase collecting duct permeability to water during calcium antagonism, as a form of NDI [243].

The PU/PD associated with hypercalcemia is resistant to exogenously administered ADH, ruling out a component of CDI, and serum osmolality is often increased in hypercalcemic patients, which additionally argues against PPD. Consequently, physiological or pathological suppression of ADH release does not appear to contribute to the PU/PD of hypercalcemia in most instances. Hypercalcemia disrupted the normal ability of the kidneys to generate and maintain a hypertonic renal interstitium as the main mechanism for PU/PD, and an increased medullary RBF was considered to be the most important mechanism to account for this reduced

interstitial solute concentration in one review. Additionally, hypercalcemia antagonized the actions of ADH on the CT such that water reabsorption was impaired at this site, but an exact mechanism how excess circulating calcium ions exerted this effect was not clear [242]. The major defect proposed in another report focused on the inability of the CT and DT to fully respond to ADH in the face of hypercalcemia. It was suggested that high extracellular concentrations of calcium ions would likely be associated with high intracellular concentrations of calcium in the CT and DT, which could then interfere with the activation of cAMP at these sites (impaired production or increased destruction of cAMP) [244, 245]. Though ADH may still properly bind to its receptor in the CT and DT, failure to activate cAMP post receptor binding would render the CT and DT impermeant to water and result in the excretion of hypotonic urine.

In a model of hypercalcemic rats, PU was found to be independent from a primary thirst mechanism, but was found to be associated with increased urinary prostaglandin E excretion. Prostaglandin inhibition using indomethacin treatment restored urinary prostaglandin excretion to lower levels and restored the kidney's ability to respond to ADH with the elaboration of more concentrated urine based on U_{osm} during hypercalcemia in this study. Increased prostaglandin synthesis was associated with PU and ADH resistance in this model of hypercalcemia that was overcome during blockade of prostaglandin synthesis [241]. There appears to be antagonism between the effects from ADH and prostaglandins within the kidney. In experimental dogs of one study, the antidiuretic effect of ADH was markedly enhanced based on an increased urine osmolality by threefold when prostaglandin synthesis was inhibited [246]. Nephrocalcinosis has been implicated in the urinary concentrating defects associated with hypercalcemia, likely following an increased concentration of calcium deposited in renal tissues, tubular dysfunction, and reduced sodium transport into the interstitium from the lumen of the ascending limb of Henle's loop. Dietary phosphorus restriction mitigated the decrease in medullary hypertonicity and mineralization of renal tissue during hypercalcemia in this study. Impaired urine concentration based on U_{osm} was seen in hypercalcemic rats consuming a normal phosphate content diet but not in hypercalcemic rats consuming a low phosphate diet. The protective effect of dietary phosphate restriction in this study likely resulted in decreased renal tubular uptake and accumulation of calcium [247].

Effects of Hypercalcemia

The effects of acutely increasing the concentration of circulating calcium were evaluated in one study of experimental dogs. In dogs with moderate total hypercalcemia (mean 15.8 mg/dL), an increased fractional excretion of calcium and sodium into urine was demonstrated, along with increased urine volume and free water excretion. In dogs with more severe total hypercalcemia (mean 27.1 mg/dL), the tubular effects of hypercalcemia were obscured by severe decreases in GFR and RBF [248].

High circulating calcium concentrations are known to exert a toxic effect on renal tubular cells either directly as excess calcium ions in the circulation interact with the basolateral membranes of the tubules or following glomerular filtration of excess calcium ions into tubular fluid that then interact with the luminal membranes of tubular cells [224, 228, 237, 249]. Intracellular toxic effects occur following tubular reabsorption of excess luminal calcium. During chronic hypercalcemia and hypercalciuria, metastatic mineralization of the kidneys occurs early in the medullary collecting ducts and the ascending loop of Henle, sites of maximal calcium tubular fluid concentration. Thickening and calcification of proximal tubular basement membranes are also features of hypercalcemic nephropathy. Mineralized renal tubular cells undergo necrosis and sloughing that contribute to the formation of obstructing calcified casts and intrarenal hydronephrosis [210, 237, 250]. Mineralization of the glomerular basement membranes can also be documented at times. The degree of mineralization will depend on the magnitude and duration of the ionized hypercalcemia as well as any enhancing effect from hyperphosphatemia. AKI during acute hypercalcemia and CKD during chronic hypercalcemia can account for the inability to maximally concentrate urine due to accrual of intrarenal structural lesions. Renal ischemia and acute renal tubular necrosis can be a consequence of hypercalcemia-induced renal vasoconstriction and renal hypoxia, due to direct effects of calcium on vascular smooth muscle, or from effects following increased angiotensin-II generated within the kidneys or from effects of angiotensin-II from the systemic circulation. Varying degrees of tubular atrophy may also occur in association with interstitial infiltration of mononuclear inflammatory cells associated with CKD [210, 237, 249].

Shrunken and collapsed glomeruli with a hyperplastic juxtaglomerular apparatus were reported in dogs with experimentally induced hypercalcemia (serum total calcium >14 mg/dL) in one study, possibly related to calcium-induced vasoconstriction of renal vascular smooth muscle, especially that of the afferent arteriole. Plasma renin activity markedly increased in this study. Segmental distribution of renal tubular lesions (ATN and cellular degeneration) suggested a role for renal ischemia in addition to any direct effect of calcium to damage the tubules [249]. Renal tubular cells undergoing degeneration or death are known to be predisposed to undergo mineralization [210], as described in this study. The mean USG ranged from approximately 1.012 to 1.027 during the 21 days studied. Two of 18 dogs with vitamin D-induced hypercalcemia had transient renal glucosuria [249], likely from a proximal tubulopathy causing impaired glucose absorption from tubular fluid secondary to calcium damage. Renal glucosuria was described in five humans with vitamin D intoxication [251], but this was considered to be an uncommon finding [252]. In general, renal glucosuria has not been noticed to be a consistent finding secondary to calcium

nephropathy in dogs or cats. Hypercalcemic nephropathy has been reviewed in the veterinary literature in some detail elsewhere for the interested reader [231, 234–237].

The Calcium Receptor and PU/PD

The mechanisms that induce PU during early stages of hypercalcemia can vary compared to those operative during later stages of hypercalcemia. Early changes in the CT and urinary concentration that occur within a few days were studied in experimental rodents of one study. The normal trafficking of phosphorylated aquaporins and urea transporter vesicles within the principal cells of the CT to the apical membrane were impaired during hypercalcemia and hypercalciuria of one study. Increased activation of the apical CaR in the CT by luminal tubular fluid calcium increased autophagy over basal levels: phagosomes imbibed AQP2, UT-A1, junctional proteins, cytoskeletal proteins, and damaged mitochondria leading to the formation of autophagosomes that subsequently fused with autolysosomes to degrade their contents. Decreased urinary concentration was then a result of decreased insertion of AQP2 and UT-A1 in the CT apical membranes. Increased autophagy appeared to occur as a result of increased enzyme or protein activity that specifically targeted AQP2 for degradation in both hypercalcemia and hypokalemia. Autophagy is considered to be a basic mechanism that provides cellular protection by removal of protein aggregates and damaged organelles; this process can be highly selective and upregulated during cellular stress [253].

In addition to the effects of tubular fluid calcium on the luminal CaR of the CT during hypercalciuria, activation of the basolateral CaR in the CT by circulating calcium may also be important in the development of PU, ADH resistance, and impaired ability to elaborate highly concentrated urine during hypercalcemia [253, 254]. During chronic hypercalcemia, the Na-K-2Cl cotransporter in the mTAL was downregulated, an occurrence that reduces the ability to generate renal interstitial hyperosmolality as part of the normal countercurrent multiplication system. Stimulation of the basolateral CaR in the mTAL by chronic hypercalcemia has been implicated as a mechanism in this downregulation and resulting decrease in urinary concentration [253].

Reduced expression of the Na-K-2Cl cotransporter in the mTAL was demonstrated as an important mechanism to explain PU and reduced urine concentration in two different models of hypercalcemia in the rat. Other sodium transporter systems in the proximal tubule such as the type-2 Na-P cotransporter and the type 3 Na-H exchanger were also downregulated, which resulted in natriuresis, and the CaR was upregulated in the mTAL in one of these studies. Upregulation of the CaR in the mTAL was considered important in reducing tubular sodium reabsorption, which contributed to reduced urinary concentration [255, 256].

Hypercalcemia activates the CaR in the basolateral membranes of the tubular cells in the loop of Henle and the luminal membrane of the CT, which leads to impaired urinary concentrating ability [254]. Stimulation of the CaR in the basolateral membrane of the mTAL by calcium ions [257] inhibits cAMP generation, resulting in less activity of the Na-K-2Cl cotransporter and a change in lumen charge that favors increased excretion of urinary calcium. Inhibition of salt transport in the mTAL following hypercalcemia is sometimes termed the "furosemide effect" [257]. The increased tubular fluid calcium from the mTAL is delivered to the CT, where it stimulates the luminal CaR that then inhibits the insertion of activated AQP vesicles into the luminal membrane. Both of these mechanisms contribute to elaboration of less concentrated urine [254].

The normal response of ADH on the CT to increase expression of AQP2 in the CT was blunted by higher concentrations of extracellular calcium through interactions with the CaR in a cell culture model using mouse cortical CT. Blockade of the CaR preserved the effect of ADH to increase AQP2 expression. High concentrations of calcium also reduced the generation of cAMP within the CT which can contribute to ADH resistance [258].

Structural disease of the CT during two models of hypercalcemia showed the disruption of tight junctions and cytostructural filaments following increased autophagy and an increased concentration of intracellular calcium in one study. In contrast to the effects of hypokalemia, early hypercalcemia did not demonstrate severe mitochondrial injury in the CT. Long-standing high renal tubular fluid calcium concentration can be associated with increased cytosolic content of calcium within the CT, which can then damage mitochondria and reduce the generation of ATP. Decreased generation of ATP could then increase autophagy as a cytoprotective response [253].

In other studies of rats, downregulation of AQP2 and reduced insertion of AQP2 into apical membranes of the CT were shown to be important in the reduction of urine concentration and PU that developed during hypercalcemia [259]. Treatment with cAMP-phosphodiesterase inhibitors that increased intracellular cAMP in the CT completely prevented the development of PU and reduced urine concentration in another rodent study of hypercalcemia. This treatment prevented the downregulation of AQP2 and AQP3 that were found to be important in this model of hypercalcemia and PU [260].

Potassium Depletion and Hypokalemia

The potential for potassium depletion, with or without the detection of overt hypokalemia, to result in the elaboration of minimally concentrated urine is not often clinically appreciated in dogs and cats. Kaliopenia is the term sometimes used to describe potassium depletion that includes both those with hypokalemia and those with normokalemia [261]. A significant body deficit of potassium can exist without the development of hypokalemia since most of the body's potassium lies within the cells. Consequently, normal serum potassium levels can underestimate total body potassium.

Similar to the NDI that develops from hypercalcemia, AQP2 undergoes autophagic degradation early in the process during hypokalemia that largely accounts for the development of PU and impaired urine concentration. It was hypothesized that depletion of intracellular potassium is associated with decreased ATP production and increased generation of reactive oxygen species that led to mitochondrial damage and selective autophagy of mitochondria (mitophagia) [253, 262].

It is likely that subacute to chronic potassium depletion in dogs and cats contributes to defective maximal urinary concentration, as well as to other primary renal effects and lesions. An effect of potassium depletion that decreases urinary concentration in dogs and cats has not been the focus of most clinical studies, and any possible effect is often obscured by or attributed to the development of progressive CKD. Though CKD can result in hypokalemia, it appears that hypokalemia can also result in the development of CKD at times, especially in cats.

Potassium depletion develops commonly during large volume losses of GI fluid. Primary hyperaldosteronism and renal potassium wasting of any origin should also be considered as causes for potassium depletion and hypokalemia [263, 264]. Additionally, diets deficient in potassium can lead to potassium depletion in dogs [263, 265] and cats [261, 266–268].

Clinical hypokalemia is common during CKD, especially in cats. The contribution of potassium depletion to impaired urinary concentration is easily obscured in those with CKD as there are multiple other mechanisms in CKD that can also account for impaired urinary concentration. Chronic hypokalemia can be the consequence of CKD, or it can be a factor in the development and progression of CKD.

Both functional and structural changes develop in the kidney during chronic potassium depletion. These changes include a reduced ability to concentrate the urine that is initially functional and structural later. Decreased GFR can initially be a result of hemodynamic changes but later due to structural changes. These effects primarily involve the renal tubules, especially the collecting duct early in the process. These renal changes are variably reversible when normokalemia has been restored especially when potassium treatment has been started early [189, 261, 263, 269]. One author contends that impaired maximal urine concentration is the most consistent and important alteration in renal function during states of chronic hypokalemia [263].

The development of primary PD during potassium depletion is a well-established phenomenon. PPD that follows a direct stimulation of the thirst center can account for PU/PD and minimally concentrated urine encountered at times in those with potassium depletion and or hypokalemia. An intrarenal urinary concentrating defect (NDI) accounts for this at other times. A return to normokalemia quickly allows the formation of more concentrated urine and the resolution of PU/PD at times [238, 263, 270].

A potassium-deficient diet fed to normal dogs resulted in increased water intake within 24 hours, even before hypokalemia had developed. Hypokalemia became more apparent when the potassium-deficient food continued to be consumed in the face of PU/PD. The peak of the PU/PD occurred at three to seven weeks of feeding the potassium-deficient diet and gradually abated to near normal values over several more weeks during the continued feeding of the same diet. The magnitude of PU/PD was not related to the circulating levels of potassium in these dogs [271].

PU in association with hypokalemia has also been attributed to reduction in renal medullary hypertonicity secondary to impaired renal tubular transport of sodium and chloride [183]. It is likely that the activity of the Na-K-2Cl transporter in the mTAL of Henle's loop is impaired when there is insufficient potassium to bind to this transporter system. This would decrease the degree of interstitial hyperosmolality generated that is needed for maximal urinary concentration. Impaired water reabsorption in the distal and CTs likely accounts for much of the PU due to the reduced interstitial osmolality, as well as decreased responsiveness of the distal and CTs to ADH at times [183, 263].

PU/PD during potassium depletion likely occurs from a combination of PPD and impaired responsiveness to ADH [269] as a form of functional NDI early in the process. During chronic potassium depletion, the development of structural renal disease will also contribute to the inability to maximally concentrate urine. Chronic potassium depletion is associated with decreased systemic vascular resistance that lowers systemic blood pressure. Additionally, potassium depletion is associated with increased renal vascular resistance that decreases the perfusion of juxtamedullary nephrons, a process mediated through angiotensin-II and thromboxane. Potassium depletion increases ammoniagenesis within renal tissue that then activates complement through the alternative pathway to promote progressive tubulointerstitial injury as part of what has been referred to as kaliopenic nephropathy [261].

A significant decrease in the water permeability of collecting ducts exposed to ADH was reported in hypokalemic rats of one study, a finding that would render the tubular fluid more hypotonic. Reduced generation of cAMP was measured in tissue from the renal papillae, which could explain the ineffective response of ADH to increase water reabsorption from tubular fluid (more dilute urine) following binding to its V-2 receptor [245].

Kaliopenic Nephropathy in Cats

Hypokalemic (kaliopenic) nephropathy has been described as a clinical syndrome in cats either as a result of CKD or resulting in CKD. Whether potassium depletion without hypokalemia can cause progressive CKD in cats has not been established. An increase in the FC for potassium at the time of hypokalemia is frequently documented in these instances. In one study of experimental cats, the development of azotemic CKD and hypokalemia was discovered at the same time in cats fed a urinary acidifying and magnesium-restricted diet that

was marginally replete for potassium [269]. Cats with normokalemic CKD also have high fractional excretion for potassium as part of the adaptive nephron response to maintain potassium balance.

The development of CKD in cats consuming high-protein acidifying diets that were marginally replete in potassium has been observed in several studies [56, 268, 269, 272–276]. The decrease in GFR induced by potassium depletion and acidification was partially corrected during potassium repletion in one study [274]. The magnitude of azotemia and kaliuresis declined in most of the CKD cats during potassium supplementation for two to eight months [261].

Hypokalemia has been reported in 20–30% of clinically azotemic CKD cats at the time of diagnosis [272, 277–279] due to some combination of anorexia (reduced intake), loss of muscle mass, vomiting, and PU. Hypokalemia is less commonly documented in azotemic CKD dogs [280]. Azotemic CKD was the most common diagnosis associated with hypokalemia in cats of one report. Cats with severe hypokalemia (<3.0 mEq/L serum potassium) were 3.5 times more likely to have a diagnosis of azotemic CKD that those with less severe hypokalemia. There was more than a 14-fold increased risk to detect hypokalemia in cats with CKD compared to other diseases [261, 267, 281]. Muscle potassium content from azotemic CKD cats with normokalemia was reduced compared to normal control cats, indicating potassium depletion without a change in circulating potassium [272]. Some cats with azotemic CKD intermittently develop hypokalemia during the course of their disease [269].

In one prospective study, the feeding of a high-protein acidifying diet that was marginally replete in potassium resulted in the development of renal lesions and azotemic CKD in some cats [266, 269]. The mean USG was 1.068 in nine experimental cats at the start before the feeding of this diet. Intermittent hypokalemia was observed in most of these cats throughout the two-year feeding study. Three cats developed isosthenuria and two were found to have severe hyposthenuria before or at the time azotemia was documented. Moderate-to-severe chronic lymphoplasmacytic tubulointerstitial nephritis was found in three cats and milder lesions in two other cats at necropsy [269].

A high urinary FC of potassium was documented in most azotemic cats with hypokalemia in cats of one study. Hypokalemia was attributed to increased urinary loss of potassium aggravated by metabolic acidosis at the same time of inadequate dietary potassium intake. It appeared that dietary supplementation with potassium was effective in slowing or reversing progressive CKD in most hypokalemic cats of this study [268]. Greater excretory renal function following correction of hypokalemia is potentially accounted for by the correction of prerenal factors and intrarenal hemodynamics or resolution of some intrarenal lesions, but these mechanisms have not been studied. Potassium supplementation for six months did not improve GFR in normokalemic CKD cats that were potassium depleted in another study [272].

A potassium-restricted diet with and without an added urinary acidifier was fed to initially normal cats for eight weeks that resulted in hypokalemia and metabolic acidosis. The addition of a urinary acidifier to the diet magnified the degree of hypokalemia and metabolic acidosis that developed and resulted in decreased GFR. Decreased GFR did not happen in cats treated solely with a potassium restricted diet. Potassium supplementation increased GFR to some degree in these instances [274].

Desoxycorticosterone Acetate (DOCA) Administration

PU/PD along with impaired maximal urinary concentration based on USG was observed in dogs treated with DOCA, often in association with hypokalemia or potassium depletion [263, 270, 282, 283]. The maximal urinary concentration based on USG was impaired by potassium depletion, whether or not associated with increased mineralocorticoid activity in one study of dogs treated with DOCA or dietary potassium deficiency [263, 265]. Potassium repletion rapidly corrected the urinary concentrating defect in some studies of dogs, but not in others [263, 265, 270]. The USG in humans with potassium depletion was usually less than 1.015 in one report [263].

Normal dogs treated with DOCA developed PU/PD and reduced urinary concentration that was attributed to primary PD in several early studies. PU/PD rapidly abated when DOCA was discontinued. Varying degrees of increased circulating sodium and decreased potassium along with deficits of intracellular potassium were also noted [270, 282, 283].

In another study, dehydrated dogs treated with DOCA and hydrocortisone exhibited less urinary concentration than prior to treatment. The elaboration of hypotonic urine continued despite the infusion of large doses of ADH indicating a form of NDI. The elaboration of hypotonic urine was attributed to failed water reabsorption by the distal and CTs after DOCA administration and/or potassium depletion, though decreased reabsorption of sodium and chloride needed to maintain renal interstitial hyperosmolality could not be excluded. DOCA enhances sodium reabsorption from tubular fluid, so the increased excretion of free water from this mechanism could also account for hypotonic urine. Hydrocortisone by itself did not affect the circulating potassium or urine concentration in this study [265].

In another study of dogs treated with desoxycorticosterone, PU was associated with the development of potassium depletion and increased urinary prostaglandins. PU was corrected when prostaglandin synthesis was inhibited. Since prostaglandins are known to block the effects of ADH by decreasing ADH-induced synthesis of cAMP, this likely accounted for the PU at least in part. The possibility that potassium depletion reset the osmotic threshold for the release of ADH was not addressed in this study [284]. Similar findings were reported in another study of dogs treated with DOCA in which the PU, but not the hypokalemia, was corrected by treatment with indomethacin. Plasma ADH was increased during this type of PU and treatment with exogenous ADH did not mitigate the PU. The osmotic threshold for the release of ADH was increased, but the rate for ADH release was not changed [285].

Liver Disease

Dogs with liver disease and hepatic encephalopathy had reduced urine concentration based on USG in one study. All dogs had highly increased urinary cortisol to urinary creatinine ratios indicative of hypercortisolism. The osmotic threshold for ADH release was increased (CDI) or there was a blunted response to ADH (NDI) in these dogs that could account for impaired ability to concentrate urine [199], similar to findings in dogs with naturally occurring HAC [42]. Dogs or cats with low circulating urea nitrogen concentrations from liver disease can have impaired ability to concentrate urine due to less availability of urea to recycle within the kidneys to maintain interstitial hyperosmolality. RBF is increased in some liver diseases, which can contribute a degree of MWO that reduces interstitial osmolality and the ability to elaborate maximally concentrated urine.

Endotoxemia

Urinary concentrating ability during sepsis and endotoxemia has not been reported in detail in veterinary medicine. In a subset of horses studied with induced endotoxemia [286], U_{osm} decreased by 10–15% (data not shown; Dr. Toribio, personal communication). Whether or not this was a specific effect of endotoxin or from systemic inflammatory response syndrome was not determined. Acute kidney injury during sepsis in humans is often nonoliguric, but the mechanisms that account for this are not clear [287]. Urine osmolality was rapidly decreased in a study of rats exposed to endotoxin despite high levels of endogenous vasopressin, demonstrating ADH resistance. Inner medullary osmolality was greatly reduced in the endotoxin treated rats compared to control rats. Also, aquaporin expression within the tubular cells of the CT was decreased and its apical localization markedly reduced in the rat endotoxin group, likely a consequence of defective V-2 receptor activation. Exogenous stimulation of the V-2 receptor with desmopressin did not restore AQP expression, but did somewhat increase medullary osmolality and urine osmolality. These findings explain, at least in part, how endotoxin acutely decreased U_{osm} and increased urine volume in this study [287]. In another rat study, the prolonged downregulation of the V-2 receptor appeared to be important in explaining a decreased response to ADH, in addition to downregulation of AQP2 during later stages of sepsis. The inflammatory response to acute endotoxin exposure was considered important in the modulation of this downregulation and prolonged impairment in urinary concentration [184].

Pyelonephritis

The notion that a low USG in dogs with bacterial UTI incriminates a diagnosis of pyelonephritis is a reasonable consideration, but studies comparing the USG in dogs or cats with pyelonephritis to those with cystitis are lacking. Upper urinary infection could result in a decreased USG secondary to inflammatory changes associated with the bacterial infection that disrupt renal interstitial hyperosmolality, or from local effects of endotoxin on the CT. It is conceivable that bacterial infection confined to the lower urinary tract could result in the absorption of endotoxin or other cytokines that are delivered to the kidneys that then impair urine concentration, but this has not been studied. Urine osmolality was determined in a large cohort of women with signs of UTI following the administration of intranasal desmopressin spray and eight hours of water deprivation. Urine osmolality was measured again four to six weeks after treatment of those with initially low U_{osm}. The renal concentrating capacity in women with urinary clinical signs and a positive culture for either *Escherichia coli* or *Staphylococcus saprophyticus* was reduced compared to those with negative bacterial cultures. Urine osmolality increased after antibacterial treatment in those with positive cultures for both those diagnosed with pyelonephritis or cystitis. Urine osmolality was similarly reduced in those diagnosed with pyelonephritis and those with cystitis, rendering the U_{osm} test unreliable in distinguishing between upper and lower bacterial UTI in this study. The finding of reduced urine concentration in those diagnosed with cystitis suggested the presence of subclinical kidney infection, but the possibility for an effect from the absorption of endotoxin or cytokines from the lower urinary tract to affect the upper urinary tract and reduce urine concentration was not considered in this study [288].

Pyometra

The urinary concentrating defect associated with pyometra in dogs has long been appreciated, often attributed to the effects of endotoxin from *E. coli* from the infected uterus. PU/PD is often the initial clinical sign noted by the owner along with vaginal discharge [289, 290] and mandates that pyometra be the top differential diagnosis in the intact bitch with PU/PD until proven otherwise due to the potential for severe illness and death when the diagnosis is delayed. The relationship of pyometra to the finding of proteinuria is discussed in Chapter 7. Impaired urinary concentration resolves following ovariohysterectomy (OHE) in most dogs with pyometra [289, 290].

Early studies attributed PU/PD and the reduced ability to elaborate concentrated urine associated with pyometra to effects within the kidneys following absorption of bacterial toxins from the infected uterus, especially those from *E. coli* [291, 292]. Toxins from *E. coli* isolated from pyometra that were injected into healthy female dogs resulted in a reversible PU and reduced urine to plasma osmolality ratio following water deprivation, supporting this concept. Exogenous ADH given to dehydrated dogs with pyometra did not correct the urinary concentrating defect, suggesting that reduced secretion of ADH from the pituitary was not part of the pathophysiology. Some of the concentrating defect and NDI in pyometra could also be accounted for by underlying glomerular and tubular lesions (CKD) that can be found in dogs with pyometra (see

Chapter 7). A component of MWO due to increased RBF following exposure to *E. coli* endotoxin was considered for its possible contribution to reduce urinary concentration. Progesterone can act an aldosterone antagonist with resulting natriuresis, but progesterone injections alone did not lower urine concentration in healthy dogs unless they developed a pyometra. Renal infection could cause reduction in urine concentration, but no bacteria were demonstrated in the kidneys of this study. The normal ability to elaborate concentrated urine was regained in most dogs within two to eight weeks following surgery to remove the pyometra [291, 292].

Eighty-nine percent of dogs with pyometra in one study had a USG <1.035 and a USG ≥1.030 was found in 19%. Twenty-five percent of the dogs in this study were azotemic all of which had a USG <1.020. Bacterial UTI was documented in 22% of these dogs and bacteria were isolated from the uterus in 64% (59% *E. coli* and 15% *Klebsiella*). A low USG was found in dogs with and without azotemia, as well as in dogs without isolation of bacteria from the uterus. The mean USG was 1.019 ± 0.010 (median USG, 1.018; range, 1.006–1.035) [293].

Dogs with pyometra and proteinuria had lower USG than normal control dogs in two studies by the same group [289, 294]. USG increased following OHE in one study, though USG remained <1.015 in 3 of 14 dogs. The median USG at the time of pyometra diagnosis was 1.016 (1.002–1.050) compared to healthy controls with a median USG of 1.030 (1.010–1.035). The median USG was lower at 1.013 (1.002–1.032) in dogs that also had a UPC >0.5 [294]. Both USG and U_{osm} were reduced when measured two days before the pyometra underwent surgical removal in another study. Most dogs (30 of 44) in this study had a USG of <1.020 at initial diagnosis [295].

In six dogs with pyometra prior to surgery, the median U_{osm} was 340 (104–1273 mOsm/kg), substantially lower than that found in control dogs (median, 1511 mOsm/kg; range, 830–1674 mOsm/kg). Desmopressin administration increased the mean U_{osm} slightly to 431 mOsm/kg (168–1491 mOsm/kg) in dogs with pyometra, but far less than urine elaborated by control dogs with a median U_{osm} of 1563 mOsm/kg (1390–2351 mOsm/kg), findings compatible with ADH resistance and NDI in dogs with pyometra. Vasopressin secretion was not impaired in dogs with pyometra of this study excluding a CDI component to the PU. These findings were compatible with interference at the level of the V-2 receptor and ADH binding, or with reduced aquaporin formation following ADH binding to the V-2 receptor. The mean urine osmolality increased significantly following pyometra surgery [290].

Treatment of pyometra with the prostaglandin synthesis inhibitors indomethacin and meclofenamate to dogs amplified the effect of ADH to increase urine concentration by as much as threefold. This supported a role for prostaglandins to antagonize the intrarenal effects of ADH [246]. Administration of the prostaglandin analog cloprostenol induced PU/PD in bitches of another study [296]. Intrarenal antagonism of ADH by prostaglandins could occur via interference with generation of cAMP following binding of ADH to the V-2 receptor on the CT or alternatively by shifting RBF away from the medulla [171].

Syndrome of Inappropriate Antidiuretic Hormone (SIADH)

The SIADH is a rare differential consideration in dogs or cats with PU/PD and mildly concentrated urine (1.018–1.029 USG) at a time of hyponatremia and low plasma osmolality. Inadequate suppression of ADH or increased activity of ADH, with resultant impaired excretion of free water, characterizes this syndrome [138, 186, 297, 298]. The release of ADH is inappropriate in SIADH, since ADH is being released at normal or higher levels without physiological stimulation from plasma hyperosmolality or from nonosmotic stimulation from hypovolemia and hypotension or drugs. A "normal" ADH during hypoosmolality demonstrates a failure to suppress ADH secretion. In humans with SIADH, ADH may be secreted independent of plasma osmolality (such as with random ectopic ADH release), the osmostat may be reset such that ADH is secreted at a lower circulating osmolality, or ADH secretion fails to be inhibited after a water load and decreased circulating osmolality (sometimes referred to as "vasopressin leak"). In some instances in humans, circulating ADH is not increased, yet more concentrated urine than expected is elaborated, possibly due to increased sensitivity of the CT to existing low levels of ADH or from the actions of some other non-ADH substance capable of activating the V-2 receptor [138, 297–299]. Activating V-2 receptor mutations (gain of function) have been reported for some human patients with SIADH [300, 301]. The increased activity of ADH V2-receptor interactions in the CT increases the expression and trafficking of aquaporins to the apical membranes, which increases the permeability of the CT to water that then enhances the reabsorption of water from the tubules into the circulation [298]. The syndrome of inappropriate antidiuresis (SIAD) has been proposed as an alternative to the use of SIADH, since increased circulating ADH is not always part of the pathophysiology [299, 301, 302].

SIADH has been associated with specific drugs that stimulate the release or enhance the action of ADH, malignancies, pulmonary diseases, central nervous system (CNS) diseases, and idiopathic forms in humans [186, 297–299]. Transient forms of SIADH can also occur following endurance exercise, general anesthesia, nausea, pain, and stress [299].

The diagnosis of SIADH is rare in dogs and even more rare in cats. In dogs, SIADH has been reported in association with dirofilariasis [303], amoebic encephalitis [304], congenital hydrocephalus [305], meningeal sarcoma in the area of the thalamus and dorsal hypothalamus [306], aspiration pneumonia [307, 308], histiocytic sarcoma [309], undifferentiated carcinoma [310], and immune-mediated liver disease [311]. Some nonazotemic dogs with babesiosis had plasma hypotonicity suspected to be caused by SIADH, but it seemed more likely that this was an appropriate compensatory response during systemic hypotension to release ADH [312]. Idiopathic forms of SIADH have been reported in dogs [313, 314].

One cat was diagnosed with SIADH in association with hypothalamic degeneration that was speculated to be caused by Rathke's cleft cyst formation [315]. In another cat suspected to have liver disease, SIADH was diagnosed following anesthesia and laparoscopy [316]. Overdose of vinblastine resulted in SIADH in another cat [317].

The finding of a USG <1.030 in dogs with SIADH will occur during states of hyponatremia and circulating hypoosmolality. The urine will be more concentrated than expected, as the normal mechanism to correct the low circulating osmolality and hyponatremia by elaborating dilute urine are overridden by the inappropriate release and actions of ADH. The excess action of ADH results in enhanced reclamation of free water that then causes mild ECFV expansion, circulating hypoosmolality, and hyponatremia. Despite the action of ADH to reclaim free water by the CT, the USG and U_{osm} are not as high as expected in health in relationship to the amount of ADH in the circulation. ECFV expansion signals elaboration of less concentrated urine and natriuresis from signals to the proximal tubules. Some of the diuresis at this time may develop following "pressure diuresis" from systemic hypertension associated with ECFV expansion. A clue to becoming aware for the diagnosis of SIADH could be the finding of minimally to moderately concentrated urine (1.018–1.029 USG) in association with low circulating osmolality and sodium, in the absence of ECFV depletion that could signal for the release of ADH or edema/ascites associated with hypervolemia that can result in hyponatremia (e.g. CHF, liver disease, nephrotic syndrome).

An important differential diagnosis for SIADH is PPD, in which mild hypoosmolality and hyponatremia can be part of the presentation for overdrinking of water, but in association with a USG that is quite dilute and often hyposthenuric (1.001–1.006 USG; U_{osm}-to-P_{osm} ratio of <1.0 during active water drinking). Elaboration of dilute urine is an appropriate response to excrete the excess water and restore normonatremia and normal plasma osmolality. Circulating osmolality and sodium concentrations can be persistently quite low in SIADH, usually more so than that encountered in PPD of dogs. USG during PPD can vary greatly between hyposthenuria and concentrated urine, depending on bursts of excess water intake. Hypoadrenocorticism due to glucocorticoid deficiency alone can easily mimic the laboratory findings of SIADH, so this diagnosis must be specifically excluded as a cause for hyponatremia [298]. A component of SIADH was incriminated in the development of marked hyponatremia in one dog diagnosed with glucocorticoid deficiency, especially since the dog responded to oral fluid restriction and demeclocycline. USG at baseline was 1.028 at the time of initial detection of hyponatremia in this report [318]. Desmopressin testing is not indicated to make the diagnosis of SIADH and not usually needed for the diagnosis of PPD unless there has been a substantial degree of MWO. An adequate degree of water restriction results in resolution of hyponatremia and hypoosmolality in both PPD and SIADH.

U_{osm} <100 mOsm/kg is expected when ADH has been completely suppressed during times of hypoosmolality. Consequently, U_{osm} >100 mOsm/kg is supportive for failure of ADH activity to be adequately suppressed during SIADH. U_{osm} >300 mOsm/kg can be elaborated during SIADH in humans at times; urine osmolality need not exceed plasma osmolality to secure this diagnosis [138, 298]. Some combination of suppression of the renin–angiotensin–aldosterone system following mild ECFV expansion, ADH-induced natriuresis, and actions of increased natriuretic peptides contribute to the natriuresis encountered in the SIADH [298]. It is important to rule out other causes of hyponatremia such as hypoadrenocorticism, myxedema from hypothyroidism, edema or ascites associated with CHF, severe liver disease, or that associated with nephrotic syndrome before SIADH can be diagnosed with certainty [298]. The finding of normal renal, adrenal, and thyroid function is needed before securing a diagnosis of SIADH [138].

The first line of treatment for SIADH in humans is usually fluid restriction, but the restoration of normal serum sodium can be slow and problematic for chronic compliance of reduced fluid intake. IV hypertonic saline and or furosemide may be needed in patients with critical hyponatremia and CNS signs [297–299, 319]. It is important to restore normonatremia gradually in order to avoid CNS demyelination.

Treatment with lithium or demeclocycline has been used successfully to treat SIADH by increasing free water clearance by the induction of NDI in humans [297, 298, 320]. Lithium enters renal tubular cells through the luminal amiloride sensitive epithelial channel. Some resulting combination of decreased V-2 receptor density, decreased expression of AQP2, and decreased generation of cAMP then creates this form of NDI [321]. Demeclocycline creates NDI by the impaired generation of cAMP and may be safer and more effective than treatment with lithium [297, 322].

Vaptans are competitive inhibitors for ADH binding to the V-receptor that are either selective V-2 inhibitors or nonselective inhibitors that affect both the V-1 and V-2 receptors. Vaptans can be considered first-line treatment at times for SIADH [138, 298] [299]. Selective V-2 receptor antagonists may be preferred as treatment for SIADH since vaptans that also affect the V-1 receptors can lower systemic blood pressure following reduction in total peripheral resistance. Free water clearance (aquaresis) increases during treatment with vaptans by decreased expression of AQP2 followed by an increase in urine volume with lower urinary concentration (USG, U_{osm}) [298]. A specific V-2 receptor antagonist (OPC-31260) was used successfully in the treatment of a dog with idiopathic SIADH for three years. Urine output increased and USG declined during treatment, but hyponatremia persisted [314]. When compliance with long-term water restriction is not possible during treatment of SIADH, treatment with vaptans is an alternative, though they are expensive. The potential utility of vaptan treatment in veterinary medicine has been reviewed [323].

The interested reader is referred to reviews detailing the treatment of SIADH and other causes of hyponatremia that are beyond the focus of this section [138, 297–299, 301, 319].

Catecholamines

Catecholamines are sometimes listed in textbooks as an uncommon differential for reduced urinary concentration and PU/PD, and mechanisms for this effect are not entirely established. Inotropic and vasoactive catecholamines are sometimes used in the emergency/critical care and anesthesia settings in order to increase cardiac output, maintain blood pressure, and provide effective tissue oxygenation [324].

The clinical effects of catecholamine administration on urinary concentrating capacity in dogs and cats are not readily available. Alpha-adrenergics, such as phenylpropanolamine, are often prescribed to control urinary incontinence in neutered female dogs with primary sphincter mechanism incompetence, but changes in urine concentration during treatment have not been reported. Effects on urine concentration or urine flow and urine concentration will vary by whether an alpha-adrenergic, beta-adrenergic, or dopaminergic catecholamine is administered [324, 325]. Increased urine production during treatment with catecholamines may be the result of impaired release of ADH (CDI), pressure natriuresis (NDI), or a direct effect that decreases ADH responsiveness in the CT following binding to the V-2 receptor (NDI).

In one canine study, there was no effect on urinary flow following high-dose injection of norepinephrine (an alpha-adrenergic) into the renal artery, but increased concentrations of circulating norepinephrine increased urinary flow without changing GFR or RBF. Increased urine flow in this instance was attributed to suppressed ADH release rather than a direct effect of the drug to change renal tubular water permeability or changes in renal hemodynamics [326], similar to findings in another study of dogs. The decreased rate for the release of ADH into the circulation was most likely mediated by baroreceptor tone via parasympathetic nerves [171, 325, 327]. Plasma vasopressin concentrations were decreased in a dose-related manner during norepinephrine infusion into normal humans of one study [328].

In a sheep model following IV 0.9% NaCl bolus administration, urine output in control animals increased, and urine output was further increased in sheep treated with phenylephrine (an alpha-adrenergic) or with dopamine. Sheep treated with isoproterenol (a beta-adrenergic) decreased urine output substantially below that of the control group. Pressure diuresis and release of atrial natriuretic peptides causing natriuresis were considered a likely explanation for the increased urine output during phenylephrine treatment in this study [324].

Rats treated with epinephrine or norepinephrine (alpha-adrenergics) developed diuresis, whereas those treated with isoproterenol (beta-adrenergic) developed antidiuresis in another study. Alpha-adrenergic stimulation is thought to inhibit the generation of cAMP within renal tissues that could impair CT responsiveness to ADH with resulting diuresis. Beta-adrenergic stimulation increases generation of cAMP, which results in greater responsiveness to ADH, leading to water conservation and greater urine concentration [171].

Iatrogenic

Iatrogenic factors that can result in PU/PD include administration of glucocorticoids, diuretics (e.g. furosemide thiazides), IV or subcutaneous fluids, nephrotoxic drugs (e.g. aminoglycosides), and high-salt diets or treats. Some inhalation anesthetics (e.g. halothane, methoxyflurane) and drugs (e.g. lithium, demeclocycline) can interfere with ADH action in the collecting ducts (NDI), as previously discussed. Increased excretion of low-molecular-weight IV radiocontrast agents can result in a transient osmotic diuresis. A thorough review of drugs, supplements, diagnostic agents, and dietary intake including salty treats is important in disclosing a definitive cause for PU/PD at times.

Colchicine and vinblastine are microtubule disrupting alkaloids that can markedly inhibit the response of the CTs to ADH as one type of NDI. The disruption of ADH effect by these compounds was marked on lessening urinary concentration, but urinary osmolality remained greater than plasma osmolality. The integrity of the microtubule assembly system is needed in order to elaborate urine of maximal osmolality [329, 330]. The specifics of urinary concentrating capacity have not been reported in dogs or cats undergoing treatment with either colchicine or vinblastine. SIADH seemed likely in a case report of vinblastine overdose in a cat [317].

CATEGORIZATION AND INTERPRETATION OF THE DEGREE OF URINE CONCENTRATION

The degree of urine concentration is precisely defined on the basis of urine osmolality in comparison to plasma osmolality. ADH release in response to plasma hyperosmolality promotes water retention and elaboration of maximally concentrated urine, whereas plasma hypoosmolality inhibits ADH release and allows for the production of maximally dilute urine. No single USG or U_{osm} can be considered normal on an absolute basis. A wide range of USG or U_{osm} is physiologically possible, but healthy dogs and cats typically elaborate moderately to highly concentrated urine, even when well hydrated. Depending on individual circumstances, a USG range of 1.001–1.070 for dogs and 1.001–1.080 for cats can be considered normal, but values that persist at the high and low ends of these ranges are not common. The average USG throughout the day should be >1.020 in dogs and >1.035 in cats.

Since there is variability in USG by refractometry among instruments (discussed earlier), it is important to NOT use rigid guidelines for interpretation of USG for those with USG near the cutoff point for classification as appropriate or not. USG that is >0.006 above or below classic cutoff points allow categorization as appropriate or not with some certainty. Those with USG near the cutoff points should have repeat USG measured to see if results are more clear-cut on subsequent samples.

It is best to try and determine if the degree of urine concentration is appropriate for the animal's hydration status (i.e. well hydrated or dehydrated), its food and water intake, and whether or not the patient is azotemic. Thus, the USG must be interpreted according to the individual situation. For example, a USG of 1.010 may be normal in a dog that recently drank a bowl of water, and the USG could be 1.038 later in the day. The finding of minimally concentrated urine in a normally hydrated animal should prompt reevaluation of USG at another time, preferably using a first morning sample before the animal has eaten food and drunk water to determine if the low USG finding is repeatable or not. USG <1.040 in a dehydrated animal is inappropriate (a USG of 1.030–1.040 would be considered equivocal), and would be cause for concern about renal dysfunction or endocrine disorders.

USG should be evaluated before treatments (e.g. glucocorticoids, diuretics, crystalloid fluids) that could affect urine concentration are started. The presence of minimally concentrated urine after such treatments is difficult to assess.

Although it potentially is possible to elaborate urine with a USG ≤1.002, such a finding is very uncommon. In such instances, it is possible the sample is not actually urine, or that the urine has been diluted with water or other fluid [2]. Such confusion is more likely to occur with voided urine samples collected by the owner. Collection of another sample is recommended to confirm or refute the finding of extremely low USG.

A USG <1.030 in dogs and <1.035 in cats is compatible with a history of PU and PD, and often the USG is <1.020. USG that fluctuates widely from low to high values sometimes occurs in normal dogs at various times of the day, and such a finding can also occur in patients with PPD of any cause (e.g. idiopathic, HAC, liver disease, conditions with hypercalcemia). A diagnosis of PPD is supported when a urine sample collected at home has a very low USG, but a sample collected in the hospital has a higher USG. In patients with suspected PU and PD, a USG >1.030–1.035 in a randomly collected urine sample should prompt the clinician to obtain additional history to eliminate other disorders that may have been confused with PU (e.g. urinary incontinence, dysuria).

In a study of 18 young dogs with PU and PD since they were puppies, the concentration of circulating ADH following stimulation with hypertonic saline did not reliably distinguish between CDI, NDI, or PPD. Exaggerated, subnormal, and nonlinear changes in ADH were found in those dogs likely to have PPD. Pulsatile secretion of ADH with and without osmotic stimulation can confound the interpretation of ADH concentration results in normal dogs and those with PU/PD. The number, duration, and magnitude of ADH pulses can vary widely in the dog [150, 151, 331]. An RIA to measure urinary AQP2 excretion was developed for use in dogs as an alternative to the measurement of ADH. Basal urinary AQP2 excretion was widely variable in normal dogs. Urinary AQP2 and circulating ADH were suppressed following water loading. AQP2 and ADH both increased following hypertonic saline infusion, and AQP2 increased following the administration of desmopressin [187]. Further studies of AQP urinary excretion in polyuric conditions appear to be warranted, but urinary AQP2 measurement is unfortunately not available from commercial laboratories.

The authors of one paper concluded that the knowledge of how concentrated urine might be above 1.030 in dogs provides no clinically relevant information [90]. This assertion is unfounded, especially for dogs with dehydration or at risk for urolithiasis in which specific USG values up to 1.060–1.070 may provide valuable information at baseline or during treatment. Also, if USG is only reported up to 1.030, the ability to detect trending decreases in USG is missed as one tool to detection of progressive CKD or in recognition of early AKI.

Hyposthenuria is the term used to describe urine that is more dilute than glomerular ultrafiltrate. The osmolality of plasma and the glomerular ultrafiltrate is approximately 300 mOsm/kg in the dog and cat. The U_{osm}/P_{osm} ratio is <1.0 in these instances. A USG <1.008 is associated with U_{osm} <300 mOsm/kg, and a USG between 1.001 and 1.007 usually indicates hyposthenuria. The finding of hyposthenuria indicates water diuresis, which can develop as a consequence of low P_{osm} and suppression of ADH secretion from the pituitary gland. Hyposthenuria is appropriate in the presence of overhydration (such as may occur with overzealous administration of IV fluids) and in patients with PPD. Pathologic hyposthenuria occurs in animals with complete CDI, NDI, HAC, pyometra, hypercalcemia, hypokalemia, and some liver diseases. Uncommonly, animals with primary intrinsic renal failure (CKD, acute kidney injury) will have hyposthenuric urine. In more difficult cases, in which the cause of hyposthenuria remains unknown, the underlying cause usually can be identified by use of a WDT and exogenous ADH response testing.

Urine osmolality that is nearly the same as that of plasma (290–310 mOsm/kg) is referred to as isosthenuric. Isosthenuria corresponds to a USG of 1.007–1.017 in dogs and cats. A range of 1.008–1.012 as used in human medicine but is not appropriate for use in dogs and cats, because P_{osm} is lower and less variable in humans. Concurrent measurement of urine and plasma or serum osmolality will allow the clinician to determine if the urine sample is truly isosthenuric. The so-called fixed USG is one that never exceeds 1.017 or falls below 1.008, a situation that often occurs in animals with advanced primary intrinsic renal disease. USG should be assessed in several other samples to determine if USG values in this range are repeatable.

Hypersthenuria (baruria) is said to be present if $U_{osm} > P_{osm}$. How much U_{osm} exceeds P_{osm}, however, is more important in the evaluation of renal function. A USG of 1.018–1.030 in dogs and 1.018–1035 in cats indicates some ability to concentrate urine above the osmolality of glomerular ultrafiltrate and is considered minimally to moderately concentrated urine. Animals that are clinically dehydrated have in effect already undergone a spontaneous WDT that should result in maximally concentrated urine if the hypothalamic–pituitary–renal axis is normal. In general, during dehydration in dogs and cats, USG >1.040 is expected, with USG 1.030–1.040 considered questionable, and USG <1.030 considered abnormal.

The interpretation of USG can be helpful in differentiating patients that have prerenal azotemia (normal but underperfused kidneys) from those with intrinsic (primary) renal azotemia (renal lesions that account for filtration failure). In the presence of azotemia, USG <1.035 for cats and <1.030 for dogs generally indicates that the kidneys are responsible for the azotemia. This conclusion is not valid for patients with postrenal azotemia, or in those with hypercalcemia, hypokalemia, or endotoxemia, conditions that can interfere with urinary concentrating ability despite otherwise normal kidneys (i.e. NDI).

High USG as part of screening before general anesthesia generally is regarded as indicative of good renal tubular function. However, in one study of young healthy dogs undergoing neutering, higher USG before general inhalational anesthesia (mean USG of 1.041) was significantly associated with lower cumulative mean arterial blood pressure and episodes of hypotension during anesthesia compared to dogs with a mean USG of 1.035. Subclinical dehydration after hospitalization and overnight fasting likely contributed to this effect, reflected by an increase in mean USG [98].

REFERENCES

1 Armstrong, J.A. (2007). Urinalysis in Western culture: a brief history. *Kidney Int.* 71: 384–387.

2 Strasinger, S.K. and Di Lorenzo, M.S. (2014). Physical examination of urine. In: *Urinalysis and Body Fluids*, 59–69. Philadelphia: F.A. Davis Company.

3 Mundt, M.A. and Shanahan, K. (2016). Physical examination of urine. In: *Graff's Textbook of Urinalysis and Body Fluids*, 3e, 79–88. Philadelphia: Wolters Kluwer.

4 Osborne, C.A., Low, D.G., and Finco, D.R. (1972). Laboratory findings in diseases of the urinary system. In: *Canine and Feline Urology* (ed. C.A. Osborne, D.G. Low and D.R. Finco), 39–61. Philadelphia, PA: W.B. Saunders C.

5 Zanghi, B.M., Gerheart, L., and Gardner, C.L. (2018). Effects of a nutrient-enriched water on water intake and indices of hydration in healthy domestic cats fed a dry kibble diet. *Am. J. Vet. Res.* 79: 733–744.

6 Armstrong, L.E., Soto, J.A., Hacker, F.T. Jr. et al. (1998). Urinary indices during dehydration, exercise, and rehydration. *Int. J. Sport Nutr.* 8: 345–355.

7 Drabkin, D.L. (1927). The normal pigment of the urine. The relationship of urinary pigment output to diet and metabolism. *J. Biolumin. Chemilumin.* 75: 443–479.

8 Ostow, M. and Philo, S. (1944). The chief urinary pigment: the relationship between the rate of excretion of the yellow pigment and the metabolic rate. *Am. J. Med. Sci.* 207: 507–512.

9 Foot, C.L. and Fraser, J.F. (2006). Uroscopic rainbow: modern matula medicine. *Postgrad. Med. J.* 82: 126–129.

10 Armstrong, L.E., Maresh, C.M., Castellani, J.W. et al. (1994). Urinary indices of hydration status. *Int. J. Sport Nutr.* 4: 265–279.

11 Macdougall, D.F. and Curd, G.J. (1996). Urine collection and complete urinalysis. In: *BSAVA Manual of Canine and Feline Nephrology and Urology*, 2e (ed. J. Bainbride and J. Elliott), 86–106. Ames, Iowa: Iowa State University Press.

12 Barlough, J.E., Osborne, C.A., and Stevens, J.B. (1981). Canine and feline urinalysis: value of macroscopic and microscopic examinations. *J. Am. Vet. Med. Assoc.* 178: 61–63.

13 Callens, A.J. and Bartges, J.W. (2015). Urinalysis. *Vet. Clin. North Am. Small Anim. Pract.* 45: 621–637.

14 Vientós-Plotts, A.I., Behrend, E.N., Welles, E.G. et al. (2018). Effect of blood contamination on results of dipstick evaluation and urine protein-to-urine creatinine ratio for urine samples from dogs and cats. *Am. J. Vet. Res.* 79: 525–531.

15 Watts, A.R., Lennard, M.S., Mason, S.L. et al. (1993). Beeturia and the biological fate of beetroot pigments. *Pharmacogenetics* 3: 302–311.

16 Blondheim, S.H., Margoliash, E., and Shafrir, E. (1958). A simple test for myohemoglobinuria (myoglobinuria). *J. Am. Med. Assoc.* 167: 453–454.

17 Gannon, J.R. (1980). Exertional rhabdomyolysis (myoglobinuria) in the racing Greyhound. In: *Current Veterinary Therapy; Small Animal Practice* (ed. E. Kirk), 783–787. Philadelphia: Saunders.

18 Davis, P.E. and Paris, R. (1974). Azoturia in a greyhound: clinical pathology aids to diagnosis. *J. Small Anim. Pract.* 15: 43–54.

19 Kohn, C.W. and Chew, D.J. (1987). Laboratory diagnosis and characterization of renal disease in horses. *Vet. Clin. North Am. Equine Pract.* 3: 585–615.

20 Giddens, W.E. Jr., Labbe, R.F., Swango, L.J. et al. (1975). Feline congenital erythropoietic porphyria associated with severe anemia and renal disease. Clinical, morphologic, and biochemical studies. *Am. J. Pathol.* 80: 367–386.

21 Glenn, B.L., Glenn, H.G., and Omtvedt, I.T. (1968). Congenital porphyria in the domestic cat (*Felis catus*): preliminary investigations on inheritance pattern. *Am. J. Vet. Res.* 29: 1653–1657.

22 Tobias, G. (1964). Congenital porphyria in a cat. *J. Am. Vet. Med. Assoc.* 145: 462–463.

23 Clavero, S., Bishop, D.F., Giger, U. et al. (2010). Feline congenital erythropoietic porphyria: two homozygous UROS missense mutations cause the enzyme deficiency and porphyrin accumulation. *Mol. Med.* 16: 381–388.

24 Klaphake, E. and Paul-Murphy, J. (2012). Disorders of the reproductive and urinary systems. In: *Ferrets, Rabbits, and Rodents: Clinical Medicine and Surgery*, 3e (ed. K.E. Quesenberry and J.W. Carpenter), 217–231. St. Louis, MO: Elsevier.

25 Macalpine, I. and Hunter, R. (1966). The "insanity" of King George 3d: a classic case of porphyria. *Br. Med. J.* 1: 65–71.

26 Banimahd, F., Loo, T., Amin, M. et al. (2016). A rare but important clinical presentation of induced methemoglobinemia. *West. J. Emerg. Med.* 17: 627–629.

27 Nordt, S.P. (2017). Pyelonephritis following phenazopyridine use. *Am. J. Emerg. Med.* 35: 805.e803–805.e804.

28 Singh, M., Shailesh, F., Tiwari, U. et al. (2014). Phenazopyridine associated acute interstitial nephritis and review of literature. *Ren. Fail.* 36: 804–807.

29 Koratala, A. and Leghrouz, M. (2017). Green urine. *Clin. Case Rep.* 5: 549–550.

30 Pak, F. (2004). Green urine: an association with metoclopramide. *Nephrol. Dial. Transplant.* 19: 2677.

31 Rogers, W. (2017) Green Urine Following IV Metochlopramide in a Dog saim@http://list.acvim.org: ACVIM.

32 Bodenham, A., Culank, L.S., and Park, G.R. (1987). Propofol infusion and green urine. *Lancet* 2: 740.

33 Rawal, G. and Yadav, S. (2015). Green urine due to propofol: a case report with review of literature. *J. Clin. Diagn. Res.* 9: OD03–OD04.

34 Flaherty, D. and Auckburally, A. (2017). Green discolouration of urine following propofol infusion in a dog. *J. Small Anim. Pract.* 58: 536–538.

35 Shim, Y.S., Gil, H.W., Yang, J.O. et al. (2008). A case of green urine after ingestion of herbicides. *Korean J. Intern. Med.* 23: 42–44.

36 Ellis, L.A., Yates, B.A., McKenzie, A.L. et al. (2016). Effects of three oral nutritional supplements on human hydration indices. *Int. J. Sport Nutr. Exerc. Metab.* 26: 356–362.

37 McStay, C.M. and Gordon, P.E. (2007). Images in clinical medicine. Urine fluorescence in ethylene glycol poisoning. *N. Engl. J. Med.* 356: 611.

38 Winter, M.L. and Snodgrass, W.R. (2007). Urine fluorescence in ethylene glycol poisoning. *N. Engl. J. Med.* 356: 2006. author reply 2006-2007.

39 Winter, M.L., Ellis, M.D., and Snodgrass, W.R. (1990). Urine fluorescence using a Wood's lamp to detect the antifreeze additive sodium fluorescein: a qualitative adjunctive test in suspected ethylene glycol ingestions. *Ann. Emerg. Med.* 19: 663–667.

40 Casavant, M.J., Shah, M.N., and Battels, R. (2001). Does fluorescent urine indicate antifreeze ingestion by children? *Pediatrics* 107: 113–114.

41 Parsa, T., Cunningham, S.J., Wall, S.P. et al. (2005). The usefulness of urine fluorescence for suspected antifreeze ingestion in children. *Am. J. Emerg. Med.* 23: 787–792.

42 Biewenga, W.J., Rijnberk, A., and Mol, J.A. (1991). Osmoregulation of systemic vasopressin release during long-term glucocorticoid excess: a study in dogs with hyperadrenocorticism. *Acta Endocrinol. (Copenh)* 124: 583–588.

43 Aycock, R.D. and Kass, D.A. (2012). Abnormal urine color. *South. Med. J.* 105: 43–47.

44 Chong, V.H. (2012). Purple urine bag syndrome: it is the urine bag and not the urine that is discolored purple. *South. Med. J.* 105: 446. author reply 446.

45 de Bruyn, G., Eckman, C.D., and Atmar, R.L. (2002). Photo quiz. Purple discoloration in a urinary catheter bag. *Clin. Infect. Dis.* 34 (210): 285–216.

46 Lin, J., Hlafka, M., Vargas, O. et al. (2016). Recurrent purple urine bag syndrome presenting with full spectrum of disease severity: case report and review of literature. *CEN Case Rep.* 5: 144–147.

47 Dealler, S.F., Belfield, P.W., Bedford, M. et al. (1989). Purple urine bags. *J. Urol.* 142: 769–770.

48 Duncan, J.R. and Prasse, K.W. (1976). Clinical examination of the urine. *Vet. Clin. North Am.* 6: 647–661.

49 Stevens, J. and Osborne, C.A. (1974). Urinalysis: indications, methodology, and interpretation. In: *American Animal Hospital Conference*, 359–403.

50 Hendriks, W.H., Moughan, P.J., Tarttelin, M.F. et al. (1995). Felinine: a urinary amino acid of Felidae. *Comp. Biochem. Physiol.* 112B: 581–588.

51 Hendriks, W.H., Tarttelin, M.F., and Moughan, P.J. (1995). Twenty-four hour felinine [corrected] excretion patterns in entire and castrated cats. *Physiol. Behav.* 58: 467–469.

52 Tarttelin, M.F., Hendriks, W.H., and Moughan, P.J. (1998). Relationship between plasma testosterone and urinary felinine in the growing kitten. *Physiol. Behav.* 65: 83–87.

53 Miyazaki, M., Yamashita, T., Suzuki, Y. et al. (2006). A major urinary protein of the domestic cat regulates the production of felinine, a putative pheromone precursor. *Chem. Biol.* 13: 1071–1079.

54 Hendriks, W.H., Rutherfurd-Markwick, K.J., Weidgraaf, K. et al. (2008). Urinary felinine excretion in intact male cats is increased by dietary cystine. *Br. J. Nutr.* 100: 801–809.

55 Futsuta, A., Hojo, W., Miyazaki, T. et al. (2018). LC-MS/MS quantification of felinine metabolites in tissues, fluids, and excretions from the domestic cat (*Felis catus*). *J. Chromatogr. B* 1072: 94–99.

56 Adams, L.G., Polzin, D.J., Osborne, C.A. et al. (1993). Effects of dietary protein and calorie restriction in clinically normal cats and in cats with surgically induced chronic renal failure. *Am. J. Vet. Res.* 54: 1653–1662.

57 Pradella, M., Dorizzi, R.M., and Rigolin, F. (1988). Relative density of urine: methods and clinical significance. *Crit. Rev. Clin. Lab Sci.* 26: 195–242.

58 Tvedten, H.W., Ouchterlony, H., and Lilliehook, I.E. (2015). Comparison of specific gravity analysis of feline and canine urine, using five refractometers, to pycnometric analysis and total solids by drying. *N. Z. Vet. J.* 63: 254–259.

59 Corcoran, A.C. (1955). Electometric urinometry; a note on comparative determinations of urinary osmolarity and specific gravity. *J. Lab Clin. Med.* 46: 141–143.

60 Hendriks, H.J., de Bruijne, J.J., and van den Brom, W.E. (1978). The clinical refractometer: a useful tool for the determination of specific gravity and osmolality in canine urine. *Tijdschr Diergeneeskd* 103: 1065–1068.

61 Penney, M.D. and Walters, G. (1987). Are osmolality measurements clinically useful? *Ann. Clin. Biochem.* 24 (Pt 6): 566–571.

62 Bovee, K.C. (1969). Urine osmolarity as a definitive indicator of renal concentrating capacity. *J. Am. Vet. Med. Assoc.* 155: 30–35.

63 Watson, A.D.J. (1998). Urinary specific gravity in practice. *Aust. Vet. J.* 76: 392–398.

64 Siemens, H.D. (2010). Multi Stix package insert.

65 van Vonderen, I.K., Kooistra, H.S., and Bruijne, J.J. (1995). Evaluation of a test strip for estimating the specific gravity of canine urine. *Tijdschrift voor Diergeneeskunde* 120: 400–402.

66 Dossin, O., Germain, C., and Braun, J.P. (2003). Comparison of the techniques of evaluation of urine dilution/concentration in the dog. *J. Vet. Med. A Physiol. Pathol. Clin. Med.* 50: 322–325.

67 Allchin, J.P., Evans, G.O., and Parsons, C.E. (1987). Pitfalls in the measurement of canine urine concentration. *Vet. Rec.* 120: 256–257.

68 Paris, J.K., Bennett, A.D., Dodkin, S.J. et al. (2012). Comparison of a digital and an optical analogue hand-held refractometer for the measurement of canine urine specific gravity. *Vet. Rec.* 170: 463.

69 Bennett, A.D., McKnight, G.E., Dodkin, S.J. et al. (2011). Comparison of digital and optical hand-held refractometers for the measurement of feline urine specific gravity. *J. Feline Med. Surg.* 13: 152–154.

70 Hardy, R.M. and Osborne, C.A. (1979). Water deprivation test in the dog: maximal normal values. *J. Am. Vet. Med. Assoc.* 174: 479–483.

71 Ayoub, J.A., Beaufrere, H., and Acierno, M.J. (2013). Association between urine osmolality and specific gravity in dogs and the effect of commonly measured urine solutes on that association. *Am. J. Vet. Res.* 74: 1542–1545.

72 George, J.W. (2001). The usefulness and limitations of hand-held refractometers in veterinary laboratory medicine: an historical and technical review. *Vet. Clin. Pathol.* 30: 201–210.

73 Voinescu, G.C., Shoemaker, M., Moore, H. et al. (2002). The relationship between urine osmolality and specific gravity. *Am. J. Med. Sci.* 323: 39–42.

74 Price, J.W., Miller, M., and Hayman, J.M. (1940). The relation of specific gravity to composition and total solids in normal human urine. *J. Clin. Invest.* 19: 537–554.

75 Siemens (2007). Clinitek Atlas with Rock Sample Handler Operating Manual. In: *Diagnostics SMS* (ed. Siemens), 1–10. Tarreytown, NY USA: Siemens Medical Solutions Diagnostics.

76 Chapelle, L., Tassignon, B., Aerenhouts, D. et al. (2017). The hydration status of young female elite soccer players during an official tournament. *J. Sports Med. Phys. Fit.* 57: 1186–1194.

77 Chadha, V., Garg, U., and Alon, U.S. (2001). Measurement of urinary concentration: a critical appraisal of methodologies. *Pediatr. Nephrol.* 16: 374–382.

78 Rubini, M.E. and Wolf, A.V. (1957). Refractometric determination of total solids and water of serum and urine. *J. Biolumin. Chemilumin.* 225: 869–876.

79 Tvedten, H.W. and Noren, A. (2014). Comparison of a Schmidt and Haensch refractometer and an Atago PAL-USG cat refractometer for determination of urine specific gravity in dogs and cats. *Vet. Clin. Pathol.* 43: 63–66.

80 Wyness, S.P., Hunsaker, J.J.H., Snow, T.M. et al. (2016). Evaluation and analytical validation of a handheld digital refractometer for urine specific gravity measurement. *Pract. Lab. Med.* 5: 65–74.

81 George, J.W. and O'Neill, S.L. (2001). Comparison of refractometer and biuret methods for total protein measurement in body cavity fluids. *Vet. Clin. Pathol.* 30: 16–18.

82 Wolf, A.V. (1962). Urinary concentrative properties. *Am. J. Med.* 32: 329–332.

83 Wolf, A.V., Fuller, J.B., Goldman, E.J. et al. (1962). New refractometric methods for the determination of total proteins in serum and in urine. *Clin. Chem.* 8: 158–165.

84 Haynes, W.M., Lide, D.R., and Bruno, T.J. (2017). *CRC Handbook of Chemistry and Physics*, 97e. Boca Raton, FL: CRC Press.

85 Lange, N.A. and Speight, J.G. (2005). *Lange's Handbook of Chemistry*, 16e. New York, NY: McGraw-Hill.

86 Rudinsky, A.J., Wellman, M., Tracy, G. et al. (2019). Variability among four refractometers for the measurement of urine specific gravity and comparison with urine osmolality in dogs. *Vet. Clin. Pathol.* 48: 702–709.

87 Mosch, M., Reese, S., Weber, K. et al. (2020). Influence of preanalytic and analytic variables in canine and feline urine specific gravity measurement by refractometer. *J. Vet. Diagn. Invest.* 32: 36–43.

88 Albasan, H., Lulich, J.P., Osborne, C.A. et al. (2003). Effects of storage time and temperature on pH, specific gravity, and crystal formation in urine samples from dogs and cats. *J. Am. Vet. Med. Assoc.* 222: 176–179.

89 Aulakh, H.K., Aulakh, K.S., Ryan, K.A. et al. (2020). Investigation of the effects of storage with preservatives at room temperature or refrigeration without preservatives on urinalysis results for samples from healthy dogs. *J. Am. Vet. Med. Assoc.* 257: 726–733.

90 du Preez, K., Boustead, K., Rautenbach, Y. et al. (2020). Comparison of canine urine specific gravity measurements between various refractometers in a clinical setting. *Vet. Clin. Pathol.* 49: 407–416.

91 Osborne, C.A. and Stevens, J.B. (1999). Urine specific gravity, refractive index, or osmolality: which one would you chose? In: *Urinalysis: A Clinical Guide to Compassionate Patient Care* (ed. C.A. Osborne and J.B. Stevens), 73–85. Shawnee Mission, KS: Bayer.

92 Steinberg, E., Drobatz, K., and Aronson, L. (2009). The effect of substrate composition and storage time on urine specific gravity in dogs. *J. Small Anim. Pract.* 50: 536–539.

93 Smart, L., Hopper, K., Aldrich, J. et al. (2009). The effect of hetastarch (670/0.75) on urine specific gravity and osmolality in the dog. *J. Vet. Intern. Med.* 23: 388–391.

94 Bouzouraa, J.M., Bonnet-Garin, M., Hugonnard, B. et al. (2017). Relationship and clincial relevance of urine osmolaltiy and specific gravity in healthy cats receiving various intravenous solutes. *J. Vet. Intern. Med.* 31: 250–251.

95 Behrend, E.N., Botsford, A.N., Mueller, S.A. et al. (2019). Effect on urine specific gravity of the addition of glucose to urine samples of dogs and cats. *Am. J. Vet. Res.* 80: 907–911.

96 Feeney, D.A., Osborne, C.A., and Jessen, C.R. (1980). Effects of radiographic contrast media on results of urinalysis, with emphasis on alteration in specific gravity. *J. Am. Vet. Med. Assoc.* 176: 1378–1381.

97 van Vonderen, I.K., Kooistra, H.S., and Rijnberk, A. (1997). Intra- and interindividual variation in urine osmolality and urine specific gravity in healthy pet dogs of various ages. *J. Vet. Intern. Med.* 11: 30–35.

98 Costa, R.S., Raisis, A.L., Hosgood, G. et al. (2015). Preoperative factors associated with hypotension in young anaesthetised dogs undergoing elective desexing. *Aust. Vet. J.* 93: 99–104.

99 DiBartola, S.P., Chew, D.J., and Jacobs, G. (1980). Quantitative urinalysis including 24-hour protein excretion in the dog. *J. Am. Anim. Hosp. Assoc.* 16: 537–546.

100 Willems, A., Paepe, D., Marynissen, S. et al. (2017). Results of screening of apparently healthy senior and geriatric dogs. *J. Vet. Intern. Med.* 31: 81–92.

101 Rudinsky, A., Cortright, C., Purcell, S. et al. (2019). Variability of first morning urine specific gravity in 103 healthy dogs. *J. Vet. Intern. Med.* 33: 2133–2137.

102 Sands, J.M. (2012). Urine concentrating and diluting ability during aging. *J. Gerontol. Ser. A* 67: 1352–1357.

103 Tian, Y., Serino, R., and Verbalis, J.G. (2004). Downregulation of renal vasopressin V2 receptor and aquaporin-2 expression parallels age-associated defects in urine concentration. *Am. J. Physiol. Renal Physiol.* 287: F797–F805.

104 Rowe, J.C., Hokamp, J.A., Braatz, J.N. et al. (2021). Interobserver reliability of canine urine specific gravity assessed by analog or digital refractometers. *J. Vet. Diagn. Invest.* 33(3): 611–614.

105 Rossi, G., Giori, L., Campagnola, S. et al. (2012). Evaluation of factors that affect analytic variability of urine protein-to-creatinine ratio determination in dogs. *Am. J. Vet. Res.* 73: 779–788.

106 West, C.D., Traeger, J., and Kaplan, S.A. (1955). A comparison of the relative effectiveness of hydropenia and of pitressin in producing a concentrated urine. *J. Clin. Invest.* 34: 887–898.

107 Hardy, R.M. and Osborne, C.A. (1982). Aqueous vasopressin response test in clinically normal dogs undergoing water diuresis: technique and results. *Am. J. Vet. Res.* 43: 1987–1990.

108 Hardy, R.M. and Osborne, C.A. (1982). Reposital vasopressin response test in clinically normal dogs undergoing water diuresis: technique and results. *Am. J. Vet. Res.* 43: 1991–1993.

109 Johnston, S.D., Root Kustritz, M.V., and Olson, P.N. (2001). The neonate- from birth to weaning. In: *Canine and Feline Theriogenology*, 1e (ed. R. Kersing), 146–167. Philadelphia: WB Saunders.

110 von Dehn, B. (2014). Pediatric clinical pathology. *Vet. Clin. North Am. Small Anim. Pract.* 44: 205–219.

111 Grundy, S.A. (2006). Clinically relevant physiology of the neonate. *Vet. Clin. North Am. Small Anim. Pract.* 36: 443–459.

112 Faulks, R.D. and Lane, I.F. (2003). Qualitative urinalyses in puppies 0 to 24 weeks of age. *J. Am. Anim. Hosp. Assoc.* 39: 369–378.

113 Laroute, V., Chetboul, V., Roche, L. et al. (2005). Quantitative evaluation of renal function in healthy Beagle puppies and mature dogs. *Res. Vet. Sci.* 79: 161–167.

114 Melandri, M., Veronesi, M.C., and Alonge, S. (2020). Urinalysis in great Dane puppies from birth to 28 days of age. *Animals (Basel)* 10: 638–648.

115 Rishniw, M. and Bicalho, R. (2015). Factors affecting urine specific gravity in apparently healthy cats presenting to first opinion practice for routine evaluation. *J. Feline Med. Surg.* 17: 329–337.

116 Kruger, J.M., Lulich, J.P., MacLeay, J. et al. (2015). Comparison of foods with differing nutritional profiles for long-term management of acute nonobstructive idiopathic cystitis in cats. *J. Am. Vet. Med. Assoc.* 247: 508–517.

117 Buckley, C.M., Hawthorne, A., Colyer, A. et al. (2011). Effect of dietary water intake on urinary output, specific gravity and relative supersaturation for calcium oxalate and struvite in the cat. *Br. J. Nutr.* 106 (Suppl 1): S128–S130.

118 Zanghi, B.M., Wils-Plotz, E., DeGeer, S. et al. (2018). Effects of a nutrient-enriched water with and without poultry flavoring on water intake, urine specific gravity, and urine output in healthy domestic cats fed a dry kibble diet. *Am. J. Vet. Res.* 79: 1150–1159.

119 Zanghi, B.M. and Gardner, C.L. (2018). Total water intake and urine measures of hydration in adult dogs drinking tap water or a nutrient-enriched water. *Front. Vet. Sci.* 5: 317.

120 Zanghi, B.M., Gerheart, L., and Gardner, C.L. (2018). Effects of a nutrient-enriched water on water intake and indices of hydration in healthy domestic cats fed a dry kibble diet. *Am. J. Vet. Res.* 79 (7): 733–744.

121 Finco, D.R., Adams, D.D., Crowell, W.A. et al. (1986). Food and water intake and urine composition in cats: influence of continuous versus periodic feeding. *Am. J. Vet. Res.* 47: 1638–1642.

122 Paepe, D., Bavegems, V., Combes, A. et al. (2013). Prospective evaluation of healthy Ragdoll cats for chronic kidney disease by routine laboratory parameters and ultrasonography. *J. Feline Med. Surg.* 15: 849–857.

123 Paepe, D., Verjans, G., Duchateau, L. et al. (2013). Routine health screening: findings in apparently healthy middle-aged and old cats. *J. Feline Med. Surg.* 15: 8–19.

124 Lees, G.E., Osborne, C.A., and Stevens, J.B. (1979). Antibacterial properties of urine: studies of feline urine specific gravity, osmolality, and pH. *J. Am. Anim. Hosp. Assoc.* 15: 135–141.

125 Thrall, B.E. and Miller, L.G. (1976). Water turnover in cats fed dry rations. *Feline Pract.* 6: 10–12.

126 Pelligand, L., Lees, P., and Elliott, J. (2011). Development and validation of a timed urinary collection system for use in the cat. *Lab Anim.* 45: 196–203.

127 Ross, L.A. and Finco, D.R. (1981). Relationship of selected clinical renal function tests to glomerular filtration rate and renal blood flow in cats. *Am. J. Vet. Res.* 42: 1704–1710.

128 Finco, D.R., Brown, S.A., Brown, C.A. et al. (1998). Protein and calorie effects on progression of induced chronic renal failure in cats. *Am. J. Vet. Res.* 59: 575–582.

129 Hoskins, J.D. (1990). Clinical evaluation of the kitten: from birth to eight weeks of age. *Comp. Contin. Educ. Pract. Vet.* 12: 1215–1225.

130 Mulnix, J.A., Rijnberk, A., and Hendriks, H.J. (1976). Evaluation of a modified water-deprivation test for diagnosis of polyuric disorders in dogs. *J. Am. Vet. Med. Assoc.* 169: 1327–1330.

131 Cowan, R.H., Jukkola, A.F., and Arant, B.S. Jr. (1980). Pathophysiologic evidence of gentamicin nephrotoxicity in neonatal puppies. *Pediatr. Res.* 14: 1204–1211.

132 Horster, M. and Valtin, H. (1971). Postnatal development of renal function: micropuncture and clearance studies in the dog. *J. Clin. Invest.* 50: 779–795.

133 Chew, R.M. (1965). Mammalian reaction to stressful environments. In: *Physiologic Mammalogy* (ed. W.W. Mayer and R.G. Van Gelder), 43. New York: Academic Press.

134 Brown, B.A., Peterson, M.E., and Robertson, G.L. (1993). Evaluation of the plasma vasopressin, plasma sodium and urine osmolality response to water restriction in normal cats and in a cat with diabetes insipidus (abstract). *J. Vet. Intern. Med.* 7: 113.

135 Crawford, M.A. (1990). The urinary system. In: *Veterinary Pediatrics: Dogs and Cats from Birth to Six Months* (ed. J.D. Haskins), 271–292. Philadelphia: W.B. Saunders.

136 Bouzouraa, T., Rannou, B., Cappelle, J. et al. (2021). Formula for the estimation of urine osmolality in healthy cats. *Res. Vet. Sci.* 135: 121–126.

137 Bruyette, D.S. and Nelson, R.W. (1986). How to approach the problems of polyuria and polydipsia. *Vet. Med.* 81 (2): 112–128.

138 DiBartola, S.P. (2012). Disorders of sodium and water: hypernatremia and hyponatremia. In: *Fluid, Electrolyte, and Acid-Base Disorders in Small Animal Practice* (ed. S.P. DiBartola), 51–85. Elsevier Saunders: St. Louis, MO.

139 Biewenga, W.J., van den Brom, W.E., and Mol, J.A. (1987). The use of arginine vasopressin measurements in the polyuric dog. *Tijdschr Diergeneeskd* 112 (Suppl 1): 117S–120S.

140 Nichols, R. and Hohenhaus, A.E. (1994). Use of the vasopressin analogue desmopressin for polyuria and bleeding disorders. *J. Am. Vet. Med. Assoc.* 205: 168–173.

141 Robinson, A.G. (1976). DDAVP in the treatment of central diabetes insipidus. *N. Engl. J. Med.* 294: 507–511.

142 Richardson, D.W. and Robinson, A.G. (1985). Desmopressin. *Ann. Intern. Med.* 103: 228–239.

143 Shiel, R.E. (2012). Disorders of vasopressin production. In: *BSAVA Manual of Canine and Feline Endocrinology* (ed. C.T. Mooney and M.E. Peterson), 15–27. Quedgeley, Gloucester: British Small Animal Veterinary Association.

144 Lundin, S. and Vilhardt, H. (1986). Absorption of intragastrically administered DDAVP in conscious dogs. *Life Sci.* 38: 703–709.

145 Aroch, I., Mazaki-Tovi, M., Shemesh, O. et al. (2005). Central diabetes insipidus in five cats: clinical presentation, diagnosis and oral desmopressin therapy. *J. Feline Med. Surg.* 7: 333–339.

146 Nichols, R. (2000). Clinical use of the vasopressin analogue DDAVP for the diagnosis and treatment of diabetes insipidus. In: *Kirk's current veterinary therapy Small animal practice*, vol. 13 (ed. J.D. Bonagura), 325–326. Philadephia PA: W.B. Saunders.

147 Harb, M.F., Nelson, R.W., Feldman, E.C. et al. (1996). Central diabetes insipidus in dogs: 20 cases (1986-1995). *J. Am. Vet. Med. Assoc.* 209: 1884–1888.

148 Biewenga, W.J., WEvd, B., and Mol, J.A. (1987). Vasopressin in polyuric syndromes in the dog. *Front. Horm. Res.* 17: 139–148.

149 Robertson, G.L. (1994). The use of vasopressin assays in physiology and pathophysiology. *Semin. Nephrol.* 14: 368–383.

150 van Vonderen, I.K., Wolfswinkel, J., Oosterlaken-Dijksterhuis, M.A. et al. (2004). Pulsatile secretion pattern of vasopressin under basal conditions, after water deprivation, and during osmotic stimulation in dogs. *Domest. Anim. Endocrinol.* 27: 1–12.

151 van Vonderen, I.K., Kooistra, H.S., Timmermans-Sprang, E.P. et al. (2004). Vasopressin response to osmotic stimulation in 18 young dogs with polyuria and polydipsia. *J. Vet. Intern. Med.* 18: 800–806.

152 van Vonderen, I.K., Wolfswinkel, J., van den Ingh, T.S. et al. (2004). Urinary aquaporin-2 excretion in dogs: a marker for collecting duct responsiveness to vasopressin. *Domest. Anim. Endocrinol.* 27: 141–153.

153 Dabla, P.K., Dabla, V., and Arora, S. (2011). Co-peptin: role as a novel biomarker in clinical practice. *Clin. Chim. Acta* 412: 22–28.

154 Grandone, A., Marzuillo, P., Patti, G. et al. (2019). Changing the diagnostic approach to diabetes insipidus: role of copeptin. *Ann. Transl. Med.* 7: S285.

155 Refardt, J. and Christ-Crain, M. (2020). Copeptin-based diagnosis of diabetes insipidus. *Swiss Med. Wkly.* 150: w20237.

156 Gupta, A. and Zimmerman, D. (2020). Hypotonic polyuria: at the cross-roads of copeptin. *Neth. J. Med.* 78: 309–314.

157 Bakhtiani, P. and Geffner, M.E. (2021). Diagnosing DI (The water deprivation test). In: *Diabetes Insipidus in Children A Pocket Guide* (ed. C.A. Alter), 9–22. Cham: Springer.

158 Verbalis, J.G. (2020). Acquired forms of central diabetes insipidus: mechanisms of disease. *Best Pract. Res. Clin. Endocrinol. Metab.* 34(5): 101449.

159 Verbalis, J.G. (2020). Disorders of water balance. In: *Brenner & Rector's The Kidney*, 11e (ed. Y. ASL, G.M. Chertow, V.A. Luyckx, et al.), 443–495.e411. Philadelphia: Elsevier.

160 Matz, R. (1986). Hypothermia: mechanisms and countermeasures. *Hosp. Pract. (Off Ed)* 21: 45–48. 54–48, 63–71.

161 Reuler, J.B. (1978). Hypothermia: pathophysiology, clinical settings, and management. *Ann. Intern. Med.* 89: 519–527.

162 Fitzgerald, F.T. and Jessop, C. (1982). Accidental hypothermia: a report of 22 cases and review of the literature. *Adv. Intern. Med.* 27: 128–150.

163 Kanter, G.S. (1959). Renal clearance of glucose in hypothermic dogs. *Am. J. Phys* 196: 866–872.

164 Debakey, M.E., Morris, G., and Moyer, J.H. (1957). Hypothermia. I. Effect on renal hemodynamics and on excretion of water and electrolytes in dog and man. *Ann. Surg.* 145: 26–40.

165 Segar, W.E., Riley, P.A. Jr., and Barila, T.G. (1956). Urinary composition during hypothermia. *Am. J. Phys* 185: 528–532.

166 Marques, P., Gunawardana, K., and Grossman, A. (2015). Transient diabetes insipidus in pregnancy. *Endocrinol. Diabetes Metab. Case Rep.* 2015: 150078.

167 Ananthakrishnan, S. (2020). Gestational diabetes insipidus: diagnosis and management. *Best Pract. Res. Clin. Endocrinol. Metab.* 34: 101384.

168 Fitzsimons, J.T. (1976). The physiological basis of thirst. *Kidney Int.* 10: 3–11.

169 Lage, A.L. (1977). Apparent psychogenic polydipsia. In: *Current Veterinary Therapy VI* (ed. R.W. Kirk), 1098–1102. Philadelphia: Saunders Co.

170 Falk, J.L. (1969). Conditions producing psychogenic polydipsia in animals. *Ann. N.Y. Acad. Sci.* 157: 569–593.

171 Schrier, R.W. and Berl, T. (1975). Nonosmolar factors affecting renal water excretion (first of two parts). *N. Engl. J. Med.* 292: 81–88.

172 Schrier, R.W. (2008). Molecular mechanisms of clinical concentrating and diluting disorders. *Prog. Brain Res.* 170: 539–550.

173 McKinley, M.J. and Johnson, A.K. (2004). The physiological regulation of thirst and fluid intake. *News Physiol. Sci.* 19: 1–6.

174 Bichet, D.G. (2019). Regulation of thirst and vasopressin release. *Ann. Rev. Physiol.* 81: 359–373.

175 Henderson, S.M. and Elwood, C.M. (2003). A potential causal association between gastrointestinal disease and primary polydipsia in three dogs. *J. Small Anim. Pract.* 44: 280–284.

176 Bichet, D.G. (2008). Vasopressin receptor mutations in nephrogenic diabetes insipidus. *Semin. Nephrol.* 28: 245–251.

177 Bichet, D.G. (2020). Genetics in endocrinology pathophysiology, diagnosis and treatment of familial nephrogenic diabetes insipidus. *Eur. J. Endocrinol.* 183: R29–R40.

178 Grünbaum, E.G., Herzog, A., Rascher, W. et al. (1995). Hereditary nephrogenic diabetes insipidus renalis in the dog. Part I: diagnosis. *Kleintierpraxis* 40: 447–464.

179 Takemura, N. (1998). Successful long-term treatment of congenital nephrogenic diabetes insipidus in a dog. *J. Small Anim. Pract.* 39: 592–594.

180 Breitschwerdt, E.B., Verlander, J.W., and Hribernik, T.N. (1981). Nephrogenic diabetes insipidus in three dogs. *J. Am. Vet. Med. Assoc.* 179: 235–238.

181 Lage, A.L. (1973). Nephrogenic diabetes insipidus in a dog. *J. Am. Vet. Med. Assoc.* 163: 251–253.

182 Luzius, H., Jans, D.A., Grunbaum, E.G. et al. (1992). A low affinity vasopressin V2-receptor in inherited nephrogenic diabetes insipidus. *J. Recept Res.* 12: 351–368.

183 Singer, I. and Forrest, J.N. Jr. (1976). Drug-induced states of nephrogenic diabetes insipidus. *Kidney Int.* 10: 82–95.

184 Grinevich, V., Knepper, M.A., Verbalis, J. et al. (2004). Acute endotoxemia in rats induces down-regulation of V2 vasopressin receptors and aquaporin-2 content in the kidney medulla. *Kidney Int.* 65: 54–62.

185 Chen, L., Jung, H.J., Datta, A. et al. (2021). Systems biology of the vasopressin V2 receptor: new tools for discovery of molecular actions of a GPCR. *Annu. Rev. Pharmacol. Toxicol.* 62: 25.01–25.22.

186 Hawkes, C.P., Herrera, A., Kohn, B. et al. (2019). Posterior pituitary disorders: anatomy and physiology, central diabetes insipidus (CDI), and syndrome of inappropriate antidiuretic hormone (SIADH). In: *Contemporary Endocrinology* (ed. B. Kohn), 201–225. Switzerland AG: Springer Nature.

187 IKv, V., Wolfswinkel, J., Ingh, T.S.G.A.M. et al. (2004). Urinary aquaporin-2 excretion in dogs: a marker for collecting duct responsiveness to vasopressin. *Dom. Anim. Endocrinol.* 27: 141–153.

188 Schrier, R.W. (2006). Body water homeostasis: clinical disorders of urinary dilution and concentration. *J. Am. Soc. Nephrol.* 17: 1820–1832.

189 Schrier, R.W. and Berl, T. (1975). Nonosmolar factors affecting renal water excretion (second of two parts). *N. Engl. J. Med.* 292: 141–145.

190 Brown, S., Atkins, C., Bagley, R. et al. (2007). Guidelines for the identification, evaluation, and management of systemic hypertension in dogs and cats. *J. Vet. Intern. Med.* 21: 542–558.

191 Peterson, M.E., Kintzer, P.P., and Kass, P.H. (1996). Pretreatment clinical and laboratory findings in dogs with hypoadrenocorticism: 225 cases (1979-1993). *J. Am. Vet. Med. Assoc.* 208: 85–91.

192 Adamantos, S. and Boag, A. (2008). Total and ionised calcium concentrations in dogs with hypoadrenocorticism. *Vet. Rec.* 163: 25–26.

193 Gow, A.G., Gow, D.J., Bell, R. et al. (2009). Calcium metabolism in eight dogs with hypoadrenocorticism. *J. Small Anim. Pract.* 50: 426–430.

194 Klein, S.C. and Peterson, M.E. (2010). Canine hypoadrenocorticism: part I. *Can. Vet. J.* 51: 63–69.

195 Lathan, P. and Tyler, J. (2005). Canine hypoadrenocorticism:path ogenesis and clinical features. *Compend. Contin. Educ. Pract. Vet.* 27: 110–120.

196 Tyler, R.D., Qualls, C.W. Jr., Heald, R.D. et al. (1987). Renal concentrating ability in dehydrated hyponatremic dogs. *J. Am. Vet. Med. Assoc.* 191: 1095–1100.

197 Chen, Y.C., Cadnapaphornchai, M.A., Summer, S.N. et al. (2005). Molecular mechanisms of impaired urinary concentrating ability in glucocorticoid-deficient rats. *J. Am. Soc. Nephrol.* 16: 2864–2871.

198 Schaer, M. (2001). The treatment of acute adrenocortical insufficiency in the dog. *J. Vet. Emerg. Crit. Care* 11: 7–14.

199 Rothuizen, J., Biewenga, W.J., and Mol, J.A. (1995). Chronic glucocorticoid excess and impaired osmoregulation of vasopressin

release in dogs with hepatic encephalopathy. *Domest. Anim. Endocrinol.* 12: 13–24.

200 Ahmed, A.B., George, B.C., Gonzalez-Auvert, C. et al. (1967). Increased plasma arginine vasopressin in clinical adrenocortical insufficeincy and its inhibition by glucosteroids. *J. Clin. Invest.* 46: 111–123.

201 Raff, H. (1987). Glucocorticoid inhibition of neurohypophysial vasopressin secretion. *Am. J. Phys* 252: R635–R644.

202 Joles, J.A., Rijnberk, A., van den Brom, W.E. et al. (1980). Studies on the mechanism of polyuria induced by cortisol excess in the dog. *Vet. Q.* 2: 199–205.

203 Toftegaard, M. and Knudsen, F. (1995). Massive vasopressin-resistant polyuria induced by dexamethasone. *Intensive Care Med.* 21: 238–240.

204 Sirek, O.V. and Best, C.H. (1952). Intramuscular cortisone administration to dogs. *Proc. Soc. Exp. Biol. Med.* 80: 594–598.

205 Galati, P.A. (2021). The use of desmopressin acetate to reduce polyuria and polydipsia associated with prednisolone administration. In: *College of Veterinary Medicine* ProQuest, 1–42. Mississippi State University.

206 Adams, W.H., Daniel, G.B., Legendre, A.M. et al. (1997). Changes in renal function in cats following treatment of hyperthyroidism using 131I. *Vet. Radiol. Ultrasound* 38: 231–238.

207 Evered, D.C., Hayter, C.J., and Surveyor, I. (1972). Primary polydipsia in thyrotoxicosis. *Metabolism* 21: 393–404.

208 Harvey, J.N., Nagi, D.K., Baylis, P.H. et al. (1991). Disturbance of osmoregulated thirst and vasopressin secretion in thyrotoxicosis. *Clin. Endocrinol. (Oxf)* 35: 29–33.

209 Epstein, F.H., Freedman, L.R., and Levitin, H. (1958). Hypercalcemia, nephrocalcinosis and reversible renal insufficiency associated with hyperthyroidism. *N. Engl. J. Med.* 258: 782–785.

210 Epstein, F.H. (1971). Calcium nephropathy. In: *Diseases of the Kidney*, 2e (ed. M.B. Strauss and L.G. Welt), 903–931. Boston: Little, Brown and Co.

211 Wang, W., Li, C., Summer, S.N. et al. (2007). Polyuria of thyrotoxicosis: downregulation of aquaporin water channels and increased solute excretion. *Kidney Int.* 72: 1088–1094.

212 Peterson, M.E., Kintzer, P.P., Cavanagh, P.G. et al. (1983). Feline hyperthyroidism: pretreatment clinical and laboratory evaluation of 131 cases. *J. Am. Vet. Med. Assoc.* 183: 103–110.

213 Broussard, J.D., Peterson, M.E., and Fox, P.R. (1995). Changes in clinical and laboratory findings in cats with hyperthyroidism from 1983 to 1993. *J. Am. Vet. Med. Assoc.* 206: 302–305.

214 Graves, T.K., Olivier, N.B., Nachreiner, R.F. et al. (1994). Changes in renal function associated with treatment of hyperthyroidism in cats. *Am. J. Vet. Res.* 55: 1745–1749.

215 DiBartola, S.P., Broome, M.R., Stein, B.S. et al. (1996). Effect of treatment of hyperthyroidism on renal function in cats. *J. Am. Vet. Med. Assoc.* 208: 875–878.

216 Becker, T.J., Graves, T.K., Kruger, J.M. et al. (2000). Effects of methimazole on renal function in cats with hyperthyroidism. *J. Am. Anim. Hosp. Assoc.* 36: 215–223.

217 Riensche, M.R., Graves, T.K., and Schaeffer, D.J. (2008). An investigation of predictors of renal insufficiency following treatment of hyperthyroidism in cats. *J. Feline Med. Surg.* 10: 160–166.

218 Williams, T.L., Peak, K.J., Brodbelt, D. et al. (2010). Survival and the development of azotemia after treatment of hyperthyroid cats. *J. Vet. Intern. Med.* 24: 863–869.

219 Peterson, M.E., Chew, D.J., and Rishniw, M. (2022). Relationship between urine concentration and development of azotemia after successful treatment of hyperthyroid cats with radioiodine. In: *ACVIM Forum Proceedings*. USA. Greenwood Village, Colorado: ACVIM.

220 Panciera, D.L. and Lefebvre, H.P. (2009). Effect of experimental hypothyroidism on glomerular filtration rate and plasma creatinine concentration in dogs. *J. Vet. Intern. Med.* 23: 1045–1050.

221 Gommeren, K., van Hoek, I., Lefebvre, H.P. et al. (2009). Effect of thyroxine supplementation on glomerular filtration rate in hypothyroid dogs. *J. Vet. Intern. Med.* 23: 844–849.

222 Midkiff, A.M., Chew, D.J., Randolph, J.F. et al. (2000). Idiopathic hypercalcemia in cats. *J. Vet. Intern. Med.* 14: 619–626.

223 Savary, K.C., Price, G.S., and Vaden, S.L. (2000). Hypercalcemia in cats: a retrospective study of 71 cases (1991-1997). *J. Vet. Intern. Med.* 14: 184–189.

224 Kruger, J.M., Osborne, C.A., Nachreiner, R.F. et al. (1996). Hypercalcemia and renal failure. *Vet. Clin. North Am. Small Anim. Pract.* 26: 1417–1445.

225 Schenck, P.A. and Chew, D.J. (2003). Determination of calcium fractionation in dogs with chronic renal failure. *Am. J. Vet. Res.* 64: 1181–1184.

226 Schenck, P.A. and Chew, D.J. (2005). Prediction of serum ionized calcium concentration by use of serum total calcium concentration in dogs. *Am. J. Vet. Res.* 66: 1330–1336.

227 van den Broek, D.H., Chang, Y.M., Elliott, J. et al. (2017). Chronic kidney disease in cats and the risk of total hypercalcemia. *J. Vet. Intern. Med.* 31: 465–475.

228 Epstein, F.H., Rivera, M.J., and Carone, F.A. (1958). The effect of hypercalcemia induced by calciferol upon renal concentrating ability. *J. Clin. Invest.* 37: 1702–1709.

229 de Brito Galvao, J.F., Schenck, P.A., and Chew, D.J. (2016). A quick reference on hypercalcemia. *Vet. Clin. North Am. Small Anim. Pract.* 47 (2): 241–248.

230 de Brito Galvao, J.F., Parker, V., Schenck, P.A. et al. (2016). Update on feline ionized hypercalcemia. *Vet. Clin. North Am. Small Anim. Pract.* 47 (2): 273–292.

231 Schenck, P.A., Chew, D.J., Nagode, L.A. et al. (2011). Disorders of calcium: hypercalcemia and hypocalcemia. In: *Fluid, Electrolyte, and Acid-Base Disorders in Small Animal Practice*, 4e (ed. S.P. DiBartola), 120–194. St. Louis: London: Saunders Elsevier.

232 Schenck, P.A. and Chew, D.J. (2008). Calcium: total or ionized? *Vet. Clin. North Am. Small Anim. Pract.* 38: 497–502. ix.

233 Schenck, P.A. and Chew, D.J. (2008). Hypercalcemia: a quick reference. *Vet. Clin. North Am. Small Anim. Pract.* 38: 449–453. viii.

234 Kruger, J.M. and Osborne, C.A. (2011). *Calcium disorders*, 642–656. Chichester: Wiley.

235 Kruger, J.M. and Osborne, C.A. (1994). Canine and feline hypercalcemic nephropathy. Part I. Causes and consequences. *Compend. Contin. Educ. Pract. Vet.* 16: 1299–1315.

236 Kruger, J.M. and Osborne, C.A. (1994). Canine and feline hypercalcemic nephropathy. Part II. Detection, cure, and control. *Compend. Contin. Educ. Pract. Vet.* 16: 1445–1458.

237 Chew, D.J. and Capen, C.C. (1980). Hypercalcemic nephropathy and associated disorders. In: *Current Veterinary Therapy VII*, 7e (ed. R.W. Kirk), 1067–1072. Philadelphia, PA: WB Saunders Co.

238 Fourman, P. and Leeson, P.M. (1959). Thirst and polyuria, with a note on the effects of potassium deficiency and calcium excess. *Lancet* 1: 268–271.

239 Levi, M., Ellis, M.A., and Berl, T. (1983). Control of renal hemodynamics and glomerular filtration rate in chronic hypercalcemia. Role of prostaglandins, renin-angiotensin system, and calcium. *J. Clin. Invest.* 71: 1624–1632.

240 Levi, M., Peterson, L., and Berl, T. (1983). Mechanism of concentrating defect in hypercalcemia. Role of polydipsia and prostaglandins. *Kidney Int.* 23: 489–497.

241 Serros, E.R. and Kirschenbaum, M.A. (1981). Prostaglandin-dependent polyuria in hypercalcemia. *Am. J. Phys* 241: F224–F230.

242 Goldfarb, S. and Agus, Z.S. (1984). Mechanism of the polyuria of hypercalcemia. *Am. J. Nephrol.* 4: 69–76.

243 Brunette, M.G., Vary, J., and Carriere, S. (1974). Hyposthenuria in hypercalcemia. A possible role of intrarenal blood-flow (IRBF) redistribution. *Pflugers Archiv.* 350: 9–23.

244 Carney, S. and Morgan, T.O. (1986). Mechanisms of polyuria of hypercalcemia. *Am. J. Nephrol.* 6: 230–231.

245 Carney, S., Rayson, B., and Morgan, T. (1976). A study in vitro of the concentrating defect associated with hypokalaemia and hypercalcaemia. *Pflugers Archiv.* 366: 11–17.

246 Anderson, R.J., Berl, T., McDonald, K.D. et al. (1975). Evidence for an in vivo antagonism between vasopressin and prostaglandin in the mammalian kidney. *J. Clin. Invest.* 56: 420–426.

247 Harris, D.C., Gabow, P.A., Linas, S.L. et al. (1986). Prevention of hypercalcemia-induced renal concentrating defect and tissue calcium accumulation. *Am. J. Phys.* 251: F642–F646.

248 Edwards, B.R., Sutton, R.A., and Dirks, J.H. (1974). Effect of calcium infusion on renal tubular reabsorption in the dog. *Am. J. Phys.* 227: 13–18.

249 Spangler, W.L., Gribble, D.H., and Lee, T.C. (1979). Vitamin D intoxication and the pathogenesis of vitamin D nephropathy in the dog. *Am. J. Vet. Res.* 40: 73–83.

250 Yendt, E.R. (1972). Disorders of calcium, phosphorus, and magnesium metabolism. In: *Clinical Disorders of Fluid and Electrolyte Metabolism*, 2e (ed. M.H. Maxwell and C.R. Kleeman), 401–503. New York: McGraw-Hill.

251 Anning, S.T., Dawson, J. et al. (1948). The toxic effects of calciferol. *Q. J. Med.* 17: 203–228.

252 Epstein, F.H. (1968). Calcium and the kidney. *Am. J. Med.* 45: 700–714.

253 Khositseth, S., Charngkaew, K., Boonkrai, C. et al. (2017). Hypercalcemia induces targeted autophagic degradation of aquaporin-2 at the onset of nephrogenic diabetes insipidus. *Kidney Int.* 91: 1070–1087.

254 Hebert, S.C. (1996). Extracellular calcium-sensing receptor: implications for calcium and magnesium handling in the kidney. *Kidney Int.* 50: 2129–2139.

255 Wang, W., Li, C., Kwon, T.H. et al. (2004). Reduced expression of renal Na+ transporters in rats with PTH-induced hypercalcemia. *Am. J. Physiol. Renal Physiol.* 286: F534–F545.

256 Wang, W., Kwon, T.H., Li, C. et al. (2002). Reduced expression of Na-K-2Cl cotransporter in medullary TAL in vitamin D-induced hypercalcemia in rats. *Am. J. Physiol. Renal Physiol.* 282: F34–F44.

257 Hebert, S.C. (2004). Calcium and salinity sensing by the thick ascending limb: a journey from mammals to fish and back again. *Kidney Int. Suppl.* 66 (91): S28–S33.

258 Bustamante, M., Hasler, U., Leroy, V. et al. (2008). Calcium-sensing receptor attenuates AVP-induced aquaporin-2 expression via a calmodulin-dependent mechanism. *J. Am. Soc. Nephrol.* 19: 109–116.

259 Earm, J.H., Christensen, B.M., Frokiaer, J. et al. (1998). Decreased aquaporin-2 expression and apical plasma membrane delivery in kidney collecting ducts of polyuric hypercalcemic rats. *J. Am. Soc. Nephrol.* 9: 2181–2193.

260 Wang, W., Li, C., Kwon, T.H. et al. (2002). AQP3, p-AQP2, and AQP2 expression is reduced in polyuric rats with hypercalcemia: prevention by cAMP-PDE inhibitors. *Am. J. Physiol. Renal Physiol.* 283: F1313–F1325.

261 Fettman, M.J. (1989). Feline kaliopenic polymyopathy/nephropathy syndrome. *Vet. Clin. North Am. Small Anim. Pract.* 19: 415–432.

262 Khositseth, S., Uawithya, P., Somparn, P. et al. (2015). Autophagic degradation of aquaporin-2 is an early event in hypokalemia-induced nephrogenic diabetes insipidus. *Sci. Rep.* 5: 18311.

263 Welt, L.G., Hollander, W. Jr., and Blythe, W.B. (1960). The consequences of potassium depletion. *J. Chronic Dis.* 11: 213–254.

264 Javadi, S., Djajadiningrat-Laanen, S.C., Kooistra, H.S. et al. (2005). Primary hyperaldosteronism, a mediator of progressive renal disease in cats. *Domest. Anim. Endocrinol.* 28: 85–104.

265 Giebisch, G. and Lozano, R. (1959). The effects of adrenal steroids and potassium depletion on the elaboration of an osmotically concentrated urine. *J. Clin. Invest.* 38: 843–853.

266 Buffington, C.A., DiBartola, S.P., and Chew, D.J. (1991). Effect of low potassium commercial nonpurified diet on renal function of adult cats. *J. Nutr.* 121: S91–S92.

267 Dow, S.W. and Fettman, M.J. (1992). Chronic renal disease and potassium depletion in cats. *Semin. Vet. Med. Surg. (Small Anim)* 7: 198–201.

268 Dow, S.W., Fettman, M.J., LeCouteur, R.A. et al. (1987). Potassium depletion in cats: renal and dietary influences. *J. Am. Vet. Med. Assoc.* 191: 1569–1575.

269 DiBartola, S.P., Buffington, C.A., Chew, D.J. et al. (1993). Development of chronic renal disease in cats fed a commercial diet. *J. Am. Vet. Med. Assoc.* 202: 744–751.

270 Ferrebee, J.W., Parker, D., Carnes, W.H. et al. (1941). Certain effects of desoxycorticosterone; the development of "Diabetes Insipidus" and the replacement of muscle potassium by sodium in normal dogs. *Am. J. Phys* 135: 230.

271 Smith, S.G. and Lasater, T.E. (1950). A diabetes insipidus-like condition produced in dogs by a potassium deficient diet. *Proc. Soc. Exp. Biol. Med.* 74: 427–431.

272 Theisen, S.K., DiBartola, S.P., Radin, M.J. et al. (1997). Muscle potassium content and potassium gluconate supplementation in normokalemic cats with naturally occurring chronic renal failure. *J. Vet. Intern. Med.* 11: 212–217.

273 Ching, S.V., Fettman, M.J., Hamar, D.W. et al. (1989). The effect of chronic dietary acidification using ammonium chloride on

acid-base and mineral metabolism in the adult cat. *J. Nutr.* 119: 902–915.

274 Dow, S.W., Fettman, M.J., Smith, K.R. et al. (1990). Effects of dietary acidification and potassium depletion on acid-base balance, mineral metabolism and renal function in adult cats. *J. Nutr.* 120: 569–578.

275 Adams, L.G., Polzin, D.J., Osborne, C.A. et al. (1994). Influence of dietary protein/calorie intake on renal morphology and function in cats with 5/6 nephrectomy. *Lab. Invest.* 70: 347–357.

276 Jones, B.R. and Gruffydd-Jones, T.J. (1990). Hypokalemia in the cat. *Cornell Vet.* 80: 13–15.

277 Elliott, J. and Barber, P.J. (1998). Feline chronic renal failure: clinical findings in 80 cases diagnosed between 1992 and 1995. *J. Small Anim. Pract.* 39: 78–85.

278. DiBartola, S.P., Rutgers, H.C., Zack, P.M. et al. (1987). Clinicopathologic findings associated with chronic renal disease in cats: 74 cases (1973-1984). *J. Am. Vet. Med. Assoc.* 190: 1196–1202.

279 Lulich, J.P., O'Brien, T.D., Osborne, C.A. et al. (1992). Feline renal failure: questions, answers, questions. *Compend. Contin. Educ. Pract. Vet.* 14: 127–152.

280 DiBartola, S.P. and DeMorais, H.A. (2012). Disorders of potassium: hypokalemia and hyperkalemia. In: *Fluid, Electrolyte, and Acid-Base Disorders in Small Animal Practice* (ed. S.P. DiBartola), 92–119. St. Louis, Missouri: Elsevier Saunders.

281 Dow, S.W., Fettman, M.J., Curtis, C.R. et al. (1989). Hypokalemia in cats: 186 cases (1984-1987). *J. Am. Vet. Med. Assoc.* 194: 1604–1608.

282 Ragan, C., Ferrebee, J.W., Phyfe, P. et al. (1940). A syndrome of polydipsia and polyurla induced in normal animals by desoxycorticosterone acetate. *Am. J. Phvsiol.* 131: 73.

283 Mulinos, M.G., Spingern, C.L., and Lojkm, M.E. (1941). A diabetes insipidus-like condition produced by small doses of desoxycorticosterone acetate in dogs. *Am. J. Phys* 135: 102.

284 Dusing, R., Gill, J.R., Gullner, H.G. et al. (1982). The role of prostaglandins in diabetes insipidus produced by desoxycorticosterone in the dog. *Endocrinology* 110: 644–649.

285 Gullner, H.G., West, D., Gill, J.R. Jr. et al. (1987). Diabetes insipidus with renal resistance to vasopressin in the desoxycorticosterone-treated dog: a possible role for prostaglandins. *Ren. Physiol.* 10: 40–46.

286 Toribio, R.E., Kohn, C.W., Hardy, J. et al. (2005). Alterations in serum parathyroid hormone and electrolyte concentrations and urinary excretion of electrolytes in horses with induced endotoxemia. *J. Vet. Intern. Med.* 19: 223–231.

287 Versteilen, A.M., Heemskerk, A.E., Groeneveld, A.B. et al. (2008). Mechanisms of the urinary concentration defect and effect of desmopressin during endotoxemia in rats. *Shock* 29: 217–222.

288 Stattin Norinder, B., Sandberg, T., and Norrby, R. (2005). Renal concentrating capacity in female outpatients with symptomatic urinary tract infection. *Scand. J. Urol. Nephrol.* 39: 483–487.

289 Maddens, B., Daminet, S., Smets, P. et al. (2010). *Escherichia coli* pyometra induces transient glomerular and tubular dysfunction in dogs. *J. Vet. Intern. Med.* 24: 1263–1270.

290 Heiene, R., van Vonderen, I.K., Moe, L. et al. (2004). Vasopressin secretion in response to osmotic stimulation and effects of desmopressin on urinary concentrating capacity in dogs with pyometra. *Am. J. Vet. Res.* 65: 404–408.

291 Asheim, A. (1965). Pathogenesis of renal damage and polydipsia in dogs with pyometra. *J. Am. Vet. Med. Assoc.* 147: 736–745.

292 Asheim, A. (1964). Renal function in dogs with pyometra. 8. Uterine infection and the pathogenesis of the renal dysfunction. *Acta Pathol. Microbiol. Scand.* 60: 99–107.

293 Stone, E.A., Littman, M.P., Robertson, J.L. et al. (1988). Renal dysfunction in dogs with pyometra. *J. Am. Vet. Med. Assoc.* 193: 457–464.

294 Maddens, B., Heiene, R., Smets, P. et al. (2011). Evaluation of kidney injury in dogs with pyometra based on proteinuria, renal histomorphology, and urinary biomarkers. *J. Vet. Intern. Med.* 25: 1075–1083.

295 Heiene, R., Moe, L., and Molmen, G. (2001). Calculation of urinary enzyme excretion, with renal structure and function in dogs with pyometra. *Res. Vet. Sci.* 70: 129–137.

296 Watts, J.R., Wright, P.J., and Parry, B.W. (2001). Sodium cloprostenol administered at a continuous low dosage induces polydipsia and suppresses luteal function in early dioestrous bitches. *Anim. Reprod. Sci.* 67: 113–123.

297 Zerbe, R., Stropes, L., and Robertson, G. (1980). Vasopressin function in the syndrome of inappropriate antidiuresis. *Annu. Rev. Med.* 31: 315–327.

298 Cuesta, M. and Thompson, C.J. (2016). The syndrome of inappropriate antidiuresis (SIAD). *Best Pract. Res. Clin. Endocrinol. Metab.* 30: 175–187.

299 Ellison, D.H. and Berl, T. (2007). Clinical practice. The syndrome of inappropriate antidiuresis. *N. Engl. J. Med.* 356: 2064–2072.

300 Ranieri, M., Tamma, G., Pellegrino, T. et al. (2019). Gain-of-function mutations of the V2 vasopressin receptor in nephrogenic syndrome of inappropriate antidiuresis (NSIAD): a cell-based assay to assess constitutive water reabsorption. *Pflugers Archiv.* 471: 1291–1304.

301 Feldman, B.J., Rosenthal, S.M., Vargas, G.A. et al. (2005). Nephrogenic syndrome of inappropriate antidiuresis. *N. Engl. J. Med.* 352: 1884–1890.

302 Robertson, G.L. (2006). Regulation of arginine vasopressin in the syndrome of inappropriate antidiuresis. *Am. J. Med.* 119: S36–S42.

303 Breitschwerdt, E.B. and Root, C.R. (1979). Inappropriate secretion of antidiuretic hormone in a dog. *J. Am. Vet. Med. Assoc.* 175: 181–186.

304 Brofman, P.J., Knostman, K.A., and DiBartola, S.P. (2003). Granulomatous amebic meningoencephalitis causing the syndrome of inappropriate secretion of antidiuretic hormone in a dog. *J. Vet. Intern. Med.* 17: 230–234.

305 Shiel, R.E., Pinilla, M., and Mooney, C.T. (2009). Syndrome of inappropriate antidiuretic hormone secretion associated with congenital hydrocephalus in a dog. *J. Am. Anim. Hosp. Assoc.* 45: 249–252.

306 Houston, D.M., Allen, D.G., Kruth, S.A. et al. (1989). Syndrome of inappropriate antidiuretic hormone secretion in a dog. *Can. Vet. J.* 30: 423–425.

307 Martinez, R. and Torrente, C. (2017). Syndrome of inappropriate antidiuretic hormone secretion in a mini-breed puppy associated with aspiration pneumonia. *Top. Companion Anim. Med.* 32: 146–150.

308 Bowles, K.D., Brainard, B.M., and Coleman, K.D. (2015). Syndrome of inappropriate antidiuretic hormone in a bulldog with aspiration pneumonia. *J. Vet. Intern. Med.* 29: 972–976.

309 Barrot, A.C., Bedard, A., and Dunn, M. (2017). Syndrome of inappropriate antidiuretic hormone secretion in a dog with a histiocytic sarcoma. *Can. Vet. J.* 58: 713–715.

310 Giger, U. and Gorman, N.T. (1984). Oncologic emergencies in small animals. Part II. Metabolic and endocrine emergencies. *Compend. Contin. Educ. Pract. Vet.* 6: 805–810. 812.

311 Kang, M.H. and Park, H.M. (2012). Syndrome of inappropriate antidiuretic hormone secretion concurrent with liver disease in a dog. *J. Vet. Med. Sci.* 74: 645–649.

312 Gojska-Zygner, O., Bartosik, J., Gorski, P. et al. (2019). Hyponatraemia and syndrome of inappropriate antidiuretic hormone secretion in non-azotaemic dogs with Babesiosis associated with decreased arterial blood pressure. *J. Vet. Res.* 63: 339–344.

313 Rijnberk, A., Biewenga, W.J., and Mol, J.A. (1988). Inappropriate vasopressin secretion in two dogs. *Acta Endocrinol. (Copenh)* 117: 59–64.

314 Fleeman, L.M., Irwin, P.J., Phillips, P.A. et al. (2000). Effects of an oral vasopressin receptor antagonist (OPC-31260) in a dog with syndrome of inappropriate secretion of antidiuretic hormone. *Aust. Vet. J.* 78: 825–830.

315 DeMonaco, S.M., Koch, M.W., and Southard, T.L. (2014). Syndrome of inappropriate antidiuretic hormone secretion in a cat with a putative Rathke's cleft cyst. *J. Feline Med. Surg.* 16: 1010–1015.

316 Cameron, K. and Gallagher, A. (2010). Syndrome of inappropriate antidiuretic hormone secretion in a cat. *J. Am. Anim. Hosp. Assoc.* 46: 425–432.

317 Grant, I.A., Karnik, K., and Jandrey, K.E. (2010). Toxicities and salvage therapy following overdose of vinblastine in a cat. *J. Small Anim. Pract.* 51: 127–131.

318 Crow, S.E. and Stockham, S.L. (1985). Profound hyponatremia associated with glucocorticoid deficiency in a dog. *J. Am. Anim. Hosp. Assoc.* 21: 393–400.

319 Tuli, G., Tessaris, D., Einaudi, S. et al. (2017). Tolvaptan treatment in children with chronic hyponatremia due to inappropriate antidiuretic hormone secretion: a report of three cases. *J. Clin. Res. Pediatr. Endocrinol.* 9: 288–292.

320 Miell, J., Dhanjal, P., and Jamookeeah, C. (2015). Evidence for the use of demeclocycline in the treatment of hyponatraemia secondary to SIADH: a systematic review. *Int. J. Clin. Pract.* 69: 1396–1417.

321 Khairallah, W., Fawaz, A., Brown, E.M. et al. (2007). Hypercalcemia and diabetes insipidus in a patient previously treated with lithium. *Nat. Clin. Pract. Nephrol.* 3: 397–404.

322 Forrest, J.N. Jr., Cox, M., Hong, C. et al. (1978). Superiority of demeclocycline over lithium in the treatment of chronic syndrome of inappropriate secretion of antidiuretic hormone. *N. Engl. J. Med.* 298: 173–177.

323 Liu, H., Chen, L., Chuang, T. et al. (2017). The effects of vasopressin on the progression of chronic kidney disease and its potential treatment using vasopressin receptor antagonists in the field of veterinary medicine. *Taiwan Vet. J.* 43: 23–28.

324 Vane, L.A., Prough, D.S., Kinsky, M.A. et al. (2004). Effects of different catecholamines on the dynamics of volume expansion of crystalloid infusion. *Anesthesiology* 101: 1136–1144.

325 Schrier, R.W., Berl, T., Harbottle, J.A. et al. (1975). Catecholamines and renal water excretion. *Nephron* 15: 186–196.

326 Johnson, M.D. and Barger, A.C. (1981). Circulating catecholamines in control of renal electrolyte and water excretion. *Am. J. Phys* 240: F192–F199.

327 Schrier, R.W. and Berl, T. (1973). Mechanism of effect of alpha adrenergic stimulation with norepinephrine on renal water excretion. *J. Clin. Invest.* 52: 502–511.

328 Shimamoto, K. and Miyahara, M. (1976). Effect of norepinephrine infusion on plasma vasopressin levels in normal human subjects. *J. Clin. Endocrinol. Metab.* 43: 201–204.

329 Dousa, T.P., Hui, Y.S., and Barnes, L.D. (1978). Microtubule assembly in renal medullary slices: effects of vasopressin, vinblastine, and lithium. *J. Lab Clin. Med.* 92: 252–261.

330 Dousa, T.P. and Barnes, L.D. (1974). Effects of colchicine and vinblastine on the cellular action of vasopressin in mammalian kidney. A possible role of microtubules. *J. Clin. Invest.* 54: 252–262.

331 Vonderen, I.K. (2004). Investigation of the role of vasopressin in dogs with polyuria. *Tijdschrift voor Diergeneeskunde* 129: 751–755.

CHAPTER 5

Chemical Properties of Urine

INTRODUCTION

Urine chemistry provides vital information as part of the complete urinalysis, in addition to physical properties (Chapter 4) and urinary sediment findings (Chapter 6). Measurement of analytes in urine may be qualitative, semiquantitative, or fully quantitative. Benchtop analyzers generate the most accurate quantitative results for specific molecules of interest, like protein. Dry reagent strip testing, often referred to as dipstick or dipstrip testing, generates results that can be qualitative (yes or no) and/or semiquantitative. Color reactions on reagent pads can be read either by manual visual inspection or by an automated reader. Semiquantitative results are assigned a score of 0, +1, +2, or +3 within a range of possible absolute values in mg/dL (see bins concept later). For each color reaction measured, there is a range of possible analyte concentrations. Abnormalities identified from urinary dipstick testing sometimes will require confirmation with a quantitative method for some molecules, especially protein, to generate a precise value. Dipstrip testing provides rapid assessment of urine chemistry and is the most commonly used method to determine urine chemistry results in clinical practice. Dipstrip measurements can be performed at cageside or in the exam room for a quick chemical screening assessment for any obvious abnormalities (glucose +, ketones+, occult blood +) when urine becomes available.

Dipstrips contain a series of chemically impregnated absorbent pads for each analyte on a cellulose or plastic strip designed to interact with urine with the potential to develop color changes (Figures 5.1 and 5.2). The intensity of the color that develops is roughly proportional to the magnitude of analyte detected, which generate semiquantitative results (Figure 5.3). This concept is different than results generated by glucose meters, in which the analyte concentration is directly proportional to the color generated following the application of blood.

Dipstrips vary by manufacturer as to the number of analytes on each strip and the color expected to develop. Some dipstrips designed for human urine chemistry contain reagent pads (e.g. urine specific gravity [USG], white blood cells [WBC] esterase, and nitrites) that are of no or limited value in veterinary patients. Some systems measure and report urobilinogen and others do not. Some urinary dipstrips also contain reagent pads to detect ascorbic acid as a quality control for possible color development interference on some reagent pads (see Section 5.4.11). The same dipstrips are used to determine color reactions during both manual and automated methods. Make sure that the dipstrip matches with the autoanalyzer from the same manufacturer when using automation.

The shelf life, depending on manufacturer, for reagent pad integrity on the dipstrip is around 18 months when the container remains unopened. Reagent strips should not be

Urinalysis in the Dog and Cat, First Edition. Dennis J. Chew and Patricia A. Schenck.
© 2023 John Wiley & Sons, Inc. Published 2023 by John Wiley & Sons, Inc.

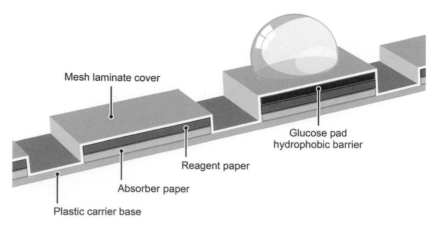

FIGURE 5.1   Structure of a typical urine chemistry dipstrip. The mesh is designed to hold and protect the reagent pad in place and to allow for the rapid and even wetting of the test pad. Note that there is a hydrophobic barrier over the glucose reagent pad that does not allow urine access from the top in some strips; in these instances, urine must enter the test pad from the side. The reagent paper contains the chemical reagents that can develop color. The presence of an inert absorber paper layer between the reagent paper and the carrier strip limits the flow of excess urine and reagents that otherwise could contaminate an adjacent pad. Some pads are thicker than others due to an additional layer that minimizes interference, as might occur with ascorbic acid during measurement of occult blood (not shown). Some pads contain a layer designed to increased sensitivity of a specific analyte (not shown). Illustration by Tim Vojt, reproduced with permission of The Ohio State University.

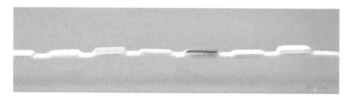

FIGURE 5.2   Side view of urinary chemistry dipstrip (ChemStrip) showing the various reagent pads prior to application of urine.

used beyond the expiration date noted by the manufacturer on the container. The shelf life for dipstrips is about three months after the container has been opened depending on the specific manufacturer and if the container has been quickly capped and the lid kept tight. The containers should be stored at room temperature and not refrigerated. Abnormal (positive) and normal (negative) quality controls for the dipstrip should be performed weekly, or at least when a new container of dipstrips is opened. Quality control liquid vials can be purchased that can be used with most brands of dipstrips. Distilled water should not be used as a negative control since its ionic concentration is markedly lower than that of urine, which affects reagent pad reactions. All reagent pad readings must be negative during use of the negative control. Positive reagent pad reactions must match up with the magnitude provided by the positive control [1].

USING THE DIPSTRIP

The urine chemistry dipstrip measurement is ideally performed on fresh warm urine before the sample is stored or refrigerated (Table 5.1) [2–4]. Refrigerated urine samples should be brought back to room temperature since the reagent pad enzymatic reactions are temperature dependent. A delay in the analysis of stored urine runs the risk for degradation of some analytes in the urine sample. Additionally,

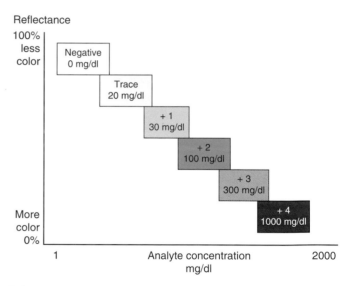

FIGURE 5.3   Hypothetical example showing the relationship between the depth of color development and its magnitude reported semiquantitatively by light reflectance. The amount of color developed is roughly proportional to the concentration of the analyte in question (see text for more details). The mg/dL noted in this example approximates the bins that are commonly measured and assigned for urinary proteins. Note that the bins overlap to some degree at the margins of the bins. This overlap can result in the assignment to either the upper or lower bin when analyte concentrations are near the margins. A second reading on the same sample using a new dipstrip may result in a different bin assignment. Different analyte concentrations within a bin range will all be reported with the same semiquantitative notation despite measured concentrations at the low end, mid-range, or high end for that bin.

lysis of red blood cells (RBC) during storage will alter the reading of how much of the color reaction is due to intact RBC or from released free hemoglobin. In general, the dipstrip measurements are performed on well-mixed urine before settling or centrifugation for urinary microscopy.

Table 5.1   Performing urinary dipstrip measurement.

Steps for performing urinary dipstrip measurement
Warm refrigerated urine to room temperature first.
Keep fresh urine sample ready (preferred over stored)
Make sure that only one brand of dipstrips is available to use throughout the hospital
Check weekly recording of negative and positive quality controls
Ensure dipstrips are not expired
Wear gloves
Ensure good room lighting
Open container and remove dipstrip
Do not touch reagent pads with fingers or gloves
Recap container immediately
Apply urine to strips (immersion of strip into urine or drop bulb technique)
Quickly remove urine from immersion
Apply dipstrip in horizontal position to absorbent paper to remove excess urine
Use stopwatch timing to know when to measure reagent pad color (times vary by pad)
Record color reactions as negative or plus and the mg/dL for most pads (not pH)

Failure to thoroughly mix the urine right before measurement will result in the underreporting of occult blood reactions due to intact RBC that have settled to the bottom of the urine container before urine can be applied to the dipstrip (true for manual or automated methods). Highly pigmented or turbid urine that interferes with accurate reading of color reactions on the reagent pads may clear upon settling or centrifugation, then allowing more accurate reading of color reactions on the pads when urine is applied from the supernatant in these instances.

Select a dipstrip from a container that has not expired. When removing the dipstrip from the container, make sure that the color of the negative blocks for each analyte matches up with the color chart provided by the manufacturer. Otherwise, discard that dipstrip as it is defective. The entire batch of strips in that bottle may be damaged, and it may be necessary to switch to a new bottle of fresh dipstrips [5]. Use only dipstrips that have been stored properly (tight lid and desiccant pad within), as exposure to air and moisture can affect the integrity of the chemicals in the reagent pad within a few hours [4]. Remember to immediately recap the dipstrip container after the dipstrip is removed. The use of only one brand and specific type of urinary dipstrip is recommended throughout the veterinary hospital (community practice, emergency room, specialty services, and in the central laboratory) in order to avoid confusion in results that are generated and to allow more meaningful comparison of serial results on the same patient. It is important to ensure that color charts are matched with the specific manufacturer of the dipstrip when determining the magnitude of color generation on the reagent pads as this is likely to vary.

Urine can be applied to the dipstrip following immersion into urine (Figure 5.4) or by using dropper bulbs or pipettes to apply urine individually to each reagent pad. Immersion of the strip into urine should be brief in order to minimize leaching out of reagents from the pads. Insufficient volume for complete immersion into urine will occur frequently with the small urine volumes often submitted for analysis in dogs and cats. Tilting a urine tube sideways will allow the urine strip to contact enough urine that will allow urine to be absorbed into the pads by wicking action as an alternative (Figure 5.5). Following urine application, the dipstrip should be turned on its side horizontally to touch a tissue or other absorbent paper to remove excessive urine volume [6]. The dipstrip should not be held vertically after urine application. This limits the contamination of urine from one pad spilling over to the other, which otherwise could allow the movement of color reacting chemicals from one pad to the other obscuring or altering the color development on the next pad.

READING THE DIPSTRIP

Urinary chemistry measurement by dipstrip is most often performed in the veterinary clinic by manual visual estimation of color development, though there appears to be a trend for the increased use of partially automated instruments in primary

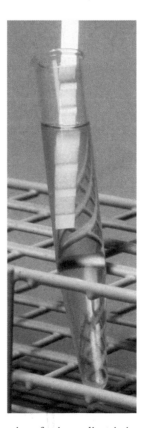

FIGURE 5.4   Immersion of urinary dipstrip in urine. Immersion is possible when a large enough urine volume has been submitted. Immersion should be brief so as to not leach out chemicals from reagent pads.

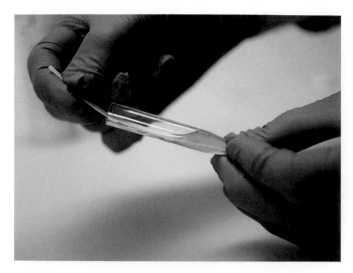

FIGURE 5.5 Insertion of a urinary dipstrip into well mixed urine in a tube before settling or centrifugation. The tube can be tilted in samples with limited urine volume in the tube so that urine that lines the side of the tube can come into contact with the dipstrip.

care practices (Figure 5.6a,b). Automated readers are usually employed by referral laboratories.

It is important to read the color reaction on the reagent pads at the manufacturer-recommended times for each pad. There may be three or four different optimal times for reading depending on the reagent pad. The optimal reading times can vary from 30 seconds to 2 minutes for some reagent pad color reactions [4]. Underdevelopment of color could occur when read too early, and overdevelopment of color could occur when read too late. Automated readers are programmed to ensure that the color reaction for each pad is read at the proper time.

The degree of color reaction on the chemistry dipstrip is generally proportional to the concentration of the analyte in the urine. A ranking for how much color has developed for each analyte is assigned during the manual visual inspection

of the dipstrip. The color on the urine exposed reagent pad is compared to a color chart provided by the specific manufacturer (Figure 5.7). Recording the intensity or depth of color change that develops on the reagent pad by visual analysis is inherently subjective, as humans have limited ability to recognize subtle gradations in color development [7, 8]. The ability of the technician to assign this ranking may vary depending on the individual's visual acuity and ambient lighting. Turbid or highly colored urine can interfere with the ability to manually read the color reaction on the reagent pad. Visibly pink or red urine from hematuria or hemoglobinuria, high amounts of bilirubin in the urine, drugs with dyes, excreted drugs that express color, or vitamins that can add color when excreted into urine can obscure color reactions on the reagent pad [8, 9].

The color of each reagent pad is aligned with the corresponding color chart to see which color block it best matches during manual visual inspection (Figure 5.8). These color blocks are also called "bins" and contain a range of values rather than a single number. It is important to ensure that the dipstrip is compared to the color block to match each analyte from the proper end of the strip. A qualitative value is assigned to most pads as 0, trace, 1+, 2+, 3+ along with a corresponding numerical value in mg/dL or µmol/L that represents each bin. Each color block or bin contains a range of values that are reported the same whether the analyte concentration is at the low or high end of that color block, despite slight differences in color generation. For example, using the protein pad, a 2+ reading that is reported in a urine sample will also report 100 mg/dL by convention. Conceptually, the actual protein content could be 80 mg/dL in one sample and 130 mg/dL in another sample, but both will be reported at 2+. The precise upper and lower limits for each bin set of values will vary somewhat by the dipstrip manufacturer.

Due to inherent variability using dipstrip methods, the same urine specimen measured twice in a row with a new

(a)   (b)

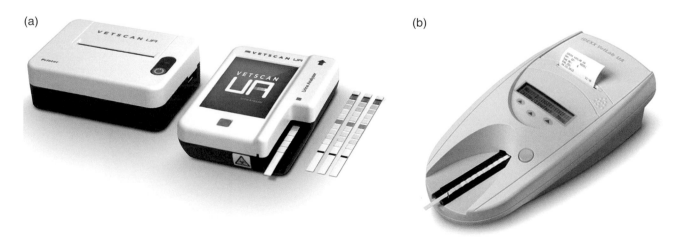

FIGURE 5.6 Two commonly used veterinary automated chemistry strip readers. (a) Zoetis VetScan® UA. Source: Zoetis. (b) IDEXX VetLab. Source: Courtesy of IDEXX Laboratories. Copyright © 2022, IDEXX Laboratories, Inc. All rights reserved. Used with permission.

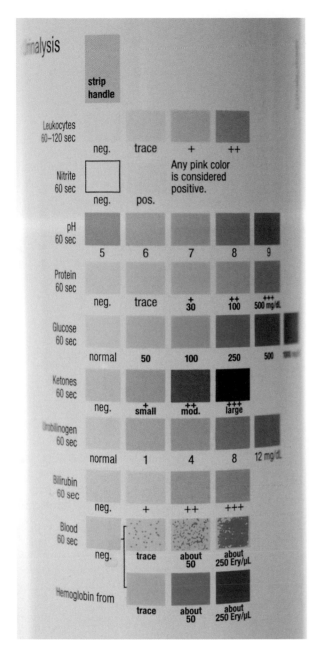

FIGURE 5.7 Color chart used to visually match color that develops on the various reagent pads on the dipstrip. Note that there is a notation to help ensure that the strip is held in the proper orientation before matching color reactions (Roche Cobas urinary dipstrip).

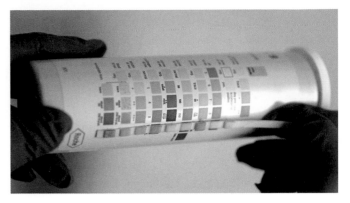

FIGURE 5.8 Matching up the reagent strip color pads with the appropriate color blocks on the chart. The reagent pads are moved over the color chart blocks to determine the best match to be reported. It is essential that the dipstrip be held in the proper orientation (with the handle to the right).

dipstrip could have different color bins reported when the actual analyte concentration is very near the margin as to how that bin is assigned. A specimen could be 0 or trace, trace or 1+, 1+ or 2+, 2+ or 3+ in these instances. It has been considered acceptable to report results that are within one color block or bin above or below the actual result [8, 10, 11]. For some analytes, the bins that are associated with the color block overlap to some degree depending on the manufacturer. A different color bin assignment can occur for two values very close in concentration to each other when one value is just above and the other value just below the margin of the bin. Analytes that measure at the margins of the bins could be read at the higher or the lower bin. In this instance, a protein reading could be 2+ or 3+ despite the same value for the measured protein in mg/dL due to the inherent variability in this method of measurement [8, 10, 11]. Always consult the manufacturer's package insert as reagent pad chemical reagents may have changed, which can have implications for clinical interpretation [5]. Factors that also affect the repeatability of reported results include the potential for varying amounts of reactive chemicals in each dipstrip pad and how urine is deposited on the pad (too little, too much, failure to wick excess after urine is applied). The temperature in the room and the temperature of the urine sample are additional considerations as enzymatic reactions within the pads are temperature dependent but most dipstrips are not temperature compensated.

Color development on an individual reagent pad is not always directly proportional to the concentration of the analyte in the urine, as color development is subject to many potential errors (Table 5.2). Technicians vary in their ability to visually match the color reactions on the reagent pads with the standard color chart on the bottle, and this ability may be adversely affected by poor lighting. Turbid urine or urine that is abnormally colored due to the presence of blood, bilirubin, or certain drugs also may affect the interpretation of color reactions on the dipstrip reagent pads. All dipstrip urinary chemistry analytes except glucose were significantly affected by the amount of blood contamination in the urine from both dogs and cats in one study [12]. Measurement of dipstrip chemistry in the supernatant of a centrifuged urine sample is recommended when obvious interference from intact RBC or turbidity prevents accurate reading of reagent pad color.

Other factors that may interfere with results of dipstrip testing include the temperature of the sample (e.g. refriger-

Table 5.2 Errors in dipstrip reagent pad results.

Urine contamination or interfering substances

Extremes of urine pH

Extremes of urine concentration or dilution

Prolonged storage before measurement

Exposure to UV light

High levels of ascorbic acid in urine (importance yet to be investigated)

Turbidity of urine obscures the pads

Highly colored urine (blood, hemoglobin, bilirubin, drugs, vitamins) obscures pad

Contamination from disinfectants, bleach, food, feces

Handler errors

Failure to return urine to room temperature after refrigeration before measurement

Reading color development on pads at incorrect times

Inadvertently matching the dipstrip colors to the color chart from the wrong end of the strip

Outdated/expired dipstrips

Failure to cap and store dipstrips properly (exposure to air lessens pad reactivity)

Failure to run positive and negative quality controls for new batch of dipstrips

Touching reagent pads with fingers (oils or contaminants interfere with reagents)

Too little or too much urine applied to dipstrip during color development

Overflow of reagent pad chemicals from one pad to another

Loss of chemicals from reagent pad after prolonged exposure in urine

Comparing results from one brand of dipstrips to another

Dipstrip color is compared to color chart from another manufacturer

Failure to match automated reader with the appropriate dipstrip for the analyzer

Poor visual acuity of the personnel reading dipstrip color generation

Poor ambient lighting

---

ated sample not allowed to return to room temperature before testing), contamination of urine by disinfectants or preservatives, interference of the color reaction by drugs in the urine sample, outdated reagent strips, contamination of reagent pads, incorrect timing for reading of reagent pad reaction, and inadvertently holding the standard color chart on the bottle of dipstrips upside down relative to the dipstrip itself. Extremes of urine pH should also be considered for possible positive or negative effects on color development of the other chemistry dipstrip pads [10, 11, 13]. This is why dipstrip readings with current technology are semiquantitative and not purely quantitative in nature.

To evaluate the effect of preservatives in urine, dipstrip chemistry reactions were determined using an autoanalyzer in free catch urine from healthy dogs at time 0, 24, and 72 hours after collection. Results obtained at time 0 from freshly collected urine samples were determined in plain tubes and in tubes with preservatives. Chemistry measurements were repeated at 24 and 72 hours in urine samples stored at room temperature in tubes that contained a preservative and in plain tubes stored in the refrigerator without preservatives. There were very high to high correlations for dipstrip chemistry analytes in all the samples at all time points. All dipstrip chemistry results from refrigerated plain tube samples or from room temperature samples with preservatives were similar to each other and to the time 0 measurements. Since no urine samples contained ketones or glucose, and few had occult blood reactions, conclusions about any effect of preservatives or storage conditions on these urine chemistry results cannot be made. 7–8-mL urine is recommended to be added to tubes containing preservatives in this system to maintain the recommended ratio of urine to preservative, which could limit its use. The effect, if any, of adding smaller urine volumes to the preservative tube has not been reported [14].

AUTOMATED URINARY DIPSTRIP READERS

Fully automated dipstrip analyzer systems are available in human medicine [15]. In these systems, urine is inserted into the instrument, and then, urine is applied to the pads on the dipstrip by the machine prior to the automated reflectance readings. Automated readers standardize the method for the reading of the color that is generated for each reagent pad at the standardized times recommended for that particular system. Automated readers objectively detect color development, which reduces interoperator variability and increases the diagnostic accuracy of the results. Partially automated analyzers are currently used in veterinary medicine, in which the technician first applies urine to the dipstrip and then inserts the dipstrip into the analyzer for measurements to commence (Figure 5.6a,b).

Automated readers direct an LED beam at the various reagent pads once the dipstrip with applied urine is inserted into the analyzer. A photoelectric cell above the reagent pad determines how much light is reflected from the reagent pad, that signal is converted from analog to digital, and then, the percent reflectance is calculated by the instrument's microprocessor. Each chemistry pad is illuminated by a specific wavelength of light, and then, the percentage that is reflected is recorded by the analyzer. Different wavelengths of light are directed to the chemistry pad depending on the specific analyte and the maker of the automated analyzer. The amount of light that is absorbed and reflected depends on how dark or light the pads are following interactions with the urine analyte. As mentioned earlier, a color change that is darker corresponds to a higher concentration of the urinary analyte. The higher the reflectance, the lower the concentration of the analyte; the lower the reflectance (greater absorbance), the greater the concentration of the urinary analyte (Figure 5.3).

Algorithms within the analyzer convert the reflectance into a numeric semiquantitative value or "bin." The reciprocal value of reflectance readings is proportional to the concentration of the measured analyte [10, 11, 16–18]. Reflectance is determined with high accuracy by these instruments, but they still generate semiquantitative results due to factors other than the concentration of the analyte that influence the development of color, as discussed above. Some automated urinary dipstrip readers used in human medicine have the ability to generate results with a specific number along a continuous scale rather than one within a semiquantitative bin [4, 15].

A color compensation pad is included on some dipstrips designed for automated urine chemistry. This pad is the same material as in the other pads but without added reagents. If there is a strong intrinsic color of the urine, the analyzer includes the compensation pad to calculate a corrected final reflectance for each pad. This correction concept is similar to background subtraction, but the algorithm employed by the analyzer is more complicated. Since this is not possible to do visually, the analyzer reading in these instances is more accurate [18].

Several in-house automated urine chemistry analyzers are now marketed to veterinarians on the premise that technician operator time will be reduced, and that the accuracy and precision of results will be greater compared to manual methods. Errors in recorded results are lessened as data are electronically captured and entered into the medical record. Variability in the reading of color pad results between different technicians is eliminated during automated chemistry measurement.

In one study at a teaching hospital, the manual reading of color reactions from the urine chemistry dipstick by the technician did not differ from those generated by the automated analyzer in any canine urine sample [19]. Similar findings were found in other studies when dipstrip reading was performed by experienced veterinary technicians [20, 21]. Such a high concordance between readings from the automated analyzer and manual reading by less experienced technicians is not as likely. In another study, a high degree of discordance was observed between visual urinary dipstrip readings and those by an automated reader using the same dipstrips in one veterinary study of pooled urine samples from dogs with varying amounts of glucose, protein, and RBC. Precision was higher during automated reading of urinary dipstrips compared to visual reading [22]. Poor precision in this study was attributed to lack of sample mixing (visual and automated), not blotting the dipstrip after dipping into the sample, and not reading the color reactions at the manufacturer-recommended time when performing visual analysis. A surprising number of operators held the strip horizontally instead of vertically while matching the color blocks [22].

The use of automated analyzers to measure urine chemistry by dipstrips is advocated over manual visual methods in order to increase the accuracy of reported results and to increase work flow efficiency, though results generated can vary by analyzer [10, 11, 21, 23]. There was high agreement between automated results using a proprietary veterinary analyzer and visual inspection results in one white paper [11]. There was good agreement between dipstrip results using a different proprietary veterinary automated reader compared with a high-end human dipstrip analyzer in another white paper [10]. Accurate reporting and transmission of results is ensured with automated methods, whereas transcription errors sometimes occur during the recording of results following manual reading [4, 11, 20, 21, 24].

There was excellent concordance between results from automated urine chemistry (Cobas u411 analyzer with Roche Chemstrip 10 UA strips) and manual methods, after altering reflectance programming for urine from the dog and cat. This automated method is used in high-throughput laboratories and is not designed for in-house analysis [25].

DIPSTRIP REAGENT PAD COLOR REACTIONS

In normal animals, most dipstrip reactions will be negative (Figure 5.9). The detection of glucose and ketones in urine often indicates excessive generation of these molecules in the body from a systemic disease process. Alterations in urinary pH, protein, and occult blood can reflect disorders of the upper and lower urinary tract, as can the presence of glucose during some types of acute kidney injury (AKI) (rarely during chronic kidney disease [CKD]). Details for individual analyte reagent pad reactions are provided in the subsections that

Chemical Properties - Normal Urinalysis

Automated Strip Reader:	Yes No
Automated White Balance:	Yes No
pH	5.5 to 7.0
Protein	Negative, Trace
	+1 (USG 1.040 to 1.050)
	+2 (USG > 1.060)
Occult Blood	Negative to Trace
Intact RBC	
Hemolyzed	
Glucose	Negative
Ketones	Negative
Bilirubin	Negative to 1+ Dogs, Especially Male
	Negative - Cats

FIGURE 5.9   Expected results from physical properties of normal urinalysis, recorded on a standardized form.

follow. Some of the urinary analytes on the dipstrip designed for humans are not accurately measured in the urine of dogs and cats, such as USG, nitrites, and LE, and are best not recorded to avoid confusion.

The magnitude of color reactions that develop on any reagent pad should be compared to those on all the other reagent pads, as color reactions on one pad could indicate factors that could influence color development on other reagent pads. Urinary physical findings (USG, color, and clarity) and urinary microscopy results should also be integrated into the interpretation of readings on the urinary chemistry dipstrip to maximize interpretation [1, 26]. It is important to remember that clinical decisions from urinary chemistry dipstrip measurements are made in the context of multiple partially flawed results (Wamsley 2020 personal communication).

Further value in the assessment of positive dipstick reactions can sometimes be gained when findings are integrated with the degree of urine concentration (USG). For example, a trace finding may be normal in a urine sample with a >1.050 USG, whereas it could assume clinical significance when the USG was 1.020. Smaller quantitative reactions in dilute urine are potentially of more significance than similar reactions in highly concentrated urine.

Abnormal results on dipstrip chemistry should be verified by repeat measurement, especially when equivocally positive results were initially identified (e.g. trace protein or trace glucose). Greater assurance for a true abnormality is gained when the second dipstrip generates a result in the same bin (both are trace or both are 1+). Some discrepancy between a dipstrip measurement and that generated from a benchtop instrument is expected due to the inherent differences in the methodologies employed (visual or reflectance color determination on a pad compared to the transmission colorimetry of urine). This discrepancy is most common for the protein value estimated on the dipstrip compared to that generated from the benchtop analyzer. Clinical decisions that require a quantitative value, such as urinary-protein-to-creatinine ratio (UPC) for proteinuria, cannot be made from the urinary dipstrip protein estimate alone. Abnormal urine chemistry results determined by dipstrip should be considered a screening procedure to be confirmed by quantitative testing using another method if precise results for that analyte are considered important.

The findings of proteinuria and hematuria on dipstrip chemistry are encountered incidentally at times during wellness screening of seemingly healthy animals that have underlying disorders not yet severe enough to create obvious clinical signs. Abnormal results for urine dipstrip measurements were common in apparently healthy geriatric and senior dogs of one study. Positive reactions for protein were detected in 79%, 84% for bilirubin, 19% for occult blood, 38% for urobilinogen, 1% for nitrite, and 5% for LE in these samples [27]. Trace positive reactions for glucose, ketones, and urobilinogen were detected in 3% of apparently healthy middle-aged and older cats. In another study of younger dogs (median five years of age), all were negative for glucose and ketones, 5% had a positive reaction for occult blood, 65% had trace (15%) or higher reactions (50%) for protein, and 55% had positive reactions for bilirubin [14]. Occult blood reactions were positive in 28%, 99% were positive for LE, while zero of these cats had reactions for bilirubin or nitrites. Based on UPC, borderline proteinuria was common in this population of cats, but comparison to dipstrip reactivity was not provided [28].

Having pet owners monitor dipstrip color reactions at home in these patients may be helpful in these cases (glucose, ketones, pH, blood), but it is also problematic to ensure the accuracy of the reading due to issues with operator training and precise timing for the reading of the dipstrip by the owner. An at-home kit with an embedded urinary dipstrip is available that allows interaction with voided urine from dogs. A smartphone and an app were used to record and score color reactions, but, unfortunately, this system provided unreliable results in one study [29].

Abnormalities on dipstrip chemistry frequently align with abnormal findings from urine microscopy. For example, with positive reactions for occult blood and protein on the dipstrip, urine microscopy will often detect RBC sometimes in association with WBC and bacteria. Protein positive status as the only abnormality on the dipstrip can occur with no microscopic abnormalities in urinary sediment, as often is the case with glomerular proteinuria. Conversely, normal findings on dipstrip chemistry do not guarantee an inactive sediment on urine microscopy. Casts, tubular epithelial cells, urothelial cells, WBC, fungal and bacterial organisms, and crystals are the findings on microscopy that are not detected by the dipstrip that can be detected during urinary microscopy (see Chapter 6). The integration of findings from physical properties, dipstick urine chemistry, and urine microscopy provides the most meaningful clinical information, more than any of these components of the complete urinalysis alone.

URINE pH

Urine pH measures only free hydrogen ions and not hydrogen ions buffered with phosphate or with ammonium in the urine [5] and can provide a crude assessment for systemic acid–base status. The appropriateness of the urinary pH measurement can provide clinically important information when integrated with other findings.

An increase in urine pH can develop when urine samples stand in open containers exposed to air at room temperature for long periods of time, allowing loss of CO_2. The pH of uncontaminated urine stored at room temperature for several hours in a sterile closed container does not change appreciably. In one study of urine from dogs, pH values determined by dipstrip did not change from time 0 (initial collection) to 24 or 72 hours later whether stored at room temperature in preservative-containing tubes or in plain glass tubes in the refrigerator. Median pH was 7 with a range of 6–8.5 in these samples [14]. In another study of dogs, there was no significant effect of storage time (0, 6, and 24 hours) or temperature (room or refrigerator) on urinary pH determined by meter in urine [30]. It is likely that increased pH would occur in urine samples that are exposed to air for long periods or that are mixed with air (allowing loss of CO_2), compared to storage under anaerobic conditions.

Extremely alkaline urine (≥8.5 pH) can also be an artifact when there is contamination of the urine, urinary container, or dipstrip with alkaline detergents (e.g. ammonium or bleach-containing) and surgical scrubs [1, 26, 31, 32]. Contamination with alcohol, benzalkonium, or betadine surgical scrub material potentially increases urinary pH when urine samples are obtained by expression while under anesthesia, but these effects have not been detailed.

Highly alkaline urine may impact findings from urine microscopy due to accelerated degeneration of free cells in the urine and cells within casts [26]. Additionally, the matrix protein within casts is more soluble under conditions of alkaline urine, which can decrease the chances to observe casts that were formed but that broke up quickly.

Urine pH Measurement by Dipstrip

The test pad on the dipstrip is impregnated with various combinations of reagents that produce color gradations depending on the urinary pH of 5–9. Most test pads include a mixture of methyl red and bromothymol blue resulting in shades of orange, yellow, green, and blue. The lowest pH (5.0) generates orange color followed by yellow and green for intermediate pH values, and the highest pH (8.5) generates blue [4, 8, 33]. The color that develops on the reagent pad is compared visually to a color chart provided by the dipstrip manufacturer immediately following the application of urine to the dipstrip. The pH that is recorded is the one that most closely matches the color block on the chart and is estimated to the nearest 0.5 or 1.0 pH unit depending on the manufacturer of the dipstrip. The measurement of pH by dipstrip is considered accurate to within 1 pH unit (±1 unit) when compared to pH meter [8, 26], a high level of discordance that is not generally appreciated in veterinary medicine. Reporting urinary pH to the nearest 0.5 pH unit can lead to the false impression that the dipstrip pH measurement provides a high level of accuracy and precision (Heather Wamsley personal communication 2019). For this reason, some urinary dipstrips are manufactured that provide pH to the nearest whole unit pH value instead (e.g. 6, 7, and 8).

Historically, urine pH by dipstrip has been considered useful in providing an approximation of urine pH during routine urinalysis [34, 35]. Unfortunately, the estimation of urine pH by dipstrip shows only poor-to-moderate agreement with pH measured by meter. The measurement of urine pH by dipstrip has been described as inherently inaccurate and its continued use is one of convenience instead of accuracy [36]. Consequently, urine pH by dipstrip often is not accurate enough to make informed clinical decisions in many disorders.

Urine pH by dipstrip in spot urine samples was compared to pH measured by an electrode in 24-hour urine samples from humans. Greater inaccuracy was found in urine samples with a spot urine pH > 6.5, but pH by dipstrip was associated with a large range in pH by electrode in this study. Based on these findings, urine pH by dipstrip from spot urine was considered unacceptable in the monitoring and management of human patients with urolithiasis [37].

The inaccurate determination of urine pH by dipstrip could also result in faulty treatment strategies to alter urinary pH to prevent urolithiasis. For example, the dipstick method tended to overestimate pH in one study of dogs suggesting the presence of alkaline urine when the urine was mildly acidic by pH meter [35]. Urinary pH by dipstrip reported acidic urine in cats when readings by pH meter indicated a neutral to mildly alkaline urine in some cats [34]. The clinical interpretation of inaccurate urinary pH readings by dipstrip is most likely to occur when pH values are near neutral [38]. Urine pH values more removed from neutral are likely to align in the same bin when measured by meter (high–high or low–low) despite differing actual values.

When measured by dipstrip, visible blood contamination lowered the score assigned to urinary pH in both dogs and cats of one study, though the magnitude of change was considered small. Urinary pH was significantly lower in red urine samples from dogs and cats, and in combined red (light pink, dark pink, and red) samples from cats [12].

Extremes in urinary pH have the potential to alter color development on other reagent pads on the dipstrip, as can occur with a high urine pH and an increased reaction for protein in urine that is highly concentrated. Also, contamination of the pH pad with acid buffer flowing from the protein reagent pad during poor technique is a consideration for a falsely low urinary pH [12, 39].

Automated readers are available to read dipstrip results and may provide more consistent and more accurate readings of urinary pH. Pooled urine samples from dogs that were acidic, neutral, or alkaline were measured by dipstrip for pH by visual and by automated methods to detect color development. Compared to urinary pH by meter as the gold standard, accuracy for pH readings was higher with the use of automated readings compared to that recorded following visual analysis assessed by multiple operators for all the samples [22]. In another study, there was good agreement between urinary pH determined by visual assessment and an automated reader in urine from dogs of one study (a pH meter was not used for comparison) [20]. Similarly, correlation between urinary pH by visual reading and those by an automated reader was considered excellent in another study of urine from dogs and cats [21].

Urine pH Measurement by a pH Meter

The gold standard for the measurement of urinary pH is provided by either benchtop or portable pH meters that have been properly maintained and calibrated [14, 30, 34–36].

If accurate measurement of urine pH is important in clinical decision-making, a pH meter should be used [26, 34–36, 38]. Relatively inexpensive portable pH meters can be used in-house, or a refrigerated urine sample can be shipped to a reference laboratory within 24 hours of collection to obtain an accurate urinary pH [30, 35].

Comparisons of Dipstrip and pH Meter Methodology

There can be significant discordance between urinary pH measured by dipstrip and pH meter. A pH meter can be used to confirm or determine more accurate results, particularly when pigmenturia obscures or alters test pad color [32].

The degree of agreement for urinary pH was compared between a benchtop pH meter, two portable pH meters, urinary dipstrip, and pH paper in urine from normal cats. The expiration of the electrodes on one of the portable pH meters accounted for a negative bias on the pH readings. The pH paper had poor agreement, and dipstrip pH readings had intermediate agreement with pH measured by the benchtop analyzer. The pH measured by dipstrip had an average negative bias of −0.12 pH units compared to the benchtop analyzer, but displayed much greater discordance at lower pH values on the dipstrip. The difference in urine pH measured by the benchtop analyzer after 24 hours of refrigeration (mean increase of 0.04) compared to time 0 was not considered clinically relevant. Electrode maintenance and daily calibration of portable pH meters is important to ensure the accuracy of test results [34]. In another study of urine from hospitalized dogs, urinary pH was compared between a benchtop pH meter, four portable pH meters, urinary dipstrip, and pH paper. Three of the four portable pH meters provided nearly identical results to that from the benchtop meter. However, there was moderate-to-poor agreement for urinary pH results determined by dipstrip or pH paper compared to the benchtop meter [35]. Mean urinary pH measured by dipstrip was significantly higher (7.11 ± 0.12) than when measured by pH meter (6.83 ± 0.12) in urine from dogs; urinary pH did not change when analyzed before or after centrifugation [40].

In cats, urinary pH by dipstrip was consistently lower compared to measurement by pH meter; a consistent error in direction of pH was not found in dogs of the same study. The authors of this study suggested that pH by dipstrip should be within ± 0.25 pH units of that measured by pH meter in order to be clinically useful, but this only occurred in 40% of the samples analyzed. A dipstrip pH of 7 corresponded to a pH meter pH of 6.2–8.2 [36]. In another study in cats, a dipstrip urinary pH of 6 corresponded to a meter pH of 5.81–7.18 [34].

Expected Urine pH in Health and Disease

The normal urinary pH of dogs and cats is generally considered to be from 5.0 to 7.5 [41, 42] or from 6.0 to 7.5 [3, 43] depending on age, nutrients in the diet, food intake (ad libitum or meal fed), and timing of the urine sample collection. The mean urinary pH of 5.1 ± 0.3 in one day old Great

Dane puppies significantly increased on day 5 of age to 5.3 ± 0.6. The initially low urinary pH was attributed to a combination of respiratory and metabolic acidosis in newborn pups [44].

Bone growth of the young is associated with the production of calcium apatite and protons that are excreted into urine, which decreases urinary pH. When bone growth is finished, urinary pH tends to increase [36, 45]. The possibility for the elaboration of slightly more acid urine following the sleeping hours and mild respiratory acidosis [42] has not been critically evaluated in dogs or cats.

The amount and type of protein, acidifying or alkalinizing minerals [46], and organic anions and cations in the diet contribute to urinary pH. Decreased urinary pH is expected when eating higher concentration of proteins, especially those with sulfur-containing amino acids, which generate acid products following metabolism (Table 5.3). The consumption of organic cations usually increases the urinary pH (Table 5.4). The ingestion of diets based on cereal or vegetables may generate alkaline urine due to the excretion of alkaline end products following metabolism. Urinary pH is lower in young cats compared to adult cats eating the same diet. Urinary pH tends

Table 5.3 Causes of acidic urine.

Causes of acidic urine
Meat-based high protein diet
Administration of acidifying agents (e.g. dl-methionine; NH_4Cl)
Metabolic acidosis
Respiratory acidosis
Paradoxical aciduria in metabolic alkalosis with hypokalemia & chloride depletion
Protein catabolic states

Table 5.4 Causes of alkaline urine.

Causes of alkaline urine
Plant-based diet (cereal or vegetable)
Urine allowed to stand open to air at room temperature (loss of CO_2)
Postprandial alkaline tide
Urinary tract infection by urease-positive organism
Contamination of urine sample with bacteria during or after collection
Administration of alkalinizing agents (e.g. $NaHCO_3$, citrate, acetate, lactate)
Thiazide diuretics
Metabolic alkalosis
Respiratory alkalosis (including stress-induced, especially in cats)
Distal renal tubular acidosis
Paradoxical alkalinuria in states of primary hyperkalemia

toward neutral to slightly acidic during fasting of normal animals, as demonstrated by the finding of a urinary pH by meter of 6.5–7 regardless of the baseline pH when normal adult cats were fasted for three days [45].

An increased urinary pH of varying magnitude following food intake is sometimes observed in dogs and cats. This transient increase in urinary pH has been attributed to the so-called postprandial alkaline tide as a response following gastric acid secretion [42], but this explanation appears too simplistic [47]. A fall in urinary acid excretion was still seen following food intake despite blockade of gastric acid secretion in one study of humans, so the mechanism for the generation of this alkaline urine remains unclear. Also, a decrease in urinary acid excretion was seen after the feeding of high compared to lower concentrations of dietary protein, fasting, or ingestion of water alone [47]. The postprandial alkaline urine effect can be protracted, and it may require 8–12 hours fasting after feeding for more acidic urine to return. For these reasons, the timing of the urine sample collection in relationship to eating or fasting should be factored into the interpretation of neutral to alkaline urinary pH.

An abnormal urine pH (>7.5 pH) was detected in 17.4% of samples from dogs and in 8.2% of samples from cats at a veterinary teaching hospital. Of these abnormal pH samples, 52.3% from the dogs and 74.4% from the cats were subsequently found to be associated with some microscopic abnormality [41]. A wide range of urinary pH was encountered in dogs evaluated at a teaching hospital, from 5.0 to 9.0 as determined by visual inspection of the color reactions. Urinary pH was 8–9 in 40% of these samples and 5.0 in 24%. A pH of 6.5–7.0 was encountered in 22% of the samples [48].

Urinary pH is not a reliable indicator for the precise assessment of acid–base status, as there are many instances where urinary pH is discordant from systemic acidemia or alkalemia. Urinary pH is influenced by acid–base balance, but this is not a simple function of the blood pH, as this can be affected by systemic disease, renal tubular health (e.g. CKD and AKI), effective circulating blood volume, and concurrent electrolyte disorders. In general, metabolic and respiratory acidosis result in aciduria, whereas metabolic and respiratory alkalosis result in alkaline urine following compensatory mechanisms. The optimal interpretation of urinary pH is made when blood gases are available to fully characterize the nature of the acid–base disturbance.

Paradoxical aciduria occurs in some dogs and cats that have metabolic alkalosis in association with the contraction of circulating blood volume, along with the depletion of sodium, potassium, and chloride as can occur during gastrointestinal (GI) obstruction. In these instances, alkalinuria develops as a compensatory response to restore normal acid–base balance following fluid therapy to restore circulating volume and chloride and potassium repletion. Paradoxical alkalinuria potentially develops in states characterized predominantly by hyperkalemia in which the translocation of potassium into and hydrogen ions out of cells occurs. Uncommonly, distal renal tubular acidosis may be responsible for alkaline urine or an inability to maximally acidify urine. Because of these variations, evaluation of urinary pH by itself can be misleading and lead to the wrong characterization of an acid–base disturbance. Intermittent alkaline urine was documented in a cat that was fed an acidifying diet, likely due to stress-induced respiratory alkalosis during visits to the veterinary hospital [49].

Drugs may affect urine pH, and the drug history of the animal should be considered when evaluating urine pH. Urinary acidifiers (e.g. ascorbic acid, d,l-methionine, and ammonium chloride) result in the production of acidic urine. The administration of alkalinizing agents, such as sodium bicarbonate or citrate, and carbonic anhydrase inhibitor diuretics (e.g. acetazolamide) causes the formation of alkaline urine.

Urinary pH often aligns with certain types of crystals in urinary sediment. For example, urate, cystine, and calcium oxalate crystals are more apt to form in acid urine, whereas struvite tends to form in alkaline urine. The prediction of the urolith type in the absence of quantitative stone analysis is facilitated by knowing the urinary pH in addition to breed, age, sex, and radiodensity of the stone. Manipulation of urinary pH is often attempted to try to prevent the recurrence of urolithiasis based on crystal type and solubility characteristics.

Urinary pH may not indicate how much acid is being excreted by the kidneys in some instances, if the urine is changed after renal processing [50]. Urinary tract infection (UTI) with urease-producing bacteria (*Proteus spp*, *Staphylococcus aureus*, *Mycoplasma spp*) can be associated with persistently alkaline urine, often with urinary pH ≥ 7.5 and as high as 9.0 in some dogs. Many bacterial UTIs, however, do not result in alkaline urine and exist in neutral or acid urine [51]. Alkaline urine may also develop if a sample of normal urine is contaminated with urease-producing bacteria. If this urine is allowed to stand at room temperature, bacteria proliferate and urea can be hydrolyzed, resulting in alkaline urine the same as happens with a real urinary infection.

URINARY PROTEIN

Protein in the urine can be measured by qualitative, semiquantitative, or quantitative methods (see Chapter 7 for details). Reagent dipstrip pads allow qualitative and semiquantitative colorimetric determination if the reaction on the pad is read at the appropriate time interval. Standard reagent strips estimate the protein concentration in urine, the magnitude of which is influenced by the degree of urine concentration (USG, U_{osm}), which is importantly dependent on the patient's state of hydration. Consequently, results from urinary reagent pads for protein only provide a rough assessment as to whether or not there is pathological proteinuria [4].

Methodology

Increasing protein concentrations in the urine cause the chemical indicator in the reagent pad (tetrabromophenol blue or tetrachlorophenol-tetrabromosulfonphthalein) to change color [1, 4, 5, 32]. A positive reaction on the reagent pad does not identify a particular protein, but the indicator is much more sensitive to albumin than to globulins, Bence Jones protein, mucoproteins, hemoglobin, myoglobin, and other nonalbumin proteins [4, 8, 32, 33, 50, 52]. The color change on the reagent pad is based on the ability of free amino groups of proteins in the urine to bind to the color indicator, which varies by specific protein. This test pad detects albumin most readily since albumin has an abundance of free amino groups compared to other proteins in urine and so develops the strongest color. Nonalbumin urinary proteins can be detected if they have enough free amino groups and the protein concentration is high enough. Consequently, a negative reagent pad reaction for protein does not automatically exclude the presence of these nonalbumin proteins [1, 5, 32, 38, 53]. Specific bins for the degree of color development on the reagent pad and the protein concentration reported vary by manufacturer, especially at the trace and maximal amount of protein that is reported.

Albumin in the urine is the protein of greatest interest in most clinical cases, as it is the predominant urinary protein in disease and in health [1, 32, 38, 54–58]. The gradations in color intensity for each block/bin of protein reagent pad on the dipstrip are subtle making it difficult at times to assign the proper block during visual inspection. It appears likely that the assignment of the proper color block for urinary protein has the most errors of any pad on the dipstrip when assessed manually using visual inspection. Any abnormal color of the urine (hemorrhage bilirubin) also makes it difficult to impossible to properly read the color that develops on the reagent pad [3].

The lower limit of sensitivity for detection of proteinuria using conventional dipstrips is approximately 10–20 mg/dL for a trace reading on the reagent pad, depending on the specific manufacturer. The ability to detect protein in urine (sensitivity) depends on the type and proportion of urinary proteins [4]. Maximal intensity color reaction occurs at protein concentrations ≥ 2000 mg/dL, ≥ 1000 mg/dL, ≥ 600 mg/dL, 500 mg/dL, or 300 mg/dL depending on the specific dipstrip manufacturer. In general, the protein concentration of urine measured by dipstrip is reported qualitatively as negative (<10 or 15 mg/dL), trace (10–20 mg/dL), 1+ (30 mg/dL), 2+ (100 mg/dL), 3+ (300 mg/dL), or 4+ (1000 mg/dL). 1+ and 2+ reactions are the most consistent reagent pad determinations among different manufacturers. Due to difficulty in the interpretation of trace protein reactions, the reporting of trace values can be suppressed by some laboratories [1].

Interferences

Visibly bloody urine can result in the reporting of false-positive protein results from discoloration of the reagent pad [8, 12]. A repeat dipstrip measurement using urine supernatant after RBC have settled by gravity or after centrifugation can lessen the discoloration of the reagent pad. The

dipstrip reagent pad for protein did not develop a positive reaction (100 mg/dL) until the hemoglobin concentration was >5 mg/dL in one study from dogs. Less than maximal reactions for hemoglobin on the dipstrip at the same time that the protein dipstrip is positive indicates that the protein being detected on the reagent pad cannot be attributed to hemoglobin [52]. According to one package insert, false-positive reactions are also noted to occur when reagent pads are exposed to strongly alkaline urine (>8.0 pH), following treatment with some intravenous (IV) blood substitutes, and when the urine sample has been contaminated with disinfectants (quaternary ammonium or chlorhexidine) that activate color development on the reagent pad (Table 5.5) [33]. False-negative results for reagent pad protein can occur in urine that is highly acidic (pH < 6.0) or urine that is minimally concentrated or dilute (1.001–1.017 USG). Results on the reagent pad do not appear to be affected by turbidity, radiographic contrast agents [59], most medications, and preservatives that are in the urine sample.

Interpretation

Small amounts of protein are excreted into urine by the normal dog and cat, which often are read as trace to 1+ on the reagent pad [32, 54, 55, 57, 58]. Highly concentrated urine magnifies the concentration of small amounts of protein normally found in the urine [3, 43]. The protein reagent pad was negative in 21%, trace in 27%, and positive at $\geq 1+$ in 52% of 97 apparently healthy senior and geriatric dogs [27]. Mean dipstrip proteinuria ≥ 30 mg/dL was not detected in any voided urine sample from healthy Great Dane puppies of 0–28 days of age. Trace reactions for protein were detected in 65.5% of these urine samples at 10 days of age [44].

Most of the protein in urine from normal and diseased animals is albumin [32, 38]; small amounts of globulins from the urethra and genital tract may be detected in samples collected by voiding from normal animals. Randomly collected,

Table 5.5 Errors in the protein measurement on dipstrip analysis.

Errors in protein measurement on dipstrip analysis
False positive
Very alkaline urine (pH > 8) overcomes acid buffer in pad
Urine contaminated with disinfectants – benzalkonium chloride or quaternary ammonium compounds
Activation of the reagent pad by cauxin in urine from cats
Highly concentrated urine (high USG) when UPC is normal
Loss of buffer reagents from pad following prolonged immersion of strip in urine
Blood substitute treatment
False negative
Very acidic or dilute urine
Non-albumin proteins in low concentration

voided urine samples from normal dogs contained 0–56 mg/dL of protein as measured by a urinary dipstrip or heat precipitation [60]. In another study of 31 normal dogs, positive urinary dipstrip reactions for protein recorded as trace (15 mg/dL) or 1+ (30 mg/dL) were common. This resulted in the recommendation that trace to 1+ reactions for protein on the dipstrip be considered within the reference range for dogs and not automatically be considered a false positive. By benchtop methods, the urinary total protein ranged from 3.0 to 39.0 mg/dL with a mean of 20.4 mg/dL, median of 15.0 mg/dL, and with the highest UPC at 0.21 [61]. When the dipstrip for urinary protein is ≥2+ regardless of USG, the UPC will usually be >0.4 for the cat or >0.5 for the dog. In minimally concentrated or dilute urine, a trace or 1+ dipstrip reaction for protein may indicate clinically relevant proteinuria when further assessed by UPC or microalbumin (MA). In samples with isosthenuria or very dilute urine (1.001–1.017), the dipstrip may register as negative or trace despite the presence of clinically relevant proteinuria due to the lower of limit of sensitivity (10–20 mg/dL) of the reagent pad.

The accurate interpretation of proteinuria necessitates integration of findings from the history, physical examination, urinary sediment activity, degree of urine concentration, and method of urine collection (Table 5.6). Postrenal proteinuria (UTI, stones, neoplasia) is most commonly encountered, renal origin is second in frequency, and prerenal proteinuria is uncommon in dogs and cats with clinical disorders. The origin of proteinuria as prerenal, postrenal, genital, glomerular, or tubular cannot be determined by the magnitude of the proteinuria in isolation on the dipstrip reagent pad. Persistent proteinuria associated with a normal urinary sediment (inactive sediment with few WBC, RBC, nonsquamous epithelial cells, no bacteria) or a sediment with excessive numbers of hyaline and granular casts is the hallmark of glomerular disease (e.g. glomerulonephritis, glomerular amyloidosis, glomerulosclerosis). Proteinuria associated with hematuria or pyuria does not allow anatomical localization, as inflammation or hemorrhage could occur anywhere along the urinary or genital tracts, allowing the entry of plasma proteins into the urine. Marked hematuria can be associated with the detection of proteinuria on the reagent pad, while disorders causing substantial pyuria can result in concomitant mild-to-moderate proteinuria by reagent pad. If the sediment is active and proteinuria is mild to moderate, consider inflammatory renal disease or disease of the lower urinary or genital tract to account for the proteinuria [62, 63].

Urine protein results should be integrated with the degree of urine concentration (USG) for the interpretation of whether the proteinuria is likely to be pathological or not. Higher protein concentrations in mg/dL are expected from urine samples with a high USG, and lower protein concentrations are expected from those with minimal urine concentration. For example, when the same amount of protein is excreted into urine, the protein may be measured by dipstrip at 30 mg/dL when the USG was 1.015 and at 300 mg/dL when the USG was 1.055. In another example, a trace or 1+ proteinuria (30 mg/dL) in a urine sample with a USG of 1.007 may be clinically relevant. The same 1+ proteinuria via reagent pad in a urine sample with a USG of 1.065 is less likely to be clinically relevant as a consequence of the concentration of urinary proteins following the removal of water by the kidneys in such a highly concentrated urine sample. Any positive protein pad color reaction in patients with minimally concentrated or dilute urine (1.001–1.020) may be clinically relevant and should be further investigated with UPC [1, 5, 32, 43, 53].

Trace and 1+ dipstrip reactions are the most problematic, regardless of the degree of urine concentration, to know if they indicate pathological proteinuria or not without confirmatory testing (UPC or MA). Dipstrip protein ≥2+ are usually associated with pathologic proteinuria and albuminuria. In some commercial veterinary laboratories, a trace or 1+ positive color reaction on the dipstrip is confirmed with sulfosalicylic acid (SSA) precipitation testing. If both are positive, then the proteinuria is deemed to be "real." Other laboratories do not confirm the dipstrip reaction with SSA, but rather recommend a UPC to verify the significance of the positive pad reaction [38]. Quantitative methods for protein determination using the UPC are recommended to confirm proteinuria detected by dipstrip reagent pads. Urinary electrophoresis can be helpful to identify globulins entering urine, especially in cases with multiple myeloma. Since urinary protein excretion can display biological variation [4], it should be determined if findings from reagent pad positive reactions for protein are repeatable on subsequent urine samples. Alternate methods to measure protein as well as causes and interpretation of proteinuria are discussed in greater detail in Chapter 7.

Table 5.6 Causes of pathologic renal proteinuria. See Chapter 7 for details about renal and nonrenal proteinuria.

Causes of pathologic renal proteinuria
Increased glomerular filtration of protein – increased permeability of glomerulus
Failure of renal tubular reabsorption of protein from tubular fluid
Tubular secretion of protein
Protein leakage from damaged tubular cells
Renal parenchymal inflammation
A combination of the above

URINARY GLUCOSE

Glucose in health is almost entirely reabsorbed from glomerular filtrate by the proximal tubules following filtration from plasma, leaving small quantities of glucose that are excreted in urine. The amount of glucose (mg/min) that appears in urine is the difference between the filtered load of glucose (circulating glucose (mg/dL) × glomerular filtration rate (GFR) (mL/min) = mg/min) and its subsequent rate of tubular reabsorption (mg/min). The filtered glucose is extensively reabsorbed by sodium-glucose cotransporters along the luminal surface of the proximal tubular cells in those with normal blood glucose concentrations and normal tubular function. The final concentration of glucose in the urine (mg/dL) depends upon this excretion rate plus the amount of water reabsorbed by the tubules during the urinary concentrating process.

The maximal ability of the proximal tubular cells to reabsorb filtered glucose is called T_{max} and is expressed as glucose reabsorbed in mg/minute. When plasma glucose is normal, the filtered load into tubular fluid in mg/minute is below T_{max}, and therefore, most of the filtered glucose will be reabsorbed. When the plasma glucose is high, the filtered load of glucose will be high and can exceed the ability of the proximal tubules to reclaim this increased level of filtered glucose. Biological splay of tubular function leads to variability in reabsorptive capacity within an individual animal's nephron population. This means that glucose can appear in the urine at a lower level of blood sugar than that associated with T_{max} and is called the renal threshold. The renal threshold will vary somewhat by the genetics of individual animals, and is generally associated with a blood sugar that exceeds 170–220 mg/dL in dogs and that exceeds 260–290 mg/dL in cats [32, 39, 43, 64, 65]. The renal threshold for glucosuria to develop in the cat occurred at approximately 270 mg/dL of circulating glucose, with near total reabsorption of filtered glucose at lower levels in one study. Unlike in other mammals, a T_{max} for glucose did not seem to exist [66]. The renal threshold for glucose in the dog was found to be considerably lower at 180–200 mg/dL in one study [67].

The renal threshold and T_{max} for glucose can differ between health and disease. As an example, T_{max} and renal threshold are increased in some humans with diabetes mellitus (DM), especially those that are elderly and with increased body mass. This means that higher levels of blood glucose are required before glucose starts appearing in the urine. Insulin treatments have variable effects in lowering tubular glucose reabsorption between humans that are normal and those with diabetes. These phenomena have not yet been investigated in veterinary patients with diabetes [68]. There are also diseases that result in a decreased T_{max} or renal threshold due to reduced expression or function of the sodium-glucose cotransporter (e.g. tubulopathy from AKI, Fanconi syndrome). In these instances, glucosuria will be apparent at lower concentrations of blood glucose. This is detailed later in this section.

Urine glucose concentrations from a hospital population of dogs demonstrated less than 40 mg/dL of glucose in over 80% of these patients when measured by methods suitable for small concentrations of glucose [69]. The mean urine glucose from 75 control bitches in another study was 0.27 ± 0.17 mmol/L (4.9 ± 3.1 mg/dL) [70]. When urine from healthy dogs was measured using a sensitive enzymatic kit, the median urinary glucose was 0.39 (0–1.55) mmol/L (7 mg/dL with range

0–27.9 mg/dL); 2.2% of the samples tested at zero. There was no effect of age, castration status, gender, obesity, or feeding in this study of normal dogs [71]. Urine glucose was measured in urine from cats without systemic disease using the same sensitive method for glucose measurement as in the dog study. All cats except one cat had detectable urinary glucose by the kit method, and no cat had glucose-positive status on the urinary dipstrip from the same sample. A median of 0.389 mmol/L (7 mg/dL) of glucose was detected with a range of <0.11 to 1.1665 mmol/L (<2 to 21 mg/dL).

In addition to the glucose oxidase reagent strip methodology for glucose detection, a copper reduction tablet methodology is available to measure glucose and other reducing substances in urine. The reduction of copper from the cupric to cuprous state results in a color change proportional to the amount of reducing substances in the urine. This method is not specific for glucose, and other reducing substances (e.g. fructose, lactose, galactose, maltose, pentoses, glucuronic acid, salicylates, penicillin, cephalosporin, formaldehyde, and chloral hydrate) also may cause a positive color reaction [5, 69]. Although ascorbic acid is also a reducing substance, it usually is not present in sufficient quantity in urine to produce a positive copper reduction reaction. This method requires ≥ 250 mg/dL glucose for detection in humans, which is less sensitive than the glucose oxidase method (100 mg/dL). This type of testing is common in human pediatric medicine to screen for metabolic defects such as galactosemia, in which the enzyme method for glucose is negative and the copper reduction test is positive for a nonglucose reducing substance [5]. This method to detect urinary reducing substances is rarely used in veterinary medicine.

Glucose Measurement by Dipstrip

Dipstrip reagent pads employ a sequential method involving glucose oxidase, peroxidase, and a chromogen that can vary by the manufacturer. The color generated corresponds to the quantity of glucose (mg/dL or %) present in the urine sample if the procedure is performed properly and read at the appropriate time interval. This method is specific for glucose because glucose oxidase will not react with other substances. As little as 50–100 mg/dL (0.05–0.1%), glucose may be detected in human urine by commercially available dipstrip tests.

Glucose and oxygen in the urine initially react with glucose oxidase in the reagent pad to generate gluconic acid and peroxide (H_2O_2). This first reaction is specific for glucose and not for other reducing substances that might be in the urine (as are detected by tablet tests). In a second sequential reaction, peroxidase catalyzes peroxide oxidation of the chromogen within the reagent pad generating a color change from blue to brown depending on the concentration of glucose in the urine [5, 32]. Potassium iodide is a commonly used chromogen in the reagent pad. The magnitude of color development should be read at 30 or 60 seconds depending on specifications by the manufacturer. It is important to read the color reaction at the proper time as delayed reading will result in continued color development and falsely increased values. Results are reported as normal (or negative) to 4+ qualitatively or semi-quantitively as normal to a maximum of 2000 mg/dL or 1000 mg/dL, with the bins of reagent readings varying somewhat by manufacturer. Tetramethylbenzidine is the chromogen in one popular urinary dipstrip that changes from yellow to green as a positive reaction to glucose [33]. Glucose oxidase readily interacts with glucose in urine samples that are more dilute; consequently, highly concentrated urine (high USG) may underestimate glucose in the urine [5, 69].

In humans, routine chemistry urine dipstrips detect glucose when urinary glucose concentration is $\geq$50 mg/dL ($\geq$2.8 mmol/L) or $\geq$100 mg/dL ($\geq$5.6 mmol/L) depending on specific brand and manufacturer [42], but 2–10 mg/dL can be measured in urine from normal humans when using benchtop methods of detection [32]. The dipstrip sensitivity for detection of glucose was noted to be from 75 to 125 mg/dL in order to be reported at the 100 mg/dL or 1+ bin by the makers of one dipstrip designed for human urine. On occasion, a trace reaction for color development that is greater than normal and <100 mg/dL can be reported as positive. Sometimes, a mottled color develops on the reagent pad at higher glucose concentrations in the urine; in these instances, the darkest color that develops on the reagent pad should be matched with the color chart provided by the manufacturer [8]. Urine glucose >40 mg/dL was reported as dipstrip positive in most human samples by another dipstrip manufacturer [33].

One recently available veterinary urinary dipstrip (Medi-Test Combi 10 VET [Machery Nagel]) can detect urinary glucose as low as 20 mg/dL (1.1 mmol/L) [71–73]; the manufacturer notes that healthy dogs usually test negative, but some have a slightly positive reading that should be considered normal [71]. It is important for clinicians to be aware that the lower limit for the detection of urinary glucose by dipstrip methods varies widely by the specific manufacturer from 20 to 100 mg/dL [72].

Large differences in sensitivity and accuracy for the detection of glucosuria exist between various brands of dipstrips and whether they are read manually or by automated methods [20–22, 74, 75]. Color development during visual inspection was reported as trace (100 mg/dL) as the lowest positive reaction that could be reported, 1+ (250 mg/dL), 2+ (500 mg/dL), 3+ (1000 mg/dL), and 4+ ($\geq$2000 mg/dL) glucose in urine from dogs and cats using one brand of dipstrip (Multistix 10SG, Bayer Diagnostics, Whippany, NJ). Urine samples analyzed by an automated reader designed to be used on the same dipstrips reported glucose as negative, trace (<75 mg/dL), 1+ (75–375 mg/dL), 2+ (376–750 mg/dL), and 3+ (>750 mg/dL) [74]. Urine glucose results determined by visual and the automated dipstrip reader were compared to the gold-standard glucose measured by a benchtop method. Automated glucose measurement from the dipstrip commonly underestimated the actual urinary glucose concentration. Visual dipstrip readings for glucose were more accurate than automated dipstrip measurements in dogs and cats of this study [74], but

in another study, the automated reader was more accurate [21]. The accuracy for the automated glucose reader was much higher in urine from cats than in urine from dogs in one study, possibly due to substances in the urine from dogs that interfered with the automated reader [74].

Interferences

The color indicators on the reagent pad can interact with molecules other than glucose (Table 5.7). Small amounts of peroxide, hypochlorite, and chlorine contamination into the urine or pad will generate a color reaction as a false positive for glucose [5, 33, 69]. In some cats with urethral obstruction, an unidentified molecule in the urine directly creates a color change on the reagent pad as a false positive for glucose (see pseudoglucosuria) [76]. The amount of blood in urine has minimal effect on dipstrip readings for glucose in the dog or cat [12].

False-negative reactions for glucose on reagent pads potentially occur in the presence of large amounts of vitamin C in urine. Ascorbic acid is oxidized by hydrogen peroxide previously generated on the reagent pad, resulting in less oxidation of the chromogen and less color formation [5]. Dogs and cats normally synthesize vitamin C (ascorbic acid), which is excreted in urine [77]. Ascorbic acid urinary concentration was most often 10 or 20 mg/dL in one study [77], but concentrations as high as 90 mg/dL have been detected in urine from dogs. A concentration of ascorbic acid of 10–30 mg/dL may interfere with the detection of a small quantity of glucose in urine [69]. In addition to a negative color reaction, a delayed color reaction may be seen in some instances with ascorbic acid interference [42]. Ascorbic acid may also enter urine from its use as a therapeutic urinary acidifier, from antibiotics with which ascorbic acid is mixed during commercial preparation, and from vitamin preparations. It appears that false-negative

Table 5.7 Causes of false results for glucosuria on dipstrip.

False positive	False negative
Contamination with peroxide, hypochlorite, chlorine	Outdated reagent strips
	Reagent strips exposed to sunlight
Prolonged time to read (greater color generation)	Failure to sufficiently wet the reagent pad with urine
	Formaldehyde contamination or generation (methenamine)
Pseudoglucosuria Some cats with urethral obstruction	Large amounts of ketones in urine
	Large amounts of bilirubin in urine
	Large amounts of ascorbic acid in urine
Cephalexin	Large amounts of enrofloxacin/ciprofloxacin in urine
	Cold urine not brought to room temperature
	Consumption of glucose by bacterial urinary infection

glucose readings on the dipstrip from ascorbic acid interference are less likely to occur when the glucose reading is 100 mg/dL or greater due to improvement in reagent pad technology in some strips [33]. Underreading of glucose by urinary dipstrip is likely to occur only in animals with high concentrations of ascorbic acid and minimal levels of increased glucose in the urine.

False-negative reactions may also occur when formaldehyde [69] or fluoride [76] is present in urine samples. These agents result in the inactivation of glucose oxidase or peroxidase in the reagent pad. Formaldehyde may be generated in urine following therapeutic administration of the urinary antiseptic methenamine or added to urine as a preservative. A large quantity of bilirubin or ketones in urine also may decrease color generation on some glucose reagent pads, but it appears that most manufacturers have eliminated the interference from a high specific gravity, ascorbic acid, or moderate levels of ketonuria [26, 43]. Refrigeration of the urine specimen also may result in failure to detect glucosuria if the specimen is not warmed to room temperature before testing. Finally, bacterial UTIs may falsely lower urinary glucose concentration due to the bacterial metabolism of glucose [5, 69].

High concentrations of enrofloxacin or cephalexin in urine from dogs can influence urinary glucose measured by some dipstrip or by tablet methods. False-positive results for glucose were recorded for both enrofloxacin and cephalexin when measured by tablet methods and for dipstrip measurement of glucose with cephalexin. Enrofloxacin in urine samples that contained added dextrose underestimated the glucose concentration. The authors of this study recommended that the glucose measurement be repeated after these drugs have been discontinued for several days [78].

Interpretation of Glucosuria

Standard dipstrip results for glucose should be negative in healthy animals. Urine is not glucose free, but glucose is not normally present in detectable quantity in urine when measured by the standard dipstrip method from normal dogs and cats. The terms normoglucuria or basal glucosuria have been used to describe the detection of small glucose quantities in urine that are not pathological. Urine from the normal dog and cat almost always contains glucose when measured by very sensitive methods. The precise urinary glucose level at which basal glucosuria escalates or transitions to levels that are considered to be pathologic have yet to be determined. Basal glucosuria does not appear to be related to circulating levels of glucose or T_{max} for the tubular reabsorption of glucose [71, 72]. Glucosuria measured by a sensitive automated wet chemistry method (lower limit of detection 0.11 mmol/L or 2 mg/dL) in urine from apparently normal dogs was detectable in over 99% of the samples. The median glucose by this method was 0.39 mmol/L (0–1.55 mmol/L range) or 7 mg/dL (0–27.9 mg/dL range). Urinary glucose >20 mg/dL occurred in 7.1% of dogs in this study measured by the wet chemistry method, which can potentially be detected as a positive reac-

tion when measured by very sensitive urinary dipstrips. There was no effect of feeding or fasting, obesity, age, or gender on the small amounts of glucose present in urine from normal dogs. A standard dipstrip reaction for glucose with a lower limit of detection for glucose at 50 mg/dL was negative in over 98% of the samples in this study from dogs at the same time [71].

The degree of glucosuria in normal cats was above the detectable limit in over 99% of cats when analyzed using the same wet chemistry method, similar to that in dogs. The median urinary glucose by this method was 0.389 mmol/L (<0.11–1.665 mmol/L) or 7 mg/dL (2–30 mg/dL range) with an upper reference limit of 1.48 mmol/L (26.7 mg/dL). Mean urinary glucose was 0.46 ± 0.32 mmol/L or 8.25 (±5.76) mg/dL. Seven percent of the normal cats in this study had a urinary glucose >20 mg/dL (>1.11 mmol/L), which might be detected when urinary glucose is measured by ultrasensitive dipstrip methods. All standard dipstrip reactions with a lower detection limit of 50 mg/dL were negative for urinary glucose in these normal cats. There was no effect of sex or neutering on urinary glucose in this study of cats, but there was a negative correlation between age and urinary glucose. There was no effect of leukocyturia on the degree of basal glucosuria, but hematuria was associated with a slight increase in measured glucosuria compared to those without hematuria [72].

Glucosuria has been considered by some to be a normal finding in puppies and kittens up to three weeks of age since maximal glucose reabsorption from tubular fluid may not occur until then [79, 80]. A greater heterogeneity of glomerular and tubular functions is generally thought to exist in the neonate compared to adults. In an early study, the renal threshold for glucose appearance in the urine was slightly lower and the degree of splay higher in the youngest puppies studied from 1 to 40 days of age [81]. Glucosuria as measured by chromatography existed in 50% of five day old puppies in one report; glucosuria was absent when puppies were evaluated at three weeks of age [82]. No puppies from 0 to 24 weeks of age had glucosuria as measured by urine dipstrips in another study [79]. Urine and blood glucose were measured by glucometer on day 1, 4, 7, and 11 after puppies were delivered. Glucosuria was common in puppies of this study for up to 14 days. Mean urinary glucose was 86.8 ± 9.02 mg/dL on day 1, 122.50 ± 55.08 mg/dL on day 4, 58.3 ± 23.62 mg/dL on day 7, and 97.11 ± 25.22 mg/dL on day 11. The magnitude of glucosuria was paradoxically higher in puppies that had hypoglycemia on day 1 [80]. Glucosuria was not detected by dipstrip in any Great Dane puppies from 0 to 28 days of age in another study [44].

The concept of indexing the urinary-glucose-to-urinary-creatinine ratio (UGCR) was introduced as potentially useful in the evaluation of urinary glucose [72], but another study concluded that the UGCR did not provide additional useful information [74]. Whether it could be clinically useful to determine increases in urinary glucose above these low physiological normal levels of glucose before glucose can be measured by dipstrip remains to be determined.

The detection of glucosuria in animals that present for the evaluation of polyuria and polydipsia is informative for diseases associated with hyperglycemia or those with normoglycemia and altered renal tubular function (Table 5.8). Glucosuria is most commonly seen as a result of hyperglycemia and the subsequent inability of normal proximal tubules to reabsorb the increased load of glucose entering the glomerular filtrate [21, 71]. It is important to determine whether hyperglycemia or normoglycemia exists at the time when glucosuria is first recognized.

DM is the most common clinical disorder resulting in significant hyperglycemia and glucosuria, though pancreatitis, hyperadrenocorticism, pheochromocytomas, and central nervous system (hypothalamus) lesions may also do so. Glucosuria may be seen following the infusion of glucose-rich IV fluid therapy. Various endocrine responses with increased release of epinephrine, cortisol, glucagon, adrenocorticotrophic hormone, and growth hormone may contribute to hyperglycemia. Cats seem to be particularly predisposed to stress of disease or stress of acute excitement resulting in transient hyperglycemia and glucosuria. Transient glucosuria has been mentioned as an occasional side effect following ketamine sedation in cats; however, possible mechanisms for this were not discussed [69].

Glucosuria may also occur with normal blood glucose concentration if the proximal tubules do not function properly to reabsorb the normal amount of glucose entering the glomerular filtrate. This may occur with primary tubular disorders, such as primary renal glucosuria, or associated with Fanconi syndrome (congenital and acquired), in which glucosuria is accompanied by phosphaturia, generalized aminoaciduria, bicarbonaturia, and proteinuria. Familial nephropathy of Norwegian Elkhounds [83] and other breeds with CKD occasionally may also show glucosuria.

Glucosuria in the presence of normoglycemia is sometimes detected in dogs with AKI of a variety of causes [84]. Mild-to-moderate glucose-positive dipstrip reactions (trace to 250 mg/L) occurred in 53% of dogs with subacute leptospirosis in an early report [85]. Glucosuria was detected in 11 of 59 dogs with renal amyloidosis and CKD, most of which had normoglycemia [86]. A positive dipstrip reaction for glucose was found in 59% of dogs with leptospirosis compared to 18% of those with other causes of AKI (p = 0.002). Also, in the same study, the median UGCR was significantly higher at 0.64 (0–26) in dogs with leptospirosis compared to 0.22 (0–13) in dogs with other causes of AKI [87]. Positive reactions for glucose on the dipstrip were found in 83% (78 of 94) of dogs with leptospirosis in another study [88]. Similarly in dogs with azotemic AKI and normoglycemia, glucosuria was reported in 19 of 84 [89]. Prior to or during azotemic renal failure in AKI, glucosuria indicates damage to proximal tubules and reduced reabsorptive function. This can be encountered during the administration of nephrotoxins such as aminoglycosides and amphotericin B, ethylene glycol intoxication, leptospirosis, and during rapid development of hypercalcemia as can happen during hypervitaminosis D. Over half of dogs diagnosed with leptospirosis had glucosuria in two studies [85, 88] and 22% of dogs and 50% of cats diagnosed with ethylene glycol intoxication had glycosuria in another report [90]. The median UGCR was 0.21 (0.01–58.19) for overall AKI in dogs, 0.32 (0.01–58.19) with intrinsic AKI, 0.09(0.01–0.93) with volume responsive AKI, and 0.03 (0.01–0.11) in control dogs [91].

High phosphorus concentrations in the diet potentially can impact the concentration of glucose in the urine. Total and soluble phosphorus content of dried meat jerky treats exceeded upper safety limits recommended for phosphorus intake in one report. The consumption of high-phosphorus treats in addition to the dietary phosphorus intake from the diet should be considered for their potential to create a proximal tubulopathy resulting in glucosuria [92] and the entry of other molecules into urine that characterize acquired Fanconi syndrome (see below). Glucosuria as well as microalbuminuria were seen in 9 of 13 experimental cats fed a high-phosphate diet in another study [93].

Glucosuria has been documented in some human patients with hypothermia, even during hypoglycemia [94]. Hypothermia in a study of experimental dogs resulted in

Table 5.8   Causes of glucosuria on dipstrip.

Hyperglycemia (transient or persistent)	Normoglycemia
Endocrine disorders	Proximal renal tubular disorders
Diabetes mellitus	Congenital Fanconi syndrome – Basenji, Irish Wolfhound
Hyperadrenocorticism	
Growth hormone excess	Acquired Fanconi syndrome
Pheochromocytoma	Copper-associated hepatitis
Hypothalamic lesions	Drugs
Acute stress or excitement, especially cats (associated with transient hyperglycemia)	Chlorambucil in cats
	Secondary to systemic disease
Parenteral administration of glucose-containing fluids	Jerky treats
	High-phosphate diets – cats
	Primary renal glucosuria (Norwegian Elkhound)
	Acute kidney injury (AKI)
	Nephrotoxins
	Ethylene glycol
	Leptospirosis
	CKD rarely; some with familial CKD
	SGLT-inhibitors (gliflozins) for diabetes mellitus control
	Hypothermia

SGLT = sodium glucose transporter.

decreased GFR and a marked increase in urine volume and the excretion of glucose into urine. The urinary glucose concentration exceeded that of circulating glucose. T_{max} for glucose was greatly reduced in this setting, which would account for the glucosuria in spite of the decreased GFR [95].

Diabetes Mellitus

The magnitude of glucosuria was historically used in veterinary medicine to help monitor DM and insulin dosage, but this method should NEVER be used by itself since the level of glucose in the urine in those with DM is not directly proportional to the blood glucose concentration. Periodic measurement of glucose in the urine can be useful to determine if it is detectable in the diabetic animal's urine or not. In those without detectable glucosuria, the blood glucose may be chronically too low or below the renal threshold with good to excellent glycemic control. High levels of urine glucose can occur in those patients with DM, in which persistent or transient hyperglycemia exists above the renal threshold for glucose, but it cannot distinguish between those with insufficient dosing of insulin and chronic hyperglycemia and those with overdoses of insulin that are suffering from posthypoglycemic rebound hyperglycemia (Somogyi effect). The measurement of urine glucose at home by the owners of diabetic patients appears to be most helpful when urine glucose is negative or highly positive, indicating a need for further evaluation. Insulin doses should not be changed based solely on urinary glucose levels, but persistently negative or high levels of glucosuria suggest closer monitoring by other methods, such as the measurement of blood sugar, fructosamine levels, or glucose versus time curves. One author recommends reduction in insulin dose when the glucose reagent pad is consistently negative, until the patient can be further evaluated [96]. The finding of glucosuria on the dipstrip should immediately prompt the clinician to refer to the ketone reagent pad. The ketone pad can be negative in early stages of untreated DM, but it can also be positive in animals that are sick and suffering from more advanced ketoacidotic diabetes.

A method to collect urine from clumping and non-clumping silica litter has been described for measuring urine glucose in diabetic cats. The "no-soak" type of litter or aquarium gravel can also be used. About one tablespoon of urine-soaked wet gravel is collected, and then, one tablespoon of tap water is added and mixed in a receptacle. The container is tipped to allow the separation of the effluent from the gravel, and then, this fluid is filtered through a 2×2 gauze sponge. The dipstrip is then dipped into this fluid, and the color recorded. The glucose dipstrip chemical measurement is about 50% of that occurring in the original urine. If the wet gravel is allowed to dry first, the glucose readings on the dipstrip are still positive, but the magnitude of the glucose reading is further reduced to 25–50% of the original urine reading [96, 97]. The effect of chemicals added to litter for odor control has not been studied.

Fanconi Syndrome

Fanconi syndrome is a well-recognized and characterized congenital disease in Basenjis [98–101]. Congenital Fanconi syndrome has also been described in the Border Terrier [102] and Irish Wolfound [103]. Fanconi syndrome results from a generalized defect in proximal renal tubular transport. Glucosuria is the most readily identified abnormality in urine that accompanies either generalized aminoaciduria or a pattern of aminoaciduria characteristic of cystinuria. Varying degrees of phosphaturia, bicarbonaturia, kaliuresis, and proteinuria can also be expected in this syndrome. Ketonuria is also occasionally described along with the glucosuria. Polyuria and polydipsia secondary to glucosuria are commonly recognized. Both AKI and CKD appear to be possible outcomes in some dogs.

Acquired Fanconi syndrome has been described in dogs from North America, Europe, Australia, and Japan that are consuming jerky treats often prepared in China [104–110]. However, a specific compound in these treats creating proximal tubular injury has not been identified.

Polyuria and polydipsia may be the only clinical signs exhibited, but sometimes the dogs are systemically ill and may have increased liver enzymes and azotemia. Glucosuria resolves within weeks to months following discontinuation for the feeding of jerky treats, but sometimes azotemia and CKD persist. A relationship between treatment with chlorambucil and the development of Fanconi syndrome has been described in cats. These cats did not have polyuria or polydipsia and glucosuria was discovered as part of laboratory surveillance during the treatment of neoplasia. Fanconi syndrome resolved in three of four cats within three months of stopping chlorambucil [111].

Copper-Associated Hepatopathy

Glucosuria as part of acquired Fanconi syndrome has been described in association with copper storage hepatic disease in a variety of breeds of dogs. Copper accumulation in the kidneys appears to result in proximal tubular dysfunction that is reversible in some dogs following treatment of the underlying hepatopathy (diet, antioxidants, chelation). In some cases, proximal tubular dysfunction may occur in part due to effects of excess bilirubin on the tubules [112]. Copper-associated hepatopathy (CAH) is a commonly diagnosed liver disease in Labrador Retrievers and was associated with proximal tubular dysfunction in 33% of cases in one review. Nine Labradors with CAH and glucosuria were reported, but confirmatory testing for Fanconi syndrome was performed only in a few of these dogs. High renal tissue levels of copper were documented in four of four Labradors in which it was measured. Heavy metals are capable of injuring the proximal tubules, so it seems likely that renal copper accumulation contributed to the proximal tubular dysfunction in these dogs. The detection of renal glucosuria in a Labrador Retriever with increased serum alanine transaminase is highly suggestive for the diagnosis of CAH; definitive diagnosis should be made on findings from hepatic histopathology [113].

Cats with Urethral Obstruction

From about 30–75% of cats with urethral obstruction were found with glucosuria when measured by reagent strip or test tape methodology at the time urethral obstruction was relieved. Glucosuria was usually transient and gone by 24–48 hours, an initial effect that was attributed to tubulopathy resulting in a decreased T_{max} for glucose reabsorption following relief of obstruction. Glucosuria, however, persisted in some cats for weeks following relief of obstruction [76, 114–117]. Blood glucose was not consistently measured in these studies, so some of these cats may have had stress-induced hyperglycemia and attendant glucosuria when the maximal amount of tubular reabsorption of glucose was exceeded [76]. One study of cats with urethral obstruction attributed the finding of proteinuria and glucosuria to hemorrhage [115], but the urine sample needs to contain about one-third blood (urocrit) before a glucose-positive reaction can be expected [76]. Blood glucose concentrations that are reported in cats with urethral obstruction are usually below the renal threshold for glucose to appear in urine. The median serum glucose was 161.5 mg/dL (65–295 range) in one study of cats with clinical urethral obstruction, but glucose in urine was not reported [118]. In 10 cats with glucose color reaction on the dipstrip, plasma glucose ranged from 99 to 270 mg/dL, with 6 of 10 cats with plasma glucose well over 200 mg/dL. Plasma glucose was considerably lower following relief of urethral obstruction in 8 of these 10 cats with glucose from 64 to 119 mg/dL [76]. In a study of cats with experimental urethral obstruction, serum glucose increased from a baseline of 90 ± 26 mg/dL to 170 ± 60 mg/dL at 48 hours before relief of obstruction [119].

Twelve of thirty cats developed a color reaction on the reagent pad for glucose in one study of cats with urethral obstruction. Urine glucose measured by a benchtop method was 36–166 mg/dL in 10 of these 12 cats, with 6 of 10 having urine glucose less than 50 mg/dL. Six of the ten cats with glucose color reaction on the dipstrip had true glucosuria, proven by ablation of the color response when fluoride was added to inactivate glucose oxidase. Color persisted following the addition of fluoride to the urine in the other four cats of this study indicating the presence of some unidentified non-glucose oxidizing substance in the urine directly interacting with the chromogen on the reagent pad, a phenomenon referred to as "pseudoglucosuria." The cats with true glucosuria on dipstrip had much higher plasma glucose concentrations than the cats with pseudoglucosuria [76].

KETONES

Ketone bodies (beta-hydroxybutyric acid [BHA], acetoacetate, and acetone) are produced by the liver and can be used as an energy source by peripheral tissues when circulating glucose is low, or glucose is not available for uptake as in DM. Peripheral tissues have a limited ability to utilize ketones, so their concentration increases in the circulation after they are generated. Ketones are normally present in the blood at low concentrations and increase during fasting and prolonged exercise in humans. Acetoacetate (acetoacetic acid) and BHA predominate, with much less acetone in the circulation [120]. Acetone is the ketone that accounts for the characteristic sweet smell to the breath of a patient with ketoacidosis as it is eliminated by the lungs [5, 32]. Normal levels of circulating ketones in humans have been defined as <0.5 mM, hyperketonemia as >1.0 mM, and ketoacidosis as >3.0 mM. Acetoacetate that undergoes a reducing reaction generates 3-hydroxybutyrate, whereas acetone results from the decarboxylation of acetoacetate. Insulin inhibits ketogenesis, whereas glucagon stimulates ketogenesis [120].

Urinary ketone levels are determined by the filtered load of ketones (plasma concentration × GFR), tubular secretion of ketones, and tubular reabsorption of ketones. Acetone is the only form of ketone that undergoes renal tubular reabsorption [43]. Ketones in plasma are filtered by the glomeruli and are incompletely reabsorbed by the renal tubular cells as a result of a readily saturated tubular transport process. The renal threshold for the excretion of plasma ketones is low, so that ketonuria develops early during the time of ketogenesis as ketone concentrations are starting to escalate in the plasma. Consequently, ketonuria often precedes detectable ketonemia [121]. Urinary ketone levels of 10 mg/dL or higher are detected in urine before circulating ketone levels have increased [8].

Urinary ketone levels are expected to be roughly proportional to increased plasma ketone concentrations, but there are exceptions. The concentration of ketones in the urine can lag behind that in the circulation during states of reduced GFR during the contraction of the effective extracellular fluid volume perfusing the kidneys. BHA accounts for the vast majority of the ketones in the circulation available to enter the urine [121], but this molecule is not detected on the urinary dipstrip. Acetoacetic acid comprises about 20% and acetone about 2% of ketones circulating in human blood [1, 5].

Methodology

The nitroprusside present in the dipstick reagent pad reacts with acetone and acetoacetate in an alkaline environment to produce a lavender color. A positive reaction is recorded when the reagent pad changes from beige to violet [33]. Nitroprusside is much more reactive with acetoacetate than with acetone [122, 123], and it does not react with BHA. However, the amount of BHA present is usually proportional to the amount of acetoacetate. Since the presence of any of these three ketones is significant, the detection of ketones in general rather than individual identification is sufficient. For clinical purposes, urinary dipstrips are considered specific for acetoacetate [122].

The nitroprusside test identifies as little as 5–10 mg/dL acetoacetate, before ketones increase in the circulation [8]. Some dipstrips also detect acetone, but none detect the presence of BHA [5]. Some commercial tests for ketone bodies add glycine to the reagent pad, which allows for the detection of both acetone and acetoacetate [120].

Color reaction on the reagent pad is reported as either negative, trace (5 mg/dL), small (15 mg/dL) moderate (40 mg/dL), or large (either 80 or 160 mg/dL) [5]. The color change from a negative reaction to a trace reaction is particularly difficult to differentiate and can be interfered with by the patient's urine color [3]. Agreement for ketones between one urinary dipstrip read by an automated method and another brand dipstrip read manually by visual inspection was considered moderate in one study of urine from dogs. The automated reader had 6% false positives compared to the manually read dipstrip as the reference method. It is possible that the trace reactions for color development detected by the automated method for ketones were not detectable by the human eye [20].

Tablet tests are available for more sensitive detection of urinary ketones than the dipstrip method and can be considered for the confirmation of dipstrip positive ketone results. A positive color reaction on the dipstrip and negative color reaction on the tablet supports that the dipstrip reaction was false positive, most often due to the color of the urine or other interfering substance [121].

Interferences

False-positive color reactions are rare, but molecules in urine that contain free sulfhydryl, aldehyde, or keto groups can interact with nitroprusside to produce color reaction on the reagent pad. In these instances, the color is not typical violet as produced from ketones (Table 5.9) [32]. The color reaction from these interfering molecules often fades upon standing, whereas color development from acetoacetic acid continues to develop over time [1, 32]. Captopril, mesna (chemoprotectant), d-penicillamine, 2-mercaptoproprionyl

glycine (tiopronin), dimercaprol (British anti-Lewisite), N-acetylcysteine, and cystine in the urine all have free sulfhydryl groups that can cause this reaction [32, 120]. Phthalein compounds such as bromsulphthalein (BSP) and phenolsulfonphthalein (PSP, phenol red) can create a false-positive reaction from the presence of diagnostic dye in the urine, but these agents are no longer used in small animal practice.

Phenylketonuria can also cause a false-positive result, but the existence of this metabolic disorder is debated in small animals. An orange–red or red–brown color change is noted on the ketone reagent pad in these instances instead of violet, which was read as positive for ketones with an automated reader in dog urine of one study. It was suggested to perform a visual inspection of the dipstrip when unexpected results for ketones are reported by automated dipstrip readers [125]. Metabolites of L-3,4-dihydroxyphenylalanine (L-DOPA) can create a false-positive reaction for ketones in urine, but this drug is not likely to be used in veterinary medicine.

Occasionally, highly pigmented urine also may result in a false-positive reaction [8, 32]. Scores for ketones were significantly higher when urine samples were classified as red in both dogs and cats when blood was added to urine compared to undiluted urine [12]. Highly acid urine can also result in a false-positive color reaction. Urine specimens with a high USG and low urinary pH are more likely to produce this false-positive reaction [5].

False-negative reactions are uncommon, but can occur during the use of dipstrips that have been improperly handled due to exposure to heat, light, or moisture (Table 5.9) [120]. *In vivo* or *in vitro* bacterial metabolism of acetoacetate, but not acetone, may cause a lower or false-negative result as this ketone is consumed. Acetoacetate is stable in sterile urine for up to 10 days [123]. Acetone is volatile and may be released from urine that is improperly stored for several hours at room temperature in an open container, which would lower the amount detected [1, 121].

Interpretation

Ketones (BHA, acetoacetate, and acetone) are not present in the urine of normal dogs [27] and cats. A trace reaction for ketones in urine was found in 3% of apparently healthy older cats [28]. Excessive ketone formation results when energy metabolism has shifted to exaggerated and incomplete oxidation of fatty acids. The inadequate consumption of carbohydrates or impaired endogenous utilization of carbohydrates for energy (e.g. DM) can increase the oxidation of fatty acids. The ability of body tissues to utilize ketones as an energy source is limited [121].

The finding of ketonuria is a significant clue to abnormal fat and energy metabolism and is most often observed in patients with poorly or uncontrolled DM (the lack of insulin activity enhances lipolysis) (Table 5.10). The finding of ketonuria obligates an immediate analysis of whether glucosuria and or hyperglycemia are concurrent. Other potential causes of ke-

Table 5.9 Interferences with ketone reaction on dipstrip.

False Positive	False Negative or Less Color Generation
Highly pigmented urine	UTI with bacteria or yeast – consumption or breakdown of acetoacetate
Urine containing phthalein molecules (BSP, PSP – atypical color develops on pad)	
Urine containing sulfhydryl group molecules– atypical color develops on pad	Production of predominantly BHA
	Volatilization of acetone in urine at room temperature exposed to air
Captopril, mesna, N-acetylcysteine, dimercaprol and penicillamine [120], 2-mercaptopropionyl glycine (tiopronin) [124]	
	Dipstrip exposure to heat, light, or moisture (improper handling)
Highly acid urine with high USG [120]	
Phenylketonuria (existence of this disease in small animals has not been confirmed)	

BHA = beta-hydroxybutyric acid.

Table 5.10 Causes of ketonuria.

Causes of Ketonuria
Uncontrolled diabetes mellitus with ketoacidosis
Starvation or prolonged fasting (Fasting dogs and cats do not become ketotic as readily as do humans)
Glycogen storage disease
Low carbohydrate diet (decreased insulin secretion increases ketone formation)
Persistent fever
Persistent hypoglycemia – insulinoma, sepsis, insulin overdose
Physiological – neonates, pregnancy, lactation[a]
Salicylate poisoning[a]

[a] Laffel [120].
Source: Adapted from Laffel [120].

tonuria include starvation or prolonged fasting, glycogen storage disease, low carbohydrate diet, persistent fever, and persistent hypoglycemia [8, 9, 32, 33]. Dogs and cats are relatively resistant to development of ketonuria during starvation unless decreased food intake has been longstanding. Ketonuria occurs more readily in young animals. Chronic catabolic diseases may occasionally demonstrate ketonuria without glucosuria due to caloric malnutrition even though intake may appear adequate [9, 32]. Salicylate poisoning stimulates ketogenesis and ketoacidosis in humans and is considered a differential diagnosis for ketoacidosis of undetermined origin [120].

The urinary dipstrip for measurement of plasma ketones has been reported to be more sensitive for the prediction of impending ketoacidotic crisis than the measurement of ketones in urine from cats with DM. There was a positive correlation between the levels of plasma and urinary ketones, but the results were significantly different [126]. The measurement of plasma ketones might be especially useful when a urine sample cannot readily be collected from a patient with diabetes.

Trace results for urinary ketones are listed as possible by one manufacturer during physiological stress that includes fasting, pregnancy, and frequent strenuous exercise [8]. Physiological ketosis occurs readily in the neonate and during pregnancy in humans.

OCCULT BLOOD

Pink-to-red urine is visually detectable when the hemoglobin concentration is greater than 30–50 mg/dL [52]. Occult blood refers to the detection of blood or blood pigments in the urine before a pink or red color change in the urine is detectable to the human eye, as occurs with dipstrip reagent pad methods. Positive color development on the urinary dipstrip for occult blood is based on the pseudoperoxidase activity of heme pigments (hemoglobin, methemoglobin, or myoglobin) to catalyze a reaction between hydrogen peroxide and a chromogen

such a tetramethylbenzidine or o-toluidine [64, 127]. Color development on this reagent pad will semiquantitatively detect the presence of intact erythrocytes, free hemoglobin, and free myoglobin in urine when read at the recommended time interval. This test is less sensitive to the detection of intact erythrocytes than to either free hemoglobin or myoglobin in urine, but is equally sensitive for the detection of myoglobin and hemoglobin [4, 8].

The occult blood reagent pad was 50 times more sensitive for the detection of canine hemoglobin than for the detection of protein by the protein reagent pad after lysed RBC, intact RBC, or whole blood from dogs were added to urine in increasing concentration in one study. The reagent pad was positive when hemoglobin in the urine was >0.1 mg/dL. Results were similar regardless of the source of hemoglobin in this study [52]. In an unpublished study, intact RBC added to urine from dogs resulted in less occult blood color reaction on the reagent pad compared to more dramatic color development when lysed RBC were added to urine (Mary Nabity, personal communication 2021). The presence of intact erythrocytes can be distinguished from the pigment of either free hemoglobin or myoglobin on some dipstrip reagent pads. Intact erythrocytes produce a spotting reaction as they lyse on the reagent pad, while either of the free pigments will produce a diffuse color change on the reagent pad [4, 8, 33, 64]. A diffuse color reaction will develop on the pad when many RBC in the sample are lysed. If it is important to determine the presence of intact RBC versus free hemoglobin, the test can be repeated on urine that has been diluted [32]. Quantitation in either case is matched with color standards provided by the manufacturer. Water must not be used during negative quality control testing of the dipstrip, as the occult blood reagent pad will develop color as a false positive [4].

The occult blood reagent pad is very sensitive in the detection of heme pigments in the urine [127] such that a small amount of blood in the urine can result in a large amount of heme pigment detected and reported [64]. Approximately 5–20 intact RBCs/μL or 150–600 μg/L of free hemoglobin are usually required to cause a positive reaction [4, 12, 64]. At times, dipstrip testing for occult blood may be too sensitive, as positive reactions can detect hemoglobin from one to two RBC per high power field (HPF) [128]. Since the occult blood reagent pad is more sensitive than the protein reagent pad, a large occult blood reaction can be detected in the absence of detectable proteinuria contributed by the heme pigment [38, 64].

Heme compounds contain iron in a porphyrin ring that result in a color reaction on the reagent pad [3]. There is usually not enough heme pigment in urine from a normal dog or cat to produce a positive reagent strip reaction. However, a trace dipstrip reaction was noted in 4%, and a 1+ dipstrip reaction was noted in 14% of apparently healthy senior and geriatric dogs of one study [27]. Similarly, in apparently healthy middle aged and old cats, 28% were dipstrip positive on the occult blood reagent pad [28]. It is possible that an underlying undiagnosed urinary disorder existed in these seemingly healthy dogs and cats. Porphyrin does not contain iron and will not result in color development on the reagent pad [32].

Interferences

False-positive results may occur in urine contaminated with bleach (sodium hypochlorite) or in urine containing large amounts of iodide or bromide (Table 5.11) [32, 129, 130]. Bromide is excreted into urine during the oral treatment of epilepsy, but there are no veterinary reports of false-positive occult blood reactions during these treatments. Contamination of voided urine samples with flea feces uncommonly may cause a positive occult blood reaction. Contamination of voided urine samples with food and feces, as often happens in metabolic cage collections from dogs, can result in positive color reactions on the occult blood reagent pad. Positive reactions for occult blood are likely due to the interaction of the reagent pad with hemoglobin or myoglobin from foods, depending on the amount of meat and blood in the diet [130].

Bacterial organisms that produce peroxidase could directly activate the color reaction on the reagent pad as another cause for a false-positive result [127, 130]. Semen and seminal fluid in urine can cause a false-positive reaction for blood on the occult blood reagent pad. Normal semen does not contain hemoglobin or myoglobin, so it is likely that other proteins in seminal fluid or spermatozoa have heme groups or peroxidase activity that can activate color generation on the reagent pad [131].

False-negative results may occur if the urine sample was not well mixed before testing, as RBC rapidly settle to the bottom of the container (Table 5.12). The presence of ascorbic acid (vitamin C) or formalin in urine may also cause

Table 5.11 Causes of dipstrip false-positive occult blood reaction.

Causes of Dipstrip False-Positive Occult Blood Reaction
Contamination of urine:
Bleach (sodium hypochlorite)
Iodide
Bromide
Semen – seminal fluid or spermatozoa
Bacterial peroxidase
Sample is water and not urine

Table 5.12 Causes of dipstrip false negative occult blood reaction.

Causes of Dipstrip False Negative Occult Blood Reaction
Urine sample is not well-mixed before being applied to dipstrip (cells settle out quickly)
Crenated RBC in urine with high USG fail to lyse
High levels of ascorbic acid in urine – some dipstrips

false-negative reactions. High levels of ascorbic acid in the urine interfere with heme detection, and some dipstrip manufactures have attempted to minimize interference from ascorbic acid by producing reagent pads that oxidize ascorbic acid [132].

Interpretation

Macroscopically visible hematuria will not occur until more than 0.5 mL of blood is added to one liter or urine or about 2500 RBC per microliter of urine [32, 42]. In one study, whole blood was added to pooled urine from dogs and cats, and then, serial dilutions were made (final dilution 1:5120). The reagent pad reaction was strongly positive in all diluted samples regardless of urine color, and most scores were 3^+ (0–3 scale). Light pink urine in the dog and the cat contained about 600 RBC/HPF, whereas dark pink urine contained about 800–950 RBC/HPF. Red urine contained from about 900–2000 RBC/HPF. Light yellow urine contained 100–200 RBC/HPF depending on dilution. Dark yellow urine contained approximately 250–430 RBC/HPF [12].

A trace result on the occult blood reagent pad detects 5–10 RBC/μL according to one manufacturer [33]. The sensitivity for the detection of hemoglobin is noted to be from 0.015 to 0.062 mg/dL for a trace color reporting, which corresponds to 5–20 intact RBC/ per μL according to another manufacturer. The presence of 0.030–0.065 mg/dL results in a 1+ positive color reaction [8, 130].

It is imperative to interpret positive dipstrip results with findings from urinary sediment microscopy. The occult blood reagent pad should be positive in those that have excessive RBC seen during urine microscopy [64]. Since the occult blood reagent pad is more sensitive than the protein reagent pad, a large occult blood reaction can be detected in the absence of detectable proteinuria contributed by the heme pigment [38, 52, 64].

Hematuria from any cause is the most common cause for a positive dipstrip reaction, free hemoglobin is the cause occasionally, and myoglobin is rarely. Positive occult blood coupled with excessive erythrocytes seen in urinary sediment confirms that hematuria is the cause of the positive reactions. Hematuria as a cause for a positive occult blood reaction can occur as a result of any lesion along the genitourinary tract that allows the entry of red cells into urine (e.g. upper and lower urinary tract trauma, inflammation, infection, infarction, neoplasia, calculi, coagulopathy).

Discordance between the finding of a positive occult blood reagent pad reaction and the finding of very few RBC during urine microscopy happens frequently. This is usually attributed to the release of free hemoglobin following lysis of RBC, presumed to happen in the bladder. The lysis of RBC from trauma as they traverse the glomerulus is a likely phenomenon at times in some glomerular diseases, though uncommonly recognized in veterinary medicine. Alternatively, the presence of myoglobin or free hemoglobin in the urine that entered from the circulation could account for this discordance (Mary Nabity, personal communication 2020).

Urine that is minimally concentrated at <1.017 USG or excessively alkaline urine [64, 129, 133] may result in lysis of RBC that entered this urine, liberating hemoglobin into the specimen and allowing a positive occult blood reaction. Ghost membranes following rupture of the erythrocytes may sometimes be seen microscopically in these instances.

When uncentrifuged or well-mixed urine is examined, hemoglobinuria often results in red but transparent urine in the supernatant, whereas hematuria results in urine that is red and cloudy. Urine containing myoglobin is often transparent and red or pink in color when fresh, but can turn brown with time as myoglobin oxidizes to methemoglobin. However, hemoglobinuria cannot be reliably differentiated from myoglobinuria on these grounds alone. If the supernatant of the urine sample clears after centrifugation, the red color was due to the presence of intact red cells. If the abnormal color remains after centrifugation, it was due to free hemoglobin or myoglobin in the urine. The presumptive differentiation of hemoglobinuria from myoglobinuria is possible using the property of differential solubility in a saturated ammonium sulfate solution in which hemoglobin is precipitated but myoglobin remains in solution [134, 135]. More definitive identification is possible using urine protein electrophoresis because myoglobin migrates more slowly than hemoglobin and can be selectively stained [136]. Hemoglobin may also be measured by the use of immunochemical methods [4, 137]. Antibodies to myoglobin do not cross react with hemoglobin and can detect small quantities of myoglobin present in normal human urine from 3 to 20 ng/mL measured by radioimmunoassay. Up to 5000 ng/mL can be encountered in humans with clinical myoglobinuria [137].

Simultaneous evaluation of the patient's serum or plasma color with the urine color is helpful in deciding whether the positive occult blood reaction is due to hemoglobin or myoglobin. The serum should be pink due to hemolysis at the time hemoglobin appears in the urine, whereas the serum should be clear if the reaction in the urine is due to myoglobin. Hemoglobin appears in the urine only after its plasma carrier haptoglobin has been saturated, free hemoglobin has been filtered, and after the capacity of the proximal tubules to reabsorb filtered hemoglobin has been exceeded. Owing to the hemoglobin binding capacity of haptoglobin, the plasma concentration of hemoglobin must exceed 50 mg/dL before hemoglobinuria is detected [32]. The increase in plasma concentration of hemoglobin is responsible for the characteristic pink color of plasma. Myoglobin released into the blood is not bound to a carrier protein and is rapidly excreted into urine by glomerular filtration before enough myoglobinemia can be achieved to result in color formation. Consequently, plasma is normal in color due to its rapid renal clearance; at the same time, myoglobinuria has caused abnormal urine color.

Hemoglobinuria may arise as a consequence of intravascular hemolysis. Hemoglobinuria has been observed in dogs with disseminated intravascular coagulation, microangiopathic hemolytic disorders, postcaval syndrome of dirofilariasis, splenic torsion, autoimmune hemolytic anemia (AIHA), and in red cell enzyme deficiencies that result in abnormal osmotic fragility of RBC membranes (Table 5.13). It is also important to remember that lysis of previously intact red cells within urine will also be detected as positive occult blood.

Myoglobinuria may occur as a consequence of severe muscle damage as in crushing trauma, prolonged seizures, infarction, severe strenuous exercise, acute myositis, and heat stroke (Table 5.14). Myoglobinuria occurs when plasma concentrations of myoglobin exceed 15–20 mg/dL [32]. Increased serum concentrations of muscle enzymes (e.g. creatine kinase and aspartate aminotransferase [also called serum glutamic-oxaloacetic transaminase]) lend support to rhabdomyolysis as the cause of myoglobinuria. Exertional rhabdomyolysis in racing Greyhounds has been reported to cause myoglobinuria [136, 140]. Exertional and nonexertional rhabdomyolysis leading to myoglobinuria in animals was detailed in one report [141], but overall the presence of myoglobinuria appears to be rare in dogs and cats. Another possibility is that myoglobinuria is underreported in veterinary medicine due to lack of a readily available laboratory

Table 5.13 Causes of dipstrip positive occult blood reaction from hemoglobinuria. See Figure 6.4 for details regarding the causes of intact RBC in urine.

Causes of Dipstrip Positive Occult Blood Reaction from Hemoglobinuria
Intact RBC in urine
Lower urinary tract disorders
Upper urinary tract disorders
Genital tract disorders
Lysis of previously intact RBC that entered urine from any cause
Renal pelvic hematoma – leeching of hemoglobin from RBC into urine
Hemolysis outside of urinary tract
Transfusion reaction
Autoimmune hemolytic anemia
Disseminated intravascular coagulation
Microangiopathic hemolysis
Postcaval syndrome of dirofilariasis
Splenic torsion
Heat stroke
Severe hypophosphatemia
Zinc toxicity
Red cell enzyme deficiencies
Pyruvate kinase
Phosphofructokinase
Flea feces contamination of urine with blood
Feces or food contamination of urine

Table 5.14 Causes of dipstrip positive occult blood reaction from myoglobinuria.

Causes of Dipstrip Positive Occult Blood Reaction from Myoglobinuria
Persistent muscular activity – status epilepticus
Crushing injury to muscle
Exertional rhabdomyolysis
Rhabdomyolysis – propofol [138, 139]
Heat stroke
Severe hypokalemia (especially in cats)
Food or feces contamination of urine

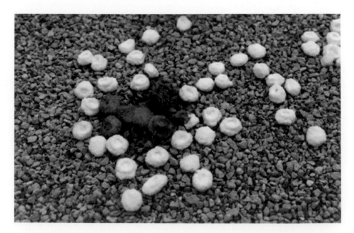

FIGURE 5.10 Hematuria Detection Technology by Blücare Litter Granules (Royal Canin). The use of these granules in the cat's litter allows the detection of RBC/hemoglobin in the urine at home. The white granules sprinkled in the litter turn blue when exposed to hemoglobin in the urine. The intensity of the blue color increases with greater amounts of RBC in the urine. The blue color change occurs within a minute following soaking with urine and persists for at least two days following exposure to hemoglobin. Granules that remain white or yellow are negative. Older granules that have been urine soaked without color development must be replaced since those granules no longer absorb urine. Source: Courtesy of Dr. Brent Mayabb, Royal Canin.

procedure enabling rapid accurate differentiation of myoglobin from hemoglobin.

Discordance between positive occult blood reactions on the reagent pad and detection of RBC during urine microscopy occurs with some frequency and is often attributed to lysis of previously intact RBC in the bladder [130]. This scenario is more likely to be encountered when urine has been examined following storage at room temperature rather than in very fresh samples. Another explanation for the finding of a greater reaction on the reagent pad than the finding of intact RBC during microscopy is that the absorbent pad examines a greater volume of urine than is evaluated during urine microscopy [1, 43]. An uncommon consideration for this discordance exists for those with glomerular disease in which RBC traverse the glomerulus and undergo lysis during traumatic passage. Many dogs with X-linked hereditary nephropathy exhibit moderate-to-large occult blood reactions on the dipstrip but consistently have <5 RBC/HPF during microscopy of a voided urine sample. The presence of dysmorphic RBC in urine sediment from most dogs in this setting supports the probability for traumatic passage of RBC during glomerular disease. Positive occult blood on the urinary dipstrip or excess RBC on urine microscopy is not commonly attributed to glomerular disease in veterinary medicine, but this connection likely is commonly missed. In addition, small numbers of RBC are often interpreted to be from trauma encountered during urine collected by cystocentesis rather than from an underlying disease process (Mary Nabity, personal communication 2021).

Uncommonly, a minimal or no reaction on the dipstrip for heme pigments can occur in those with increased RBC observed on urinary microscopy. This false-negative reagent pad reaction potentially can be attributed to the presence of crenated RBC from highly concentrated urine that fail to lyse on the reagent pad as one explanation [1].

A hematuria detection test (Blücare®, Royal Canin) is available for use in cat litter that allows an owner to detect hemoglobin in a cat's urine at home (Figure 5.10). Small white granules that contain the indicator dye 3,3′,5,5′-tetramethylbenzidine are sprinkled on top of the litter. These granules turn blue following a pseudo-peroxidation reaction with hemoglobin in urine that soaks the granules. When hemoglobin is detected, the blue color develops within a minute and lasts for at least 48 hours. Any type of cat litter can be used, but it appears to work best in clumping clay litter. Granules soiled with urine should be removed each day as these granules will no longer absorb new urine. These granules are considered sensitive since they detect a lower limit of about 12 RBC/HPF or 100 RBC/μL. There is less sensitivity for the granules to develop color when the urinary pH is ≥8.5 or when the USG is >1.050. The greater the amount of RBC in the urine, the greater the depth and intensity of blue color that develops that is scored from 0 to 3+. A score of 1+ is associated with about 12 RBC/HPF or 100 RBC/μL, a 2+ score with 45 RBC/HPF or 800 RBC/μL, and 3+ with TNTC RBC/HPF or >32 000 RBC/μL [142, 143]. A positive blue color reaction on these granules should prompt a visit to the veterinary hospital in order to obtain a complete urinalysis and possibly other diagnostics.

BILIRUBIN

Deep amber (yellow–brown or green–brown) color may be the result of either highly concentrated urine or increased amounts of bile pigments in the urine. Urine with excessive bilirubin may turn green upon standing as bilirubin is oxidized to biliverdin. A small quantity of white foam is produced when normal urine is shaken, though a large amount of white foam that persists after shaking may occur if the patient has severe proteinuria. A yellow, yellow–green, or brown foam often develops in shaken urine samples that are positive for bilirubinuria. The presence of bilirubinuria alters the surface tension of urine allowing the foam to more easily form [5]. The appearance of this foam is a crude predictor of bilirubinuria and does not replace more definitive testing with urinary chemistry dipstrips that deliver a semiquantitative report for bilirubin in the urine. False-positive results for bilirubin-discolored foam can occur if the urine contains large quantities of urobilinogen [144].

Metabolism and Excretion

Bilirubin is the normal end product of senescent RBC broken down by macrophages in the liver and spleen [3, 43, 145] and is derived from the catabolism of the heme part of hemoglobin. In health, most of the circulating bilirubin consists of unconjugated bilirubin [5]. Unconjugated bilirubin (indirect-reacting bilirubin) is bound to plasma proteins and transported to the liver where it is conjugated with glucuronic and sulfuric acids and excreted in the bile [144]. Most of the direct reacting bilirubin (conjugated bilirubin) is conjugated in the liver as a diglucuronide, while a small fraction is conjugated as a monoglucuronide [146]. Bilirubin is primarily excreted into bile and then into the intestines in healthy animals, but some conjugated bilirubin backflows from the liver into the circulation at low concentrations [5, 32].

Conjugated bilirubin is water soluble and freely filtered across the glomerulus, whereas unconjugated bilirubin does not pass through the glomerular capillaries due to its protein binding [39, 144]. Only conjugated bilirubin appears in the urine [146]. Circulating conjugated bilirubin is excreted into urine predominantly following glomerular filtration with little contribution from tubular secretion [147].

Dogs have a particularly low renal threshold for the appearance of bilirubin in urine, which allows bilirubinuria to be detected before the observation of hyperbilirubinemia or icterus [39, 144]. Cats appear to have a higher renal threshold for the appearance of bilirubinuria than dogs; the appearance of bilirubinuria in cats is never normal [53, 148].

For unknown reasons, male dogs excreted twice as much bilirubin on a 24-hour basis as did female dogs in one study [149]. Marked bilirubinuria is often associated with free hemoglobin in plasma (after hemoglobin has saturated its haptoglobin carrier) and urine following systemic hemolysis, despite no increase in plasma bilirubin levels. In dogs, this bilirubinuria appears to develop after plasma hemoglobin undergoes glomerular filtration, and then, some is reabsorbed by the renal tubules from tubular filtrate. Bilirubin is then produced by the catabolism of hemoglobin within the renal tubule that then enters tubular fluid. There appears to be a large difference by sex in the renal handling of filtered hemoglobin in dogs for reasons that are not clear. Bilirubin was the end product of hemoglobin catabolism in the kidney of all males and 20% of the females in one study. The bilirubin from tubular origin is predominantly excreted in the tubular lumens of male dogs, whereas it is returned to the circulation in females [149].

Methodology

The reagent pad designed to detect bilirubin in urine contains diazotized 2,4-dichloroaniline in a strongly acid medium for one brand of urinary chemistry strip. The sensitivity of this strip is from 0.4 to 0.8 mg/dL bilirubin. This reaction is specific for bilirubin and does react with other molecules normally excreted into urine [8]. Bilirubin in the urine reacts with this reagent to form azobilirubin, which causes a color change to a light tan or light brown. This methodology is much more sensitive to measurement of conjugated bilirubin than it is to unconjugated bilirubin [5, 8, 32, 39, 144]. In another dipstrip brand, 2,6-dichlorobenzene diazonium tetrafluoroborate reacts with bilirubin in an acid environment to generate a pink to red violet color change [33, 144].

Ideally, the test should not be performed on centrifuged urine. Urine samples analyzed for bilirubin should be fresh to avoid hydrolysis of conjugated to unconjugated bilirubin or oxidation of bilirubin to biliverdin in the presence of light [33]. Neither unconjugated bilirubin nor biliverdin is detected by the reagent pad. If dipstrip measurement within 30 minutes is not possible, refrigeration of the urine sample and then warming the sample to room temperature followed by well mixing is recommended [33]. There was a very high correlation for measurement of urinary bilirubin in samples stored at room temperature in preservative containing tubes or in plain glass tubes that were refrigerated for up to 72 hours compared to the time 0 fresh sample of one study [14].

The lower limits for detection of bilirubinuria by dipstrip are 0.2–0.4 mg/dL, though the practical limit of sensitivity is 0.5 mg/dL for some dipstrips [144]. A tablet method (Siemens Ictotest®; Ictero-Check Biorex Labs LLC) can detect as little as 0.05–0.1 mg/dL of bilirubinuria [5, 150].

Interferences

False-negative and false-positive results may occur for bilirubinuria (Table 5.15). Bilirubinuria is expected in patients with hyperbilirubinemia in general. In those with hyperbilirubinemia and zero bilirubinuria, a false-negative reaction for bilirubin should be suspected. Bilirubin can undergo spontaneous oxidation to biliverdin and intermediary metabolites that do not react with the reagent pad for bilirubin. Conjugated bilirubin in urine can spontaneously hydrolyze to free bilirubin (unconjugated), which is not detected by standard methods. These phenomena are most likely to happen in urine stored at room temperature and exposed to light potentially resulting in a false-negative report for bilirubinuria [33]. It has been suggested that urine should not be centrifuged prior to the measurement of bilirubin, as some bilirubin could adhere to crystals that have settled out. This is an uncommon consideration for a false-negative reading for bilirubin due to a preanalytical error [64, 144]. The presence of mostly unconjugated or free bilirubinemia during acute intravascular hemolysis is not associated with a positive bilirubin reaction on the urinary reagent pad, as this form of bilirubin does not traverse the intact glomerulus.

Table 5.15 False negative and false-positive reactions for bilirubinuria.

False Negative for Bilirubinuria
Urine stored at room temperature and exposed to light
High concentration of ascorbic acid in urine
High concentration of nitrites (sometimes in bacterial UTI)
Bilirubin crystals interference on reagent pad
Analysis of centrifuged urine with bilirubin trapped in dependent crystals

False Positive for Bilirubinuria
Highly colored urine
Highly concentrated urine (dark color).
Pink or red urine
Prolonged time beyond that recommended to match color block
Chlorpromazine
Phenazopyridine
Etodolac (NSAID) metabolite
Indican absorption following GI tryptophan metabolism

False-negative results or artifactually low readings may occur in urine samples that contain large amounts of ascorbic acid or nitrites that may be encountered with bacterial UTI. False-negative reactions for bilirubinuria occurred in 31% of dipstrip testing and in 48% of tablet testing in dogs that had high serum bilirubin levels, suggesting the presence of an unidentified inhibitor of the color reaction, possibly ascorbic acid [32]. The presence of bilirubin crystals in the urine may also interfere with the bilirubin reagent pad, resulting in false-negative results [3].

The interpretation of color development on the bilirubin reagent pad is often more difficult to interpret than other reagent pad reactions as the color generated is influenced to a greater degree by other pigments in the urine. Atypical colors generated on this reagent pad are common and reported as positive for color reaction by manual visual and automated methods [1]. There was only moderate agreement for bilirubin measured between automated strip reader results and manual visual methods in one study [20].

Difficulty in reading the color reaction of the bilirubin reagent strip may occur in urine samples that are discolored or highly concentrated; in these instances equivocal results should be further tested by reagent tablet methods [9]. Dipstrip scores reported for bilirubin using visual assessment of the dipstrip were significantly higher in samples that were categorized as dark pink and red for both dogs and cats, compared with scores for samples undiluted with blood [12]. In a study of urethral obstruction in cats, 12% of the cats were reported with bilirubinuria in the absence of hemolysis, hepatic disease, or posthepatic obstruction. It was likely that the

bilirubin positive reading of the reagent pad was an artifact due to the color of the urine from hematuria [117].

Indoxyl sulfate (indican) in urine can generate an atypical yellow–orange to red color on the pad that does not match up with any negative or positive color block on the color chart that can make it impossible to read the result as positive or negative [8, 32]. Metabolites of the nonsteroidal anti-inflammatory drug (NSAID) etodolac can result in either atypical color generation or a false-positive reaction on the reagent pad. Atypical colors on the reagent pad can indicate the presence of other bile pigments in the urine that are masking the detection of bilirubin [8]. False-positive reactions for bilirubin on the dipstrip can occur in those treated with chlorpromazine or phenoazopyridine [5, 151].Tryptophan metabolism within the intestine by bacteria can produce indican that is absorbed into the circulation and excreted into urine resulting in false-positive color generation on the reagent pad [43]. False-positive color reactions on the reagent pad can also occur if the color block is checked after the specified amount of time for that strip to be read [5].

Interpretation

A small or trace reaction for bilirubin is frequently reported in concentrated urine of healthy dogs (1.025–1.040 USG). Trace to +1 reactions for bilirubin may be measured in urine from normal dogs (especially males), particularly if the urine specimen is concentrated to a specific gravity of 1.040 or greater [64, 144]. As many as 60% of normal dogs have measurable bilirubinuria [42]. About 25% of normal male dogs with a normal serum bilirubin had a positive color reaction for bilirubin on the urine reagent strip, while 50% were positive for bilirubin with tablet testing [64]. The finding of bilirubinuria was common in apparently healthy geriatric and senior dogs of another study, occurring with a trace reaction in 45/97 (46%), a positive reaction in 36/97 (37%), and negative reaction in 16/97 (16%) [27]. In dogs, even though up to 1+ bilirubin in concentrated urine is considered normal and is common, the finding must correlate with other clinical abnormalities in other to exclude underlying disease [53, 148].

Dipstrip reactions for bilirubin that are +2 to +3 are likely to be abnormal in concentrated urine samples from dogs (USG 1.020–1.035), and trace to +1 reactions may be abnormal in dogs with dilute urine [42, 152]. Positive readings from more dilute urine samples may also be clinically relevant in dogs. Bilirubinuria in cats was never normal in some reports, even when the urine was highly concentrated (high USG). Bilirubinuria was not detected by dipstrip in 99 apparently healthy middle-aged or old cats in one study [28] and in no urine samples tested by tablet from 82 adult normal experimental male cats [153]. Bilirubinuria is always considered a pathological finding in cats [144, 153, 154], unless readings are an artifact of urine color. Bilirubinuria was detected by the tablet test in 4% of urine samples from 808 client-owned cats; most with bilirubinuria were diagnosed with underlying liver disease in those that were sick [153].

Table 5.16 Causes of bilirubinuria.

Causes of Bilirubinuria
Hemolysis – intravascular
Autoimmune hemolytic anemia
Liver dysfunction 2° to anemia, hemosiderosis
Hemoglobinuria transformed to bilirubin by renal tubules (dogs)
Liver disease – primary hepatic
Extrahepatic biliary obstruction
Fever
Prolonged starvation

The evaluation of bilirubinuria is not generally helpful in the evaluation of renal disease or function, though low GFR for any reason may lessen the amount of conjugated bilirubin filtered across the glomerulus.

The finding of bilirubinuria often indicates the presence of hemolytic disease or liver disease (mostly cholestatic) (Table 5.16) [53, 148]. Bilirubinuria may be detected before clinically detectable jaundice or hyperbilirubinemia and so may be valuable in the early diagnosis of diseases that can increase circulating bilirubin [39, 64, 144, 154]. It should be noted, however, that significant hepatic and posthepatic lesions may exist without the detection of bilirubinuria. The interpretation of bilirubinuria or its absence is difficult if severe renal dysfunction occurs as that decreases filtration of bilirubin.

Bilirubinuria occurs as a consequence of primary intrahepatic diseases and biliary obstruction, but the bilirubinuria associated with extrahepatic biliary obstruction is usually more severe [152]. Small amounts of bilirubinuria may occur in any febrile disorder, particularly when testing is done with the reagent tablet method. Similar reactions may occur during prolonged starvation [42, 144].

Bilirubinuria also occurs as a consequence of hemolysis (e.g. AIHA). Chronic extravascular hemolysis may result in hepatic dysfunction due to anemia and hemosiderosis, leading to regurgitation of conjugated bilirubin from the liver into plasma with subsequent excretion of large amounts of bilirubin into urine [42]. Acute intravascular hemolysis results in hemoglobinuria. In dogs, renal tubular reabsorption of filtered hemoglobin can result in metabolism to bilirubin, conjugation within the tubular cell, and excretion of conjugated bilirubin into the urine. In this instance, serum bilirubin concentration remains unchanged and liver function may be normal.

UROBILINOGEN

Dipstrips commonly used in veterinary medicine were designed for use in human medicine. In humans, urobilinogen in urine has been used to screen for hepatic disorders, hemolytic disorders, and patency of the bile ducts; better tests are available to evaluate the hepatobiliary tree [151]. In humans, the evaluation of bilirubin and urobilinogen together on the same urine sample can provide additional clinical information to help in the evaluation of jaundice and disorders of the liver and biliary tree [8].

The measurement of urobilinogen in urine has been generally considered to be unreliable or of little clinical value in small animals [3, 32, 38, 43, 64, 148, 155], but there have no modern reports examining its possible clinical utility. Some veterinary laboratories do not report urobilinogen as part of their standard urinalysis findings, but some commercial veterinary laboratories continue to report urobilinogen results.

Metabolism of Bilirubin and Urobilinogen

The urinary concentration of urobilinogen generally reflects the concentration of urobilinogen in plasma, in addition to the level of excretory renal function. The concentration of plasma urobilinogen depends on the magnitude of conjugated bilirubin delivered from the liver and bile duct into the intestine, the activity of large intestinal bacterial organisms that transform bilirubin into urobilinogen (which includes mesobilirubin and stercobilinogen), the degree of absorption of urobilinogen into the circulation, and the degree of removal of urobilinogen from the circulation by the liver (enterohepatic recirculation). The amount of urobilinogen in urine then depends on the filtered load of urobilinogen (GFR × plasma urobilinogen concentration) followed by the degree of tubular secretion and reabsorption of urobilinogen [32].

Senescent or damaged RBC are removed from the circulation primarily by the macrophages of the spleen, but also degraded in the liver and bone marrow [156]. This process releases hemoglobin that is further processed into heme and globin. Under the influence of heme oxygenase, heme is converted to biliverdin and then unconjugated bilirubin, which enters the circulation. Unconjugated bilirubin is bound to plasma albumin and undergoes glucuronidation in the presence of glucuronyl transferase in the liver, which generates bilirubin diglucuronide (conjugated bilirubin).

Conjugated bilirubin is secreted into bile and transported through the bile duct to the small intestine where this polar compound is poorly absorbed. In the colon, most conjugated bilirubin is reduced by dehydrogenases of anaerobic bacteria to several related colorless compounds, including urobilinogen and stercobilinogen. Stercobilinogen is not reabsorbed and is oxidized to stercobilin. Urobilinogen and its oxidation products stercobilin and urobilin are then largely excreted in feces. Urobilin and stercobilin are responsible for the normal dark color to feces. Some urobilinogen (10–15%) is absorbed into the portal circulation, picked up by the liver and then excreted into bile (enterohepatic recirculation). A small fraction (1–5%) of absorbed urobilinogen is not processed by the liver and circulates to the kidneys where it is excreted [1, 5, 32, 39, 64, 145]. Urobilinogen is a weak acid that enters urine by a combination of glomerular filtration, tubular secretion, and pH-dependent nonionic diffusion in the distal tubules of the dog [157]. Less than 1 mg/dL is considered normal for urinary urobilinogen in humans [1, 5].

Alkaline urine (pH 8.0) dramatically increased urobilinogen excretion into urine in one study of dogs. Urobilinogen exists in an ionized state in alkaline urine, rendering it less reabsorbable across tubular membranes. An increase in urinary flow rate markedly increased urobilinogen excretion when the urine was acid, but not when the urine was alkaline. Optimal clinical interpretation of urinary urobilinogen status necessitated consideration of both the urinary flow rate and urinary pH in addition to its plasma concentration and level of renal function [157].

Methodology

Reagent pads may contain either benzaldehyde compounds (Ehrlich's test) in Multistix® [8] or a stable diazonium salt in Chemstrip® [33]. A cherry-red light to dark pink color is generated with the Ehrlich's test when urobilinogen is present [1, 32, 39, 64]. Ehrlich's test is not specific for urobilinogen and may detect the presence of porphobilinogen, sulfisoxazole, p-aminosalicylic acid, and indole as well. This method can detect urobilinogen as low as 0.2 mg/dL and up to a maximum of 8 mg/dL [1, 8, 43]. Urobilinogen must be determined on fresh samples since it is a very unstable compound [33] and may readily oxidize to urobilin, which will not be detected by reagent strip methodology [43].

White to pink color is generated on the reagent pad during the interaction of the diazonium salt with urobilinogen. This reaction is more specific for urobilinogen than that measured with Ehrlich's reagent [1]. This method detects urobilinogen as low as 0.4 mg/dL and to a maximal 12 mg/dL [1, 33, 64]. Up to 1 mg/dL of urinary urobilinogen is considered normal [8, 33]; ≥2 mg/dL is considered abnormal and should trigger considerations for hemolytic and hepatic diseases [43].

Very concentrated highly colored urine specimens may make it difficult to read the color reaction on the reagent strip resulting in a false-positive report. A green color may be produced on the reagent pad when large quantities of bilirubin are present due to the conversion of bilirubin to biliverdin again making it difficult to report color generation on the reagent pad. Color development on the reagent pad increases as ambient and urine temperature increase and could result in a false-positive amount reported for urobilinogen at temperatures ≥80 °F.

False-positive color reactions (brown to red) for urobilinogen can occur in the presence of para-aminosalicylic acid, p-aminobenzoic acid, sulfonamides, and other compounds with aromatic amines [8]. Phenazopyridine can result in the generation of red color on the pad [33]. Indoles, skatole, and indican found at times in normal urine can also generate a false-positive color reaction. The oxidation of urobilinogen to urobilin while the sample is standing too long can result in a false negative, as can the presence of formaldehyde >200 mg/dL (urinary preservative or from methenamine metabolism), or high concentrates of urinary nitrites >5 mg/dL [8, 32, 33].

Urobilinogen in urine that is exposed to ultraviolet (UV) light can be converted to urobilin, which is not detected on the reagent strip as another consideration for a false-negative result; the urine may show shades of green in this instance [32, 43]. Dilute urine samples may preclude the detection of urobilinogen on a random urine sample. The excretion of urobilinogen into urine is variable in health and is noted to be diurnal in humans [33, 39]. Consequently, the absence of detectable urobilinogen on a single sample should not be overinterpreted.

Interpretation

Normal dog or cat urine usually contains small amounts of urobilinogen, but none may be reported since it requires 1 mg/dL or more to register as an increased amount. A dipstrip result that records normal urobilinogen means that its concentration is ≤1 mg/dL, but it cannot be used to detect decreased concentrations of urinary urobilinogen as there is no negative color block for this molecule [8, 32, 33, 64]. The frequency for positive urobilinogen results on urinary dipstrip was very uncommon in one report from a teaching hospital, noted at 0.015% (0.006% at ≥1+) in over 10 000 urine specimens from dogs and 0.015% (0.007% at ≥1+) in over 2000 urine specimens from cats [32].

The measurement of urinary urobilinogen may be valuable in the early detection of disease as hemolytic diseases or diseases with reduced functional liver mass can result in an increased amount of urobilinogen in urine [1, 39]. With reduced hepatic mass and function, there is bile flow, but less urobilinogen absorbed from the large intestine into the circulation is removed by dysfunctional or reduced numbers of hepatocytes from portal blood. This leaves an excess of urobilinogen in the plasma than then undergoes renal excretion [1, 39].

When decreased re-excretion of urobilinogen into bile occurs following its reabsorption from the large intestine into the circulation, increased concentrations of urobilinogen in urine may be encountered [1, 5]. A combination of increased urine urobilinogen, normal fecal urobilinogen, and negative urinary bilirubin can also be seen in some disorders of the liver; bilirubin conjugation and excretion into bile are normal, but the liver is not able to remove urobilinogen from the circulation [5].

Excessive urobilinogenuria may suggest liver disease when all other liver tests are normal [42]. When animals have a disease that should cause an abnormal urobilinogen result, the dipstrip reaction is frequently normal, possibly due to the instability of urobilinogen that is rapidly converted to urobilin. The correlation between hepatobiliary disease and urinary urobilinogen has been noted to be poor in animals [39].

Hemolysis in the dog can result in high urinary urobilinogen levels, but this does not happen consistently in other species [39, 43]. Hemolytic disorders result in increased delivery of unconjugated bilirubin to the liver, and then, delivery of conjugated bilirubin to the intestine via the bile duct. Increased production of urobilinogen in the large intestine occurs, and some urobilinogen undergoes enterohepatic circulation. Some of the urobilinogen that has entered the circulation will undergo further processing and excretion by the liver, and some will be available to undergo renal excretion into urine. Urobilinogenuria in hemolytic disorders results from this increased urobilinogen production and from decreased hepatic function that can occur as a consequence of the anemia [42]. In a model of onion-induced hemolysis in dogs, urinary urobilinogen increased substantially by day 2 and achieved its highest concentration on day 4. Increased urinary bilirubin at 3+ on the dipstrip persisted from day 2 to day 9 after onion ingestion [158]. Though urobilinogenuria is expected during hemolysis, it has not consistently been found [64]. Increased formation of urobilinogen may also occur in the intestine during severe constipation [1], enteritis, intestinal obstruction or in bowel disorders where increased bacterial fermentation may occur [42].

Urobilinogen is present in urine when the bile duct is patent [39], though its concentration may be below the level of detection on the regent pad at <1 mg/dL categorized as normal. Complete bile duct obstruction causes an absence of urobilinogen in urine [1]; however, this absence of urobilinogen is recorded as urobilinogenuria "normal" (<1 mg/dL) on the reagent pad color block. Consequently, dipstrip reagent pads cannot be used to diagnose biliary obstruction when the reading is normal [39]. The absence of urobilinogen may also be noted as a consequence of reduced bile formation by the liver, and when the intestinal flora necessary for bilirubin reduction to urobilinogen have been eradicated by antibiotic therapy [42]. Urobilinogen was absent in urine and feces of experimental germ-free animals that lacked intestinal bacteria in one study [159].

LEUKOCYTE ESTERASE

The LE dipstrip reagent pad was designed to indirectly detect leukocytes in the urine of humans associated with urinary tract inflammation or urinary infection. The LE test is often used in concert with the nitrite reagent pad to make a decision as to the likelihood of a bacterial UTI, and whether the urine should undergo microscopy and/or urine culture in human medicine. The combination of a negative LE test and a negative nitrite test can be used to exclude the need to perform urine microscopy or urine culture in human medicine for patients suspected of a bacterial UTI [4].

The reagent pad contains a buffered mixture of derivatized pyrrole amino acid ester and a diazonium salt. Indoxyl esterases released from granulocytic leukocytes (neutrophils, eosinophils, and basophils), macrophages, and monocytes catalyze the pyrrole amino acid to liberate 3-hydroxy-5-phenylpyrrole, which produces a purple color when it reacts with the diazonium salt. Lymphocytes in urine are not be detected by this method. A positive color reaction detects a lower limit of 5–15 WBC per microliter in human urine. False-negative or less color development on the reagent pad can

occur in the presence of glucosuria, proteinuria, very high USG, and when cephalexin, cephalothin, tobramycin, or high amounts of oxalic acid are in the urine of humans. Alkaline urine with low USG favors lysis of WBC, which can result in discordance between positive dipstrip color development and a low number of WBC observed during urine microscopy. False-negative LE results can also happen in those with highly concentrated urine that prevents lysis of WBC. This results in less color development on the reagent pad despite WBC observed on urine microscopy [4, 8, 32, 33, 50, 160].

The use of results from the LE dipstrip reagent pad cannot be recommended for urine from either the dog or the cat and should not be used to replace urine microscopy to detect the presence of WBC in urine [28, 39, 161, 162]. Compared to urine microscopy in one study of cats, there was no significant association between >5 WBC/HPF and a positive LE test for color reaction. In this study, the LE test strip had a sensitivity of 77%, specificity of 34%, positive predictive value of 14%, negative predictive value of 91%, and overall test efficiency of 39% [162]. The LE test was positive in 98 of 99 apparently healthy middle-age and old cats of another study indicating a very high rate for false-positive reactions [28]. The freezing of urine samples eliminated the false-positive LE reactions in one report; it was speculated that cat urine contains esterases of nonleukocyte origin [32].

In contrast to findings in cats, the LE test was negative in 95% of apparently healthy senior and geriatric dogs in one study [27]. In another study of dogs, the LE test was specific for the detection of pyuria at 93.2% (few false positives) but was poorly sensitive at 46.0% (many false negatives) compared to urine microscopy enumeration. Therefore, a positive LE reaction indicates pyuria in dogs, but a negative result is not reliable. It was speculated that canine urine might contain an esterase inhibitor or that canine leukocytes do not contain the same quantity or type of esterases as in human leukocytes [161]. In an unpublished study, positive quantitative bacterial urine culture results were highly correlated with positive LE reactions on the reagent pad in dogs [32].

NITRITE

Many gram-negative bacteria produce nitrate reductase, which facilitates the conversion of nitrate in the urine to nitrite [8, 50, 160]. Nitrates are normally found in urine [77], but the amount will vary largely by dietary intake of vegetables [160]. A positive test for nitrite supports the likelihood for a bacterial UTI in humans. The nitrite reagent pad only detects nitrites in urine, and a positive nitrite reagent pad color reaction is designed to indicate the presence of $\geq 10^5$ cfu/mL from quantitative bacterial urine culture [8].

The nitrite reagent pad contains arsanilic acid and a quinolol. The arsanilic acid combines with nitrite in the urine to create a diazonium salt. The diazonium salt then combines with a quinolol to produce a pink color on one strip [8] or combines with sulfanilamide that generates a red–violet color on another test strip [33]. The lower limit for the detection of nitrite on one manufacturer's dipstrip is as low as 0.05 mg/dL and will generate a positive test result with slightly pink color [33]. Sensitivity for detection of urinary nitrate is 0.06–0.1 mg/dL on a competitor's dipstrip [8].

Color generation on the nitrite reagent pad is less in human urine samples with a high USG and in urine with greater than 25 mg/dL ascorbic acid, an effect that is greater when the nitrite concentration in the urine is low [4]. Bacterial UTI can still exist in the presence of a negative nitrite reagent pad reaction if the bacteria produce little or no nitrate reductase, such as *Pseudomonas* species, *Staphylococcus spp*, and *Enterococcus* species, or in situations with minimal dwell time before urine is voided [50, 160]. Medications that turn the urine red can result in a false-positive nitrite reagent pad reading [33].

A positive test for nitrite requires urine that contains adequate nitrate for conversion to nitrite, bacteria that elaborate nitrate reductase, a critical number of bacteria (cfu/mL) to generate nitrite, and enough dwell time within the bladder to allow for the conversion of nitrate to nitrite occur. The development of a positive color reaction on the nitrite reagent strip may require four to eight hours of urine dwell time within the bladder in order for enough nitrite to be generated from nitrate to be detected in the face of bacterial UTI [33]. In instances in which bladder urine is not held for very long (as in cystitis with pollakiuria), there will be less time to generate nitrite to be measured on the reagent pad resulting in a negative test result [4].

In one report in dogs and cats, nitrite positive reactions on a dipstrip did not accurately detect clinically significant bacteriuria based on cfu/mL and was found to be unsuitable to use for screening of UTI. The nitrite reaction was negative in all samples tested, including those with bacterial growth greater than 10 000 cfu/mL. It was speculated that high levels of urinary ascorbic acid may have inhibited the development of the nitrite color reaction on the reagent pad [77]. Ascorbic acid at 5 mg/dL or greater resulted in a negative nitrite pad reaction when known quantities of nitrite at less than 1 mg/dL were added to water. Ascorbic acid at 5–40 mg/dL did not cause interference in the detection of nitrite when its concentration was greater than 1 mg/dL in water. Ascorbic acid was detected in 95% of urine samples from dogs and cats when measured by a reagent pad dipstrip designed to measure this molecule. Ascorbic acid was detected at 5–40 mg/dL in these urine samples with most at 10 or 20 mg/dL [77].

URINE SPECIFIC GRAVITY BY DIPSTRIP

Measuring the USG on a dipstrip is designed as a screening test in human medicine, but this has not replaced measuring urine concentration with USG by refractometry or osmometry. For USG dipstrip measurement, the reagent pad contains a polyelectrolyte indicator system (polymethylvinyl ether/maleic acid with bromthymol (bromothymol) blue and hydrogen peroxide in Multistix Siemens [8] and ethylene glycol-bis-tetra-acetic acid in Chemistrip® Roche [32]), which is sensitive to urinary ionic strength. The urinary ionic concentration (strength) determines how much color develops on the reagent pad, which is proportional to the specific gravity in humans. As the USG increases, so does the ionic (cationic) strength of the urine, which is associated with release of protons from the reagent pad that then causes a color change in the indicator dye [33, 121, 163].

Dipstrip reagent pads that develop a color change are designed to measure USG of 1.000–1.030 [8, 33] in increments of 0.005. Thus, a USG by refractometer of 1.008 would be reported as either 1.005 or 1.010 when measuring by dipstrip reagent pad. The USG by pad generally correlates within 0.005 USG by refractometer in human urine [8, 33].

For precise investigation into urine concentration and dilution, refractometry or osmometry should be used as has been shown in a number of studies with human urine [163–165]. Dipstrip USG measurement may be higher or lower than measurement by refractometry, depending on what is present in urine. When a dipstrip is used for USG measurement, other nonionic components in urine such as proteins and organic acids, may not contribute to USG estimation [165], even though dipstrip inserts maintain that moderate concentrations of protein in the urine (100–500 mg/dL) will increase the reported USG on the reagent pad [8, 33]. According to the package insert of one manufacturer, radiocontrast dyes in the urine do not impact color development on the USG reagent pad; however, USG measured by refractometer can be substantially increased by radiocontrast dyes [8]. Human patients with ketoacidosis tend to have higher USG measured by reagent pad than by refractometer [33]. High urinary concentration of glucose or urea in urine results in the report of a lower USG by pad than by refractometer [4, 33]. Highly buffered alkaline urine samples can result in lower USG readings on the reagent pad. Consequently, urine samples with a pH > 6.5 [8] or ≥ 7.0 [33] can be "corrected" by adding 0.005 to the USG when read either manually or automatically with strip readers.

The screening of USG by urine dipstrip is considered unsuitable for use in dogs or cats due to poor correlation with USG determined by refractometry or urine concentration by osmolality. The average urine concentration in healthy dogs and cats is considerably higher than that encountered in human urine, so the measurement of a maximal USG of 1.030 on a dipstrip reagent pad cannot detect "adequate" urinary concentrating capacity under many circumstances (see Chapter 4). Additionally, the reagent pads for USG do not correlate well enough with USG by refractometry to be clinically useful even when USG results are ≤1.030.

In one study of dog urine, the USG measurement by dipstrip differed from that determined by refractometry by more than 0.005 in 77.5% of urine samples; a difference in 60% still existed when a correction of 0.005 was added to results from urine with a pH≥6.5 [166]. In another study of urine from healthy Beagle dogs, there was marked disagreement between USG by dipstrip compared to that determined by refractometry. All USG by reagent pad were lower than that by refractometry, and the difference in reported USG was >0.005 in 28 of 30 samples [163]. The systematic underestimation of USG in urine from dogs by reagent pad compared to refractometry in another study led the author to conclude that dipstrip methods to measure USG should never be used in dogs [167]. The USG in dog urine measured by dipstrip and an automated reader showed severe disagreement with USG measured by refractometer; similar USGs by reagent pad results were generated following visual or automated reading of the dipstrip [165]. Conversely, there was good correlation between USG measured by a refractometer compared to an automated dipstrip reader for both cats (R = 0.83) and for dogs (R = 0.78) in another study. However, in this study, there was a wide range in the reported USG value by refractometry compared to the dipstrip reading. For example, a 1.015 automated dipstrip USG reading was associated with a refractometer USG reading of 1.010–1.040 in cats and 1.010–1.035 in dogs [21].

ASCORBIC ACID

Some urinary dipstrips contain a reagent pad to measure ascorbic acid. This serves as a quality control to detect variable concentrations of ascorbic acid in urine that could interfere with color reactions on some reagent pads. In human medicine, there is concern for the reporting of false-negative urinary dipstrip results most commonly for glucose, occult blood, LE, nitrite, and bilirubin due to interference from ascorbic acid [168–171]. There was concordance in reading color reactions between two brands of dipstrips when ascorbic acid levels were negative, but discordance was often high when ascorbic acid levels were positive in one study of human urine [169]. Despite the ability of the dog to synthesize vitamin C, plasma and urinary concentrations of ascorbic acid were low under basal conditions in experimental dogs. Increased plasma and urinary levels of vitamin C followed exogenous supplementation with vitamin C. Compared to humans, dogs have less capacity to reabsorb ascorbic acid following its filtration into tubular fluid [172, 173]. There is the possibility that animals being treated with vitamin C could similarly develop false-negative dipstrip reactions, but Vitamin C urinary levels in clinical dogs and cats at basal levels or after supplementation have not been reported.

REFERENCES

1 Strasinger, S.K. and Di Lorenzo, M.S. (2014). *Chemical Examination of Urine. Urinalysis and Body Fluids*, 71–97. Philadelphia: F.A. Davis Company.

2 Rizzi, T.E., Valenciano, A., Bowles, M. et al. (2017). *Sample Collection and Handling Atlas of Canine and Feline Urinalysis*, 3–46. Hoboken, N.J.: Wiley.

3 Rizzi, T.E., Valenciano, A., Bowles, M. et al. (2017). *Urine Chemistry Atlas of Canine and Feline Urinalysis*, 53–65. Hoboken, N.J.: Wiley.

4 Lamb, E.J. and Jones, G.R.D. (2018). Kidney function tests. In: *Tietz Textbook of Clinical Chemistry and Molecular Diagnostics*, 6e (ed. N. Rifai, A.R. Horvath and C.T. Witter), 479–516. St. Louis, MO: Elsevier.

5 Mundt, M.A. and Shanahan, K. (2016). *Chemical Analysis of Urine Graff's Textbook of Urinalysis and Body Fluids*, 3e, 89–110. Philadelphia: Wolters Kluwer.

6 Barger, A.M. (2015). Urinalysis. In: *Clinical Pathology and Laboratory Techniques for Veterinary Technicians*, 1e (ed. A. Barger and A.L. MacNeil), 141–175. Wiley.

7 Welles, E.G., Whatley, E.M., Hall, A.S. et al. (2006). Comparison of Multistix PRO dipsticks with other biochemical assays for determining urine protein (UP), urine creatinine (UC) and UP:UC ratio in dogs and cats. *Vet. Clin. Pathol.* 35: 31–36.

8 Siemens, H.D. (2010). Multi Stix package insert.

9 Duncan, J.R. and Prasse, K.W. (1976). Clinical examination of the urine. *Vet. Clin. North Am.* 6: 647–661.

10 Lem, L. and Rosenfeld, A. (2018). VetScan® UA Urine Analyzer Clinical Performance. https://www.abaxis.com/sites/default/files/resource-papers/888-6207%20Rev.%20B%20UA%20White%20Paper%20-%20UA%20Clinical%20Performance.pdf. 1–5.

11 LePage, W., Corey, S., Hunt, T., et al. (2006). Validation of IDEXX Vet-Lab® UA™ Analyzer and IDEXX UA™ Strips for Veterinary Samples: https://www.idexx.no/files/idexx-vetlab-ua-validation-study-en.pdf.

12 Vientos-Plotts, A.I., Behrend, E.N., Welles, E.G. et al. (2018). Effect of blood contamination on results of dipstick evaluation and urine protein-to-urine creatinine ratio for urine samples from dogs and cats. *Am. J. Vet. Res.* 79: 525–531.

13 Pugia, M.J. (2000). Technology behind diagnostic reagent strips. *Lab. Med.* 31: 92–98.

14 Aulakh, H.K., Aulakh, K.S., Ryan, K.A. et al. (2020). Investigation of the effects of storage with preservatives at room temperature or refrigeration without preservatives on urinalysis results for samples from healthy dogs. *J. Am. Vet. Med. Assoc.* 257: 726–733.

15 Oyaert, M. and Delanghe, J.R. (2019). Semiquantitative, fully automated urine test strip analysis. *J. Clin. Lab. Anal.* 33: e22870.

16 Oyaert, M. and Delanghe, J. (2019). Progress in automated urinalysis. *Ann. Lab. Med.* 39: 15–22.

17 Abaxis (2017). VetScan UA User's Manual.

18 IDEXX (2014). IDEXX VetLab UA Analyzer Operator's Guide English. https://ca.idexx.com/en-ca/veterinary/support/documents-resources/vetlab-ua-resources.

19 Ayoub, J.A., Beaufrere, H., and Acierno, M.J. (2013). Association between urine osmolality and specific gravity in dogs and the effect of commonly measured urine solutes on that association. *Am. J. Vet. Res.* 74: 1542–1545.

20 Bauer, N., Rettig, S., and Moritz, A. (2008). Evaluation the Clinitek status automated dipstick analysis device for semiquantitative testing of canine urine. *Res. Vet. Sci.* 85: 467–472.

21 Defontis, M., Bauer, N., Failing, K. et al. (2013). Automated and visual analysis of commercial urinary dipsticks in dogs, cats and cattle. *Res. Vet. Sci.* 94: 440–445.

22 Ferreira, M.D.F., Garcia Arce, M., Handel, I.G. et al. (2018). Urine dipstick precision with standard visual and automated methods within a small animal teaching hospital. *Vet. Rec.* 183: 415.

23 Mie, K., Hayashi, A., Nishida, H. et al. (2019). Evaluation of the accuracy of urine analyzers in dogs and cats. *J. Vet. Med. Sci.* 81: 1671–1675.

24 Morissette, E. (2018). Evaluation of urine by automatic and manual methods ABX-00145: Zoetis.

25 Evans, S.J.M., Sharp, J.L., and Vap, L.M. (2020). Optimizing the u411 automated urinalysis instrument for veterinary use. *Vet. Clin. Pathol.* 49: 106–111.

26 Alleman, R. and Wamsley, H.L. (2017). Complete urinalysis. In: *BSAVA Manual of Canine and Felne Nephrology and Urology*, 2e (ed. J. Elliott, G.F. Grauer and J.L. Westropp), 60–83. Gloucester, UK: BSAVA.

27 Willems, A., Paepe, D., Marynissen, S. et al. (2017). Results of screening of apparently healthy senior and geriatric dogs. *J. Vet. Intern. Med.* 31: 81–92.

28 Paepe, D., Verjans, G., Duchateau, L. et al. (2013). Routine health screening: findings in apparently healthy middle-aged and old cats. *J. Feline Med. Surg.* 15: 8–19.

29 Krimer, P.M., Tanner, M.C., and Camus, M.S. (2019). Evaluation of a home urinalysis kit in dogs. *J. Am. Anim. Hosp. Assoc.* 55: 144–151.

30 Albasan, H., Lulich, J.P., Osborne, C.A. et al. (2003). Effects of storage time and temperature on pH, specific gravity, and crystal formation in urine samples from dogs and cats. *J. Am. Vet. Med. Assoc.* 222: 176–179.

31 Wamsley, H.L. and Alleman, R. (2007). Complete urinalysis. In: *BSAVA Manual of Canine and Felne Nephrology and Urology*, 2e (ed. J. Elliott and G.F. Grauer), 87–116. Gloucester, UK: BSAVA.

32 Osborne, C.A. and Stevens, J.B. (1999). Biochemical analysis of urine: indications, methods, interpretation. In: *Urinalysis: A Clinical Guide to Compassionate Patient Care* (ed. C.A. Osborne and J.B. Stevens), 86–124. Shawnee Mission, KS: Bayer.

33 Roche, D. (2015). Chemstrip Package Insert.

34 Raskin, R.E., Murray, K.A., and Levy, J.K. (2002). Comparison of home monitoring methods for feline urine pH measurement. *Vet. Clin. Pathol.* 31: 51–55.

35 Johnson, K.Y., Lulich, J.P., and Osborne, C.A. (2007). Evaluation of the reproducibility and accuracy of pH-determining devices used to measure urine pH in dogs. *J. Am. Vet. Med. Assoc.* 230: 364–369.

36 Heuter, K.J., Buffington, C.A., and Chew, D.J. (1998). Agreement between two methods for measuring urine pH in cats and dogs. *J. Am. Vet. Med. Assoc.* 213: 996–998.

37 Omar, M., Sarkissian, C., Jianbo, L. et al. (2016). Dipstick spot urine pH does not accurately represent 24 hour urine PH measured by an electrode. *Int. Braz. J. Urol.* 42: 546–549.

38 Fry, M.M. (2011). Urinalysis. In: *Nephrology and Urology of Small Animals* (ed. J. Bartges and D. Polzin), 46–57. Chichester: Wiley.

39 Tripathi, N.K., Gregory, C.R., and Latimer, K.S. (2011). Urinary system. In: *Duncan and Prasse's Veterinary Laboratory Medicine: Clinical Pathology*, 5e (ed. K.S. Latimer), 253–294. Ames, Iowa: Wiley-Blackwell/Wiley.

40 Athanasiou, L.V., Katsoulos, P.D., Katsogiannou, E.G. et al. (2018). Comparison between the urine dipstick and the pH-meter to assess urine pH in sheep and dogs. *Vet. Clin. Pathol.* 47: 284–288.

41 Barlough, J.E., Osborne, C.A., and Stevens, J.B. (1981). Canine and feline urinalysis: value of macroscopic and microscopic examinations. *J. Am. Vet. Med. Assoc.* 178: 61–63.

42 Chew, D.J. (1984). Urinalysis. In: *Canine Nephrology* (ed. K.C. Bovee), 235–274. Media, PA: Harwal Publishing Co.

43 Sink, C.A. and Weinstein, N.M. (2012). *Routine Urinalysis: Chemical Analysis Practical Veterinary Urinalysis*, 29–53. Ames, Iowa: Wiley.

44 Melandri, M., Veronesi, M.C., and Alonge, S. (2020). Urinalysis in great Dane puppies from birth to 28 days of age. *Animals (Basel)* 10: 636.

45 Buffington, C.A., Rogers, Q.R., and Morris, J.G. (1994). Effects of age and food deprivation on urine pH of cats. *Vet. Clin. Nutr.* 1: 12–17.

46 Kienzle, E., Schuknecht, A., and Meyer, H. (1991). Influence of food composition on the urine pH in cats. *J. Nutr.* 121: S87–S88.

47 Johnson, C.D., Mole, D.R., and Pestridge, A. (1995). Postprandial alkaline tide: does it exist? *Digestion* 56: 100–106.

48 Rudinsky, A.J., Wellman, M., Tracy, G. et al. (2019). Variability among four refractometers for the measurement of urine specific gravity and comparison with urine osmolality in dogs. *Vet. Clin. Pathol.* 48: 702–709.

49 Buffington, C.A. and Chew, D.J. (1996). Intermittent alkaline urine in a cat fed an acidifying diet. *J. Am. Vet. Med. Assoc.* 209: 103–104.

50 Wald, R. (2019). Urinalysis in the diagnosis of kidney disease. *UpToDate*.

51 Chew, D.J. and Kowalski, J. (1981). Urinary tract infections. In: *Pathophysiology of Surgery in Small Animals* (ed. M.J. Bojrab), 255–270. Lea & Febiger.

52 Jansen, B.S. and Lumsden, J.H. (1985). Sensitivity of routine tests for urine protein to hemoglobin. *Can. Vet. J.* 26: 221–223.

53 Meuten, D. and Sample, S. (2022). Laboratory evaluation and interpretation of the urinary system. In: *Clinical Chemistry of Common Domestic Species*, 2e (ed. M.A. Thrall, G. Weiser, R.W. Allison, et al.). In Press.

54 Grauer, G.F. (2011). Proteinuria: measurement and interpretation. *Top. Companion Anim. Med.* 26: 121–127.

55 Grauer, G.F. (2007). Measurement, interpretation, and implications of proteinuria and albuminuria. *Vet. Clin. North Am. Small Anim. Pract.* 37: 283–295, vi–vii.

56 Reine, N.J. and Langston, C.E. (2005). Urinalysis interpretation: how to squeeze out the maximum information from a small sample. *Clin. Tech. Small Anim. Pract.* 20: 2–10.

57 Harley, L. and Langston, C. (2012). Proteinuria in dogs and cats. *Can. Vet. J.* 53: 631–638.

58 Langston, C. (2004). Microalbuminuria in cats. *J. Am. Anim. Hosp. Assoc.* 40: 251–254.

59 Feeney, D.A., Osborne, C.A., and Jessen, C.R. (1980). Effects of radiographic contrast media on results of urinalysis, with emphasis on alteration in specific gravity. *J. Am. Vet. Med. Assoc.* 176: 1378–1381.

60 Hendriks, H.J., Haage, A., and de Bruyne, J.J. (1976). Determination of the protein concentration in canine urine. *Zentralbl. Veterinarmed. A* 23: 683–687.

61 Tvedten, H. (2016). Urine total protein concentration in clinically normal dogs. *Vet. Clin. Pathol.* 45: 395–396.

62 Dibartola, S.P. and Westropp, J.L. (2020). Diagnostic tests for the urinary system. In: *Small Animal Internal Medicine* (ed. R. Nelson and G. Cotuto), 658–674. St. Louis, MO: Elsevier.

63 Chew, D.J., DiBartola, S.P., and Schenck, P.A. (2011). Urinalysis. In: *Canine and Feline Nephrology and Urology*, 2e (ed. D.J. Chew, S.P. DiBartola and P.A. Schenck), 1–31. Elsevier Saunders.

64 Stockham, S.L. and Scott, M.A. (2008). *Urinary System. Fundamentals of Veterinary Clinical Pathology*, 708–840. Ames, IA: Blackwell Publishing.

65 Kruth, S.A. and Cowgill, L.D. (1982). Renal glucose transport in the cat. *Am. Coll. Vet. Intern. Med. Sci. Proc.* 78.

66 Eggleton, M.G. and Shuster, S. (1954). Glucose and phosphate excretion in the cat. *J. Physiol.* 124: 613–622.

67 Miki, Y., Mori, A., Hayakawa, N. et al. (2011). Evaluation of serum and urine 1,5-anhydro-D-glucitol and myo-inositol concentrations in healthy dogs. *J. Vet. Med. Sci.* 73: 1117–1126.

68 Pereira-Moreira, R. and Muscelli, E. (2020). Effect of insulin on proximal tubules handling of glucose: a systematic review. *J. Diabetes Res.* Epub.

69 Osborne, C.A., Stevens, J.B., Rakich, P. et al. (1980). Clinical significance of glucosuria. *Minn. Vet.* 20: 16.

70 de Schepper, J., van der Stock, J., Capiau, E. et al. (1987). Renal injury in dogs with pyometra. *Tijdschr. Diergeneeskd.* 112 (Suppl 1): 124S–126S.

71 Zeugswetter, F.K. and Schwendenwein, I. (2020). Basal glucose excretion in dogs: the impact of feeding, obesity, sex, and age. *Vet. Clin. Pathol.* 49 (3): 428–435.

72 Zeugswetter, F.K., Polsterer, T., Krempl, H. et al. (2019). Basal glucosuria in cats. *J. Anim. Physiol. Anim. Nutr. (Berl.)* 103: 324–330.

73 Macherey-Nagel (2018). Medi-Test Glucose: Macherey-Nagel GmbH & Co. KG.

74 Aldridge, C.F., Behrend, E.N., Smith, J.R. et al. (2020). Accuracy of urine dipstick tests and urine glucose-to-creatinine ratios for assessment of glucosuria in dogs and cats. *J. Am. Vet. Med. Assoc.* 257: 391–396.

75 Fletcher, J.M., Behrend, E.N., Welles, E.G. et al. (2011). Glucose detection and concentration estimation in feline urine samples with the Bayer Multistix and Purina Glucotest. *J. Feline Med. Surg.* 13: 705–711.

76 Loeb, W.F. and Knipling, G.D. (1971). Glucosuria and pseudoglucosuria in cats with urethral obstruction. *Mod. Vet. Pract.* 52: 40–41.

77 Klausner, J.S., Osborne, C.A., and Stevens, J.B. (1976). Clinical evaluation of commercial reagent strips for detection of significant bacteriuria in dogs and cats. *Am. J. Vet. Res.* 37: 719–722.

78 Rees, C.A. and Boothe, D.M. (2004). Evaluation of the effect of cephalexin and enrofloxacin on clinical laboratory measurements of urine glucose in dogs. *J. Am. Vet. Med. Assoc.* 224: 1455–1458.

79 Faulks, R.D. and Lane, I.F. (2003). Qualitative urinalyses in puppies 0 to 24 weeks of age. *J. Am. Anim. Hosp. Assoc.* 39: 369–378.

80 Molina, C., Bosch, L., Rigau, T. et al. (2020). Urine glucose concentration: a useful parameter as a surrogate for glycaemia on the first day of life in canine neonates. *Res. Vet. Sci.* 133: 59–62.

81 Arant, B.S. Jr., Edelmann, C.M. Jr., and Nash, M.A. (1974). The renal reabsorption of glucose in the developing canine kidney: a study of glomerulotubular balance. *Pediatr. Res.* 8: 638–646.

82 Bovee, K.C., Jezyk, P.F., and Segal, S.C. (1984). Postnatal development of renal tubular amino acid reabsorption in canine pups. *Am. J. Vet. Res.* 45: 830–832.

83 Heiene, R., Bjorndal, H., and Indrebo, A. (2010). Glucosuria in Norwegian elkhounds and other breeds during dog shows. *Vet. Rec.* 166: 459–462.

84 Ross, L. (2011). Acute kidney injury in dogs and cats. *Vet. Clin. North Am. Small Anim. Pract.* 41: 1–14.

85 Rentko, V.T., Clark, N., Ross, L.A. et al. (1992). Canine leptospirosis. A retrospective study of 17 cases. *J. Vet. Intern. Med.* 6: 235–244.

86 DiBartola, S.P., Tarr, M.J., Parker, A.T. et al. (1989). Clinicopathologic findings in dogs with renal amyloidosis: 59 cases (1976-1986). *J. Am. Vet. Med. Assoc.* 195: 358–364.

87 Zamagni, S., Troia, R., Zaccheroni, F. et al. (2020). Comparison of clinicopathological patterns of renal tubular damage in dogs with acute kidney injury caused by leptospirosis and other aetiologies. *Vet. J.* 266: 105573.

88 Knopfler, S., Mayer-Scholl, A., Luge, E. et al. (2017). Evaluation of clinical, laboratory, imaging findings and outcome in 99 dogs with leptospirosis. *J. Small Anim. Pract.* 58: 582–588.

89 Vaden, S.L., Levine, J., and Breitschwerdt, E.B. (1997). A retrospective case-control of acute renal failure in 99 dogs. *J. Vet. Intern. Med.* 11: 58–64.

90 Thrall, M.A., Grauer, G.F., and Mero, K.N. (1984). Clinicopathologic findings in dogs and cats with ethylene glycol intoxication. *J. Am. Vet. Med. Assoc.* 184: 37–41.

91 Troia, R., Gruarin, M., Grisetti, C. et al. (2018). Fractional excretion of electrolytes in volume-responsive and intrinsic acute kidney injury in dogs: diagnostic and prognostic implications. *J. Vet. Intern. Med.* 32: 1372–1382.

92 Fleeman, L.M., Dobenecker, B., Foster, S. (2021). Is Glucosuria in Dogs Fed Jerky Treats Associated with Excessive Intake of Soluble Phosphorus? Abstract NU07. 2021 ACVIM Virtual Forum.

93 Dobenecker, B., Webel, A., Reese, S. et al. (2018). Effect of a high phosphorus diet on indicators of renal health in cats. *J. Feline Med. Surg.* 20: 339–343.

94 Fitzgerald, F.T. and Jessop, C. (1982). Accidental hypothermia: a report of 22 cases and review of the literature. *Adv. Intern. Med.* 27: 128–150.

95 Kanter, G.S. (1959). Renal clearance of glucose in hypothermic dogs. *Am. J. Physiol.* 196: 866–872.

96 Schaer, M. (2001). A justification for urine glucose monitoring in the diabetic dog and cat. *J. Am. Anim. Hosp. Assoc.* 37: 311–312.

97 Schaer, M. (1994). A method for detecting glycosuria in urine soaked cat litter. *Fel. Pract.* 22: 6–9.

98 Bovee, K.C., Joyce, T., Reynolds, R. et al. (1978). Spontaneous Fanconi syndrome in the dog. *Metabolism* 27: 45–52.

99 Bovee, K.C., Joyce, T., Blazer-Yost, B. et al. (1979). Characterization of renal defects in dogs with a syndrome similar to the Fanconi syndrome in man. *J. Am. Vet. Med. Assoc.* 174: 1094–1099.

100 Bovee, K.C., Anderson, T., Brown, S. et al. (1982). Renal tubular defects of spontaneous Fanconi syndrome in dogs. *Prog. Clin. Biol. Res.* 94: 435–447.

101 Yearley, J.H., Hancock, D.D., and Mealey, K.L. (2004). Survival time, lifespan, and quality of life in dogs with idiopathic Fanconi syndrome. *J. Am. Vet. Med. Assoc.* 225: 377–383.

102 Darrigrand-Haag, R.A., Center, S.A., Randolph, J.F. et al. (1996). Congenital Fanconi syndrome associated with renal dysplasia in 2 border terriers. *J. Vet. Intern. Med.* 10: 412–419.

103 Bommer, N.X., Brownlie, S.E., Morrison, L.R. et al. (2018). Fanconi syndrome in Irish wolfhound siblings. *J. Am. Anim. Hosp. Assoc.* 54: 173–178.

104 Hostutler, R.A., DiBartola, S.P., and Eaton, K.A. (2004). Transient proximal renal tubular acidosis and Fanconi syndrome in a dog. *J. Am. Vet. Med. Assoc.* 224: 1611–1614, 1605.

105 Hooper, A.N. and Roberts, B.K. (2011). Fanconi syndrome in four non-basenji dogs exposed to chicken jerky treats. *J. Am. Anim. Hosp. Assoc.* 47: e178–e187.

106 Major, A., Schweighauser, A., Hinden, S.E. et al. (2014). Transient Fanconi syndrome with severe polyuria and polydipsia in a 4-year old Shih Tzu fed chicken jerky treats. *Schweiz. Arch. Tierheilkd.* 156: 593–598.

107 Hooijberg, E.H., Furman, E., Leidinger, J. et al. (2015). Transient renal Fanconi syndrome in a Chihuahua exposed to Chinese chicken jerky treats. *Tierarztl. Prax. Ausg. K Kleintiere Heimtiere* 43: 188–192.

108 Igase, M., Baba, K., Shimokawa Miyama, T. et al. (2015). Acquired Fanconi syndrome in a dog exposed to jerky treats in Japan. *J. Vet. Med. Sci.* 77: 1507–1510.

109 Yabuki, A., Iwanaga, T., Giger, U. et al. (2017). Acquired Fanconi syndrome in two dogs following long-term consumption of pet jerky treats in Japan: case report. *J. Vet. Med. Sci.* 79: 818–821.

110 Bates, N., Sharman, M., Lam, A. et al. (2016). Reporting cases of Fanconi syndrome in dogs in the UK. *Vet. Rec.* 178: 510.

111 Reinert, N.C. and Feldman, D.G. (2016). Acquired Fanconi syndrome in four cats treated with chlorambucil. *J. Feline Med. Surg.* 18: 1034–1040.

112 Appleman, E.H., Cianciolo, R., Mosenco, A.S. et al. (2008). Transient acquired fanconi syndrome associated with copper storage hepatopathy in 3 dogs. *J. Vet. Intern. Med.* 22: 1038–1042.

113 Langlois, D.K., Smedley, R.C., Schall, W.D. et al. (2013). Acquired proximal renal tubular dysfunction in 9 Labrador retrievers with copper-associated hepatitis (2006-2012). *J. Vet. Intern. Med.* 27: 491–499.

114 Carbone, M.G. (1965). Phosphocrystalluria and urethral obstruction in the cat. *J. Am. Vet. Med. Assoc.* 147: 1195–1200.

115 Rich, L.J. and Kirk, R.W. (1969). The relationship of struvite crystals to urethral obstruction in cats. *J. Am. Vet. Med. Assoc.* 154: 153–157.

116 Burrows, C.F. and Bovee, K.C. (1978). Characterization and treatment of acid-base and renal defects due to urethral obstruction in cats. *J. Am. Vet. Med. Assoc.* 172: 801–805.

117 Segev, G., Livne, H., Ranen, E. et al. (2011). Urethral obstruction in cats: predisposing factors, clinical, clinicopathological characteristics and prognosis. *J. Feline Med. Surg.* 13: 101–108.

118 Eisenberg, B.W., Waldrop, J.E., Allen, S.E. et al. (2013). Evaluation of risk factors associated with recurrent obstruction in cats treated medically for urethral obstruction. *J. Am. Vet. Med. Assoc.* 243: 1140–1146.

119 Finco, D.R. and Cornelius, L.M. (1977). Characterization and treatment of water, electrolyte, and acid-base imbalances of induced urethral obstruction in the cat. *Am. J. Vet. Res.* 38: 823–830.

120 Laffel, L. (1999). Ketone bodies: a review of physiology, pathophysiology and application of monitoring to diabetes. *Diabetes Metab. Res. Rev.* 15: 412–426.

121 Osborne, C.A. and Stevens, J.B. (1999). *Biochemical Analysis of Urine: Indications, Methods, Interpretation. Urinalysis: A Clinical Guide to Compassionate Patient Care*, 86–124. Shawnee Mission, KS: Bayer.

122 Chertack, M.M. and Sherrick, J.C. (1958). Evaluation of a nitroprusside dip test for ketone bodies. *JAMA* 167: 1621–1624.

123 Free, A.H. and Free, H.M. (1958). Nature of nitroprusside reactive material in urine in ketosis. *Am. J. Clin. Pathol.* 30: 7–10.

124 Osborne, C.A. and Stevens, J.B. (1999). Biochemical analysis of urine: indications, methods, interpretation. In: *Urinalysis: A Clinical Guide to Compassionate Patient Care* (ed. C.A. Osborne and J.B. Stevens), 86–124. Shawnee Mission, KS, Bayer.

125 Cartwright, J. and Green, R.M. (2010). Tyrosine-derived 4-hydroxyphenylpyruvate reacts with ketone test fields of 3 commercially available urine dipsticks. *Vet. Clin. Pathol.* 39: 354–357.

126 Zeugswetter, F. and Pagitz, M. (2009). Ketone measurements using dipstick methodology in cats with diabetes mellitus. *J. Small Anim. Pract.* 50: 4–8.

127 Fogazzi, G.B. and Ponticelli, C. (1996). Microscopic hematuria diagnosis and management. *Nephron* 72: 125–134.

128 Cohen, R.A. and Brown, R.S. (2003). Clinical practice. Microscopic hematuria. *N. Engl. J. Med.* 348: 2330–2338.

129 Stevens, J. and Osborne, C.A. (1974). Urinalysis: indications, methodology, and interpretation. In: *American Animal Hospital Conference*, 359–403.

130 Aulbach, A.D., Schultze, E., Tripathi, N.K. et al. (2015). Factors affecting urine reagent strip blood results in dogs and nonhuman primates and interpretation of urinalysis in preclinical toxicology studies: a Multi-Institution Contract Research Organization and BioPharmaceutical Company perspective. *Vet. Clin. Pathol.* 44 (2): 229–233.

131 Mazouz, B. and Almagor, M. (2003). False-positive microhematuria in dipsticks urinalysis caused by the presence of semen in urine. *Clin. Biochem.* 36: 229–231.

132 Nagel, D., Seiler, D., Hohenberger, E.F. et al. (2006). Investigations of ascorbic acid interference in urine test strips. *Clin. Lab.* 52: 149–153.

133 McIntyre, M. and Mou, T.W. (1965). Persistence of leukocytes and erythrocytes in refrigerated acid and alkaline urine. *Am. J. Clin. Pathol.* 43: 53–57.

134 Blondheim, S.H., Margoliash, E., and Shafrir, E. (1958). A simple test for myohemoglobinuria (myoglobinuria). *JAMA* 167: 453–454.

135 Kohn, C.W. and Chew, D.J. (1987). Laboratory diagnosis and characterization of renal disease in horses. *Vet. Clin. North Am. Equine Pract.* 3: 585–615.

136 Davis, P.E. and Paris, R. (1974). Azoturia in a greyhound: clinical pathology aids to diagnosis. *J. Small Anim. Pract.* 15: 43–54.

137 Ingelfinger, J.R. (2021). Hematuria in Adults. *N. Engl. J. Med.* 385: 153–163.

138 Mallard, J.M., Rieser, T.M., and Peterson, N.W. (2018). Propofol infusion-like syndrome in a dog. *Can. Vet. J.* **59** (11): 1216–1222.

139 Cervone, M., Nectoux, A., and Pouzot-Nevoret, C. (2022). Rhabdomyolysis and myoglobinuria following single induction dose of propofol in a dog. *J Vet Emerg Crit Care.* 1–5.

140 Gannon, J.R. (1980). Exertional rhabdomyolysis (myoglobinuria) in the racing greyhound. In: *Current Veterinary Therapy; Small Animal Practice* (ed. E. Kirk), 783–787. Philadelphia: Saunders.

141 Shelton, G.D. (2004). Rhabdomyolysis, myoglobinuria, and necrotizing myopathies. *Vet. Clin. North Am. Small Anim. Pract.* 34: 1469–1482.

142 Khenifar, E. (2019). Early screening for feline hematuria. *Veterinary Focus* https://vetfocus.royalcanin.com/en/doc-228.html: Royal Canin.

143 Scherk, M., Buffington, C.A.T., Carozza, E. et al. (2018). Blücare® Granules: A Novel Tool for the Early Detection and Monitoring of Urinary Tract Disorders in Cats. Recommendations from an Expert Panel. https://my.royalcanin.com/UserFiles/Images/vet/Hematuria%20Detection%20by%20BluCare/Blücare%20Granules%20-%20A%20Novel%20Tool%20for%20the%20Early%20Detection%20and%20Monitoring%20o. . . . pdf: Blucare. 1–8.

144 Osborne, C.A., Stevens, J.B., Lees, G.E. et al. (1980). Clinical significance of bilirubinuria. *Comp. Cont. Educ. Pract. Vet.* 2: 897–902.

145 Kreutzer, K.V., Turk, J.R., and Casteel, S.W. (2008). Clinical biochemistry in toxicology. In: *Clinical Biochemistry of Domestic Animals*, 6e (ed. J. Kaneko, J. Harvey and M. Bruss), 821–827. Imprint: Academic Press.

146 Schmid, R. (1956). Direct-reacting bilirubin, bilirubin glucuronide, in serum, bile and urine. *Science* 124: 76–77.

147 Fulop, M. and Brazeau, P. (1964). The renal excretion of bilirubin in dogs with obstructive jaundice. *J. Clin. Invest.* 43: 1192–1202.

148 Meuten, D. (2012). Laboratory evaluation and interpretation of the urinary system. In: *Veterinary Hematology and Clinical Chemistry*, 2e (ed. M.A. Thrall, G. Weiser, R.W. Allison and T.W. Campbell), 323–377. Chichester: Wiley.

149 DeSchepper, J. (1974). Degradation of Haemoglobin to bilirubin in the kidney of the dog. *Tijdschr. Diergeneeskd.* 99: 699.

150 Siemens (2021). Siemens Ictotest Reagent Tablets On Line Siemens.

151 Greenberg, A. (2018). Urinalysis and urine microscopy. In: *National Kidney Foundation Primer on Kidney Diseases*, 7e (ed. S.J. Gilbert and D.E. Weiner), 33–41. Philadelphia, PA: Elsevier.

152 Chew, D.J. and DiBartola, S.P. (1998). *Handbook of Canine and Feline Urinalysis*. Wilmington, DE: Ralston Purina Co./The Gloyd Group.

153 Lees, G.E., Hardy, R.M., Stevens, J.B. et al. (1984). Clinical implications of feline bilirubinuria. *J. Am. Anim. Hosp. Assoc.* 20: 765–771.

154 Skeldon, N. and Ristić, J. (2016). Urinalysis. In: *BSAVA Manual of Canine and Feline Clinical Pathology (BSAVA British Small Animal Veterinary Association)*, 3e (ed. E. Villiers and J. Ristic), 183–218.

155 Meuten, D. (2012). Laboratory evaluation and interpretation of the urinary system. In: *Clinical Chemistry of Common Domestic Species*, 2e (ed. M.A. Thrall, G. Weiser, R.W. Allison, et al.), 323–377.

156 Knutson, M. and Wessling-Resnick, M. (2003). Iron metabolism in the reticuloendothelial system. *Crit. Rev. Biochem. Mol. Biol.* 38: 61–88.

157 Levy, M., Lester, R., and Levinsky, N.G. (1968). Renal excretion of urobilinogen in the dog. *J. Clin. Invest.* 47: 2117–2124.

158 Tang, X., Xia, Z., and Yu, J. (2008). An experimental study of hemolysis induced by onion (Allium cepa) poisoning in dogs. *J. Vet. Pharmacol. Ther.* 31: 143–149.

159 Gustafsson, B.E. and Lanke, L.S. (1960). Bilirubin and urobilins in germfree, ex-germfree, and conventional rats. *J. Exp. Med.* 112: 975–981.

160 Fogazzi, G.B., Verdesca, S., and Garigali, G. (2008). Urinalysis: core curriculum 2008. *Am. J. Kidney Dis.* 51: 1052–1067.

161 Vail, D.M., Allen, T.A., and Weiser, G. (1986). Applicability of leukocyte esterase test strip in detection of canine pyuria. *J. Am. Vet. Med. Assoc.* 189: 1451–1453.

162 Holan, K.M., Kruger, J.M., Gibbons, S.N. et al. (1997). Clinical evaluation of a leukocyte esterase test-strip for detection of feline pyuria. *Vet. Clin. Pathol.* 26: 126–131.

163 Allchin, J.P., Evans, G.O., and Parsons, C.E. (1987). Pitfalls in the measurement of canine urine concentration. *Vet. Rec.* 120: 256–257.

164 Ciulla, A.P., Newsome, B., and Kaster, J. (1985). Reagent strip method for specific gravity: an evaluation. *Lab. Med.* 16: 38–40.

165 Paquignon, A., Tran, G., and Provost, J.P. (1993). Evaluation of the Clinitek 200 urinary test-strip reader in the analysis of dog and rat urines in pre-clinical toxicology studies. *Lab. Anim.* 27: 240–246.

166 van Vonderen, I.K., Kooistra, H.S., and Bruijne, J.J. (1995). Evaluation of a test strip for estimating the specific gravity of canine urine. *Tijdschr. Diergeneeskd.* 120: 400–402.

167 Dossin, O., Germain, C., and Braun, J.P. (2003). Comparison of the techniques of evaluation of urine dilution/concentration in the dog. *J. Vet. Med. A Physiol. Pathol. Clin. Med.* 50: 322–325.

168 Nikolac Gabaj, N., Miler, M., Unic, A. et al. (2020). Ascorbic acid in urine still compromises urinalysis results. *Ann. Clin. Biochem.* 57: 64–68.

169 Unic, A., Nikolac Gabaj, N., Miler, M. et al. (2018). Ascorbic acid-A black hole of urine chemistry screening. *J. Clin. Lab. Anal.* 32: e22390.

170 Ko, D.H., Jeong, T.D., Kim, S. et al. (2015). Influence of vitamin C on urine dipstick test results. *Ann. Clin. Lab. Sci.* 45: 391–395.

171 Lee, W., Kim, Y., Chang, S. et al. (2017). The influence of vitamin C on the urine dipstick tests in the clinical specimens: a multicenter study. *J. Clin. Lab. Anal.* 31.

172 Berger, L., Gerson, C.D., and Yu, T.F. (1977). The effect of ascorbic acid on uric acid excretion with a commentary on the renal handling of ascorbic acid. *Am. J. Med.* 62: 71–76.

173 Sherry, S., Friedman, G.J., Paley, K. et al. (1940). The mechanism of the excretion of vitamin C by the dog kidney. *Am. J. Physiol.* 130: 276.

CHAPTER 6

Examination of Urinary Sediment

INTRODUCTION

Clinically important abnormalities have been observed by microscopy of urinary sediment in human medicine for over 400 years[1, 2]. Microscopic examination of the urine sediment should always be performed as part of the complete urinalysis, especially in animals that are sick and those that have abnormal color or clarity, abnormalities detected on chemical dipstrip testing (see Chapter 5), lower than expected urine specific gravity (USG) (Chapter 4), or on physical examination findings. It is preferable to perform the complete urinalysis in-house, though urine microscopy was considered optional by one veterinary author if the urinary chemistry reagent pads were all normal and there were no abnormalities in color or clarity of the urine specimen [3].

Unfortunately, urinary microscopy is often omitted in veterinary practice, which can result in failure to identify important diagnostic information. White blood cells (WBC), bacteria, fungal organisms, epithelial cells, crystals, and casts are not detected using dry-reagent strip pad analysis. Failure to perform urine sediment microscopy can be attributed to the perception that it takes too much time (approximately 20 minutes to perform a complete urinalysis) and concern about the skill level and experience necessary for in-clinic technicians to proficiently perform a urinalysis [4]. In veterinary medicine, standard manual urine microscopy has a within-run coefficient of variation (CV)

Urinalysis in the Dog and Cat, First Edition. Dennis J. Chew and Patricia A. Schenck.
© 2023 John Wiley & Sons, Inc. Published 2023 by John Wiley & Sons, Inc.

of 30–40% for red blood cells (RBC) and WBC [5]. How the urine is mixed, what volume is centrifuged, the force of centrifugation, and the volume of sediment examined all should be standardized to obtain repeatable and accurate results.

Urine sediment examination has been referred to as the "liquid kidney biopsy" [6], but it also often reflects disorders of the lower urinary tract, so the moniker "liquid urinary tract biopsy" may be more apt. Macroscopic screening of urine based on its physical and chemical properties is sometimes used in human medicine to decide if urine sediment examination will be cost-effective [7]. Abnormal elements in urine sediment are more likely to be found during microscopy when urine has an abnormal color (colorless, very dark yellow, red, brown), if the urine is cloudy, if the USG is lower than normal, if USG is extremely high, or if the reagent pads on the dry reagent strip pad are positive for abnormalities (e.g. blood, protein, glucose). In human medicine, the leukocyte esterase test pad is valuable to prompt microscopic sediment evaluation, but this reaction is not useful in veterinary medicine (see Chapter 5). In human medicine, the need for trained specialists to perform urine sediment examination as a biomarker for kidney disease continues to be emphasized, especially in patients with acute kidney injury (AKI) [8]. Nephrologists examining urine sediment are more likely to identify clinically important findings as compared to laboratory technicians in some disease settings [9]. Some believe that the best doctors examine fresh urine sediment themselves during evaluation of sick patients and, thus, gain immediate information that can be clinically useful [9, 10].

If the urine is of normal color and clear, and the chemical reagent dipstrip chemistry reactions are all normal, results of microscopic examination of the urine sediment will be normal in most instances [3, 11]. The likelihood that urine sediment examination will disclose abnormalities in urine samples from apparently healthy dogs and cats (i.e. normal history and physical examination) is low. Approximately 3% of dogs without a history of genitourinary disease had no macroscopic urine abnormalities but had abnormal urine sediment findings (i.e. were falsely negative on macroscopic screening) [12]. In another study, failure to examine the urine sediment of macroscopically normal urine samples would have yielded false-negative results in 16.5% of the dogs and 5.7% of the cats [13]. All animals with clinical signs or physical examination findings compatible with disease of the genitourinary tract should have a complete urinalysis that includes urine sediment examination even if macroscopic screening is normal. Animals that are sick at initial presentation in general practice, at referral to specialty practice, or during examination at emergency presentation are more likely to have abnormal findings on urine sediment examination, even in the absence of abnormal color, clarity, or urine concentration. It is our impression that patients that have received intravenous fluids and drugs during hospitalization are more likely to have abnormal findings in their urine sediment after suspected and unsuspected renal damage (casts and renal tubular epithelium [RTE]). Abnormal urine sediment from sick animals can include increased numbers of RBC, WBC, epithelial cells, casts, infectious agents (bacterial and fungal), parasite ova or larvae (*Capillaria plica*, *Dioctophyma renale*, *Dirofilaria immitis*), and crystals. Reagent pads do not detect epithelial cells, WBC, casts, infectious agents, parasites, or crystals.

METHODOLOGY

PREPARING URINE SEDIMENT FOR EXAMINATION

Procedures for processing and evaluating urine sediment vary by laboratory, which likely contributes to differences in numbers and types of elements reported. A surprising lack of standardization in the evaluation of urine sediment also exists in human medicine [14]. An outline for the preparation of urinary sediment for microscopy is presented in Table 6.1. Reasons for errors in reporting elements in urinary sediment are outlined in Table 6.2.

Storage and Preservation

Prompt examination of fresh urine (at body temperature) is recommended to maximize the ability to properly identify abnormal elements in the urine and to minimize artifacts that develop over time in some samples. Ideally, urine sediment should be examined at room temperature within 30–60 minutes after collection [15, 16]. Microscopic examination of very fresh urine favors preservation of fragile cellular elements and minimizes chances for cellular degeneration, which enhances identification of abnormal elements in the sediment. Up to 12 hours of refrigeration before analysis has traditionally been considered acceptable, but we recommend less than four hours of refrigeration before urine sediment examination if possible. Refrigeration of urine for up to eight hours before performing microscopy likely compromises the ability to accurately identify RBC casts, dysmorphic RBC, and other formed elements because they may be degraded with time and refrigeration [9]. In sick or critically ill patients, it is best to examine the urine sediment within 15 minutes of collection to increase the likelihood of identifying and enumerating cellular casts and RTE. Cooling and storage of urine favor crystal precipitation, cellular degeneration, and dissolution or disintegration of casts. The degradation of urinary elements is more likely in alkaline and dilute urine samples [17], a process that may be particularly important for casts [18]. Warming a stored urine sample to room temperature does not necessarily result in the dissolution of all crystals that formed as artifacts during cooling of the sample. A first morning sample, collected before emptying the bladder by voiding, may contain more formed elements as a consequence of the longer time of urine formation overnight, but cellular detail may be lacking because of longer residence time in the bladder that could allow degeneration of elements before urine sediment examination. In some situations, it may be advantageous to examine a urine sample that has been collected after the first voiding in the morning so as to allow better cellular detail to be observed. In human medicine, more accurate identification and classification of urinary elements

Table 6.1 Preparing urinary sediment for microscopy.

1. Collect at least 3 mL of urine to ensure enough volume to perform the USG, urine chemistry dipstrip, and microscopy of urine sediment. A larger urine volume that is collected allows further testing on the remaining urine after the urinalysis has been performed, such as UPC or quantitative urine culture.
2. Examine fresh warm urine whenever possible, soon after urine collection. This is especially important for sick animals or those with obvious urinary signs.
3. If urine has been refrigerated, bring to room temperature before proceeding.
4. Measure USG using a refractometer; record the value.
5. Well-mix the urine sample and then measure urine chemistry on a standard urine dipstrip; record the values.
6. Preparations for microscopy of urine sediment **without stain**:
   a. Well-mix the remaining urine volume after USG and dipstrip testing have been performed. Invert the tube several times. This is to avoid a potentially large pre-analytical error when elements have settled out while sitting.
   b. Immediately transfer 1 mL of the well-mixed urine to a 3-mL plastic conical centrifuge tube. Save the remaining urine volume in case more measurements are needed later.

      A larger urine volume of well-mixed urine (e.g. 3 mL) is removed per some veterinary laboratory protocols, but recent evidence suggests that any degree of amplification or concentration of elements in urine sediment is not enhanced when comparing a larger to a smaller urine volume that is processed.
   c. Centrifuge at 400 × g for 5 mins

      Consult manufacturer booklet or calculate g using RPM and length of centrifuge arm.

      Do NOT centrifuge at high speeds or g forces used to process serum or plasma tubes, as this can damage delicate urinary elements.
   d. Do NOT use any braking function on the centrifuge. Braking can resuspend the sediment.
   e. Using a 1 mL bulb plastic pipette, aspirate 0.8 mL of the supernatant to another tube, in case more testing such as UPC is needed later or discard. Use the etched lines (¼, ½, ¾, and 1 mL) to estimate the volume within the pipette. Leave the 0.2 mL of sediment below. Be careful to NOT resuspend the sediment during removal of the supernatant.

      Decanting of the supernatant as performed in some laboratories, makes it more difficult to achieve an accurate residual volume and provides a greater risk for resuspending some sediment, especially following centrifugation of small volumes.
   f. Re-suspend the sediment in the 0.2 mL remaining by gently tapping or flicking the tube several times. Alternatively, aspirate the sediment gently up and down a few times with the plastic pipette, while avoiding any vortexing that can disrupt fragile elements.
   g. Aspirate a drop of the re-suspended sediment with a 1 mL plastic bulb pipette and apply to a standard glass microscope slide. The goal is for the drop to fully distribute under the coverslip without overflow. Too much fluid under the coverslip generates distracting motion of elements during microscopy.
   h. Apply a 25 × 25 mm coverslip, taking care to not introduce air bubbles.
   i. Let the slide sit for one to two minutes. This allows elements in the sediment to come into the same plane of view and then start urine microscopy.
   j. Lower the microscope condenser and close the iris as needed to improve contrast of elements with similar optical density of urine (e.g. hyaline casts).
   k. Examine urinary sediment per LPF (100× total magnification from a 10× ocular and 10× objective) initially to discover areas of interest and to determine if elements are uniformly distributed. Enumerate casts as the average number per LPF in 10 fields, or report range.
   l. Further evaluate urinary elements per HPF (400× total magnification from a 10× ocular and a 40× objective) and record their numbers and character for RBC, WBC, epithelial cells, crystals, and bacteria. Casts are usually best characterized under HPF. Enumerate elements as the average number per HPF in 10 fields. A range is often also reported (e.g. 5–10 RBC per HPF)
   m. The 100× objective (1000× total magnification using oil immersion and 10× ocular) is not used during routine wet-mount microscopy.
7. Preparations for microscopy of urine sediment **with supravital stain**:
   a. Take one drop of the well-mixed urinary sediment as above and add one drop of Sedi-Stain or new methylene blue to enhance detail and contrast within the cytoplasm and nuclei of cells.
   b. Apply one drop of the stained sediment to the same glass slide as the one with the unstained sediment and add coverslip.
   c. Ensure enough distance between the stained and unstained sediment samples so that there is no chance for cross flow between fluid under each cover slip
   d. Enumerate elements on the unstained (and less dilute) sample as described above.
   e. Further evaluate morphology on the stained sediment.
   f. The author prefers to evaluate BOTH stained and unstained sediment.
   g. Make a dry mount slide from the unstained sediment if further morphological detail is needed depending on findings from the urine sediment wet mount. Process and evaluate this slide as one would for standard cytology.

This is one standardized protocol for urinary microscopy using 1 mL of well-mixed urine that undergoes manual centrifugation and microscopy. This protocol is used by some veterinary laboratories. Alternatively, a larger volume (e.g. 3 mL or 5 mL) of well-mixed urine could be used in which 80% of the supernatant is removed, and the sediment is then resuspended in the remaining 20% of the initial volume.

Standardization of all aspects of setting up the slide for urinary microscopy will improve the quality and accuracy of the results that are generated and available for interpretation. This includes the volume of urine analyzed, the volume of supernatant used to resuspend the sediment, centrifuge tube size and shape, plastic bulb pipettes, microscope glass slides and coverslips, and the same high-quality microscope.

(including casts) is made possible by analysis of the second morning specimen. This approach decreases the likelihood of lysis or degeneration of urinary elements that might otherwise occur in urine that has remained in the bladder overnight [18].

Preservatives do not need to be added to urine samples when urine sediment examination can be performed within a few hours of collection. When urine cannot be examined soon after collection, the sample should be refrigerated to minimize

Table 6.2 Reasons for inaccurate enumeration or failure to replicate reported numbers of elements per HPF, LPF, and μL.

Storage or preparation of urine
    Failure to well-mix urine sample before adding to tubes
      Reduced number of elements observed following settling
    Glass versus plastic sedimentation tubes
    Variable volume of urine processed
    Mucous threads that trap casts and cells

Centrifugation
    Use of conical versus round bottom tubes
    Centrifugation versus sedimentation by gravity
    Centrifugation force (x G)
    Braking to end centrifugation
      Elements resuspended in supernatant
      Fragile elements disrupted or lysed
    Aspiration versus decanting of supernatant

Preparation of slide and staining
    Variable dilution of sediment from fluid lining tube
    Variable dilution of supernatant used to resuspend sediment
    Variable dilution of sediment by stain
    Failure to adequately resuspend sediment – decreased reporting of elements
    Variation in size of drop of sediment added to glass slide
    Variation in coverslip size and thickness

Microscopy
    Microscopic field of view (FOV) not standardized
    Insufficient microscopic fields are counted
    Margins of coverslip not examined – heavier elements may migrate there
    Slide randomly rather than systematically examined
    Poor microscopy skills
      Too much illumination, iris diaphragm opened too much
      Failure to recognize elements with very similar optical density to urine (e.g. hyaline casts)
      Dirty objectives
      Fine focus "rocking" skill lacking – failure to find or ID elements

Reporting of elements
    Inability to recognize and report common elements
    Brownian motion of small elements confused with bacteria
    Punctate debris confused with cocci
    Confusion of stain precipitate with bacteria or pathological crystals
    Mucous with punctate appearance after staining reported as bacteria
    Bacterial or environmental contamination of stain
    Confusion of small lipid droplets or crystals with bacteria

degeneration of elements in the urine sediment and to inhibit bacterial multiplication. WBC, casts, epithelial cells, and bacteria are well preserved when boric acid alone or boric acid in combination with formic acid has been added to the urine sample container, but RBC may become smaller and unstable. One drop of formalin may be added per 30 mL of urine to preserve urine sediment [19]. Preservatives can also alter the chemical dry reagent strip pad reactions. When used, lyophilized preservatives in containers are preferred so that urine dilution does not occur [17, 20]. The beneficial or damaging effects of routinely adding preservatives to urine samples before analysis have been recently evaluated in veterinary medicine (see later).

When using preservatives to send urine samples to a reference laboratory, we recommend dividing the initial urine sample into two aliquots. The aliquot with preservative is used for urine sediment examination, and the second aliquot without preservative is used for urine dry reagent strip pad chemical analysis. Alternatively, for confusing or complicated cases, an unstained dry-mount preparation of urine sediment can be sent along with a urine sample in ethylenediaminetetraacetic acid to the reference laboratory [21]. The dry mount is prepared in the usual manner as for cytology; it does not involve allowing the wet mount to dry. The dry mount preparation using fresh urine sediment will allow identification of RBC, WBC, epithelial cells, and bacteria (cocci, cocci in chains, short rods, coccobacilli) that have not undergone degeneration, but crystals and casts usually do not adhere to the slide and, thus, cannot be evaluated using routine techniques. A technique that employs cytocentrifugation of fresh urine followed by Papanicolaou staining has been described and allows permanent dry mount slides to be prepared for evaluation of urine casts. The evaluation of such slides can allow more precise identification and enumeration of casts, especially cellular casts [22].

Thorough mixing of urine before centrifugation is essential in order to avoid a preanalytical error, in which important elements are not included in the sample transferred to the centrifuge tube, as a consequence of elements falling by gravity to the bottom of the container. The effect on the recovery of various urinary elements varies by time for urine mixing, time elapsed for aspiration after mixing, and the location in the tube from which the sample is of aspirated (top, middle, or bottom), but these aspects of sample handling have not been standardized in veterinary medicine [23]. One study determined that the lowest crystal counts were observed when more settling time was allowed before aspiration of the urine sample and when urine was aspirated from a higher position in the tube. Sinking of urinary elements by gravity apparently occurs more rapidly than generally appreciated. A mathematical model was developed that predicted noncrystalline elements to settle at 1 μm per second and crystals to settle at 10–60 μm per second, depending on crystal size and density. Based on these observations, sample aspiration immediately after mixing is necessary to ensure consistent and accurate reporting of urinary elements [23]. After mixing, the sample should be aspirated from a position near the bottom of the container to ensure that a representative urine sample is obtained.

Centrifugation

Traditionally, a standardized volume of urine is gently centrifuged in a conical tube (Figure 6.1). Glass centrifuge tubes were

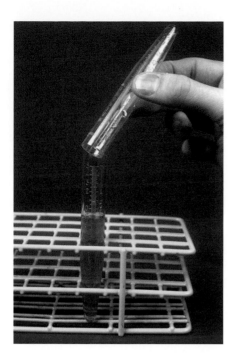

FIGURE 6.1 A standard volume of urine (often 1–3 mL) is placed into a conical centrifuge tube. Following centrifugation, the tube is inverted, and the supernatant is drained into a second tube and saved for further evaluation if needed (e.g. urinary protein-to-creatinine ratio or electrolyte chemistry). There may or may not be anything visible at the bottom of the tube following centrifugation. Sediment can still be present in the bottom of the tube even when there is no visible evidence to the naked eye. Following decanting and repositioning of the tube to a vertical position, sediment will be resuspended in a small volume of urine lining the side of the tube.

not recommended for urine sedimentation in one report, since cells and casts were noted to readily adhere to glass [24]. The accepted rationale for the use of centrifugation is that this procedure concentrates or amplifies the detection of small numbers of elements in urine that would otherwise not be observed. The examined volume usually is 10 or 15 mL in human medicine [7], but this volume is not consistently available for urine samples collected from dogs and cats. Although a minimum of 5 mL is recommended in veterinary medicine [25, 26], a sample size of 1–3 mL of urine is routinely examined by some veterinary laboratories. Although it seems intuitive that a larger volume of urine would allow more elements in urinary sediment to be concentrated, retrieved, and identified, this assumption has recently been challenged (see below). It has been considered important to centrifuge the same sample volume in all patients so as to compare quantitative results in a consistent manner. Corrected enumeration of urine sediment elements (based on multiplication factors) are reported by some human medical laboratories depending on the volume that is centrifuged and the volume of sediment examined [7], but such corrections are not made by veterinary laboratories.

Excessive force can disrupt fragile elements during centrifugation, especially casts. Debris and free RBC, WBC, or nonsquamous epithelial cells that are identified may appear following disintegration of casts. The hemolysis of RBC in urine will cause under-reporting of RBC numbers. Traumatic handling of the sample can cause rupture of nucleated cells that also results in under-reporting of WBC and epithelial cells. Too much force can also cause crystals to aggregate and appear less numerous than when nonaggregated. Similarly, too much force can cause clumps of WBC and RBC that can be difficult to evaluate and may be confused with casts. A relative centrifugal force (RCF) of less than 400 appears to be optimal to generate sediment without damaging urinary elements [7]. The use of RCF for a specific centrifuge is preferred to revolutions per minute (rpm) because the radius of the centrifuge rotor also contributes to force. Some centrifuge manuals provide both rpm and RCF. RCF is used interchangeably with gravity force (g). The following formula can be used to convert rpm to RCF: RCF $= 1.118 \times 10^{-5} \times$ rotor radius (cm) $\times$ rpm^2 [7]. The use of centrifuges at settings used to separate serum and plasma exert too high an RCF to be useful for urine sediment. Braking of the centrifuge should not be used since doing so can cause turbulence and resuspension of lighter elements into the supernatant, which will result in less enumeration of urinary elements during sediment microscopy. The force from braking also has the potential to disrupt fragile elements in the urine such as casts (Figure 6.2) [27].

Commercial veterinary laboratories vary in the techniques they use to evaluate urine sediment. At one commercial veterinary reference laboratory (IDEXX), a small volume (60 μL) of mixed urine is placed into one well of a multiple well plate so that a technician using an inverted microscope can easily read urine sediments from different patients (Figure 6.3). Neither centrifugation nor coverslips are used with this technique, because the urine sample sits in the well at $1 \times g$ for at least 10 minutes to allow sedimentation before microscopy [28]. Another commercial laboratory (ANTECH Diagnostics) centrifuges 2–3 mL of urine at $400 \times g$, after which the supernatant is

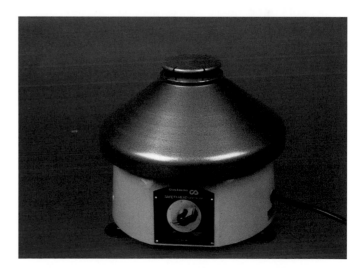

FIGURE 6.2 A centrifuge capable of lower force (radius × RPM) is selected for urine sediment preparation so that delicate elements in urine are not damaged. The brake function on the centrifuge should not be used; otherwise, fragile elements may be disrupted or resuspended in the supernatant.

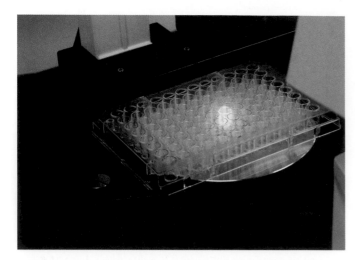

FIGURE 6.3 Multiple well plate on the microscopic stage of the inverted microscope. Sediment accumulates by gravity and not centrifugation. Light is shining through each individual well of urine sediment sequentially for evaluation under high- and low-powered lens objectives below. Source: Courtesy of IDEXX Laboratories. Copyright © 2022, IDEXX Laboratories, Inc. All rights reserved. Used with permission.

decanted and the sediment resuspended for wet mount microscopy. Further discussion of microscopy results using different methods to prepare urine for microscopy is provided below.

More WBC, RBC, squamous epithelial cells, and non-hyaline casts were identified and enumerated using a modified technique for analysis of urinary sediment compared to a "standard" technique in one study from human medicine. The modified technique employed centrifugation of 10 mL urine in round bottom tubes at $1358 \times g$, and decanting of the supernatant, compared to centrifugation of 5 mL of urine in conical tubes at $400 \times g$, with aspiration of the supernatant [29].

In an early report using urine samples from dogs, three methods of urine handling were used to compare the enumeration of urinary elements during urine sediment examination after centrifugation. Results were compared among large volume samples handled with low force (5 mL at $400 \times g$ for 5 minutes), small volume samples handled with low force (1.5 mL at $250 \times g$ for 5 minutes), and low volume samples handled with high force (1.5 mL at $3900 \times g$ for 45 seconds; Statspin®). Similar results for numbers of cells, casts, and crystals were noted, but the samples used did not contain sufficient numbers of casts or crystals to perform a meaningful statistical evaluation. Similar studies of this type using urine samples with larger numbers of casts should be performed [30]. In a more recent study, four different methods of preparing canine urine for microscopy were evaluated using urine with added RBC and compared centrifuge force and time of centrifugation. High volume low force (5 mL at $390 \times g$ for 5 minutes), low volume high force (1.5 mL at $3900 \times g$ for 45 seconds), 60 μL in a microtiter plate well with no centrifugation, and 30 μL on a microscope slide with coverslip were examined and compared. The microtiter plate performed best with a CV of 14%, and the 1.5 mL $3900 \times g$ centrifugation method performed worst with a CV of 71% for RBC. No so-called amplification benefit of centrifugation was identified, whereas substantial variability in results for all of these methods used for microscopic examination was found [28].

A standard volume of urine is chosen for centrifugation based on the laboratory standard operating procedure (SOP). Textbooks often mention to add 5–10 mL of well-mixed urine to the centrifuge tube, but far smaller volumes of urine are often provided to the laboratory from dogs and cats. Following urine sedimentation by gravity or centrifugation during manual analysis, the supernatant is poured off (decanted) or aspirated by dropper or pipette, and the supernatant can be submitted for other required analyses (e.g. urine protein/creatinine ratio) if necessary. The sediment must be resuspended before microscopy to ensure equal distribution of elements in the sediment. The sediment is diluted by a variable fluid volume lining the tube (estimated at 0.2–0.4 mL) following decanting, which contributes to variations in reports of the number of elements per low-power field (LPF) or high-power field (HPF). Similarly, the urine sediment is also diluted to a variable degree when liquid stain is added to the tube. Resuspension can be accomplished by gentle aspiration into a pipette or by tapping gently on the tube using the index finger. Vigorous agitation should be avoided because it can damage some elements in the sediment. It is recommended to remove 80% of the supernatant following centrifugation, followed by resuspension of the sediment in the remaining 20% of the supernatant in an effort to standardize the degree of sediment dilution (Dr. Jessica Hokamp, personal communication, 2020).

EXAMINATION OF URINARY SEDIMENT

Manual microscopy has been the gold standard to which automated microscopy is compared, but there can be considerable operator variability in the identification of findings in urine sediment. The amount of interobserver variability (imprecision) in the evaluation of urinary sediment raises concern about the reliability of this method as the gold standard [31]. The level of agreement in the identification of casts among human nephrologists was 59% in one study; an estimated level of agreement for other findings in urinary sediment was 69% [32]. Casts were not accurately identified by community laboratories in one study; there was minor variation in casts detected by nephrologists in the same study [33]. In another study, only slight-to-moderate agreement for the identification of urinary sediment elements was found by nephrologists during evaluation of digital images; agreement was not associated with seniority [34].

An excellent core curriculum on urinalysis that emphasizes urinary sediment examination in human medicine is available for the interested reader [35, 36]. A detailed technical review of morphological findings from human urine microscopy is also available with many high-quality images of urinary elements [37]. Automated methods for urine chemistry and urine microscopy have become common at centralized laboratories in human medicine; a trend has resulted in a decreased number of urinary sediment evaluations by nephrologists. There is still value in nephrologist-performed urine microscopy, especially in those with AKI in which valuable information is provided that is not typically generated from automated urinalysis by laboratory technicians. The gold standard in the evaluation of human renal patients is still regarded by some to be the performance of manual microscopy by a highly trained and motivated examiner [35, 36].

Routine microscopy of urine sediment employs bright-field microscopy, but phase microscopy can be helpful to facilitate the identification of cells, casts, and bacteria [18, 38]. Polarizing light microscopy can further aid in the identification of crystals [39]. Elements in the urine sediment can be reported as number per mL or number per HPF (40× objective) or LPF (10× objective). Most veterinary laboratories report using the number of elements per high- or low-power microscopic field. To report as numbers per milliliter, the number of milliliters centrifuged divided by the milliliter of sediment volume evaluated equals the concentration factor [7]. It is best to record all the observations on a standard form for inclusion in the medical record (Figure 6.4).

Staining

Many experienced laboratory technicians prefer to evaluate unstained urinary sediment, but the added cellular detail obtained using supravital stains (e.g. Sternheimer-Malbin, Sedi-Stain™, KOVA*, new methylene blue) can facilitate proper identification of cells in a wet mount preparation [40–45], especially for the less experienced observer. There are advantages of examining urine sediment with and without stain (Table 6.3). The use of supravital stain for urine sediment examination enhances the examiner's ability to properly identify RTE, casts, and WBC [45]. Stains are designed to change the refractive index of cells and provide nuclear contrast. Urine sediment that has been stained currently cannot be used in automated systems for sediment examination because stain disrupts the recognition algorithms that allow the identification of cell borders. For conventional microscopy, stain is added at a volume equal to the volume of sediment remaining in the bottom of the tube after centrifugation (usually one to two drops) (Figure 6.5), with gentle mixing (Figure 6.6). Doing so adds a dilutional factor that ideally should be considered in how many elements per microscopic field are reported. When stain is used, it is recommended that an unstained portion of the initial sediment be examined at the same time. Both stained and unstained sediment can be examined side by side on the same slide using two coverslips [15]. Enumeration of elements should be determined on the unstained preparation, whereas definitive identification of elements can be made on the stained preparation. Precipitates of stain sometimes can be observed during sediment examination if outdated stain is used. Bacterial and fungal elements sometimes are present as contaminants in the urinary stain [3]. Sedi-Stain and KOVA contain stabilizing agents to

Microscopic sediment evaluation - normal urinalysis

Automated Microscopy: Yes No   Sediment Stain: Yes No

Casts / LPF

Hyaline	0, 0 to 2 Highly concentrated urine
Granular	0, 0 to 1 Highly concentrated urine
Waxy	0
Cellular	
RBC	0
WBC	0
Renal Epi	0

WBC / HPF

Voided	< 10
Catheterized	< 7
Cystocentesis	< 3
Free	Yes
Clumped	No

RBC / HPF

Voided	0–10
Catheterized, Routine	0–5
Catheterized, Traumatic	> 50
Cystocentesis, Routine	< 10
Cystocentesis, Traumatic	> 50

Epithelial Cells / HPF

Squamous	0 to Few
Transitional	0 to Few
Free	Yes
Clumped	No
Strap Cells	No
Stirrup Cells	No
Renal Tubular	No
Renal Caudate (tails)	No

Crystals / LPF

	0 in Fresh Warm Urine
	Few to Mod, Refrigerated & Stored

Bacteria / HPF

Voided Catch	0 to Few
Post Void - Surface	0 to Moderate
Catheterized	0 to Few
Cystocentesis	0

Miscellaneous:
0 Ova/Parasites
0 Fungal Organisms
Lipid droplets in cats YES

FIGURE 6.4 Form for recording observations from microscopic sediment evaluation and expected results from normal dogs and cats.

prevent precipitation that occurred with the original Sternheimer-Malbin stain. Staining of mucus sometimes can result in confusion with casts. Punctate forms that resemble cocci sometimes are seen as an artifact when stain is used for examination of feline urine sediment. Special stains that can be used include 0.5% toluidine blue to enhance nuclear detail (metachromatic) and Oil Red O or Sudan stain to identify triglycerides or neutral fats. The combination of negative lipid staining and positive polarization (Maltese cross appearance) provides supporting evidence to identify cholesterol in urine sediment [7, 46].

Table 6.3 Advantages and disadvantages for staining or not staining urine for microscopy.

	Advantage	Disadvantage
Stained	Enhanced nuclear detail of cells	Artifacts resembling bacteria
		Stain precipitation – crystals
	Cytoplasmic staining	Dilution of sediment
		Emphasizes mucus strands
Unstained	No dilution of sediment counts	Elements optical density similar to urine at times – some elements missed
	No artifacts that resemble bacteria	

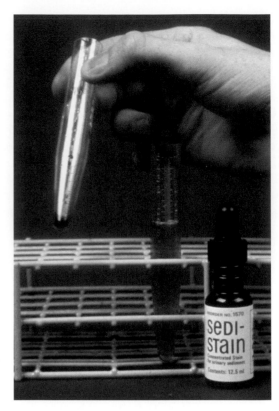

FIGURE 6.6 The sediment and stain are mixed by gentle tapping or agitation of the tube.

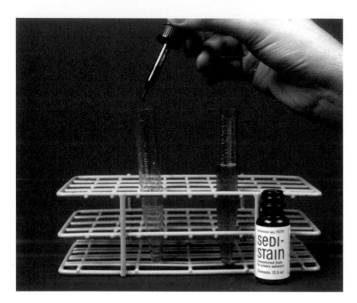

FIGURE 6.5 One to two drops of supravital stain (Sternheimer-Malbin; Sedi-Stain) are added to match the volume of the sediment in the bottom of the tube (optional). A drop of unstained sediment can be removed at this time instead of adding stain, or this can be used in addition to the stained sediment. The unstained sediment can be examined as described further below or can be submitted for dry-mount cytology if needed.

A consistent volume (one drop or 50 μL) of resuspended urine sediment (Figure 6.7) is transferred to a microscope slide using a pipette and a coverslip is applied (22 × 22 mm) [31] (Figure 6.8). A single view during LPF microscopy (100× total magnification) evaluates 3.14 mm² under the coverslip and 0.196 mm² during HPF microscopy (400× total magnification). This corresponds to 7.27 μL of uncentrifuged urine during LPF and 0.45 μL during HPF microscopy [37].

An excessively large drop that spreads beyond the coverslip has the potential to carry heavier elements beyond the cover slip and prevent their identification [7] and also promotes distracting Brownian motion of urinary elements. Care should also be taken to avoid including air bubbles during the placement of the coverslip. Likewise, care is also taken to ensure that immersion oil does not contaminate the slide and create oil droplets. We recommend waiting for approximately

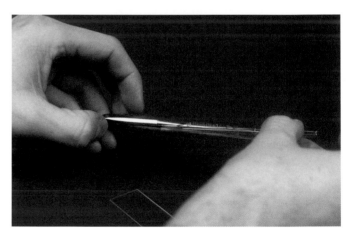

FIGURE 6.7 Urinary sediment, stained or unstained, is gently aspirated by glass or plastic pipette. In this example, a glass pipette is used to collect urine sediment by capillary action.

90 seconds before starting microscopy to allow urinary sediment and artifacts to cease Brownian motion and achieve the proper plane for examination (Figure 6.9).

Wet mount microscopy necessitates the use of different techniques for placement of the microscope condenser and the intensity of the lighting compared to dry mount bright-field microscopy used for blood films and cytology where the light is in focus with the plane of focus for the microscopic specimen. Because the optical density of urine is very close to that of some of the elements in the urine sediment, the microscope lighting

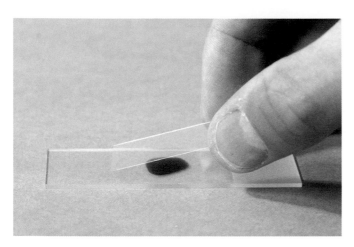

FIGURE 6.8 One drop of aspirated urine sediment is added to a glass microscope slide and a coverslip applied. Care is taken to not overfill the area under the coverslip and to avoid the introduction of air bubbles.

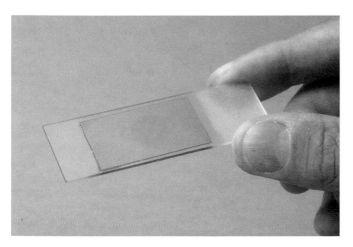

FIGURE 6.9 The coverslip has been applied. We recommend allowing the sediment to settle to the same level on the slide for about 90 seconds before starting microscopy. Smaller coverslips are used by some laboratories. Larger cover slips can allow for more fields to be examined when there is suspicion for small number of abnormal elements.

should be out of focus to render the formed elements as refractile as possible, which, in turn, will optimize their identification. Adjusting or "rocking" the fine focus of the microscope up and down can facilitate the examination of cellular elements in the sediment. Several other techniques can be used to improve microscopic examination of the urine sediment: The light intensity can be decreased, the iris diaphragm slightly closed, and the condenser slightly lowered. These adjustments should be made while microscopically viewing the urine sediment to identify the optimal settings for the specimen being evaluated.

The numbers of elements reported during urine sediment examination of normal dogs and cats are affected by the extent of trauma to the urinary tract and the amount of contamination from the environment or genitourinary tract that occur depending on the method of urine collection that is used (e.g. initial stream voided, midstream voided, endstream voided, catheterized, cystocentesis, from the floor or table top (see Chapter 3)). Urinary elements can be retained on items from which the urine sample is collected (e.g. cage pads, diapers), which potentially can lead to under-reporting of some elements (e.g. casts). Such collection methods also may add artifacts such as fibers to the sediment [47].

The average number of elements observed is counted in 10 HPF (400×) for RBC, WBC, epithelial cells, crystals, and bacteria. Casts are counted per LPF (100×) but further evaluated and the type characterized at HPF (as described below). Clumps of WBC and epithelial cells should be specifically reported (as described below). Bacteria should be reported as cocci, rods, or mixed populations, and bacteria in chains or those engulfed by WBC should be noted. The margins of the cover slip should be examined carefully because heavier elements such as casts often are found there. Sometimes, a large number of RBC (designated "too numerous to count") dominate the urine sediment, making it impossible to identify other elements. In such instances, 2% acetic acid can be added to the sediment to lyse RBC and allow other elements to be observed more easily [7]. The addition of acetic acid, however, has a dilutional effect that makes it difficult to accurately estimate the number of elements that originally were present. Addition of dilute acetic acid can also be used to dissolve the large numbers of calcium carbonate crystals in the urine of horses that can obscure other elements in the sediment [48, 49].

Standardization of Enumeration During Urinary Microscopy

Enumeration of elements in urinary sediment per HPF or LPF has traditionally been utilized in clinical practice and in the veterinary literature. Unfortunately, what constitutes an LPF or HPF has not been standardized. In this method, the number of observed elements is counted within the surface area (mm^2) and depth (mm) of the wet mount (between the coverslip and the glass microscope slide) examined. Most elements under the coverslip fall into the same plane of focus within a short time. Consequently, the use of LPF and HPF enumeration is a crude estimate of elements per volume of urine examined.

Historically using the most commonly available equipment at the time, it was assumed that an LPF was that area observed using a 10× ocular (eye piece) and a 10× objective (100-fold magnification); an HPF was that area observed with the use of a 10× ocular and a 40× objective (400-fold magnification). The higher the total magnification, the smaller the area (mm^2) examined in that field. The traditional 100× objective is designed to be used with oil and the 10× ocular to achieve 1000-fold magnification, but this is not part of a routine examination of urinary sediment. Oil immersion microscopy can be used at times to gain greater detail and magnification of wet mount preparations, but the mechanics of oil interacting with the coverslip over liquid and the resulting movement within the field of view (FOV) is challenging to achieve an optimal view as the slide position is changed. Dry mount cytology from urine sediment is recommended in these instances. Alternatively, the use of newer generation oil-free 100× objectives (1000× total magnification) can be used to examine details of organisms or intracellular features; oil should not be used with these objectives. This facilitates shifting the objectives readily between higher and lower magnification fields without blurring from oil on the coverslip. Focusing collars on the 40×, 60×, and 100× objectives in some microscopes allows greater resolution and clarity to be achieved, as the operator coordinates the fine focus with one hand and rotating the focusing collar on the objective with the other hand.

Numerous advances in the manufacturing of microscopes now allow access to microscopes with several different magnifications for the ocular (7×, 10×, and 15×) and for the objectives (4×, 10×, 25×, 40×, 45×, 50×, 65×, and 100×). The total magnification (ocular × objective) is loosely associated with the area (mm²) examined, but field area can vary by 33–200% depending on the field number (FN) of the ocular, even with the same objective magnification [3, 50–53]. The diameter of the FOV is calculated by the formula: FN ocular/objective magnification (e.g. 20 mm FN/40× objective = 0.5 mm) [54]. If the same objective is used, then the limiting factor of the size of the area viewed is the diameter (mm) of the opening in the field diaphragm of the ocular. Early microscopes had an ocular FN of 18 mm, but modern scopes now use oculars with FN up to 28 mm to widen the field viewed. If a tube lens was present between the ocular and the objective, that would need to be considered to determine the final FOV; however, most modern day scopes do not have a tube lens and have infinity objective lens such that the tube length is constant as well [50, 51]. The FN is often engraved on the side of the ocular indicating how many millimeters of diameter are under view (approximately 18–26.5 mm). If a number is engraved on the side of the objective, it is the *numerical aperture*, which improves resolution but is not needed to calculate the FOV.

The higher the FN of the oculus, the greater the diameter (mm) that will be examined and, thus, more opportunity to observe and report an element per "field." Small changes in the diameter (d) of the field lead to relatively large changes in area (mm²) according to the formula Area $= \pi(d/2)^2$ [55]. Precise denotation of the field size examined is pivotally important during mitotic counts and evaluation of suspected neoplastic tissue and in histomorphometry for the enumeration of osteoclasts or osteoblasts per unit examined during the evaluation of bone [50, 56]. Such precise definition of the area of the field to be examined from a wet mount is not likely to be of such great importance, since the number of elements from urine sediment is often near zero or there are many elements. It is unlikely that there will be much variation between the FOV encountered with microscopes commonly used in veterinary private practices when the same magnification objective is used. When the number of elements is near the upper cutoff for the reference range, elements could be reported to be increased or in the reference range when LPF or HPF areas are examined by different microscopes. In such instances, it is advisable to examine more than the usual 10 microscopic fields in order to increase the accurate classification as increased or not by LPF or HPF methods.

Since reporting the average number of elements per LPF and HPF is potentially misleading, it has been suggested to instead report the number of elements by total magnification of 100× for LPF and 400× for HPF [56]. For precise work, the number of elements reported per area (mm²) or diameter of field (mm) avoids confusion as to the field evaluated. Periodic calibration of your microscope system by measuring the FOV diameter (mm) with a stage micrometer that is within 0.02 μm is recommended (Meuten personal communication 2020). A paradigm shift from the well-entrenched reporting as per LPF and per HPF for urine sediment in veterinary medicine to the more accurate method of per μl of well-mixed urine before sedimentation is advocated. This change would then align with how elements are generally enumerated quantitatively in other veterinary body fluids as in a CBC or cytological evaluation of body fluids [27].

The decislide method to examine and quantify urine sediment is preferred by some veterinary clinical pathologists for generation of the most accurate results for enumeration (Dr. Mary Nabity and Dr. Jessica Hokamp, personal communication, 2020). The decislide contains 10 individual acrylic chambers that standardize the volume per area examined and prevents cross contamination between the multiple samples. This method allows greater certainty that the volume of urine examined will be known and the same each time urine microscopy is performed. In one method, a standardized volume of well-mixed whole urine is added to the chamber and allowed to sediment to the bottom by gravity and then examined. In another method more commonly used in veterinary medicine when precise enumeration of elements is desired, the urine is centrifuged first, the supernatant is resuspended in 20% of the original volume of the processed urine, and then 25 μL is added to the chamber (Dr. Jessica Hokamp, personal communication). More cells are usually identified with the use of this system compared to the microscopy of glass slides with coverslips (Mary Nabity, personal communication).

Considerable variability in the volume of urine examined can occur with the use of glass slides and coverslips associated with the use of small or large coverslips, as the same volume applied will spread across the coverslip. Additional variables that effect the enumeration of elements include the volume of sediment applied to the glass slide and the dilutional effect of urine added to the sediment for resuspension, if any. Resuspension of sediment with supernatant is sometimes accomplished by using a volume of urine using 10–20% of the total urine volume that was processed. In some laboratories, the volume of urine is preset at 1 mL, but this is not optimal (Jessica Hokamp, personal communication). Another recommendation has been to add 0.5 mL of supernatant to resuspend the sediment regardless of the original urine volume processed [27]. Due to all of these variables, converting the numbers of elements reported per HPF or per LPF to per μL is problematic, as there can be substantial variation in the volume of urine under the coverslip that will vary by how the slides are prepared.

Urine microscopy results reported as per HPF or per LPF are inherently semiquantitative and can lead to false-negative or false-positive bins that result in both overdiagnosis and underdiagnosis of upper and lower urinary tract diseases compared to the per μL method of reporting [27]. Increased WBC in urine sediment reported at >40/μL using volumetric chamber counting compared well to the finding of >5WBC/HPF in one report. In the same report, much greater variability for the enumeration of WBC per HPF was noted compared to chamber counts, an effect that was attributed to differences in the volume of supernatant used to resuspend sediment and the size of the drop applied to the microscope slide [57]. Dramatic differences in the number of elements reported per HPF from the same urine sample were illustrated in one white paper depending on the volume of urine processed and the volume of supernatant used for resuspension of sediment [58]. The initial urine volume that was processed in one example was either 5, 2.5, or 1mL, and then, all sediments were resuspended in 500μL of supernatant. Elements were reported at 12, 6, and 2–3 per HPF, respectively, with the lowest numbers reported due to greater dilution in the analysis of the smallest urine volume analyzed with a preset amount of supernatant used for resuspension. In a second example, 2.5mL of urine was analyzed using 500-μL supernatant to resuspend the sediment generating a report of six cells per HPF. When 5mL from the same sample were analyzed but resuspended in 250μL of supernatant, 24 cells per HPF were reported. Results from these two examples could be considered normal or abnormal, depending on the methods of preparation for microscopy.

Unidentified Elements in Sediment – What to Do?

It is not always possible to accurately identify all the elements in a urine sediment sample because the morphology of cellular elements can be altered as a consequence of the relatively wide pH and osmolality range of normal and abnormal urine, as well as the storage conditions employed before microscopy. Inexperienced laboratory technicians may have more difficulty identifying elements in the sediment, but experienced laboratory personnel and veterinary nephrologists can also encounter difficulty at times. When the definitive identification of elements in the urine sediment is in doubt, consultation with more experienced personnel is warranted. Urine sediment examination by an experienced nephrologist often yields clinically important information that is not reported by routine hospital laboratory personnel in human medicine [9, 39, 59, 60]. A nephrologist is more likely to recognize the presence of RTE, granular casts, renal tubular epithelial cellular casts, and dysmorphic RBC in urine than are certified medical technologists in human medicine [9].

Cells may enter the urine either by desquamation of epithelial cells along the course of the genitourinary tract or by entry from the circulation through the urinary tissues into urine (WBC and RBC). Cells that enter the urine are exposed to a potentially hostile environment of variable osmolality and pH that also may contain enzymes, toxins, and sometimes bacteria. Changes in cell size, morphology, and staining characteristics may occur when cells undergo permeability changes and degenerate [61]. Clinical experience and science must often be integrated to accurately identify elements observed in the urine sediment [39].

Adding a drop of formalin to urine sediment (unstained or stained) can preserve elements until another observer can offer an opinion. A digital picture of a confusing or interesting urine sediment finding taken through the microscope eyepiece using a smart phone or other digital camera can provide excellent images that can be sent to specialists for further assessment. Digital images of abnormal urinary sediment can also be included as part of the patient's medical record. The camera is placed approximately 0.5–1.0cm above the microscope eyepiece, and automated focus and exposure are used to capture the image [62]. The use of smart phone or camera adapters that mount the digital device to the microscope eyepiece can make this process easier, because the stable attachment no longer requires fine eye–hand motor coordination. Several brands of adapters are made for this purpose and can be found during a routine web search. Digital cameras for permanent attachment to the microscope as well as digital microscopes themselves are becoming more affordable and, therefore, more common in the average veterinary practice. Multiple digital images of urinary sediment are acquired by automated sediment analyzers that allow the sharing of images for further review.

Dry mount slides can be prepared by spreading a drop of urine sediment on a microscope slide and allowing the film to air dry, a technique similar to that used for preparing samples for cytologic evaluation. The prepared slide can then be stained using Diff-Quik® on site or submitted to a reference laboratory for Wright-Giemsa (Romanowsky) staining to allow a more detailed evaluation of cells and bacteria. Casts and crystals usually are not preserved by this technique [61], but crystals may be faintly visible. Finding intracellular bacteria indicates that the bacteria are not merely contaminants. Slides prepared for cytology should not be heat fixed, frozen, or exposed to temperature extremes, condensation, or formalin fumes [63]. Dry mount films can also be made from sediment that previously has been stained using a supravital stain. Such a preparation can be examined as is or can undergo additional staining with Wright-Giemsa (method of Dr. Gary Kociba). One veterinary author recommends submission of urine sediment in a small Eppendorf tube® that is tightly sealed, rather than whole urine, in addition to films on glass slides [63].

Semipermanent wet mounts of urinary sediment provide another method to keep urine sediment elements available for further on-site evaluation or for training of laboratory personnel. Coverslipped glass slides of urine sediment can be kept for several hours in a covered Petri dish humidified by moist filter paper on the bottom [64]; the glass slide is separated from the bottom of the Petri dish by wooden applicator sticks while being refrigerated [11]. Permanent wet mounts of urine sediment may be made on glass slides if a portion of the sediment is mixed with gelatin, glycerin, and phenol [65] or with formaldehyde and gelatin [66]. The sediment can be placed on the microscope slide first, but placement on the cover slip is preferred because doing so minimizes the entry of air bubbles and is more likely to establish an airtight seal when lowered onto the microscope slide.

The coverslip is then sealed with Vaseline, balsam, or methacrylate polymer (Shandon-Mount®; Shandon, PA, USA). Refrigeration of these wet mounts also may enhance long-term preservation of the sample. Excellent cellular detail and integrity of casts were maintained for over six months when a drop of formaldehyde was added to the urine sediment after centrifugation. The preparation was then allowed to sit overnight at room temperature to kill microorganisms and preserve elements in the sediment. 2–3 mL of 15% liquid gelatin is then applied, and a few drops of supravital stain are added to this mixture (optional). A drop of this sediment mixture is placed on a coverslip, applied to a glass slide, and sealed [65]. This method was adapted from a similar one designed to preserve urine sediment stored in tubes for future teaching of students and technicians [64]. With the tube technique, formalin is added to the sediment in a small tube and supravital stain is added (optional). Adding serum to the sediment is also an option, as described in the original report. The tube is capped or sealed and stored in the refrigerator. We have used this tube method to store interesting urine sediments for teaching purposes for up to one year.

Automated Microscopy

Automated microscopy has been used increasingly in human medicine to improve laboratory efficiency as well as accuracy and reproducibility in identifying and enumerating elements in urine sediment [18] and is now considered economically feasible for routine use. In human medicine, these methods are reproducible, faster, and more accurate than results provided by manual microscopy [67, 68]. Use of automated in-house microscopy is likely to provide more standardization than is possible using manual microscopy in veterinary practices. Automated microscopy in veterinary medicine offers a method to standardize how urine is processed (e.g. volume analyzed, speed of centrifugation), how the sediment is examined, and how the elements are counted. Increased accuracy for identification of elements in sediment can be provided in veterinary practices where highly trained and experienced laboratory personnel are not available. An additional advantage of automated microscopy in veterinary medicine, where the amount of urine available a dog or cat is often small, is that a very small volume of urine is required for analysis.

An automated microscopy system for veterinary use (IDEXX SediVue®) has been adapted from a human medicine using veterinary-specific algorithms to recognize elements in urine from dogs and cats (Figures 6.10 and 6.11) [69]. A urine sediment examination report is generated in approximately three minutes after urine is added to the cartridge and the analysis started. This system has been used in private veterinary practices since 2015. The algorithms employed by a convolutional neural network in this analyzer have continued to evolve to allow a more accurate identification of elements in urine sediment. In this proprietary system, an automatically loaded cartridge is filled with 165 μL of urine using a pipette to aspirate from the bottom of the sample tube

immediately after thorough mixing. SediVue® captures 70 digital images that correspond to about 45 HPF. Each digital image is nearly two-third of an HPF at 400× total magnification. Approximately 10 μL of the 165 μL inserted into the cartridge is analyzed [31].

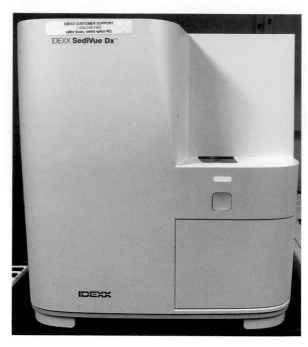

FIGURE 6.10 Front view, closed door of IDEXX SediVue Dx® Urine Sediment Analyzer. Source: Courtesy of Dr. Ronald Lyman, Ft. Pierce, FL.

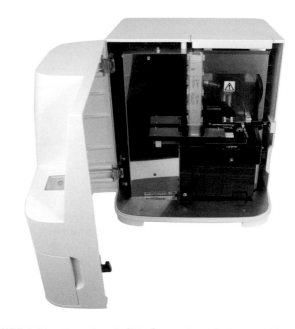

FIGURE 6.11 Open-door SediVue®. Overview of urine cartridge handling system, light source, microscope lens, and centrifuge. Source: Courtesy of IDEXX Laboratories. Copyright © 2022, IDEXX Laboratories, Inc. All rights reserved. Used with permission.

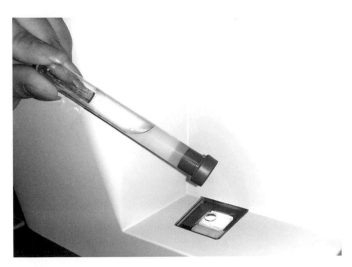

FIGURE 6.12 It is essential that urine be well mixed just prior to placing the urine sample into the urine cartridge. Picture is showing the urine tube being gently inverted and back to its original position a few times before the urine sample is aspirated. Source: Courtesy of Dr. Ronald Lyman, Ft. Pierce, FL.

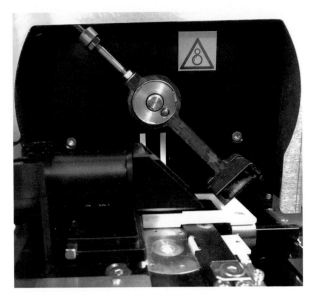

FIGURE 6.13 Long arm of low force centrifuge in back. Note chamber that accepts the urine cartridge to be spun and then delivered to the stage for sediment viewing. Source: Courtesy of Dr. Ronald Lyman, Ft. Pierce, FL.

It is crucial to mix the urine sample immediately before pipetting it into the cartridge, [70] because settling may occur within 15 seconds after mixing (Figure 6.12) [23]. If the urine sample has not been well mixed, aspiration from the top of the tube will underestimate the number of elements, whereas the overestimation of cells will occur if the sample is aspirated from the bottom of the tube. This factor is important during both manual and automated microscopy. Alternatively, urine can be added to the cartridge using a specialized syringe adapter. Overfilling of the cuvette results in an analysis error, and another cartridge must be properly filled in order to start the analyzer. The filled cartridge is delivered to an onboard gentle centrifugation system using a perpendicular arm at 260 RCF for 30 seconds (Figure 6.13). This centrifugation is well below the maximal 400 RCF that is recommended, providing a technique that provides less acceleration and force that otherwise could contribute to breakage of sensitive elements. No pellet of urine sediment is achieved using this method because the sediment rapidly settles to the floor of a 1-mm-deep horizontal chamber in the cartridge. Also, no coverslip margin is present to examine for preferential delivery of sediment elements. In most cases, lipids accumulate above this level and are out of the field of microscopy, eliminating confusion between RBC and lipid droplets. Light is directed through the top of the cartridge to the inverted microscope below, and 70 high-resolution, grayscale images are captured for analysis. Urine sediment samples that are highly cellular result in an error notice so that the element numbers per field are not reported until the sample has been diluted and the analysis rerun.

This technology uses face recognition algorithms to accurately identify and enumerate elements in urinary sediment (Figure 6.14). Each image captured represents two-thirds

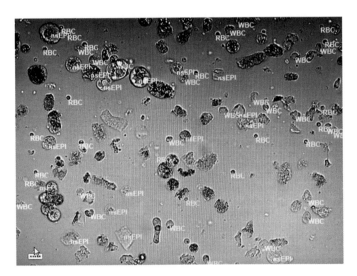

FIGURE 6.14 Screen shot capture showing representative identification and labeling of elements in urine sediment identified by SediVue® (IDEXX). The labels can be turned off and on. For quality control, it is a good practice to examine several fields to see how well the face recognition technology matches up the labeled element with what you see in the captured image. Not all elements are labeled. RBC = red blood cells; WBC = white blood cells; nsEpi = nonsquamous epithelial cell. Source: Courtesy of Dr. Ronald Lyman, Ft. Pierce, FL.

of a typical HPF (400×) examined during standard manual microscopy; a total of 46 HPFs are analyzed. The number of elements per HPF is averaged from evaluation of all 70 images. This instrument measures the number of elements per μL and converts this number to elements per HPF (400×) or per LPF (100×) and provides options to report elements per μL, per

HPF or LPF, or both. A report is generated that details the numbers per HPF of RBC, WBC, squamous epithelial cells, nonsquamous epithelial cells, and crystals (struvite, calcium oxalate dihydrate, or nonclassified crystals) identified during the analysis. Casts are reported per LPF as hyaline and non-hyaline. Additionally, bacteria are reported as rods or cocci and as none seen or rare, as well as suspected presence or present. Laboratory technicians and the supervising veterinarian still must have the necessary skills to identify specific types of urine sediment elements that are not completely characterized by this automated system. The 70 high-resolution digital images are captured and available for manual review for a limited time, after which only the best six images selected by the system will be archived [69, 71]. Each image is scored relative to the clinical relevance of the formed elements present. For example, an image with a nonhyaline cast that is present in only a few of the 70 images will have a higher score than an image with RBC or WBC, which should be present in most of the images. The best three images based on clinically relevant score are incorporated into the final report for review and permanently stored on IDEXX servers. All 70 images are initially available for review or for distribution to other individuals for review; an additional three images can be selected and added to the permanent patient record. To maintain quality control, it is recommended that a laboratory technician routinely checks at least the three selected images to further ensure the accuracy of what the analyzer has reported. Further clarification of reported items can include clumps of WBC if they are seen on the images, the specific type of non-hyaline cast (i.e. granular, cellular, waxy), the type of non-squamous epithelium (transitional or RTE) if these cells are found in clumps, and a specification of "other" for nonspecified crystal types.

In some instances, automated microscopy outperforms manual microscopy, possibly due to the higher number of microscopic fields evaluated and method of centrifugation (less time and lower g forces). In other instances, automated microscopy is outperformed by manual microscopy possibly related to larger volumes of urine that are evaluated and failure of algorithms to accurately identify urinary elements.

Initial studies of the SediVue® for RBC and WBC using Kova® commercial controls displayed excellent precision [5]. Kova controls are well established for microscopic evaluation of RBC and WBC, and they have excellent stability for more than 12 months. Using the original software, automated microscopy of dog and cat urine had moderate sensitivity and high specificity for detecting >5 WBC or RBC/HPF when compared to manual microscopy, accurately identifying clinically relevant increases in these elements [4]. Positive and negative agreement between manual and automated methods was slightly higher for WBC than RBC in another study. Occasional false-positive and false-negative results for RBC and WBC were reported during automated microscopy in this study, but many of these occurred as a result of differences of only a few cells on either side of the cutoff threshold [72]. In

another study by the same group, results from SediVue® were compared to those of manual microscopy as the gold standard for determination of elements in urine from dogs and cats. Positive results were defined when ≥6 cells per HPF were identified as WBC or RBC. Moderate-to-high sensitivity and specificity for the detection of urine RBC and WBC numbers were possible using this automated method of urine sediment microscopy (dog and cat urine combined) [73]. Updated software for this analyzer resulted in an increase in sensitivity for the detection of RBC and WBC with a slight decrease in specificity [74]. Using the current software, sensitivity and specificity for detection of RBC in dog urine or cat urine is good to excellent. For detection of WBC, the sensitivity and specificity in dog urine is good, but the apparent sensitivity in cat urine was less. The specificity of WBC in cat urine is excellent [74].

Automated microscopy by SediVue® categorizes crystals at ≥1 crystal/HPF into struvite, calcium oxalate dihydrate, or unclassified. Positive and negative agreement between manual and automated methods was very high for crystal identification in this study. False-negative and false-positive classification of crystals was uncommon. Struvite and calcium oxalate dihydrate crystals occasionally were categorized as unclassified [75]. In another study by the same group, urine sediment samples were considered positive for struvite or for calcium oxalate dihydrate crystalluria when ≥1 per HPF of either crystal was detected. Use of the updated software greatly improved the sensitivity (>97%) for recognition of struvite, but a mild decrease in specificity (81%) was observed. Sensitivity for detection of calcium oxalate dihydrate was close to 80% and specificity was >98% using either the old or new software [76]. Another study that examined urine from dogs (80%) and cats (20%) defined positive as >1 crystal per HPF for either struvite or calcium oxalate dihydrate by either method. Using manual microscopy, reported crystals were divided into semi-quantitative categories: none-rare, 1–5/HPF, 6–20/HPF, 21–50/HPF, and >50/HPF. Using the updated software, automated microscopy had a sensitivity of 91% and a specificity of 84% for detection of struvite. Sensitivity for detection of calcium oxalate dihydrate was 75% and specificity was 99% using the updated software compared to manual microscopy [74, 77].

Clinical interpretation of epithelial cells was similar between automated SediVue® and manual methods of urine sediment examination in one study [78]. In another study, ≥1 squamous epithelial cell per HPF or ≥1 nonsquamous epithelial cell per HPF was defined as positive by either manual or automated microscopy. Manual microscopy detected squamous epithelial cells in 5% of the samples and nonsquamous epithelial cells in 11% of the samples [79]. Using updated software, automated microscopy had a sensitivity of 33.3% for the detection of squamous epithelial cells and 99.4% specificity [74]. False negatives for detection of squamous epithelial cells by the automated method seemed to occur when the number was just above the minimal definition of ≥1.0 per HPF. Sensitivity was 71% and specificity was 87% for the detection of nonsquamous epithelial cells using automated microscopy. Categorization of nonsquamous epithelial cells requires the technician to review the digital images to further classify these cells.

Bias for the identification of RBC and WBC in urine was compared between manual and automated microscopy in another study. High bias was identified with the automated analyzer at 21.2% for RBC and 15.1% for WBC. Bias was considerably reduced following a manual review of the digital images acquired by the automated analyzer to 2.5% for RBC and 3.1% for WBC [80].

The detection of casts during manual microscopy was compared to detection by automated microscopy using Sedi-Vue® in urine from dogs at a veterinary teaching hospital. Casts were identified by manual microscopy as the gold standard comparator in 112 of 455 samples (24.6% prevalence). The automated sediment reader had a sensitivity of 72% and a specificity of 94% in this study. A review of digital images allowed for a correction in the number of false-positive and false-negative results reported by automated microscopy. It is anticipated that improvements in the neural net used in the algorithm for cast identification will improve over time [81]. A review of digital images is needed to confirm the accuracy for the reporting of hyaline and nonhyaline casts, serving as a quality control for results generated by automated urine microscopy. Additionally, further categorization of casts as granular, waxy, and or cellular is needed when nonhyaline casts are reported by automated methods.

Results from one automated urinary sediment analyzer (SediVue®) were compared to manual microscopy on the same sample as the gold standard for the identification of casts in urine from dogs. The identification of any cast (>0/LPF) by either method was considered positive. This automated method showed poor-to-moderate sensitivity (53.7%; 43.85–63.35%) in the detection of casts, as there were many false negatives [31]. Failure to identify casts might be attributed to low cast numbers, small sample volume, and an inability of the automated method to focus through different planes of urinary sediment. Moderate-to-high specificity (86.0%; 81.78–89.51%) was demonstrated by the automated method, indicating few false positives. Mucous strands, squamous epithelial cells, debris, and environmental contamination were occasionally identified as casts. Excellent specificity (>99%) for the analyzer compared to the manual method was found when the threshold for casts was modified to ≥1/LPF instead of >0/LPF, but the sensitivity did not improve. The automated analyzer generated 47 false-positive and 50 false-negative results prior to digital image review. Interestingly, a review of digital images collected by the analyzer identified casts in 36.2% (17 of 47) of cases originally classified as "false positive" that were not detected during manual microscopy (6 hyaline and 14 nonhyaline casts), so these were reclassified as true positives. In these instances, the analyzer performed better than the human operator, challenging the concept of manual microscopy as the gold standard reference for all urinary elements. This study concluded that there was moderate

agreement between the automated and manual methods for the identification of casts [31]. Whenever the analyzer reports casts, a visual review of the captured digital images should be undertaken to confirm their presence and type. Additionally, the digital images should be reviewed in cases with suspected AKI, in which casts were not reported. Manual urine microscopy is also an alternative to confirm the presence or absence of casts in these instances.

Another automated urinary sediment analyzer became available for use in veterinary medicine in 2018 (Zoetis VETSCAN® SA Sediment Analyzer) (Figure 6.15). This analyzer uses similar technology to identify elements in urine sediment as described above for SediVue® but does not use centrifugation before the enumeration of the elements. A probe outside the analyzer aspirates 650 μL of urine into a counting chamber. Urine then sits in this chamber for three minutes to allow sediment to fall by gravity before elements are counted. Elements are identified and then counted as the average occurring per μL from 192 fields and 96 high-resolution digital images. Ninety-six images are pulled forward and are available for review at the time of analysis if desired and are stored in the cloud for later review if needed. The urine sediment report displays six images with the most rare or important elements (such as casts) displayed first. The displayed images are approximately the size of what would be viewed during HPF manual microscopy (Figure 6.16). Urine sediment results are reported as the number per μl instead of per HPF or LPF. Reporting the number of elements per μL is considered a more accurate method, but this has not yet become widely accepted in private general practice. Reference ranges using per μL have been developed for use with this

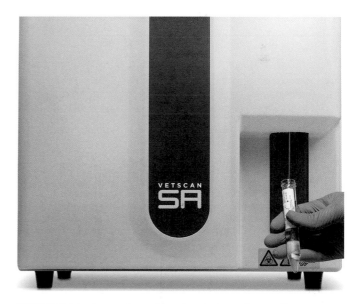

FIGURE 6.15 Front view of Zoetis VETSCAN® SA Sediment Analyzer. Automated urine sediment analyzer aspirates urine from probe on the outside of the analyzer (below shelf on right). Source: Courtesy of Zoetis.

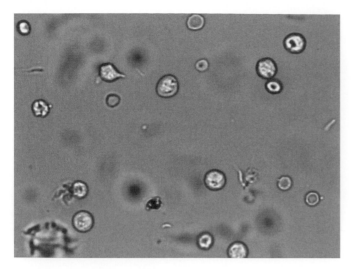

FIGURE 6.16 WBC and RBC. Note that RBC are about one-third to one-half the size of the WBC. WBC are identified by their nucleus, most of which appear polymorphonuclear. Some bacteria that are out of focus are in the background. Image acquired by VETSCAN® SA Sediment Analyzer. Source: Reproduced with permission of Zoetis.

analyzer. Comparisons of the urinary sediment results from this analyzer to that of manual microscopy or to SediVue® automated microscopy have yet to be published.

In general, automated microscopy agrees well with manual microscopy for the identification of RBC and WBC in human [82–84] and veterinary medicine (dogs and cats). Automated urine sediment microscopy appears to be well suited for screening healthy individuals with minimally active urine sediment and less accurate for those with more unusual pathology [83, 84]. Crystals and squamous epithelial cells are identified with moderate accuracy, but the accurate identification of nonsquamous epithelial cells, bacteria, and casts was poor at times [83].

Enumeration of RBC, WBC, and epithelial cells was very similar when comparing results from manual to automated urine microscopy in one report from human medicine. In contrast, there was no concordance in these methods for the identification and reporting of casts. Manual microscopic examination by trained personnel was recommended to improve the accuracy of reporting for dysmorphic RBC, bacteria, yeast, crystals, and casts. Automated urine microscopy was still advocated to save time and to provide the standardization of methods [84]. Review of the digital images of urine sediment harvested by the automated analyzer may be of high enough quality for laboratory personnel to assess in lieu of manual microscopy in these instances.

The accuracy of automated methods of urine sediment evaluation has continued to improve, but still needs further improvement [18]. Lack of agreement between manual and automated methods for identification of casts was particularly problematic in one study of humans [84]. A review of results flagged during automated microscopy requires a review of the digitally captured pictures or manual microscopy of the urine sediment to assign definitive identification for the final

report [83, 84]. The quality of the digital images is usually sufficient to identify questionable elements without the need to perform manual microscopy. For elements still in question, digital images can be sent to consultants for further review and rendering of an opinion.

Recent advances in recognition software can allow for the identification of malignant or atypical epithelium by some analyzers in human medicine. One of the weakest points in automated microscopy remains accurate recognition for small cocci. Some analyzers now include phase contrast in addition to routine bright-field microscopy to improve the identification of some urinary elements [85].

The accurate detection of bacteriuria remains difficult using automated analyzers [86]. Of 191 feline urine samples analyzed for bacteriuria, 36% were determined to be free of bacteria by both an observer and an automated analyzer, and no bacterial growth was detected in these samples. Of the samples, 14% were determined to have bacteriuria, and 24 of these 27 samples were culture positive. In 50% of the samples, a clear identification was not possible; 85% of those that did not have a clear identification were culture negative.

SediVue® reports bacteria as rods or cocci and enumerates them as none to rare, suspect present, or present [87]. Concordant negative findings were found in 36% (69 of 191) of samples from cats as no bacteria were reported by an automated sediment analyzer (SediVue®), none were observed following human review of digital images from the analyzer, and urine culture was negative; WBC count was low in most samples. Bacteria were identified by the analyzer and review of digital images along with positive urine culture (>10 colony-forming units (cfu)/mL [3]) in 24 of 27 cases. In the review of digital images, bacteria were placed into the same category as cocci or rods by both the analyzer and a human observer. In the remaining 95 cases, there was discordance between the report of bacteria by the analyzer and the observer in 50% of the samples; 81 samples were culture negative. Disagreement was more frequent in categorization of bacteria as cocci (91 samples) compared to rods (41 samples). Cocci are more difficult to identify with certainty and were frequently noted as suspected to be present by the analyzer and the human observer. WBC counts were >5/HPF in 82% of those samples with positive urine culture results. Dry mount cytological evaluation of urine sediment or urine culture is recommended to confirm bacteriuria when there is discordance between bacteria identified by the analyzer and the human observer [87].

Automated urine sediment examination in veterinary medicine has the potential to increase the number of complete urinalyses performed in private practice, as has been observed in human medicine due to an environment of improved workflow and decreased turnaround time [18, 82, 84]. Increased performance of complete urinalyses in-house provides both a means to increase the quality of diagnostic information that is generated and an appropriate source of income for the practice. Automated methods standardize the method of analysis (volume of urine, centrifugation force and time) while decreasing the time required to generate a report. Captured high-resolution images still should be reviewed by the veterinarian and technician to assure the accuracy of results reported by the analyzer before providing final approval for entry into the medical record. Review of images can also provide an opportunity for ongoing technician training. In general, the review of digitally acquired urine sediment images can replace standard microscopy. However, manual microscopy using LPF and HPF magnification still remains the gold standard for evaluation of urine sediment despite increased availability and accuracy of automated urine sediment analyzers [18].

ELEMENTS IN URINE SEDIMENT

Small numbers of RBC, WBC, and epithelial cells are often identified during the urine sediment examination of healthy animals (i.e. inactive urine sediment), but casts (hyaline and granular) are rare in normal animals. The number of these elements (per HPF or per LPF) identified during urine sediment examination of sick animals (i.e. active sediment) is higher and associated with various upper and lower urinary tract disease processes. Generalized reference ranges for urinary sediment evaluation are not easily provided because of methodological differences among laboratories. These differences include the sample volume processed, time and force of centrifugation, amount of resuspended sediment used to make the coverslip preparation, and whether or not the sediment is stained. The average numbers of RBC, WBC, and epithelial cells are reported per HPF, whereas the numbers of casts are reported per LPF. The presence or absence of bacteria, crystals, amorphous material, lipid droplets and sperm (in males) are also noted. Positive findings should be further characterized as few, moderate, or many. Results from an average of 10 microscopic fields are reported. Adherence to a standardized method of urine sediment examination allowed the quantification of numbers of RBC and WBC per HPF that correlated well with numbers of WBC and RBC excreted per day as the gold standard in human medicine [88]. The WBC and RBC estimates on examination of wet mount preparations also agreed well with hemocytometer counts performed using urine from dogs and cats [89].

CELLULAR ELEMENTS

Red Blood Cells

Detailed causes and the suggested diagnostic approaches for symptomatic and asymptomatic hematuria in human medicine have been reviewed [90–94]. Despite intense investigation, the cause of isolated microscopic hematuria frequently remains unidentified in human medicine [90]. Table 6.4 lists the causes for excessive numbers of intact RBC in urinary sediment in dogs and cats. Some of the differentials overlap with that for the causes of hemoglobinuria shown in Table 5.11.

RBC measure approximately 5–7 μM in diameter and are smaller than WBC (Figure 6.17) [63]. RBC appear as non-nucleated pale yellow discs in unstained urine sediment preparations (Figure 6.18). If RBC have been present in urine for a

Table 6.4 Causes for excessive number of intact RBC in urinary sediment. Some of the causes for increased RBC will also be associated with variably increased numbers of WBC in the urinary sediment.

Upper or lower urinary tract

Trauma
  Urine collection by catheter or cystocentesis
  Renal biopsy
  Blunt or sharp abdominal trauma
    Hit by vehicle
    Fall from height (high-rise syndrome)
  Gunshot wound
  Penetrating knife wound
  Highly intense exercise
  Inflammatory disease – variable numbers of WBC in sediment also
    UTI – bacterial or fungal
    Urolithiasis
    Feline idiopathic/interstitial cystitis – sterile
    Cyclophosphamide-induced cystitis – sterile
Nephritis
  Pyelonephritis
  Glomerulonephritis – including rapidly progressive GN
  Acute Interstitial – immune drug reactions (allergic)
  Tubulo-Interstitial – Leptospirosis
  Nephrosis – acute tubular necrosis (ATN, AKI) – ischemia, nephrotoxins
  Parasites (e.g., *Dioctophyma renale*, *Capillaria*).
Neoplasia
  Kidney
  Ureter – rare
  Bladder – most common
  Urethra
Renal infarction – rare
Renal pelvic hematoma
Renal vascular malformation
  Renal telangiectasia (Welsh Corgi)
  Idiopathic renal hematuria
Coagulopathy
  Thrombocytopenia (<50 000 platelets)
  Warfarin intoxication
  Disseminated intravascular coagulation
Genital tract
  Prostatic disease
    Benign prostatic hyperplasia
    Prostatitis – with WBC
    Abscess – with WBC
    Neoplasia
  Penile disease
  Preputial contamination – mostly WBC
  Estrus
  Vaginal, vestibular, or vulvar inflammation – with WBC
  Uterine disease (e.g. pyometra, endometritis) – with WBC

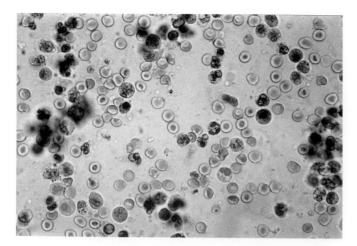

FIGURE 6.17 Urine sediment from a dog. Numerous RBC, all of which are light orange in color. The concave nature of these RBC is apparent based on the central darkened area. A few RBC are seen on-end, further demonstrating this concavity. Three WBC in the central field are easy to identify due to the distinct lobulation of the neutrophil; these stain red and are slightly larger than the RBC next to them. There are numerous degenerating WBC that are considerably larger than the RBC, have a bluish stain, and have less recognizable nuclei. No obvious bacteria are identified.

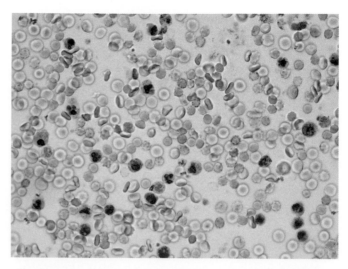

FIGURE 6.19 Urine sediment from the cystocentesis syringe as shown in Figure 6.26. This sample was from a young Great Dane with botryoid rhabdomyosarcoma. Note a large number of pale staining RBC, many of which display a concave shape. There are moderate numbers of neutrophils. Most of the WBC display red staining to the nucleus, while same show a blue stain. No tumor cells or bacteria were identified.

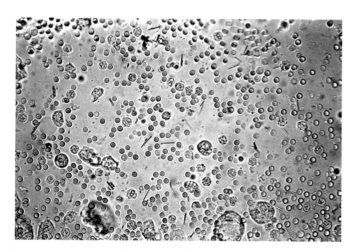

FIGURE 6.18 Note three types and sizes of round cells in this unstained urine sediment. The most numerous cell is the RBC; it is the smallest and has some inherent color without stain. Next most common are moderate numbers of neutrophils, which are defined by their being about 2–2.5 times the size of the RBC and having a lobulated nucleus. The largest of the round cells are transitional epithelial cells (nonsquamous epithelium). Sporadically throughout the field are needle-like struvite (amorphous) crystals.

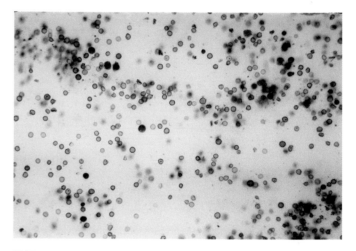

FIGURE 6.20 Urine was obtained by free catch from a middle aged intact male dog. Urine sediment at 104×. Too numerous to count (TNTC) RBC with rare WBC, and no bacteria identified. Hematuria was from bleeding associated with benign prostatic hyperplasia (BPH).

relatively long time, they may appear colorless because hemoglobin is leached from the cells over time (Figure 6.19) [95]. RBC are variably stained by Sedi-Stain® and may vary in appearance from light pink to dark red (Figure 6.20). Feline RBC often stain darker than do canine RBC (Figure 6.21). Staining can vary among RBC in a single urine sediment

sample or among different urine sediment samples. RBC in highly concentrated urine are smaller than normal as a result of crenation [96] caused by water movement out of the RBC as a consequence of the osmotic gradient (Figure 6.22).

Very dilute urine will result in swelling of RBC, [96], and some RBC may rupture, leaving "ghost" membranes behind if the cell membranes have not completely disintegrated. Ghost RBC are not readily detected by routine light microscopy, but can often be observed using phase microscopy. In a study of dogs, RBC survival in urine was correlated with osmotic stress.

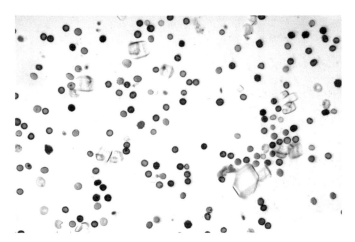

FIGURE 6.21 Numerous RBC in urine sediment from a cat with idiopathic cystitis (100×). Note light and dark staining RBC and the complete absence of WBC. There are some struvite crystals that are of questionable significance in this disease. It is important to know how the urine was handled as crystals often appear following storage that were not there when freshly collected.

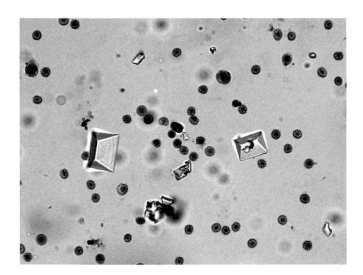

FIGURE 6.22 Struvite crystals. Many crenated RBC and rare WBC in the background.

RBC survival markedly decreased when urine was highly concentrated and decreased to a lesser extent when urine was dilute [97]. Survival time of ^{51}Cr-labeled RBC was determined in water-restricted dogs excreting concentrated urine and again in the same dogs after a six-week period of ad libitum water consumption. During water restriction, RBC survival was decreased to 14% of normal. In rats with untreated diabetes insipidus, ^{51}Cr-RBC survival was decreased 30% as compared to the same rats treated with antidiuretic hormone.

Unrefrigerated urine causes a relatively rapid lysis of erythrocytes and leukocytes [98]. Leukocytes persisted without significant decrease in numbers or altered morphology for at least 45 days in some refrigerated urine samples that were acidic

of one study of human urine [98]. In contrast to WBC, the enumeration of RBC and squamous epithelial cells was better maintained in tubes at room temperature containing preservatives [99]. Alkaline urine also contributes to the lysis of RBC [98].

Crenated RBC are sometimes confused with WBC because the spicules on crenated RBC can look like granules [63]. Lipid droplets are occasionally confused with RBC (especially in cats), but lipid droplets vary markedly in size, are highly refractile, and are in a plane of focus just below the coverslip (Figure 6.23) [100]. If in doubt, a drop of 10% acetic acid can be added to the edge of the coverslip to lyse the RBC. Lipid droplets also take up Sudan stain (Figure 6.24). Precipitated hemoglobin (in patients with intravascular hemolysis and hemoglobinuria) may appear as distinctive orange–brown globules that initially resemble RBC

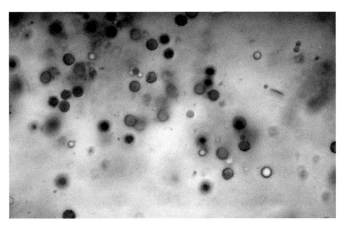

FIGURE 6.23 Stained urine sediment from a cat. RBC are all the same size and stain orange-red. Note a few refractile droplets (lipid), one of which is about the same size as RBC. Lipiduria is normal in cats. Source: Reproduced by permission Dr. Richard Scott, Animal Medical Center, NY.

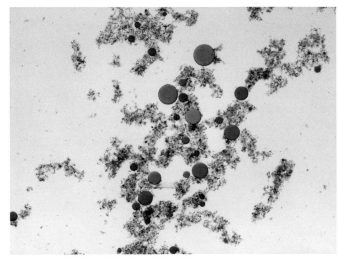

FIGURE 6.24 Lipid droplets in urinary sediment from a cat. Sudan stain has resulted in strong uptake of red color into droplets. The amorphous material in the background is possibly stain precipitate.

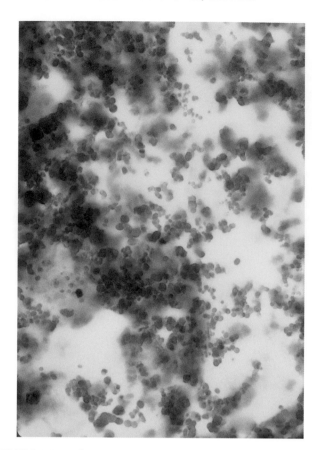

FIGURE 6.25 The report on this dog initially returned with TNTC RBC as the major finding. More careful inspection of this microscopic field reveals multiple size spherical structures that have their own peculiar color. These are the precipitates of hemoglobin that entered urine from this animal following a splenic torsion and hemolysis of systemic RBC.

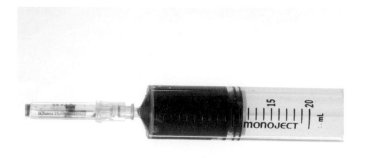

FIGURE 6.26 Dark red urine from a young Great Dane with botryoid rhabdomyosarcoma that presented for signs related to bone pain.

(Figure 6.25). Careful examination will disclose wide variation in particle size, whereas RBC are of more uniform size.

The finding of occasional RBC is considered normal in the urine sediment of healthy dogs and cats. The origin of these RBC in healthy individuals is not known. Healthy dogs and cats may have 0–8 RBC/HPF in voided urine, 0–5 RBC/HPF in urine obtained by catheterization, and 0–3 RBC/HPF in urine obtained by cystocentesis [70, 100, 101]. Hematuria is the common term used to describe increased numbers of RBC in urine [95]. Hematuria can be macroscopic (or "gross") when easily identified by the naked eye (Figure 6.26) or may be microscopic (invisible to the naked eye). The number of RBC/HPF needed to impart red color to a urine sample has been described in dogs [102], as discussed in Chapter 4. One group of investigators considered even 1 RBC/HPF indicative of hematuria in the second midstream voided urine sample of the morning in people [95, 103].

The extent of trauma that occurs during urine collection must always be considered when evaluating possible causes for hematuria (see Chapter 3). Although 0–3 RBC/HPF originally was defined as the normal range for RBC in urine collected by cystocentesis from normal dogs and cats [100], 0–10 RBC/HPF is often considered normal, and up to 50 RBC/HPF [104] may

be encountered in some urine samples as a result of the largely unavoidable trauma associated with this method of urine collection, regardless of operator expertise. An alternative consideration is that the trauma of cystocentesis more readily allows RBC to enter the sample when the bladder is diseased.

It is often advised to evaluate first morning urine samples for the presence of RBC because RBC are better preserved in more acidic and relatively concentrated urine. However, RBC that have remained in the bladder overnight can undergo some lysis as a result of prolonged contact time in urine [1]. Lysis of RBC in the sample should be considered when the occult blood chemistry dipstrip reaction is highly positive for heme pigment despite a paucity of RBC observed microscopically.

The finding of hematuria in itself does not identify where in the urogenital tract the excessive entry of RBC has occurred. The kidney is incriminated when free RBC are observed simultaneously with casts that also contain RBC (see section on casts below). In human medicine, free RBC in the presence of granular casts increases the likelihood of loss of RBC through the glomeruli [95]. Renal parenchymal bleeding can result in the presence of erythrophagocytes, which develop when renal tubular cells phagocytize RBC that pass through the nephron. Bleeding from the renal pelvis, ureter, bladder, or urethra was considered more likely when RBC were observed along with larger epithelial cells arising from deeper layers of the uroepithelium [95]. In human medicine, hematuria of renal origin is considered more likely when renal proteinuria, cylindruria, renal tubular epitheliuria, and dysmorphic RBC are also identified [105].

Hematuria has many potential causes (Table 6.4). RBC in urine may arise from the kidney, ureter, bladder, urethra, prostate gland, uterus, vestibule, vagina, vulva, penis, prepuce, or perineum, in part depending on how the urine sample was collected. The causes of hematuria can be grouped in categories such as renal parenchymal disease, renal vascular disease, lower urinary tract disorders (including trauma), and systemic coagulation disorders [88]. Findings from the history, physical examination, and method of urine collection must all be analyzed and integrated in order to properly local-ize the origin of hematuria. Hematuria is most often identified after trauma (e.g. cystocentesis, urolithiasis, and injury), bac-terial infection, and neoplasia in veterinary medicine.

Hematuria in lower urinary tract disorders occurs as a consequence of small-to-large vessel damage and subsequent bleeding. RBC in the urine sediment that arise from the lower urinary tract have been called "isomorphic" (i.e. a homoge-neous population of normochromic oval and biconcave cells) as opposed to "dysmorphic" RBC [106]. The presence of so-called dysmorphic RBC in the urine sediment indicates renal origin in humans, likely following transglomerular passage. RBC in the urine sediment of human patients with glomerulo-nephritis sometimes have distorted morphology with characteristic membrane blebs and are referred to as dysmor-phic RBC, whereas RBC in the urine sediment of patients with urologic disorders typically have normal morphology and are referred to as isomorphic RBC [90, 91, 95, 106]. It is important to not confuse crenated RBC with spicules that form in con-centrated urine [91]. Isomorphic RBC in the urine sediment can have either normal (dark cells) or decreased (clear cells) hemoglobin content [95]. The occurrence of dysmorphic RBC has not yet been reported from urine microscopy of dogs or cats with glomerular disease. Close inspection of urine sedi-ment from dogs with XLHN, however, routinely reveals the presence of RBC that have the characteristics described for human dysmorphic RBC. These dogs always have moderate-to-large blood on the dipstrip reagent pad in association with <5 RBC/HPF in urinary sediment from voided samples, sug-gesting that most RBC lyse as they pass through the diseased glomerulus (Mary Nabity, personal communication 2020).

How dysmorphic RBC are formed is not known, but they could arise from some combination of physical trauma during passage through the glomeruli, exposure to osmotic stress in the distal nephron, and alteration after phagocytosis by RTE [105]. In rats with experimental glomerulonephritis and hematuria, RBC traversed the glomerular capillary between gaps in the dis-continuous basement membranes as demonstrated by scanning and transmission electron microscopy [107]. In a similar study of rabbits with experimental glomerulonephritis with hematu-ria and RBC casts, RBC were found in the glomerular urinary space in 50% of the glomeruli evaluated by scanning EM as well as passage of RBC and neutrophils crossing the glomerulus through gaps in the basement membrane [108].

Wide variation in size (anisocytosis) and shape (poikilo-cytosis) characterized dysmorphic RBC that were recognized during bright-field microscopy. Dysmorphic RBC are often hypochromic (ghost cells) with a large amount of central pal-lor. Spherocytes, target cells, schistocytes, acanthocytes, and crenated cells are also sometimes observed [90, 91, 105]. Dys-morphic RBC may be more readily recognized by phase microscopy [95]. RBC morphology should be normal on examination of a peripheral blood smear in a patient with dys-morphic RBC in the urine [105, 106].

Hematuria in humans was considered to be of glomerular origin when >40 or > 80% of the RBC were dysmorphic, and

nonglomerular when the RBC were isomorphic [95, 103]. The proteinuria was considered mixed in origin when equal pro-portions of dysmorphic and isomorphic RBC were identi-fied [95]. This classification system was not always accurate because isomorphic RBC can also be found in patients with glomerular disease [95], and dysmorphic RBC can be found in patients with nonglomerular (renal tubular) bleeding [106]. A less subjective indicator for the presence of glomerular bleeding is the finding of ≥5% acanthocytes during urine sedi-ment examination. These acanthocytes are described as ring formations of RBC with ≥1 protrusions of variable shape and size. RBC that originate from glomerular bleeding (as com-pared to those originating from urologic disorders) are consid-erably smaller when measured by Coulter counter methods [95]. Glomerular-origin RBC have a high predictive value for the presence of glomerular disease, even when they occur as an isolated finding. In humans, three urine speci-mens from the same patient, each collected at least one week apart, may need to be evaluated before the renal origin of hematuria can be identified [103]. It is not clear if glomerular hematuria is only a consequence of glomerular disease or if transglomerular passage of RBC contributes to the progression of chronic kidney disease (CKD) [90]. We recommend the evaluation of dry mount urine sediment preparations to further evaluate for the presence of dysmorphic RBC in veteri-nary patients with suspected renal origin hematuria.

White Blood Cells

WBC in urine are spherical and usually 1.5–2.0 times as large as RBC (Figure 6.27). The diameter of a WBC in urine sedi-ment usually is 10–14 μM, depending on the type of WBC (e.g. polymorphonuclear, mononuclear) and conditions in the

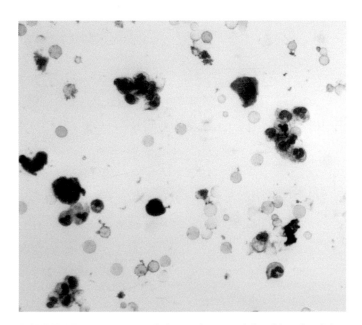

FIGURE 6.27   Four areas of clumped neutrophils with red staining nuclei. There are increased numbers of pale staining RBC, with small numbers of what appears to be punctate bacteria.

urine (e.g. osmolality, pH, presence of bacterial toxins) [63]. Neutrophils are the most commonly reported type of WBC in urine sediment, but it is likely that lymphocytes and eosinophils are underreported because of difficulty in making definitive identification using wet mount microscopy. Neutrophils with distinct nuclear lobulation are easily identified. However, cellular degeneration with loss of nuclear detail frequently occurs and makes it difficult to distinguish neutrophils, lymphocytes, small renal tubular epithelial cells, and small transitional epithelial cells from one another. Fusion of the segmented nucleus of the neutrophil is an early degenerative change and is followed by nuclear fragmentation that contributes to the overall granular appearance of these cells. Other degenerative changes in WBC observed during urine microscopy can include the presence of foamy cytoplasm and nuclear dissolution, swelling, necrosis, and decreased stain uptake (karyolysis) [109]. Phagocytosis of bacteria by neutrophils also may contribute to the granular appearance of the cytoplasm (Figure 6.28), but such cells are readily lysed and frequently not detected. This distortion of morphology is most marked in the presence of bacterial infection. Neutrophils in the same urine sediment sample stained with Sedi-Stain® can exhibit variable nuclear staining, ranging in color from pink to blue or dark purple (Figure 6.29).

In dilute urine, neutrophils may swell (Figure 6.30), stain poorly, have Brownian movement of cytoplasmic granules, and are often referred to as "glitter" cells [61]. Glitter cell forms of WBC were noted to frequently be associated with pyelonephritis, but specificity for this finding is low [37]. The glitter

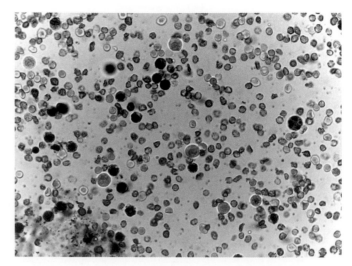

FIGURE 6.29 Stained urine sediment from a cat with *Corynebacterium* UTI associated with urethral obstruction and a perineal urethrostomy. There is punctate "debris" in the background that could be bacteria or cellular detritus. The nuclei of some WBC stain deep red and others are light blue. The light blue staining WBC are slightly larger than the ones staining red. One WBC to the mid far right shows nuclear fragmentation. Many RBC are in this field, some which stain light red while others stain light orange and some do not take up stain. Encrusting cystitis associated with *Corynebacterium* was the diagnosis.

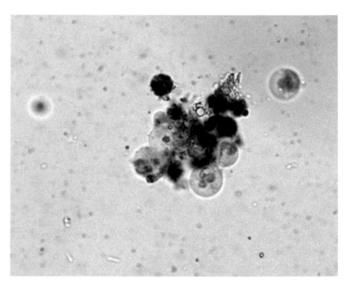

FIGURE 6.30 Clump of neutrophils with blue staining nuclei and swollen cytoplasm. The cytoplasm can swell when the USG is less than 1.015 or from toxic effects on the neutrophil. One WBC with red staining has shrunken cytoplasm near top of image. Particulate matter that is not identified is seen at the top of this clump.

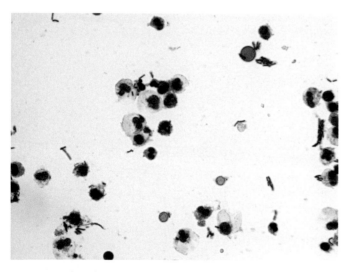

FIGURE 6.28 Stained urine sediment from a dog with a bacterial pyelonephritis. Renal involvement cannot be suspected based on the findings of this urine sediment alone. Note small clumps of WBC, which often indicate the presence of an organism causing the WBC to clump. Rod forms of bacteria are seen free and in clumps between WBC and free floating. A few of the WBC appear to have intracellular bacteria. Several of the WBC have swollen cytoplasm. A few RBC in the background allow the microscopist to make a comparison of size.

phenomenon may also be observed in patients with USG < 1.015. Leukocytes readily lyse in dilute (hypotonic) urine. Highly concentrated urine specimens may result in shrinkage of WBC with scant visibility of cytoplasm surrounding the nucleus, making definitive identification difficult (Figure 6.31) [35].

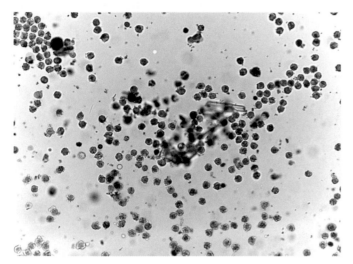

FIGURE 6.31 Urine sediment showing numerous WBC with some in clumps. Notice the lack of cytoplasm around most of the neutrophils – this can happen in highly concentrated urine that has been in contact with the WBC for some time. Clumping of WBC often indicates an underlying inciting bacterial organism. There are many punctate particles in the background that could be bacteria. It would be best to convert the urine sediment to a dry mount cytology slide for further evaluation to more definitively determine if the bacteria are real or not. A few amorphous struvite crystals appear in the center of the field.

Phase microscopy may be useful to more definitively identify the nature of the WBC nucleus. Adding a drop of dilute acetic acid to the edge of the coverslip may enhance the nuclear detail of neutrophils [96]. In some instances, staining may change the shape of WBC so that they are more easily recognized [45]. Peroxidase staining of urine sediment from humans turns neutrophils greenish-blue and allows positive identification because peroxidase is abundant in mature neutrophils and absent in other cells [110]. Cytological evaluation of dry mount slides may also be helpful in the further evaluation of morphology, either using unstained sediment or processing previously stained wet mount sediment preparations. In a study of dogs and cats, differential WBC counts could not be performed because of poor preservation of WBC in air-dried urine sediment preparations [89].

Small numbers of WBC may be found in urine from healthy dogs and cats, but their anatomical origin is not known. Neutrophils are the predominant type of WBC reported on urine sediment examination. Lymphocytes and monocytes are not easily differentiated from small epithelial cells and, thus, are likely underreported. The ratio of RBC to WBC (neutrophils) in normal urine is approximately 1:1, much different from the ratio in peripheral blood (approximately 500 : 1). Up to 8 WBC/HPF in voided urine, 5 WBC/HPF in urine obtained by catheterization, and 3 WBC/HPF in urine obtained by cystocentesis are considered normal. Up to 5 WBC/HPF is considered normal by several veterinary laboratories. WBC are not added to urine as contaminants during trauma associated with urine collection, as are RBC. In a study of urine from apparently healthy dogs, enumeration of WBC in urinary sediment measured in fresh urine at time 0 was better maintained in urine samples stored in plain glass tubes in the refrigerator for up to 72 hours compared to urine samples stored at room temperature in tubes with preservatives [99]. Leukocyturia and pyuria are the terms used to describe pathological increases in the number of WBC observed in the urine sediment. Table 6.5 lists the possible causes for detection of pyuria in dogs and cats.

Abnormal numbers of WBC in urine sediment indicate urinary tract inflammation or inflammation of (or contamination by) the genital tract (i.e. vulva, vestibule, vagina, uterus, prostate gland, testes, epididymis, vas deferens, penis, prepuce, or perineum). The anatomical origin of excessive numbers of WBC (i.e. kidney, ureter, bladder, urethra, extraurinary) cannot conclusively be determined unless WBC are found in casts, which incriminates the kidney. Although not

Table 6.5 Causes of pyuria.

Urinary Tract – kidneys, ureters, bladder, urethra

Inflammation

  Infectious – upper or lower urinary tract, or both

    UTI – bacterial or fungal infection

    Struvite urolithiasis – urease positive bacterial UTI

  Noninfectious – sterile urine

    Urolithiasis

    Neoplasia – lower urinary tract predominantly

      Minimal increases in WBC compared to increases in RBC

    Feline idiopathic/interstitial cystitis

      Minimal increases in WBC compared to increases in RBC

    Nephrosis

      Minimal increases in WBC

    Nephritis

      Pyelonephritis

      Acute tubulo-interstitial – immune-mediated drug allergy (eosinophils and neutrophils)

    Chemically-induced cystitis (e.g. cyclophosphamide)

Trauma

  Not from cystocentesis or one-time urinary catheter pass

  Indwelling urinary catheter

  Abdominal trauma

    Minimal increases in WBC compared to increases in RBC

Genital tract – inflammation (infection and sterile), neoplasia, trauma

  Prostate

  Testicles, epididymis, vas deferens

  Penis or prepuce

  Vagina, vestibule, vulva

  Perineum

  Estrus – mostly RBC

  Uterine disease (e.g. pyometra, endometritis)

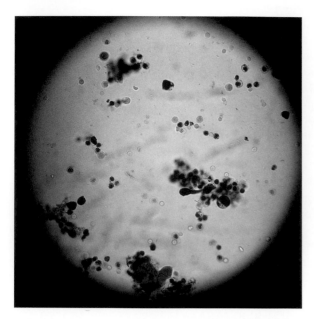

FIGURE 6.32 Image captured through the microscope eye piece using a hand-held iPhone. The smallest poorly staining cells are RBC. Both blue and red staining nuclei are seen in the numerous neutrophils (larger than the RBC). Note that some large clusters of WBC are seen, often indicating the presence of an infectious organism. Occasional bacteria are near the WBC or are free-floating. Occasional free nonsquamous epithelial cells are observed and one clump of the same type of epithelial cells can be seen at the bottom of the field. One epithelial cell is seen with a prominent tail, near the lower middle of the field. Epithelial cells are considerably larger than WBC.

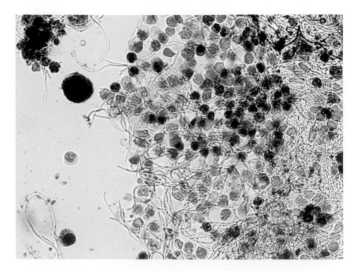

FIGURE 6.33 Stained urine sediment. Notice sheets of WBC clumping together. Most WBC are light blue staining and somewhat larger than those that are red staining. RBC to the left in this field stain light orange. Rare epithelial cells are seen.

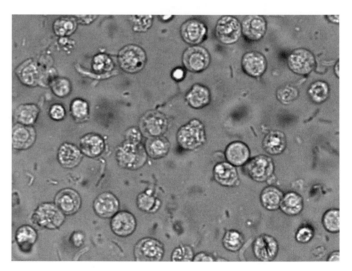

FIGURE 6.34 Many WBC (neutrophils) with easy to recognize polymorphonuclear nuclei. There is abundant cytoplasm in these neutrophils and the nuclei are well preserved. Bacterial rods are in the background. Image acquired by VETSCAN® SA Sediment Analyzer. Source: Reproduced with permission of Zoetis

pathognomonic for bacterial infection, urine samples with the most severe pyuria typically are obtained from animals that have bacterial urinary tract infection (UTI). Sterile pyuria may accompany other urinary disorders, including urolithiasis and neoplasia. Because pyuria usually accompanies bacterial infection in patients with clinical signs, a finding of excessive numbers of WBC in the urine sediment should prompt a search for a possible infectious agent. Clumps of WBC often occur with bacterial infection although bacteria may not be readily visible (Figure 6.32). Careful examination of the spaces between clumped WBC often discloses bacterial organisms. Bacteria can often be identified adhering to the surface of WBC whether these cells are clumped or solitary. Bacteria may also be found within the cytoplasm of neutrophils after phagocytosis or may be seen free in the urine sediment (Figures 6.33 and 6.34) WBC can also clump in an alkaline environment [98], and alkaline urine frequently occurs in conjunction with UTI caused by urease-producing bacteria.

Eosinophils seemingly occur rarely in urine, but have the potential to be identified in patients with some types of AKI, including acute interstitial nephritis [111]. Eosinophiluria and eosinophilia were described in one dog with azotemic AKI with an underlying diagnosis of acute tubulointerstitial nephritis, likely secondary to an immune-mediated reaction to ormetoprim-sulfa. Urine sediment contained >500 WBC per HPF, >50 RBC/HPF, and 15–20 epithelial cells/HPF. The nature of the WBC and epithelial cells were not further characterized during urine microscopy. Cytology of urine sediment revealed that 60% of the WBC were eosinophils and the remainder were neutrophils. The occurrence of eosinophiluria appeared to be uncommon when evaluated by urine cytology in other veterinary urinary disorders associated with pyuria. The authors of this report recommended the increased use of urine cytology in cases with AKI and pyuria in order to further characterize the WBC beyond neutrophils [112]. It is likely that the occurrence of eosinophiluria is under-reported when AKI patients with pyuria do not undergo cytological evaluation, as it is difficult to definitively identify WBC other than as neutrophils during wet mount urine microscopy.

Organisms

Bacteria

Bacteria should not be seen in the urine sediment of normal dogs and cats when samples are collected by cystocentesis. Normal bladder urine is sterile (based on conventional bacterial culture techniques), but the distal urethra, genital tract, and skin harbor bacteria that can enter urine when samples are collected by voiding or catheterization. Urine samples collected from the tabletop, cage floor, cage pads, hospital floors, litter box, or containers of urine submitted by owners often have bacteria that are identified in the urine sediment. If allowed to incubate at room temperature, these contaminant bacteria may proliferate, doubling in number after 45 minutes [100, 113, 114], which allows the observation of bacteria in the absence of pyuria (Figure 6.35). Contamination with normal bacterial flora from the urethra in voided or catheterized specimens usually does not result in large enough numbers of bacteria to be visualized microscopically in urine sediment that has been refrigerated. Most often, pyuria accompanies bacteriuria in animals with UTI, but pyuria can be absent in immunosuppressed patients (e.g. exogenous or endogenous corticosteroids, diabetes mellitus, cancer, and chemotherapy) and CKD (Figure 6.36). The absence of visible bacteria in the sediment does not rule out UTI, because approximately 10 000 rods/mL or 100 000 cocci/mL of urine must be present to be seen by the human eye in wet mount preparations of urine sediment [100]. False-positive results for bacteria may occur because of confusion with amorphous particulate debris (e.g. cellular debris, small crystals, lipid

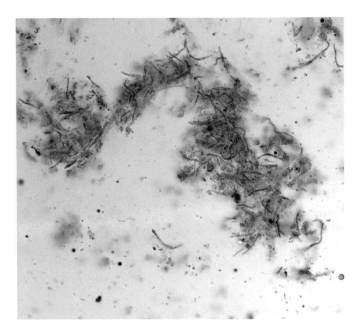

FIGURE 6.36 Urine sediment with many rod bacteria in the complete absence of any WBC. This is from a dog that is receiving chemotherapy. It was considered likely that the chemotherapy was immunosuppressing the dog so that a pyuric response was not elicited.

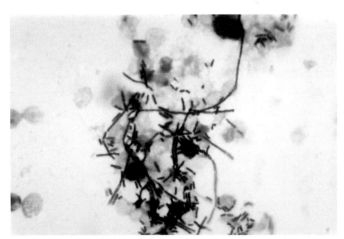

FIGURE 6.37 Urine cytology confirming large numbers of bacterial rods, some of which are quite long. It is important not to confuse this with the presence of fungal organisms. There are a few RBC in the background, but no WBC which is unusual in the presence of a true urinary infection.

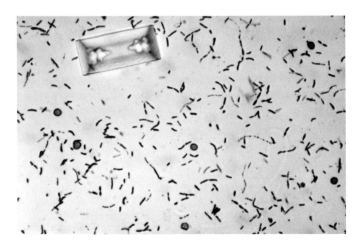

FIGURE 6.35 Numerous rod bacteria are obvious in this urinary sediment. Some cocci are also seen. Occasional RBC and one struvite crystal are observed in this field. The mixed population of bacteria and the absence of WBC suggest that the bacterial growth occurred secondary to contamination of the sample and perhaps improper storage before urine microscopy.

droplets, and stain precipitate), especially when these particles experience Brownian motion. Some coliform organisms assume a filamentous morphology when growing in urine. These bacteria should not be confused with fungal hyphae (Figure 6.37). The gold standard for the diagnosis of bacterial UTI is the isolation of organisms in clinically relevant quantities based on numbers of cfu per mL of urine [115]. Examination of urine sediment that has been prepared as a dry mount and stained with Gram [116] or Wright's-Giemsa stain for cytology will facilitate confirmation of suspected bacterial organisms [117–119].

The use of Gram stain on a dry mount from urinary sediment to identify bacteria had increased sensitivity, specificity, positive predictive value, and negative predictive value compared to standard evaluation with urine microscopy in one report [116]. In another report, one drop of uncentrifuged well-mixed urine was added to a slide using a Pasteur pipette, allowed to air dry without spreading, and then Gram stained. Significant bacteriuria was defined as the finding of ≥2 bacteria under oil immersion microscopy (1000×). Identification of bacteriuria from dogs using this method agreed closely with results of quantitative bacterial culture, demonstrating a specificity of 98.4% and a sensitivity of 96.2% [120]. Though Gram staining can be considered to confirm suspected bacteriuria while awaiting culture results, this is not recommended to be performed in-house due to difficulty in standardizing the method of Gram staining in order to generate consistent results; standardization at commercial laboratories is also difficult (Dr. Heather Wamsley, personal communication, 2020).

Rod-shaped bacteria (Figure 6.38) are more easily identified with certainty on urine sediment examination than are cocci (Figure 6.39). Smaller cocci (e.g. enterococci) can be very difficult to see during bright-field microscopy. They are more readily detected using phase contrast microscopy. Protoplasts (long rod-shaped bacteria with central swellings) can form after antibiotic damage to bacterial cell walls [121]. Sometimes, short chains of small cocci, such as enterococci, are mistaken for rods, and large refractile forms of staphylococci can be misidentified as crystals. Stain contaminated with bacteria sometimes can be the source of the observed organisms.

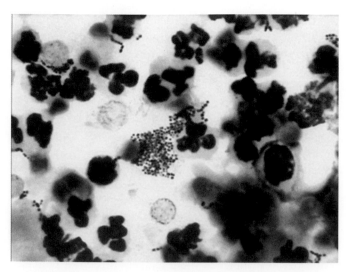

FIGURE 6.39 Wrights-Giemsa stain. Oil immersion dry mount cytology. Cocci are easily identified among the polymorphonuclear WBC. Occasional RBC. Dry mount cytology of urine sediment is very helpful in confirming that small cocci-like elements identified in wet mount microscopy really are bacteria.

Misidentification of elements in urine sediment as bacteria is common, especially when cocci-like findings are described. Cellular detritus, fibers, contaminants from the environment, lipid droplets, and small crystals can resemble bacteria at times. It is common for tiny struvite crystals in urine sediment to highly resemble rods. Supravital stain of urine sediment can result in over-reporting of bacteria at times (Dr. Jessica Hokamp, personal communication, 2020). Chemicals in old stain may precipitate in the sediment, mucus sometimes takes up stain in a punctate fashion, and bacterial contamination of the stain creates confusion during the reporting of "bacteria." Periodically, a drop of stain should be examined by itself to eliminate consideration for the presence of bacterial contamination in the bottle. The presence of bacteria in the stain is often blamed for the reporting of "bacteria" in stained urinary sediment; however, this appears to be uncommon. Comparison of unstained to stained urinary sediment is helpful in these instances to more accurately detect artifacts from the use of stain that potentially arise.

Standard microscopy of unstained sediment for the identification of bacteria from dogs and cats had a sensitivity of 89% and a specificity of 91% in the prediction of quantitative urine culture results in one study. Higher specificity for the identification of bacteriuria was achieved following examination of air-dried urinary sediment using Gram or Wright-Giemsa stain in this study. It appeared that small lipid droplets were misidentified as bacteria during wet mount microscopy in some instances, contributing to false-positive results. Results from a Gram or Wright-Giemsa stain of dried urinary sediment predicted urine culture results with greater accuracy than following evaluation of wet mount microscopy, though neither stain was found to be better than the other [118].

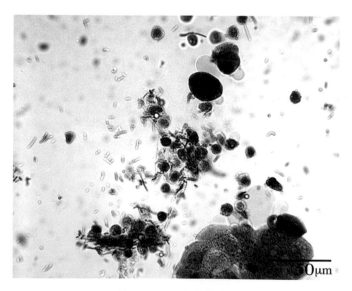

FIGURE 6.38 Moderate number of WBC most of which are in clumps. Linear bacteria in large quantity are between two clumps. At the bottom right of the field is a large clump of transitional epithelium with prominent nucleoli that is considered to be "reactive" to urinary tract infection based on the WBC and bacteria. Source: Reproduced with permission of Dr. Michael Horton, Fairborn, OH.

In a study from cat urine, bacteriuria detected by routine urine microscopy (unstained wet mount) was compared to that detected on modified Wright staining (dry mount urinary sediment) and quantitative urine culture. The sensitivity for detection of bacteria compared to urine culture results was increased slightly with the use of dry mount-stained slides compared to wet mount microscopy, whereas the specificity was greatly increased by the use of dry mount microscopy. The presence or absence of bacterial growth in urine was not associated with pyuria in this study; pyuria was documented in only 34% of cats with significant bacteriuria in this study [119]. Similar findings were reported from the urine of dogs in which improved sensitivity and specificity were documented during the use of dry mount stained sediment compared to wet mount unstained microscopy. Unlike the cat study, pyuria was significantly associated with bacteriuria, as was positive occult blood and lower USG in dogs [117].

In one study of dogs with inactive urinary sediment (≤5 RBC/HPF, ≤5 WBC/HPF, and 0 bacteria), very few samples had positive growth on urine culture (3.4% with either quantitative or qualitative growth). The authors of this study suggested that culture of urine from dogs with an inactive sediment should not be routinely performed due to the low yield of positive results and the high cost of urine culture with susceptibility testing [122]. A 6% rate of positive bacterial growth was reported in another study of dogs with inactive urinary sediment findings. Culture of urine from dogs without clinical lower urinary tract signs was not recommended; culture of urine from dogs with clinical signs and an inactive urinary sediment were recommended in this study [123].

A proprietary regent kit is available from IDEXX (Sedi-Vue Bacterial Conformation Kit®) that can be used when results generated by the SediVue® sediment autoanalyzer are suspicious but not conclusive for the presence of bacteria (reported by the analyzer as "Suspect Presence" or if the manually inspected digital images are not definitive). These reagents are added to a fresh urine sample and are designed to dissolve most cells or crystals that otherwise obscure or interfere with the accurate determination for the presence of bacteria. Sperm and epithelial cells may not be fully dissolved, so there still may be uncertainty in these instances. This treatment of urine is likely to be of most value in further evaluation of urinary sediment for bacteria that was initially crowded with cells or crystals. Results following this second analysis are reported for bacteria as "None detected" or "Present" [124, 125].

Fungal Organisms and Yeast

Fungal organisms and yeast (Figure 6.40) may occasionally be a cause of pyuria. Fungal organisms or yeast that are detected during urine sediment examination sometimes are contaminants. Contamination during collection, in the transport container, or from the bottle of stain, if used, all should be considered. A second urine sample should be examined to determine if the finding is reproducible. Periodically, a drop of stain alone should be microscopically examined to

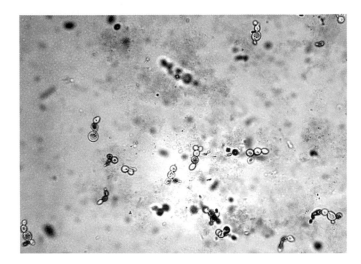

FIGURE 6.40 Urine sediment from a cat with an upper motor neuron bladder. This was taken as surveillance for development of bacterial UTI. Note budding yeast without other cells reacting to this organism.

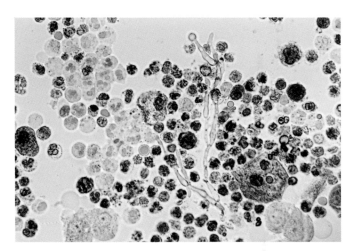

FIGURE 6.41 There are numerous WBC in this field, and most are in clumps. The light blue staining neutrophils appear to be more well-preserved than those staining red. There is one squamous epithelial cell located at the right third of this image just above a small clump of nonsquamous epithelial cells (transitional or urothelial cells) at the bottom of the image. The branching septate organism was identified as Candida.

verify that contaminated stain is not the source of bacteria or fungal organisms.

Candida UTI occurs rarely in dogs and cats, often in a clinical setting of urinary tract obstruction, structural urinary tract disease, and prolonged use of antimicrobials or immunosuppressive drugs (Figure 6.41) [126]. Systemic mycoses (e.g. blastomycosis, aspergillosis) may occasionally be diagnosed by evaluation of urine sediment if the urogenital tract has been colonized by the fungus (Figure 6.42). *Blastomyces dermatitidis* was identified in the urine sediment in 3 of 20 dogs with systemic blastomycosis [127].

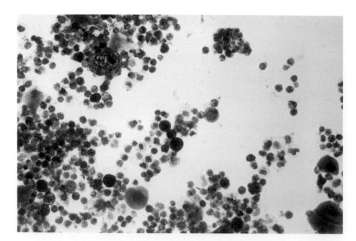

FIGURE 6.42 Notice many degenerate WBC in this field along with occasional transitional epithelial cells. The wall and size of the round structures in the center field are characteristic for *Blastomyces* organisms. This dog had systemic blastomycosis and the urine was the first finding from the laboratory that suggested the diagnosis. Source: Reproduced with permission of Dr. James Brace, Knoxville, TN.

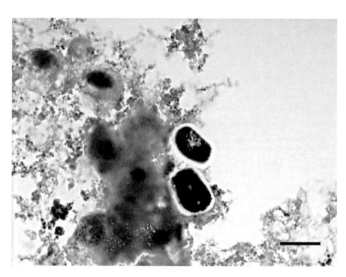

FIGURE 6.43 *Prototheca* sp. in a cytospin urine sediment preparation from a dog with systemic prototheciosis. Diff-Quik stain, 600×. Bar 5 = 10 μm. Source: Pressler et al. [128].

Prototheca spp. are saprophytic algae that can disseminate systemically in immunocompromised animals (Figure 6.43). In these instances, Protothecal organisms may appear in the urine sediment as thick-walled ovoid structures that sometimes are confused with pollen. In one study, urine sediment was positive for *Prototheca* in four of eight dogs with prototheciosis in which urine sediment was examined. Very-few-to-moderate numbers of organisms were identified [128]. Examination of dry mount or cytospin preparations of urine sediment will allow more definitive identification of these organisms. Urine culture should be performed for definitive identification of suspected prototheceal organisms.

Epithelial Cells

Urine sediment from normal dogs and cats contains few, if any, epithelial cells, usually as a result of normal cell turnover. Epitheliuria is the term used to describe the presence of abnormal numbers or types of epithelial cells in the urine sediment [129]. Squamous, transitional, and renal tubular epithelial cells may be identified and enumerated. Squamous epithelial cells are most commonly observed, especially in voided urine specimens. An occasional transitional cell can be observed per HPF as a consequence of normal cellular senescence and desquamation. RTE is never observed in the urine sediment of normal dogs and cats (described further below). Epithelial cells in wet mount preparations sometimes are reported as squamous or nonsquamous because of difficulty in accurately differentiating renal from transitional epithelial cells [63]. An approach to epitheliuria characterized by increased numbers of small-to-large-size nonsquamous epithelial cells is shown in Figures 6.44 and 6.45. The causes of epitheliuria are presented in Table 6.6.

Though the numbers of elements retrieved from urine sediment may be increased when urine has been forming and stored in the bladder over longer times, results from urine microscopy and urine cytology may be suboptimal due to cellular degeneration and loss of detail. For similar reasons, it is important to prepare the urine sediment for microscopy and cytology quickly after the urine is collected. Irrigation of the bladder with sterile saline through a urinary catheter can retrieve fresh cells with excellent preservation of cellular morphology and detail of uroepithelium. The addition of a drop of albumin or autologous serum to the urinary sediment before smearing and drying on a glass slide potentially improves the diagnostic experience. Cell clusters can be found in urine sediment following desquamation in animals with neoplasia, inflammation, and urolithiasis. Some drugs excreted into urine, including following chemotherapy, can cause urothelial cell hyperplasia and loss of cell differentiation. Squamous metaplasia can be identified in some cases with chronic inflammation and with transitional cell carcinoma (TCC) [109].

Squamous Epithelial Cells

Squamous cells are seen as large, flat, polygonal epithelial cells that tend to fold on themselves (Figure 6.46). They are 30–60 μM in diameter [63] and can be observed alone or in sheets. When folded or rolled into a tubular configuration, epithelial cells may be confused with WBC or casts, but squamous epithelial cells are much wider than casts [100].

Rolled up squamous epithelial cells sometimes have irregular margins as a consequence of shearing of the epithelium. When present, the nucleus is relatively small and round to oval (Figure 6.47). These cells arise from the distal urethra, vagina, and prepuce. Small numbers of squamous cells per HPF may be seen normally in voided or catheterized urine samples as a result of vaginal, vestibular, or urethral

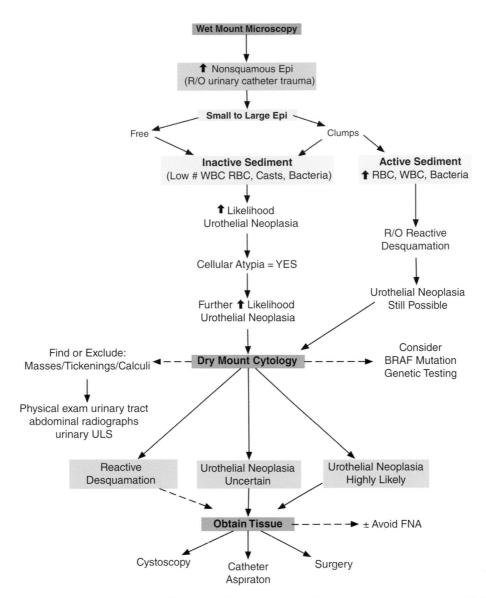

FIGURE 6.44 Approach to epitheliuria characterized by increased numbers of small-to-large-size nonsquamous epithelial cells discovered during urine microscopy. ± FNA refers to the risk for planting malignant cells along the needle tract when the diagnosis is urothelial carcinoma.

Epi – epithelial (urothelial) cells, WBC – white blood cells, RBC – red blood cells, R/O – rule out, ULS – ultrasonography, FNA – fine needle aspiration, BRAF – gene that encodes for the protein called B-Raf also called the proto-oncogene B-Raf.

contamination (Figure 6.48). Estrus may markedly increase the number of squamous cells observed in a voided urine sample. Squamous epithelial cells sometimes are observed in the sediment of urine samples obtained by cystocentesis, presumably as a result of aspiration of epithelial cells from skin. They are usually of no diagnostic relevance.

The finding of squamous epithelium in urine sediment samples obtained from cystocentesis can sometimes be explained by the occurrence of squamous metaplasia from underlying chronic inflammation or urothelial neoplasia. Some of the cells can have characteristics of malignant squamous cells in those with TCC. Squamous cell carcinoma of the urinary or genital tracts should be considered as a differential diagnosis when large numbers of keratinized squamous epithelial cells are identified in urine sediment [109]. Alternatively, squamous epithelial cells could be added to the urine during aspiration through the hypodermic needle on the way in or out through the skin during cystocentesis.

Small Epithelial Cells

Small epithelial cells are slightly larger than WBC and may arise either from RTE or from transitional epithelium at more distal sites, a distinction that is difficult to make using wet

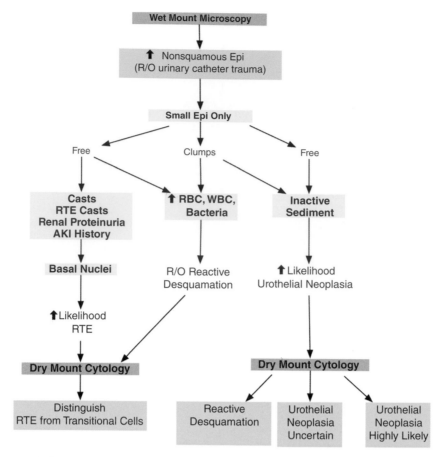

FIGURE 6.45   Approach to epitheliuria characterized by increased numbers of small nonsquamous epithelial cells.
Epi – epithelial (urothelial) cells, RTE – renal tubular epithelium, WBC – white blood cells, RBC – red blood cells, R/O – rule out, AKI – acute kidney injury

mount microscopy. WBC with degenerating nuclei can sometimes resemble small epithelial cells. Only small epithelial cells originate from the kidneys (i.e. transitional cells from the renal pelvis or RTE), but small transitional cells can also originate from the ureter, bladder, and urethra when they originate closer to the laminar layer of the mucosa. Large epithelial cells do not arise from the kidney. Larger epithelial cells can only arise from the urothelium and should not be confused with the smaller renal tubular epithelial cells. Stirrup or strap cells are small epithelial cells with lateral extensions that are thought to originate from deeper in the epithelial layer of the bladder, closer to the basement membrane (Figure 6.49). Their presence is thought to indicate a process that involves the deeper layers of the mucosa.

Transitional Epithelial Cells

Transitional epithelial cells (Figure 6.50) line the urinary tract (urothelium) from the renal pelvis to the urethra. Their nuclei are round centrally located, and occasionally, the cells are binucleate. The size of transitional epithelium varies considerably, even when arising from the same anatomic location, but transitional epithelial cells are considerably smaller than squamous epithelial cells. Nonneoplastic transitional epithelial cells are slightly larger to twice the size of WBC and are seen as individual cells (i.e. not in clumps). The shape of transitional epithelial cells varies from round or oval to cuboidal.

The size of transitional epithelial cells depends on the depth from which they originate in the mucosa, with the smallest cells from the basilar layer and the largest cells from the surface epithelium [63]. Transitional cells that originate near the basilar layer are approximately 20 μM in diameter and tend to be cuboidal to columnar in shape [63]. More rounded transitional epithelial cells with a tapered or tail-like appearance are thought to originate from the middle layers of the mucosa. These cells have a diameter of approximately 30 μM and are sometimes described as "caudate cells" (Figure. 6.51). By convention, they have been considered to arise from the renal pelvis, but one author considers them to be more indicative of the depth of origin from transitional epithelium rather than a specific anatomic location [63]. Transitional cells from the surface epithelium are approximately 40 μM in diameter, but these cells are flattened and tend to be polygonal [63].

Table 6.6   Causes of epitheliuria.

Lower Urinary Tract

  Urothelial cells – transitional cells

    Inflammation with infection – bacterial or fungal

    Urolithiasis – abrasion

    Neoplasia

    Sterile inflammation

      Feline idiopathic/interstitial cystitis

      Chemical cystitis – cytoxan induced

    Parasitic inflammation– *Capillaria plica* in bladder

    Urinary catheter passage – abrasion

    Indwelling urinary catheter – abrasion

  Squamous cells

    Usually contamination

Renal Origin

  Renal tubular epithelium (RTE)

    Ischemic AKI

    Nephrotoxic AKI

    Pyelonephritis – bacterial

    Glomerulonephritis – rapidly progressive, acute

    Leptospirosis

    Dioctophyma renale

  Urothelial cells – transitional cells

    Renal pelvic inflammation – caudate cells

    Renal pelvic neoplasia

    Renal pelvic urolithiasis

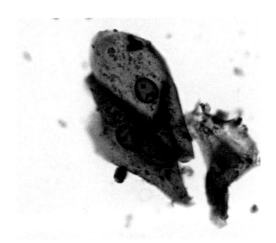

FIGURE 6.47   Two squamous epithelial cells attached to each other and one free squamous cell. Note the tendency for these large cells to fold or roll onto themselves.

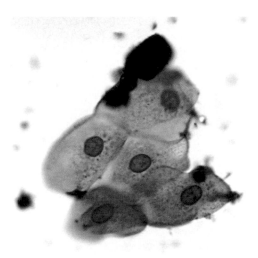

FIGURE 6.48   Clump of large squamous epithelial cells. Note the relatively small central nucleus.

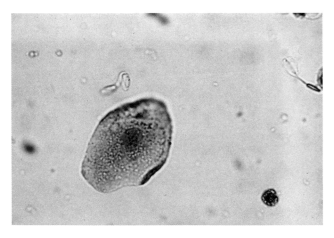

FIGURE 6.46   Single large squamous epithelial cell. Note the linear borders and the tendency for the edge to roll. A single WBC is in the lower right and two sperm are seen. Voided urine sample collected from a male dog.

Transitional Cell Carcinoma

Excessive numbers of transitional cells may enter the urine as a consequence of infection, inflammation, mechanical abrasion (e.g. urolithiasis and catheterization), neoplasia, or chemical irritation (e.g. cyclophosphamide). Transitional cells may exfoliate into the urine singularly or in clumps, depending on the process. Prominent clumps of epithelial cells as a major finding during urine sediment examination should prompt the consideration of neoplasia as the most important differential diagnosis.

TCC of the lower urinary tract may result in exfoliation when the tumor burden is sufficiently large (Figures 6.52 and 6.53), whereas renal tumors rarely exfoliate neoplastic cells into the urine. Clumps of transitional cells, often called sheets or rafts, may occur in neoplastic conditions, (Figure 6.54) but also may reflect reactive epithelial hyperplasia as may occur in patients with bacterial UTI or urolithiasis (Figures 6.55 and 6.56). Reactive epithelial cells also may be shed as a consequence of underlying neoplasia. WBC and RBC often accompany rafts of epithelial cells in association with inflammation; however, inflammatory cells (WBC and RBC), protein, and bacteria are also commonly observed

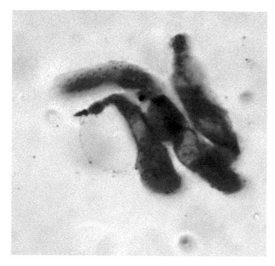

FIGURE 6.49 Urine sediment from a cat with FIC (feline interstitial/idiopathic cystitis). Rafts of epithelium were also in this sediment (not shown). A small cluster of epithelial cells with tails is identified. These cells are sometimes referred to as strap or stirrup cells. Epitheliuria is far less common than the finding of RBC in FIC.

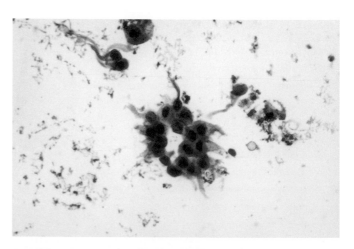

FIGURE 6.51 Cluster of small epithelial cells with tails. Urine sediment obtained from a dog by voiding. Small epithelial cells with tails can originate from the kidneys that are sometimes called caudate renal epithelium. Caudate cells may originate from the renal pelvis.

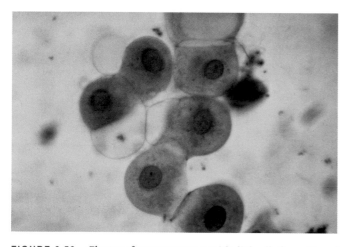

FIGURE 6.50 Cluster of nonsquamous epithelial cells (transitional cells). Sample was collected by urinary catheter from a normal male dog. Clump of epithelial cells is attributed to dislodgement of cells by the catheter.

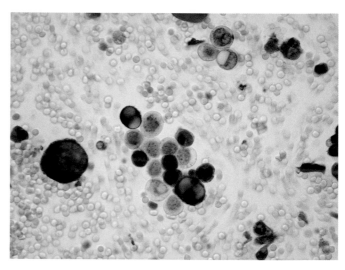

FIGURE 6.52 Numerous RBC and moderate numbers of transitional epithelial cells in the absence of WBC. This urine sediment is from an older female spayed Sheltie. Shelties are one of the high-risk breeds to develop TCC of the urinary bladder, which was the diagnosis in this case. Slight swirl of RBC around the central clump of epithelial cells occurred because the urine sediment had not fully settled on the slide before examination under the microscope.

during urinary microscopy from those with urothelial neoplasia. The finding of reactive epithelium (hyperplastic or dysplastic) can be created by inflammation in this setting, but they can also be seen in those with urothelial malignancy making definitive diagnosis between reactive and malignant difficult to impossible at times [63, 130, 131]. Urothelial neoplasia is more confidently diagnosed when cytological criteria for malignancy are present in the epithelial cells and inflammation is minimal [63].

Large nuclei, multiple nucleoli, coarse nuclear chromatin, mitotic figures, and cytoplasmic basophilia are cytological features of neoplasia that can be observed in wet

mount preparations of stained urine sediment (Figure 6.57), but these abnormalities are best identified using dry mount cytology. Nuclear detail is not always sufficient to differentiate neoplasia from severe inflammatory or reactive changes when evaluating wet mount sediment preparations. Cytology can be performed on dry mount preparations of urine sediment that has been processed with or without supravital staining.

The term "atypia" is often used to indicate diagnostic uncertainty. In these instances, no clear-cut evidence for malignancy is present, but the cells are not entirely normal.

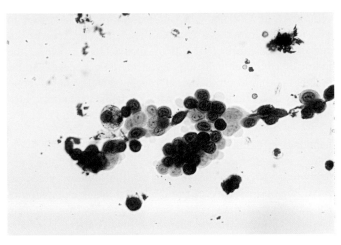

FIGURE 6.53   Clumps of small epithelial cells with large nuclei. A diagnosis of TCC was confirmed in this dog.

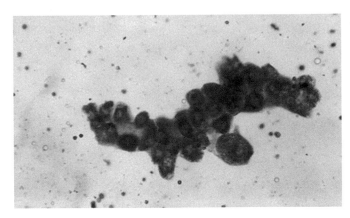

FIGURE 6.55   Clump of transitional epithelium in urine sediment from a cat with interstitial/idiopathic cystitis. Desquamation of this many epithelial cells is not common in this condition.

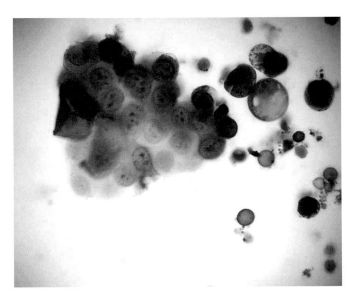

FIGURE 6.54   Image captured using digital camera in cell phone. There is a large raft of epithelial cells near center of filed. There are also some free nonsquamous epithelial cells and RBC. The combination of clumps of epithelium and RBC with no to few WBC is frequently encountered in animals with a diagnosis of TCC (UCC).

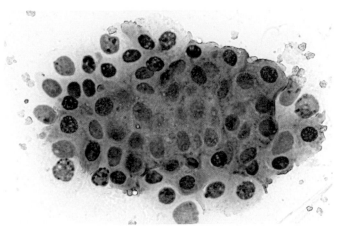

FIGURE 6.56   Large clump of epithelium in the urine from an older sick cat. There was concern about urothelial cancer, but no urinary tract masses were identified following ultrasonography and the cat recovered. The cat did not have reported clinical signs related to the urinary tract.

Umbrella cells comprise the single layer of superficial uroepithelium and are often seen in urine cytology samples from human patients who have undergone urinary catheterization, bladder washing, or cystoscopy. Umbrella cells are usually seen as single large cells with scalloped margins and abundant cytoplasm. They may contain a single large nucleus, but can often be binucleate or multinucleate. The nucleus is centrally located, is round to oval in shape, and has a smooth nuclear membrane. These cells are recognized as benign by their low nuclear-to-cytoplasmic ratio, scalloped margins, and smooth nuclear membrane. Clusters of transitional epithelial cells raise concern about the possibility of urothelial carcinoma, but they can be found after instrumentation and can occur in patients with urolithiasis. When epithelial cell clusters occur with urolithiasis, the presence of a rim of cytoplasm around the nucleus (collars or collarettes) decreases the likelihood of malignancy. Bacterial UTI can cause reactive changes in transitional epithelial cells. Reactive epithelial cells can be single or occur in clumps and often have prominent nucleoli accompanied by many WBC. Systemic or intravesicular chemotherapy with cyclophosphamide, thiotepa, or mitomycin results in characteristic reactive changes to the urothelium [132].

Lipid degeneration of urothelial cells can cause cells to appear swollen (Figure 6.58) or have a signet ring appearance (Figure 6.59). Degeneration of urothelial cells can also produce pink intracytoplasmic inclusions (Melamed–Wolinska bodies) that can be single and large, or multiple and small. These inclusions may be ovoid, club-shaped, rod-shaped, curvilinear, or branching. These inclusions are rarely identified in

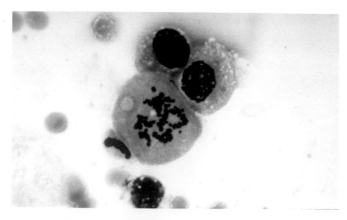

FIGURE 6.57 Cytology from urine sediment. Clump of epithelial cells with malignant character of mitotic figure, coarse nuclear chromatin, and prominent nucleoli. The diagnosis in this dog was transitional cell carcinoma.

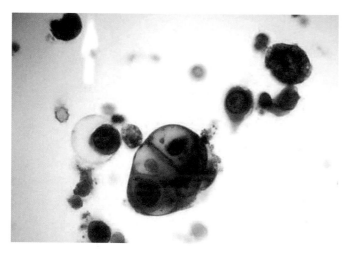

FIGURE 6.58 Clump of epithelial cells with lipid degeneration of cytoplasm in center field. Free nonsquamous epithelial cells and RBC are also seen.

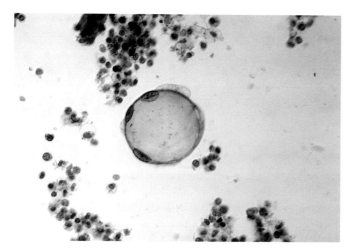

FIGURE 6.59 Signet ring cells. This is thought to be lipid-laden degeneration of nonsquamous epithelial cells. Many WBC in clumps and bacteria are in the background.

well-preserved epithelial cells and are commonly identified in exfoliated cells from those with TCC. Their presence was considered a unique feature of TCC in one review [130]. However, the finding of urothelial inclusions is considered nonspecific and is thought to occur as urothelial cells degenerate. Epithelial inclusions may be found in patients with urothelial carcinoma, various inflammatory conditions, and in healthy controls [133].

Diagnosis of TCC by Cytology

In human medicine, positive results from urine cytology are highly correlated to the finding of high-grade urothelial carcinoma on histology, but much less so for urinary tumors with lower malignant potential. The value from finding "atypical" urothelial cells identified on urine cytology was challenged in one study, in which this category did not distinguish between patients with a diagnosis of urothelial malignancy to those with benign disease. Cytological evaluation of urine obtained by voiding was more specific than samples acquired by instrumentation, likely due to less clustering of cells that tend to occur during instrument-acquired methods. The criteria to distinguish reactive from neoplastic atypia have not been clearly defined, but it appears that urine cytology is most helpful in the detection of high-grade urothelial lesions [134, 135]. In another study by the same group, the finding of >10 atypical cells was significantly associated with an eventual diagnosis of high-grade urothelial carcinoma. Hyperchromatic atypical cells with a nuclear to cytoplasmic ratio of ≥0.7, irregular nuclear membranes, single cells, and pleomorphism aligned with a surgically acquired diagnosis of high-grade urothelial carcinoma, whereas prominent nucleoli, eccentric nuclei, and nuclear to cytoplasmic ratio of 0.5–0.7 were not associated with this diagnosis [135].

Cytology of urine sediment is often diagnostic for urothelial neoplasia in dogs and cats, especially since they are most often presented with high-grade urothelial malignancy, rather than at earlier stages [136–138]. Well-differentiated TCC is less likely to add cells to urine than those with higher degree malignancy [130]. The finding of an inflammatory urinary sediment can render a definitive diagnosis of TCC as equivocal, since urinary inflammation is associated with hyperplastic or dysplastic epithelium that can be confused with malignant epithelium. High-grade TCC frequently exfoliates individual cells or clusters (so-called rafts) of epithelium with distinct junctions between cells and other cytological features that meet many criteria for malignancy [130].

Thirty percent of dogs were diagnosed with TCC (urothelial cell carcinoma [UCC]) by findings from urinary sediment in one study. Lower urinary tract TCC was definitively diagnosed following observation of results from fine-needle aspiration (FNA) of a mass or from prostatic/urethral washing in many more instances than from urinary sediment in this study [131].

Another veterinary review focused on the cytological evaluation of urinary sediment for its utility to diagnose conditions associated with infection, inflammation, or neoplasia. Irritation and inflammation can add urothelial cells (transitional) to urine that are considered "reactive" and are often found in sediment along with WBC, RBC, and bacteria. Unfortunately, there is no single criterion that allows reactive cells to be definitively distinguished from malignant cells. In the absence of evidence for much inflammation (low numbers of WBC and RBC), increased numbers of urothelial cells as the main or only cell type assume more significance for the probability of malignancy. The findings of many urothelial cells with variation in size, nuclear size, nucleoli size and number, mitotic figures, and cells with multiple nuclei support the diagnosis of malignancy [63].

The utility of cytology to establish a diagnosis following FNA of urinary tract masses (kidney, bladder, urethra), traumatic (diagnostic) catheterization of bladder and urethral masses, and urine has been recently reviewed for dogs and cats [63, 130]. Cytologic evaluation of urine from those with underlying neoplastic lesions of the urinary tract was frequently found to be inconclusive, so that in these instances, cytology from other sources or histopathology of tissue was required to achieve a definitive diagnosis [130]. Ultimately, biopsy of affected tissue is necessary to definitively differentiate urinary tract neoplasia, polyp, hyperplasia, and inflammation. Tissue for histopathology can be retrieved using conventional surgery, catheter aspiration biopsy [139], ultrasound guidance [140], or by cystoscopy.

Diagnosis of TCC by Molecular Testing

Recently, a urine test (CADET* BRAF; Sentinel Biomedical, Raleigh, NC, USA) has been marketed for the early diagnosis of noninfiltrating urothelial carcinoma, potentially allowing much earlier diagnosis than is possible by urine sediment examination. A positive BRAF mutation test on urine provides definitive evidence for urothelial carcinoma because no false-positive tests are thought to occur with this test. Surveillance for the early development of TCC (urothelial carcinoma) is warranted in high-risk breeds (e.g. Scottish Terrier, Shetland Sheepdog, West Highland White Terrier, Beagle, American Eskimo). Although many cases of TCC occur in females, no female sex predisposition for TCC seems to exist in high-risk breeds.

CADET* BRAF testing is an extremely sensitive molecular diagnostic test based on polymerase chain reaction (PCR) for the detection of the BRAF mutation in cells shed into voided urine in dogs with urothelial or prostatic carcinoma [141–145]. Urothelial carcinoma is associated with the BRAF mutation in approximately 85% of dogs [144], whereas 15% of dogs with urothelial carcinoma develop the disease by another mechanism. Test results are both qualitative and quantitative; the highest possible percentage of nucleated cells with the mutation is 50% because the mutation is only on one allele. Dogs with clinical signs usually have larger amounts of the BRAF mutation detected. False-positive test results do not occur in the presence of blood, inflammatory cells, bacteria, glucose, or protein as occurred in earlier tests for the diagnosis of TCC using a different technology [146–148]. Negative test results from the older test were useful to exclude a diagnosis of TCC [148]. Negative BRAF mutation test results can occur if

the urothelial carcinoma is not associated with the BRAF mutation (approximately 15% of cases), if the urothelial tumor burden is extremely low, or if the dog does not have a urothelial tumor (i.e. true negative). A positive BRAF mutation test indicates the presence of urothelial carcinoma somewhere in the urinary tract, with or without the presence of clinical signs or urine sediment changes indicating epithelial cell atypia. A positive BRAF mutation test result can occur months before clinical signs of urothelial proliferation are apparent and long before epithelial cell atypia in urine sediment, thickening of the urinary tract wall, or masses are detectable. The numbers of BRAF-positive cells appear to decline in dogs with urothelial carcinoma during effective treatment. Different gene mutations may be detected through the use of digital drop PCR molecular methods that detect DNA copy number aberrations in canine urothelial carcinoma [145].

Differential Diagnosis of TCC

Other conditions potentially can be confused with TCC (UCC). Inflammatory myofibroblastic tumors (a subset of inflammatory pseudotumors) are reported rarely in dogs. They are usually found as single intravesicular masses in various locations in the bladder and are associated with an inflammatory urine sediment, but not with atypical epithelial cells. The prognosis is considered good with complete excision of the lesion [149].

Polypoid cystitis occurs mainly in female dogs, and these bladder masses typically are located in the cranioventral bladder wall, as opposed to the trigone bladder neck area for TCC [150]. RBC and WBC are commonly found with or without bacteriuria in urinary sediment from dogs with polypoid cystitis, but details related to epithelialcyturia have not been reported. Mild pyuria was found by urine sediment examination in 50% of affected dogs, and moderate-to-severe pyuria was observed in the remaining 50% of cases. Urine cultures were frequently positive. The nature of the epithelial cells in urine sediment was not described in one large case series of dogs with polypoid cystitis [150]. Hyperplastic transitional epithelium that develops in polypoid cystitis can exfoliate in large clusters at times. In one review, the cytology of urine sediment in those with polypoid cystitis often revealed transitional cells that were round to cuboidal with distinct cellular junctions in clusters, moderate basophilia, a single round nucleus with coarse chromatin, and nucleoli that were not prominent [130].

TCC was diagnosed in two of 17 dogs in addition to the diagnosis of polypoid cystitis in one study [150]. TCC in the bladder of a dog was diagnosed eight months after chronic polypoid cystitis had been diagnosed and treated, suggesting malignant transformation in another report [151]. Based on these findings, it appears that the finding of polypoid cystitis can be a preneoplastic lesion that can occur months to years before a diagnosis of TCC emerges in some dogs with ongoing inflammation from this disorder.

Proliferative urethritis is a chronic inflammatory and infiltrative disease of the urethra in female dogs that sometimes causes urethral obstruction [152–155]. Proliferative urethritis is characterized by mass lesions in the urethra and vestibule with multiple finger-like extensions. TCC is a much more common cause of urethral thickening in the dog, but proliferative urethritis should be considered in the differential diagnosis because the prognosis is better than that of TCC. Various combinations of proteinuria, hematuria, pyuria, and bacteriuria are expected findings from urinalysis in dogs with proliferative urethritis; more cells are anticipated to be reported in urine samples collected by voiding compared to cystocentesis, but abnormalities still occur in samples collected by cystocentesis presumably from the reflux of cells from the urethral into bladder urine. Proliferative urethritis was previously referred to as granulomatous urethritis, but proliferative urethritis more accurately reflects the underlying histopathology. Details from urine microscopy or urine cytology describing epitheliuria in dogs with proliferative urethritis have not been provided [152, 153]. A mild-to-severe increase in the number of epithelial cells during urine microscopy was described in the first report of chronic active urethritis (proliferative urethritis) in 10 dogs; cellular atypia was absent [155]. Pyuria and proteinuria in the absence of hematuria were noted in two dogs, without mention of epithelial cells in urine sediment of another early report [154].

The extent of transitional cell exfoliation, clumping, and cytoplasmic and nuclear features should be compared before and after treatment for TCC. Remission and partial remission are reflected in fewer epithelial cells in the urine sediment. Currently, in veterinary medicine, most cases of TCC are diagnosed at an advanced stage of the disease [156, 157].

Renal Epithelial Cells

It is difficult to reliably differentiate small epithelial cells of renal tubular origin from small transitional epithelial cells. Presumptive identification of small epithelial cells as renal in origin can be made if epithelial cells are also seen within casts or if numerous noncellular casts are present to indicate renal injury. The location of the cell nucleus as central (transitional cell) versus eccentric or basal (RTE) also provides information as to the identity of the epithelial cells (Figures 6.60 and 6.61).

Renal epithelial cells originate from RTE, from the renal pelvis (caudate transitional cells), or may represent podocytes. In our experience, the finding of renal tubular epithelial cells in urine sediment is always abnormal, but one veterinary author described them as normal in low numbers as a consequence of normal cell turnover [63]. Renal tubular epithelial cells are observed most often in patients with AKI (ischemic, nephrotoxic, inflammatory, or degenerative) (Figure 6.62). Renal tubular epithelial cells were reported in 67% of dogs and 41% of cats at the time of clinical diagnosis of ethylene glycol poisoning in one study (Figures 6.63 and 6.64) [158]. Severely decreased renal arterial perfusion should be considered an uncommon differential diagnosis when RTE is observed in the urine sediment. Sheets of RTE were observed in dogs as early as 30 minutes after unilateral renal artery occlusion in one study [129]. The detection of

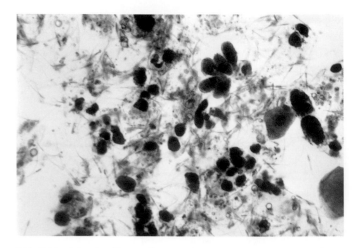

FIGURE 6.60 Small round to ovoid epithelial cells. Many nuclei are basal suggesting renal tubular origin for these epithelial cells. One clump of elongated small epithelial cells is at the top of this field, but the nuclei have degenerated. The two largest cells are squamous epithelium. Two short coarsely granular casts are in the right middle field. Many sperm are in the background. Yellow background debris is not identified but can be compatible with tubular necrosis and detritus. This young male German Shepherd was evaluated for acute illness associated with azotemia. Urine sediment evaluation was performed by the emergency service to try to determine if ethylene glycol had recently been ingested, but no calcium oxalate crystals were observed. The diagnosis in this dog was ischemic nephropathy (AKI) due to the entrapment of abdominal contents within a pericardial-diaphragmatic hernia.

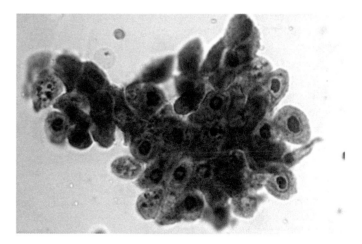

FIGURE 6.61 Cluster of small epithelial cells. The central location of most nuclei suggests urothelial rather than renal tubular origin.

podocytes in urine sediment indicates severe podocyte injury encountered in some types of glomerular injury. Podocyturia dissipates during successful treatment and may be a prognostic indicator [159]. The podocyte is identified by positive immunofluorescent reactions to podocalyxin. Podocalyxin has been detected within casts, as fine granules, and within intact cells in urinary sediment [160]. Identification of podocyturia has not yet been reported in veterinary patients.

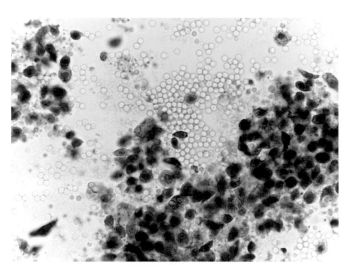

FIGURE 6.62   The predominant cell type is the small epithelial cell. There are also numerous RBC and moderate numbers of WBC without detectable bacteria. This urine sediment is from a cat with necropsy-confirmed acute renal injury.

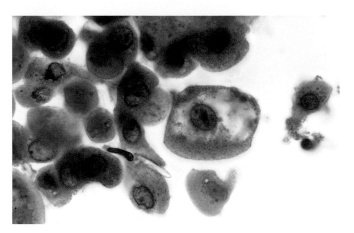

FIGURE 6.64   Large clump of renal tubular epithelium (RTE) in urine sediment from a dog with early ethylene glycol poisoning. RTE are round, oval, and cuboidal in shape. Note RTE that are free, and also in clumps. The nuclei are basal in most of the cells. A few of the RTE have tails. A single calcium oxalate monohydrate crystal is seen near the bottom of the clump.

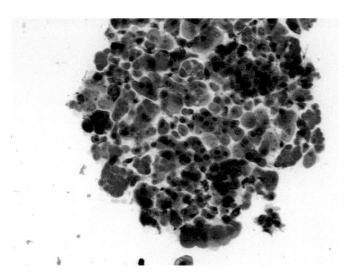

FIGURE 6.63   Large clump of renal tubular epithelium (RTE) in urine sediment from a dog with early ethylene glycol poisoning. RTE are round, oval, and cuboidal in shape. Many nuclei appear in the basal position of the cell.

In humans, oval fat bodies are lipid-laden renal tubular cells that have sloughed into urine from patients with tubular damage from a variety of causes. These cells form after partial reabsorption of lipids filtered into tubular fluid and then taken up into lysosomes. Transmission electron microscopy has been used to further describe these structures [161]. Oval fat bodies occasionally are observed in animals.

Definitive identification of RTE during wet mount or dry mount cytology urine sediment examination in veterinary medicine has not been emphasized. Renal tubular cells and WBC can easily be confused with transitional epithelial cells during wet mount microscopy, [63] and often such cells are reported as transitional epithelial cells. Staining of sediment improves the identification of renal tubular epithelial cells that are free or in casts. Renal tubular epithelial cells can be shed into urine as single cells, or sometimes in rows [63]. When renal tubular epithelial cells are identified in casts (see Casts section), free small epithelial cells are often are classified as RTE because of their association with the observed casts. When renal tubular epithelial cells are incorporated into casts, they indicate renal tubular pathology, such as pyelonephritis or renal tubular necrosis. Renal tubular epithelial cells are larger than WBC and tend to be oval to round, ranging in size from 10 to 50 μM [63]. A cytoplasmic tail from a renal tubular epithelial cell is sometimes observed [63]. Renal tubular epithelial cells from the proximal tubules are large and rectangular or columnar [7] but can assume a round shape once released from the tubular basement membrane. Identification of microvilli on the surface of a renal tubular epithelial cell confirms its origin from the proximal tubule, but this identification is rarely made during wet mount microscopy [63]. The brush border (i.e. microvilli) of a proximal renal tubular epithelial cell is more likely to be identified during dry mount cytological examination. The cytoplasm of renal tubular epithelial cells from the proximal tubule is often coarsely granular and easy to confuse with a cast [7], but a cast does not have a single nucleus. Renal tubular epithelial cells from other sites are smaller than those from the proximal tubule and can be round or oval; they are often mistaken for WBC and spherical transitional cells. The eccentric location of the nucleus distinguishes renal tubular epithelial cells from transitional cells (Figure 6.65). Renal tubular epithelial cells from the collecting tubules are cuboidal and never round, often having one straight side [7]. All suspected renal tubular epithelial cells observed on wet mount evaluation of urine sediment should be further evaluated using dry mount cytology.

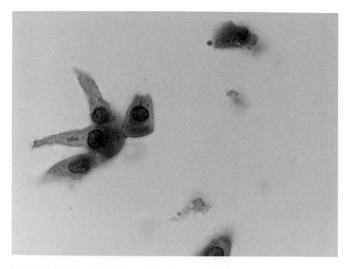

FIGURE 6.65 Urine sample is from the same dog in Figure 6.64 with ethylene glycol poisoning. RTE are seen in a clump and free. In this view, it is easy to determine the basal positioning on the nuclei in RTE that are cuboidal.

It is difficult at times to distinguish small renal tubular epithelial cells from neutrophils, especially when cellular detail is lacking. A stain was developed based on the peroxidase reaction, which permitted accurate and rapid identification of neutrophils. This stain was prepared with a specific combination of diaminofluorene, phloxine B, ethanol, sodium acetate, acetic acid, and hydrogen peroxide. Neutrophils stained a deep blue–black, while RTE stained pink and RBC stained red. The cytoplasm of the neutrophil is initially clear, which then becomes slightly blue with the nuclei appearing dark blue. The nuclei and cytoplasm of the neutrophil progressively take up stain and become darker to the point that the entire cell appears blue–black [162].

CASTS

Casts are cylindrical molds that form within the renal tubular lumen and then are excreted into urine. A spectrum from nearly all matrix protein precipitation to nearly all cells or granules may occur, depending on the specific disease and its activity associated with cast formation. Casts are identified as large cylindrical structures with well-defined parallel sides that usually maintain the same diameter throughout their length. The length of a cast is generally expected to be several times its width. The width of casts varies according to the segment of the nephron in which they were formed, and the ends of casts are often rounded. The convoluted appearance of a cast reflects the course of the distal convoluted tubule in which it was formed. Casts may be eliminated in the urine immediately after formation or may remain in the tubules for variable periods of time, undergoing a variable amount of degeneration [100]. The use of phase contrast microscopy and polarizing light during urine sediment microscopy allows additional morphological detail to be observed and allows

more accurate identification of casts as compared to bright-field microscopy alone [18]. The causes of cylindruria are presented in Table 6.7.

Table 6.7 Causes of cylindruria.

Hyaline casts

≤2 per LPF in concentrated urine can be normal

Abnormal >2 per LPF, or any in minimally concentrated or alkaline urine

Increased Tamm-Horsfall protein precipitation in tubular lumen

    Glomerular proteinuria/albuminuria

      Pathologic – persistent

      Physiologic – transient

        Fever

        Passive congestion to kidney

        Dehydration + acidic urine

    Hemoglobinuria/myoglobinuria

    Increased secretion of Tamm-Horsfall protein by tubules

Granular casts

≤1 per LPF in concentrated urine can be normal

Abnormal >1 per LPF, or any in minimally concentrated urine

Increased rate of tubular degeneration – coarse and finely granular casts

    AKI – nephrotoxic, ischemic, leptospirosis, rapidly progressive GN

Glomerular proteinuria – precipitation of plasma proteins into tubular fluid – finely granular

Waxy Casts

0 is normal

Final transformation of intrarenal granular casts to translucent protein (classic theory)

Transformation of intrarenal hyaline casts to translucent protein (alternate theory)

Substantial intrarenal time required for this cast to form – implies tubular fluid stasis

± Poor prognosis

Cellular casts

0 is normal; any cellular cast is abnormal and indicates an active intrarenal process

RBC casts

    Glomerulonephritis

    Renal trauma

WBC casts

    Pyelonephritis

    AKI –WBC mixed with epithelial cells and RBC

    Glomerulonephritis

    Acute tubulo-interstitial nephritis – allergic

Renal tubular epithelial cell casts

    AKI – nephrotoxic, ischemic, leptospirosis, rapidly progressive GN

    Acute tubulo-interstitial nephritis – allergic – mixed with WBC

    Conglutination of RTE indicates more severe process than agglutination of RTE

The prevalence of casts identified during manual urine microscopy was 24.4% (108 of 443) in samples submitted to a teaching hospital in one study. Most of the samples had only hyaline casts (83.3%; 90 of 108), 18 (11.1%) samples had both hyaline and nonhyaline casts, and 6 of 108 (5.6%) had only nonhyaline casts. Nonhyaline casts had a prevalence of 4.0% and accounted for 16.7% (18 of 108) of identified casts. All samples with nonhyaline casts contained granular casts (18 of 18), 2 of 18 were characterized with RTE casts, and 1 of 18 was characterized as a WBC cast. Further characterization as finely or granular casts was not provided [31].

"Pseudocasts" are sometimes erroneously identified as casts (Figure 6.66). Linear strands of mucus or fibrin can resemble casts, but they do not have parallel sides and at times are twisted. Fibers and plant material at times can appear linear, but often they have internal structure not seen in casts. Clumps of RBC, WBC, and epithelial cells can also resemble cellular casts, but the width of such aggregates is not uniform and often they are much wider than casts (Figure 6.67). Squamous epithelial cells can look surprisingly like acellular casts when they are rolled up, but they are much larger than casts.

Casts are classified as hyaline, cellular (RBC, WBC, epithelial), granular (fine or coarse), or waxy, based on their predominant composition. The presence of casts in the urine sediment localizes the disease process to the kidneys, and their type and number may provide information about the nature and severity of the disease process. All elements (cells, crystals, bacteria) embedded in the cast matrix are derived from the kidney because the cast forms in the lumen of the renal tubule [18]. The term cylindruria denotes abnormal numbers of casts in the urine sediment [22]. The persistence of even low numbers of casts in the urine sediment can indicate ongoing renal pathology that should be further investigated. Identification of casts during examination of the urine sediment is a well-accepted indicator of kidney disease [8, 18, 163,

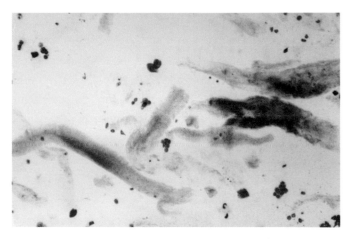

FIGURE 6.66 Pseudocasts. Some of these structures look like casts due to their parallel walls, but they are too big to be casts forming within tubular lumens. Several of these structures have rapidly tapering fine ends (wispy) that often occur with mucus strands.

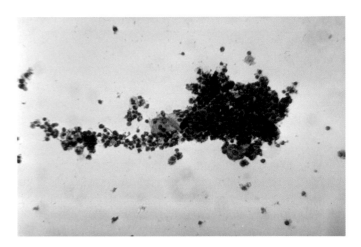

FIGURE 6.67 Pseudocast. At first glance this looks like a WBC cast, especially toward the left side of the liner array of cells. The walls of the "cast" are not as parallel as needed to be certain that this is a cast and the very wide accumulation of WBC to the right cannot fit into a cast. This is an example of a "pseudocast" in which WBC have assumed a linear fashion along a mucus thread.

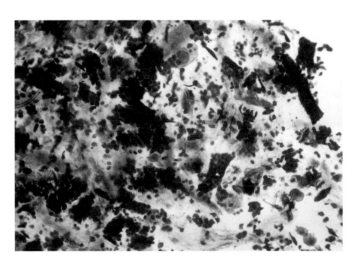

FIGURE 6.68 Cellular casts, renal tubular epithelial in origin. Low power magnification shows numerous cellular casts and abundant free round epithelial cells that look the same as those trapped within the cats. Urine sediment from a nonazotemic young Yorkshire Terrier with lead poisoning.

164]. The number of casts in urine is not necessarily correlated with glomerular filtration rate, but patients with large numbers of casts often have severe renal disease (Figure 6.68). Large numbers of casts are more likely to be observed during acute decompensation of CKD or during AKI. The presence of large numbers of casts is alarming and often indicates an aggressive or severe intrarenal disease process. Small numbers of casts can be seen in either AKI or CKD. Alternatively, no casts may be observed despite the presence of substantial intrarenal disease.

Casts were reported in 28 of 89 (31%) dogs with a diagnosis of azotemic AKI in one report, with one cast type in 25 and two types of casts in three dogs. Rare and 0–5 casts per LPF accounted for 25 of 31(81%), 5–20 casts per LPF for 5 of 31 (16%), and >20 casts per LPF for 1 of 31 (3%). The cast type was finely granular in 12, coarsely granular in 12, and hyaline in 7; no cellular casts were noted in this report [165]. The presence of granular cylindruria was presumably present following necrosis of RTE. Glomerular proteinuria could also have contributed to the development of finely granular casts and hyaline casts.

Cylindruria may occur intermittently, and examination of urine sediment from several samples over time may be helpful. As mentioned previously, automated urine microscopy reports casts merely as hyaline and nonhyaline (Figure 6.69). Consequently, the technician or veterinarian must review the acquired digital images to determine that hyaline casts were identified properly and to assign the proper type to casts classified as nonhyaline by the automated process (granular, cellular, waxy).

Casts typically are not observed during microscopic examination of urine sediment from normal dogs. An occasional cast can be encountered in highly concentrated or acidic urine (up to 2 hyaline casts per HPF and up to 1 granular cast per HPF). Low numbers of granular casts are excreted as a part of the normal senescence of RTE. More than 1000 hyaline casts can be excreted during a 12-hour period of urine collection in normal humans, but typically very few casts are identified in a single sample during urine sediment microscopy. Many thousands of casts can be excreted over a 12-hour period in human patients with certain types CKD, and representative casts will be identified during routine sediment examination of a single urine sample [166]. Granular and cellular casts are more likely to be identified during examination of fresh urine sediment obtained from hospitalized veterinary patients. The cover slip edges tend to accumulate more casts and should be included as a part of the sediment field examination [35].

The clinical relevance of casts is not necessarily associated with the absolute number of casts observed per LPF. For example, a single granular cast per LPF observed in a patient with a USG of 1.015 likely is more important than one granular cast per LPF observed in a urine sample with a USG of 1.050. Casts are named according to their predominant element. For example, a cast that is one-third hyaline and two-thirds coarsely granular would be described as a granular cast on the urinalysis report. Alternatively, such a cast could be called a mixed hyaline-granular cast (Figure 6.70). The term "showers of casts" refers to the excretion of a large number of casts, often of more than one type.

Formation of Casts

Tamm-Horsfall protein (THP; uromodulin) precipitation is the initial event in the formation of casts, except for renal fragments (described later). THP is the most abundant protein in human urine under normal physiological conditions [167] and has also been identified in normal dogs [168]. Uromodulin has been determined to be identical to THP, and these terms can be used interchangeably. The term uromodulin is now preferred, although THP is more commonly used [169]. THP remains in solution in the tubular fluid of normal individuals [170]. Casts form after precipitation of this mucoprotein and trapping of any intact cells, intracellular organelles, brush border (microvilli), or cellular debris that may be present in the tubular lumen at the same time (Figure 6.71 and 6.72). THP is secreted in small quantity by normal RTE in the loop of Henle, distal tubule, and collecting tubule, and most casts form in these regions of the nephron [164, 168, 171–173]. THP is comprised of a meshwork of fibrils. Based

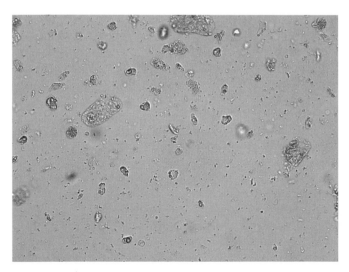

FIGURE 6.69 Note two nonhyaline casts (granular) identified during SediVue® automated microscopy (left center and middle top of image). This urine sample was from an eight-year-old Labrador Retriever with glucosuria, proteinuria, and bacteriuria. Source: Courtesy of Dr. Ronald Lyman, Ft Pierce, FL.

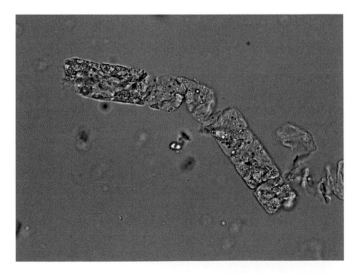

FIGURE 6.70 Mixed waxy and granular cast. Source: Reproduced with permission of Dr. Heather L. Wamsley, Bradenton, FL, USA.

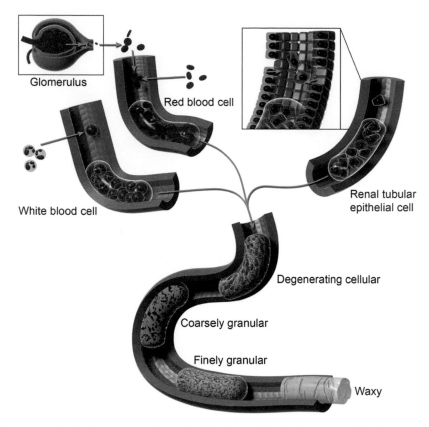

FIGURE 6.71 Addis and Lippman classic theory of cast formation. In this model, cellular casts (RBC, WBC, renal tubular epithelial) form as these cells enter tubular lumens. In an acute process, these cellular casts would be excreted as such into urine. In less acute processes, cellular casts undergo breakdown first into a degenerating cellular cast, and then to granular casts (coarse and granular), and then to a final transformation to a waxy cast. The time a cast spends within the kidney determines what degeneration or transformation will take place from the original cellular cast. Source: Illustration by Tim Vojt, reproduced with permission of The Ohio State University.

on ultrastructural studies, all casts seem to share a similar underlying fibrillar structure. Hyaline casts consist entirely of this structure. The same fibrillar structure was also found to be closely associated with epithelial cells and RBC within cellular and waxy casts [174]. Factors that increase the secretion or concentration of THP favor its precipitation and increase the likelihood of cast formation. Increased concentration of THP in renal tubules can occur during exercise and dehydration [170]. Some renal diseases may result in increased secretion of THP, but this effect of renal disease has not been well studied [171]. Decreased urinary excretion of THP has been described in dogs with progressive CKD, presumably as a result of less renal tubular mass available for THP synthesis [168]. Less THP excretion into urine could result in less generation of casts in patients with more advanced CKD.

Casts form most readily in the distal tubules as a consequence of maximal acidity, highest solute concentration, and lowest tubular flow rate in this segment of the nephron. Results of microdissection studies indicated that most hyaline casts formed in the distal and collecting tubules [164]. Processes in the proximal tubule, however, can contribute to cellular and granular cast formation (described further below).

During severe AKI, proximal tubular cast formation (cellular and granular) is sometimes observed during histopathological evaluation of renal tissue from dogs and cats (Figure 6.73). Such intrarenal casts may not be excreted intact into urine, but they can add debris to the tubular lumen that favors cast formation more distally.

Unusually wide casts of any type are referred to as "broad casts" or "renal failure casts" (Figure 6.74). They form either in the collecting tubule or in pathologically dilated portions of the distal tubule [163]. The diameter of a broad cast is several times that of other casts. Tubular flow normally is rapid in the collecting tubules, making cast formation difficult in this segment of the nephron. Thus, the presence of broad casts suggests severe intrarenal stasis or tubular obstruction. Broad casts often are waxy in nature because of the associated intrarenal stasis required for this cast type to form, but any kind of cast can be classified as a broad cast. Their presence should be noted during urine sediment microscopy, because the more severe type of disease process that can account for the formation of these wide casts may warrant a worse prognosis. The abrupt appearance of broad casts may be a favorable prognostic sign when oliguria resolves and normal urine

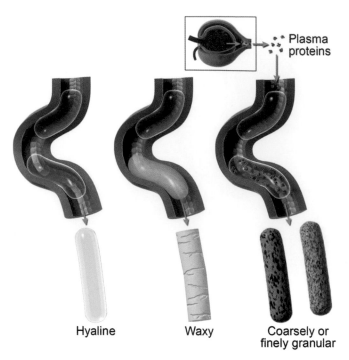

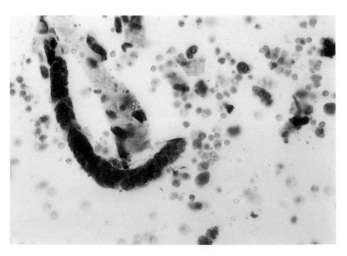

FIGURE 6.74 A long coarsely granular cast is seen in the left field. A "broad cast" is seen just to the right of the coarsely granular cast. This broad cast is quite wide and has a large hyaline component with some coarse granules (mixed cast). The width of the broad cast is about twice the width of other casts. The finding of broad casts may indicate a more severe renal process since they form in the wide collecting tubule or a pathologically dilated portion of the distal nephron. Increased numbers of WBC and RBC and occasional nonsquamous epithelial cells are seen throughout the background in this field.

FIGURE 6.72 The image to the left shows the genesis of a hyaline cast as pure precipitation of Tamm-Horsfall mucoprotein (THP). The middle panel shows an alternative explanation for the genesis of a waxy cast forming directly from a hyaline cast (no cellular degeneration involved). The image on the right shows another mechanism to explain the generation of granular casts in which plasma proteins cross the glomerulus and enter tubular fluid where they precipitate along with THP. Source: Illustration by Tim Vojt, reproduced with permission of The Ohio State University.

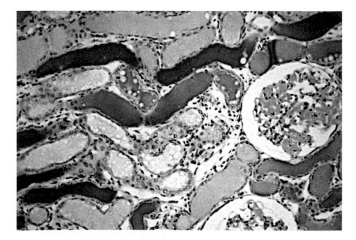

FIGURE 6.73 Renal histopathology from a dog with high level of renal proteinuria (H&E stain). Note extensive dark and light pink staining of the tubular fluid. This staining is characteristic of tubular fluid that contains substantial amounts of protein within the tubular fluid. This stain does not specifically stain Tamm-Horsfall mucoprotein (THP), but the presence of intratubular protein favors precipitation of THP and hyaline cast formation. It also favors the precipitation of these plasma proteins into granules that can be found in granular casts. Source: Reproduced with permission of Dr. Donald Meuten, North Carolina State University College of Veterinary Medicine, Raleigh NC.

output or polyuria develops and previously formed broad casts are excreted in the urine. Very thin casts referred to as "cylindroids" may form in areas of tubular compression associated with interstitial inflammation, edema, or tubular swelling. Cylindroids are usually a form of hyaline cast that is longer and thinner than usual, and they may have tapered ends [175].

The duration of time a cast is retained inside the kidney before being excreted into urine determines the type of cast that will be observed during urine sediment microscopy. Local stasis occurs during decreased flow of urine through certain nephrons and allows cellular casts to degenerate [163]. Urinary casts and other formed elements found in the sediment may reflect specific kidney diseases, but their presence lacks specificity for a definitive diagnosis. An exception to this rule is the identification of bacterial casts, which strongly supports a diagnosis of acute pyelonephritis [176].

Detection of increased number of casts (cylindruria) in the urine sediment generally indicates the presence of renal tubular injury, which certainly is the case for the presence of RTE in cellular casts and mixed cellular casts that contain RTE. Granular casts can indicate renal tubular injury if they arise from cellular degeneration within the kidney before they are excreted in urine. Hyaline and granular casts can sometimes form as a result of glomerular disease and the associated proteinuria; thus, their presence is not a specific indicator of renal tubular injury. In these instances, the granules in granular casts are precipitates of circulating proteins that traverse the glomerulus. Hyaline casts can also form in the absence of any structural disease in the kidney.

Hyaline Casts

Hyaline casts are the most common type of cast observed and can be seen in low numbers in normal dogs and cats (0–2/ LPF) with concentrated urine and in higher numbers in patients with kidney disease. Hyaline casts are transparent and may contain a few granules or lipid droplets (Figure 6.75), but the largest portion of the cast typically is clear and nonrefractive (Figure 6.76). Hyaline casts are likely under-reported during routine urine sediment microscopy because their optical density is very low and similar to that of urine, making them hard to see (Figure 6.77). Failure to identify hyaline casts is much more likely when the microscope condenser and diaphragm have not been adjusted to allow less light

transmission through the wet mount to provide adequate contrast (Figure 6.78). Hyaline casts are easily identified during phase microscopy [177]. Supravital staining imparts a light pink to lavender color to hyaline casts. Hyaline casts are sometimes confused with waxy casts, which are translucent but darker staining (see waxy casts below). Care must be taken not to confuse hyaline casts with mucus threads. Hyaline casts are less likely to be seen in urine that is highly

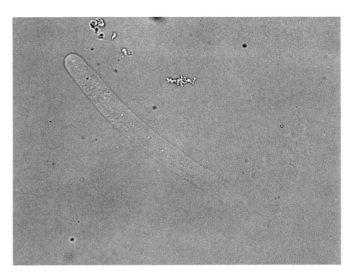

FIGURE 6.77 Pure hyaline cast. The portion of this cast at the upper left of this image is more easily seen. Faint outlines of the walls of this cast are more difficult to see in the lower portion of this image. Hyaline casts are transparent. Source: Reproduced with permission of Dr. Heather L. Wamsley, Bradenton, FL, USA.

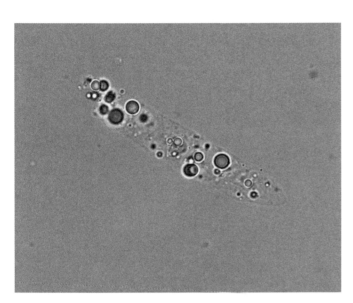

FIGURE 6.75 Hyaline cast with lipid droplets. Unstained sediment. The walls of this cast are very close in optical density of the surrounding urine. Source: Reproduced with permission of Dr. Heather L. Wamsley, Bradenton, FL, USA.

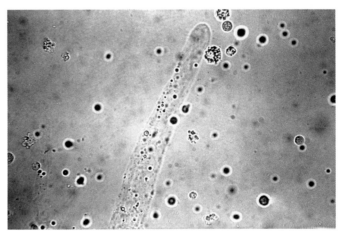

FIGURE 6.78 Hyaline cast (unstained). A single hyaline cast is seen in the central part of this image. Notice that this cast is transparent. The lighting has been decreased and the condenser moved to optimize contrast visualization of the hyaline cast which has similar optical density to that of urine. It is easy to overlook hyaline casts when the lighting is not adjusted. This hyaline cast contain a few small granules, but the cast would be called hyaline since precipitated matrix protein is the predominant feature of this cast.

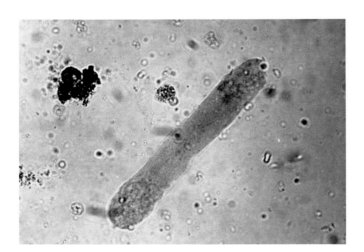

FIGURE 6.76 A single hyaline cast. This hyaline cast lightly takes up purple color from the stain. Notice that elements on the other side of the cast can be seen.

alkaline or dilute. We have occasionally documented hyaline casts in horses despite their normally high urine pH.

Previously, hyaline casts were thought to be precipitates of serum proteins. This notion unfortunately still persists, although now it is known that hyaline casts are composed principally of THP with small contributions from serum proteins [164, 178]. The presence of serum proteins in tubular fluid, especially albumin, contributes to the precipitation of THP and is associated with the formation of hyaline casts [164]. THP was originally identified in hyaline casts that formed in patients with chronic glomerulonephritis and acute renal failure [172]. Precipitation of THP in the matrix of casts is favored by acidic pH, high tubular fluid solute concentration, and low tubular flow rates. THP rapidly dissolves in an alkaline environment and can reprecipitate when the sample is acidified [164]. Hyaline casts have different appearance and complexity under bright-field, immunofluorescence, and electron microscopy. Convoluted hyaline casts can have enough complexity to cause confusion with cellular casts, especially when they assume a wrinkled appearance [18, 179].

The presence of hyaline casts does not always indicate primary renal disease, because processes such as fever, passive congestion of the kidney, and seizures can be associated with hyaline cylindruria that resolves after the underlying nonrenal condition abates. Dehydration and the associated high osmolality of tubular fluid favor precipitation of THP. Increased excretion of hyaline casts has been observed after fever, strenuous exercise, and furosemide therapy in healthy humans [170]. Loss of glomerular polyanion (negative charges that normally repel serum proteins) during dehydration can lead to temporary glomerular proteinuria that favors THP precipitation. Hemoglobin or myoglobin in tubular fluid also favors THP precipitation and transient hyaline cast formation.

Persistent hyaline cylindruria indicates primary kidney disease that is often associated with proteinuria that favors THP precipitation (Figure 6.79). In these instances, the reagent dipstrip will be positive for protein, and the urine protein/creatinine ratio will be increased. Hyaline casts are commonly seen in patients with primary glomerular disease (e.g. amyloidosis, glomerulonephritis) characterized by marked proteinuria. Hyaline casts can also be present with other types of CKD and AKI, as can other types of casts. They are sometimes seen in patients with renal tubular diseases that decrease renal tubular reabsorption of proteins or add inflammatory proteins to urine. Hyaline casts are found in most humans with glomerulonephritis and acute interstitial nephritis [18]. Although hyaline casts are usually found along with other types of casts in humans with renal disorders, they are often the only type of cast identified in patients with nonrenal conditions. [18]

Granular Casts

Granular casts are the second most commonly observed type of cast, and 0–1/LPF granular casts can be seen in normal dogs and cats with concentrated urine. Larger numbers can be identified in patients with active kidney disease. Care must be

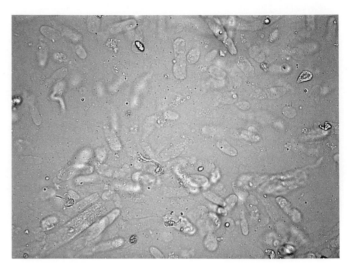

FIGURE 6.79 Showers of hyaline casts captured by SediVue® automated microscopy. Large numbers of hyaline casts as the single abnormal finding in the urine sediment are often associated with renal proteinuria. Source: Courtesy of IDEXX Laboratories. Copyright © 2022, IDEXX Laboratories, Inc. All rights reserved. Used with permission.

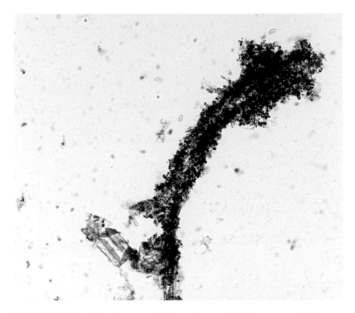

FIGURE 6.80 Pseudocast. At first glance, this linear array looks like a granular cast. Upon closer inspection, this is not a cast but alignment of crystals and particulate debris and sperm. The sudden widening of this array at the top is not compatible with a true cast. Struvite crystals are seen free and embedded in the linear array.

taken that degenerating RTE and transitional epithelial cells are not misidentified as granular casts. In these instances (socalled pseudocast), the margins of the suspected cast are not uniformly parallel, and these cells are shorter and rounder than actual casts (Figure 6.80). Granules in casts have traditionally been thought to arise as a result of progressive degenerative changes in RTE that initially result in the appearance of coarsely granular and then finely granular casts over time [163, 172] Identification of casts that appear to be in transition from cellular to granular morphology supports this assumption (Figure 6.71). In a study using immunofluorescence, granules in casts were found to contain serum proteins in patients with glomerulonephritis, but granules did not fluoresce when the diagnosis was AKI. Filtered serum proteins adhered to the THP and appeared as granules when glomerular disease had resulted in leakage of serum proteins across the glomerulus into tubular fluid. During severe AKI, the granules arose from cellular necrosis and degeneration within the nephron (presumably RTE) [172]. Another study of granular casts also identified THP staining in the matrix of the cast and staining of granules in the cast for several serum proteins [173]. Granular casts can appear quickly in urine after exercise in normal humans, a finding compatible with direct incorporation of filtered serum proteins into the cast matrix, because sufficient time would not elapse in such a situation for granules to arise from degeneration of cells [173]. If bilirubin is present in urine, a characteristic yellow-to-brown pigment can be observed in granular casts. Bilirubin crystals also may be incorporated into casts that form under these conditions [7].

The clinical relevance of coarse (Figure 6.81) or finely granular casts (Figure 6.82) generally has been considered the same, but recently this notion has been questioned. Coarse granules were thought to be more likely to arise from degeneration of cells in casts, although some filtered proteins can also as coarse granules [180]. In one study, fine granules in casts from proteinuric patients were considered more likely to occur as a result of filtration of plasma proteins across the glomerulus, whereas coarse granules in nonproteinuric patients were thought more likely to develop from degeneration of cellular elements [18]. Granules have been reported to originate from leukocytes, RTE, unidentified mucopolysaccharide, or bacteria in another study [181]. Shedding of brush border

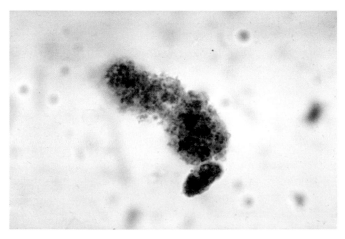

FIGURE 6.81   Coarsely granular cast. Source: Reproduced with permission of Dr. Richard Scott, Animal Medical Center, New York, NY, USA.

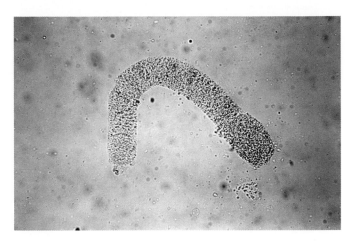

FIGURE 6.82   Finely granular cast. Unstained urinary sediment from a dog. Finely granular cast (400×). Granular casts represent renal cellular degeneration (Addis Theory) or precipitation of filtered plasma proteins.

(swollen microvilli) from proximal RTE, as may occur in some types of AKI [182, 183], may represent another source of granules in casts. Granules in granular casts could also be composed of degenerating intracellular organelles from proximal tubular cells, as has been demonstrated in dogs with early ethylene glycol toxicity [184]. Amorphous granular casts and necrotic debris were also described in the proximal tubular lumina of dogs with gentamicin toxicity [185].

Rarely identified sources of granules in casts include bacteria [176], bacterial variants, [186], and crystals. Bacteria in casts may be densely or sparsely packed. Calcium crystal casts have been described in humans with hyperparathyroidism [187], and calcium oxalate casts have been reported in ethylene glycol poisoning [188]. Methotrexate, sulfadiazine, and immunoglobulin light chains have also been encountered in urinary casts that appear granular [188]. Bacteria in casts were difficult to identify in unstained sediment but were easily seen using phase or interference contrast microscopy [176]. Intravascular hemolysis can result in large amounts of hemoglobin being filtered across the glomerulus into tubular fluid, favoring precipitation of THP and trapping of variably sized precipitates of hemoglobin that can be incorporated into coarsely or finely granular casts (Figure 6.83).

Fatty casts are an uncommon type of coarsely granular cast containing lipid granules (Figure 6.84). Fat accumulation in RTE and the subsequent shedding and degeneration of these cells lead to the formation and appearance of this type of cast. Humans with glomerular disease or diabetes mellitus are at higher risk of developing this type of cast. The fat droplets are highly refractile and may be determined to contain cholesterol by use of polarizing microscopy (i.e. Maltese-cross formation) or triglycerides by Sudan staining [7, 175].

Excessive numbers of granular casts indicate renal pathology, but not a specific disease (Figure 6.85). Excessive numbers of granular casts are associated with disease processes (e.g. AKI) that cause accelerated degeneration of

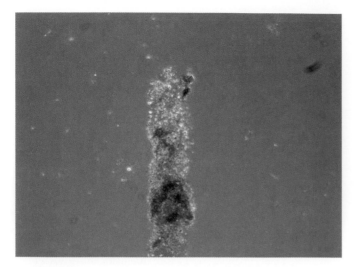

FIGURE 6.83 Granular cast (phase microscopy). Granules within this cast are precipitates of hemoglobin. This cast was originally misidentified as an RBC cast due to the orange-red color of the granules. These granules vary in size substantially. This dog had systemic hemolysis and hemoglobinuria that precipitated into this cast. Source: Reproduced with permission of Dr. Michael Horton, Fairborn, OH, USA.

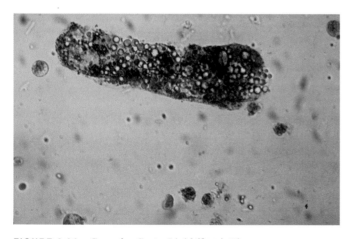

FIGURE 6.84 Granular Cast – Lipid (fatty). The numerous granules in this cast are highly refractile and are likely to be lipid in nature. Lipid droplets are the result of cellular degenerative processes. A few swollen WBC with red-staining nuclei are also seen in the background. Source: Reproduced with permission of Dr. Richard Scott, Animal Medical Center, New York, NY, USA.

renal tubular cells. Granular casts can also develop in patients with glomerular disease when large amounts of filtered plasma proteins precipitate into a protein matrix in tubular fluid. Hyaline and granular casts were reported during urine sediment examination of all dogs with renal amyloidosis in one study. These casts were associated with severe proteinuria and formed in isosthenuric and hyposthenuric urine [189]. Daily cast counts (hyaline and granular) using randomly collected urine samples can provide an inexpensive means of identifying early renal tubular damage in critically ill human

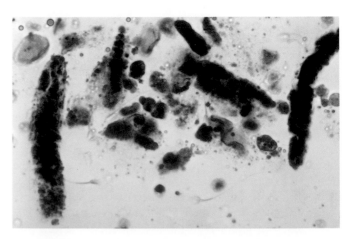

FIGURE 6.85 "Shower" of coarse granular casts (high power view). Some WBC can be identified in the background. Several large round cells cannot be identified due to degenerative changes; some of these could be renal tubular epithelium. A few sperm are also seen.

patients, regardless of specific cause. This technique can be used to evaluate patients receiving nephrotoxic drugs when serum creatinine concentration has not yet increased above baseline and may be especially important because cast numbers have been reported to decrease by the time serum creatinine concentration increases during AKI [190]. We have used the sudden appearance of casts or increasing numbers of casts to make clinical decisions in veterinary patients with AKI.

The number of RTE and granular casts identified during microscopy of fresh urine sediment by a nephrologist has been used in a scoring system to predict worsening AKI associated with acute tubular necrosis or prerenal AKI in hospitalized human patients. The presence of granular casts or RTE was associated with high positive and negative predictive value for a final diagnosis of acute tubular necrosis [191–193]. A similar assessment and scoring system has not been evaluated yet in veterinary medicine.

Waxy Casts

Waxy casts (Figure 6.86) are the third most common type of casts after hyaline and granular casts. Unlike other types of casts, waxy casts are relatively stable over time in dilute and alkaline urine. They are easily identified because of their high refractive index and homogenous translucent appearance. They can be convoluted and often contain cracks and blunt ends, thought to be associated with their brittle nature (Figure 6.87). Staining of waxy casts is variable, but they may appear pink to dark purple when the urine sediment is stained using Sedi-Stain (Figure 6.88).

According to one hypothesis, waxy casts represent the final stage of the degeneration of finely granular casts in the kidney. Any renal disorder that results in the formation of epithelial or granular casts may, thus, result in formation of waxy casts if sufficient time for degeneration occurs within the

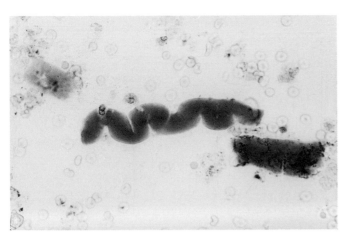

FIGURE 6.86 Two waxy casts. Intense uptake of stain into the casts with faint staining of RBC in the background. Note the crack on the bottom wall of the larger cast to the right – this occurs due to the brittle nature of the protein that comprises this cast. Waxy casts are classically thought to represent the final transformation of cellular breakdown products within the renal tubules to this homogeneous translucent protein.

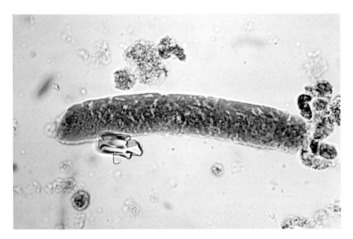

FIGURE 6.87 Waxy cast. Notice the translucent, but not transparent, nature of this cast. The cast is blue to purple from stain uptake. Also notice that there are several small cracks along the border of this cast; this is a common occurrence in waxy casts. There are several WBC in the background. A cluster of crystals just beneath the cast is likely to be struvite.

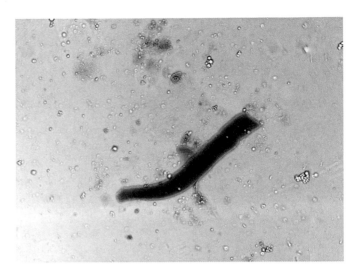

FIGURE 6.88 Waxy cast (stained). Same sediment as in Figure 6.87. This waxy cast intensely took up blue stain.

kidney. In this scenario, the cast undergoes fusion of all of its granules into a waxy mass of high refractive index [163]. Another group was unable to find evidence of the evolution of waxy casts from cellular and granular casts. The same group determined that waxy casts consisted of condensed amorphous material associated with a fibrillar matrix and speculated that waxy casts represent a further transformation of hyaline casts [174, 181].

The presence of waxy casts in urine sediment is never normal. Compatible with both hypotheses described above, the presence of waxy casts suggests substantial chronic intrarenal stasis because waxy casts take considerable time to form.

They have often been described in azotemic patients with CKD and, consequently, have been called "renal failure casts." They are associated with advanced CKD, and their presence is usually considered an ominous finding. In early reports, the presence of waxy casts strongly suggested a diagnosis of renal amyloidosis in dogs [70], but in one large case series of dogs with renal amyloidosis, hyaline and granular casts were reported in all dogs during urine sediment microscopy, but no waxy casts were identified [189]. Cylindruria was observed in 42% of dogs with renal amyloidosis in another report. These casts were hyaline in 22%, granular in 35%, hyaline and granular in 17%, and a combination of hyaline, granular, and waxy in 26% [194]. It is likely that these casts formed as a result of the proteinuria that characterizes glomerular amyloidosis and development of CKD.

The clinical situations in which waxy casts appear are not well documented in human medicine. Waxy casts were observed, often in low numbers, in approximately 14% of human patients with known glomerular disease. They were more likely to be observed in patients with postinfectious glomerulonephritis and renal amyloidosis as compared patients with other glomerular diseases. Waxy casts were also encountered more commonly in patients with higher serum creatinine concentrations and in patients who had other types of casts in the urinary sediment [195].

Cellular Casts

Cellular casts are the least common type of cast found in urine sediment, and they are never observed in normal animals. Observation of even a single cellular cast signifies an underlying kidney disease process and prompts further patient evaluation. Cellular casts can be comprised of RBC, WBC, or RTE or may contain combinations of these cell types and be referred to as mixed cellular casts. Cellular casts are reported far less frequently in veterinary medicine than in human medicine. Conditions during preanalytical handling of the urine specimen likely account for this discrepancy because in veterinary medicine, urine samples are not often analyzed immediately after collection. The cells in cellular casts degenerate rapidly, and the casts themselves disintegrate quickly. Casts in which cellular outlines are still visible but the cell type cannot be identified are reported as degenerative casts. In these instances, degeneration may have occurred within the kidney or after urine sample collection. When the identity of the cell type in the cast is uncertain, the observer is often biased by the predominant cell type in the urine sediment when reporting the cast type.

Cellular casts disintegrate rapidly when urine sediment examination is delayed, and the cells from the cast are released into the urine as free elements. Excessive force during centrifugation also may disrupt cellular casts, especially RBC and WBC casts that can be easily damaged. Nephrologists in human medicine often evaluate fresh urine sediment examination while the patient waits. Examination of urine sediment from sick dogs and cats within 15 minutes of collection sometimes yields a surprising number of cellular casts (Chew – personal observations). Remote reference laboratories to which urine samples have been shipped rarely report cellular casts.

Epithelial Cell Casts

Epithelial cell casts are the most common type of cellular cast identified in veterinary medicine. These casts are easily identified when the morphology of the constituent renal tubular epithelial cells is maintained. Renal epithelial cells in casts and those that are free in the urine undergo rapid degeneration after excretion, making their identification difficult. Renal epithelial cells are considerably larger than WBC and much larger than RBC. Distinct cell outlines with basal nuclei typify this type of cast, which may consist nearly entirely of RTE (Figure 6.89), or variable numbers of renal tubular epithelial cells can be separated by matrix protein (Figure 6.90). Even if only a few renal tubular cells can be identified in a hyaline matrix, the cast should be reported as an epithelial cell cast. If a cast contains large degenerating cells that still have distinct cell outlines and few large granules, the cast should be reported as a degenerating cellular cast. Fatty degeneration of damaged RTE can occur before desquamation of these cells into tubular fluid [163]. The presence of free renal tubular epithelial cells in urine facilitates the definitive identification of renal tubular cellular casts [18].

The common type of epithelial cellular cast forms as individual renal tubular epithelial cells from various segments of the nephron become entrapped by precipitated matrix proteins. Fibrils of matrix protein may attach to damaged renal tubular cells in the tubular lumen and draw the cells into the cast [174]. No serum protein fractions were identified in renal tubular cell casts in one study [172].

Renal fragments are a type of epithelial cell cast that is identified less commonly than are renal epithelial cellular

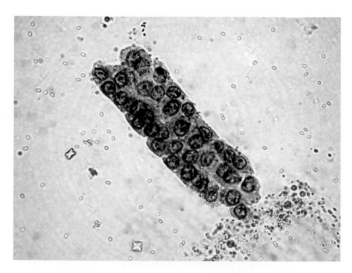

FIGURE 6.89 Renal tubular epithelial cast. Cellular casts were observed on day 5 of a "cast watch" in which urine microscopy was performed daily during treatment with the potentially nephrotoxic aminoglycoside gentamicin. Note that this is an example of conglutination rather than agglutination of renal tubular epithelial cells. During conglutination, whole segments of the renal tubular structure are sloughed into the urine. During agglutination, renal tubular cells are shed separately into the matrix protein. The presence of renal epithelial cell casts often indicates severe acute renal tubular injury whereas the finding of renal fragments indicates an even more severe process. A few calcium oxalate dihydrate crystals are seen in the background; other apparent crystalline material cannot be identified with certainty. A digital camera was placed over the microscope eye piece to acquire this image. Source: Reproduced with permission of Dr. Brian Luria, Florida Veterinary Specialists Tampa, FL, USA.

casts. Renal fragments form by the process of conglutination, whereas RTE casts form by the agglutination of cells in the tubular lumen. Renal fragments form when blocks of RTE desquamate from the tubular basement membrane (conglutination). These tubular cells maintain their epithelial connections with one another, and the resulting renal fragments do not contain matrix protein, as observed in other types of casts. These fragments often appear as sleeve-like cylinders, and they contain at least three cells that have maintained intercellular connections [196]. The three-dimensional circumferential appearance helps to identify this cast. Sometimes, a lumen can be seen within the sleeve-like renal fragment (Figure 6.91). Often, it is not possible during wet mount urine sediment examination to determine the precise location in the nephron from which the RTE was shed. Cytologic features of free RTE, however, may suggest its site of origin as proximal tubule, collecting tubule, or other nephron segment [7, 106]. It is unlikely that intact RTE from the proximal tubules can traverse the thin loops of Henle and appear in the urine. It is important to report renal fragments when they occur because their presence indicates disruption of tubular basement membranes and more severe renal injury.

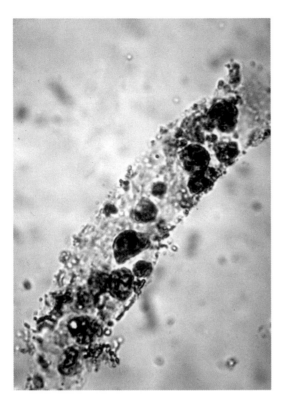

FIGURE 6.90 Renal tubular epithelial cell cast (unstained). This cast is predominantly hyaline in nature, but it contains several renal tubular epithelial cells. This cast is named for its most important element, that of the renal tubular cell. Source: Reproduced with permission of Dr. Richard Scott, Animal Medical Center, New York, NY, USA.

FIGURE 6.91 Renal tubular epithelial cell cast. This cast is an example of "conglutination" in which a fragment of tubular epithelial cells has been lost together, rather than by individual sloughing of RTE into the cast matrix. Notice the three-dimensional nature of this cast in which a lumen can be seen with an opening to the left.

The finding of RTE casts in urine sediment indicates that the casts spent little time in the kidney after formation; otherwise, they would have been transformed into granular casts. The finding of renal tubular epithelial cellular casts or

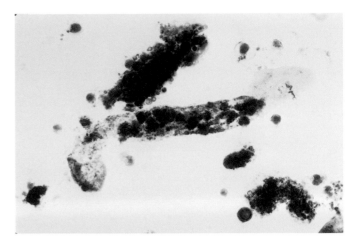

FIGURE 6.92 Coarsely granular cast at top of field, degenerating cellular cast in middle, and coarse to finely granular cast at bottom of field. Cellular outlines can be seen in the degenerating cellular cast but the origin of the cells cannot be determined with certainty due to lack of cellular detail. Source: Reproduced by permission of Dr. Richard Scott, Animal Medical Center, New York, NY, USA.

renal fragments indicates a severe ongoing process that is actively damaging the kidney. Renal tubular epithelial cellular casts can be identified in dogs and cats with ischemic or nephrotoxic renal injury. Acute interstitial nephritis and pyelonephritis can be associated with renal tubular epithelial cellular casts. Leptospirosis in dogs is an example of AKI and interstitial nephritis, in which renal tubular epithelial cellular casts can be observed, and they also may be seen with renal infarction. Renal tubular epithelial cellular casts may be the only type of cast observed or they may be observed in combination with granular and hyaline casts, depending on the extent of renal injury. They can also be observed along with WBC casts. Degenerating renal tubular epithelial cellular casts that have spent more time in the kidney before excretion likely have the same clinical relevance as do more well-preserved renal tubular epithelial cellular casts (Figure 6.92).

White Blood Cell Casts

WBC casts sometimes are called "pus casts" (Figure 6.93). They are easy to identify in fresh urine sediment in which cellular detail is well preserved. WBC are larger than RBC and usually smaller than renal tubular epithelial cells. As with free WBC in urine, peroxidase staining may facilitate the positive identification of WBC in casts. WBC casts are fragile and unlikely to be observed when urine sediment examination is delayed. In these instances, WBC that initially were trapped within the cast are liberated into urine as the WBC cast disintegrates. Supravital stains highlight nuclear detail and promote identification of WBC in these casts. Phase microscopy can also facilitate the identification of WBC in casts. WBC can be densely packed in the cast or they may occupy only a small portion of the cast. Degenerative changes in such casts can make it impossible to differentiate WBC from renal tubular

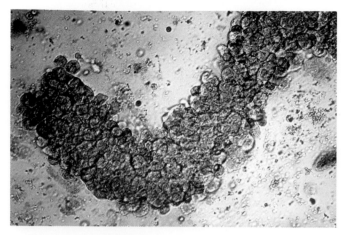

FIGURE 6.93 WBC cast. Note densely packed WBC in this cast with parallel walls. It is difficult to identify the WBC when many cells are layered on top of each other, but neutrophils can be more easily identified near the periphery of this cast.

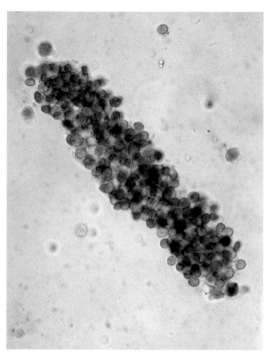

FIGURE 6.94 RBC Cast. Note the preponderance of RBC packed within the parallel walls of this cast. There are a few WBC interspersed among the RBC. The cast is named for the predominating cell.

epithelial cells. It is important to be certain that what has been identified as a WBC cast is not actually a pseudocast arising from WBC adhering in a linear fashion to a mucus or fibrin strand during centrifugation (Figure 6.67).

The presence of WBC casts is never normal and indicates active renal inflammation that is often associated with pyelonephritis. WBC enter the renal tubular lumen between and through tubular epithelial cells during active renal interstitial inflammation. The diagnosis of bacterial pyelonephritis is more certain when WBC casts are observed in the urine sediment along with pyuria and bacteriuria. The presence of large numbers of WBC casts is compatible with the diagnosis of acute pyelonephritis, but not pathognomonic. The specific diagnosis of acute pyelonephritis is associated with the identification of bacterial casts [176]. Phase contrast microscopy can be useful to identify bacterial casts, which otherwise can be difficult to identify and result in the misidentification of observed casts as granular in nature [18]. WBC casts can also occur in patients with nephrosis and other types of inflammatory renal disease, such as acute glomerulonephritis and acute interstitial nephritis [176].

Red Blood Cell Casts

RBC casts are the most fragile type of the cellular casts and the least commonly identified in the urine of dogs and cats. It is impossible to identify RBC casts when urine sediment examination is delayed, because RBC are rapidly lost from these casts. Failure to examine fresh urine sediment may explain the lack of descriptions of RBC casts in veterinary medicine. RBC casts may consist entirely of RBC or may contain primarily RBC mixed with a few WBC or renal tubular epithelial cells (Figure 6.94). When similar numbers of RBC, WBC, and renal tubular epithelial cells are found within a cast, it is called a mixed cellular cast. Hemoglobin casts that form with hemolysis and hemoglobinuria may contain hemoglobin

precipitates that resemble RBC, but, unlike RBC, the size of these precipitates varies markedly (Figure 6.83).

RBC casts identified during urine sediment examination are never normal. The aggregation of RBC into casts indicates intrarenal bleeding. They may be seen with acute glomerulonephritis, renal trauma (e.g. renal biopsy), renal infarction, acute tubulointerstitial nephritis, or after strenuous exercise. In acute interstitial nephritis, RBC from the renal interstitium enter the tubular lumina through disruptions in the tubular basement membrane [18, 197]. RBC traversing the glomerulus have been demonstrated in Bowman's space and in RBC casts in models of glomerular disease [107, 108]. RBC casts must be differentiated from free RBC arranged in a linear fashion in the urine sediment. Blood casts are variants of RBC casts in which the RBC have lost their distinct cell membrane outlines, but in which hemoglobin persists. Blood casts are best seen in unstained urine sediment and have the same clinical relevance as do intact RBC casts.

Mixed Casts

Not all casts have a single defining characteristic. Some casts fall into a mixed category in which the cast has features of two different primary types of casts (Figure 6.95). Most often, the cast is named for the process or cell type that predominates within the cast, but such casts can also be called mixed casts (Figure 6.96). The most common type of mixed cast is the hyaline-granular cast (Figure 6.74). Granular-cellular, granular-fatty, waxy-granular, and waxy-cellular mixed casts are also sometimes identified [18, 70]. The clinical relevance of a

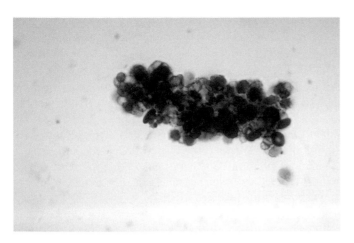

FIGURE 6.95 WBC and RBC cast-mixed. Note that neutrophils are most readily seen along the edges of the cast. There are also several RBC within the cast. It is called a mixed cast as both the WBC and RBC components of the cast are important.

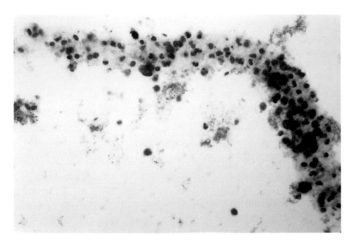

FIGURE 6.96 Mixed cellular cast. RBC and WBC predominate as the cell type on the left upper end of this cast. RTE predominate as the cell type at the right and lower part of this cast. Urine sediment from a young female Doberman with acute onset of polyuria and polydipsia, likely due to pyelonephritis.

mixed cast is related to the two types of processes or cells found in the cast.

Crystalline Casts

Casts comprised of crystalline material rarely have been noted in veterinary medicine. Many uric acid crystalline casts were reported in a dog with lymphoma one day after treatment with l-asparaginase; serum uric acid was increased at the same time (Figure 6.97). Large amounts of free amorphous crystals observed during urine microscopy were identified as 100% uric acid dihydrate by infrared spectroscopy. These findings were attributed to tumor lysis syndrome [198]. Calcium carbonate crystalline casts of unknown significance are sometimes observed during urine microscopy from horses (DJC personal observation).

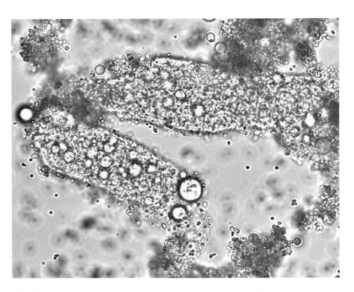

FIGURE 6.97 Uric acid crystal casts, high power (60× objective) in unstained sediment. The urine was cloudy and contained these casts one day after treatment of lymphoma with l-asparaginase. Crystals within the cast appear to be the same type as in the background. Source: Image from figure 3 in Tvedten et al. [198]. John Wiley & Sons. Used with permission.

CRYSTALS

Considerable confusion exists about the clinical relevance of crystalluria in dogs and cats, regardless of the presence or absence of clinical signs. Microscopic crystalluria is often of no diagnostic importance when discovered in urine of otherwise healthy dogs and cats. Crystalluria often occurs in the absence of disease, especially in highly concentrated urine that has been stored under refrigeration.

Urine pH, temperature, solubility of the crystalloid, concentration of the crystalloid (degree of saturation), urine osmolality, presence of crystal promoters and inhibitors, and the time between urine collection and analysis act together to determine whether or not a crystal will precipitate from solution and be visible during urine sediment examination. The concentration of crystalloids in urine is influenced by diet, systemic acid–base balance, and specific metabolic abnormalities (e.g., hypercalcemia, portosystemic shunting, cystinuria). Evaporation of water from the urine sample during storage also contributes to crystal formation.

The time elapsed from sample collection to urine sediment examination and whether or not refrigeration was used are important to note during the interpretation of crystals reported on urine sediment examination. Crystals are commonly observed during urine sediment examination, especially in samples that have been stored in the refrigerator before analysis. Cooling of urine to room temperature occurs quickly after sample collection, and refrigeration likely increases the precipitation of all types of crystals in supersaturated urine. The clinical relevance of crystalluria in urine that has been refrigerated is dubious because such crystals might not have been present in the urine when it was at body temperature. Crystals observed in urine may form de novo during transport to the laboratory or during storage at room or refrigerator temperature. Rewarming and remixing of cold urine do not necessarily cause crystals to go back into solution.

Crystals formed more often in the refrigerated samples without preservative compared to samples maintained at room temperature with preservative at 24 hours in one study. Crystal formation further increased by 72 hours of urine storage in the refrigerator affecting 25% of the samples, similar to findings in other studies of *ex vivo* crystal formation [99].

Struvite crystals formed during storage in 28% of urine samples that did not have struvite crystals identified at body temperature [199]. Calcium oxalate crystals formed more commonly during storage than did struvite crystals in another study [200]. In general, more numerous and larger crystals formed during longer storage times and during refrigeration. The mean size of crystals increased during refrigeration as compared to storage at room temperature, an effect that was more pronounced for calcium oxalate than for struvite. Urine should be evaluated within 60 minutes of collection to minimize temperature- and time-dependent effects on *in vitro* crystal formation [200]. If the presence or absence of specific crystal types in urine is important in the clinical decision making process, conclusions should be based upon prompt evaluation of a fresh urine sample that has not been stored at room or refrigerator temperature.

Most crystals in urine sediment can be identified by considering crystal morphology, urine pH, and the nature of birefringence under polarized light [201]. Phase microscopy can also be useful to identify crystals [202]. Unusual crystals can be further characterized by a variety of qualitative and quantitative methods. Electron microscopy, infrared spectroscopy, and high-performance liquid chromatography may be needed for definitive identification of unusual crystals [201]. The chemical composition of unusual crystals sometimes can be determined by polarizing microscopy or optical crystallography employing oils of known refractive index. X-ray microanalysis, Fourier transformation infrared spectroscopy, or scanning electron microscopy can be used for further analysis of unusual crystals if optical crystallography does not provide definitive identification [203]. Detailed descriptions of the morphology of the most commonly encountered crystal types in dogs and cats are available for further review [204, 205].

Crystalluria is not synonymous with urolithiasis [16, 205]. Crystalluria can be absent in patients with urolithiasis, present in patients without urolithiasis, and a patient with urolithiasis can have crystals of one type in the urine sediment and a calculus composed of another type of crystal [205, 206]. However, crystalluria in freshly examined warm urine from an animal with a previous history of urolithiasis should be considered to have potential clinical relevance for increased risk of recurrent urolithiasis. Also, evaluation of crystalluria in fasting and postprandial states may be warranted in patients with recurrent urolithiasis.

Struvite, amorphous phosphate, and calcium oxalate are examples of crystals that may be found in urine samples from normal dogs and cats. The finding of persistent crystalluria in fresh urine samples may indicate risk for urethral plug formation and recurrent urolithiasis in male cats with other underlying risk factors. Crystals that are usually seen in alkaline urine include magnesium ammonium phosphate ($MgNH_4PO_4 \cdot 6H_2O$) or struvite (also called "triple phosphate"), amorphous phosphate, calcium phosphate, calcium carbonate, and ammonium urate. Crystals typically associated with acid urine include urates, cystine, calcium oxalate monohydrate, and calcium oxalate dihydrate.

Crystalluria was reported in 41% of urine microscopy results from 99 apparently healthy middle-aged and old cats in one study. Amorphous crystals were described in 80% of these reports, often noted to be mild in severity [207]. Crystalluria was reported in 65% of urine microscopy results from apparently healthy senior and geriatric dogs. The crystals were noted to be amorphous in most instances [208]. Urine was analyzed within 30 minutes of collection in both of these studies.

Occasionally, detection of crystalluria can indicate exposure to drugs or toxins (e.g. ethylene glycol, pet food contaminated with melamine and cyanuric acid) or the presence of metabolic disorders or organ dysfunction (e.g. cystinuria, bilirubinuria). Characteristic crystals may be observed in the urine sediment of animals being treated with certain drugs, especially sulfonamides (Figure 6.98).

Crystals should be reported according to type (i.e. chemical composition), quantity, size, and whether they are aggregated or individual (i.e. crystal habit) [70, 205]. Crystals in urine sediment usually are quantified subjectively as none, few, moderate, or many. In one arbitrary scheme, few refers to 1–2 crystals per LPF, moderate to 3–9 per LPF, and many as >10 per LPF. Clumps of crystals should be noted as should the presence of budding daughter crystals, because these features

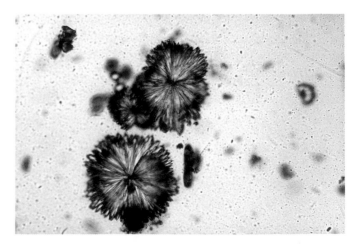

FIGURE 6.98 Sulfa crystals in urine sediment from a dog. Crystals are in round configuration radiating from the center. Epithelial cells are out of focus in the background.

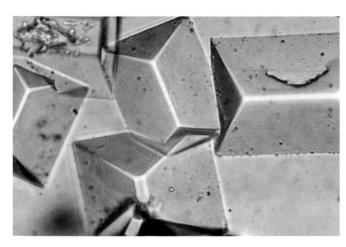

FIGURE 6.99   Struvite crystals (high power view). Crystals are in clusters, which may be more significant than isolated crystals. Source: Reproduced with permission Dr. Michael Horton, Fairborn, OH, USA.

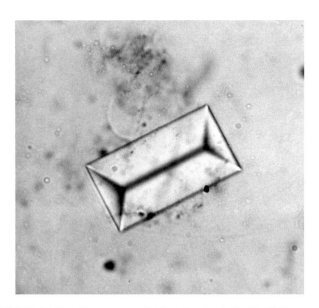

FIGURE 6.100   Struvite crystal. Note the classic "coffin-lid" appearance.

could indicate increased risk of urolithiasis. Although not specifically studied, large-sized crystals could be important in calculogenesis. Crystal size should be reported, especially if the crystals are very large or small. Large numbers of crystals, crystals that are very large, and crystals that are aggregated (Figure 6.99) have more clinical relevance for possible urolith formation when observed in the sediment of a fresh urine sample at body temperature. Definitive identification of crystals during bright-field microscopy is not always possible because the same type of crystal can assume different physical conformations under different conditions in urine.

Struvite Crystals

Struvite crystals are colorless, refractile, and of variable size. They exist as three-dimensional prisms usually with three to six or even eight sides [15, 204]. The structure is described as orthorhombic (three unequal axes intersecting at right angles) [204]. They sometimes are described as "coffin lids" or "picture frames" when they have blunt ends (Figure 6.100). Amorphous needle-like forms can also be identified (Figure 6.101). Sometimes struvite crystals appear flat, but usually some three-dimensional character is observed after adjusting the fine focus of the microscope. The prisms can also have pointed, oblique ends (Figure 6.102). More rarely, struvite crystals can aggregate and assume a fern leaf appearance [7, 21, 204]. Struvite crystals can also take on a feather-like or moth-eaten appearance as they dissolve [21, 205]. Six-to-eight-sided flat prisms of struvite can be confused with cystine crystals (Figure 6.103) [205].

Struvite crystals may be observed in urine sediment of normal dogs and cats and in the urine of cats with idiopathic or interstitial cystitis without necessarily having pathophysiologic importance. They may also occur in the urine of cats with urethral obstruction, dogs or cats with struvite urolithiasis, or dogs or cats with nonstruvite urolithiasis. Cats with

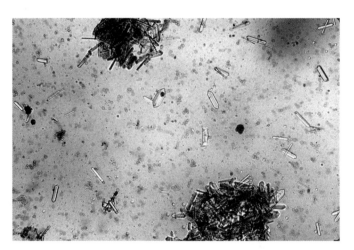

FIGURE 6.101   Struvite crystals and RBC. Two large clusters of struvite crystals are seen at the top and bottom of this image. Most of these crystals are relatively flat and with six sides. They appear needle-like when viewed from their side. Some display internal structure. Numerous RBC in the background.

urethral obstruction often have struvite crystalluria that likely arises as a consequence of urinary stasis and increased urine pH. Alkaline urine promotes precipitation of struvite crystals. Consequently, increased numbers of struvite crystals are expected postprandially, in the presence of urease-positive bacterial UTI, and in animals with persistently alkaline urine of other cause (e.g. plant-based diet, metabolic disorder).

Struvite crystals are much more common in the urine of cats fed dry foods as compared to cats eating primarily canned food. This difference is presumably due to the effect of lower urine osmolality and decreased concentration of crystalloids in cats with higher total daily water intake while consuming canned food [209–211]. In cats fed both dry and canned food

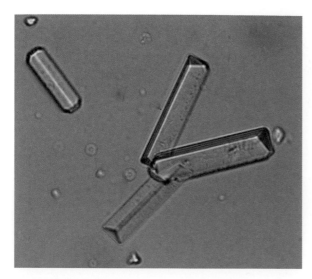

FIGURE 6.102 Struvite crystals. A few WBC and RBC are seen in the background. The WBC are larger than the RBC. Image acquired by VETSCAN® SA Sediment Analyzer. Source: Reproduced with permission of Zoetis

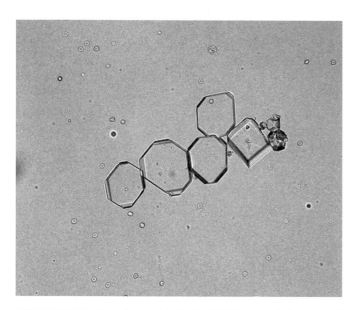

FIGURE 6.103 Struvite crystals. Refractile lines reveal the internal three-dimensional nature of this crystal. Source: Reproduced with permission of Dr. Heather L. Wamsley, Bradenton, FL.

diets, struvite crystals were more numerous in urine samples after storage at room temperature or in the refrigerator, as compared to fresh urine samples. Urine samples that had marked struvite crystalluria after storage were also likely to have crystals identified in fresh urine samples. Interestingly, no cats in this study that were fed canned food had crystalluria, regardless of the type of urine storage (i.e. freshly examined urine, urine stored at room temperature, and refrigerated urine) [199]. The type, number, and size of crystals observed during urine sediment examination were determined within 60 minutes of urine collection, after room temperature storage

for 6 and 24 hours, and after refrigeration for 6 and 24 hours in a study of urine from dogs and cats with USG > 1.025. Longer storage times and refrigeration resulted in more numerous and larger crystals [200].

Calcium Oxalate Crystals

Calcium oxalate crystals can be identified in urine sediment from normal dogs, cats, and horses, especially in animals with concentrated urine. Calcium oxalate crystals can also be found as an artifact after cooling, and thus, it is important to know how the urine sample was handled and stored. The presence of calcium oxalate crystals in the urine sediment of systemically ill animals supports a diagnosis of ethylene glycol intoxication, especially when the urine is hyposthenuric or isosthenuric and the patient has oligo-anuric AKI. Calcium oxalate crystals can be observed in the urine of animals with calcium oxalate urolithiasis, but often no crystals are observed or a different type of crystal is observed. Calcium oxalate crystalluria was infrequently found during urine microscopy of dogs with calcium oxalate urolithiasis of one study. It was concluded that calcium oxalate crystalluria status could not be used to predict which dogs had calcium oxalate stones from those that did not [212]. Chocolate intoxication can be associated with hyperoxaluria and hypercalciuria [213] that can result in formation of calcium oxalate monohydrate crystals [15].

Calcium oxalate crystals can assume monohydrate (whewellite) (Figure 6.104) and dihydrate (weddelite) (Figure 6.105) forms. Crystal size varies from extremely small to very large. Both forms of calcium oxalate crystals are birefringent under polarizing light [7].

Calcium oxalate dihydrate crystals often appear as square envelope-shaped octahedrals. This rhomboid form often is said to have a "Maltese cross" appearance (Figure 6.106). The X of the Maltese cross becomes prominent

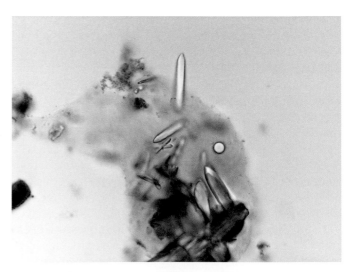

FIGURE 6.104 Oxalate monohydrate crystals are seen as a cluster of "picket fence" like structures at the bottom of the field and also free. Ethylene glycol poisoning in a dog.

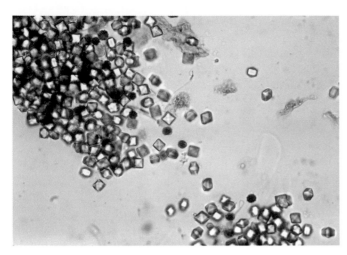

FIGURE 6.105   Calcium oxalate dihydrate crystals. Many small calcium oxalate dihydrate crystals in clusters. Several WBC and rare sperm are in the background.

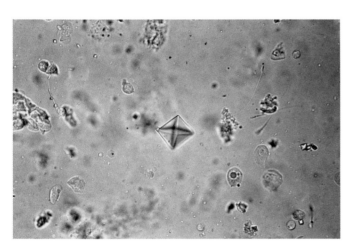

FIGURE 6.106   Calcium oxalate dihydrate crystals. A large crystal is in the center of this image (rhomboid with Maltese cross in center) and two small crystals are to the far right. Nonsquamous epithelial cells and sperm are in the background. Rare WBC are present. A clump of nonsquamous epithelial cells that cannot be further characterized is to the far left middle of this image.

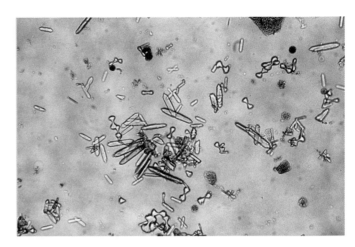

FIGURE 6.107   Calcium oxalate monohydrate crystals. Many dumbbell and picket fence-shaped crystals are in this field.

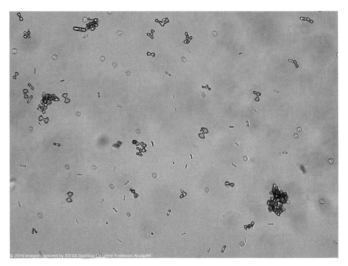

FIGURE 6.108   Calcium oxalate monohydrate crystals. Image acquired by SediVue®. Several dumbbell-shaped crystals are seen in this field. These crystals are relatively small being slightly larger than RBC in the background. Source: Courtesy of IDEXX Laboratories. Copyright © 2022, IDEXX Laboratories, Inc. All rights reserved. Used with permission.

when focusing up and down on this crystal during microscopy [46]. Calcium oxalate dihydrate crystals have been described as bipyramidal tetragons in urine sediment and during crystallographic evaluation of calculi [214].

Calcium oxalate monohydrate crystals can assume different appearances in urine sediment and are less easily identified than calcium oxalate dihydrate crystals [215]. Two common morphologies for calcium oxalate monohydrate include narrow rectangles with pointed ends (so-called picket fence appearance) (Figure 6.107) and "dumbbell" appearance (Figure 6.108). The "picket fence" crystals appear flat, which distinguishes them from struvite crystals, which have a more three-dimensional appearance. The "dumbbell" shape appears to occur as a result of twinning of thin flat sheets of calcium oxa-

late monohydrate crystals [214]. Calcium oxalate monohydrate crystals are birefringent under polarizing light and appear yellow or blue, depending on the angle at which they are examined [216]. Daughter crystals (flakes) that bud from the parent six-sided crystal can be seen in some instances of calcium oxalate monohydrate crystalluria [217, 218]. Calcium oxalate monohydrate crystals can also appear sheath-shaped [216, 218]. Elongated spindle- or needle-shaped crystals (Figure 6.109) as well as "hemp seed" or oval-shaped calcium oxalate monohydrate crystals have also been described (Figure 6.110) [158]. Oval crystals have been described as having the shape of orzo pasta [219]. At times, small calcium oxalate monohydrate crystals resemble calcium carbonate crystals, which can cause confusion if the urine sample is from a rabbit or horse.

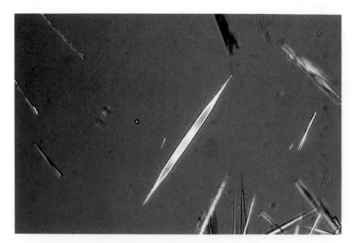

FIGURE 6.109 Calcium oxalate monohydrate crystals. Spindle-shape crystals under polarizing light. Urine sediment from a dog with suspected ethylene glycol poisoning.

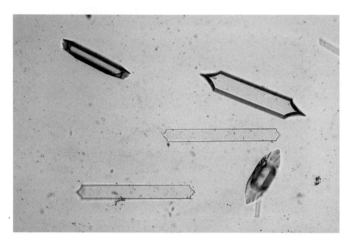

FIGURE 6.110 Calcium oxalate monohydrate crystals. Crystal at right bottom of this field has a hemp seed appearance with a budding daughter crystal.

The recognition of atypical forms of calcium oxalate crystalluria is important for the early diagnosis of ethylene glycol poisoning. It has been our experience that "unidentified" crystals are often reported in the urine of dogs and cats that have been poisoned with ethylene glycol. Likely, many of these "unidentified" crystals represent forms of calcium oxalate monohydrate that are difficult to identify accurately.

Six-sided prismatic crystals were reported to be hippurate or "hippurate-like" in appearance in early reports of ethylene glycol poisoning in dogs [158, 217, 220]. It is likely that these previously described "hippurate-like" crystals actually were calcium oxalate monohydrate, based on further evaluation by X-ray diffraction techniques [218]. Interestingly, the morphology of calcium oxalate dihydrate crystals can change to that of calcium oxalate monohydrate in urine that has been stored up to 24 hours [218, 221].

Large quantities of calcium oxalate crystals were observed during the urine sediment microscopy of dogs with experimental ethylene glycol poisoning. Mild crystalluria was detected at 5 and 7 hours postingestion in some dogs, with many crystals per HPF identified after 8–24 hours. Equal numbers of six-sided "hippurate-like" prisms (i.e. calcium oxalate monohydrate) and "envelope" forms (i.e. calcium oxalate dihydrate) were identified. Dumbbell- or sheaf-shaped crystals were seen less commonly, and hemp-seed-shaped crystals were rarely seen. Many of the six-sided prismatic crystals had budding crystals [218]. In an earlier experimental study of dogs, calcium oxalate crystals (mono- versus dihydrate not distinguished) first were observed at six hours after exposure to ethylene glycol and increased in frequency at 9 and 12 hours [222]. Although calcium oxalate dihydrate crystalluria occurs during ethylene glycol poisoning clinically, calcium oxalate monohydrate crystalluria is more common [158, 217]. Calcium oxalate crystalluria was identified in 66% of dogs and 32% of cats with clinical ethylene glycol poisoning in one report. The monohydrate form ("hippurate-like") of calcium oxalate occurred in 67% of the dogs and in 56% of the cats [158]. Calcium oxalate crystalluria occurs during ethylene glycol poisoning despite the presence of dilute urine [220]. It is important to carefully examine urine sediment from patients suspected to have ethylene glycol exposure, because these crystals sometimes are very small and easy to miss during casual urine sediment microscopy.

Calcium oxalate crystal formation was studied *in vitro* after mixing various proportions of potassium oxalate and calcium chloride solutions. When precipitates occurred, calcium oxalate monohydrate crystals predominated at all concentrations. Calcium oxalate dihydrate crystals only formed in solutions with a high concentration of both calcium and oxalate. Crystal morphology (size and configuration) was determined by both the relative supersaturation of calcium oxalate and the ratio of calcium to oxalate in the solution. Aggregation of crystals was dependent on both time and relative supersaturation and was more pronounced in samples with the greatest supersaturation [221]. In another study, sodium oxalate and calcium chloride solutions were added to normal human urine in quantities that caused spontaneous calcium oxalate crystallization. Increasing supersaturation of calcium oxalate resulted in much larger numbers of crystals, and further increases in supersaturation resulted in larger crystals. Calcium oxalate dihydrate crystals predominated in this study. X-shaped crystals were identified at very high calcium oxalate supersaturation [223].

Calcium Phosphate

Calcium phosphate crystals in urine potentially can occur in three forms: basic calcium phosphate (apatite), calcium hydrogen phosphate dihydrate (brushite) (Figure 6.111), or tricalcium phosphate (whitlockite) [214]. The many different forms of colorless calcium phosphate crystals are sometimes referred to as amorphous phosphates. Amorphous phosphate crystals are usually spherical and often observed in association with struvite crystalluria [205]. These crystals can also develop

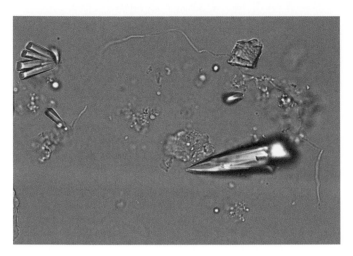

FIGURE 6.111 Calcium phosphate (brushite) crystals. Also in view is what appears to be a piece of sheared epithelium at the top and linear bacteria. Source: Reproduced with permission of Dr. Heather L. Wamsley, Bradenton, FL, USA.

as long thin needles or elongated thin prisms [21, 205]. They have been identified in normal animals, in patients with calcium-containing uroliths, and in those with persistently alkaline urine from any cause [205]. The presence of calcium phosphate crystalluria may be more important than previously appreciated, because calcium phosphate promotes the nucleation of calcium oxalate. Interestingly, calcium phosphate has the ability to dissolve and recrystallize as calcium oxalate [214].

Ammonium Urate (Biurate), Amorphous Urates, and Uric Acid

Urate crystals are spherical and have a characteristic yellow–brown color. The spheres can be smooth or have projections from the surface sometimes referred to as "thorn apple" in appearance (Figure 6.112) [15, 21, 219]. Some spherical urate crystals have internal radial striations [21]. If only spherical crystals are present, it can be difficult to definitely identify the crystals, but the animal species affected and urine pH can help in such instances. Amorphous urates appear as yellow–brown to colorless fine granules.

Ammonium urate and amorphous urates (Figure 6.113) are common in the urine sediment of Dalmatians and English bulldogs [15, 21]. Urate crystals can be observed in dogs of these breeds whether or not urate urolithiasis is present because of breed-specific genetic mutations for synthesis of uric acid transporters in the kidney and liver [206].

The presence of ammonium biurate crystals in the urine of other breeds of dogs and in cats can be associated with high blood ammonia concentrations as a consequence of congenital or acquired portosystemic shunting or severe hepatic disease. Cats with urate urolithiasis most often have urate crystalluria that is not associated with hepatic disorders [224]. The Egyptian Mau, Birman, and Siamese breeds are at increased risk for urate urolithiasis [225], and presumably this predisposition is associated with increased urate crystalluria observed on urine sediment examination.

Uric acid crystals are far less common in dogs and cats than are ammonium urates or amorphous urates. Uric acid crystals are diamond- or rhomboid-shaped and yellow–brown in color. Some uric acid crystals have concentric rings. They sometimes have six sides and can be confused with cystine crystals [21]. Uric acid crystals form under the same conditions as do urates (Figure 6.114). Amorphous urates and ammonium urate are transformed into uric acid crystals when 10% acetic acid is added to urinary sediment which can then be reexamined after 20–30 minutes [205].

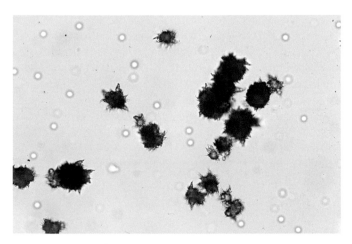

FIGURE 6.112 Urate crystals. Several faint RBC are in the background slightly out of focus. Source: Reproduced with permission of Dr. Joe Bartges, University of Georgia, Athens, GA.

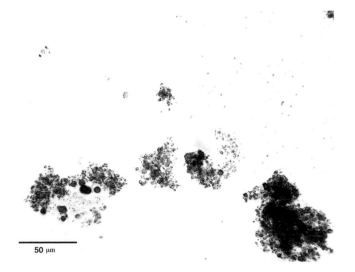

50 µm

FIGURE 6.113 Amorphous urate crystals. Source: Reproduced with permission Dr. Michael Horton, Fairborn, OH, USA.

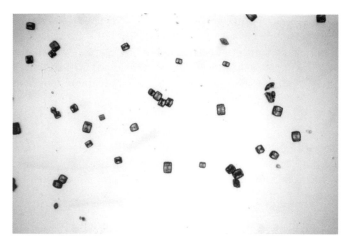

FIGURE 6.114 Uric acid crystals. Source: Reproduced with permission of Dr. Richard Scott, Animal Medical Center, NY, NY, USA.

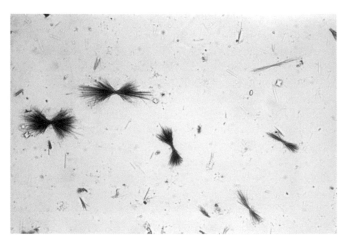

FIGURE 6.116 Bilirubin crystals. Bilirubin crystals can be normal in dogs, especially males. There are also a few small calcium oxalate crystals in the background. Urine sediment from a dog.

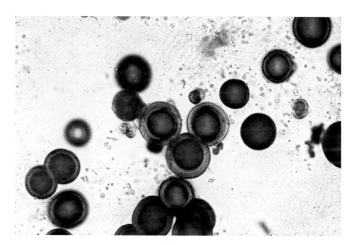

FIGURE 6.115 Xanthine crystals. Urine sediment from a dog on allopurinol treatment to help prevent recurrence of urate urolithiasis. Source: Reproduced with permission of Dr. Joe Bartges, University of Georgia, Athens, GA.

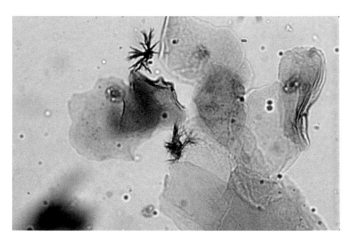

FIGURE 6.117 Bilirubin crystals in urine sediment from a cat. Sheets of squamous epithelial cells are in the background. Bilirubin crystals are never normal in urinary sediment from a cat. Source: Reproduced with permission of Dr. Michael Horton, Fairborn, OH, USA.

Xanthine

Xanthine crystals are brown to yellow–brown spheres of variable size (Figure 6.115), but they can also appear as amorphous crystals. Light microscopy does not allow the definitive identification of xanthine crystals, and they resemble ammonium urate and amorphous urates [21]. Xanthine crystalluria most likely will be encountered in dogs being treated with allopurinol to prevent recurrent urate urolithiasis. Inadequate restriction of dietary purines increases the chance of observing xanthine crystals in the urine during allopurinol treatment [206]. Rarely, xanthinuria has been observed in untreated dogs (usually King Charles spaniels) and young cats [206].

Bilirubin

Bilirubin crystals occur as single needles or clusters (sheaves) of needles (Figure 6.116). These crystals are dark orange to

golden brown in color. Dogs normally have a low renal threshold for excretion of conjugated bilirubin, and male dogs excrete more bilirubin into their urine than do females. Consequently, small numbers of bilirubin crystals are considered normal in concentrated urine samples from dogs, but not in cats (Figure 6.117) [226, 227]. The finding of increased numbers of bilirubin crystals has the same clinical relevance as does a positive dipstrip chemical reactions for bilirubin (i.e. hemolytic, primary hepatic, and posthepatic diseases) (see Chapter 5) [15, 21, 219].

Cystine

Cystine crystals appear as colorless flat hexagonal sheets [214] of variable thickness (Figure 6.118). The sides of these crystals may be of equal or unequal length [15, 21]. Flat forms of struvite and cholesterol crystals can be confused with cystine

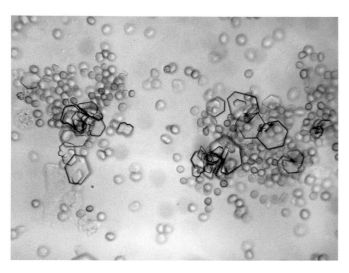

FIGURE 6.118 Cystine crystals. Urine sediment from a female Newfoundland with urolithiasis. The laboratory originally misidentified these crystals as struvite. Numerous RBC are in the background.

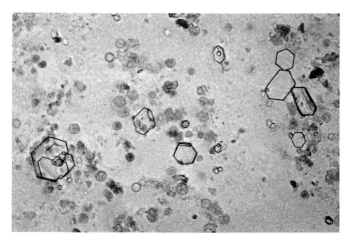

FIGURE 6.119 Cystine crystals in a male Bassett Hound with cystine urolithiasis. Six-sided flat clear crystals are seen in this field. There is a cascade of cystine crystals on top of each other in the far-left field. Cystine crystals are sometimes confused with struvite, but cystine crystals lack internal three-dimensional structure. Numerous degenerating WBC seen in the background are taking on more red stain than usually occurs. Some RBC are also identified. Source: Courtesy of Dr. Stephen DiBartola, The Ohio State University College of Veterinary Medicine.

crystals (Figure 6.119). Cystine crystals are not birefringent under polarizing light, unless the crystals are very thick [7]. Cystine crystals can also form in sheets that cascade on top of one another.

The observation of cystine crystals in urine sediment is never normal as it indicates the presence of the metabolic disorder of cystinuria. In health, nearly all cystine is reabsorbed from tubular fluid by transporters along the proximal tubule. Cystinuria is caused by a congenital or acquired defect in these transport systems [228–231]. Cystine may be the sole

amino acid affected by a genetic defect (e.g. Newfoundland, English Bulldog, Dachshund, Chihuahua, Mastiff, Australian Cattle Dog, Bullmastiff, American Staffordshire terrier) or a generalized amino acid transport disorder can occur as in familial Fanconi syndrome (Basenji) [232] or Fanconi syndrome associated with the ingestion of chicken jerky treats [233]. Cystinuria can occur with or without cystine urolithiasis. Siamese and American Domestic Shorthair cats are at increased risk for cystinuria and cystine uroliths [229, 234, 235]. Because cystine is much less soluble than other amino acids reabsorbed by the proximal tubule, the identification of cystine crystals serves as a surrogate for the presence of other amino acids that may also be affected by a renal tubular transport disorder. Confirmation that cystinuria is an indication of more generalized aminoaciduria can be made by the measurement of a panel of amino acids in urine (PennGen, University of Pennsylvania, School of Veterinary Medicine). Preliminary confirmation of cystinuria can be made using a cyanide-nitroprusside test [7] that produces a red to purple color in urine samples that contain cystine.

Unusual or Rare Crystals

Calcium Carbonates

Calcium carbonate crystals are not observed in the urine of dogs and cats, but are commonly present in large quantities in the urine of horses, rabbits, and guinea pigs (Figure 6.120) [49, 236].

Cholesterol

Cholesterol crystals appear as colorless large rectangular plates, often with a notch in one or more margins. They can appear linear when viewed on end [7, 21, 219] (Figure. 6.121). Cholesterol crystals are highly birefringent under polarized light [7] and can exhibit a variety of colors as well as a Maltese cross pattern [46]. The clinical relevance of finding cholesterol crystals in the urine sediment of domestic animals is not

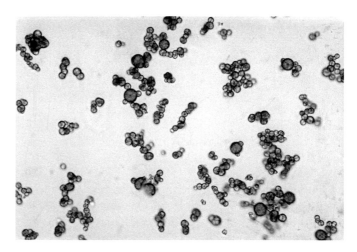

FIGURE 6.120 Calcium carbonate crystals. Note aggregates of brown round crystals typical of calcium carbonate. Urine sediment from a horse.

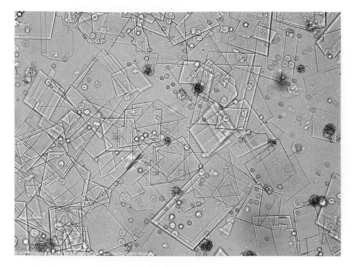

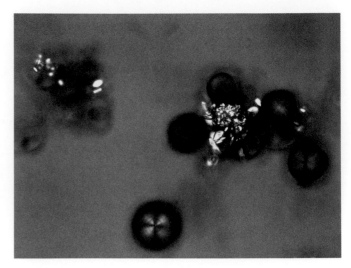

FIGURE 6.121 Cholesterol crystals. Image acquired by SediVue®. Rectangular sheets of cholesterol crystals dominate this field. Numerous RBC and occasional WBC are in the background. Source: Courtesy of IDEXX Laboratories. Copyright © 2022, IDEXX Laboratories, Inc. All rights reserved. Used with permission.

FIGURE 6.122 Leucine crystals in biliary fluid (polarizing microscopy). The dark round crystals are leucine. The radiating interior pattern is typical of leucine during polarizing microscopy. The smaller white refrengent crystals were not identified though they resemble calcium oxalate monohydrate. Source: Reproduced with permission of Dr. Heather L. Wamsley, Bradenton, FL.

known, and they can sometimes be identified in the urine of apparently normal dogs. An association may exist between protein-losing nephropathy [21, 219] and lipiduria in humans. The presence of cholesterol crystals in urine has been associated with accelerated tissue breakdown during active renal inflammation and also with chyluria caused by obstruction of lymphatic drainage in the thorax or abdomen [46]. In humans, cholesterol crystals are more likely to be observed in urine that has been refrigerated because refrigeration allows the transformation of lipid droplets into crystals [7]. Cholesterol crystals may be observed more commonly as a film on the surface of the urine rather than in the urine sediment [46]. Cholesterol crystals are identified uncommonly during urine sediment examination of dogs and cats.

Leucine and Tyrosine

Leucine and tyrosine crystals are rarely observed during urine sediment examination in dogs or cats. Their presence indicates severe hepatic dysfunction. Tyrosine crystals are observed as highly refractile fine needles, often in clusters. Leucine crystals are observed as yellowish-brown spheres with radial and concentric striations sometimes described as resembling a cut grapefruit with a thick rind (Figure 6.122) [21, 46]. Spherical leucine crystals have a typical Maltese cross pattern when observed under polarized light [46].

Melamine and Cyanuric Acid

Melamine and cyanuric acid crystals are usually small, round, and light brown to yellow or golden brown in color. They often have striations that radiate from the center of the crystal. Their color may also vary from light green to blue. They can be observed as aggregates of crystals that form small clumps or linear extensions (Figure 6.123). Experimental cats fed a diet

FIGURE 6.123 Melamine–cyanuric acid crystals. Round light brown crystals with concentric rings observed in some. These crystals were often confused with urate or carbonate crystals before a syndrome of food contamination with melamine and cyanuric acid leading to renal injury was discovered. Urine sediment from a cat with CKD and AKI eating contaminated food.

containing both melamine and cyanuric acid excreted fan-shaped crystals [237]. Melamine–cyanuric acid crystals look similar in all species. Small, needle-like crystals frequently align themselves radially to form spheres. These spheres vary from 10 to 100 μm in diameter, with most in the 20–40 μm range [238]. Melamine–cyanuric acid crystals are birefringent under polarizing light (Figure 6.124). At times, these crystals can resemble small oxalate crystals observed in patients with ethylene glycol poisoning, but melamine–cyanuric acid crystals are brown in

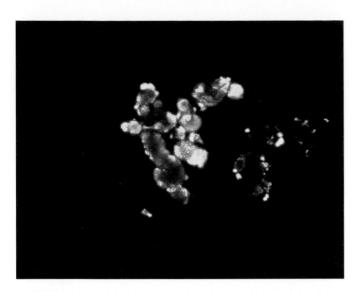

FIGURE 6.124   Melamine–cyanuric acid crystals (polarizing light microscopy).

color and often have a radiating linear pattern that is not present in oxalate crystals.

Melamine–cyanuric acid crystals were originally thought to be similar to a form of urate [238] or calcium carbonate, before they were definitely determined to contain mostly melamine and cyanuric acid [239]. Melamine is a nitrogen-rich compound that is used in the manufacture of plastics and as a fertilizer. Cyanuric acid is a byproduct of melamine manufacturing or degradation that is also nitrogen-rich [237] and used to stabilize chlorine in swimming pools [240]. Melamine and cyanuric acid were intentionally added to feed ingredients in China to increase nitrogen content. Increasing nitrogen content gives the appearance of a product with a higher protein content, which has more monetary value as a "higher quality" product [237, 239]. This practice is common in some regions of the world [241]. The contaminated additives were mostly associated with wheat gluten and rice protein concentrate [239] (Food and Drug Administration website, www.fda.org) provided in the form of vegetable protein concentrates [241]. Canned or semimoist pet foods had more food contamination than did dry products.

Melamine–cyanuric crystals were not recognized until clusters of cases of renal failure cases (AKI and CKD) in dogs and cats associated with contaminated food were recognized in North America in 2007 [238, 241]. Clusters of renal failure cases in Asia in 2004 were originally thought to have been caused by mycotoxins, but reevaluation of these cases indicates the more likely cause to be melamine–cyanuric acid [241]. This condition has been referred to as "food-associated renal failure" and, more specifically, "crystal-associated nephropathy." When melamine is exposed to cyanuric acid in solution, melamine and cyanuric acid crystals precipitate in urine and in the distal renal tubules and collecting tubules [237, 241, 242]. Cyanuric acid or melamine alone does not precipitate from solution. Melamine and cyanuric

acid together form a stable structure held together by multiple hydrogen bonds [239]. It appears that acidic urine enhances the formation of insoluble melamine–cyanuric acid complexes in cats [237] and in humans [243].

Crystals are rarely observed in kidney FNAs; however, both calcium oxalate monohydrate crystals and melamine–cyanuric acid crystals have been reported [130]. Compression of kidney slices on glass slides readily provides crystals for wet mount identification of melamine–cyanuric acid crystals from affected animals at necropsy [237]. We also have observed crystals characteristic of melamine–cyanuric acid on cytological examination of material aspirated from the kidney of an affected cat (Figure 6.125).

Identification of unusual crystals during urine sediment examination provided the initial clue to the cause of an epidemic of AKI and CKD in dogs and cats that subsequently was determined to be associated with the consumption of contaminated pet food. Melamine–cyanuric acid crystalluria could reappear if a lapse in food safety practices were to occur [238, 243]. In this situation, astute observation and interpretation of newly recognized crystals in urine provided a crucial clue to toxic environmental exposure.

Daisy-Like Crystals

Daisy-like crystals recently were described in the urine sediment of one dog and nine humans. The chemical composition of these crystals has not been determined, and their clinical relevance is uncertain (Figure 6.126) [201].

Therapeutic or Diagnostic Agents

Therapeutic and diagnostic agents can result in the formation of crystals in urine sediment that are not easily identified.

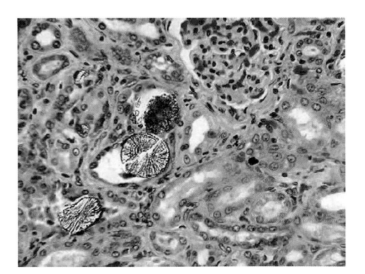

FIGURE 6.125   Photomicrograph of a hematoxylin–eosin–stained section of kidney removed from a 12-year-old mixed-breed dog that had acute renal failure. Note the characteristic appearance of the melamine/cyanuric acid crystals within the tubular lumens. The crystals were highly birefringent when examined by polarizing light microscopy. Source: Osborne et al. [244] Used with permission.

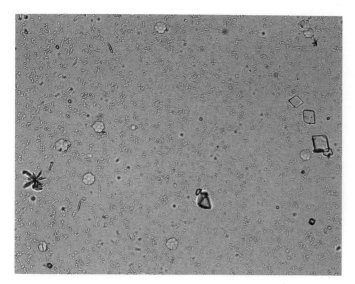

FIGURE 6.126 Six petaliform crystals are observed in this field of urine sediment from a cat. The identity of these crystals is not known. These crystals resemble "daisy-like" crystals which were reported in humans and one dog in 2017 [201]. There are three struvite crystals in the upper right field. Numerous structures in the background look like bacteria, but they could also be small crystals. Source: Reproduced with permission of Dr. Heather L. Wamsley, Bradenton, FL, USA.

A review of the patient's drug exposure history often discloses the offending compound. Any agent that achieves high concentration in urine (e.g. many drugs used to treat bacterial UTI) has the potential to precipitate in the urine as crystals, especially in urine that is highly concentrated and refrigerated. Administration of sulfonamide drugs can result in urinary crystals in humans [202] and in veterinary patients. Even at standard therapeutic doses, the activity product of sulfonamides in urine can exceed the solubility product so that crystals form in urine. As with all solutes, the precipitation of sulfonamides is more likely to occur in concentrated urine [202]. Sulfonamide crystals can assume a variety of forms, commonly including sheaves and rosettes (Figures 6.127 and 6.98) [21]. Sulfonamide crystals dissolve when acetone is added to the urine sample [46]. The lignin test can be used to identify sulfonamide crystals in urine. A drop of urine sediment mixed with one to two drops of dilute hydrochloric acid and dripped onto newspaper will turn bright yellow to orange if sulfonamides are present [219].

Ampicillin [7, 42] and amoxicillin crystals [245] are sometimes observed during urine sediment examination. Ciprofloxacin crystals have been identified in human urine [246, 247], and it is likely that fluoroquinolone crystals can form in samples from animal urine, based on the high urinary concentrations that fluoroquinolones can achieve. High urinary concentrations of enrofloxacin and very high concentrations of ciprofloxacin are achieved (after metabolism of enrofloxacin) in dogs [248]. High concentrations of radiocontrast agents occur urine after excretory urography or contrast cystography

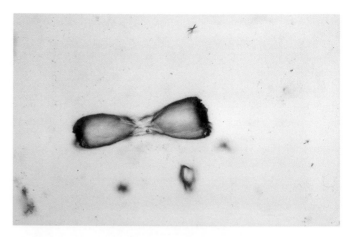

FIGURE 6.127 Sulfa crystal in urine sediment from a dog. Sheath configuration is seen in this field.

and may lead to formation of crystals that are birefringent. These crystals have been described as being similar in appearance to cholesterol crystals [7] or as pleomorphic needles occurring singly or in sheaves [46].

MISCELLANEOUS ELEMENTS AND ARTIFACTS

Oil or fat droplets (lipiduria) (Figure 6.128) occasionally are seen in urine sediment and may be confused with RBC, but, unlike RBC, lipid droplets are highly refractile. They are more

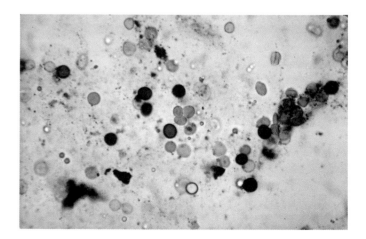

FIGURE 6.128 Stained urine sediment from a cat. Note RBC of similar size but varying intensity of stain uptake. Some are red to dark red, while others are pale. Some RBC show faint outlines without color uptake. The intensity of the color is likely related to the hemoglobin content of the RBC, as hemoglobin has leached out from the RBC with faint or no staining. One RBC on its side shows a concave appearance. Also note several highly refractile droplets that are smaller than RBC; these are lipid droplets. Lipid droplets are found commonly in urine sediment from normal cats but should not be confused with RBC. Lipid droplets are in a different plane from cells in urine sediment and can be more readily identified while rocking the fine focus during microscopy. Source: Reproduced by permission Dr. Richard A. Scott, Animal Medical Center, New York, NY, USA.

commonly seen in urine from cats, but there appears to be no specific clinical relevance in dogs or cats [100].

Spermatozoa are present in 25% [249] to 88% of urine samples collected by cystocentesis from male dogs (Figure 6.129) [250]. Occasionally, spermatozoa will be encountered in the sediment of urine samples collected by cystocentesis from normal intact male cats [251]. Some regurgitation of spermatozoa into bladder urine is considered normal in male dogs [100]. Recently, bred females may have spermatozoa in urine sediment evaluation prepared from voided samples.

Amorphous debris can be a normal finding in some urine samples as a result of normal cell turnover (Figure 6.130). An increased amount of amorphous debris can also be observed when there are upper and lower urinary tract disor-ders causing breakdown of an increased number of cells in the urine. Amorphous granular precipitate in the sediment may adhere to the surface of hyaline casts, imparting a granular appearance to them [252].

Mucous threads occasionally are encountered in urine from normal animals (Figure 6.131), and they may increase in number with inflammatory conditions of the urinary tract. Fibrin strands are not normal and are associated with inflammatory or hemorrhagic lesions.

Foreign material often enters urine samples, especially voided samples. Plant matter (Figures 6.132 and 6.133), straw, hair, surgery glove powder, and fecal contamination may be seen (Figure 6.134). Lubricants used to facilitate

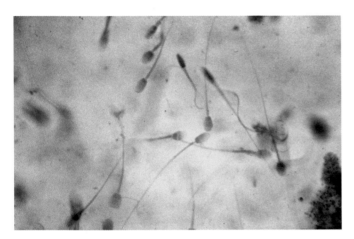

FIGURE 6.129 Sperm. Sperm can be a normal finding in urine, likely to be more common in voided urine. Sperm can reflux into bladder urine and also be identified from cystocentesis samples taken from intact male dogs.

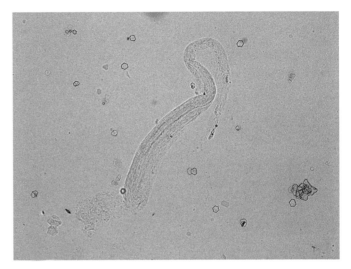

FIGURE 6.131 Pseudocast. Notice the large mucous strand that varies greatly in its width. Small cystine crystals are in the background. Source: Reproduced with permission of Dr. Heather L. Wamsley, Bradenton, FL, USA.

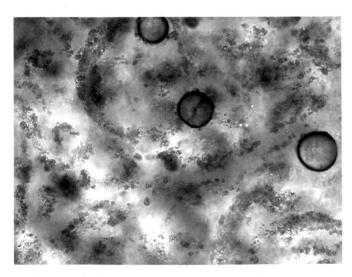

FIGURE 6.130 Calcium carbonate crystals – rabbit urine. There are three large round crystals with concentric rings and central striations. Amorphous crystals predominate in this field.

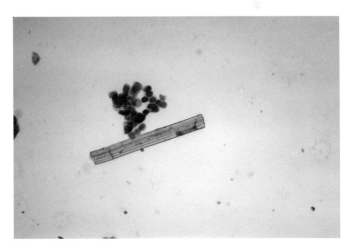

FIGURE 6.132 Pseudocast. Note the extremely rigid wall structure with blunt ends. There are several parallel lines within this structure that are characteristic of plant material. The cells to the top of the pseudocast are not identified.

FIGURE 6.133 Pseudocast and waxy casts. A long narrow fiber (pseudocast) is seen in the upper left of this field. In the middle field is a waxy cast. A smaller waxy cast is seen between the pseudocast and the larger waxy cast.

catheterization may add refractile droplets to urine sediment. (Figure 6.135).

Precipitates in stains used for urine sediment examination may occur and cause confusion with bacteria or crystals (Figure 6.136). Contaminants in the stain (e.g. bacteria, fungi) can also occur. Aged supravital stain (Sedi-Stain) may contribute to the presence of unusual crystals in the urine sediment, especially near the coverglass edge.

"Pseudocasts" occur when conditions in the urine create what appears to be a cast from the kidney. Squamous epithelial cells may roll on themselves and resemble casts. Fibrin and mucous strands in urine may cause cells in the sediment to appear in a linear fashion resembling a cellular cast (Figure 6.137). However, usually, the strand itself can be seen, and the borders of what has been interpreted as a "cast" are ill-defined. Highly cellular sediment (with many WBC and RBC) may be subject to compression artifact during centrifugation, causing cellular clumps that appear to be casts. Close inspection will reveal the irregularity of these clumps; often

(a)

(b)   (c)

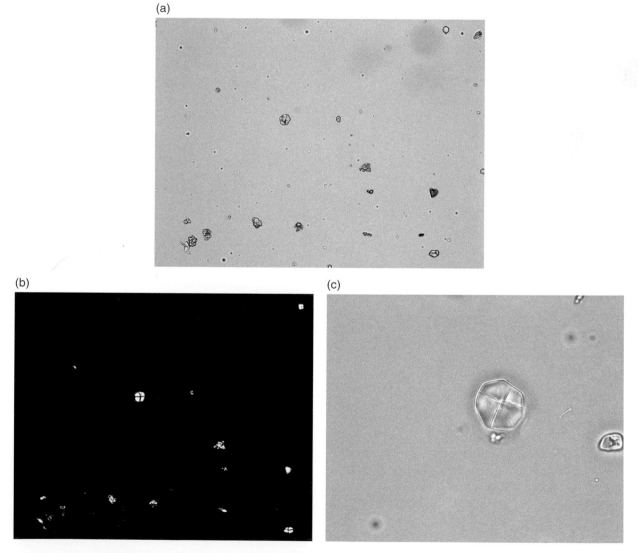

FIGURE 6.134 A, B, C. Starch granule contamination of urine sediment from glove powder. A. 200× light microscopy. B. 200× polarizing light microscopy. C. 600× (oil) microscopy. Source: Reproduced with permission of Dr. Heather L. Wamsley, Bradenton, FL, USA.

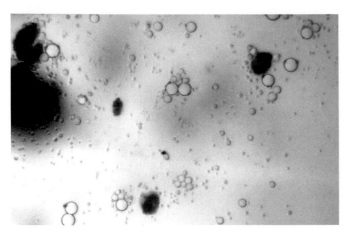

FIGURE 6.135 Aqueous lubricant droplets. These droplets are from contamination of the urine sample with lubricant during the passage of a urinary catheter. These droplets can be confused with lipid droplets or air bubbles.

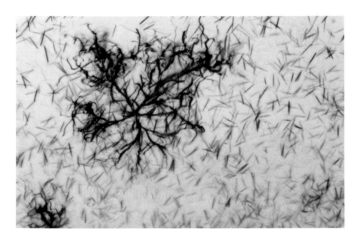

FIGURE 6.136 Precipitates of crystals from supravital stain (Sedi-Stain). This can occur when the stain is old and dehydrated. This can also occur under the coverslip as the urine evaporates from the sample and often is more prominent at the edges of the coverslip.

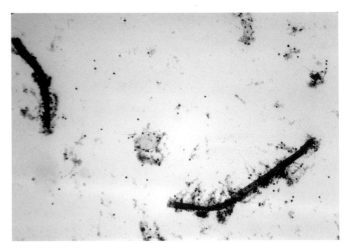

FIGURE 6.137 Pseudocasts. Two fibers are seen that are linear and easily confused with a cast. Note that debris and cells are lining up next to the fibers. It appears that the fiber has an internal linear structure that casts do not have.

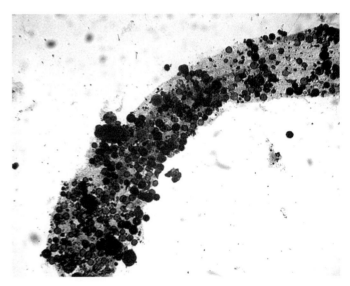

FIGURE 6.138 400× view of a pseudocast. Prostatic plug from a dog with prostatic bleeding. This plug contains many RBC and a few epithelial cells. The size of this plug is considerably larger than the usual renal cast.

the clumps are too large and nonlinear to be casts. Examination of uncentrifuged urine is helpful in equivocal cases to determine if the presumed casts can be identified before centrifugation. Pseudocasts have been identified in some humans with prostatic disease when WBC cells line up along or are embedded in prostatic secretions [253]. Such pseudocasts have rarely been suspected in dogs with prostatic conditions that result in large plugs of cast-like material (Figure 6.138).

Ova from the nematode bladder worm *C. plica* (*Pearsonema plica*) in the dog and *Capillaria feliscati* in the cat (Figure 6.139) occasionally are recognized in urine sediment. They may be identified in animals with signs of lower urinary tract disease [254] or may be identified incidentally in animals without clinical signs [255, 256]. Inflammatory changes at the site of worm attachment typically are mild. Over 50% of dogs from two kennels (predominantly Whippets) were noted to harbor *C. plica* in one study. Hematuria, dysuria,

and pollakiuria were commonly noted in dogs from these kennels in the absence of secondary bacterial urinary infection. Diagnosis in this study was based on the characteristic appearance of eggs or degenerate worms (some of which were gravid). Ova usually were accompanied by numerous clumps of transitional epithelial cells along with some RBC, but increases in WBC or bacteria were not observed. Puppies less than eight months of age did not excrete *C. plica* eggs in their urine. Failure to observe ova in urine sediment is likely to occur in animals with a light worm burden, in those with a recently resolved infection, or in those infected only with nongravid females or males. Infection may be self-limiting if exposure to the source of the intermediate life cycle host (earthworm) is removed. Multiple examinations of urine

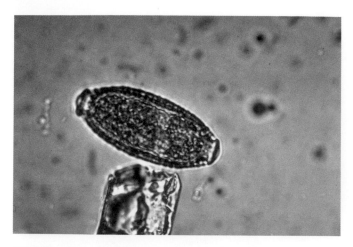

FIGURE 6.139 *Capillaria* in unstained urine sediment. Source: Reproduced with permission of Dr. Richard A. Scott, Animal Medical Center, New York, NY, USA.

sediment may be required to establish the diagnosis in animals with low worm burdens.

Dogs do not normally eat earthworms, and thus, it is likely that soil containing the earthworms was ingested. Direct dog-to-dog transmission in these kennels was also considered possible. The presence of ova in urine was negative in 85% of dogs after 30 days of treatment with albendazole [254]. Levamisole was effective against *C. plica* infection in a single dog that had failed treatment with fenbendazole, moxidectin, and ivermectin [257].

During cystoscopy, we have on occasion discovered *Capillaria* worms in cats that had normal urinalyses (Figure 6.140). When evaluating urine for ova, care must be taken to ensure that fecal contamination of urine has not occurred. Whipworm (*Trichuris*) ova from fecal contamination can easily be confused with *Capillaria* ova. *C. plica* eggs are

oval and colorless with a thick, slightly pitted, shell, and bipolar plugs, ranging in size from 22 to 32 µM wide by 50–69 µM long in one report, [254] and 55–68 µm by 24–29 µm in another study [257]. *Capillaria* eggs are amber-colored in unstained urine and have a granular [15] sculpted character [258] to the outer shell (wall). The bipolar plugs of *Capillaria* are not directly opposite each other, but slightly askew [15], a feature that distinguishes them from *Trichuris*. *Capillaria* eggs are wider and have more parallel walls compared to the more concave appearance of *Trichuris* [258]. Immature eggs were described in three of six dogs [255] and lacked shells, were smaller, and had rudimentary polar plugs [257]. Two flotation techniques have recently been developed for use in urine to provide more quantitative results for the number of *Capillaria* ova as compared to the qualitative results provided by urine sediment microscopy [259].

Dioctophyme renale (*Dioctophyma renale*) is the largest known species of nematode and is commonly referred to as the "giant kidney worm." Distribution is worldwide, with increased incidence in the Caspian Sea region, Brazil, and in some areas of North America (e.g. Ontario and Minnesota). Infections can be found in both rural and urban areas. Adult worms are red in color and female worms can grow to 103 cm long with a width of 10–12 mm. Ova of *Dioctophyme renale* (Figure 6.141) rarely are identified in the urine of dogs. The eggs are oval-shaped, brownish-yellow in unstained sediment, with thick shells that are pitted except at the poles [260]. The eggs are oval and measure 60–84 µm × 39–52 µm. [257, 261].

Carnivores (including dogs, mink, raccoons, wolves, foxes, weasels, and cats) are definitive hosts (Centers for Disease Control and Prevention website https://www.cdc.gov/dpdx/dioctophymiasis/index.html). Infected hosts shed unembryonated eggs in urine, and L1 larvae develop after about

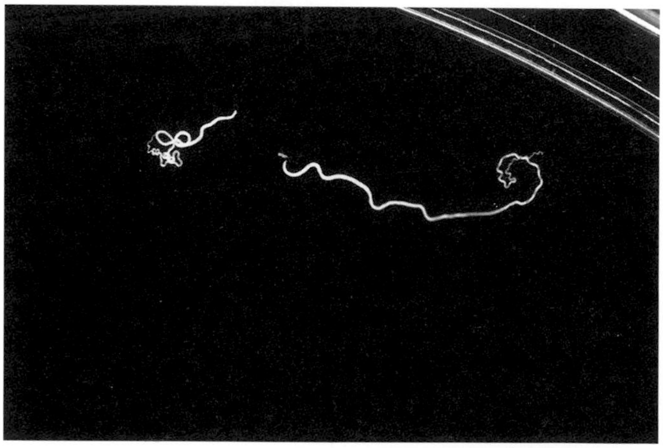

FIGURE 6.140 Two *Capillaria* worms in a Petri dish. These worms were discovered and removed during cystoscopy of a "normal" female cat. This cat had no clinical signs and the urinalysis was normal. No ova or larvae were observed in the urine sediment. Source: Reproduced with permission of Dr. Jody Westropp, The Ohio State University College of Veterinary Medicine.

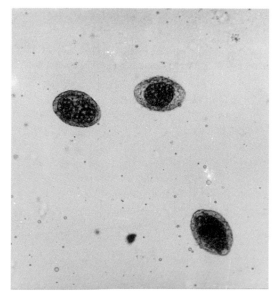

FIGURE 6.141 Three ova of *Dioctophyma renale* from a dog; stained urine sediment.

one month in water, but this process may take up to seven months depending on environmental conditions. An invertebrate annelid host (including the earthworm) consumes the L1 larvae; the larvae then hatch in the small intestine and mature into L3 larvae in approximately three months. If a paratenic host (e.g. fish, amphibians) consumes an annelid containing the L3 larvae, the larvae encyst and do not develop further. A definitive host can become infected from eating either the annelid intermediate host or a paratenic host. Once larvae enter the definitive host, they migrate through the gastric wall to the liver and eventually to the kidney. It takes approximately six months for the larvae to mature into adults in the definitive host. Humans can become infected by consuming raw or undercooked paratenic hosts (e.g. fish, amphibians). In humans, the larvae often encyst in subcutaneous nodules.

In order for ova to be detected, at least one gravid female worm must be present in the kidney. *Dioctophyme renale* most often are found in the right kidney, possibly due to the close proximity of the right kidney to the liver and duodenum. In the dog and cat, adult worms more commonly may be found free in the peritoneal cavity [261]; they may also be found in the ureters or urinary bladder. Hematuria may occur or no clinical signs may be observed. Abdominal distention may be present when worms are present in the peritoneal cavity. Affected dogs are not likely to be systemically ill when the contralateral kidney is normal. Renomegaly occurs as a consequence of hydronephrosis caused by the adult worms in the kidney. Sometimes, hematuria is so severe that large blood clots form in the bladder. Renal enlargement can be documented by radiographs, but ultrasonography and computed tomography can identify hydronephrosis and characteristic patterns for the parasites within the kidney [262, 263]. Often, the worms can be identified within the renal pelvis in conjunction with renal parenchymal atrophy. The diagnosis is confirmed when characteristic eggs are identified on urine sediment examination (Figure 6.142). Ova were identified during urine sediment examination in 8 of 15 dogs with confirmed *Dioctophyme renale* infection. Female worms were identified in those dogs that were shedding ova into urine, but an additional two female dogs were identified that did not shed ova, presumably because the worms were not gravid. All of the giant kidney worms in this study were located in the right kidney [262].

In dogs infected with *Dioctophyme renale*, nephrectomy or nephrotomy with the removal of the worms from the urinary tract (Figure 6.143) may be of value if irreversible renal insufficiency has not yet occurred. During surgery, the peritoneal cavity should be thoroughly examined for parasites. Susceptible hosts should be prevented from consuming paratenic hosts or invertebrate intermediate hosts. If fish or amphibians are consumed, they should be thoroughly cooked to prevent infection.

Rarely, heartworm microfilaria (*Dirofilaria*) can be observed in urine sediment [264, 265]. They can be distinguished from plant material by their curved end (Figure 6.144).

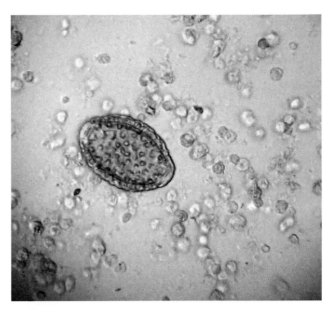

FIGURE 6.142 Ova of *Dioctophyma renale* in unstained urine sediment from a dog evaluated for macroscopic hematuria. Note the rough or corrugated character of the shell. Numerous degenerating WBC and RBC in background. Source: Courtesy of Dr. Marcia Kogika, University of São Paulo, São Paulo, Brazil.

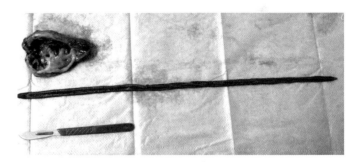

FIGURE 6.143 *Dioctophyma renale* (the giant kidney worm) after surgical removal of the right kidney and then incision into the hydronephrotic kidney. This worm has a greater preference to end up in the right kidney. Source: Courtesy of Dr. Marcia Kogika, University of São Paulo, São Paulo, Brazil.

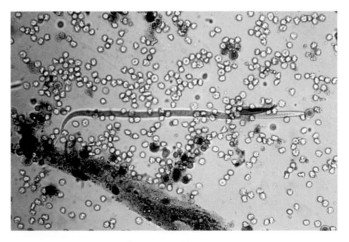

FIGURE 6.144 Heartworm microfilaria in center of image. Many RBC, rare WBC, and one granular cast.

REFERENCES

1 Fogazzi, G.B. and Cameron, J.S. (1996). Urinary microscopy from the seventeenth century to the present day. *Kidney Int.* 50: 1058–1068.

2 Magiorkinis, E. and Diamantis, A. (2015). The fascinating story of urine examination: from uroscopy to the era of microscopy and beyond. *Diagn. Cytopathol.* 43: 1020–1036.

3 Meuten, D. and Sample, S. (2022). Laboratory evaluation and interpretation of the urinary system. In: *Clinical Chemistry of Common Domestic Species*, 2e (ed. M.A. Thrall, G. Weiser, R.W. Allison, et al.). IN PRESS.

4 Hernandez, A.M., Bilbrough, G.E.A., DeNicola, D.B. et al. (2016). Comparison of the Sedivue Dx(TM) analyzer with manual microscopy for detection of red blood cells and while blood cells in urine sediments. In: *American College Veterinary Pathology/American Society Veterinary Clinical Pathology Concurrent Annual Meeting*, 5–6. New Orleans: http://asvcp.org/meeting/pdf/2016_Abstracts.pdf.

5 Hammond, J., Moisan, L., Bilbrough, G. et al. (2015). 26: erythrocyte and leuocyte count precision with an in-clinic automated urine sediment microscopy system. *Vet. Clin. Pathol.* 44: E-13.

6 Luciano, R.L., Castano, E., Fogazzi, G.B. et al. (2014). Light chain crystalline kidney disease: diagnostic urine microscopy as the "liquid kidney biopsy". *Clin. Nephrol.* 82: 387–391.

7 Strasinger, S.K. and Di Lorenzo, M.S. (2014). Microscopic examination of urine. In: *Urinalysis and Body Fluids*, 99–146. Philadelphia: F.A. Davis Company.

8 Perazella, M.A. (2015). The urine sediment as a biomarker of kidney disease. *Am. J. Kidney Dis.* 66: 748–755.

9 Tsai, J.J., Yeun, J.Y., Kumar, V.A. et al. (2005). Comparison and interpretation of urinalysis performed by a nephrologist versus a hospital-based clinical laboratory. *Am. J. Kidney Dis.* 46: 820–829.

10 Kincaid-Smith, P. (1982). Haematuria and exercise-related haematuria. *Br. Med. J. (Clin. Res. Ed)* 285: 1595–1597.

11 Wamsley, H.L. and Alleman, R. (2007). Complete urinalysis. In: *BSAVA Manual of Canine and Felne Nephrology and Urology*, 2e (ed. J. Elliott and G.F. Grauer), 87–116. UK: BSAVA, Gloucester.

12 Fettman, M.J. (1987). Evaluation of the usefulness of routine microscopy in canine urinalysis. *J. Am. Vet. Med. Assoc.* 190: 892–896.

13 Barlough, J.E., Osborne, C.A., and Stevens, J.B. (1981). Canine and feline urinalysis: value of macroscopic and microscopic examinations. *J. Am. Vet. Med. Assoc.* 178: 61–63.

14 Chawla, L.S., Dommu, A., Berger, A. et al. (2008). Urinary sediment cast scoring index for acute kidney injury: a pilot study. *Nephron Clin. Pract.* 110: c145–c150.

15 Alleman, R. and Wamsley, H.L. (2017). Complete urinalysis. In: *BSAVA Manual of Canine and Feline Nephrology and Urology*, 2e (ed. J. Elliott, G.F. Grauer and J.L. Westropp), 60–83. Gloucester, UK: BSAVA.

16 Callens, A.J. and Bartges, J.W. (2015). Urinalysis. *Vet. Clin. North Am. Small Anim. Pract.* 45: 621–637.

17 Delanghe, J. and Speeckaert, M. (2014). Preanalytical requirements of urinalysis. *Biochem Med (Zagreb)* 24: 89–104.

18 Caleffi, A. and Lippi, G. (2015). Cylindruria. *Clin. Chem. Lab. Med.* 53 (Suppl 2): s1471–s1477.

19 Mundt, M.A. and Shanahan, K. (2016). Collection and preservation of urine. In: *Graff's Textbook of Urinalysis and Body Fluids*, 3e, 72–78. Philadelphia: Wolters Kluwer.

20 Delanghe, J.R. and Speeckaert, M.M. (2016). Preanalytics in urinalysis. *Clin. Biochem.* 49: 1346–1350.

21 Rizzi, T.E., Valenciano, A., Bowles, M. et al. (2017). *Urine Sediment Atlas of Canine and Feline Urinalysis*, 67–179. Hoboken, N.J: Wiley.

22 Schumann, G.B., Harris, S., and Henry, J.B. (1978). An improved technic for examining urinary casts and a review of their significance. *Am. J. Clin. Pathol.* 69: 18–23.

23 Hammond, J., Ericson, C., Myrick, C. et al. (2016). Impact of urine formed element settling and sample aspiration location on microscopic urinalysis. In: *American College Veterinary Pathology/American Society Veterinary Clinical Pathology Concurrent Annual Meeting*, 32. New Orleans http://asvcp.org/meeting/pdf/2016_Abstracts.pdf.

24 Kim, Y., Jin, D.C., Lee, E.J. et al. (2002). Quantitative analysis of urine sediment using newly designed centrifuge tubes. *Ann. Clin. Lab. Sci.* 32: 55–60.

25 Braun, J.P., Bourges-Abella, N., Geffre, A. et al. (2015). The preanalytic phase in veterinary clinical pathology. *Vet. Clin. Pathol.* 44: 8–25.

26 Gunn-Christie, R.G., Flatland, B., Friedrichs, K.R. et al. (2012). ASVCP quality assurance guidelines: control of preanalytical, analytical, and postanalytical factors for urinalysis, cytology, and clinical chemistry in veterinary laboratories. *Vet. Clin. Pathol.* 41: 18–26.

27 Morissette, E. (2018). Evaluation of urine by automatic and manual methods ABX-00145: Zoetis.

28 Chase, J., Hammond, J., Bilbrough, G. et al. (2015). 27: examination of imprecision and effectiveness of different centrifugation and uncentrifugation methods for urine sediment microscopic evaluation. *Vet. Clin. Pathol.* 44: E-13.

29 Bunjevac, A., Gabaj, N.N., Miler, M. et al. (2018). Preanalytics of urine sediment examination: effect of relative centrifugal force, tube type, volume of sample and supernatant removal. *Biochem. Med. (Zagreb)* 28: 010707.

30 Layssol, C., Geffr, A., Braun, J.P. et al. Comparison of three different methods of urine canine sediment preparation for microscpic analysis *European Society of Veterinary Clinical Pathology (ESVCP) and European College of Veterinary Clinical Pathology (ECVCP) 11th Annual Congress. Thessaloniki, Greece – October 7–9, 2009, 2009;E-40*.

31 Vasilatis, D.M., Cowgill, L.D., Farace, G. et al. (2021). Comparison of IDEXX SediVue dx([R]) urine sediment analyzer to manual microscopy for detection of casts in canine urine. *J. Vet. Intern. Med.* 35: 1439–1447.

32 Palsson, R., Colona, M.R., Hoenig, M.P. et al. (2020). Assessment of Interobserver reliability of nephrologist examination of urine sediment. *JAMA Netw. Open* 3: e2013959.

33 Rasoulpour, M., Banco, L., Laut, J.M. et al. (1996). Inability of community-based laboratories to identify pathological casts in urine samples. *Arch. Pediatr. Adolesc. Med.* 150: 1201–1204.

34 Wald, R., Bell, C.M., Nisenbaum, R. et al. (2009). Interobserver reliability of urine sediment interpretation. *Clin. J. Am. Soc. Nephrol.* 4: 567–571.

35 Cavanaugh, C. and Perazella, M.A. (2019). Urine sediment examination in the diagnosis and Management of Kidney Disease: Core curriculum 2019. *Am. J. Kidney Dis.* 73: 258–272.

36 Fogazzi, G.B., Verdesca, S., and Garigali, G. (2008). Urinalysis: core curriculum 2008. *Am. J. Kidney Dis.* 51: 1052–1067.

37 Committee E (2017). Urinary sediment examination. *Jpn. J. Med. Tech.* 66: 51–85.

38 Becker, G.J., Garigali, G., and Fogazzi, G.B. (2016). Advances in urine microscopy. *Am. J. Kidney Dis.* 67: 954–964.

39 Fogazzi, G.B. and Garigali, G. (2003). The clinical art and science of urine microscopy. *Curr. Opin. Nephrol. Hypertens.* 12: 625–632.

40 Sternheimer, R. and Malbin, B. (1951). Clinical recognition of pyelonephritis, with a new stain for urinary sediments. *Am. J. Med.* 11: 312–323.

41 Chew, D.J. and DiBartola, S.P. (1998). *Handbook of Canine and Feline Urinalysis.* Wilmington, DE: Ralston Purina Co. The Gloyd Group.

42 Osborne, C.A. and Stevens, J.B. (1999). *Urinalysis: A Clinical Guide to Compassionate Patient Care.* Shawnee Mission, KS: Bayer.

43 Mundt, M.A. and Shanahan, K. (2016). *Graff's Textbook of Urinalysis and Body Fluids*, 3e. Philadelphia: Wolters Kluwer.

44 Strasinger, S.K. and Di Lorenzo, M.S. (2014). *Urinalysis and Body Fluids.* Philadelphia: F.A. Davis Company.

45 Chu-Su, Y., Shukuya, K., Yokoyama, T. et al. (2017). Enhancing the detection of dysmorphic red blood cells and renal tubular epithelial cells with a modified urinalysis protocol. *Sci. Rep.* 7: 40521.

46 Mundt, M.A. and Shanahan, K. (2016). *Microscopic Examination of Urine Graff's Textbook of Urinalysis and Body Fluids*, 3e, 89–110. Philadelphia: Wolters Kluwer.

47 Sink, C.A. and Weinstein, N.M. (2012). Routine urinalysis: chemical analysis. In: *Practical Veterinary Urinalysis,* 29–53. Ames, Iowa: Wiley.

48 Fish, P.A. (1906). *The Examination of the Urine of the Horse and Man.* Ithaca, N.Y: Taylor and Carpenter.

49 Kohn, C.W. and Chew, D.J. (1987). Laboratory diagnosis and characterization of renal disease in horses. *Vet. Clin. North Am. Equine Pract.* 3: 585–615.

50 Meuten, D.J., Moore, F.M., and George, J.W. (2016). Mitotic count and the field of view area: time to standardize. *Vet. Pathol.* 53: 7–9.

51 George, J.W. (1999). Ocular field widths and platelet estimates. 28:126.

52 Bonert, M. and Tate, A.J. (2017). Mitotic counts in breast cancer should be standardized with a uniform sample area. *Biomed. Eng. Online* 16: 28.

53 Ellis, P.S. and Whitehead, R. (1981). Mitosis counting--a need for reappraisal. *Hum. Pathol.* 12: 3–4.

54 Davidson, M.R. (2021). Field of View *MicroscopyU.* https://www.microscopyu.com/microscopy-basics/field-of-view:Nikon.

55 Kirkham, N., Braye, S.G., and Cotton, D.W.K. (1984). Magnifications and mitoses counts. *Histopathology* 8: 1085.

56 Meuten, D.J., Moore, F.M., and George, J.W. (2017). Mitiotic count. In: *Tumors in Domestic Animals*, 5e (ed. D. Meuten), 944–945. Ames, IA: Wiley.

57 Vail, D.M., Allen, T.A., and Weiser, G. (1986). Applicability of leukocyte esterase test strip in detection of canine pyuria. *J. Am. Vet. Med. Assoc.* 189: 1451–1453.

58 Zoetis. Why are you changing my urinalysis? I want my HPF! What are cells/uL? ABX-00151, 2018.

59 Fogazzi, G.B. and Grignani, S. (1998). Urine microscopic analysis–an art abandoned by nephrologists? *Nephrol. Dial. Transplant.* 13: 2485–2487.

60 Fogazzi, G.B., Grignani, S., and Colucci, P. (1998). Urinary microscopy as seen by nephrologists. *Clin. Chem. Lab. Med.* 36: 919–924.

61 Sternheimer, R. (1975). A supravital cytodiagnostic stain for urinary sediments. *JAMA* 231: 826–832.

62 Mutter, W.P. and Brown, R.S. (2011). Point-of-care photomicroscopy of urine. *N. Engl. J. Med.* 364: 1880–1881.

63 Vap, L.M. and Shropshire, S.B. (2017). Urine cytology: collection, film preparation, and evaluation. *Vet. Clin. North Am. Small Anim. Pract.* 47: 135–149.

64 Lehman, R.M. (1968). Preservation of urine sediments. *Tech. Bull. Regist. Med. Technol.* 38: 268–269.

65 Zabor, L. (1970). Preservation of urine sediments on slides. *Am. J. Med. Technol.* 36: 544–545.

66 Love, B.F. and Petracca, T.R. (1964). Preparation of permanent mounts of stained and unstained urinary sediments. *Tech. Bull. Regist. Med. Technol.* 34: 48–49.

67 Zaman, Z., Fogazzi, G.B., Garigali, G. et al. (2010). Urine sediment analysis: analytical and diagnostic performance of sediMAX – a new automated microscopy image-based urine sediment analyser. *Clin. Chim. Acta* 411: 147–154.

68 Zaman, Z. (2015). Automated urine screening devices make urine sediment microscopy in diagnostic laboratories economically viable. *Clin. Chem. Lab. Med.* 53 (Suppl 2): s1509–s1511.

69 Hammond, J., Myrick, C., McCrann, D.J. et al. (2015). 1: application of current automated microscopy technology to qualitative identification of urine formed elements in veterinary medicine. *Vet. Clin. Pathol.* 44: E-5.

70 Osborne, C.A. and Stevens, J.B. (1999). Urine sediment: under the microscope. In: *Urinalysis: A Clinical Guide to Compassionate Patient Care* (ed. C.A. Osborne and J.B. Stevens), 125–150. Shawnee Mission, KS: Bayer.

71 DeNicola, D.B., Hammond, J., Bayer, G. et al. (2015). 25: application of current automated urine microscopy in veterinary medicine. *Vet. Clin. Pathol.* 44: E-13.

72 Alleman, R., Bilbrough, G., Hammond, J. et al. (2016). C-35: Qualitative evaluation of erythrocyte and leukocyte numbers with an in-clinic automated urine sediment microscopy system. In: *2016 American College Veterinary Pathology/American Society Veterinary Clinical Pathology Concurrent Annual Meeting*, 35–36. New Orleans http://asvcp.org/meeting/pdf/2016_Abstracts.pdf.

73 Allcman, R., Bilbrough, G., Hammond, J. et al. (2017). Evaluation of an in-house automated urine sediment analyzer for qualitative evaluation of erythroctye and leukocyte numnbers. American society. *Vet. Clin. Pathol..*

74 Hernandez, A.M., Bilbrough, G.E.A., DeNicola, D.B. et al. (2019). Comparison of the performance of the IDEXX SediVue dx(R) with manual microscopy for the detection of cells and 2 crystal types in canine and feline urine. *J. Vet. Intern. Med.* 33: 167–177.

75 Alleman, R., Bilbrough, G., Hammond, J. et al. (2016). C-33:Qualitative evaluation of calcium oxalate dihydrate and struvite crystal numbers with an in-clinic automated urine sediment microsocopy systtem.

In: *2016 American College Veterinary Pathology/American Society Veterinary Clinical Pathology Concurrent Annual Meeting*, 34. New Orleans: http://asvcp.org/meeting/pdf/2016_Abstracts.pdf.

76 Alleman, R., Bilbrough, G., Hammond, J. et al. (2017). Evaluation of an in-house automated urine sediment analyzer for qualitative evaluation of struvite and calcium oxalate dihydrae cyrstals. Proceedings of American Society Veterinary Clinical Pathology.

77 Hernandez, A.M., Bilbrough, G.E.A., DeNicola, D.B. et al. (2017). Evaluation of an automated urine sediment analyzer for detection of struvite and calcium oxalate dihydrate crystals. Proceedings of European Society of Veterinary Clinical Pathology.

78 Alleman, R., Bilbrough, G., Hammond, J. et al. (2016). C-34:Qualitative evaluation of squamous and nonsquamous epithellial cell numbers with an in-clinic automated urine sediment microscopy system. In: *2016 American College Veterinary Pathology/American Society Veterinary Clinical Pathology Concurrent Annual Meeting*, 35. New Orleans: http://asvcp.org/meeting/pdf/2016_Abstracts.pdf.

79 Hernandez, A.M., Bilbrough, G.E.A., DeNicola, D.B. et al. (2017). Evaluation of an automated urine sediment analyzer for detection of epithelial cells. Proceedings of European Society of Veterinary Clinical Pathology.

80 Blanco, T., Hernandez, A., DiNicola, D., Myrick, C., Nabity, M. (2019). Analysis of Bias Between the Sedivue Dx(TM) and Manual Microscopy in Detecting Urine Sediment Cells NU-19. *J. Vet. Intern. Med.* 33(5): 2527.

81 Vasilatis, D.M., Cowgill, L., Yerramilli, M. et al. (2019). Comparison of IDEXX SediVue dx® with manual microscopy for detection of casts in canine urine. *J. Vet. Intern. Med.* 33: 2524.

82 Bottini, P.V., Martinez, M.H., and Garlipp, C.R. (2014). Urinalysis: comparison between microscopic analysis and a new automated microscopy image-based urine sediment instrument. *Clin. Lab.* 60: 693–697.

83 Bogaert, L., Peeters, B., and Billen, J. (2017). Evaluation of a new automated microscopy urine sediment analyser – sediMAX conTRUST(R). *Acta Clin. Belg.* 72: 91–94.

84 Ince, F.D., Ellidag, H.Y., Koseoglu, M. et al. (2016). The comparison of automated urine analyzers with manual microscopic examination for urinalysis automated urine analyzers and manual urinalysis. *Pract. Lab. Med.* 5: 14–20.

85 Oyaert, M. and Delanghe, J. (2019). Progress in automated urinalysis. *Ann. Lab. Med.* 39: 15–22.

86 Neubert, E. and Weber, K. (2021). Using the Idexx SediVue dx to predict the need for urine bacteriologic culture in cats. *J. Vet. Diagn. Invest.* https://doi.org/10.1177/10406387211038918.

87 Neubert, E. and Weber, K. (2021). Using the Idexx SediVue Dx to predict the need for urine bacteriologic culture in cats. *J. Vet. Diagn. Invest.* 33: 1202–1205.

88 Fogazzi, G.B., Passerini, P., Bazzi, M. et al. (1989). Use of high power field in the evaluation of formed elements of urine. *J. Nephrol.* 2: 107–112.

89 O'Neil, E., Burton, S., Horney, B. et al. (2013). Comparison of white and red blood cell estimates in urine sediment with hemocytometer and automated counts in dogs and cats. *Vet. Clin. Pathol.* 42: 78–84.

90 Ingelfinger, J.R. (2021). Hematuria in Adults. *N. Engl. J. Med.* 385: 153–163.

91 Cohen, R.A. and Brown, R.S. (2003). Clinical practice. Microscopic hematuria. *N. Engl. J. Med.* 348: 2330–2338.

92 Grossfeld, G.D., Litwin, M.S., Wolf, J.S. Jr. et al. (2001). Evaluation of asymptomatic microscopic hematuria in adults: the American urological association best practice policy--part II: patient evaluation, cytology, voided markers, imaging, cystoscopy, nephrology evaluation, and follow-up. *Urology* 57: 604–610.

93 Grossfeld, G.D., Litwin, M.S., Wolf, J.S. et al. (2001). Evaluation of asymptomatic microscopic hematuria in adults: the American urological association best practice policy – part I: definition, detection, prevalence, and etiology. *Urology* 57: 599–603.

94 Grossfeld, G.D., Wolf, J.S. Jr., Litwan, M.S. et al. (2001). Asymptomatic microscopic hematuria in adults: summary of the AUA best practice policy recommendations. *Am. Fam. Physician* 63: 1145–1154.

95 Fogazzi, G.B. and Ponticelli, C. (1996). Microscopic hematuria diagnosis and management. *Nephron* 72: 125–134.

96 Morgan, H.C. and Ellington, L. (1967). Practical evaluation of urine sediment. *Vet. Med. Small Anim. Clin.* 62: 984–988.

97 Alexander, C.S., Swaim, W.R., and Garcia, M.C. (1975). Urine concentration and dilution: effect on red cell survival. *Proc. Soc. Exp. Biol. Med.* 150: 295–298.

98 McIntyre, M. and Mou, T.W. (1965). Persistence of leukocytes and erythrocytes in refrigerated acid and alkaline urine. *Am. J. Clin. Pathol.* 43: 53–57.

99 Aulakh, H.K., Aulakh, K.S., Ryan, K.A. et al. (2020). Investigation of the effects of storage with preservatives at room temperature or refrigeration without preservatives on urinalysis results for samples from healthy dogs. *J. Am. Vet. Med. Assoc.* 257: 726–733.

100 Ling, G.V. and Kaneko, J.J. (1976). Microscopic examination on of canine urine sediment. *Calif. Vet.* 30: 14–18.

101 Zinkl, J.G. (1995). Urine sediment examination. In: *Lower Urinary Tract Diseases of Dogs and Cats* (ed. G.V. Ling), 29–36. St. Louis Mosby-Year Book, Inc.

102 Vientos-Plotts, A.I., Behrend, E.N., Welles, E.G. et al. (2018). Effect of blood contamination on results of dipstick evaluation and urine protein-to-urine creatinine ratio for urine samples from dogs and cats. *Am. J. Vet. Res.* 79: 525–531.

103 Fogazzi, G.B., Edefonti, A., Garigali, G. et al. (2008). Urine erythrocyte morphology in patients with microscopic haematuria caused by a glomerulopathy. *Pediatr. Nephrol.* 23: 1093–1100.

104 Barsanti, J.A. and Finco, D.R. (1979). Protein concentration in urine of normal dogs. *Am. J. Vet. Res.* 40: 1583–1588.

105 Thal, S.M., DeBellis, C.C., Iverson, S.A. et al. (1986). Comparison of dysmorphic erythrocytes with other urinary sediment parameters of renal bleeding. *Am. J. Clin. Pathol.* 86: 784–787.

106 Schumann, G.B. and Schumann, J.L. (1992). Microscopic examination of the urinary sediment to differentiate high from low renal bleeding. In: *International Yearbook of Nephrology* (ed. V.E. Andreucci and L.G. Fine), 337–352. London, England: Springer-Verlag.

107 Makino, H., Nishimura, S., Soda, K. et al. (1986). Mechanism of hematuria. I. Electron microscopic demonstration of the passage of a red blood cell through a glomerular capillary wall in rat masugi nephritis. *Virchows Arch. B Cell Pathol. Incl. Mol. Pathol.* 50: 199–208.

108 Makino, H., Nishimura, S., Takaoka, M. et al. (1988). Mechanism of hematuria. II. A scanning electron microscopic demonstration of the passage of blood cells through a glomerular capillary wall in rabbit Masugi nephritis. *Nephron* 50: 142–150.

109 Ling, G.V. (1995). Techniques of urine collection and handling. In: *Lower Urinary Tract Diseases of Dogs and Cats* (ed. G.V. Ling), 23–27. St. Louis Mosby-Year Book, Inc.

110 Kaye, M. (1958). A peroxidase-staining procedure for the identification of polymorphonuclear leukocytes and leukocyte casts in the urinary sediment. *N. Engl. J. Med.* 258: 1301–1302.

111 Muriithi, A.K., Nasr, S.H., and Leung, N. (2013). Utility of urine eosinophils in the diagnosis of acute interstitial nephritis. *Clin. J. Am. Soc. Nephrol.* 8: 1857–1862.

112 Hadrick, M.K., Vaden, S.L., Geoly, F.J. et al. (1996). Acute tubulointerstitial nephritis with eosinophiluria in a dog. *J. Vet. Intern. Med.* 10: 45–47.

113 Osborne, C.A. and Stevens, J.B. (1999). Baacteriuria and urinary tract infections: definition of terms and concepts. In: *Urinalysis: A Clinical Guide to Compassionate Patient Care*, 17–30. Shawnee Mission, KS: Bayer.

114 Chew, D.J. and Kowalski, J. (1981). Urinary tract infections. In: *Pathophysiology of Surgery in Small Animals* (ed. M.J. Bojrab), 255–270. Lea & Febiger.

115 Westropp, J.L., Sykes, J.E., Irom, S. et al. (2012). Evaluation of the efficacy and safety of high dose short duration enrofloxacin treatment regimen for uncomplicated urinary tract infections in dogs. *J. Vet. Intern. Med.* 26: 506–512.

116 Way, L.I., Sullivan, L.A., Johnson, V. et al. (2013). Comparison of routine urinalysis and urine gram stain for detection of bacteriuria in dogs. *J. Vet. Emerg. Crit. Care (San Antonio)* 23: 23–28.

117 Swenson, C.L., Boisvert, A.M., Kruger, J.M. et al. (2004). Evaluation of modified Wright-staining of urine sediment as a method for accurate detection of bacteriuria in dogs. *J. Am. Vet. Med. Assoc.* 224: 1282–1289.

118 O'Neil, E., Horney, B., Burton, S. et al. (2013). Comparison of wet-mount, Wright-Giemsa and gram-stained urine sediment for predicting bacteriuria in dogs and cats. *Can. Vet. J.* 54: 1061–1066.

119 Swenson, C.L., Boisvert, A.M., Gibbons-Burgener, S.N. et al. (2011). Evaluation of modified Wright-staining of dried urinary sediment as a method for accurate detection of bacteriuria in cats. *Vet. Clin. Pathol.* 40: 256–264.

120 Allen, T.A., Jones, R.L., and Purvance, J. (1987). Microbiologic evaluation of canine urine: direct microscopic examination and preservation of specimen quality for culture. *J. Am. Vet. Med. Assoc.* 190: 1289–1291.

121 Gutman, L.T., Turck, M., Petersdorf, R.G. et al. (1965). Significance of bacterial variants in urine of patients with chronic bacteriuria. *J. Clin. Invest.* 44: 1945–1952.

122 Strachan, N.A., Hales, E.N., and Fischer, J.R. (2022). Prevalence of positive urine culture in the presence of inactive urine sediment in 1049 urine samples from dogs. *J. Vet. Intern. Med.*.

123 Liebelt, R. and Pigott, A. (2019). The prevalence of positive urine cultures in 100 dogs with an inactive urine sediment. *Vet. Evid.* 4: 273.

124 IDEXX (2021). SediVue Bacterial Confirmation Kit Quick Reference Guide. https://image.success.idexx.com/lib/fe8d13727c62077f70/m/4/7a28e3a0-4624-4a7a-a826-0e072d66f096.pdf.

125 IDEXX (2021). Advanced bacterial detection https://pages.idexx.com/advancedbacteriadetection?utm_source=sales&utm_medium=vdc&utm_campaign=sedivue_abd_2020&utm_content=clarity: IDEXX.

126 Pressler, B.M., Vaden, S.L., Lane, I.F. et al. (2003). Candida spp. urinary tract infections in 13 dogs and seven cats: predisposing factors, treatment, and outcome. *J. Am. Anim. Hosp. Assoc.* 39: 263–270.

127 Rudinsky, A.J., Guptill-Yoran, L., Wheat, L.J. et al. (2013). Urine sediment identification of Blastomyces dermatitidis organisms in dogs with confirmed systemic infection (ID-12). *J. Vet. Intern. Med.* 27: 723–724.

128 Pressler, B.M., Gookin, J.L., Sykes, J.E. et al. (2005). Urinary tract manifestations of prototheosis in dogs. *J. Vet. Intern. Med.* 19: 115–119.

129 Warner, R.S., Tessler, A.N., and Andronaco, R.B. (1982). Epitheliuria: aid in early diagnosis of renal artery embolus. *Urology* 19: 628–629.

130 Wycislo, K.L. and Piech, T.L. (2019). Urinary tract cytology. *Vet. Clin. North Am. Small Anim. Pract.* 49: 247–260.

131 Norris, A.M., Laing, E.J., Valli, V.E. et al. (1992). Canine bladder and urethral tumors: a retrospective study of 115 cases (1980-1985). *J. Vet. Intern. Med.* 6: 145–153.

132 Wojcik, E.M. (2015). What should not be reported as atypia in urine cytology. *J. Am. Soc. Cytopathol.* 4: 30–36.

133 Melamed, M.R. and Wolinska, W.H. (1961). On the significance of intracytoplasmic inclusions in the urinary sediment. *Am. J. Pathol.* 38: 711–719.

134 Brimo, F., Vollmer, R.T., Case, B. et al. (2009). Accuracy of urine cytology and the significance of an atypical category. *Am. J. Clin. Pathol.* 132: 785–793.

135 Brimo, F., Xu, B., Kassouf, W. et al. (2015). Urine cytology: does the number of atypical urothelial cells matter? A qualitative and quantitative study of 112 cases. *J. Am. Soc. Cytopathol.* 4: 232–238.

136 Knapp, D.W., Glickman, N.W., Denicola, D.B. et al. (2000). Naturally-occurring canine transitional cell carcinoma of the urinary bladder a relevant model of human invasive bladder cancer. *Urol. Oncol.* 5: 47–59.

137 Knapp, D.W., Richardson, R.C., Chan, T.C. et al. (1994). Piroxicam therapy in 34 dogs with transitional cell carcinoma of the urinary bladder. *J. Vet. Intern. Med.* 8: 273–278.

138 Griffin, M.A., Culp, W.T.N., and Rebhun, R.B. (2018). Lower urinary tract neoplasia. *Vet. Sci.* 5 (4): 96.

139 Holt, P.E., Lucke, V.M., and Brown, P.J. (1986). Evaluation of a catheter biopsy technique as a diagnostic aid in lower urinary tract disease. *Vet. Rec.* 118: 681–684.

140 Lamb, C.R., Trower, N.D., and Gregory, S.P. (1996). Ultrasound-guided catheter biopsy of the lower urinary tract: technique and results in 12 dogs. *J. Small Anim. Pract.* 37: 413–416.

141 Decker, B., Parker, H.G., Dhawan, D. et al. (2015). Homologous mutation to human BRAF V600E is common in naturally occurring canine bladder cancer – evidence for a relevant model system and urine-based diagnostic test. *Mol. Cancer Res.* 13: 993–1002.

142 Mochizuki, H. and Breen, M. (2015). Comparative aspects of BRAF mutations in canine cancers. *Vet. Sci.* 2: 231–245.

143 Mochizuki, H., Kennedy, K., Shapiro, S.G. et al. (2015). BRAF mutations in canine cancers. *PLoS One* 10: e0129534.

144 Mochizuki, H., Shapiro, S.G., and Breen, M. (2015). Detection of BRAF mutation in urine DNA as a molecular diagnostic for canine urothelial and prostatic carcinoma. *PLoS One* 10: e0144170.

145 Mochizuki, H., Shapiro, S.G., and Breen, M. (2016). Detection of copy number imbalance in canine urothelial carcinoma with droplet digital polymerase chain reaction. *Vet. Pathol.* 53: 764–772.

146 Henry, C.J., Tyler, J.W., McEntee, M.C. et al. (2003). Evaluation of a bladder tumor antigen test as a screening test for transitional cell carcinoma of the lower urinary tract in dogs. *Am. J. Vet. Res.* 64: 1017–1020.

147 Billet, J.P., Moore, A.H., and Holt, P.E. (2002). Evaluation of a bladder tumor antigen test for the diagnosis of lower urinary tract malignancies in dogs. *Am. J. Vet. Res.* 63: 370–373.

148 Borjesson, D.L., Christopher, M.M., and Ling, G.V. (1999). Detection of canine transitional cell carcinoma using a bladder tumor antigen urine dipstick test. *Vet. Clin. Pathol.* 28: 33–38.

149 Bohme, B., Ngendahayo, P., Hamaide, A. et al. (2010). Inflammatory pseudotumours of the urinary bladder in dogs resembling human myofibroblastic tumours: a report of eight cases and comparative pathology. *Vet. J.* 183: 89–94.

150 Martinez, I., Mattoon, J.S., Eaton, K.A. et al. (2003). Polypoid cystitis in 17 dogs (1978-2001). *J. Vet. Intern. Med.* 17: 499–509.

151 Butty, E.M., Hahn, S., and Labato, M.A. (2021). Presumptive malignant transformation of chronic polypoid cystitis into an apical transitional cell carcinoma without BRAF mutation in a young female dog. *J. Vet. Intern. Med.* 35 (3): 1551–1557.

152 Borys, M.A., Hulsebosch, S.E., Mohr, F.C. et al. (2019). Clinical, histopathologic, cystoscopic, and fluorescence in situ hybridization analysis of proliferative urethritis in 22 dogs. *J. Vet. Intern. Med.* 33: 184–191.

153 Emanuel, M., Berent, A.C., Weisse, C. et al. (2021). Retrospective study of proliferative urethritis in dogs: clinical presentation and outcome using various treatment modalities in 11 dogs. *J. Vet. Intern. Med.* 35: 312–320.

154 Hostutler, R.A., Chew, D.J., Eaton, K.A. et al. (2004). Cystoscopic appearance of proliferative urethritis in 2 dogs before and after treatment. *J. Vet. Intern. Med.* 18: 113–116.

155 Moroff, S.D., Brown, B.A., Matthiesen, D.T. et al. (1991). Infiltrative urethral disease in female dogs: 41 cases (1980-1987). *J. Am. Vet. Med. Assoc.* 199: 247–251.

156 Mutsaers, A.J., Widmer, W.R., and Knapp, D.W. (2003). Canine transitional cell carcinoma. *J. Vet. Intern. Med.* 17: 136–144.

157 Knapp, D.W., Ramos-Vara, J.A., Moore, G.E. et al. (2014). Urinary bladder cancer in dogs, a naturally occurring model for cancer biology and drug development. *ILAR J.* 55: 100–118.

158 Thrall, M.A., Grauer, G.F., and Mero, K.N. (1984). Clinicopathologic findings in dogs and cats with ethylene glycol intoxication. *J. Am. Vet. Med. Assoc.* 184: 37–41.

159 Nakamura, T., Ushiyama, C., Suzuki, S. et al. (2000). The urinary podocyte as a marker for the differential diagnosis of idiopathic focal glomerulosclerosis and minimal-change nephrotic syndrome. *Am. J. Nephrol.* 20: 175–179.

160 Nakamura, T., Ushiyama, C., Suzuki, S. et al. (2000). Urinary excretion of podocytes in patients with diabetic nephropathy. *Nephrol. Dial. Transplant.* 15: 1379–1383.

161 Blackburn, V., Grignani, S., and Fogazzi, G.B. (1998). Lipiduria as seen by transmission electron microscopy. *Nephrol. Dial. Transplant.* 13: 2682–2684.

162 Prescott, L.F. and Brodie, D.E. (1964). A simple differential stain for urinary sediment. *Lancet* 2: 940.

163 Lippman, R.W. (1952). Significance of the urine examination. *Surg. Gynecol. Obstet.* 95: 369–371.

164 McQueen, E.G. (1962). The nature of urinary casts. *J. Clin. Pathol.* 15: 367–373.

165 Vaden, S.L., Levine, J., and Breitschwerdt, E.B. (1997). A retrospective case-control of acute renal failure in 99 dogs. *J. Vet. Intern. Med.* 11: 58–64.

166 Addis, T. (1926). The number of formed elements in the urinary sediment of normal individuals. *J. Clin. Invest.* 2: 409–415.

167 Kumar, S. and Muchmore, A. (1990). Tamm-Horsfall protein—uromodulin (1950-1990). *Kidney Int.* 37: 1395–1401.

168 Chacar, F., Kogika, M., Sanches, T.R. et al. (2017). Urinary Tamm-Horsfall protein, albumin, vitamin D-binding protein, and retinol-binding protein as early biomarkers of chronic kidney disease in dogs. *Physiol. Rep.* 5 (11): 1–9.

169 Rampoldi, L., Scolari, F., Amoroso, A. et al. (2011). The rediscovery of uromodulin (Tamm-Horsfall protein): from tubulointerstitial nephropathy to chronic kidney disease. *Kidney Int.* 80: 338–347.

170 Imhof, P.R., Hushak, J., Schumann, G. et al. (1972). Excretion of urinary casts after the administration of diuretics. *Br. Med. J.* 2: 199–202.

171 McQueen, E.G. (1966). Composition of urinary casts. *Lancet* 1: 397–398.

172 Orita, Y., Imai, N., Ueda, N. et al. (1977). Immunofluorescent studies of urinary casts. *Nephron* 19: 19–25.

173 Rutecki, G.J., Goldsmith, C., and Schreiner, G.E. (1971). Characterization of proteins in urinary casts. Fluorescent-antibody identification of Tamm-Horsfall mucoprotein in matrix and serum proteins in granules. *N. Engl. J. Med.* 284: 1049–1052.

174 Haber, M.H. and Lindner, L.E. (1977). The surface ultrastructure of urinary casts. *Am. J. Clin. Pathol.* 68: 547–552.

175 Cannon, D.C. (1979). The identification and pathogenesis of urine casts. *Lab. Med.* 10: 8–11.

176 Lindner, L.E., Jones, R.N., and Haber, M.H. (1980). A specific urinary cast in acute pyelonephritis. *Am. J. Clin. Pathol.* 73: 809–811.

177 Brody, L., Webster, M.C., and Kark, R.M. (1968). Identification of elements of urinary sediment with phase-contrast microscopy. A simple method. *JAMA* 206: 1777–1781.

178 Tamm, I. and Horsfall, F.L. (1950). Characterisation and separation of an inhibitor of viral hemagglutination present in urine. *Proc. Soc. Exp. Biol. Med.* 74: 108–114.

179 Lindner, L.E. and Haber, M.H. (1983). Hyaline casts in the urine: mechanism of formation and morphologic transformations. *Am. J. Clin. Pathol.* 80: 347–352.

180 Israni, A.K. and Kasiske, B.L. (2008). Laboratory assessment of kidney disease: clearance, urinalsis, and kidney biopsy. In: *Brenner and Rector's the Kidney*, 8e, 724–756. Philadelphia: Saunders Elsevier.

181 Lindner, L.E., Vacca, D., and Haber, M.H. (1983). Identification and composition of types of granular urinary casts. *Am. J. Clin. Pathol.* 80: 353–358.

182 Arbeit, L.A. and Weinstein, S.W. (1981). Acute tubular necrosis. *Med. Clin. North Am.* 65: 147–163.

183 Donohoe, J.F., Venkatachalam, M.A., Bernard, D.B. et al. (1976). Tubular leakage and obstruction in acute ischemic renal failure. *Kidney Int.* 10: 567–567.

184 Smith, B.J., Anderson, B.G., Smith, S.A. et al. (1990). Early effects of ethylene glycol on the ultrastructure of the renal cortex in dogs. *Am. J. Vet. Res.* 51: 89–96.

185 Spangler, W.L., Adelman, R.D., Conzelman, G.M. Jr. et al. (1980). Gentamicin nephrotoxicity in the dog: sequential light and electron microscopy. *Vet. Pathol.* 17: 206–217.

186 Domingue, G.J., Woody, H.B., Farris, K.B. et al. (1979). Bacterial variants in urinary casts and renal epithelial cells. *Arch. Intern. Med.* 139: 1355–1360.

187 Albright, F. and Bloomberg, E. (1935). Hyperparathyroidism and renal disease: with a note as to the formation of calcium casts in this disease. *J. Urol.* 34 (1): 1–7.

188 Luciano, R.L. and Perazella, M.A. (2015). Crystalline-induced kidney disease: a case for urine microscopy. *Clin. Kidney J.* 8: 131–136.

189 Slauson, D.O., Gribble, D.H., and Russell, S.W. (1970). A clinicopathological study of renal amyloidosis in dogs. *J. Comp. Pathol.* 80: 335–343.

190 Schentag, J.J., Gengo, F.M., Plaut, M.E. et al. (1979). Urinary casts as an indicator of renal tubular damage in patients receiving aminoglycosides. *Antimicrob. Agents Chemother.* 16: 468–474.

191 Perazella, M.A., Coca, S.G., and Hall, I.E. (2010). et al., Urine microscopy is associated with severity and worsening of acute kidney injury in hospitalized patients. *Clin. J. Am. Soc. Nephrol.* 5: 402–408.

192 Perazella, M.A., Coca, S.G., Kanbay, M. et al. (2008). Diagnostic value of urine microscopy for differential diagnosis of acute kidney injury in hospitalized patients. *Clin. J. Am. Soc. Nephrol.* 3: 1615–1619.

193 Perazella, M.A. and Parikh, C.R. (2009). How can urine microscopy influence the differential diagnosis of AKI? *Clin. J. Am. Soc. Nephrol.* 4: 691–693.

194 DiBartola, S.P., Tarr, M.J., Parker, A.T. et al. (1989). Clinicopathologic findings in dogs with renal amyloidosis: 59 cases (1976-1986). *J. Am. Vet. Med. Assoc.* 195: 358–364.

195 Spinelli, D., Consonni, D., Garigali, G. et al. (2013). Waxy casts in the urinary sediment of patients with different types of glomerular diseases: results of a prospective study. *Clin. Chim. Acta* 424: 47–52.

196 Schumann, G.B., Johnston, J.L., and Weiss, M.A. (1981). Renal epithelial fragments in urine sediment. *Acta Cytol.* 25: 147–152.

197 Fogazzi, G.B., Ferrari, B., Garigali, G. et al. (2012). Urinary sediment findings in acute interstitial nephritis. *Am. J. Kidney Dis.* 60: 330–332.

198 Tvedten, H., Lilliehook, I., Ronnberg, H. et al. (2019). Massive uric acid crystalluria and cylinduria in a dog after l-asparaginase treatment for lymphoma. *Vet. Clin. Pathol.* 48 (3): 425–428.

199 Sturgess, C.P., Hesford, A., Owen, H. et al. (2001). An investigation into the effects of storage on the diagnosis of crystalluria in cats. *J. Feline Med. Surg.* 3: 81–85.

200 Albasan, H., Lulich, J.P., Osborne, C.A. et al. (2003). Effects of storage time and temperature on pH, specific gravity, and crystal formation in urine samples from dogs and cats. *J. Am. Vet. Med. Assoc.* 222: 176–179.

201 Fogazzi, G.B., Anderlini, R., Canovi, S. et al. (2017). "Daisy-like" crystals: a rare and unknown type of urinary crystal. *Clin. Chim. Acta* 471: 154–157.

202 Fogazzi, G.B. (1996). Crystalluria: a neglected aspect of urinary sediment analysis. *Nephrol. Dial. Transplant.* 11: 379–387.

203 Koehler, L.A., Osborne, C.A., Buettner, M.T. et al. (2009). Canine uroliths: frequently asked questions and their answers. *Vet. Clin. North Am. Small Anim. Pract.* 39: 161–181.

204 Osborne, C.A., Davis, L.S., Sanna, J. et al. (1990). Identification and interpretation of crystalluria in domestic animals: a light and scanning electron microscopic study. *Vet. Med.* 85: 18–37.

205 Osborne, C.A., Lulich, J.P., Ulrich, L.K. et al. (1996). Feline crystalluria. Detection and interpretation. *Vet. Clin. North Am. Small Anim. Pract.* 26: 369–391.

206 Bartges, J.W. and Callens, A.J. (2015). Urolithiasis. *Vet. Clin. North Am. Small Anim. Pract.* 45: 747–768.

207 Paepe, D., Verjans, G., Duchateau, L. et al. (2013). Routine health screening: findings in apparently healthy middle-aged and old cats. *J. Feline Med. Surg.* 15: 8–19.

208 Willems, A., Paepe, D., Marynissen, S. et al. (2017). Results of screening of apparently healthy Senior and geriatric dogs. *J. Vet. Intern. Med.* 31: 81–92.

209 Buffington, C.A., Chew, D.J., and DiBartola, S.P. (1994). Lower urinary tract disease in cats: is diet still a cause? *J. Am. Vet. Med. Assoc.* 205: 1524–1527.

210 Markwell, P.J., Buffington, C.T., and Smith, B.H. (1998). The effect of diet on lower urinary tract diseases in cats. *J. Nutr.* 128: 2753S–2757S.

211 Willeberg, P. (1984). Epidemiology of naturally occurring feline urologic syndrome. *Vet. Clin. North Am. Small Anim. Pract.* 14: 455–469.

212 Kennedy, S.M., Lulich, J.P., Ritt, M.G. et al. (2016). Comparison of body condition score and urinalysis variables between dogs with and without calcium oxalate uroliths. *J. Am. Vet. Med. Assoc.* 249: 1274–1280.

213 Nguyen, N.U., Henriet, M.T., Dumoulin, G. et al. (1994). Increase in calciuria and oxaluria after a single chocolate bar load. *Horm. Metab. Res.* 26: 383–386.

214 Khan, S.R., Pearle, M.S., Robertson, W.G. et al. (2016). Kidney stones. *Nat. Rev. Dis. Primers.* 2: 16008.

215 Terlinsky, A.S., Grochowski, J., Geoly, K.L. et al. (1981). Identification of atypical calcium oxalate crystalluria following ethylene glycol ingestion. *Am. J. Clin. Pathol.* 76: 223–226.

216 Hanouneh, M. and Chen, T.K. (2017). Calcium oxalate crystals in ethylene glycol toxicity. *N. Engl. J. Med.* 377: 1467.

217 Kramer, J.W., Bistline, D., Sheridan, P. et al. (1984). Identification of hippuric acid crystals in the urine of ethylene glycol-intoxicated dogs and cats. *J. Am. Vet. Med. Assoc.* 184: 584.

218 Thrall, M.A., Dial, S.M., and Winder, D.R. (1985). Identification of calcium oxalate monohydrate crystals by X-ray diffraction in urine of ethylene glycol-intoxicated dogs. *Vet. Pathol.* 22: 625–628.

219 Sink, C.A. and Weinstein, N.M. (2012). Routine urinalysis: microscopic elements. In: *Practical Veterinary Urinalysis*, 55–112. Ames, Iowa: John.

220 Grauer, G.F. and Thrall, M.A. (1982). Ethylene glycol (antifreeze) poisoning in the dog and cat. *J. Am. Anim. Hosp. Assoc.* 18: 492–497.

221 Burns, J.R. and Finlayson, B. (1980). Changes in calcium oxalate crystal, morphology as a function of concentration. *Invest. Urol.* 18: 174–177.

222 Grauer, G.F., Thrall, M.A., Henre, B.A. et al. (1984). Early clinico-pathologic findings in dogs ingesting ethylene glycol. *Am. J. Vet. Res.* 45: 2299–2303.

223 Carvalho, M. and Vieira, M.A. (2004). Changes in calcium oxalate crystal morphology as a function of supersaturation. *Int. Braz J Urol* 30: 205–208; discussion 209.

224 Dear, J.D., Shiraki, R., Ruby, A.L. et al. (2011). Feline urate urolithiasis: a retrospective study of 159 cases. *J. Feline Med. Surg.* 13: 725–732.

225 Appel, S.L., Houston, D.M., Moore, A.E.P. et al. (2010). Feline urate urolithiasis. *Can. Vet. J.* 51: 493–496.

226 Lees, G.E., Hardy, R.M., Stevens, J.B. et al. (1984). Clinical implications of feline bilirubinuria. *J. Am. Anim. Hosp. Assoc.* 20: 765–771.

227 DeSchepper, J. (1974). Degradation of Haemoglobin to bilirubin in the kidney of the dog. *Tijdschr. Diergeneeskd.* 99: 699.

228 Ruggerone, B., Marelli, S.P., Scarpa, P. et al. (2016). Genetic evaluation of English bulldogs with cystine uroliths. *Vet. Rec.* 179: 174.

229 Mizukami, K., Raj, K., Osborne, C. et al. (2016). Cystinuria associated with different SLC7A9 gene variants in the cat. *PLoS One* 11: e0159247.

230 Brons, A.K., Henthorn, P.S., Raj, K. et al. (2013). SLC3A1 and SLC7A9 mutations in autosomal recessive or dominant canine cystinuria: a new classification system. *J. Vet. Intern. Med.* 27: 1400–1408.

231 Casal, M.L., Giger, U., Bovee, K.C. et al. (1995). Inheritance of cystinuria and renal defect in Newfoundlands. *J. Am. Vet. Med. Assoc.* 207: 1585–1589.

232 Bovee, K.C., Joyce, T., Reynolds, R. et al. (1978). The fanconi syndrome in basenji dogs: a new model for renal transport defects. *Science* 201: 1129–1131.

233 Hooper, A.N. and Roberts, B.K. (2011). Fanconi syndrome in four non-basenji dogs exposed to chicken jerky treats. *J. Am. Anim. Hosp. Assoc.* 47: e178–e187.

234 DiBartola, S.P., Chew, D.J., and Horton, M.L. (1991). Cystinuria in a cat. *J. Am. Vet. Med. Assoc.* 198: 102–104.

235 Mizukami, K., Raj, K., and Giger, U. (2015). Feline cystinuria caused by a missense mutation in the SLC3A1 gene. *J. Vet. Intern. Med.* 29 (1): 120–125.

236 Redrobe, S. (2002). Calcium metabolism in rabbits. *Semin. Avian Exot. Pet. Med.* 11: 94–101.

237 Puschner, B., Poppenga, R.H., Lowenstine, L.J. et al. (2007). Assessment of melamine and cyanuric acid toxicity in cats. *J. Vet. Diagn. Invest.* 19: 616–624.

238 Puschner, B. and Reimschuessel, R. (2011). Toxicosis caused by melamine and cyanuric acid in dogs and cats: uncovering the mystery and subsequent global implications. *Clin. Lab. Med.* 31: 181–199.

239 Dobson, R.L., Motlagh, S., Quijano, M. et al. (2008). Identification and characterization of toxicity of contaminants in pet food leading to an outbreak of renal toxicity in cats and dogs. *Toxicol. Sci.* 106: 251–262.

240 Bischoff, K. and Rumbeiha, W.K. (2012). Pet food recalls and pet food contaminants in small animals. *Vet. Clin. North Am. Small Anim. Pract.* 42: 237–250, v.

241 Brown, C.A., Jeong, K.S., Poppenga, R.H. et al. (2007). Outbreaks of renal failure associated with melamine and cyanuric acid in dogs and cats in 2004 and 2007. *J. Vet. Diagn. Invest.* 19: 525–531.

242 Cianciolo, R.E., Bischoff, K., Ebel, J.G. et al. (2008). Clinicopathologic, histologic, and toxicologic findings in 70 cats inadvertently exposed to pet food contaminated with melamine and cyanuric acid. *J. Am. Vet. Med. Assoc.* 233: 729–737.

243 Bhalla, V., Grimm, P.C., Chertow, G.M. et al. (2009). Melamine nephrotoxicity: an emerging epidemic in an era of globalization. *Kidney Int.* 75: 774–779.

244 Osborne, C.A., Lulich, J.P., Ulrich, L.K. et al. (2009). Melamine and cyanuric acid-induced crystalluria, uroliths, and nephrotoxicity in dogs and cats. Vet. Clin. North Am. Small Anim. *Pract.* 39 (1): 1–14.

245 Fogazzi, G.B., Cantu, M., Saglimbeni, L. et al. (2003). Amoxicillin, a rare but possible cause of crystalluria. *Nephrol. Dial. Transplant.* 18: 212–214.

246 Fogazzi, G.B., Garigali, G., Brambilla, C. et al. (2006). Ciprofloxacin crystalluria. *Nephrol. Dial. Transplant.* 21: 2982–2983.

247 Thorsteinsson, S.B., Bergan, T., Oddsdottir, S. et al. (1986). Crystalluria and ciprofloxacin, influence of urinary pH and hydration. *Chemotherapy* 32: 408–417.

248 Daniels, J.B., Tracy, G., Irom, S.J. et al. (2014). Fluoroquinolone levels in healthy dog urine following a 20-mg/kg oral dose of enrofloxacin exceed mutant prevention concentration targets against Escherichia coli isolated from canine urinary tract infections. *J. Vet. Pharmacol. Ther.* 37: 201–204.

249 Hubbert, W.T. (1972). Bacteria and spermatozoa in the canine urinary bladder. *Cornell Vet.* 62: 13–20.

250 Ferguson, J.M. and Renton, J.P. (1988). Observation on the presence of spermatozoa in canine urine. *J. Small Anim. Pract.* 29: 691–694.

251 Herron, M.A., Barton, C.L., and Applegate, B. (1986). A modified technique for semen collection by electroejaculation in the domestic cat. *Theriogenology* 26: 357–364.

252 Glenn, B.L. (1970). Facts and artifacts in the microscopic examination of urine sediment. *J. Am. Vet. Med. Assoc.* 157: 1667–1671.

253 Petersdorf, R.G. and Turck, M. (1970). Some current concepts of urinary tract infections. *Dis. Mon.* 1–30.

254 Senior, D.F., Solomon, G.B., Goldschmidt, M.H. et al. (1980). Capillaria plica infection in dogs. *J. Am. Vet. Med. Assoc.* 176: 901–905.

255 Mariacher, A., Millanta, F., Guidi, G. et al. (2016). Urinary capillariosis in six dogs from Italy. *Open Vet. J.* 6: 84–88.

256 Bedard, C., Desnoyers, M., Lavallee, M.C. et al. (2002). Capillaria in the bladder of an adult cat. *Can. Vet. J.* 43: 973–974.

257 Basso, W., Spanhauer, Z., Arnold, S. et al. (2014). Capillaria plica (syn. Pearsonema plica) infection in a dog with chronic pollakiuria: challenges in the diagnosis and treatment. *Parasitol. Int.* 63: 140–142.

258 Fugassa, M.H. (2010). Trichuris or Capillaria? *Parasitol. Int.* 59: 104.

259 Maurelli, M.P., Rinaldi, L., Rubino, G. et al. (2014). FLOTAC and mini-FLOTAC for uro-microscopic diagnosis of Capillaria plica (syn. Pearsonema plica) in dogs. *BMC. Res. Notes* 7 (591).

260 Osborne, C.A., Stevens, J.B., Hanlon, G.F. et al. (1969). Dioctophyma renale in the dog. *J. Am. Vet. Med. Assoc.* 155: 605–620.

261 Pedrassani, D., Lux Hoppe, E.G., Avancini, N. et al. (2009). Morphology of eggs of Dioctophyme renale Goeze, 1782 (Nematoda: Dioctophymatidae) and influences of temperature on development of first-stage larvae in the eggs. *Rev. Bras. Parasitol. Vet.* 18: 15–19.

262   Rahal, S.C., Mamprim, M.J., Oliveira, H.S. et al. (2014). Ultrasonographic, computed tomographic, and operative findings in dogs infested with giant kidney worms (Dioctophyme renale). *J. Am. Vet. Med. Assoc.* 244: 555–558.

263   Ferreira, V.L., Medeiros, F.P., July, J.R. et al. (2010). Dioctophyma renale in a dog: clinical diagnosis and surgical treatment. *Vet. Parasitol.* 168: 151–155.

264   Monobe, M.M., da Silva, R.C., Araujo Junior, J.P. et al. (2017). Microfilaruria by Dirofilaria immitis in a dog: a rare clinical pathological finding. *J. Parasit. Dis.* 41: 805–808.

265   Kaewthamasorn, M., Assarasakorn, S., and Niwetpathomwat, A. (2008). Microfilaruria caused by canine dirofilariasis (Dirofilaria immitis): an unusual clinical presence. *Comp. Clin. Pathol.* 17: 61–65.

Urinalysis in the Dog and Cat, First Edition. Dennis J. Chew and Patricia A. Schenck.
© 2023 John Wiley & Sons, Inc. Published 2023 by John Wiley & Sons, Inc.

INTRODUCTION

Normal urine from dogs and cats contains very little, if any, protein (mg/dL) when measured by conventional urine chemistry dipstrip methods. Albumin is the predominant protein detected in urine from normal dogs [1] and cats as well as those with renal disease [2]. Some dogs [3] and cats with chronic kidney disease (CKD) have predominantly nonalbumin proteinuria characteristic of tubular proteinuria.

Small quantities of urinary protein can be detected in urine from healthy individuals using more sensitive analytical methods such as sulfosalicylic acid (SSA), urinary protein-to-creatinine ratio (UPC), microalbuminuria (MA), and urinary protein electrophoresis. Plasma proteins <40kD are considered low-molecular-weight (LMW) proteins that easily cross the glomerular barrier. Intermediate-weight proteins that are approximately the size of albumin at 65kD do not readily cross the glomerulus based on size and charge, whereas high-molecular-weight (HMW) proteins >100kD do not cross the normal glomerular barrier at all. Immunoglobulin G (IgG), immunoglobulin M (IgM), and immunoglobulin A (IgA) are examples of HMW proteins that do not cross the glomerulus unless it is damaged [4–6].

"Proteinuria" is the general term used to describe the detection of an abnormally high quantity of protein in the urine due to a pathological condition. Proteinuria can be caused by prerenal, postrenal, and primary renal disorders (Table 7.1). Trauma or contamination from the method of urine collection must be considered as a possibility of adding plasma proteins along with red blood cells (RBC) to urine (catheterization, cystocentesis, or voiding). Proteinuria may indicate a pathologic process anywhere in the urinary tract (i.e. kidney, ureter, urinary bladder, urethra) in addition to that from iatrogenic trauma or contamination from the genital tract.

The finding of proteinuria provides a diagnostic clue for disorders of the upper and lower urinary tract. The findings from urine specific gravity (USG) and urinary sediment microscopy are important components of the complete urinalysis that help determine the importance of the proteinuria and its likely origin. A combination of findings from history, physical examination, imaging, hematology, routine serum biochemistry, and urinalysis may be needed to determine the origin of the proteinuria. Sometimes, the cause of the proteinuria is readily identified in animals with inflammatory lower urinary tract disease based on history and physical exam (e.g. urinary tract infection [UTI], urolithiasis, and neoplastic masses). Renal biopsy, with special techniques of light microscopy, electron microscopy (EM), and immunofluorescent antibody (IFA), is needed to determine with certainty the underlying lesions resulting in renal proteinuria [26, 27] in patients in which prerenal and postrenal causes have been eliminated as a differential consideration.

GLOMERULAR AND TUBULAR HANDLING OF PROTEIN IN HEALTH

The concentration of proteins in urine leaving the kidney in health depends on the extent that protein was filtered across the glomerulus, the extent of tubular reabsorption, any additions of protein from tubular secretion of Tamm–Horsfall protein (THP) or from cellular or intracellular contents [6, 16, 20], and the degree of water removed by the tubules during the process of urine concentration. The glomerulus performs the first step in urine formation (as reviewed in Chapter 1, Figure 1.10). A detailed review of the molecular structures and functions of the glomerular basement membrane (GBM), including GBM assembly, maintenance, and repair, is available for the interested reader [28]. The glomerular capillary membrane functions to readily allow an ultrafiltrate of plasma (water, nonprotein bound electrolytes, and small-molecular-weight waste products) to appear in Bowman's space, while restricting the passage of cells and large-molecular-weight plasma proteins across the glomerulus at the same time. The glomerulus displays a sophisticated system of structural and functional effects that limit the entry of larger plasma proteins and cells into Bowman's space. Normal glomerular barrier function, sometimes called permselectivity, involves resistance to the passage of molecules based on their size and charge. The unique arrangement and function of the glomerular endothelium, endothelial fenestrae, basement membrane (lamina rara interna, lamina densa, and lamina rara externa), podocyte foot processes, slit pore membranes, and podocyte cell bodies provide an integrated system that maintains normal glomerular barrier function and glomerular filtration (Figures 7.1 and 7.2).

Type IV collagen, laminin, nidogen, and perlecan, a proteoglycan, are the major protein constituents of GBM [29]. Collagen IV is the main structural component of the framework of the GBM, which is important for the permselective barrier [30, 31]. The anionic charge of the GBM is important in hindering the filtration of negatively charged plasma proteins [31].

A large amount of protein enters the glomerular capillaries (6–8g/dL) from the systemic circulation, but very little passes through the glomerulus into the urinary space and then into the proximal tubule for further processing. Albumin is the predominant circulating protein (3–4g/dL) that enters the glomerulus. Albumin constitutes 40–60% of the proteins in normal urine due to incomplete proximal tubular reabsorption of the small amount of albumin filtered from plasma across the glomerulus into tubular fluid [32, 33]. The remaining 40–60% of the protein in normal urine originates from protein secreted by the distal tubule and collecting duct (THP), as well as protein contributed by the urothelium of the lower urinary tract and genital tract [33, 34].

Normal glomerular barrier function impedes the passage of proteins across the glomerulus due to the unique interaction and function of the endothelial cells, basement membrane, and the podocytes that comprise the glomerulus. The podocyte is important in the development of the glomerular endothelium and maintenance of its fenestrations [31]. The morphology and function of the podocyte is largely determined by its complex cytoskeleton and interactions with proteins in the slit pore diaphragm (Figure 7.3) [35, 36]. The slit pore membrane is a zipper-like structure with a constant width [31]. Podocytes help to control shape, structure, and spatial orientation of the glomerulus through contractility, which is important in maintenance of glomerular filtration rate (GFR) [35].

Table 7.1 Classification of proteinuria based on site or mechanism.

Category	Subcategory	Mechanism	Causes/Examples	Comments
Prerenal - Rare		Glomerular barrier function is normal – selectivity maintained for molecular size and charge	Myoglobinuria – rhabdomyolysis	Myoglobin has no plasma carrier – clear plasma; high CK supportive
			Hemoglobinuria – systemic hemolysis	Hemoglobin has a carrier protein that must first become saturated before free hemoglobin can enter urine – pigmented plasma
		Overload of small MW molecules in plasma that can cross the normal glomerulus into urine (overflow)	Bence Jones Proteinuria (light chains) Multiple Myeloma or Paraproteinemia (lymphoma)	
			Lysozymuria (muramidase) – acute monocytic/ myelocytic leukemia	
Postrenal	Urinary	Glomerular barrier is normal	Trauma, Cystocentesis, Urolithiasis, Urothelial neoplasia, Urinary infection	History – LUT urgency or trauma; physical exam, imaging, urine culture, urine cytology, histopathology
	Very Common	Blood loss into urine – capillary bleeding or inflammation	Cystitis (including interstitial) urethritis, urethral obstruction, ureteral obstruction	
		Ureter, bladder, urethra		
	Genital	Glomerular barrier is normal	Prostatitis, prostatic neoplasia, benign Prostatic hypertrophy (BPH)	History, physical exam, imaging, urine cytology, histopathology
	Occasional	Blood loss into urine	Estrus, pyometra, metritis, balanoposthitis, TVT	
		Prostate, penis, prepuce, uterus, vagina vestibule, vulva	Mating, ejaculation, normal retrograde urine flow	
		Semen - normal intact males		
Renal	Functional	No structural renal lesions. Transient dysfunction of the glomerular barrier results in mostly albuminuria. Renal vascular congestion and adrenergic system activation result in proteinuria	Fever, seizures, exposure to extreme heat or cold, strenuous exercise (nonconditioned dogs), congestive heart failure, large tumors obstructing blood return from vena cava	UPC often <1.0
				History, physical exam, thoracic and abdominal imaging, echocardiogram
				Transient nature of proteinuria

Table 7.1 (Continued)

Category	Subcategory	Mechanism	Causes/Examples	Comments
	Pathological	Result of functional or structural lesions within any region of the kidney		Proteinuria is persistent
	Glomerular	Abnormal glomerular barrier	Systemic hypertension (any cause)	UPC often >0.5–1.0
		Loss of glomerular permselectivity	Primary glomerulonephritis, hereditary nephropathy or glomerulopathy, glomerulosclerosis (CKD), amyloidosis	UPC > 1.0 and often >2.0 at time of diagnosis
			Secondary glomerulonephritis: chronic infectious or parasitic disease, acute and chronic inflammation, neoplasia, immune-mediated disease, drug reactions, leptospirosis (rarely), any disease with circulating chronic antigen excess (immune complexes)	
			Exogenous glucocorticosteroid, (D), Cushing's disease (D), hyperthyroidism (C), diabetes mellitus, critical illness	
	Tubular	Glomerular barrier is normal	AKI, ATN, ARF	UPC < 2.5
		Tubulopathy: Decreased tubular reabsorption of small MW molecules:	Leptospirosis	UPC often 0.5–1.0
			Fanconi syndrome – congenital (D) – Basenji	Glucosuria and aminoaciduria if generalized proximal tubulopathy
		α1-microglobulin	Fanconi syndrome – acquired: jerky treats (D), drugs; sometimes part of AKI; Cooper associated hepatitis (D); chlorambucil (C)	
		β2-microglobulin		
		Retinol-binding protein	CKD – tubules fail to reabsorb small amounts of albumin and nonalbumin proteins that are normally reabsorbed by proximal tubules	
		Lysozyme		
		Some moderate MW molecules (albumin)	CKD – proximal tubular reabsorptive capacity exceeded by glomerular leakage of plasma proteins	
		Increased tubular secretion (THP)		
		Decreased THP CKD		
		Leakage of intracellular or luminal tubular cell proteins (enzymuria; GGT, NAG)		
	Interstitial	Glomerular barrier is normal	Allergic drug reactions (acute interstitial nephritis)	Tubules and interstitium are often involved with the same disease process at the same time
		Exudate or plasma enters tubular lumens from peritubular capillaries	Leptospirosis	Tubulo-interstitial disease is the term often used
			Pyelonephritis (bacterial)	

MW – molecular weight, MA – microalbuminuria, LUT – lower urinary tract, UPC – urinary protein to urinary creatinine ratio, TVT – transmissible venereal tumor, AKI – acute kidney injury, ATN – acute tubular necrosis, ARF – acute renal failure. Source: Vaden and Elliott [7]; Grauer [8]; DiBartola [9]; Grauer [2]; Harley and Langston [10]; Whittemore [11]; Whittemore [13]; Lees et al. [14]; Langston [15]; Harrison et al. [17]; Aguado et al. [18]; Osserman and Lawlor [19]; Delaney and Lamb [20]; Summers [21]; Hedgespeth and Harrell [22]; Benzing [23]; Albright [24]; Norden et al. [25];

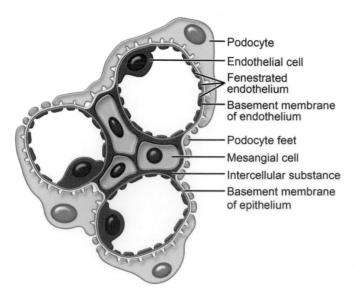

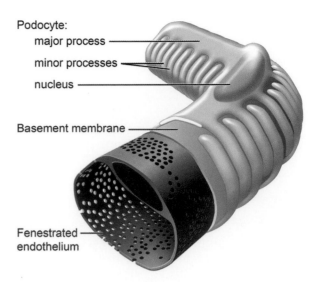

FIGURE 7.1   Schematic representation of the glomerulus as seen in transverse section. The urinary space lies outside the podocytes where ultrafiltrate accumulates on its way to the proximal tubules for further processing. The basic layers of the glomerulus are shown (from within the capillary lumen to the urinary space) as the endothelial cells and their fenestrations, basement membrane of the endothelial cells and podocytes, podocytes (also called visceral epithelium) and their foot processes. The mesangium consists of mesangial cells and mesangial matrix. Note that there is only one layer of basement membrane around the mesangium. Mesangial cells can proliferate and lay down more mesangial matrix during some kidney diseases. Mesangial cells also have contractile properties that can alter the available surface area for glomerular filtration in health and disease. The podocyte provides cytoskeletal support for normal glomerular architecture. Not shown is the slit pore membrane between the podocyte feet. Proper slit pore function is necessary to retard passage of plasma proteins across the glomerulus. Glomerular origin proteinuria can occur when any of these anatomical sites are disturbed. Source: Illustration by Tim Vojt, reproduced with the permission of The Ohio State University.

Nephrin, the first slit pore protein to be identified [31], appears to be the most important molecule within the slit pore membrane for the maintenance of normal podocyte function [37]. Nephrin is a major component of the 40-nm slit diaphragm protein complex between adjacent podocyte foot processes. Nephrin and Neph1 are transmembrane proteins with extracellular domains that form the slit membrane. They also importantly regulate the actin cytoskeleton, which controls the shape and ultrastructure of the podocyte and foot process apposition to the GBM. Nephrin and Neph1 interact with the membrane protein podocin, which influences the expression of transient receptor potential cation channel 6 as a mechanosensitive channel in the slit diaphragm. Genetic or acquired defects in any proteins comprising the slit membrane or podocyte membrane consistently result in proteinuria [23, 36].

Endothelial cells of the glomerulus have numerous fenestrated openings of 70–100 nm diameter [31]. The normal glomerulus does not generally allow plasma proteins with a

FIGURE 7.2   Schematic three-dimensional view of the glomerulus as would be observed during scanning electron microscopy. The filtration barrier consists of capillary endothelium, glomerular basement membrane, and visceral epithelial cells (podocytes). The glomerular endothelium is highly fenestrated (relatively unique to the kidney), and these openings of 50–100 nm in diameter are larger than those in systemic capillaries. These openings restrict the passage of cells (WBC, RBC, and platelets) based on their large size. The endothelium and basement membranes are coated with negatively charged glycocalyx (sialoglycoproteins) that repel plasma proteins that have a net negative charge. A breakdown in this coating is associated with transglomerular passage of plasma proteins. Podocytes with major and minor foot processes are shown in relationship to the glomerular basement membrane. The slit pore (not shown) is between the minor foot processes. Source: Illustration by Tim Vojt, reproduced with permission of The Ohio State University.

size equal to or greater than albumin (MW 67 kD and 3.5 nm diameter) to cross into Bowman's space and then into tubular fluid [16]. Very small molecules, such as inulin, creatinine, urea, glucose, and nonprotein bound electrolytes, are freely filtered across the glomerulus into the urinary space, as is water. Normal glomerular barrier function opposes the passage of negatively charged plasma proteins as the various structural layers of the glomerulus are negatively charged. The surface of endothelial cells has a negative electric charge because of the presence of glycoproteins, glycosaminoglycans, and the glycocalyx [28, 38–40]. This negative charge acts as a barrier to the interaction of anionic proteins such as albumin with endothelial cells. Normally, circulating negatively charged albumin is repelled from the endothelial surface due to electrical repulsion, decreasing the permeability of albumin. Larger molecules that are negatively charged and globular in shape (such as albumin and IgG) will not readily cross the normal glomerulus and are retained within the circulation [16, 20].

The normal GBM and podocytes counteract luminal pressure from within the glomerular capillary. The interdigitating podocyte foot processes normally compress the gel-like

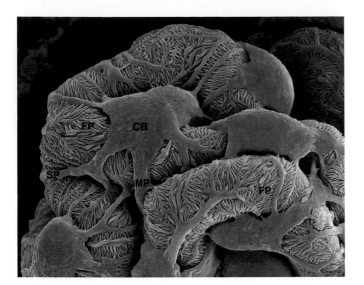

FIGURE 7.3 Podocytes in the glomerulus as seen on scanning electron microscopy, looking at the glomerulus from the urinary space in Bowman's capsule – 800×. Podocytes have narrow cell extensions (processes) that give rise to secondary extensions called pedicels. The podocytes completely surround the capillary system. CB – cell body; MP – major foot process; SP- secondary foot process; FP – finely interdigitating foot process. Source: Dennis Kunkel Microscopy / Science Photo Library.

composition of the GBM. Buttressing force from the podocytes that compress the GBM helps to maintain the shape of the GBM and restrict the passage of macromolecules such as albumin across the GBM (permselectivity). As podocytes are injured, the buttressing forces from the podocyte foot processes are decreased, which results in less compression of the GBM. This results in a shape change of the GBM and increased permeability to molecules of the size of albumin and larger across the GBM. Injury to podocytes also reduces the length of the slit diaphragm, which reduces the surface area available for glomerular filtration of water and small molecules at the same time that increased permeability to proteins happens. This reduction in GFR is counteracted to some degree by the effect of angiotensin-II (AG-II) to increase the vasoconstriction of the efferent arteriole, which increases GFR. This "compensatory" increase in GFR is associated with increased glomerular capillary pressure that is no longer able to be counteracted (buttressed) by the diseased podocytes, resulting in more proteinuria. Since podocytes are mechanically sensitive, an increased GFR in single nephrons (hyperfiltration) with decreased surface area exposes the podocytes to more damage or podocyte detachment from sheering stress that occurs from increased fluid flow across the glomerulus [23, 36]. Though podocytes exert a pivotal role in maintaining glomerular barrier integrity, alterations in the structure and function of the GBM or glomerular endothelial cells also result in albuminuria, so it is important to consider all three of these possibilities as mechanisms resulting in glomerular proteinuria [23].

Once the glomerular ultrafiltrate reaches the proximal tubule, it undergoes changes in composition due to water and solute reabsorption. The final urinary excretion of proteins largely depends on the interaction of protein with proximal tubular epithelial cells. The proximal tubular epithelial cells have a prominent layer of microvilli, which is the site for megalin-receptor-mediated endocytosis of negatively charged proteins. The megalin receptor and its interaction with cubulin is important in the proximal tubular reabsorption of albumin and some other molecules like vitamin-D-binding protein (VDBP) [6, 20, 38, 41–44]. Albumin binds to this specific membrane receptor complex and is internalized by membrane vesicles [45–47]. These endocytic vesicles fuse with lysosomes that degrade the protein into amino acids, which are released at the basolateral surface of the tubular cell into the interstitium and peritubular capillaries [20]. The very small amount of plasma albumin that was sieved across the normal glomerulus into tubular fluid undergoes 99% reabsorption by the proximal tubule in health. The plasma proteins of lower molecular weight that freely crossed the glomerular filter are also reabsorbed by normal tubules [16, 20].

Tamm–Horsfall mucoprotein (THP, Tamm–Horsfall glycoprotein [THG], uromodulin) is an HMW globulin (90–130 kD) produced by the distal tubules and collecting ducts as well as the thick ascending limb of the loop of Henle [3, 32, 48, 49]. The tubular secretion of THP or THG by the thick ascending limb of Henle's loop and the early distal tubule contribute to the small amount of protein content in normal urine [3, 16, 20, 50]. THP was found in normal dog urine at a concentration of 0.5–1.0 mg/dL, similar to that in humans in one study [32], and at these low levels, it is not detected by conventional semiquantitative urinary tests. The median urinary THP (ng/mL measured by ELISA; 2.5–500 ng/mL standard curve) to urinary creatinine (mg/dL)×10^{-2} ratio was 101 (58–172) in healthy dogs and 0 (0–88) in dogs with CKD of one study [51]. The ratio of THP (measured by quantitative Western Blot) to urinary creatinine was also reduced in CKD dogs with moderate-to-severe azotemia and proteinuria of another study. The median THP-to-urinary-creatinine ratio in nonazotemic and nonproteinuric dogs was 15.2 mg/g (9.62–65.2) [49]. Decreased urinary THP was also demonstrated in another study of dogs with CKD [3].

LOCALIZATION AND CLASSIFICATION OF PROTEINURIA

Proteinuria may be classified as prerenal, renal (functional renal, pathologic tubular, pathologic interstitial, or pathologic glomerular), or postrenal in etiology (Figure 7.4 and Table 7.1 [2, 7–16]. Proteins in urine can appear following the increased filtration of plasma proteins across the glomerulus, the failure of proximal tubular epithelial cells to reabsorb protein, the addition of proteins from tubulointerstitial inflammation and degeneration, and the addition of plasma proteins to urine from anatomical sites below the kidney. When postrenal proteinuria has been excluded, the presence of medium-to-high-molecular-weight

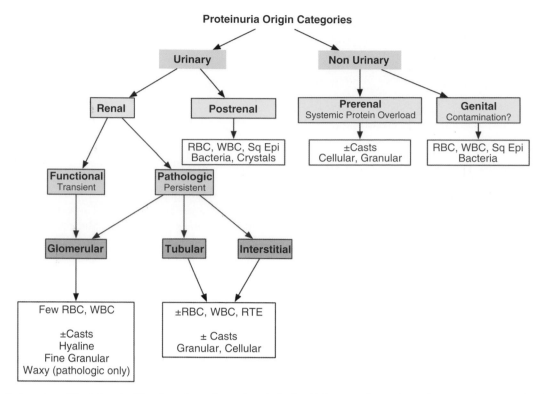

FIGURE 7.4 Categories of Proteinuria. The detection of proteinuria by itself does not determine where it originated. The first decision is whether the proteinuria is from the urinary tract or from nonurinary tract sources. Prerenal proteinuria is uncommon. Genital tract sources for proteinuria occasionally occur during prostatic or uterine/vaginal disease. Postrenal sources of proteinuria from lower urinary tract disorders are very common. Renal proteinuria that is persistent is pathological and most commonly occurs due to glomerular diseases.

proteins (such as albumin) in urine usually indicates the loss of normal glomerular barrier function. For renal origin proteins with LMW, the defect causing proteinuria is likely related to decreased function of proximal renal tubular cells. Mixed patterns of renal proteinuria can include a varying degree of glomerular and tubular origin proteinuria.

PRERENAL PROTEINURIA

Prerenal proteinuria is uncommon in dogs and cats. The glomerular barrier function is normal. It occurs following hemoglobinemia during systemic hemolysis, myoglobinemia from traumatized muscle, and production of light chains (Bence Jones proteins) associated with multiple myeloma or other paraproteinemia. These small-molecular-weight proteins readily filter through the normal glomerulus from plasma to enter the urine [2, 9, 14].

Prerenal proteinuria can be considered an overload or overflow of LMW molecules not normally present in plasma that are freely filtered across the glomerulus. These proteins enter tubular fluid in an amount that exceeds the ability of tubules to reabsorb the particular protein [16]. There are no changes in the urinary tract anatomy, and the urinary sediment contains very few elements supporting inflammation. Granular casts containing hemoglobin, myoglobin, or Bence

Jones proteins can sometimes form. Acute kidney injury (AKI) can occur in these conditions, which would add a component of tubular proteinuria and possibly cellular casts (see below) to the prerenal proteinuria.

Pigmented plasma may be present due to binding of hemoglobin to a carrier, whereas myoglobinemia is not associated with pigment in the plasma as there is no plasma carrier for myoglobin [52]. A screening test to distinguish myoglobin from hemoglobin uses ammonium sulfate to precipitate and remove hemoglobin, but the definitive measurement of myoglobin requires the use of immunochemical methods [16]. Bence Jones proteins are suspected in urine when the heat test is positive for precipitation [53], but urinary electrophoresis with immunofixation is considered definitive [16].

POSTRENAL PROTEINURIA

Postrenal proteinuria is the most common type of proteinuria in veterinary medicine [2, 10]. In postrenal proteinuria, glomerular barrier function is normal. Protein enters the lower urinary tract from the circulation following hemorrhage or during inflammation at anatomic sites below the kidneys, including the lower urinary and genital tracts. The history may include signs of lower urinary tract urgency (dysuria, stranguria, pollakiuria). Results from physical examination and imaging often reveal structural changes to the lower urinary tract anatomy. Urinary sediment is abnormal with varying combinations of hematuria, pyuria, bacteriuria, epitheliuria, and crystalluria. The most common causes for postrenal proteinuria include trauma, obstruction, urinary infection, inflammation, neoplasia, or urolithiasis.

RENAL PROTEINURIA

Renal proteinuria occurs when plasma proteins excessively cross the glomerulus, the proximal renal tubules fail to reabsorb filtered proteins, or protein is added to the urine as a result of tubulointerstitial bleeding and inflammation. Renal proteinuria develops as a consequence of many primary renal diseases and also when a systemic disorder secondarily involves the kidneys. Prerenal and postrenal sources of proteinuria must be ruled out before renal proteinuria can be diagnosed with certainty.

Renal functional or physiological proteinuria is attributed to changes in glomerular vascular tone without structural renal disease that result in albuminuria. Fever, seizures, extremes of heat and cold, renal congestion, and severe stress can lead to this type of proteinuria. Functional proteinuria is transient and disappears when the underlying condition resolves as there is no permanent change to the glomerulus [2, 9].

Pathological renal proteinuria can originate from glomerular, tubular, or tubulointerstitial causes (Table 7.2). Primary glomerular diseases include glomerulonephritis (GN), amyloidosis, glomerulosclerosis, and hereditary nephropathy (HN). Secondary glomerular barrier dysfunction can occur in systemic diseases characterized by chronic antigen excess and antibody formation, endocrinopathy, and during critical illness.

Renal tubular proteinuria can occur during AKI and in those with congenital or acquired Fanconi syndrome (FS) (see Chapter 5 and Table 7.2). Though glucosuria is often the major initial feature discovered in the generalized proximal tubular defect in FS, renal proteinuria can also be found. LMW proteinuria following the failure of proximal tubules to reabsorb freely filtered plasma proteins is commonly documented. HMW proteinuria that includes albumin can also be identified in humans with FS. LMW tubular protein markers accounted for about 50% and albumin accounted for about 30% of the proteins in urine in one report of FS in humans. Proteinuria was attributed to the failure of receptor-mediated endocytic reabsorption by proximal tubules to reclaim the small quantities of these proteins that are normally present in proximal tubular fluid [25]. Though aminoaciduria has been well characterized in FS in dogs, the magnitude and nature of proteinuria as to tubular or glomerular origin has not [90, 91]. Angiotensin-converting enzyme inhibitor (ACE-I) treatment reduced the magnitude of albuminuria in children with FS associated with cystinosis but alpha-1 microglobulinuria did not change [92].

Abnormal glomerular barrier function is the most common mechanism leading to pathological renal proteinuria. Interactions between glomerular capillary pressure, the GBM, and podocytes importantly determine glomerular permeability to circulating proteins including albumin. Damaged podocytes result in proteinuria (albuminuria) as the podocyte assumes a simplified architecture characterized as foot-process effacement (fusion of foot processes) and a shortening of the slit pore diaphragm; this early lesion is potentially reversible. Podocyte loss due to detachment or necrosis is irreversible since podocytes are postmitotic cells with limited ability to regenerate themselves, which results in fibrosis. Most types of podocyte injury are acquired, and many are created by immune injury to various podocyte target antigens in human medicine. Podocyte injury is associated with changes in the GBM in most instances. Decreased GFR occurs in renal diseases, in which the glomerular surface area available for filtration is reduced or when intrinsic glomerular permeability is decreased. The protection of the podocyte as a means to prevent the progression of CKD was described as a main treatment goal in human medicine [23, 36].

Experimentally injured podocytes allow molecules of the size of albumin and larger to enter the GBM that are then taken up into the podocytes. Some circulating molecules traverse the GBM but do not pass through the slit diaphragm leading to the notion that the GBM is a coarse filter and the slit diaphragm is a fine filter. It appears that podocyte injury is central to all proteinuric renal diseases [23].

A variety of systemic and primary renal disease processes can decrease glomerular barrier integrity so that there is less resistance to the passage of plasma proteins (mostly albumin early in the disease) into Bowman's space. The hallmark of glomerular-origin proteinuria (regardless of specific disease) is the documentation of excess urinary protein in association with a noninflammatory urinary sediment (≤10 RBC/high-power field (HPF), ≤5 white blood cells (WBC)/HPF, <2 nonsquamous epithelial cells/HPF). Glomerular proteinuria can be associated with increased excretion of casts, especially hyaline casts and sometimes a few granular casts in which filtered proteins precipitate as granules (see Chapter 6 for more details). It should be noted that newer thinking suggests that lower urinary tract inflammation or hemorrhage contributes less to the measurement of urinary proteins than has been traditionally considered to be important [93, 94].

Primary glomerular disease with heavy renal proteinuria is far less common in cats than in dogs [26, 54, 95]. CKD in cats is generally idiopathic, and tubulointerstitial lesions with fibrosis predominate. Episodic renal hypoxia has been speculated to play an important role in the development and progression of these types of CKD lesions in cats [95].

In 58 cats with renal proteinuria, the origin of the proteinuria was glomerular in 42, tubular in 11, and other or both in 5 cats [96]. Immune-complex glomerulonephritis (ICGN) (31 of 42 cats) was the most common diagnosis in cats with glomerular proteinuria; other glomerular diseases were diagnosed in 11 cats. UPC was borderline increased (0.2–0.3, median 0.26) in four cats with tubulointerstitial disease, and significantly increased (1.0–5.8, median 2.2) in seven cats with

Table 7.2 Differential diagnoses associated with renal proteinuria.

Glomerular – Primary

  Glomerulonephritis

    Immune-mediated disease

    Anti-GBM disease (rare)

  Familial/hereditary nephropathy (D)

  Juvenile renal disease (D)

  Familial GN – sibling cats

  Minimal change glomerular disease

  Idiopathic hypertriglyceridemia

  Amyloidosis

  Glomerulosclerosis

Glomerular – Secondary

  Systemic hypertension – most secondary to CKD; idiopathic is rare

  Endocrine

    Diabetes mellitus

    Hyperadrenocorticism (D)

    Hyperthyroidism (C)

    Acromegaly (C)

    Exogenous glucocorticosteroids

  Critical illness

    Acute pancreatitis

    Pancreatic fat necrosis (C)

    Sepsis

    SIRS

    Pyometra (D)

  Immune-mediated

    Immune-mediated hemolytic anemia (IMHA)

    Immune-mediated thrombocytopenia (ITP)

    Immune-mediated polyarthritis (IMPA)

    Systemic lupus erythematosus (SLE)

Infectious

  Vector-borne diseases (D)

    Anaplasma, Babesia, Bartonella, *Borrelia burgorferi*, Ehrlichia, *Hepatazoon americanum*, Leishmania, Rocky Mountain Spotted Fever

  Leptospirosis

  Endocarditis

  Brucella canis (D)

  FeLV, FIV, FIP, Morbillivirus (C)

  Canine adenovirus type 1 – Hepatitis (D)

  Mycoplasma spp (D)

  Mycoplasma gatae (C) chronic progressive polyarthritis

  Blastomycosis (D)

  Histoplasmosis (D)

  Coccidiomycosis (D)

  Chronic bacterial infections

  Chronic pyoderma

  Chronic prostatitis (D)

Parasitic

  Heartworm disease (dirofilariasis)

  Trypanosomiasis

  Schistosomiasis (*Heterobilharzia americana*)

  Cytauxzoon felis (C)

Neoplastic

  Lymphoma

  Mast cell tumor

  Osteosarcoma

  Polycythemia rubra vera (primary erythrocytosis)

Functional

  Fever, seizures, passive renal congestion, CHF, temperature extremes, exercise (severe in the nonathlete)

Miscellaneous

  Cyclic hematopoiesis (Gray Collie syndrome)

  Renal thromboembolic disease

  High dietary phosphate (C)

Tubulo-interstitial

  Fanconi syndrome

    Congenital: Basenji (D)

    Acquired: drugs, jerky treats (D)

    Chlorambucil (C)

  Leptospirosis (D)

  Pyelonephritis

  AKI/ARF: nephrotoxins, renal ischemia

  Allergic drug reactions (interstitial nephritis)

Refer to the text for more detailed information about specific differentials, but not all disorders listed in the table are discussed in the text. References for several of the causes of renal proteinuria are provided here (Harley and Langston [11]; Roura [54]; Syme and Elliott [55]; Vaden and Grauer [56]; Vaden [57]; DiBartola et al. [58]; Dibartola and Westropp [59]; Cianciolo et al. [27]; Schneider [60]; Cianciolo et al. [61]; Crisi et al. [62]; Wright and Cornwell [63]; Crowell and Barsanti [64]; Nash and Wright [65]; Zeugswetter et al. [66]; Bennett and Nash [67]; Johnson and Mackin [68]; Johnson and Mackin [69]; Furrow et al. [70]; Smith et al. [71]; Crowell and Leininger [72]; Vilafranca et al. [73]; Aresu et al. [74]; Gori et al. [75]; Paltrinieri et al. [76]; Ibba et al. [77]; Winiarczyk et al. [78]; Brown et al. [79]; Backlund et al. [80]; Grauer et al. [81]; Grauer et al. [82]; Page et al. [83]; Dobenecker et al. [84]; Alexander et al. [85]; Laflamme et al. [86]; Grauer et al. [87]; Clinkenbeard et al. [88]; Yang [89]; Norden et al. [25]; Bovee et al. [90]; Yearley et al. [91]).

tubulointerstitial disease. In 42 cats with protein-losing nephropathy (PLN), median UPC was 8.38 (0.45–30). The median UPC was significantly lower at 6.5 (1.81–13.3) in cats with ICGN compared to cats with other glomerular diseases that exhibited a median UPC of 14.5 (10.1–30). Interestingly, 4 of 12 cats with tubulointerstitial disease had a UPC > 2.0 and 5 of 43 cats with primary glomerular lesions had a UPC < 2.0. This demonstrates that the general notion that a UPC > 2.0 is associated with primary glomerular disease is not absolute [96].

In another study of 68 cats with proteinuric CKD, slightly greater than half the cats had ICGN (37/68); the remaining cats were classified as having non-ICGN. Membranous or membranoproliferative glomerular lesions were those most commonly described in those with ICGN. The mean UPC at the diagnosis of ICGN was 7 ± 3.2 (median: 2.6; 2.4–18.6). The magnitude of UPC was lower in cats with non-ICGN compared to those with ICGN. Mean UPC in the non-ICGN cats increased with the severity of the tubulointerstitial lesions (mean range of 1.5–3.1). A UPC > 3.8 was considered the best cutoff point to distinguish those with ICGN from those with other causes of glomerular disease in this study [97].

In one study from the USA, 501 dogs with renal proteinuria suspected to have GN underwent renal biopsy (Figure 7.5). ICGN was the diagnosis in 48.1% of these dogs, 20.6% had primary glomerulosclerosis, 15.2% had amyloidosis, 9% had nonimmune-complex glomerulopathy, 4.8% had nonimmune-complex nephropathy, and 2.4% had primary tubulointerstitial disease [27]. An accurate diagnosis required analysis using light, immunofluorescent, and EM [27, 60, 61]. In a study from mainland Europe, 162 renal biopsies from dogs suspected to have glomerular disease were evaluated by light and EM. ICGN was the final diagnosis in 50.6%, 36.4% as nonimmune-complex-mediated GN, and 13% nonspecified renal lesions. The number of cases with the diagnosis of ICGN increased substantially over that made by light microscopy alone when results from EM were used as the gold standard for the presence of immune complexes [74]. The diagnosis of ICGN was less frequent in 62 dogs with renal proteinuria from the UK compared to those in the USA or mainland Europe. ICGN occurred in 27% of the dogs, glomerulosclerosis in 35%, nonspecific glomerulopathy in 13%, amyloidosis in 11%, and unspecified renal lesion in 13% following evaluation by light, immunofluorescent, and EM [98].

DEVELOPMENT OF RENAL PROTEINURIA

Renal proteinuria develops long before overt loss of excretory renal function is identified in humans with a variety of glomerular diseases [99]. Renal proteinuria is also observed before the onset of azotemic CKD in dogs and cats in general [10] and in dogs with X-linked HN [100]. Clinical studies have shown various degrees of proteinuria or albuminuria (none, borderline, overt) at the time of diagnosis of CKD in dogs and cats, but the temporal role of proteinuria preceding the diagnosis and its role in development of CKD has not been determined in most forms of CKD.

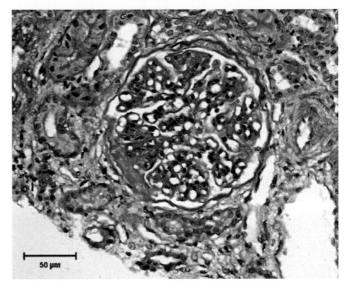

FIGURE 7.5 Membranoproliferative glomerulonephritis. Renal biopsy by light microscopy 40X PAS, consensus report from the International Veterinary Renal Pathology Service (IVRPS). Note thickened glomerular capillary loops and glomerular adhesion between visceral and parietal epithelium. This is from a three-year-old Boxer with azotemic CKD and PLN. The dog had a two-to-three-week history of anorexia, vomiting and weight loss. She had mild hypoalbuminemia (2.2 g/dL), serum creatinine of 3.9 mg/dL, and UPC of 12.7 in urine with an inactive sediment. Mildly hyperechoic kidneys with mild pyelectasia were seen on ultrasonography. Serologic testing for heartworms, leptospirosis, and tick-borne diseases were negative. There were no body effusions or edema despite the marked proteinuria and hypoalbuminemia. Systolic blood pressure was 150–160 mmHg initially, but occasionally, it was 180–190 mmHg.

A variety of immunological and nonimmunological mechanisms can be important in the development of glomerular proteinuria [31, 99, 101]. All layers of the glomerulus work together in an integrated way to maintain glomerular barrier function, which normally prevents proteinuria. Consequently, proteinuria is an expected consequence of damage or change in function for any component or layer of the glomerulus [38]. A net negative charge of the endothelial cells, GBM, and the visceral epithelial cells (podocytes) is important in thwarting transglomerular passage of negatively charged plasma proteins [99, 102]. A loss of this net negative charge can occur during many diseases of the glomerulus, which then favors the development of glomerular proteinuria (albuminuria) [102]. Loss of the negative charge of the glycocalyx also exposes the podocytes to damaging effects of albumin and other macromolecules [101].

The downregulation of megalin receptor expression occurs when tubular fluid albumin content is high, and this can contribute to increased tubular cell apoptosis [20]. The capacity of the proximal tubules to reabsorb proteins from the tubular fluid is also limited as receptor binding can become saturated during tubular fluid protein overload. T_{max} for protein reabsorption by the proximal tubule can be exceeded when diseases lead to an increase of filtered proteins presented for binding to the proximal tubule.

A vicious cycle of nephron loss and development of intraglomerular hypertension in surviving adapting nephrons leads to proteinuria during CKD [102–104]. Additional adaptations include glomerular hypertrophy, increased single-nephron GFR, and mesangial matrix expansion that contribute to proteinuria in dogs and cats [105, 106].

MEASUREMENT OF PROTEINURIA

Protein in urine can be measured by qualitative, semiquantitative, or quantitative methods. The gold standard for the evaluation of proteinuria is the quantitative measurement of total protein and or albumin from an accurately timed and collected 24-hour urine specimen. Quantitative results are reported in total mg/day or mg/kg/day [9, 16]. A 24-hour urine collection is uncommonly performed in clinical practice, due to the difficulty in accurately collecting all urine during this time and from the effects of stress from hospitalization needed for the procedure [16].

It is more difficult to measure total proteins in urine than in serum due to low concentration of urinary proteins and high concentrations of potentially interfering substances in urine, which affect the precision and accuracy of these methods. Methods to measure total proteins vary in their sensitivity and specificity to detect all proteins. Most methods to measure total protein favor the detection of albumin over globulins and nonalbumin proteins [16].

The measurement of urinary protein on the chemistry dipstrip is the most common method to initially evaluate proteinuria (see Chapter 5). The finding of dipstrip positive proteinuria can be detected in those in which no urinary disease was originally suspected, during the screening of patients with known CKD or AKI, or in those with lower urinary tract signs (postrenal proteinuria). The evaluation of proteinuria with other methods such as SSA, UPC, or MA should be used to confirm and further characterize the presence or absence of renal proteinuria. Renal proteinuria provides diagnostic information as supporting the presence of renal disease, but it also serves as a prognostic indicator since survival of dogs and cats with CKD is related to the degree of renal proteinuria. The evaluation of protein by dipstrip, SSA, UPC, and MA at the same time on the same urine sample has the potential to provide more clinically useful information than from any of these tests individually, but this is not yet considered standard of approach. Individual proteins in urine are best measured by immunoassay [16], but this is beyond the scope of this chapter.

DIPSTRIPS

The cellulose pad on the dipstrip contains the inert base tetrabromphenol blue (3′,3″,5′,5″-tetrachlorophenol-3,4,5,6-tetrabromosulfophthalein) buffered with citrate to a pH of 3.0 [16, 107, 108]. The color that develops in the presence of protein is based on the "protein error of indicators" [16, 109]. The protein error of indicators refers to the ability of protein to change the color of the acid–base indicator (tetrabromphenol blue) without altering the pH. In the absence of detectable protein, tetrabromphenol blue buffered to a pH of 3 remains yellow. Light green and then darker green to blue color develops in the presence of increasing concentration of detected protein [16, 108, 110].

The standard semiquantitative reagent test strip for protein measures total proteins in urine, but is most sensitive for the detection of albumin. Urinary albumin is usually the protein of most interest in CKD. Albumin readily binds to the indicator dye and generates the strongest color change per gram of any protein [111]. The reagent pad is less sensitive to overflow (prerenal) and tubular origin proteins that include globulins, Bence Jones protein, mucoproteins, myoglobin, hemoglobin, lysosomes, acute phase proteins, THP, and cauxin. Consequently, dipstrip protein pads better measure urinary albumin than urinary total protein or nonalbumin proteins [16, 108, 110, 112–117]. Since "other" nonalbumin proteins can bind to the indicator dye at times, a positive dipstrip reaction does not always mean that this is all due to albumin [111].

The intensity of the color reaction that develops on the dipstrip pad is determined by how much protein is in the urine [107], and by the number and affinity of binding sites on a specific urinary protein [113, 115]. At least six different binding regions for albumin have been identified and three of these regions appear to be very specific [118]. It appears that the dye and protein form a specific ionic complex that depends on positive charges within the albumin molecule [119]. The degree of color development may depend in part on the dynamics of indicator dye binding to the NH_3 groups on the protein. Positively charged groups on proteins are thought to increase binding to the dye [120]. The presence of positive charges and protein binding to high-affinity sites appear to be more important than the structure of the amino acids possessing the positive charge (lysine, arginine, or histidine). Variation in dye binding to various proteins has been attributed to nonspecific electrostatic interactions [119].

Protein measurements from dipstrips are both qualitative and semiquantitative [110], if the colorimetric reaction is read on urine at room temperature at the appropriate time interval as discussed in Chapter 5. Standard urine chemistry dipstrips contain one pad that detects total protein; some dipstrips measure microalbumin. Optimal results are generated when color reactions on the dipstrip are read by an automated strip reader, which objectively reads the degree of color reaction at the prescribed time interval. An exact mg/dL of protein is not provided; the reported value represents a range (or bin) that the sample concentration is within. The degree of protein in urine is reported as 0, trace, 1+, 2+, and 3+, which corresponds to <15, 15, 30, 100, and 300 mg/dL semiquantitative values, respectively. The exact bins or cutoff values vary somewhat by manufacturer especially at the lower limits of detection [16].

Hydration status and the concentration of urine can impact protein measurement. Highly concentrated urine overestimates the degree of proteinuria/albuminuria determined on the dipstrip color reaction compared to other methods. A positive color reaction on the pad could be due to excessive protein added to the urine by some disease or it could reflect normal small amounts of protein in highly concentrated urine. False-negative reactions for protein on the dipstrip are less common, but do occur at times in urine that is very acidic or not well concentrated (Table 7.3).

The sensitivity and specificity for urine dipstrip protein reactions are low in dogs and cats [2, 8]. False-positive reactions on dipstrip (decreased specificity) reactions to protein (compared to more quantitative bench top reference methods) are common for dipstrip reactions in both the dog and cat, but especially so for cats [2, 15]. The high occurrence of false-positive dipstrip reactions in the cat is possibly due to the presence of cauxin. Cauxin is a carboxyesterase secreted by renal tubules into urine in high concentration in cats. Cauxin acts as an enzyme in urine to hydrolyze felinine precursors to felinine. Markedly higher urinary cauxin concentrations are encountered in intact male cats compared to neutered male, intact, or neutered female cats [127]. It appears that even low concentrations of cauxin in feline urine can activate the tetraphenol blue color indicator on the urine chemistry dipstrip. This reaction with cauxin may be the reason why so many cats without albuminuria have a dipstrip color reaction (false positive for albuminuria). Positive dipstrip reactions in this instance indicate a form of nonalbumin proteinuria that appears to be physiologically normal in cats. The selective removal of cauxin from normal feline urine resulted in negative readings during urinary dipstrip protein testing in one study [128].

There is concern and confusion in the interpretation of a positive dipstrip reagent pad reaction for protein when there is also a positive reagent pad reaction for occult blood. Based on a study of dogs with hemoglobin added to urine, it required

Table 7.3   Interpretation of urine total protein results from urine dipstrip chemistry.

Positive reaction	False positive reaction	Negative reaction	False negative reaction
Albuminuria ≥30 mg/dL (Trace = 10–20 mg/dL)	Highly alkaline urine (pH ≥ 8.5)	Albumin <30 mg/dL (microalbuminuria)	Low urine pH
			Very dilute urine
Most sensitive to albumin	Highly pigmented urine	Non albumin proteins may or may not be detected:	
		Myoglobin	
Less detection of nonalbumin proteins	Blood substitutes (Oxyglobin®)	Hemoglobin	
		Immunoglobulins	
Cauxin (cats)	Phenazopyridine (urinary analgesic)	Bence Jones Proteins	
		Acute Phase Proteins	
		Mucoproteins	
>1.050 USG trace or 1+ (protein concentration increased by water removal from urine)	Disinfectants	Tamm–Horsfall (uromodulin)	
	Chlorhexidine (Skin cleanser)		
	Quaternary ammonium (compounds)		
Blood contamination – if pink or red urine (plasma proteins and hemoglobin)		Pad contaminated by finger touching	
	Oversaturation of pad dilutes buffer – prolonged immersion	Pad not exposed to enough urine volume	
	Pad exposure to air and moisture – loss of reagent or reactivity from improper storage		
	pH pad runover to adjacent protein pad		
	Semen		

Source: Lamb and Jones [16], Strasinger and Di Lorenzo [121], Sink and Weinstein [122], Sink and Weinstein [123], Rizzi et al. [124], Roura [54], Bertholf [110], Tripathi et al. [125], Miyazaki et al. [126], Miyazaki [127], Miyazaki [128], Stockham and Scott [129], Moore [130], Elliott and Sargent [131].

a maximal reaction on the occult blood reagent pad before the protein reagent pad turned positive from the presence of hemoglobin in the urine. This demonstrated that the dipstrip pads for protein detection were not that sensitive for the detection of protein contained in hemoglobin. In the same study, the SSA test was not sensitive for the detection of hemoglobin as it required ≥40 mg/dL of hemoglobin in order to generate a positive test [132].

Highly concentrated urine samples sometimes result in trace to 1+ protein readings that are not confirmed when measured by other methods to detect proteinuria. False-positive reactions for protein can occur in samples with highly alkaline urine (pH >8), urine containing phenazopyridine or blood substitutes (polyvinyl compounds), and urine contaminated with benzalkonium chloride, quaternary ammonium compounds, or chlorhexidine [108, 133]. Bloody urine can obscure the interpretation of color development on the pad resulting in a false-positive reading [116]. Dogs and cats with gross hematuria or pyuria are likely to have positive reactions for protein on dipstrip and by UPC and MA. Dipstrip reactions for protein were significantly increased in urine samples that were light pink to red in dogs and dark pink to red in cats following the addition of whole blood in one study [134]. The proteinuria or albuminuria that is reported cannot be assessed as originating from the kidneys until after gross hematuria or pyuria clears. Microscopic hematuria or pyuria is not always associated with albuminuria in the dog and cat as has frequently been considered to be true in the past. The presence of an active sediment and a large amount of urinary protein in the same sample can still be associated with renal proteinuria, but an accurate assessment is better made after analysis when the sediment is inactive [2, 93, 135].

The submission of a bacterial urine culture has been recommended to exclude a bacterial UTI that is adding postrenal proteins to urine during the evaluation for possible renal proteinuria [136]. In one study of dogs with proteinuria (UPC > 0.5), positive quantitative bacterial growth was uncommon (30/451). Sixty percent of those with positive culture had an active urinary sediment, and some combination of pyuria, bacteriuria, and a history of lower urinary tract disease predicted positive bacterial growth in most instances. A positive urine culture from dogs with proteinuria and an inactive urinary sediment was very uncommon. This finding suggests that it may not be necessary to submit a quantitative urine culture in dogs to rule out postrenal urinary infection in all instances. Submission of urine culture is still recommended when the urinary sediment is active or in those with a history of lower urinary tract disease [137].

The contamination of urine samples with semen from sexually intact dogs can increase the color reactions for protein and blood on the urine chemistry dipstrip. Sperm are sometimes found in the urine of sexually intact male dogs and cats collected by voiding, catheter, or cystocentesis. Retrograde flow of sperm into the urinary bladder occurs during ejaculation, during the use of some sedatives, and at times during routine urinary voiding [138–141]. The addition of dilutions of whole ejaculate or seminal fluid to urine of dogs increased the magnitude of dipstrip proteinuria over that from baseline. The addition of ejaculate or seminal fluid to urine also resulted in positive reactions for blood on the dipstrip in the absence of RBC in urinary sediment [142].

A negative color reaction for protein on dipstrip reliably indicates the absence of pathological proteinuria based on UPC in most instances. A negative dipstrip reaction for protein will align with a UPC < 0.5 in dogs and <0.4 in cats most of the time, regardless of USG. Dipstick protein ≥2+ are usually associated with pathologic proteinuria and albuminuria [2, 10, 11, 94].

A dipstick positive result ≥trace for protein should be confirmed with another method to measure protein irrespective of urine concentration based on USG. Trace and 1+ dipstick reactions are the most problematic to know if they indicate pathological proteinuria without confirmatory testing (UPC or MA) [11, 15]. USG and positive protein dipstrip reactions were weakly correlated in one study of dogs but USG did not add value for accurate prediction of abnormal UPC [94]. In a study of clinically normal dogs, trace (15 mg/dL) or 1+ (30 mg/dL) reactions for protein on the urine chemistry dipstrip were common. The highest UPC was 0.21 and the highest total urinary protein was 39.0 mg/dL in this population. The authors of this paper concluded that dipstrip reactions for protein at this level should be considered unremarkable instead of a falsely positive finding [143].

A substantial difference in the assigned bin for proteinuria occurred at times following visual inspection and color assessment by the technician performing the test in one study [112]. The bin for proteinuria assigned was consistent when performed by the same technician, but discordance was relatively high between technicians in human medicine. Some of the variability between protein content reported on serial urine samples can be accounted by different technicians reading the color reaction on the strip. Variation by technologist was substantial even when color blindness was excluded. Most of the discordant readings were in urine samples that were negative, trace or 1+. There was greater concordance when reading samples with stronger color reactions [112]. It is also important to remember that variation in urinary dipstrip protein readings can sometimes be attributed to different brands of reagent dipstrip used to perform the measurement [115].

PRECIPITATION TESTING FOR URINARY PROTEINS

Turbidimetric assays based on protein precipitation using SSA, trichloracetic acid, or heat and acetic acid are additional methods for the semiquantitative measurement of proteinuria. These methods detect albumin, globulins, and Bence Jones proteins, whereas the urinary dipstrip primarily detects mostly albumin. SSA is not sensitive for the detection of hemoglobin or myoglobin in urine. The lower limit of sensitivity of these assays is 5–10 mg/dL. Radiographic contrast agents and large doses of penicillins, cephalosporins, or sulfisoxazole as well as thymol urine preservative may result in false-positive reactions during SSA testing. False-negative reactions may occur with highly alkaline urine [2].

Some veterinary laboratories perform confirmatory SSA testing on urine samples that have trace or 1+ positive on dipstrip reactions for protein. Both should be positive at the same time if there is albuminuria [2]. SSA testing was abandoned by one veterinary laboratory due to its inferiority to dipstrip pro-

tein results when compared to automated microprotein assay [144]. SSA testing for urinary proteins is uncommonly performed in veterinary commercial laboratories.

If the urine supernatant is not clear following centrifugation, SSA testing will overestimate the amount of urinary proteins. In one version of this test, equal amounts of supernatant and 3–5% SSA are mixed in glass tubes [2]. One part of urine is added to three parts of 3% SSA in another method. The degree of turbidity of urine supernatant that develops after the addition of SSA is subjectively estimated from 0 and trace to 4+ (Figure 7.6). 0 is perfectly clear with no turbidity

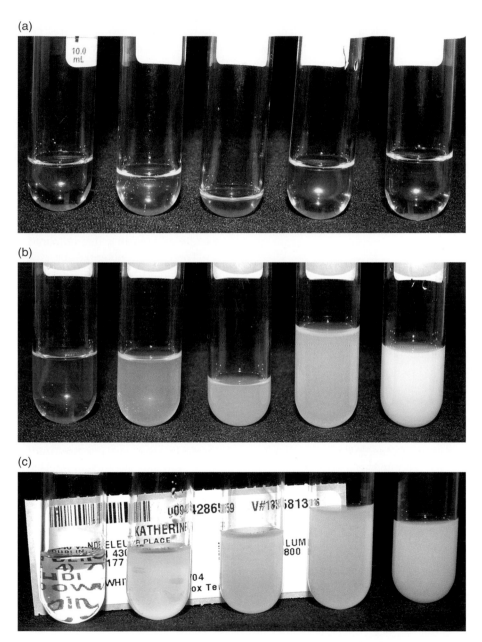

FIGURE 7.6   (a)–(c) Visual inspection of urine supernatant following centrifugation, before (a) and after addition of SSA (b) and (c). The sample on the far left is negative and would be reported as 0 or <5 mg/dL; note that it is easy to read print through the sample. The sample next to the right would be trace to 1+. The sample at the far right would be 4+. Source: Used with permission of Dr. Catherine Langston, Columbus, Ohio.

(<5 mg/dL), trace has slight turbidity (5–15 mg/dL), 1+ has some turbidity but print can still be read through it (>15–30 mg/dL), 2+ is diffusely white but heavy print can still be seen (>30–100 mg/dL), 3+ is heavy white with fine precipitates and print cannot be seen (>100–300 mg/dL), and 4+ has flocculent precipitates (>300 mg/dL). A set of standard tubes with SSA reactions from 5 to 100 mg/dL increases the accuracy for the subjective scoring of the SSA reaction for proteins [2, 54, 133, 145–149]. The subjectivity during visual reading the amount of turbidity that develops in urine following the addition of SSA can be removed by turbidimetric analyzers that do not depend on visual inspection [130].

If the dipstrip test for protein is negative and the SSA test is positive, nonalbumin proteinuria is a consideration that includes light chains (Bence Jones proteins) and tubular proteinuria [114]. Lysozymuria is a rare type of overflow proteinuria (prerenal proteinuria) that can be detected following SSA and urinary dipstick testing [16, 150]. Increased production and urinary excretion of lysozymes can occur in some human patients with acute monocytic or myelocytic leukemia. A persistently positive urine dipstick for proteinuria in the absence of albuminuria can suggest the presence of lysozymuria, particularly in the absence of other signs of the nephrotic syndrome (NS) [150]. A positive dipstrip reading is considered falsely positive when the SSA reading is negative; the dipstrip positive readings are usually minimal or slight in these instances [107].

URINARY PROTEIN-TO-CREATININE RATIO

The measurement of UPC is useful to confirm or deny proteinuria/albuminuria initially suspected on dipstrip results, but it can also be used initially to screen for proteinuria. In the case where UPC is increased (>0.2) but the dipstrip protein reaction is minimal or zero and the MA is negative, prerenal and tubular proteinuria must be considered.

UPC is a unitless number following the division of urinary protein in mg/dL by urinary creatinine in mg/dL. Urinary creatinine excretion varies little in an individual stable dog or cat over a 24-hour period allowing for the use of this ratio. Having urinary creatinine in the denominator corrects for urine that is highly concentrated or highly diluted, as urinary creatinine concentration will be correspondingly high or low. For example: if the dipstrip is 1+ protein, urine protein on the benchtop is 70 mg/dL, and the urinary creatinine is 350 mg/dL, the UPC calculates as 0.2. If the same 70 mg/dL urinary protein were associated with a 100 mg/dL urinary creatinine, the UPC is now 0.7.

Benchtop analyzers measure total protein that includes albumin and other proteins. Pyrogallol red molybdate (PRM) and Coomassie brilliant blue (CBB) are the most commonly used methods to measure urinary total proteins. Values for total urinary protein are higher when measured by PRM compared to CBB. Differences between protein concentrations measured by PRM and CBB affected International Renal Interest Society (IRIS) substaging of CKD in dogs when protein concentrations

were near the cutoffs for overt proteinuria [151]. In another study, UPC was determined in proteinuric and nonproteinuric cats by either CBB or PRM methods to measure protein. Both methods were precise, but higher protein values were generated in urine measured with CBB. The coefficient of variation (CV) on replicates for CBB was higher than that for PRM. Misclassification of IRIS substaging based on UPC was similar by either CBB or PRM when values were close to the cutoff points (< 0.2 or >0.4) [152]. Aminoglycosides and gelatin volume expanders can also falsely increase the urinary total protein reported [16].

There is no universal agreement on the methods for measurement of urinary creatinine in human or veterinary medicine; all urinary methods have been modified from those initially designed to measure creatinine in serum or plasma [153]. Urinary creatinine concentrations can vary on the same urine sample when measured by different methods and analyzers. The optimal dilution for the measurement of urinary creatinine was recommended at 1:20 in general and 1:100 for samples with a USG > 1.030 in one study [154]. In a study of dog urine diluted 1:20 with distilled water, urinary creatinine concentrations were not different when measured on an autoanalyzer using the kinetic Jaffe or enzymatic methods; the degree of inaccuracy was <5% using human creatinine as a control. A trivial difference in urinary creatinine concentration determined by Jaffe and enzymatic methods is expected since interference from noncreatinine chromogens is usually very low in urine compared to that in serum.

There is the potential for analytical error during the measurement of both urinary protein and urinary creatinine used to calculate the UPC, which can make the diagnostic interpretation of results less reliable. The use of benchtop analyzers has been reported to underestimate the amount of urinary creatinine for dogs (as discussed in Chapter 1). In such instances, the lower creatinine in the denominator results in an increased UPC without any change in the amount of urinary protein. This phenomenon can result in an increase of UPC such that the categorization of proteinuria is escalated from normal to borderline, and from borderline to overtly increased at times [153]. Benchtop analyzers likely to be used in-house by veterinary practices underestimated urinary creatinine especially at concentrations >200 mg/dL; urinary creatinine concentrations were 25% lower when determined by one analyzer [153]. Consequently, it is important to base the interpretation of UPC on results obtained from reliable measurements. Urine creatinine results from benchtop analyzers may not be acceptable for clinical use, and results should not be compared to those generated from automated methods used by commercial laboratories.

Both analytical and biological variability can occur during the measurement of UPC at different times on different samples from the same animal. Consequently, it is especially important to consider these factors when the reported UPC is slightly above or below the defined decision-making points of <0.2 in the dog and cat as nonproteinuric and ≥0.4 in the cat or ≥0.5 in the dog as overtly proteinuric. The coefficients of variation for UPC in urine from dogs during repeated measurements from the same sample were 10–20% when the UPC was 0.2 (0.15–0.25) and 10% when the UPC was 0.5 (0.45–0.55) [151, 154, 155]. Consequently, a UPC slightly above or below these tipping points (UPC 0.15–0.25 for dogs and cats; 0.35–0.45 for cats and 0.45–0.55 for dogs) could result in the wrong assessment as to whether there is proteinuria or not based on this level of analytical imprecision for both urinary creatinine and urinary total protein (Figure 7.7) [154, 155]. In instances where UPC values are near defined cutoff values, the UPC should be measured at another time on another sample to determine if the UPC values are repeatable and found to be in the same category or bin of proteinuria (none, borderline, or overt) or if there is discordance.

The method of urine storage can impact UPC measurement. Prolonged storage at high temperature for 30 days decreased urinary creatinine in a study of human urine, but minimal decreases were detected when stored at the same high temperature (55 °C) for two days [156]. UPC was unchanged in urine samples from dogs stored up to four hours at room temperature before measurement but UPC increased after storage at room temperature or refrigeration (4 °C) for 12 hours. There was no change in UPC when samples from dogs were immediately frozen and stored up to 3 months at −20 °C. Freezing of urine is recommended if samples cannot be immediately measured [154]. Stored samples should be analyzed after reaching room temperature and thorough mixing [16].

UPC results can also be generated from urinary dipstrips used in human medicine that contain a pad to measure urinary creatinine concentration using automated strip readers [16]. This allows UPC to be calculated and reported in semiquantitative bins. UPC screening was found to be useful in dogs but not cats in one study using a dipstrip autoanalyzer that measured urinary creatinine and protein [149]. Some discordance between UPC determined by benchtop and dipstrip analyzers is expected as they employ different methods to measure protein and creatinine. The use of urine dipstrips to accurately estimate bins for UPC needs further clinical validation in veterinary medicine.

UPC is generally not influenced by feeding or fasting, and whether urine is collected by cystocentesis or voiding in normal dogs and cats [8, 10]. Exposure to plastic nonabsorbent spherical pellet cat litter for one hour had no impact on feline UPC measurements [157]. In addition, UPC and urine albumin-to-creatinine ratio (UAC) were not different between dogs that were overweight or obese compared to those that had ideal body weight and body condition score (BCS) [158]. UPC may be influenced by the time of day that urine is collected in children [159]. In humans, there is less variation in samples collected early in the morning, as compared to samples collected at bedtime.

Mean UPC measured by the CBB method in kittens from 4 to 32 weeks of age ranged from 0.14 ± 0.03 to 0.34 ± 0.18 from week to week, findings similar to that in adult cats. The UPC for cats ≥9 weeks of age correlated well to 24-hour urinary protein excretion [160]. Mean quantitative urinary protein excretion was 52.30 ± 25.70 mg/day or 17.43 ± 9.05 mg/kg/day (4.1–42.9 mg/kg/day) in healthy adult cats as measured by the CBB method of one study, with no difference found between males and females. There was considerable variation in protein excretion in some cats on consecutive days by as much as 25 mg/kg/day [161].

Mean quantitative protein excretion in sexually intact healthy adult cats was 12.65 ± 5.45 mg/kg/24 hours and proteinuria was significantly greater in male cats (16.62 mg/kg/24 hours) compared to female cats (8.69 ± 4.09 mg/kg/24 hours). Protein in urine was measured by the CBB method. Less than 29 mg/kg/day of protein excretion is expected from healthy adult cats based on mean ± 3 SD in this study. A single UPC was highly correlated with the 24-hour protein loss. In voided samples, the mean UPC was 0.317 ± 0.132 for all cats, 0.222 ± 0.110 in female cats, and 0.413 ± 0.065 in male cats but this did not achieve statistical significance. There was no significant difference in UPC in urine samples obtained by cystocentesis compared to voiding. The UPC of normal cats should be ≤0.7 or ≤0.65 as derived in this paper [162], which is quite a bit higher than the <0.2 currently endorsed as nonproteinuric by IRIS.

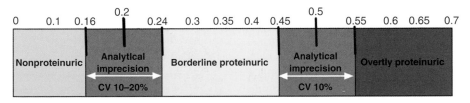

FIGURE 7.7 Imprecision in the measurement of UPC in the dog. The CV for the repeated measurement of UPC was approximately 10–20% when the UPC was 0.2 and about 10% when the UPC was 0.5. For a UPC of 0.2, the value could vary from 0.16 to 0.24. This degree of imprecision could result in assignment of the bin as either nonproteinuric or borderline proteinuric. For a UPC of 0.5, the value could vary from 0.45 to 0.55 resulting in assignment of the bin as borderline proteinuric or overtly proteinuric. It is important to consider this level of imprecision in any UPC value near the cutoff values of 0.2 or 0.5 in the dog. The UPC should be repeated to see if the same bin is assigned on subsequent samples with UPC values near the cutoffs. Similar concerns are likely for cats with cutoff values of 0.2 or 0.4 UPC. Assignment to a particular proteinuria bin should not be based on a single UPC value that is close to the cutoff, due to this degree of analytical uncertainty. Source: Adapted from Scarpa [155] and Rossi et al. [154].

Sexually intact male cats can have a higher UPC than is generally accepted as normal for neutered male and female cats. UPCs up to 0.6 were found in 124 normal young sexually intact male cats maintained in a research laboratory. All urine samples were collected by cystocentesis. The increase in UPC was likely attributed to an abundance of cauxin in the urine of intact male cats. All UPCs were <0.2 within two weeks following castration (Dr. Scott Brown, personal communication April 2020). Castration of normal dogs decreased the urinary protein detected by dipstrip and by UPC in one study (urine collected by cystocentesis) [163]. Dipstrip protein was negative in 9 and ≥1+ for 10 of 19 sexually intact normal male dogs studied prior to castration. The dipstrip for protein was negative in 13 and ≥1+ in 6 dogs after at least 15 days following castration in the same dogs. UPC was <0.5 in all the sexually intact male dogs of this study and <0.2 following castration for all except one dog. Spermaturia was found in 15 of 19 dogs before castration and in no dogs following castration, but there was no significant association between the number of spermatozoa in the urine and the UPC prior to castration. The UPC decreased in 18 of 19 dogs following castration; mean UPC was 0.12 prior to castration and significantly decreased to a mean UPC of 0.08 following castration [163].

The magnitude of creatinine excretion into urine has not been studied in detail for dogs and cats based on age. Urinary protein excretion (mg/kg/day) and UPC increased between 4 and 14 weeks of age for normal kittens in one study [160]. Trace to 1+ dipstrip protein reactions were recorded from voided or postvoided urine samples in most puppies from an animal shelter or commercial pet stores up to 24 weeks of age [164]. In a small number of Beagle puppies, mean UPC (0.21 versus 0.10) and protein excretion (5.73 mg/kg versus 2.80 mg/kg) were higher at 9 weeks than that at 27 weeks old [165]. Total daily protein excretion was lower in puppies (6.0 ± 1.9 mg/kg) compared to mature dogs (48 ± 68.4 mg/kg) in another study [166]. It is known that the excretion of creatinine into urine declines with age in humans, which can increase the UPC despite no change in protein excretion into urine [16].

Extremes of muscle mass for any individual must be considered for its effect on the UPC. UPC may increase when urinary creatinine excretion declines with loss of muscle mass, as frequently occurs with CKD [167]. In these instances, the UPC will increase despite the fact that urinary protein excretion has not increased at the same time. Those with a very high muscle mass and an increased urinary creatinine excretion will exhibit a decrease in the UPC [16].

The variability in UPC within a normal patient is expected to be minimal from day to day. Renal proteinuria based on UPC can be observed in apparently healthy animals. Borderline or overt proteinuria based on UPC (0.2–0.5 and >0.5 respectively) were found in 25–32% of apparently healthy senior and geriatric dogs [168, 169]. Borderline proteinuria (UPC 0.2–0.4) was encountered in 44.1% and overt proteinuria

(>0.4 UPC) in 4.7% of seemingly healthy geriatric cats of one study [170]. This could indicate random biologic variability of protein filtration or an underlying disorder that has not yet been diagnosed.

Variability in UPC may be more dramatic in dogs with underlying glomerular disease, as shown in one study of female dogs with stable X-linked HN, in which UPC was measured once daily for three consecutive days. The variability in UPC was greatest in this study as the magnitude of proteinuria increased. To prove a significant difference between serial UPC, UPC had to change by at least 35% when the UPC was near 12 and by 80% when the UPC was near 0.5. One sample was considered adequate to evaluate the UPC when it was <4.0, whereas multiple samples were needed to reliably evaluate UPC with higher values [171]. Whether or not the variability in UPC demonstrated in this study also exists in other populations of dogs with glomerular disease has yet to be reported.

Multiple UPCs are sometimes recommended to evaluate proteinuria in dogs with stable glomerular disease in an effort to limit the effect of random biological variability. There is inherent biological variability in the excretion of urine total protein and albumin among individual animals, so reliance on one single measurement of urinary protein can be problematic. It has been recommended to demonstrate that glomerular proteinuria is persistent and repeatable [2, 7, 8, 14, 54]. Some of this individual variability might be accounted for by genetic influences on tubular reabsorption of albumin via the cubulin receptor [16].

There was high correlation between the average of UPC from three separate urine collections and the UPC of pooled urine from samples in one study of dogs. A maximum ±20% difference in UPC from the pooled urine compared to the individual average of samples was observed in this study. Pooling of urine samples from sequential first morning urine provides a reliable cost affordable method for clients to collect voided urine specimens at home from dogs for evaluation of proteinuria [172]. UPC did not appear to differ between measurements from a single sample compared to a pooled sample in another study of dogs with proteinuria [173].

Proteinuria of renal origin is one finding that can be useful in making a decision if a patient should be staged as IRIS CKD stage 1. Patients in IRIS Stage 1 are nonazotemic and have a serum creatinine <1.6 mg/dL (C) and <1.4 mg/dL (D) and symmetrical dimethyl arginine (SDMA) <18 μg/dL. The decision for Stage 1 is not usually made on the isolated finding of renal proteinuria, but often in some combination of findings that show reduced urinary concentrating ability, abnormal renal structure on palpation or imaging, trending increases of serum creatinine, SDMA, or renal biopsy results. IRIS CKD substaging is based on UPC and not the degree of MA [174]. IRIS recommends the use of UPC to substage CKD in dogs and cats as nonproteinuric (<0.2), borderline proteinuric (0.2 to <0.4 [cats]; 0.2 to <0.5 [dogs]), and overtly proteinuric (>0.4 [cats]; >0.5 [dogs]) (Table 7.4).

Table 7.4 Proteinuria assessed by urine protein/creatinine ratio for the assignment of IRIS substage of CKD in dogs and cats.

Urine protein/urine creatinine ratio (UPC)	Classification
<0.2 (dogs) <0.2 (cats)	Nonproteinuric
0.2–0.5 (dogs) 0.2–0.4 (cats)	Borderline proteinuric
>0.5 (dogs) >0.4 (cats)	Proteinuric

There is the possibility that the presence of RBC, WBC, and bacteria in urine may have an impact on measured protein, due to the presence of hemoglobin and plasma proteins in the urine. Urinary tract hemorrhage and inflammation are commonly considered to be causes for proteinuria [93, 183]. Clinically relevant increases in UPC developed following the addition of whole blood (urocrit 10% by volume) to urine in one study. UPC increased in urine following cystotomy and after the creation of *Escherichia coli* UTI in experimental dogs in the same study. The increase in UPC from lower urinary tract inflammation was not predictable based on the urinary sediment enumeration of RBC or WBC however [183]. In another study that added blood to canine urine, the UPC did not exceed 0.4 at any dilution even when urine was pink to red, and albuminuria (>1 mg/dL) did not occur until the urine was pink (RBC TNTC or >250/HPF) [93]. Median UPC values increased to >0.5 in cats and dogs when the urine samples were pink and further increased when samples were dark pink (>0.7) and red (>1.2) in another study [134]. Blood contamination led to different categorizations of proteinuria as normal, borderline, or increased based on UPC even without obvious color change to the urine in this study. A false-positive assessment for proteinuria occurred when there were ≥250 RBC/HPF [134]. The effect of blood contamination on the UPC was more prominent in this study than in the study mentioned previously [93] prompting caution to be exercised when interpreting blood contaminated urine samples and proteinuria.

Many clinical samples from dogs with pyuria did not have albuminuria or an increase in total urinary protein based on UPC in one study. There was no significant relationship between the degree of pyuria (>5 WBC/HPF) and UPC or MA [93]. The UPC was <0.5 in 41% of dogs with heavy bacterial growth in another study [94, 184]. Based on these findings, caution should be used in routinely attributing increases in albuminuria or total proteinuria to inflammation with associated pyuria or to hemorrhage (sample not red or pink). In these instances, glomerular origin proteinuria is still possible and should be reassessed following resolution of pyuria and hematuria to know with more certainty.

MICROALBUMINURIA

The term "microalbuminuria" has historically been used to described increased urinary albumin excretion or concentrations in urine that are not detectable with routine urinary chemistry dipstrips. The continuing use of this term is discouraged by some in favor of the term "albuminuria" since this term refers to increased loss of albumin of any amount [16].

The measurement of MA is useful to determine loss of protein into urine below the detection of urine on dipsticks and to confirm results of positive dipstick reactions for protein [2, 12, 13]. Urine from normal dogs and cats contains <1.0 mg/dL of albumin. MA is defined as 1–29 mg/dL of urinary albumin; ≥30 mg/dL is considered overt proteinuria or albuminuria [135]. Low concentration of urinary albumin may be reported as <2 or <2.5 mg/dL depending on the laboratory and method of analysis due to lower limits of detection. Variability in MA over the same day or between days in the same patient has not been studied, as it has with UPC in some populations of dogs.

Urinary albumin can be detected by both colorimetric and immunological methods [16]. Many laboratories offer urinary albumin measured by immunoturbidimetric methods designed as the gold standard for use in human urine [16, 185]. The use of species-specific antibodies toward dog and cat albumin is not routinely employed by veterinary reference laboratories. Early studies to measure MA in dogs and cats employed a point-of-care analyzer using species-specific antibodies toward albumin, but this analyzer is no longer marketed. In this method, the urine was first diluted to a USG of 1.010 to remove artifact from varying degrees of urine concentration [12, 13, 15, 145, 186]. Though the performance of this analyzer was generally acceptable as a screening test, subjectivity in the visual assessment of color development sometimes resulted in discordance with benchtop methods for MA or when compared to positive reactions on UPC or dipstrip.

Reagent strips for the specific detection of human urinary albumin using colorimetry or immunoassays are available. This method can provide false-negative results when the urine is dilute; positive albuminuria results from the dipstrip for MA should be confirmed with the standard benchtop laboratory measurement of urinary albumin and UPC [16]. One such dipstrip performed poorly when protein in urine from dogs was assessed using a dipstrip reader [187]. MA was measured by VetScan UA 14 strips with an automated analyzer that employs fluorescein dye as a nonspecific binder for proteins. MA is reported as either <2.5 mg/dL (negative) or ≥2.5 mg/dL (positive). All quality control materials that were negative or positive generated results that were in the correct bin for MA, but demonstrated a negative bias at lower albumin concentrations. Immunoturbidimetric or ELISA testing that generates a numerical value was recommended instead of relying on these two bins of MA assignment.

MA measured at a referral laboratory is needed to determine a specific value for MA between 2.5 and 29 mg/dL and to determine a baseline to document trends. It is more appropriate to follow UPC when MA values exceed 29 mg/dL [135].

MA positive status was found in 25% of apparently healthy dogs [188] and 9–14% of apparently healthy cats [15, 186]; this increases with age and when a dog or cat is ill. MA positive status was found in 31% of dogs and 26% of cats with various clinical conditions [12, 13]. MA occurred in greater than 50% of critically ill dogs, a finding that was more frequent than an increased UPC [189].

MA positive status develops in dogs and cats early on in many disease processes, often before UPC is overtly increased. The same diseases shown to be associated with increased UPC usually have MA positive status at the same time. It appears likely that MA becomes positive first, followed by UPC, and then dipstrip positive for protein in diseases with progressive glomerular injury [135]. Based on the UAC, MA (UAC ≤ 0.3) was detected in 32.5% of dogs with CKD and macroalbuminuria (UAC > 0.3) in 50% of dogs with CKD [190]. In general, a UPC > 1.0 was associated with macroalbuminuria, UPC of 0.5–1.0 was associated with MA, and a UPC < 0.5 was not associated with albuminuria in this study [190].

MA occurred before overt proteinuria was detected by UPC in dogs with X-linked nephritis in both male [191] and female dogs [192]. Similarly, the prevalence of MA was high in soft-coated Wheaton terriers (SCWTs) genetically predisposed to develop glomerular disease and MA increased with age. MA occurred more frequently than a UPC > 0.5 in this population [193].

The detection of MA can indicate the presence of early glomerular damage not detectable by other methods [11]. Albuminuria that is persistent or of increasing magnitude may be the earliest clinical indicator of glomerular disease [93]. Systemic inflammation can be associated with the endothelial leakage of protein and MA. Dogs with severe inflammatory response syndrome (SIRS) frequently have increased UPC and MA due to glomerular barrier dysfunction [194]. Deposition of immune complexes within the glomerulus, as well as decreased blood flow to the kidneys and injurious molecules synthesized by tumors, is thought to contribute to glomerular injury and proteinuria in patients with neoplasia [195]. The long-term effects or associations of stable MA or borderline UPC levels on renal function or survival during primary glomerular disease or systemic disease are not known [15]. Clearly, not all MA positive animals develop CKD, as there are many more MA positive status dogs and cats than are diagnosed with CKD.

Nearly 25% of over 3000 dogs owned by veterinary hospital personnel were found to have MA positive status in one study. MA positive status increased in frequency with age from 4% at 1 year to 55% at 15 years of age. Of the 572 dogs with MA positive status that were followed, 56.3% were diagnosed with underlying infectious, inflammatory, neoplastic, or metabolic disease. Dogs with renal disease accounted for 31%, 12.1% had no specific diagnosis, and 0.6% had multiple diagnoses or ones not related to proteinuria [12, 188]. Forty-five percent of apparently healthy dogs were found to be MA positive using a dipstrip automated reader to measure albumin and creatinine in another study [196].

In another study of dogs examined at a teaching hospital that were negative for protein on dipstrip chemistry, the association between MA status and diagnosis within three months was determined. MA positive status was shown in 111 of 352 (31.5%) dogs with one diagnosis. Of dogs with positive quantitative MA status, 6% were diagnosed as healthy, 31% with neoplasia, 20% with infectious-inflammatory-immune-mediated diseases, 14% with urinary disorders, and 29% had diseases that did not fall into any of the other categories. Quantitative MA had a sensitivity of 35.6% and specificity of 85.4% for the detection of systemic disease in dogs [12].

MA was documented in 14% of 611 apparently healthy cats, and its frequency increased with age [15]. At a teaching hospital, MA positive status was shown in 85 of 324 (26%) cats. Of cats with MA positive status, 2% were diagnosed as healthy, 11% with neoplasia, 20% with infectious-inflammatory-immune-mediated diseases, 33% with urinary tract disease, 16% with endocrine disease, and 18% with other diseases that did not fall into any of the other categories. Quantitative MA had a sensitivity of 37% and a specificity of 94% for the detection of systemic disease in these cats [13]. MA by semiquantitative strip testing was found in 36% of sick cats and 9% of healthy cats in another study. MA was positive in more samples than for increased UPC as expected, but there were instances in which UPC was increased but MA was negative. Either the MA was falsely negative or proteins other than albumin accounted for the increased UPC [186].

MA status was evaluated in 599 canine and 347 feline urine samples from apparently healthy animals [145]. The ability of positive dipstrip protein reactions to predict MA was high in the dog and very high in the cat, but false positives on dipstrip for protein were frequent, especially in the cat. The finding of positive results for both SSA and dipstick for protein decreased the number of false-positive results but did increase the number of false negatives in both species compared to MA. When ≥2+ protein reactions were considered as the cutoff for positive protein on the dipstrip, very few false positives were diagnosed, but false negatives based on MA increased [145].

A total of 239 urine samples from 37 cats with CKD were evaluated for proteinuria. Positive results from dipstick and SSA together, SSA alone, or dipstick ≥2+ were indicative of albuminuria. The higher the dipstick reaction for protein, the lower the number of false positives. Conversely, lower dipstick reactions for protein increased the number of false negatives. The performance of dipstick and SSA positive reactions in combination was better in CKD cats than in apparently healthy cats for the identification of MA positive status. Highly concentrated urine can result in false-positive reactions for protein on the dipstick that are not associated with MA positive status, a situation which is more likely to occur in healthy cats as CKD cats often have much less concentrated urine. A UPC of ≥0.2 as a cutoff performed well for the identification of MA in CKD cats of this study [148].

URINARY PROTEIN ELECTROPHORESIS

The concentration of total urinary protein or urinary albumin is measured clinically, but specific proteins can be quantitated by immunoassay or specialized electrophoresis at times. Urinary proteins can be separated according to mass and electrical charge using high-resolution gel electrophoresis techniques (SDS-PAGE). This method allows urinary proteins to be separated into origin as glomerular, tubular, or mixed pattern [16]. As glomerular damage increases, the permeability of the glomerulus to plasma proteins increases. This allows intermediate-molecular-weight proteins, such as albumin (67 kD), to appear in the urine first followed by the appearance of higher weight proteins (HMW ≥ 100 kD, such as immunoglobulins) as more glomerular damage occurs [6]. Urinary protein electrophoresis was helpful in classifying renal proteinuria as glomerular or tubular in origin in dogs of one study. Glomerular origin protein was likely when >41.4% of the total proteins in urine consisted of albumin and when the ratio of urinary albumin to alpha-1 globulin was >1.46 [197]. Urine protein banding patterns were correlated with the degree of histopathological glomerular or tubulointerstitial injury in another study [5].

LMW proteinuria at <69 kD typifies patients with tubular proteinuria. LMW proteins are freely filtered across the glomerulus and would normally be reabsorbed by healthy proximal tubules, so the detection of these proteins reflects the failure of tubular reabsorption [3, 5, 16, 135, 198]. When excess albumin enters tubular fluid from glomerular disease, LMW proteinuria can also occur following the saturation of proximal tubular mechanisms for the absorption of proteins, resulting in both albuminuria and the appearance of LMW proteins in urine. Additionally, persistent high-level exposure to protein in proximal tubular fluid can induce toxic lesions to proximal tubular cells, which further impairs their ability to reabsorb protein [6, 199]. Tubular proteinuria is expected in some forms of AKI and CKD from impaired proximal tubular reabsorptive function independent of tubular fluid protein toxicity.

INTERPRETATION AND MONITORING OF RENAL PROTEINURIA

Progressive glomerular damage often results in some combination of renal proteinuria, reduced GFR, and glomerular lesions that can be identified on renal histopathology (microscopy by light, EM, and IFA), but the finding of renal proteinuria (urine reagent strip, UPC, or MA) is the most sensitive indicator of early renal disease, in which glomerular permeability to primarily albumin has increased [200]. The magnitude of glomerular proteinuria is considered a marker for the severity of glomerulopathy (Table 7.5) [20, 201, 202]. Though not conclusively proven in dogs and cats with CKD, it is likely that renal proteinuria serves as a marker of underlying glomerular disease as well as a contributor to the progression

of further renal injury. Similarly, the magnitude of proteinuria indicates the degree of glomerular involvement rather the diagnosis of a specific glomerular disease [203–205].

A UPC < 0.2 is normal for most dogs and cats. Borderline values are from 0.2 to <0.4 for the cat and from 0.2 to <0.5 for the dog. Values ≥0.4 for the cat and ≥0.5 for the dog are considered overtly proteinuric according to IRIS guidelines. Proteinuria based on the UPC generally increases with an increase in CKD stage.

It is often accepted that a UPC > 2.0 in CKD is associated with primary glomerular disease and HMW proteinuria that includes albuminuria [2, 14, 136]. The notion that dogs with UPC > 2.0 usually have glomerular proteinuria does not always hold true. In dogs with biopsy proven CKD, those with tubulointerstitial disease had a median UPC of 3.9 (0.6–8.6). Some of the increase in UPC in these instances was attributed to secondary damage to glomeruli [60]. The finding of a low UAC or low MA could be helpful in supporting tubular proteinuria in those with a high UPC. Similarly, the analysis of SDS-PAGE can be used to confirm a preponderance of lower molecular weight

Table 7.5 Hypothetical interpretation of various combinations of proteinuria results by dipstrip, SSA, UPC, and MA.

Dipstrip	SSA	UPC	MA[a]	Interpretation
0	0	<0.2	Neg	No proteinuria
0 or trace	0	<0.2	Positive	Albuminuria
				Mild or early proteinuria
Trace to 1+	0	<0.2	Neg	No proteinuria
Trace to 1+	0 to 1+	>0.4(c)	Neg	False-negative MA – uncommon
		>0.5(d)		Tubular proteinuria – most Likely
1+	1+	<0.2	Positive	Albuminuria – mild
Trace to 2+	0	<0.2	Negative	False-positive dipstrip
2+	2+	0.2–0.4 (c)	Positive	Albuminuria
		0.2–0.5 (d)		Mild-to-moderate proteinuria
3+	2+	>0.4 (c)	Positive	Albuminuria
		>0.5 (d)		Moderate-to-severe proteinuria
3+	3+	>2.5	Positive	Severe proteinuria
				Primary glomerular disease likely
				Protein-losing nephropathy
				Rule out nephrotic syndrome – Evaluate serum albumin and clotting cascade

UPC – urinary protein to creatinine ratio; d – dogs; c – cat.
[a] MA – microalbuminuria; negative <2.5 mg/dL; MA positive ≥2.5 mg/dL.

proteins that occur with tubular origin proteinuria. Tubular proteinuria alone should not result in decreased circulating albumin as can occur with high-magnitude albuminuria.

In another study, dogs with IRIS CKD stages 3 and 4 had a predominant pattern of tubular proteinuria based on electrophoretic pattern. In the same study, some dogs with CKD IRIS stage 4 and a UPC > 2.0 had predominantly LMW proteinuria characteristic of tubular proteinuria, indicating that current UPC guideline suggestions can result in a flawed interpretation for the origin of the proteinuria at times [3]. THP significantly decreased as the severity of CKD increased based on the IRIS CKD stage suggesting that THP could be used as an indicator for the progression of CKD in dogs [3].

Cats with advancing CKD have less proteinuria than in dogs with CKD since cats appear to have less glomerular disease and more tubulointerstitial disease. Despite less proteinuria for cats compared to dogs with CKD, survival was significantly related to the degree of proteinuria based on UPC in two studies. Cats with UPC < 0.2 lived the longest, and cats with > 1.0 or > 0.4 UPC lived the shortest times [167, 206]. Dogs with UPC ≥ 1.0 at the time of CKD diagnosis did not live as long as dogs with UPC < 1.0 and were at greater risk for a uremic crisis [207].

It is not clear if acute stress can increase the UPC in veterinary patients, though this notion has been considered possible [2, 10]. Increases in circulating cortisol are one aspect of the stress response that could have an impact on the UPC. Chronic increases in circulating cortisol from hyperadrenocorticism (HAC) or from exogenous administration of glucocorticosteroids can increase the UPC in dogs [208]. Healthy dogs were more stressed when in the hospital compared to when at home as assessed by the urinary cortisol-to-creatinine ratio and results of a client questionnaire, but stress had no impact on the UPC in this study. The UPC determined in voided samples from healthy dogs with low level UPC did not differ between samples collected in the hospital (median 0.03) or at home (median 0.02), and there was no relationship between time spent in the hospital, travel time to the hospital, or elapsed time until sample collection on UPC [209]. In dogs with a UPC > 0.5 in another study, the collection of voided urine in the hospital was associated with an increase of UPC compared to samples collected at home, but an index of stress was not evaluated. There was no impact of the urine collection site when the UPC was <0.5. The magnitude of increase in the UPC in some of the in-hospital collected samples was substantial [210] and would affect IRIS CKD substaging based on the UPC. In dogs with PLN receiving at least one month of treatment with ACE-I, angiotensin II receptor blocker (ARB), or both, the effect of urine collection at home or in the hospital on the magnitude of UPC was reported. The UPC was higher when urine samples were collected in the hospital compared to urine samples collected by owners at home, both when the UPC was >4.0 and ≤4.0. The determination of a UPC from a single sample, the average of multiple samples, or from a pooled sample was considered comparable in this study [173].

Serial UPC is helpful to monitor the efficacy of dietary or drug therapy to mitigate proteinuria during CKD. The magnitude of proteinuria and trends for increasing or decreasing proteinuria over time are important considerations in determining how aggressive the diagnostic approach and treatment should be (Figure 7.8a, b). In nonazotemic dogs and cats, proteinuria should be monitored when MA is positive and/or UPC ≥ 0.5 to <1.0, investigated when the UPC is between 1 and 2, and intervention should occur when the UPC is 2 or above. In azotemic dogs and cats, proteinuria should be monitored and investigated when MA is positive and/or the UPC is between 0.2 and 0.4 in the cat, and 0.2 and 0.5 in the dog. Intervention should occur when the UPC is 0.4 or above in the cat and 0.5 or above in the dog [14]. Progressive increases in albuminuria characterize many active glomerular diseases. It should be noted that severe reductions in GFR from loss of nephron mass potentially can limit the degree of expected rise in proteinuria due to loss of glomerular surface area available for the filtration of plasma proteins as nephron mass is lost [167]. In these instances, a reduction in UPC is not associated with improvement in glomerular barrier function, but this phenomenon is uncommon.

Persistence of protein positive status based on UPC or MA ideally should be confirmed three times two or more weeks apart (Figure 7.9a) [7, 14]. If MA is positive and UPC is overtly positive, UPC (and not MA) is monitored in the future. If MA is positive and UPC is normal, MA should be followed to see if the magnitude of MA is increasing over time. A low level of MA that is not increasing may reflect previous damage or a disease process that is no longer active. A low level of MA that increases over time is a cause for concern that a primary or secondary disease process may be progressively damaging the kidneys. In a patient with MA positive status on qualitative dipstrip screening, it can be advantageous to send an MA to a reference laboratory to get a specific value (1–29 mg/dL) rather than just knowing it is ≥ 2.5 mg/dL from the dipstrip. The finding of MA during routine clinical visits offers the clinician a chance to investigate and diagnose systemic and primary renal disease processes before the patient is clinically ill and before UPC is increased (Figures 7.9a, b). The risk for persistent MA positive status to result in progressive CKD is not known.

More effort is directed to the investigation and treatment of renal proteinuria that is persistent, of high magnitude, and that is sequentially increasing in magnitude even when not yet above the reference range (Figure 7.9b) [7, 10, 14]. It has been suggested that dogs with higher level MA > 20 mg/dL and those that have increasing levels of MA over time are at the greatest risk to develop further glomerular injury [219]. When renal proteinuria persists or escalates from lower levels, the patient should be evaluated for CKD, and systemic processes ruled out. Once CKD is suspected as the cause for the proteinuria, a renal biopsy could be performed for a definitive diagnosis. Following the diagnosis of CKD, an IRIS stage should be assigned, and treatment for renal disease, systemic disease, renal proteinuria, and hypertension initiated.

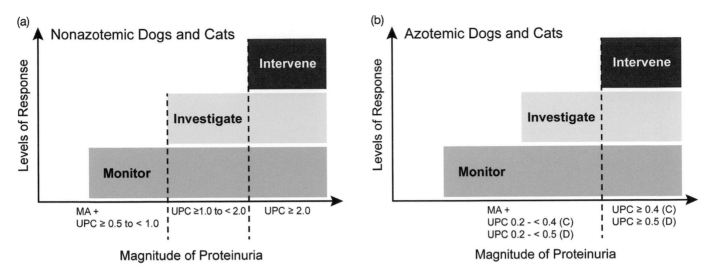

FIGURE 7.8 (a) Recommended scheme of responses for clinicians based on the magnitude of proteinuria in nonazotemic dogs and cats (2005 ACVIM Consensus Statement) [14]. The intensity of monitoring proteinuria, investigating the cause of renal proteinuria, and treatment of renal proteinuria increases as the magnitude of proteinuria increases. Note that no decisions are based on proteinuria determined by urine chemistry dipstrip. The effect of renal proteinuria on survival in nonazotemic animals is not known in dogs, but has been reported to have a negative impact on survival in cats [211]. The documentation of renal proteinuria in nonazotemic dogs and cats can be used as one factor in deciding if IRIS CKD stage 1 should be assigned. There is no evidence that intervention at lower levels of proteinuria change outcome. MA – microalbuminuria; UPC – urinary protein to urinary creatinine ratio. Source: Figure redrawn from Lees et al. [14]. Illustration by Tim Vojt, reproduced with permission of The Ohio State University. (b) Recommended responses for clinicians based on the magnitude of proteinuria in azotemic dogs and cats (2005 ACVIM Consensus Statement) [14]. Note that the threshold for responses is based on lower levels of proteinuria when the dog or cat is azotemic than when nonazotemic. MA – microalbuminuria; UPC – urinary protein to urinary creatinine ratio. Source: Figure redrawn from Lees et al. [14] by Tim Vojt © College of Veterinary Medicine – The Ohio State University. Illustration by Tim Vojt, reproduced with permission of The Ohio State University.

DISORDERS CHARACTERIZED BY RENAL PROTEINURIA

GENETIC DISORDERS

Familial nephropathy is not a single disease, but the use of this term provides an umbrella to include renal dysplasia, renal cortical hypoplasia, juvenile renal disease, glomerulopathy, HN, some forms of renal amyloidosis, polycystic kidney disease, and tubular transport dysfunctions [30, 220–222]. Familial glomerulopathy is used to include all conditions with a predominantly glomerular component. Familial glomerulopathy has been described in over 24 dog breeds, and the genetics involved in dogs and cats has been extensively reviewed [30, 221, 223, 224]. Early onset renal origin proteinuria characterizes these diseases. Many of these diseases are discovered during the documentation of proteinuria and progressive CKD in related young patients, but in some the diagnosis is made in older animals. Genetic mutations can alter the molecular composition of the GBM and the podocyte slit pore membranes leading to proteinuria and progressive CKD, the severity of which will vary based on the specific genetic defect. Much remains to be discovered about the molecular and biochemical alterations within the glomerulus that result in proteinuria and progression of CKD and the specific associated genetic defects.

HEREDITARY NEPHROPATHY

HN occurs in a few dog breeds. HN is the term used to describe a rare form of progressive CKD due to a genetic defect in type 4 collagen of the GBM. Progressive renal proteinuria occurs as the first clinical abnormality during the development of HN. Multilaminar splitting and thickening of the GBM on EM and abnormal immunolabeling of alpha chains from type 4 collagen characterize HN. Mutations in gene translation result in abnormalities that prevent the assembly of the full complex of side chains that are needed for normal GBM structure and function [221, 225]. Samoyed [226] and mixed-breed dogs in Navasota, Texas [221, 227] have an X-linked form of HN, whereas English Cocker Spaniels [228] and English Springer Spaniels [229] have an autosomal recessive form of HN. Canine HN is a rare disease that should be considered whenever a dog exhibits a juvenile-onset kidney disease characterized partly by proteinuria [221].

Early reports of Cocker Spaniels with apparent familial nephropathy and proteinuria were described to have renal cortical atrophy. At that time, it was not determined if the cortical atrophy and reduced number of nephrons were from hypoplasia at birth or an acquired loss of renal tissue later [230–233]. It was later discovered that this syndrome was not from a congenital lack of renal cortical tissue, but that it was associated with a primary glomerular disease and progressive proteinuria [234, 235]. Primary renal glucosuria was also occasionally documented in this syndrome [232]. The incidence of HN in English Cockers has dramatically declined since the development of a genetic test that identifies carriers in this breed [221]. A specific polymerase chain reaction (PCR) test is available to identify English cocker spaniel carriers at www. pawprintgenetics.com [30].

There is an X-linked dominant HN in male Samoyed dogs characterized by renal proteinuria and renal failure. The characteristic ultrastructural lesion is multilaminar splitting of the lamina densa of the GBM [236, 237]. This disease is caused by a single gene mutation that leads to a severe reduction in alpha-5 chains of collagen type 4 in the GBM [226]. Defective cross linking of collagen type 4 appears to lead to weakening of the GBM [238]. A PCR test for this mutation is available and can be ordered at www.vetgen.

com; www.pawprintgenetics.com. The use of genetic testing results allows the removal of carrier dogs from a breeding program [30].

PODOCYTOPATHY

Detailed reviews of the structure and function of podocytes as well as their response to injury and development of proteinuria are available for the interested reader [23, 36]. Stretching of podocytes is now recognized as a central mechanism contributing to podocyte injury, proteinuria, and progressive CKD. Stretching and shear forces within the glomerulus contribute to foot process simplification, foot process effacement, detachment of podocytes, and loss of podocytes, all of which contribute to the development of proteinuria [23, 36].

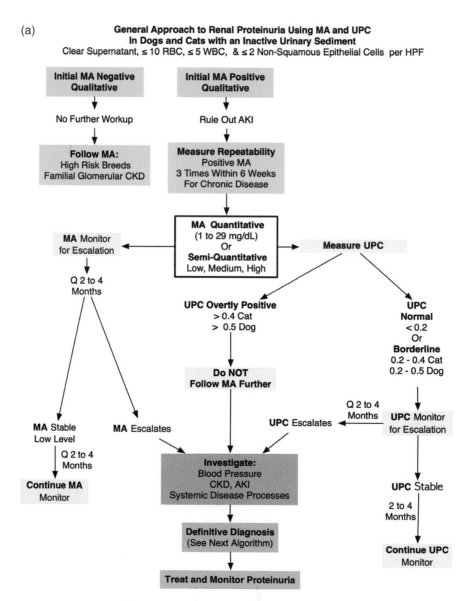

(a)

General Approach to Renal Proteinuria Using MA and UPC In Dogs and Cats with an Inactive Urinary Sediment
Clear Supernatant, ≤ 10 RBC, ≤ 5 WBC, & ≤ 2 Non-Squamous Epithelial Cells per HPF

FIGURE 7.9   (Continued)

(b) **Approach to Establish a Definitive Diagnosis and Monitoring of Renal Proteinuria**

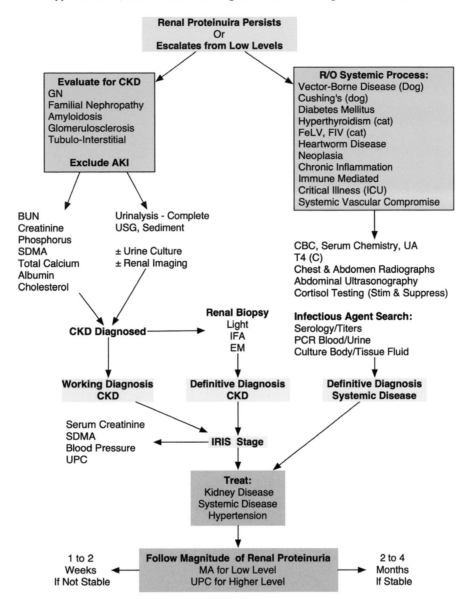

FIGURE 7.9 (a) Algorithm for a general approach to renal proteinuria. Qualitative MA has historically been measured by point-of-care devices (Heska® ERD) that are no longer in the veterinary market. The qualitative measurement of MA (negative or positive) for dogs and cats is under current exploration by some veterinary laboratories and may be feasible as a screening test on expanded urinary chemistry dipstrips. The accuracy of this measurement compared to benchtop quantitative measurement has not been established. Alternatively, this algorithm can be started when MA is determined quantitatively. Source: Lees et al. [14], IRIS [174], Whittemore et al. [13], Whittemore et al. [12], Harley and Langston [11]. Note: RBC – Red blood cells, WBC – white blood cells, HPF – high powered microscopic field, MA – microalbuminuria (dipstrip and bench methods), UPC – urinary protein to urinary creatinine ratio, CKD – chronic kidney disease, AKI – acute kidney injury. (b) Algorithm showing an approach to determine the diagnosis for renal proteinuria. * Renal biopsy is not advocated for all patients with CKD, especially if the kidneys are small and there is advanced disease. Renal biopsy is helpful to disclose immunological and nonimmunological causes for those with renal proteinuria before there is obvious azotemia and extensive renal fibrosis. Pathological findings from the combination of light microscopy using special stains, immunofluorescent microscopy, and electron microscopy are needed in order to properly assess underlying renal pathology causing renal proteinuria. Glomerular causes of renal proteinuria are most common. The prognosis for patients with renal proteinuria varies by the specific pathological diagnosis. Aggressive treatment protocols using immunosuppressive drugs are best directed in patients that have undergone renal biopsy providing evidence for an immune process (e.g. immune-complex deposition within the glomeruli). Source: Cianciolo et al. [27]; Segev et al. [212]; Brown et al. [136]; Schneider et al. [60]; Littman et al. [213]; Goldstein et al. [214]; Pressler et al. [215]; Cowgill and Polzin [216]; Cianciolo et al. [61]; Klosterman et al. [217]; Lees et al. [14]; Dambach et al. [218],. The International Veterinary Renal Pathology Service (IVRPS) processes renal tissues and examines them with the special techniques mentioned above, and then a group of veterinary nephropathologists consult to deliver a final diagnosis. Further information about how to handle and submit renal tissue and fees can be accessed on line form the IVRPS at https://vet.osu.edu/vmc/international-veterinary-renal-pathology-service-ivrps. Note: AKI – acute kidney injury, BUN – blood urea nitrogen, SDMA – symmetrical dimethyl arginine, USG – urine specific gravity, FeLV – feline leukemia virus, FIV – feline immunovirus, CKD – chronic kidney disease, IRIS – International Renal Interest Society, Light – light microscopy, IFA – Immunofluorescent antibody, EM – electron microscopy, MA – microalbuminuria, UPC – urinary protein to urinary creatinine ratio.

The earliest podocyte lesions include foot process simplification and effacement; later lesions are associated with death and loss of podocytes. Live and dead podocytes can be identified at times in the urine in these instances. Typical kidney biopsy lesions in humans include minimal change glomerular disease and focal segmental glomerulosclerosis (FSGS) [36].

Several types of mechanical shear forces are thought to contribute to podocyte injury and fragility. Initial hydrostatic forces during glomerular filtration create circumferential stress on podocyte foot processes, followed by shear stress on the lateral aspects of foot processes, and then lateral flow force across the podocyte cell body. Higher hydraulic pressures develop in single nephrons as part of the adaptive/maladaptive response to loss of nephron mass (intraglomerular hypertension and hyperfiltration) in those with progressive CKD, which increases shearing forces. Loss of podocytes reduces the density of the podocyte population within glomeruli which increases shearing forces transmitted to the remaining podocytes. Also, an increased amount of protein in Bowman's space in those with proteinuria increases the oncotic pressure and fluid drag that favors a higher single-nephron GFR, adding to the magnitude of glomerular hypertension and shearing force [36].

Loss or altered function of nephrin and podocin molecules within the slit pore membrane and loss of podocytes (podocytopenia) contribute to proteinuria in some glomerulopathies affecting humans [31, 36, 99, 101]. The slit pore membrane can also be damaged by immunological mechanisms in addition to that caused by genetic defects. Genetic podocytopathy has recently been identified in dogs.

Following podocyte loss and exposure of denuded GBM, surviving podocytes undergo hypertrophy in an attempt to cover the GBM. The development of hypertrophic podocytes, however, is considered a maladaptive response at times when foot process structure and function do not develop, allowing increased shearing forces to be transmitted. Parietal podocytes in Bowman's capsule can deliver some podocyte progenitors, potentially contributing to recovery of podocyte function within the glomerulus, but this process can be inefficient and maladaptive with scar formation [36].

An adult-onset PLN is estimated to involve 5–15% of SCWT dogs. More females are affected than males, but this is not sex-linked genetically [219, 239, 240]. The mode of inheritance is considered complex, as both recessive and dominant inheritance patterns can be observed and environmental triggers for gene expression may be important. PLN is the result of an inherited podocytopathy in some SCWT dogs that involves mutations of a single nucleotide in the genes NPHS1 and KIRREL2. These genes control the synthesis of nephrin and Nephr3/filtrin that are important proteins required for normal structure and function of the podocyte slit pore membrane. Dogs that are homozygous for both mutations are more seriously affected [239]. Alterations in these slit pore proteins reduce the integrity of the glomerular barrier with resulting proteinuria. FSGS along with podocyte degeneration and loss are the most consistent renal lesions on light microscopy due to

genetic podocytopathy and slit diaphragm protein defects. These defective podocytes are considered at increased risk for injury by other mechanisms (inflammation or circulating immune complexes) [30, 219]. PLN most often is diagnosed alone, but it can be preceded by protein-losing enteropathy (PLE), or diagnosed concurrently with PLE in this breed. SCWT with both PLE and PLN have a higher degree of proteinuria based on UPC compared to PLN alone, suggesting that proteinuria can be aggravated by other insults in carriers [30]. Some affected dogs with MA at low levels can be observed without progression to overt renal disease, whereas other dogs with higher levels of MA show more rapid progression of CKD [219]. Early studies of PLN in this breed reported dogs with advanced CKD, hypoalbuminemia, and a poor prognosis [240]. Very early reports of familial nephropathy in this breed did not have proteinuria, and it appears that the likely diagnosis was renal dysplasia [241]. Genetic testing for variant genes affecting podocytes can be ordered at http://www.scwtca.org/health/dnatest.htm [30]. Of 214 breeds screened, only Airedale Terriers were found to have the same genetic defect associated with podocytopathy and risk for the development of CKD as described for SCWT. There are many opportunities for genetically mediated podocytopathy to develop not involving the specific genes shown to affect SCWT and Airedale Terriers [30, 224, 242].

FSGS was described at necropsy in eight related Miniature Schnauzers with persistent renal proteinuria (UPC 1.2–6.5) and minimal to absent azotemia. Proteinuria was usually adult onset and hypoalbuminemia rare. The progression of CKD was slow and systemic hypertension mild to moderate. These dogs were part of a long-term study investigating renal disease in this breed. Glomerular synechia and hyalinosis were commonly identified by light microscopy. Extensive effacement of podocyte foot processes was characteristic. There was no splitting of the GBM or identification of electron dense deposits in the GBM. Glomeruli contained varying amounts of lipid in sclerotic areas and unusual electron dense aggregates were prominent within podocytes. A genetic podocytopathy with resulting podocytopenia was suggested to cause FSGS in these dogs. An underlying podocytopathy could render the glomeruli "fragile" and predispose to further renal injury from hyperlipidemia, glomerular hypertension, or other unidentified stressors. Renal-related death did not occur in this population [243]. Schnauzers with proteinuria accounted for 3% of all renal biopsies that were submitted from dogs with proteinuria for comprehensive evaluation in another study; FSGS was the diagnosis in 78% of these biopsies [60].

FSGS has been reported in 20.6–33% of dogs undergoing comprehensive renal biopsy for renal proteinuria, second in frequency to immune-complex-mediated glomerulopathy [60, 74]. A similar incidence for the diagnosis of FSGS was reported in 26% (77 of 299) of dogs in another study detailing clinical pathology and prognosis. Significantly more females were affected than male dogs. Systemic hypertension was common, but azotemia and severe hypoalbuminemia were uncommon.

The median UPC of 5.9 (1.4–22) was not associated with survival, but the degree of renal proteinuria and systemic hypertension control during treatment could not be determined in this study. Decreased survival was related to serum creatinine >2.1 mg/dL and serum albumin <2.0 g/dL. The magnitude of proteinuria based on UPC did not differentiate immune-complex from nonimmune-complex glomerular disease [244].

IMMUNE COMPLEXES, GLOMERULAR DISEASE, AND RENAL PROTEINURIA

Mechanisms of renal damage leading to glomerular proteinuria include deposition of immune complexes, complement activation, cytokine activation, and precipitation of complexes within glomeruli [245]. When complement activation is unrestricted, it overcomes the protection of complement regulators, leading to cellular injury [246]. Immune-complex deposition from the circulation is likely the most common process within the glomerulus.

It appears that a delicate balance between antigen and antibody concentrations is required in order to form the antigen–antibody complexes likely to be deposited in the glomerulus. A mild excess of circulating antigens favors the formation of antigen–antibody complexes [247]. Rarely, autoantibodies can react with normal antigens within the glomerulus, which appear as a smooth linear pattern on immunofluorescent microscopy. Alternatively, antibodies from the circulation can combine with antigens previously planted within the basement membrane (Figures 7.10a, b), resulting in "lumpy-bumpy" immune complexes on immunofluorescent microscopy in both examples. Rarely, autoantibodies can react with normal antigens within the glomerulus, which appear as a smooth linear pattern on immunofluorescent microscopy. Cytokines and oxygen radicals are generated along with an influx of inflammatory cells in reaction to these immune complexes. Proteinuria results as these processes disturb the delicate relationship between the various components of the glomerulus that are needed to maintain glomerular barrier integrity [99].

The size and solubility of circulating immune complexes impact where they can be deposited within the glomerulus. Small soluble complexes tend to be deposited just below the visceral epithelium (subepithelial) within the GBM though they can be deposited deeper within the GBM also (intramembranous). Intermediate size complexes are more likely to be deposited within the mesangium, whereas large immune complexes never make it to the kidney since they are removed by phagocytosis [248, 249].

Definitive diagnosis for ICGN requires the evaluation of microscopy by transmission EM and immunofluorescence (Figure 7.11) [27, 60]. Even when it is known that ICGN is the underlying renal lesion, antigens within the immune complex are rarely identified [213, 250].

Idiopathic membranous nephropathy was reported in 11 cats and 5 dogs that underwent the extensive evaluation

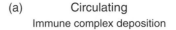

(a) Circulating
Immune complex deposition

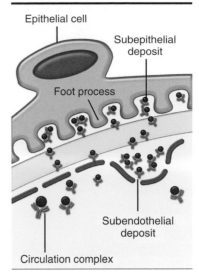

(b) **In Situ**
Anti-GBM

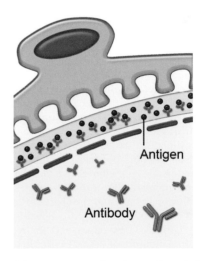

FIGURE 7.10 (a) Immune-complex glomerulonephritis. Circulating immune complexes become trapped as subendothelial deposits, within the basement membrane, or subepithelial deposits. The location of the deposits depends on the size of the complex and the nature of the antigen. Chronic mild antigenic excess is considered necessary in order to stimulate the right ratio of antibody to antigen for this to occur (infectious agents, neoplasia). The location of the complex within the glomerulus can determine how inflammatory a reaction will develop. Source: Illustration by Tim Vojt, reproduced with permission of The Ohio State University. (b) In this scheme, antigens were planted within the basement membrane from the circulation first and then circulating antibodies bound to the antigen in situ. Alternatively, the antigen within the basement membrane is normally there and antibodies develop to this antigen as part of an autoimmune disease, though this is rare in dogs and cats. Source: Illustration by Tim Vojt, reproduced with permission of The Ohio State University.

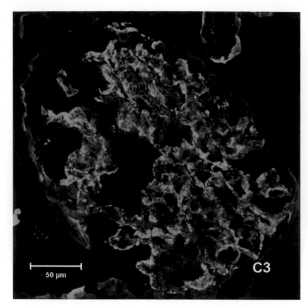

FIGURE 7.11 Immune-complex glomerulonephritis (ICGN). IFA renal biopsy 40× –pathology consensus report from the International Veterinary Renal Pathology Service (IVRPS). Global diffuse granular mesangial staining against C3 (lumpy bumpy, granular discontinuous pattern). Not shown: Equivocal fine granular staining for IgG. Diffuse global mesangial staining for IgM. Negative staining for IgA. Based on the finding of IFA positive results and electron dense deposits on TEM (not shown), the diagnosis of immune-complex glomerulonephritis was concluded. The nature of the antigen is not known, but there were some features on EM (not shown) that suggested a condition similar to lupus nephropathy in humans. An ANA titer or LE prep were never analyzed. Over the next 15 months, the dog was treated with enalapril and spironolactone for proteinuria control, amlodipine to achieve normal blood pressure, and anti-platelet treatment with Plavix® to help prevent thromboembolism. She initially received immunosuppressive therapy with prednisone tapered over two months, and then was maintained on chlorambucil. Over that last year, she gained 3–5 kg from her lowest weight and the degree of her azotemia declined (serum creatinine of 1.9 mg/dL). She is still proteinuric but to a lower magnitude (UPC of 3.6) and her hypoalbuminemia abated (serum albumin of 3.3 g/dL). Her hypertension is well controlled (systolic blood pressure of 140 mmHg), which helps to lessen proteinuria in addition to the immunosuppressive treatments.

of renal tissue by light microscopy, immunofluorescence, transmission EM, and scanning EM. Most of these animals were presented in the NS, and some had azotemic CKD. Proteinuria was heavy with most animals having >1000 mg/dL. Immunofluorescence for IgG and C3 as well as electron dense glomerular deposits was demonstrated in all the renal tissues studied, but the antigen(s) were not identified [251].

An underlying genetic podocytopathy, disorder of GBM, or immunodysregulatory defect may trigger abnormal immune-complex handling within the kidneys [30]. This could predispose animals to infection-associated GN, as immune complexes could more readily accumulate at these abnormal sites in the glomerulus. Animals with an underlying genetic podocytopathy conceivably could have a very sensitive or fragile podocyte population that when exposed to an accumulation of immune complexes would result in greater proteinuria and progression of CKD. It has been speculated that the alteration of the molecular structure or the quantity of proteins within the slit pore diaphragm could cause abnormal folding of that protein, leading to subtle or overt proteinuria depending on the magnitude of the defect (Littman, personal communication 2019; Cianciello, personal communication 2019).

ACUTE KIDNEY INJURY

AKI can result in a varying magnitude and type of renal proteinuria, though CKD and chronic glomerular injury most commonly cause renal proteinuria. Tubular origin proteinuria can develop during AKI secondary to nephrotoxins, renal ischemia, or leptospirosis. The magnitude of this proteinuria is usually considered as mild to moderate (0.5–2.0 on UPC) and occurs secondary to proximal tubular injury.

UPC > 0.5 occurred in 77% of dogs with AKI in one series with a variety of underlying causes and 58% had a UPC > 2.0. The median UPC in these dogs was 1.68 (0.1–18). Fluid overload and systemic hypertension were common in this population [252] and likely accounted for some of the renal proteinuria. Predominantly glomerular involvement in AKI is not common, so a very high degree of albuminuria is not expected to increase the UPC in typical AKI in which tubular damage is expected to predominate. AKI can decrease the proximal tubular reabsorption of the small quantities of albumin as well as LMW proteins in tubular fluid. Tubular proteinuria is expected to increase during nephrotoxic, ischemic, and some infectious causes of AKI that could account for an increased UPC in some instances, in addition to glomerular injury.

In a study of dogs with different causes of AKI, the median UPC in survivors was 1.4 (0.1–14.7) and 2.7 (0.2–72) in nonsurvivors was significantly different. The median UPC was 1.62 (0.09–72.00) for all dogs with AKI, 2.21 (0.09–72.00) for those with intrinsic AKI, 1.00 (0.10–10.15) in those with volume response AKI, and 0.07 (0.04–0.28) in controls. Further characterization for the nature of the proteinuria was not reported [253].

The median UPC was 2.14 (0.40–184) in dogs with AKI due to leptospirosis compared to 2.38 (0.09–72) in those with other causes of AKI and 0–0.5 in controls. The nature of the proteinuria was not characterized further [254]. The median UPC in 64 dogs with leptospirosis was 2.1 (0.24–18.4) in survivors and 2.5 (0.45–11.3) in nonsurvivors of another study. UPC was increased in 78% of dogs, but the nature of the proteins as glomerular or tubular was not studied further [255].

High-level proteinuria based on UPC is occasionally found in dogs with azotemic leptospirosis, but prominent glomerular involvement is usually lacking as this is predominantly a tubulointerstitial disease. The UPC was a mean of 2.59 ± 2.79 (0.2–9.3) in 6 of the 10 dogs with leptospirosis in which it was measured in one study; most of the dogs were azotemic. The increased excretion of LMW proteins (<69 kD) in all 10 dogs with leptospirosis likely accounted for the increased UPC, as LMW proteins comprised 72.1% of the total urinary proteins measured. A unique band of HMW protein (80–90 kD) was seen in 6 of 10 dogs with leptospirosis, and HMW immunoglobulins were identified in 3 of 10 of these dogs, indicating glomerular origin to urinary proteins in some instances. Albuminuria was not specifically measured [256].

Acute glomerular injury is less commonly the cause of AKI and renal proteinuria in dogs or cats compared to acute tubulointerstitial disease. Rapidly progressive glomerulonephritis (RPGN) often associated with Borrelia positive serology, cutaneous and renal glomerular vasculopathy (CRGV) and hemolytic uremic syndrome (HUS) are associated with predominantly glomerular lesions, renal proteinuria, and AKI in dogs that are discussed in detail below. Based on the nature of these glomerular lesions, glomerular origin proteinuria is expected, but acute tubular necrosis (ATN) is sometimes a component of these diseases, so tubular proteinuria may also be documented.

Active acute GN is rarely recognized in veterinary medicine, but a syndrome of RPGN (or ICGN) has been described. *Borrelia* infection associated with chronic glomerular disease and proteinuria was initially reported in one dog [257]. RPGN has been reported mostly in young dogs in Lyme endemic areas. Less than 2% of Lyme seropositive dogs develop this aggressive form of Lyme nephritis, and 9–28% of affected dogs have a history of concurrent or prior lameness [258]. Nearly all dogs with RPGN are *Borrelia* seropositive, but coinfections with other tick-borne organisms may also be encountered with *Ehrlichia, Anaplasma, Babesia, Bartonella*, other *Borrelia* spp., Rocky Mountain spotted fever, heartworm (HW), or leptospirosis [259]. Membranoproliferative GN was the most commonly documented renal lesion (88%) followed by membranous GN (10%) of affected dogs. Subendothelial deposits of IgG, IgM, and C3 were frequently observed within the glomerulus [218]. The antigen in the immune complexes has not yet been identified, and the relationship of *Borrelia* seropositivity and the development of RPGN is not clear [259].

The combination of GN with tubular necrosis and regeneration along with interstitial inflammation are distinctive and unique lesions of RPGN. Silver staining of renal tissue may identify the presence of small numbers of spirochetes, but this finding is uncommon. The direct invasion of *Borrelia* into renal tissue does not appear to be a primary driver for the development of RPGN. The necrosis of glomerular tufts, glomerular crescents, periglomerular fibrosis, and fibrinoid necrosis of small-to-medium-sized renal vessels are observed in some cases [218, 258, 260].

Severe proteinuria in dogs with RPGN is often associated with the development of progressive renal failure and hypoalbuminemia, peripheral edema, and body cavity effusions that are fatal; oligoanuria develops in some cases. Evidence for hypercoagulability and thromboembolic disease may be documented in some affected dogs as consequences of the proteinuria and hypoalbuminemia. Hematuria, glucosuria, and cylindruria (granular and hyaline) are also seen in some dogs [218, 258, 260, 261]. Early renal biopsy is advocated in dogs with severe proteinuria, declining serum albumin, and progressive azotemia in order to evaluate for the presence of immune complexes (documentation of electron-dense deposits on transmission EM and/or positive immunofluorescent glomerular staining) that factor into a decision whether to treat with immunosuppressive agents [212, 258].

Labrador Retrievers, Golden Retrievers, and possibly Shetland Sheepdogs are over-represented in this form of RPGN [30]. A podocytopathy has been suspected, but not yet confirmed for Golden Retrievers and Labrador Retrievers with "Lyme" nephritis (RPGN) associated with a high C6 Borrelia titer and high-level renal proteinuria. These two breeds may have more severe disease from an underlying podocytopathy when infected with Borrelia or other infectious agents compared with other breeds. It should be noted that ICGN has been frequently documented in Goldens and Labradors with proteinuria from the International Veterinary Renal Pathology Service (IVRPS) database without a specific diagnosis of Lyme disease (Ciancello, personal communication, 2019). Other breeds with documented ICGN related to infectious diseases or drug sensitivities include American Foxhounds, Basenjis, Doberman Pinschers, German Shepherd Dogs, and SCWT [262]. A complement C3 deficiency may cause a secondary GN in the Brittany [262].

CRGV was originally described in the USA as a disease of unknown etiology involving the skin and kidneys of affected kenneled and racing Greyhounds, a syndrome initially called Alabama Rot [263]. This syndrome has recently been extensively reviewed [264]. Acute disease of small blood vessels in the skin and kidneys of dogs appears to uniquely define CRGV [265]. Ulcerated skin lesions without systemic signs occurred with most frequency in an early report. Skin lesions in association with azotemic CKD occurred in 44 of 168 dogs in one study. Glomerular necrosis and coagulation within the glomerular capillaries were distinctive lesions in eight dogs that underwent necropsy. The afferent glomerular arteriole was more affected than the efferent arteriole. Hyaline, granular, and RBC casts were observed within some renal tubular lumens. Some of the RBC casts contained fragmented RBC. Thrombocytopenia and anemia were described in some dogs [263]. At the time of CRGV diagnosis in another series of 18 racing Greyhounds, 10 were azotemic, 16 were anemic, 11 were hypoalbuminemic, and all had thrombocytopenia. None of the azotemic dogs in this series survived (8 of 10 were anuric or oliguric); seven of the eight nonazotemic dogs survived. UPC was ≥1.0 in two of six nonazotemic dogs and five of five azotemic dogs (1.19–7.0) [266]. Median UPC was 0.85 (0.56–1.14) and 3.42 (1.81–7.64) in nonazotemic and azotemic dogs, respectively, in another study [267]. Over 95% of the azotemic AKI dogs had occult blood (hemoglobin or myoglobin) on their urine chemistry dipstrip, and about 1/3 had glucosuria and some had hyaline or granular cylindruria [267].

Changes in glomerular endothelial cells were prominent during EM of 12 Greyhounds with CRGV that had some combination of characteristic ulcerated skin lesions, azotemia, and thrombocytopenia [268].

Many different breeds of dogs in the UK were found to be affected with CRGV, in contrast to only greyhounds in the USA [265, 269]. Working dogs (hounds and gun dogs) were at increased risk compared to terriers; no toy breeds were reported. Females and neutered dogs were at increased risk, and seasonal outbreaks of this disease were characteristic [269]. Most dogs of one report were initially evaluated for a skin lesion(s) followed by signs of systemic illness. Nearly all dogs (26 of 30) were azotemic at the time of diagnosis and the remaining four developed azotemia shortly thereafter. In 17 dogs with a UA, the mean USG was 1.020, occult blood positive in 16, protein positive on dipstrip in 11, and glucose positive in 6. It was not determined if the occult blood reactions were from hemoglobin in RBC or from myoglobin. The median UPC was 5.6 with a range of 1.35–16.6 in 11 dogs in which it was measured. Moderate-to-severe thrombocytopenia was common. Thrombotic microangiopathy (TMA) was the characteristic glomerular lesion along with fibrinoid necrosis of glomerular arterioles. Endothelial cell hypertrophy and swelling were common (17 of 30). Tubular lumens were frequently filled with protein casts and sometimes with RBC casts. Glomeruli were distended with RBC, some of which were fragmented. Lesions of ATN were identified in 29 of 30 dogs, presumably secondary to renal ischemia from glomerular thrombosis. Twenty-four dogs either died or were euthanized due to the extent of their disease; an additional six were euthanized due to owner concerns about prognosis or financial constraints. Oligoanuria and progressive azotemia were the most common reasons for death or euthanasia in this study [265]. In azotemic CRGV dogs of another study in which urine output was measured, oliguria occurred in 30/61 and anuria in 13/61 [264].

HUS has been described in a small number of dogs with azotemic AKI that is often preceded by hemorrhagic diarrhea. HUS is defined by the combination of azotemic AKI, thrombocytopenia, and microangiopathic hemolytic anemia. Abnormal RBC morphology from shearing has been described, as well as hemoglobinemia and hemoglobinuria [270–272]. Renal proteinuria in HUS is expected as described above for CRGV due to the severity of glomerular lesions. In one dog with a silent urinary sediment, the occult blood reaction was 4+ and protein 3+ on dipstrip chemistry in association with a USG of 1.027. The occult blood reaction is presumed to be from hemoglobinuria. The proteinuria reaction could result from a combination of renal proteinuria and prerenal protein measured in the filtered hemoglobin [271]. In another case with a USG of 1.018, the dipstick chemistry was positive for occult blood and protein, but it was not characterized further. It has not been determined if HUS and CRGV are variants of a disease with the same cause or not. HUS in dogs has not been described in association with skin lesions, whereas characteristic skin lesions are commonly encountered in dogs with CRGV [264, 265].

TMA is a characteristic lesion common to both CRGV and HUS. Definitive diagnosis requires identification of TMA on renal histopathology. TMA is characterized by vascular inflammation and microthrombi of small vessels that result in ischemia, necrosis, and infarction [270–272]. Consumptive thrombocytopenia, hemolytic anemia with red cell shearing, and multiple organ disruption can also be part of this pathology [264, 265, 273–275]. TMA is an uncommon renal lesion as it was encountered in <1% of renal biopsies evaluated by the IVRPS.

OTHER FAMILIAL GLOMERULOPATHIES

Collagen type 3 glomerulopathy (collagenofibrotic glomerulopathy) was described in a mixed-breed family of dogs. This glomerular disease was characterized by a massive accumulation of collagen type 3 in the glomeruli. This disease appears to be inherited in a simple autosomal recessive pattern, but the specific gene defect was not identified [276]. Progressive high-magnitude proteinuria, systemic hypertension, azotemia, and NS developed in four of seven puppies following cross-mating of parents that had previously produced affected puppies [277]. Four of nine Drever puppies developed this glomerulopathy at a young age as confirmed by EM and immunohistochemistry. Collagen type 3 predominated, but there was also the presence of collagen type 5 and rare collagen type 1 [278]. A similar disease was described in three of eight Newfoundland dog littermates with severe proteinuria, hypoalbuminemia, and progressive azotemic CKD. Mesangial glomerulosclerosis and glomerular fibrosis were prominent histopathological findings on light and EM. Collagen fibrils within the GBM, within the mesangium, and below the visceral epithelium were described. Lesions of glomerulosclerosis were far more severe than in other familial nephropathies in dogs. It was proposed that a metabolic defect of endothelial or mesangial cells could result in collagen formation. Immunochemistry to confirm the presence of collagen type 3 was not performed [279].

An autosomal dominant glomerular disease associated with proteinuria and a variable rate for progression of CKD has been described in Bull Terriers [280, 281] and Dalmatians [282]. Males and females were equally affected in both breeds, and the GBM was thickened, lamellated, vacuolated, and displayed some subepithelial frilling on ultrastructure. Similar changes on EM are described as in those with HN, but with normal immunostaining of collagen type 4 side chains. The gene mutation leading to abnormal synthesis of GBM proteins or collagen has not been identified [281, 282].

Familial renal disease has been described in Doberman Pinschers [283–285], Beagles [286], and Rottweilers [287] in association with renal proteinuria, progressive CKD, and electron micrographic changes within the GBM similar to that observed in HN, but the genetics and type 4 collagen composition have not been evaluated [221]. There is currently no genetic test available to screen for HN in these breeds [30].

In Doberman Pinschers, mesangioproliferative GN [285] or glomerulosclerosis [284] was described as the underlying light microscopic glomerular lesions associated with familial nephropathy, but the method of inheritance was not determined. In another study, the EM of renal tissue from eight Dobermans affected with juvenile renal disease and membranoproliferative GN by light microscopy was evaluated. The lamellation of GBM was identified as one distinct lesion (five of eight dogs). The accumulation of cross-banded fibers likely to be non-type-4 collagen within the GBM was identified (three of eight dogs) as a second distinct ultrastructural lesion in this study, but the nature of the collagen was not further characterized. These lesions suggested that the glomerulus was damaged as a result of a metabolic defect in collagen synthesis or metabolism [283]. Ultrastructural lesions of what appears to be primary glomerular fibrosis in these Dobermans are similar to those reported in Newfoundland [279] and in dogs with collagen type 3 glomerulopathy [277].

A progressive familial nephropathy characterized by glomerular proteinuria and azotemia has been described in French (Bordeaux) Mastiffs. It appeared likely that this was an autosomal recessive genetic disorder. EM did not reveal splitting or lamellation of GBM as described for HN but did show nonspecific changes featuring podocyte foot process fusion; no immune complexes were identified. Light microscopy revealed changes compatible with membranoproliferative GN [288, 289]. Bull Mastiffs appear to have an autosomal recessive familial nephropathy with light microscopic changes similar to that seen in French Mastiffs [288]. This disorder is characterized by proteinuria associated with glomerular lesions, but further evaluation with EM was not performed [290]. Familial nephropathy was described in three of nine Bedlington Terrier puppies from the same litter with advanced CKD, but the protein content of urine was not reported [291].

Membranoproliferative GN associated with glomerular proteinuria and progressive renal disease has been described in Bernese Mountain dogs as an autosomal recessive disorder [292, 293]. Immune complexes associated with IgM and complement were frequently identified, but an antigen was not identified. EM showed subepithelial electron dense deposits and duplication of GBM [293], but not splitting of GBM as seen in HN.

A progressive familial CKD in association with isosthenuria and proteinuria affecting young Golden Retrievers has been reported as juvenile renal disease [294] or renal dysplasia [295]. Cystic glomerular atrophy and periglomerular fibrosis were extensive and fetal glomeruli were observed in some of these dogs. The mode of inheritance was not established nor was an ultrastructural study performed.

Familial renal disease was suspected in Norwegian Elkhound dogs of both sexes based on analysis of pedigree in an early report, but the mode of inheritance was not established. Isosthenuria or hyposthenuria was present in all nine dogs. Moderate proteinuria by dipstrip (2+ or 3+) was seen in three dogs, trace in two dogs, and zero in three dogs. Glucosuria was noted for some dogs and aminoaciduria in one dog. Histopathology showed advanced changes of fibrosis and cystic glomerular atrophy along with thickening of Bowman's capsule, and some glomerular adhesions to Bowman's capsule. Fibrosis was accompanied by minimal lymphoplasmacytic inflammation [233]. Over one-third of dogs from a specific line of inbred Norwegian Elkhounds were diagnosed with renal disease between 4 and 48 months of age in another study, but proteinuria was not detailed; aminoaciduria was detected in a few dogs [296]. Renal biopsy at 3–14 months of age from this same line showed periglomerular fibrosis as the earliest renal lesion, a finding that developed prior to the onset of azotemia and urinary concentrating defects. Nephron number and size were normal during early study of these Norwegian Elkhounds, which does not support a diagnosis of renal cortical hypoplasia [222]. Abnormality in genes coding for collagen type IV side chains (alpha 3 and alpha 4) were not found in one study [297].

RENAL DYSPLASIA

Renal dysplasia results from disorganized development and defective differentiation of renal tissues. Histopathology reveals various combinations of asynchronous differentiation of nephrons, persistent mesenchyme, persistent metanephric ducts, atypical tubular epithelium, and dysontogenic metaplasia. Lhasa Apsos and Shih Tzus were overrepresented in one large series of dogs. Many abnormalities of glomerular structure exist in those with renal dysplasia [298] so the finding of renal proteinuria is expected. Proteinuria, isosthenuria, and progressive CKD were described in Shih Tzu dogs with renal dysplasia due to a suspected simple recessive mode of inheritance in one study. The presence of fetal glomeruli was the most consistent finding; no ultrastructural evaluation was performed [299]. In an earlier study of young Lhasa Apso and Shih Tzu dogs with progressive CKD, proteinuria was not a consistent feature. No cause or specific renal lesion was identified though the presence of fetal glomeruli was common. The evaluation of renal tissue was limited to light microscopy. The mode of possible inheritance was not determined in this study, but a pilot study indicated that it was not a simple autosomal recessive disorder. Variable proteinuria was reported in this small number of dogs [300].

A familial renal disease was suspected in two litters of related Standard Poodles. Isosthenuria and proteinuria were detected when urinalysis findings were available from a small number of dogs. Immature glomeruli and collapse of capillary lumens were seen on light microscopy suggestive for renal dysplasia. Ultrastructural evaluation was not performed, and the mode of possible inheritance was not further investigated [301]. Isolated cases of renal cortical hypoplasia were described in a single Malamute puppy (protein not reported on urinalysis) [302] and in a litter of Keeshonds with proteinuria and advanced CKD [303].

There are many other sporadic case reports of CKD in young dogs associated with proteinuria, but most of these have not been well characterized as to a likely genetic origin or specific lesion leading to proteinuria. Not all breeds with a familial predisposition for renal proteinuria will have proteinuria attributed to a genetic defect. Consequently, it is important to also evaluate these patients for the possibility of ICGN and glomerular amyloidosis (Rachael Cianciolo, personal communication, 2019).

RENAL AMYLOIDOSIS

Renal amyloidosis results in variable amounts of amyloid fibril deposition in the glomerulus and interstitium (Figures 7.12 and 7.13) and can be either genetic or acquired. Amyloidosis is a less common cause for PLN in dogs than GN, affecting 7–23% of dogs with biopsy proven glomerular lesions [60, 74, 304]. Most dogs and cats have a reactive form of renal amyloidosis, which develops secondary to chronic inflammation or neoplasia and

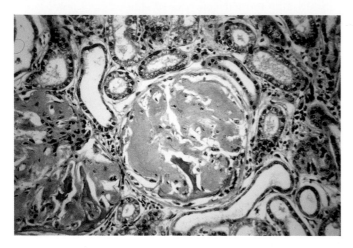

FIGURE 7.12 Extensive glomerular amyloid in a dog with PLN and azotemia; H&E. Note the homogeneous eosinophilic (pink) extracellular amyloid material and hypocellularity of the glomerulus in the center of this field. Source: Courtesy of Dr. Steven DiBartola, The Ohio State University CVM.

stimulation of acute phase proteins [305–311]. Animals with substantial glomerular deposits of amyloid will have moderate-to-severe proteinuria, whereas those with mostly interstitial deposits have minimal to no proteinuria. In one series of dogs with histopathologic evidence for glomerular disease, the magnitude of increased UPC, severity of hypoalbuminemia, and frequency of azotemia were greater in those with amyloidosis compared to those with GN [304]. In another study, mean urinary protein excretion was highest for dogs with renal amyloidosis, but there was overlap in the ranges between these values in dogs with GN and those with glomerular atrophy making a definitive diagnosis impossible based on the magnitude of proteinuria alone; renal biopsy was required to make these distinctions [205]. Acute renal failure sporadically happens in dogs and cats with renal amyloidosis due to papillary necrosis [312, 313], presumably due to medullary deposits contributing to medullary hypoxia.

Beagles, Collies, and Walker Hounds were found to be at increased risk for development of renal proteinuria due to amyloidosis [305]. A hereditary predisposition for reactive renal amyloidosis diagnosed during middle age was suspected in related beagles [314] and in related English foxhounds [312]. Beagles and English foxhounds had both glomerular and interstitial amyloid fibril deposits, in addition to proteinuria and CKD. The mode of inheritance was not determined. Familial secondary renal amyloidosis has been described in related Chinese Shar-Pei dogs; mean age at diagnosis was 4.1 years. All of the dogs in one study had medullary amyloid deposits, whereas 64% had glomerular involvement. Moderate-to-severe proteinuria was apparent in most of these dogs; two dogs with only medullary amyloid had zero to trace proteinuria. The histopathology in Chinese Shar-Peis was similar to that described for Abyssinian cats (Figure 7.14) [315]. Between 25% and 50% of Shar-Pei littermates are expected to develop renal amyloidosis if one parent had renal amyloidosis or a history of recurrent

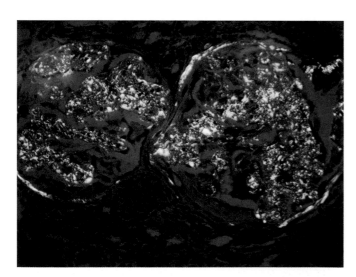

FIGURE 7.13 Glomerular amyloidosis. Note the green birefringence within the glomeruli as viewed under polarized light, after Congo red staining. Source: Courtesy of Dr. Stephen DiBartola, The Ohio State University CVM.

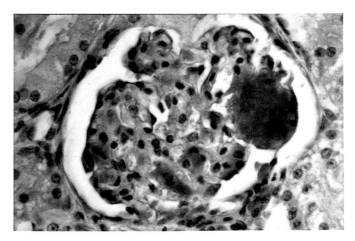

FIGURE 7.14 Amyloid material in glomerulus from an Abyssinian cat with CKD and proteinuria; Congo Red. Congo Red positive uptake supports the diagnosis of glomerular amyloid. Source: Courtesy of Dr. Stephen DiBartola, The Ohio State University CVM.

fever of unknown origin (Shar-Pei fever). It appears that this disorder is autosomal recessive and affects Shar-Pei dogs at an earlier age than non-Chinese Shar-Pei dogs [316].

Renal proteinuria was described in eight related young-to-middle-aged Bracchi Italiani dogs (median, five years; 2–10 range) diagnosed with familial nephropathy. All of the dogs were proteinuric and four were azotemic at the time of diagnosis. The median serum creatinine was 4.1 mg/dL (range, 0.8–7.8 mg/dL). Serum albumin was below the reference interval in all dogs but did not correlate with the magnitude of the proteinuria; serum cholesterol was increased in one of eight dogs. Clinical signs were variable and nonspecific, with inappetence being the most common in three of eight dogs. The median UPC was 8.3 (range, 1.3–30) in five dogs in which it was measured; dipstrip protein was positive at 2+ to 3+ in the remaining three dogs. The underlying glomerular lesion was glomerular amyloidosis in six dogs, nephrosclerosis in one, and nonamyloidotic fibrillar glomerulopathy in one dog. The prognosis was poor once clinical signs were manifested [317].

Related Abyssinian cats have been described with secondary renal amyloidosis and renal papillary necrosis [308, 313, 318]. Medullary and glomerular amyloid deposits occur together, but medullary deposits can predominate. Some combination of renal proteinuria, minimally concentrated urine, and azotemia leads to the diagnosis.

CONSEQUENCES AND PROGRESSION OF GLOMERULAR PROTEINURIA

It appears that longstanding proteinuria of glomerular origin can lead to further glomerular injury, tubular damage, tubulointerstitial inflammation, and progressive nephron loss (Figure 7.15) [93, 103, 104, 167, 199, 207, 325–328]. Despite a reduced global GFR (mL/min) in CKD, glomerular permeability increases to macromolecules, especially albumin during the early stages of disease. Single-nephron glomerular capillary hypertension develops as an adaptation to substantial nephron loss in CKD regardless of cause. This then favors increased filtration of plasma proteins across the glomerulus following increases in single-nephron GFR and transglomerular pressure [23, 329, 330]. Studies in dog and cat models of subtotal nephrectomy CKD support this scheme [105, 106]. It appears that further renal injury is greatest when systolic blood pressure (BP) is >160 mmHg in the dog and cat [331], but renal injury with systolic BP <160 mmHg is still possible in CKD when systemic pressure is transmitted to the glomeruli from failed vasoconstriction of the afferent arteriole [105, 106, 332].

Glomerular hypertension and subsequent mechanical stretching can directly damage the glomerulus [102]. An increased filtration of plasma proteins across the glomerulus results in passage of proteins into the mesangial space, into tubular fluid, and accumulates within podocytes with damaging consequences. There is close interaction between endothelial cells, mesangial cells, and podocytes such that injury in one cell population has the potential to adversely affect the other two.

Increased protein trafficking across the glomerulus results in a local accumulation of plasma protein within the mesangial space that promotes mesangial cell proliferation and deposition of extracellular matrix. The obliteration of glomerular tufts and further reduction in GFR characterize the glomerulosclerosis that develops. The altered mesangial space allows immune-complex accumulation and subsequent generation of inflammatory mediators, further contributing to glomerular injury [102]. The intrarenal effects of systemic or locally generated angiotensin II also contribute to further podocyte injury and albuminuria, promoting progression to end-stage kidney disease.

Dysfunction and loss of podocytes importantly contribute to the progression of glomerulopathy in human medicine. Podocytes are not replaced as they are lost, as podocytes have limited ability to replicate [333]. The excess trafficking of plasma proteins across the glomerulus can directly damage podocytes (visceral epithelium). This loss of podocytes lessens coverage of the GBM, which further increases glomerular permeability to plasma proteins and development of a higher level of proteinuria. Podocyte damage leads to cellular and intercellular junction alterations that include actin filament disorganization and distortion of podocyte shape, which affect cell adhesion to the extracellular matrix. Podocyte detachment decreases the number of functional podocytes resulting in the apoptosis of podocytes. Increased glomerular capillary hydraulic pressure that is part of the adaptive response to nephron loss can also lead to podocyte damage that includes vacuolization, fusion of podocyte foot processes, and detachment of epithelial cells from the basement membrane [23, 31, 35, 38, 99, 101, 102, 201, 319–322].

Renal proteinuria is associated with increased circulating phosphate and FGF23 in studies of humans, rats, and mice. Increases in plasma phosphate were a consequence of increased tubular fluid phosphate reabsorption following greater expression of the Na-Pi-IIa transporters in the proximal tubule. Albuminuria was an independent risk factor for higher levels of circulating phosphate in this study, but albumin did not directly cause proximal tubular cells to increase phosphate reabsorption. Albuminuria was associated with higher FGF23 and PTH concentrations and less renal Klotho expression. The expected effect from increased FGF23 is to decrease the expression of Na-Pi cotransporters and lower circulating phosphorus. This effect was not seen, likely due to a decreased expression of renal Klotho as a needed cofactor for full biological activity of FGF23, leading to FGF23 resistance [323, 324]. In another study, proteinuria (albuminuria) caused early downregulation of Klotho expression and increased circulating phosphorus in rodent models of CKD. Klotho is an obligate coreceptor for FGF23 that promotes phosphaturic effects as proximal tubules reabsorb less phosphorus from tubular fluid. Decreased expression of renal Klotho during CKD dampens the phosphaturic effect of FGF23, resulting in increased circulating levels of phosphorus, which then contribute further to the progression of CKD. FGF23 also further increases in the face of Klotho deficiency, which is then considered maladaptive [334].

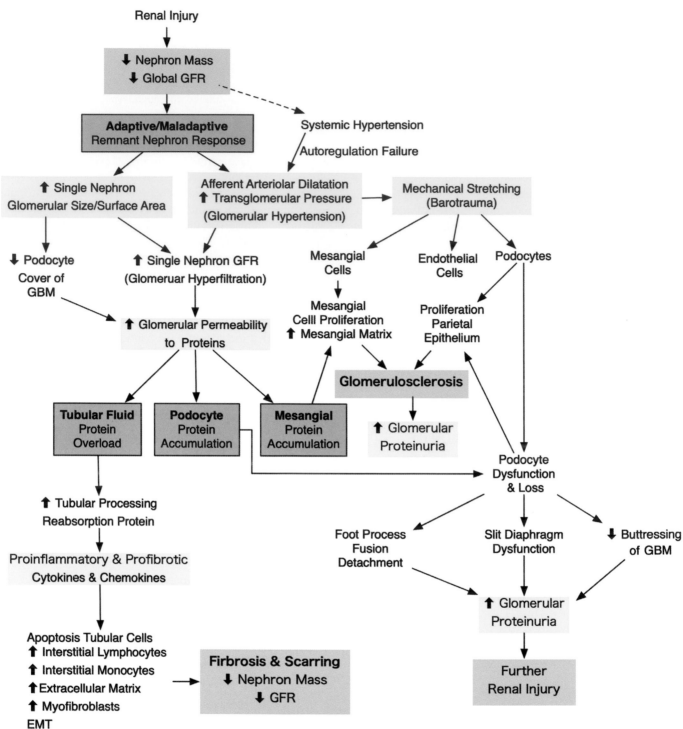

FIGURE 7.15 Glomerular proteinuria and progression of CKD. This figure emphasizes the role that glomerular origin proteinuria can play in the progression of CKD, though there are other important factors that that are not considered here. Increased passage of transglomerular proteins from plasma into the mesangium and tubular fluid can promote glomerulosclerosis and tubulo-interstitial inflammation and fibrosis. The role of podocytes in the development of proteinuria and CKD progression is also featured. Systemic hypertension from any cause can contribute to progression of CKD but it is most often found in association with CKD. Many of the concepts for this figure were derived from Cravedi and Remuzzi [201]; Perico et al. [102]; Kramer [319]; Remuzzi and Bertani [103]; Remuzzi [104]; Zoja et al. [44]; Zandi-Nejad et al. [199]; Toblli et al. [101]; Perico et al. [320]; Shankland and Mathieson [321]; Benzing and Salant [23], 44; Taal [322]; Roura et al. [54]. Glomerular proteinuria can lead to less renal expression of Klotho which then translates into a higher circulating phosphate concentration. This can occur since the full effect of FGF-23 to induce phosphaturia by the proximal tubules requires Klotho interaction. The potential role for higher circulating phosphate that is associated with mineralization of vasculature and renal tissue (de Seigneux et al. [323, 324]) is NOT shown in this graphic. Also, the specifics of an activated RAAS in promoting renal proteinuria and progression of CKD are not detailed. CKD – chronic kidney disease, GFR – glomerular filtration rate, EMT – epithelial to mesenchymal transitioning, GBM – glomerular basement membrane.

It is generally accepted that naturally occurring CKD is progressive in dogs and cats when azotemia exists at the time of diagnosis [95, 167, 206, 207, 335–346]. The progression of CKD is identified when further renal lesions accumulate and or decreases in GFR and loss of other renal functions are documented. The persistence of the initial cause of renal injury (immune-complex disease, amyloid, toxins, infection, and idiopathic) results in progressive CKD. There also appears to be an "inexorable progression" of CKD that occurs after a critical threshold for loss of renal mass has occurred, whether or not the original cause of the injury is still present [347].

It is less clear as to how much progression, if any, develops in animals with nonazotemic CKD at the time of initial diagnosis (IRIS CKD Stage 1) as it is difficult to define this stage with certainty and to find these early cases for study. Some with IRIS CKD stage 1 are likely to progress, whereas others are not. No one factor by itself adequately predicts the progression of CKD in clinical dogs and cats, but serum phosphorus, Ca × P product, renal proteinuria based on UPC, low USG, indoxyl sulfate, and FGF23 can do so at times alone or in combination [86, 167, 340, 341, 344, 348–352]. Algorithms that use a combination of commonly measured laboratory parameters that include the magnitude of proteinuria over time have been developed for use in cats to predict a future diagnosis of CKD [353].

The threshold for the magnitude of renal mass loss that is required before CKD progression continues by self-perpetuation (inexorable progression) varies by species based on data from the remnant kidney model. Self-perpetuation of renal disease occurs in rats with the remnant kidney model (subtotal nephrectomy) of CKD [347]. Rats with ≥75% reduction in nephron mass consistently undergo progressive loss of renal function and renal lesions. In aged dogs with 50% reduction in renal mass (unilateral nephrectomy), GFR did not progressively decline over the next four years though mild renal lesions did develop. UPC was increased over baseline following unilateral nephrectomy, but did not increase further; some UPC were >1.0 [354]. Dogs with 75% nephron mass reduction did not progress based on loss of excretory renal function, but they did develop mild renal lesions in another study; a few dogs fed the highest dietary protein had more severe glomerular lesions. Mean urinary protein excretion was higher in the surgical ligation model for dogs consuming the highest dietary protein intake in this study, but this difference was not statistically significant. A pattern for increasing magnitude of proteinuria was not observed over 48 months regardless of dietary protein intake. There was no relationship between the degree of proteinuria and severity of renal lesions [355, 356]. In dogs with more extensive mass reduction (11/12 nephrectomy), the development of renal lesions and an increased tendency to undergo progression similar to rats were shown [347, 357]. In a study of 60 dogs with 11/12 nephrectomy, the UPC approached significance for its association with decreases in GFR (P = 0.087). The UPC was associated with the magnitude of decline in GFR for non-survivors, but not for survivors. Proteinuria increased when progressive decline in GFR was rapid [347].

The progression of CKD was observed in some dogs of one study with CKD created by 7/8 renal mass reduction [357]. Twenty-four-hour urinary protein excretion increased following nephrectomy compared to controls and progressively increased in some dogs at 18 and 34 months. Postsurgical reduction in GFR was stable in most dogs, but GFR further decreased in 3 of 10 dogs at 21–24 months. Proteinuria and glomerular structural lesions were detected before GFR declined in these dogs. Glomerular lesions progressed from focal mesangial hyperplasia or focal glomerulosclerosis to focal and segmental sclerosis or glomerular obsolescence as the most advanced lesions in this model. Progression of CKD in experimental dogs appears to be slower than in rats as shown in this study and others in dogs [357]. In a study of dogs with 7/8 nephrectomy studied for two years, renal function was stable or increasing for the first 40 weeks following nephron mass reduction. Thereafter, GFR progressively decreased in a small number of dogs by the end of the study and proteinuria increased before GFR declined in this small subset [358].

Adaptive changes in remaining nephrons that could contribute to progressive CKD include glomerular hypertrophy, increased single-nephron GFR, increased transglomerular pressure and capillary flow, and increased glomerular proteinuria based on studies of animals with experimental CKD. Oxidative stress and the generation of oxygen free radicals in CKD and tubulointerstitial reactions are also considerations among others that could be important for progression. The relative importance for these factors in the progression of naturally occurring CKD has not been determined [347].

Studies from remnant kidney models of CKD in dogs and cats provide insight as to possible mechanisms that contribute to progression, but these models may not reflect how progression occurs in clinical patients. Progressive azotemia, uremia, and death appear to be common following an initial clinical diagnosis of CKD in dogs with azotemia [207, 335, 336, 347]. Some cats with naturally occurring CKD undergo progression, but others apparently do not. Progression occurs at a slower rate for cats than dogs in general [95, 340–342]. Subtotal nephrectomy models of CKD in dogs [354, 355, 357, 359] and cats [360, 361] demonstrate the progression of CKD to a variable degree. Failure to identify progression based on GFR could be obscured by adaptations in surviving nephrons that increase single-nephron GFR. In these instances, global GFR would be maintained despite lower numbers of nephrons until the CKD is further advanced. Experimental studies also varied in the degree of nephron mass reduction, time the animal was followed, and nature of dietary intake. Attributing an effect to one component of dietary intake is not possible since intake of protein, phosphorus, calcium, salt, lipids, antioxidants, and calories varied among these studies.

FIBROSIS

The development of renal fibrosis occurs in progressive CKD regardless of cause and is characterized by excessive accumulation of extracellular matrix in the interstitium. Damaging reactions to excess protein trafficking across the glomerulus can result in development of tubulointerstitial inflammation and fibrosis following the entry of these proteins into tubular fluid of the proximal tubule [44, 103, 104]. A similar response may occur when the more distal nephron is exposed to high concentrations of luminal albumin that result when the reabsorption of albumin by the proximal tubules has become saturated. This increased exposure to albumin results in signals that are important in inflammation and fibrosis from the collecting tubule [362]. An overload of albumin in the tubules leads to a decrease in the expression of megalin and clathrin receptor-mediated endocytosis of proteins [102]. This results in albumin-induced epithelial injury and apoptosis of tubular cells. These activated tubular cells release molecules that recruit lymphocytes and macrophages into the interstitium. Subsequent cytokine and chemokine release ultimately lead to peritubular inflammation and fibrosis [41, 54, 95, 363–367].

There are many mediators of fibrosis, but the activation of NF-kappa-B with subsequent formation and action of transforming growth factor beta appears to be particularly important in this process [41, 54, 363, 364, 368]. There is a recruitment of myofibroblasts and fibroblasts that lead to cell proliferation and fibrosis [102, 366]. Renal epithelial to mesenchymal cell transitioning to myofibroblasts also appears to be important in the development of fibrosis [41, 365, 366]. Additionally, glomerular endothelial cell health depends on close cross talk with podocytes [102]. Podocyte loss following injury from proteinuria adversely affects endothelial fenestrae formation and endothelial cell apoptosis. Injured podocytes from any cause, including proteinuria, may send signals that activate parietal epithelial cell proliferation in Bowman's capsule [102].

Another important mediator of fibrosis is the activation of the complement cascade. The increased glomerular filtration of complement C3 during compromised glomerular barrier function can lead to renal tubule damage and an increase in proinflammatory mediators [246]. Tubular cells also synthesize C3 and other complement factors in response to protein in the ultrafiltrate, further enhancing the inflammatory response. The secreted cytokines and accumulating complement components recruit inflammatory cells and lymphocytes into the interstitium, which contributes to progressive fibrosis. Monitoring the level of complement may be a method to predict the severity and outcome of renal disease [246].

SPECIFIC DISEASE SYNDROMES AND PROTEINURIA

SYSTEMIC HYPERTENSION

Systemic hypertension from any cause can be associated with glomerular proteinuria. The ability of the afferent arteriole to vasodilate or vasoconstrict and respond to changes in systemic BP is decreased during CKD. The afferent arteriole in advanced CKD has been characterized as fixed and dilated with loss of autoregulatory function. In these instances, increased systemic BP is more easily transmitted to the glomerulus, which then increases glomerular pressure that leads to glomerular injury and glomerular proteinuria [332]. With progressive vascular narrowing, the preglomerular circulation has limited ability to constrict or dilate in response to systemic pressure. Any change in arterial pressure results in a proportional change in GFR in the absence of effective autoregulation. Thus, a small degree of systemic hypertension can lead to an exaggerated response that increases glomerular pressure [369]. This mechanism could account for the development of proteinuria or its accentuation in those already exhibiting glomerular proteinuria.

Systemic hypertension is most commonly diagnosed in association with CKD (dogs and cats) [331, 370–372], HAC (dogs) [373], or hyperthyroidism (cats) [370]. In cats, systemic hypertension was associated with albuminuria in a surgical model of CKD [374] and also in naturally occurring CKD [167].

Systemic hypertension has the potential to increase glomerular capillary pressure and transglomerular forces that favor proteinuria/albuminuria, especially in patients with CKD that already have glomerular hypertension [2, 338]. Higher systemic BP was associated with an increased magnitude of proteinuria, lower GFR, and more substantial renal histopathologic lesions in dogs with experimental reduction of nephron mass of one study [375]. Dogs with CKD and systolic BP ≥ 180 mmHg (24 of 40) had more proteinuria (median UAC 1.72) than CKD dogs with lower BP (median UAC: 0.10) [190]. The magnitude of renal proteinuria was greater in hypertensive CKD dogs compared to those that were normotensive in one clinical study [335], but not in another study of dogs with glomerular disease associated with Leishmaniasis [376].

In dogs with various disorders including CKD, there was a weak positive correlation between systemic BP and UPC [338]. Hypertension was encountered independent of proteinuria, and proteinuria was found independent of hypertension in some dogs. In dogs of the same study with azotemic CKD, systemic hypertension and proteinuria (≥ 1.0 UPC) were associated with shorter survival time [338], similar to previous reports in dogs with initial systemic hypertension or proteinuria (UPC > 1.0) [207, 335].

Dogs with high systemic BP at the time of CKD diagnosis were more likely to develop a uremic crisis, had decreased survival time, and had greater progression of CKD and loss of excretory renal function based on 1/serum creatinine [335]. The role of renal proteinuria was further evaluated in a subsequent report utilizing the same dogs [207]. CKD dogs with a UPC ≥ 1.0 had greater loss of renal function and a higher risk to die or develop a uremic crisis. Dogs with UPC ≥ 1.0 had significantly higher systolic BP (164 ± 23 mmHg) compared to dogs with UPC < 1.0 (139 ± 18 mmHg) [207]. Similar outcomes were seen in CKD dogs with high systolic BP and those with high UPC at the time of initial CKD diagnosis in these two studies.

UPC and UAC in nonazotemic and azotemic CKD cats were greater in those with systolic hypertension than those with normotension [167]. Decreased survival was related to higher levels of renal proteinuria in this study of CKD cats, but survival was not significantly related to BP as had been reported in CKD dogs. One explanation for this difference could be that a return to normotension is more easily accomplished during antihypertensive treatment in cats than in dogs [167]. Proteinuria before and after the treatment of systolic hypertension with amlodipine was strongly associated with survival in cats of another study. UPC was higher in cats with higher quartile levels of systolic BP compared to those in the lower quartile [377].

Systemic BP should be measured in all patients with glomerular proteinuria since successful lowering of BP can lessen this type of proteinuria. It is difficult to decide how proteinuria should be classified in those with systemic hypertension, as it could be considered functional [21] or pathological glomerular proteinuria depending upon specific circumstances and stage of CKD.

CONGESTIVE HEART FAILURE (CHF)

The degree of proteinuria, if any, has not been detailed in dogs or cats with CHF or other heart conditions. Proteinuria was reported before and after treatment for CHF in humans of one study. Modest 24-hour proteinuria measured by SSA precipitation and urinary electrophoresis was noted to frequently occur in this population; proteinuria quickly resolved when CHF treatment was successful. If proteinuria did not resolve following the successful treatment of CHF, intrinsic renal disease emerged as a more likely cause. High-magnitude proteinuria was an unlikely finding in humans with CHF in this study [24]. In another study, proteinuria was found in 88% of human patients with CHF, in which the degree of proteinuria paralleled the severity of the heart failure. There was no relationship between the magnitude of proteinuria and systolic or diastolic BP [378]. Chronic heart failure in humans of another study was associated with no proteinuria in 58%, 30% with MA, and 11% with macroalbuminuria, and proteinuria was not mitigated during treatment with an ARB. An increased UAC was a strong independent predictor of prognosis in this study [379]. There is a clear association of proteinuria with adverse outcomes in humans with a variety of cardiovascular diseases, so the mitigation of renal proteinuria in this population is warranted [380].

The mechanism for the development of renal proteinuria during CHF is not well established [381], but it appears to fall into the functional proteinuria category because the proteinuria usually abates during the successful treatment of CHF and renal histopathology reveals either normal or minimally affected renal tissue [378]. Renal proteinuria resulted following renal venous congestion created by the clamping of the renal vein in experimental dogs. The urinary protein excretion rate increased quickly as renal venous pressure increased ($\geq 250\,mm$ water pressure) following clamping and the proteinuria abated quickly when pressure on the renal vein was released [382]. In a canine model of chronic heart failure and renal insufficiency, urinary protein increased from 37 ± 7 to $83 \pm 12\,mg/dL$ at eight weeks in another study [383]. The magnitude of proteinuria was inversely related to RBF in humans with heart failure of one study [379].

It is likely that veterinary cardiologists do not frequently assess urinalysis before and after treatment for severe cardiac disease due to medications like furosemide that substantially decrease USG. More dilute urine samples are unlikely to test positive on the urinary dipstrip for protein, but it is possible that assessment of UPC or MA could disclose previously unrecognized proteinuria. Whether proteinuria has any predictive value in veterinary patients with CHF has not been evaluated. Anecdotally, dogs with third-degree heart block often have proteinuria that occurs in association with passive congestion, but the mechanism(s) for this proteinuria has not been further explored (John Bonagura, personal communication, 2011).

CRITICAL CARE

MA occurred in greater than 50% of critically ill dogs of one study, a finding that was more frequent than an increased UPC [189]. The activation of cytokine cascades and ischemia-induced disruption of the glomerular endothelial cells and basement membrane are potential mechanisms that contribute to endothelial dysfunction and increased glomerular permeability to plasma proteins during critical illness [384]. Albuminuria was negatively associated with 7- and 30-day survival in 78 critically ill dogs admitted to two teaching hospital intensive care units (ICUs) [385]. Microalbumin was measured in urine samples from 32 dogs admitted to the ICU and 73 dogs that were recovering from general anesthesia at a veterinary teaching hospital in another study. MA was documented in 72% of the dogs admitted to the ICU and in 55% of the dogs recovering from anesthesia. MA from 1 to $<15\,mg/dL$ was more commonly detected than levels of microalbumin from 15 to $<30\,mg/dL$ or overt proteinuria in dogs admitted to the ICU. Albuminuria was suggested to be a risk factor for death in dogs, but not in cats, that were admitted to the ICU in this study [384].

Dogs with SIRS frequently had increased UPC, MA, and retinol-binding protein (RBP) in urine, indicating both glomerular and tubular dysfunction in one study. UPC > 0.5 occurred in 69% and MA was detected in 64% of the dogs in this study. Urinary electrophoresis showed that 58% of bands were in the LMW range ($<60\,kD$), and 42% were in the middle ($60-80\,kD$) or HMW range ($>80\,kD$). Increased RBP in urine could indicate either saturation of reabsorption sites for RBP in the tubules by other proteins such as albumin or tubular injury in dogs with SIRS [194].

Urinary protein by dipstrip was negative in 65% and positive at +1 to +3 in 35% of dogs that survived acute pancreatitis in one study. For dogs that did not survive, dipstrip protein was negative in 42% and positive at +1 to +3 in 58%, which was not statistically different from the survivors (P = 0.09). UPC ≥ 2.0 was associated with mortality when dogs with urinary casts were removed from consideration [75].

NEOPLASIA

The deposition of immune complexes within the glomerulus, as well as decreased blood flow to the kidneys and injurious molecules synthesized by the tumor, is thought to contribute to glomerular injury and proteinuria in patients with neoplasia [195]. Of 60 dogs presenting to a university oncology service, 51% were found to have proteinuria based on UPC. Borderline proteinuria with a UPC of 0.2–0.5 was noted in 22 dogs and overt proteinuria with a UPC of >0.5 in 9 dogs. Very few dogs had a UPC ≥ 2.0. Systemic hypertension likely contributed to the proteinuria in some of these dogs. Cutaneous mast cell tumor and multicentric high-grade lymphoma were the most common tumors, followed by squamous cell carcinoma and soft tissue carcinoma in this study [386].

Based on UPC, dogs with lymphoma were more likely to have proteinuria than age-matched controls in one study, but the proteinuria was not usually severe nor was it associated with tumor stage [387]. Dogs with lymphoma or osteosarcoma often were MA positive in the face of a normal UPC, but it is not known if this relates to tumor burden or remission status [189, 388]. Preoperative proteinuria identified on dipstrip and SSA testing was identified as a negative prognostic factor in dogs with appendicular osteosarcoma [389].

Interference with vascular endothelial growth factor (VEGF) signaling to glomerular endothelial cells results in albuminuria following anti-VEGF chemotherapy in humans with cancer and in humans with preeclampsia [23].

EXERCISE

Transient reversible albuminuria may occur in people following exercise. A study of facial cooling and moderate exercise in men over two weeks reported ketonuria and "marked" proteinuria, but details about the proteinuria were not provided [390]. This transient albuminuria does not appear to commonly develop in dogs. In an early study, urine protein (biuret method) increased by 47% following heavy treadmill exercise (30 minutes, 5 mph, and a 15% incline) in four mongrel female dogs [391]. Swimming increased albuminuria in some normal dogs, an effect that was greater in splenectomized dogs. It is possible that proteinuria in this model was more related to stress than to exercise, as albuminuria decreased with repeated swimming experience. Treadmill running did not affect albuminuria or lysozymuria in the same study [392]. MA was present before and after another treadmill exercise in 15% of normal dogs, but the magnitude of MA did not increase following exercise [393]. Well-conditioned Alaskan Sled Dogs did not have MA before or following runs over four days under extreme weather conditions in Alaska [394]. The effect of exercise on proteinuria or albuminuria in sick dogs has not been evaluated, so it is possible that those with underlying changes in glomerular barrier integrity will experience an increase in proteinuria following exercise. The intensity of exercise influences proteinuria in people, so the possibility remains that very intense or prolonged exercise could result in proteinuria especially in nonconditioned animals [393].

HYPERTHERMIA AND HYPOTHERMIA

Mild glomerular proteinuria developed in one-third of apparently healthy human volunteers after experimental hyperthermia for up to two hours in one study. This proteinuria was considered functional due to transient changes in glomerular hemodynamics initiated by the high body temperature. The development of high-magnitude proteinuria following hyperthermia exposed unsuspected underlying glomerular or tubulo-interstitial renal disease in a few subjects [395].

Heat stroke can lead to rhabdomyolysis and myoglobinuria in dogs that can be detected as proteinuria in some instances. A high CK and SGOT released from damaged muscles and the presence of nucleated RBC in the circulation are useful to support this diagnosis [396]. Heat stroke occurs in the absence of pyrogens and can be caused by exertional activity, exposure to high ambient temperature environments if not acclimated, confinement within a vehicle, and during grooming and hospitalization that result in a high body core temp >41 °C (>105.8 F). Body temperature may not be elevated at the time of evaluation, especially when cooling measures have been previously administered [396–400]. Though the presence or absence of proteinuria has not been featured in studies of heatstroke in dogs, significant heat retention can cause glomerular hemodynamic changes early on that are likely to result in glomerular proteinuria (albuminuria). AKI that develops during heat retention can also cause tubular proteinuria from damage to renal tubules, either from direct thermal injury or from secondary to reduced renal perfusion [401, 402]. Some of the glomerular proteinuria that develops is likely to occur as part of SIRS and endothelial damage that allow protein leakage across the glomerulus. Endothelial cells are quite susceptible to direct thermal damage [396, 400] that can result in glomerular proteinuria. Up to 3+ positive reactions for urinary protein by urinary chemistry dipstrip were noted in association with minimally concentrated urine in an early report of heatstroke in dogs [403]. The median UPC at presentation was 4.8 (0.4–46.0) in naturally occurring heat stroke in dogs of one study, likely reflecting both glomerular and tubular origin proteinuria and potentially that from myoglobinuria also. UPC was >0.4 in 62% of dogs with heatstroke at presentation, > 2.0 in 42%, and >5.0 in 35%, but UPC did not distinguish survivors from nonsurvivors. Increased concentrations of urinary C-reactive protein in dogs of the same study indicated increased glomerular permeability, whereas biomarkers for renal tubular injury were substantially increased in this same study. The notion that the combination of exercise and hyperthermia could have contributed to the development of functional and reversible glomerular proteinuria was advocated by authors of this study [401]. The severity of the heat stroke, organ injury/failure, and survival was related to the magnitude of the temperature elevation and how long that lasted in experimental dogs of one study [404].

Reduced GFR and RBF occur during hypothermia so that blood urea nitrogen (BUN) and creatinine can be increased, likely due to changes in the balance between vascular tone of the afferent and efferent glomerular arterioles. Proximal renal tubular dysfunction can also occur that results in glucosuria without increased circulating glucose concentrations [405, 406]. Though not detailed in these reports, it is conceivable that reduced proximal tubular reabsorption of proteins in tubular fluid would also occur along with the renal glucosuria since the reabsorption of both molecules occurs in the proximal tubule. Also, since vasoconstriction characterizes hypothermia, changes in glomerular hemodynamics could contribute to the development of glomerular proteinuria. The development of AKI during hypothermia could account for proteinuria at times too.

ENDOCRINE DISORDERS

Hyperadrenocorticism

Proteinuria and hypertension are commonly recognized in dogs with spontaneous HAC [196, 304, 373]. The mechanisms for proteinuria during excess glucocorticosteroid exposure are not well understood. There are several mechanisms that could result in renal proteinuria in patients with HAC that involve glomerular and or tubular mechanisms that create proteinuria. In one study of dogs with HAC, it was determined from results of urinary electrophoresis that LMW urinary proteins were predominant, indicating a tubular origin [407]. Some of the renal proteinuria is likely a consequence of systemic hypertension associated with HAC. Multiple possible mechanisms for proteinuria during spontaneous HAC and during exogenous administration of glucocorticosteroids that include functional and structural renal changes have been reviewed in detail elsewhere [196, 408–413].

The incidence of increased UPC varies among studies, but UPC > 1.0 is common. A UPC > 1.0 was reported in 43.7% of dogs with untreated pituitary-dependent hyperadrenocorticism (PDH) [208], and in 69.2% of dogs with HAC and systemic hypertension in another study [414]. In those with hypertension, 100% had albuminuria. In the same study, dogs with HAC and normal BP had a UPC > 1.0 in 47.1% and albuminuria in 64.3% [414]. Of nine dogs with HAC in another study, three had a UPC > 1.0 and two had a UPC > 2.0 [407].

In an early study, systemic hypertension and proteinuria based on UPC were commonly encountered in dogs with untreated or poorly controlled HAC [415]. In untreated dogs with PDH, the mean UPC was 1.47; after successful treatment, the mean UPC was 0.64. Dogs with inadequate control of PDH had a mean UPC of 1.53. In untreated dogs with HAC due to adrenal tumor, the mean UPC was 2.74; after successful treatment, the mean UPC was 1.11. Blood pressure was higher in dogs with untreated HAC, and UPC was significantly correlated with systolic, mean, and diastolic BPs in all dogs [415]. MA and overt albuminuria occurred with greater frequency in dogs with HAC compared to normal dogs in another study, but was not associated with systemic BP [196]. In another study, the median UPC in dogs with PDH was 0.7 (0.03–4.2). Seven of 16 dogs had a UPC > 1.0. Following successful treatment with mitotane, median UPC was 0.36, but UPC remained high in five dogs. Structural disease of the glomerulus may account for failure to resolve proteinuria following the successful treatment of HAC. Renal biopsy was recommended for those whose proteinuria continued to escalate despite normal adrenal gland function during treatment [416].

Exogenous Glucocorticosteroids

Proteinuria is also known to develop in some dogs being clinically treated with exogenous glucocorticosteroids. In one study, prednisone was administered at 2.2 mg/kg twice daily by mouth for 42 days to nine normal young adult male dogs [412]. The median UPC increased from a baseline of 0.29 ± 0.10 to a maximal mean value at day 28 of 1.27 ± 1.02 and 0.92 ± 0.56 at day 42. No dog exceeded a UPC of 3.0 in this study. The finding of hypercellular glomerular tufts compatible with mesangial cell hyperplasia was the most common light microscopic lesion at necropsy. Four of nine dogs had adhesions of the glomerulus to Bowman's capsule. No deposits of immunoglobulins were found with immunofluorescent microscopy. GBMs exhibited mild segmental thickening, fusion of foot processes, and glomerular adhesions. Clinically relevant proteinuria and evidence for glomerular damage related to long-term prednisone administration was documented in this study [412]. A group of experimental dogs were given hydrocortisone orally at 8 mg/kg twice daily for 12 weeks and compared to a placebo. A maximal median UPC of 0.38 (0.18–1.78) was shown at day 28 in dogs receiving hydrocortisone. Quantitative albuminuria developed in all dogs during hydrocortisone treatment with maximal values on day 84. After the discontinuation of hydrocortisone, the mild proteinuria that had developed completely resolved within one month [373]. In a group of dogs with a specific glomerulopathy (carrier females with X-linked HN), a clinically relevant increase in UPC was documented within two weeks of the start of prednisone treatment (2.2 mg/kg/day) [413]. In these dogs, UPC increased from a mean of 1.5 at baseline to 5.6 after four weeks of prednisone treatment. The UPC returned to baseline within four weeks after stopping prednisone treatment. The ability of prednisone or other glucocorticosteroids to exacerbate the magnitude of renal proteinuria and its potential reversibility has not been determined in populations of dogs with other glomerulopathies.

Diabetes Mellitus

Proteinuria may also develop in animals with diabetes mellitus (DM). The mechanisms for proteinuria are not fully understood but may involve glomerular hypertension and hyperfiltration in addition to systemic hypertension. The risk for proteinuria to cause progressive CKD in animals with diabetes is not well understood. Proteinuria was identified as the major vascular complication of DM in 11 dogs that were followed for two years [417]. The highest prevalence for MA ≥2.5 mg/dL was 73%, and the highest prevalence for UPC ≥0.5 was 55% in dogs of this study. Three of the 11 dogs had MA without an increase in UPC at the start of the study. The initial median UPC was 0.41 (0.10–5.06) and overt proteinuria (>30 mg/dL albumin) was found in 7 of 16 (44%) dogs. The magnitude of proteinuria did not increase during this study. No significant interactions between BP, urine albumin concentration, UPC, and retinopathy were detected. The time since diagnosis and the degree of glycemic control had no significant effect on proteinuria or BP over the two years of this study [417]. MA status was positive in 47.1% of dogs with DM in another study. The magnitude of MA was higher in dogs with a longer history of diabetes, but was not influenced by systemic hypertension [418].

Systemic hypertension and proteinuria were also commonly found in an earlier study of spontaneous DM in dogs. The UPC was >1.0 in 7 of 35 (20%) at the time of diagnosis. Albuminuria was significantly higher in diabetic dogs compared to healthy controls. The presence of systemic hypertension was related to the duration of DM and the presence of proteinuria in this study [419]. Albuminuria and increased UPC were common in a study of dogs with DM or with HAC in another study. A maximal UPC of 6.6 occurred in dogs with DM and 7.1 in dogs with HAC. The mean urinary albumin was 20 mg/dL in dogs with DM and 52 mg/dL in dogs with HAC [420].

Proteinuria is commonly detected in diabetic cats [421, 422]. A UPC > 0.4 was detected in 70% of diabetic cats, in 35% of sick nondiabetic cats, and in 9% of healthy cats [421]. In another study, UPC > 0.4 was reported in 39% of diabetic cats compared to 30% of cats with CKD [422]. The prevalence of MA measured by semiquantitative methods was 70% in diabetic cats, 39% in sick nondiabetic cats, and 18% in apparently healthy cats [421]. Seventeen of 45 (38%) cats with a UPC < 0.4 were positive for MA. An unexpected 20 of 48 (42%) cats were negative for MA with a UPC > 0.4, suggesting the presence of nonalbumin proteinuria [421]. When UPC of >0.5 was used as the cutoff for proteinuria, 21% of cats in this study were negative for MA, as was found in 12% of a more general population of cats in another study [186].

Hyperthyroidism

Mild renal proteinuria develops in some cats with hyperthyroidism that is caused by a combination of increased global and single-nephron GFR, intraglomerular hypertension, and systemic hypertension. Decreased proteinuria often follows the restoration of euthyroidism following treatment [423–428]. The degree of pretreatment proteinuria in hyperthyroid cats was associated with survival, but it did not predict the development of posttreatment azotemia [425, 429]. A median UPC of 0.53 (0.01–13.44) was reported at the time of diagnosis of hyperthyroidism, which then significantly decreased after treatment in one study [425]. The UAC did not significantly decrease at the same time in this study [425], but did decrease in another [429]. Discordance between UPC and UAC could indicate that the type of proteinuria arose from the excretion of nonalbumin proteins in some hyperthyroid cats [425]. Median UPC was 0.52 (0.17–1.14) in cats with hyperthyroidism in one study [430], and the median UPC was 0.49 pretreatment, which decreased to 0.23 following treatment in another study [429]. UPC > 0.5 occurred in 52% and >1.0 in 20% of hyperthyroid cats in this study. Proteinuria resolved in most cats following treatment of hyperthyroidism regardless of azotemia or nonazotemia [429]. In another study of hyperthyroid cats, proteinuria (UPC > 0.4) was detected in 18 of 21 cats prior to treatment [428]. UPC significantly decreased by four weeks after treatment with radioiodine (median UPC: 0.2–0.4). Proteinuria resolved (UPC < 0.2) in 17 of the 18 cats by 24 weeks after treatment. It was proposed that the initial renal proteinuria was likely due to a functional change in the glomerular barrier due to the rapid decrement of proteinuria by four weeks after treatment [428].

Acromegaly

Renomegaly is detectable both early and late in the disease progression of cats with acromegaly [431]. Acromegaly was associated with late developing azotemic CKD in 50% of cats in an early study [432]. Renomegaly was palpable in all of these cats. Proteinuria ≥2+ based on dipstrip was positive in 9 of 14 cats with submaximally concentrated urine and negative urine culture. In cats that developed CKD, persistent proteinuria was observed, but UPC was not determined. At necropsy, renomegaly was documented in 9 of 10 cats. Light microscopic examination revealed moderate to marked mesangial matrix expansion and variable periglomerular fibrosis. Tubular lumens contained pink staining homogeneous material compatible with proteinaceous material (glomerular origin proteinuria), and interstitial inflammatory changes were minimal or absent. It was speculated that some of the glomerular lesions were a consequence of poorly controlled DM in these cats, but similar glomerular lesions in diabetic cats with CKD without acromegaly are not known to occur [432].

Palpable renomegaly and CKD were considered common in another review of acromegaly in cats, but proteinuria was not reported [433]. Proteinuria was detected in two of eight cats, but CKD was noted as uncommon in another study [434]. Persistent proteinuria characterized by mild increases in UPC and positive MA status was considered common in one review [435]. This proteinuria was speculated to arise from changes in hemodynamics causing glomerular hyperfiltration. It is not clear if there is a unique pattern of proteinuria in cats with diabetes and acromegaly since proteinuria based on UPC and MA is common in cats with DM without acromegaly [421]. Nephropathy with azotemia has been noted to be common in cats with acromegaly, but the magnitude of azotemia was not different between diabetic cats with or without acromegaly in one study [431].

IDIOPATHIC HYPERTRIGLYCERIDEMIA

Idiopathic hypertriglyceridemia (HTG) and renal proteinuria associated with HTG are common in Miniature Schnauzers [436]. HTG will affect >75% of Miniature Schnauzers by 10 years of age [71]. In one study of 34 Miniature Schnauzers with fasting HTG and 23 without HTG, there was a strong correlation between serum triglyceride concentration and UPC. Proteinuria, defined as a UPC ≥ 0.5, was found in 60% of dogs with HTG and in no dogs without HTG. Proteinuria occurred in 41% of dogs with mild HTG and in 85% of dogs with moderate-to-severe HTG. UPC was most often ≥ 2.0 in proteinuric dogs with HTG. Increased cholesterol also correlated with proteinuria but was a less common finding than that with HTG. Proteinuric dogs were not associated with azotemia or hypoalbuminemia in this study. The authors speculated that renal proteinuria was associated with a subclinical lipid-induced glomerular injury, but renal histopathology was not reported in this study [70]. A retrospective study of Miniature Schnauzers with renal proteinuria revealed some combination of lipid thromboemboli in glomerular capillary loops by light microscopy and osmophilic globules consistent with lipid by EM in most of these dogs. The presence of lipid thromboemboli has only been described in renal biopsies from Miniature Schnauzers [437]. A good prognosis for a small number of Miniature Schnauzers with HTG and proteinuria was found for 18 months in a prospective case-controlled study. It is not known if proteinuria should be specifically targeted for treatment in dogs with HGT and proteinuria, but treatment to lower triglycerides is indicated for other possible comorbidities [71].

SYSTEMIC LUPUS ERYTHEMATOSUS (SLE)

Deposits of circulating autoantibody complexes in various tissues including the kidneys account for many of the lesions in SLE. In a study of 75 dogs with SLE, nonerosive polyarthritis was the most common clinical manifestation followed by renal involvement and then mucocutaneus disorders; hemolytic anemia was less common. Positive antinuclear antibody (ANA) titers were found in all dogs diagnosed with SLE in this study; high-level ANA titers were often encountered that were associated with the severity and stage of the disease. Male German Shepherds were overrepresented in this study, and irregular cycles of fever were typical. Renal glomerular involvement was commonplace when the disease was severe and sometimes was the cause for death due to the development of advanced renal failure, but detailed description from histopathology was not provided. Proteinuria at >50 mg/dL was present in all cases and was generally >100 mg/dL with a maximum of 700 mg/dL; UPC was not determined. Microscopic hematuria was observed in some

cases, but RBC morphology was not described as to a possible renal origin with dysmorphic RBC [438]. A positive ANA titer is helpful in the diagnosis of SLE along with other criteria, but it can also be positive in dogs with infectious disease, other non-SLE autoimmune disease, and in some controls [439, 440].

Positive ANA titers in dogs diagnosed with SLE were much less frequent in another study; thrombocytopenia occurred in 25% of these SLE cases. Hypoalbuminemia and proteinuria occurred in about 20% of SLE cases, but UPC was not determined [440]. Dogs with lupus GN of one series were noted to have proteinuria from 100 to 1000 mg/dL; UPC was not determined [441]. In a series of 42 dogs diagnosed with SLE, proteinuria was documented in 52%, but UPC was not determined. A common renal lesion at necropsy in some of dogs with SLE was that of glomerular mesangial matrix expansion [442].

Membranous glomerulopathy has also been described in other dogs with SLE [438, 441]. Renal amyloidosis and proteinuria rarely are associated with SLE in the dog [443]. SLE is rarely diagnosed in cats. Three cats diagnosed with SLE over a 14-year period were described that had erosive polyarthritis as the major presenting sign, along with positive ANA titers, enlarged kidneys on radiographs, azotemia, isosthenuria, and proteinuria (UPC: 2.1, 2.5, and 4.1). Chronic GN was reported at necropsy in all three cats; one was specifically noted with membranous glomerulopathy [444].

CYCLIC HEMATOPOIESIS (GRAY COLLIE SYNDROME)

The cyclic development of neutropenia at about 12-day intervals characterizes Gray Collie syndrome, though other blood elements are also affected (cyclic hematopoiesis). This is caused by a recessive autosomal gene defect involved in the regulation of hematopoietic stem cells. Infectious insults during states of neutropenia are continual and cumulative that lead to renal and other organ lesions [89, 445, 446]. Amyloidosis of several organs including the kidneys developed in all Gray Collies with cyclic hematopoiesis that survived to adulthood in one early study, but details regarding proteinuria were not provided [447]. In a later study, amyloidosis of liver, lung, spleen, and lymph nodes was a prominent feature in Gray Collies over 30 weeks of age in one study, but renal involvement with amyloid was less frequent and occurred only in dogs most severely affected. Membranoproliferative GN was diagnosed in 75–100% of the more severely affected dogs. Lesions of chronic interstitial nephritis and nephrosis were also common in older dogs, whereas lesions of pyelonephritis were common in younger dogs [448]. All of these underlying renal lesions are expected to be associated with renal proteinuria (glomerular, tubular, and/or interstitial).

PYOMETRA

Proteinuria has frequently been reported in studies of dogs with pyometra, but the relationship between pyometra in dogs and the development of glomerular lesions and proteinuria is not entirely clear. Mild-to-moderate proteinuria is commonly encountered in dogs with pyometra; severe proteinuria is less common [449, 450]. It is important to exclude postrenal sources of proteinuria before attributing its origin to the kidney. The contamination of urine with bacteria and inflammatory proteins from the infected uterus can occur during urine collection by voiding or catheterization. Contamination can also occur from uterine content reflux into the bladder urine before collection by cystocentesis.

In an early study, increased protein in urine measured by benchtop methods was reported in 36 of 58 urine samples, 10 with and 26 without azotemia [451]. For this laboratory, <40 mg/dL was considered to be normal urinary protein concentration. In nonazotemic dogs with pyometra, mean urinary protein was 20–24 mg/dL in 22 dogs and 138–202 mg/dL in 26 dogs. Mean urinary protein in the 10 azotemic dogs was 130 mg/dL [451].

Transient renal proteinuria from glomerular and tubular origins has been associated with pyometra in the dog [449, 452]. The glomerular lesions and renal proteinuria are reversible within weeks to months following the removal of the pyometra [452–454]. Tubular and glomerular biomarkers were increased in the urine of dogs with pyometra, and all decreased to levels that were not different from controls by six months after the surgical removal of the pyometra [452]. At the time of diagnosis, the median UPC of 0.48 (0.05–8.69) was significantly higher in 47 dogs with pyometra compared to intact female controls. UPC > 0.5 occurred in 22, >1.0 in 12, and >2.0 in 7 dogs of this study. UPC by three weeks following ovariohysterectomy (OHE) decreased to a median 0.11 (0.02–4.46) [449]. In another study, UPC measured in urine collected by cystocentesis at the time of OHE surgery was compared between 6 azotemic and 21 nonazotemic dogs with pyometra and 11 controls. The median UPC was 0.95 (0.02–5.53) in the nonazotemic dogs and 1.67 (0.52–3.02) in the azotemic dogs, which was significantly higher than the median 0.23 (0.14–0.49) in the control dogs [450]. In 18 dogs with pyometra, UPC was >0.5 in 10 and ≤0.5 in 8; UPC was ≥1.0 in five dogs at the time of diagnosis [455]. Proteinuria usually resolves following OHE but can persist in some dogs [456]. Zero to two days prior to OHE, the mean UPC was 2.4 ± 5.4 (voided and by cystocentesis). Following OHE, the UPC was >1.0 in 20 of 34 dogs at day 12 and >1.0 at two to four months following OHE in 7 of 26 dogs [457]. Proteinuria was not observed in one study of nonazotemic dogs with pyometra when evaluated by 24-hour protein excretion, but UPC was not determined [458].

Most dogs with pyometra are infected with *E. coli* [457–460]. UTI was documented following cystocentesis with the isolation of high numbers of bacteria in 22%, 25%, and 72% of dogs with pyometra in separate studies [457, 458, 460]. In one study, bacterial infection appeared to be limited to the lower urinary tract as no bacteria were isolated from the kidneys of dogs with pyometra [459]. However, in another study, strong immunofluorescence directed toward the same strain of *E. coli* as in the uterus was often detected in tubular casts, and

intact *E. coli* were found attached to renal tubular epithelium and lower urinary tract epithelium in some cases [460].

Lesions of GN have been described during chronic purulent processes in the dog, including that associated with pyometra [454, 459]. All the bitches with pyometra in one early study were reported to have membranous GN or mixed proliferative and membranous GN when evaluated with light microscopy. Findings on EM in a small subset of these dogs supported this diagnosis. Immune-complex injury was suspected to be associated with a bacterial antigen or an antigen from damaged uterine tissue. Discrete electron dense deposits consistent with the deposition of immune complexes were not described on EM, and immunofluorescence studies were not performed [453, 461]. Immunofluorescence was positive for immune complexes within the glomeruli in 12 dogs with pyometra of another study. Bright and distinct staining was seen during early phases of pyometra, whereas fluorescence was faded and linear in more advanced cases. The antigen in the immune complexes of this study was not identified [460].

In another study of pyometra, mild lesions of tubulointerstitial nephritis were commonly observed, but overall glomerular lesions were considered minimal to moderate during microscopy by light, electron microscope, and immunofluorescence. Foot process fusion and mesangial proliferation were reported as minimal to moderate. Immunofluorescence of the mesangium was detected in 18%, and electron dense deposits within the GBM and mesangium were occasionally identified. Authors of this study considered the glomerular lesions in dogs with pyometra to be age related [458]. Similarly in another report, glomerular lesions beyond that expected in association with age were not demonstrated in dogs with pyometra studied by light microscopy when compared to age matched controls. Interstitial inflammation and tubular atrophy were more common in dogs with pyometra in this study. Glomerulosclerosis was the predominant glomerular lesion in both groups [456]. In another study, renal biopsy was performed in 10 dogs with pyometra that had 2+ or 3+ proteinuria measured by chemistry dipstrip [449]. Renal tissue evaluated by light, immunofluorescence, and electron microscopic examination revealed glomerulosclerosis and tubulointerstitial nephritis as common lesions in these dogs. Dogs with a UPC > 1.0 were more likely to have clinically relevant renal lesions [449]. It appears that early reports describing GN in dogs with pyometra had lesions more consistent with glomerulosclerosis using updated classification schemes [456, 458].

INFECTIOUS CAUSES

Infectious agents can also be responsible for proteinuria; infections with *Leptospira* and *Borrelia* species have been previously discussed in the AKI section. The frequency for the detection of exposure to vector-borne organisms was evaluated in a population of dogs with renal proteinuria. Proteinuria was defined by a UPC ≥ 1.0 or 1+ protein on dipstick in addition to hypoalbuminemia. Exposure was determined by results of serologic assay or PCR in this study. Exposure to one or more organisms occurred in 34% (72 of 209) of proteinuric dogs, most commonly positive for *Rickettsia spp.*, *Ehrlichia spp.*, and *Borrelia burgdorferi*. Exposure to ≥2 vector-borne organisms occurred in 23 of 72 dogs with proteinuria. Far fewer dogs were detected with exposure when evaluated using an in-house rapid ELISA analyzer. Exposure to vector-borne disease was greater in dogs with lower serum albumin and with higher serum creatinine concentrations. Higher exposure to vector-borne pathogens was found in proteinuric dogs compared to that encountered from the general population evaluated by the same laboratory [250]. The relationship of exposure to vector-borne pathogens and subsequent development of renal proteinuria related to the formation and deposition of immune complexes or glomerular amyloidosis has not been conclusively proven in clinical patients [250]. In another study of dogs, proteinuria with inactive urine sediment was frequently detected with naturally occurring *Ehrlichia ewingii* infection [462].

Heartworm Disease

HW disease due to *Dirofilaria immitis* has been associated with the development of membranoproliferative GN, ICGN, and renal proteinuria in dogs [82, 463–468]. Mild-to-moderate mesangial expansion and thickening of the GBM have been described, and microfilaria has been seen within glomerular capillaries and tubular lumens [463, 464, 466, 469]. The presence of microfilaria within the glomeruli could result in both physical and immune injury. Dogs with marked microfilaremia had more severe glomerular histopathological findings that were attributed to physical damage from the presence of motile microfilaria within the glomeruli of one study [470]. In some instances, microfilaria has been observed connected to glomerular endothelium by narrow cytoplasmic bands. It was proposed that this could be a method to deliver microfilarial antigens within the glomerular membrane that then allow in situ immune-complex formation as antibodies bind to these planted antigens. The number of immune complexes appeared to be related to the number and duration of microfilaremia in this study [464]. In another report, dogs infected with HW but without circulating microfilaria had a greater degree of proteinuria that those dogs with circulating microfilaria. HW-infected dogs with microfilaria had urinary protein of 130 ± 120 mg/dL SEM (30–760 mg/dL) and those without microfilaria had urinary protein of 560 dL ± 240 mg/dL SEM (30–1400 mg/dL) [465]. Dogs infected with HW but without circulating microfilariae may have previously been immunized to the microfilaria. Dogs without microfilaria can have higher antibody titers toward microfilaria compared to dogs with circulating microfilaria [471, 472].

In an early study following the induction of HW infection in dogs, a pattern of linear fluorescence and fine electron dense deposits were described within glomeruli suggesting in situ antibody reaction with antigen within the glomerulus to form the immune complex. A second pattern was also described for discrete nonlinear immunofluorescent and electron dense deposits of immune complexes predominantly within the mesangium. Elution studies from the immune-complexes identified antibodies toward the worm and microfilaria. Antibodies were variably directed toward the adult filarial wall, microfilarial surface, and uterine fluid of the worm. Antibodies against the adult filarial wall were most commonly found in those with the linear fluorescent pattern, whereas the discrete nonlinear complexes were associated with antibodies against the uterine fluid. Antimicrofilarial antibodies were encountered in both groups. There were no antibasement antibodies demonstrated. IgG was demonstrated by immunofluorescence in all glomeruli studied as were variable amounts of IgM and C3 [463, 464].

In a later study, all dogs developed high concentrations of circulating antibodies to dirofilarial antigens and remained microfilaremic following the injection of infective larvae into Beagles. Mean 24-hour urinary protein excretion was increased at 58 mg/kg/day. Membranoproliferative GN was described in all dogs along with positive immunofluorescence, mostly in a fine granular pattern along the glomerular wall. EM confirmed the presence of electron dense deposits. Antibodies directed against specific dirofilarial antigens were confirmed by elution studies from the immune complexes. The combination of these findings heavily leaned toward an immune-mediated glomerular injury. Aqueous soluble adult HW antigen adhered to the glomerular wall following injection into the renal artery of HW naïve dogs, supporting the possibility for in situ immune-complex formation after planting of antigen there. This study did not distinguish whether immune complexes were deposited from the circulation or developed following in situ planting of antigens [82].

Antigens from adult *D. immitis* were found in serum and urine of all experimentally infected dogs of another study. Serum antibodies against these antigens were also detected in all infected dogs. It is likely that antigens and antibodies against these antigens could be measured at the same time due to conditions of antigen excess. Elution of renal tissue revealed antibody toward these specific HW antigens, providing support for an immune-mediated glomerulopathy. Findings from this study suggested that soluble HW antigens adhere to the glomerulus prior to the formation of immune complexes. In this scenario, immune complexes would form within the glomerulus after circulating antibodies react with the planted antigens [473].

Dogs mounted a circulating antibody response following immunization with antigens from adult *D. immitis* in another study. Dirofilarial antigen was then infused into the renal artery of one kidney and the renal tissue examined 14 days later. Substantial glomerular lesions were found in this kidney compared to normal histology found in the preinfusion renal biopsy of the same kidney. Histopathological changes described on light, immunofluorescent, and EM in the infused kidney were similar to glomerular lesions described during naturally occurring HW disease in the dog. Renal eluates from the infused kidney isolated antibodies against antigens associated with *D. immitis*. These findings further support the notion that immune complexes associated with HW antigens can form in situ along the glomerulus after the antigens are planted there. Renal lesions in the noninfused contralateral kidney were mild and likely reflected deposits of circulating immune complexes that formed following immunization [87]. In another study using a similar model, treatment with a thromboxane synthase inhibitor significantly lessened the development of glomerular lesions based on light microscopy, but did not alter the detection of IgG, IgM, C3, dirofilarial antigen, electron dense deposits, or levels of antibodies against Dirofilaria. Immune-complex formation or deposition was not altered by this treatment [474].

In client-owned dogs with HW disease, a UPC > 0.5 was found in 19.2% and a UPC 0.2–0.5 in 17%. The UPC was higher in dogs with higher adult parasite loads as well as in those with microfilaremia. Pulmonary hypertension was associated with greater proteinuria, but systemic hypertension had no effect on proteinuria. All dogs with increased plasma proteins had either borderline or overt proteinuria in this study [468]. Young male Beagle dogs that were inoculated with infective HW larvae developed MA (>1 mg/dL) that progressively increased over time and preceded development of overt proteinuria (> 30 mg/dL) in one report. MA developed in 75% and overt proteinuria in 7% of dogs in this report [81].

Cats may also be infected with *D. immitis*. Positive urine chemistry dipstrip reactions for protein were found in 90% of cats with natural HW infections; 10% were negative, 52% 1+, 23% 2+, and 16% 3+. Age- and sex-matched control cats without HWs showed 65% negative, 26% 1+, 10% 2+, and 0% 3+. No cats had 4+ dipstrip proteinuria detected. Cats with HW disease had a nearly threefold increase in urinary protein based on the chemistry dipstrip of this study [475]. Urine protein was also measured in urine from cats that were experimentally and naturally infected with *D. immitis*. Ten of 64 experimentally infected cats were MA positive at eight months post infection. Mean UPC in these 10 cats was 0.57 ± 0.91 and was >0.4 in 9 of 10 cats. The development of renal proteinuria required the presence of adult heart worms but was not influenced by the presence or absence of microfilaremia. The detection of circulating HW antigen, HW antibody, or HW antigenuria did not predict which cats would have renal proteinuria in this study. Cats with low numbers of adult HWs were no less likely to develop proteinuria than cats with a higher adult worm burden. All cats with induced infection had HW antigenuria, indicating renal exposure to these antigens [475].

Recent studies indicate that *Wolbachia* infection associated with canine HW disease can contribute to the development of immune-mediated renal disease [476, 477]. All the stages of dirofilariasis are infected with this intracellular rickettsial endosymbiont, including microfilaria, and it appears that dead and dying worms and microfilaria release Wolbachia antigens that result in a specific IgG response against Wolbachia surface proteins [476, 477]. Dogs with circulating microfilaria had a greater level of proteinuria and higher levels of anti-Wolbachia antibodies compared to those without circulating microfilaria in one study [477]. Antibodies to Wolbachia surface proteins have also been documented in cats naturally infected with HW as have rising titers in experimentally infected cats following larval death of HW [477, 478]. The relationship of an immune response to *Wolbachia* and the development of glomerular lesions and glomerular proteinuria have not yet been established in cats.

Histoplasmosis

Mild proteinuria based on dipstrip urine chemistry was detected at trace to 1+ in five dogs and 2+ in one dog with disseminated histoplasmosis and concurrent hypoalbuminemia, but proteinuria was not further evaluated by UPC or MA. It is likely that gastrointestinal (GI) loss of albumin and reduced synthesis of albumin by the liver also contributed to the genesis of hypoalbuminemia in addition to any urinary protein losses in this study [88].

Leishmaniasis

Leishmaniasis is a common endemic disease of dogs encountered in Mediterranean countries [479, 480]. Renal lesions and proteinuria are commonly found in dogs with leishmaniasis following immune-mediated injury within the glomeruli and tubules. Nonazotemic and azotemic renal disease can be encountered depending on the stage of leishmaniasis. Death due to advanced renal disease is common and is influenced by the degree of proteinuria before and after anti-leishmanial treatment [480]. GN was found in all dogs infected with *Leishmania infantum* of one study. Focal or diffuse mesangial cell proliferation or membranoproliferative GN were characteristic lesions in association with IFA-positive granular deposits of IgG, IgM, and C3 and electron dense deposits characteristic for immune complexes. Quantitative total proteinuria varied from a mean of 20 to 160 mg/dL with greater proteinuria significantly related to the type and severity of glomerular involvement. Immune-complex deposits were also present in the tubular basement membrane in over 90% of infected dogs, a finding that could account for mild-to-moderate tubulointerstitial disease that commonly occurred in this population [481]. In another study, nearly all infected dogs had nonselective glomerular proteinuria (albumin and other bands >69 kD including transferrin and IgG), and a few dogs had mixed glomerular and tubular proteinuria based on qualitative proteinuria assessment. Glomerular lesions were described in all dogs and nonprimary lesions of tubulointerstitial nephritis in 55% based on light microscopy. Glomerular lesions consisted of mesangial GN, membranous GN, membranoproliferative GN, and focal segmental GN [482].

Dogs with leishmaniasis had a significantly higher mean UPC (2.6 ± 4.2) compared to control dogs (0.3 ± 0.1) in an early study; UPC was also significantly related to hypoalbuminemia [483]. UPC significantly decreased (median: 0.35 to 0.26) in a study of naturally infected nonazotemic dogs treated with one cycle of allopurinol and miltefosine. Based on UPC before treatment in 20 dogs, 9 were nonproteinuric, 7 were borderline proteinuric, and 4 were overtly proteinuric. Following treatment, two of four dogs changed from overt proteinuria (UPC > 0.5) to nonproteinuric (UPC < 0.2) and three of seven dogs with borderline proteinuria (0.2–0.5) converted to nonproteinuric status [484]. Four patterns of proteinuria were identified in one study of infected dogs using urinary electrophoresis (SDS-PAGE). Patterns for albuminuria (26%), glomerular (albumin + higher molecular weight proteins at 8%), tubular (LMW proteins at 10%), and a mixed pattern (albumin plus LMW proteins at 56%) were described in this population. It was proposed that a high urinary gamma-glutamyl transferase (GGT)-to-urinary-creatinine ratio (UGGT/Ucr) could be used as a surrogate for those dogs that had some form of mixed or tubular proteinuria that is associated with advanced leishmaniasis [77]. A method for combining the assessment of UPC and UGGT/Ucr was proposed to more fully evaluate the origin of proteinuria before and after treatment with N-methylglucamine antimoniate. No significant difference in mean UPC was seen at six weeks following treatment, since the UPC increased in half and decreased in the other half of the dogs. However, the UGGT/Ucr decreased at six weeks indicating that the tubular component to the renal proteinuria had resolved in most of the dogs. The initial tubular proteinuria could be caused in part by the flooding of plasma proteins across the glomerulus that impaired proximal tubular uptake of LMW proteins. Additionally, some of the tubular proteinuria could be caused by immune mechanisms affecting the tubular basement membrane. Glomerular and tubular proteinuria persisted in some patients following therapy indicating more severe renal damage [76].

Canine Adenovirus 1 (CAV-1)

Viral infections can create nephropathy following the replication of the virus in renal tissues or following immune-mediated injury to the glomerulus. If the dog survives an initial infection with CAV-1, a transient proliferative ICGN can develop that is followed by tubulointerstitial nephritis. CAV-1 virus was mostly demonstrated within mesangial cells and some within glomerular endothelial cells, associated with mesangial cell proliferation and mesangial expansion with a partial or complete occlusion of capillary loops of one study. Granular deposits of IgG, C3, and viral antigen as well as electron dense deposits were shown in the mesangium. The most striking ultrastructural changes were observed in the visceral podocytes with the obliteration and bulbous swelling of tertiary foot processes. Despite striking glomerular changes, proteinuria was minimally increased at 15–80 mg/dL [63].

Feline Leukemia Virus (FeLV)

Membranous glomerulopathy has commonly been associated with leukemia virus infection (FeLV) in cats [485–488]. Early studies employing anti-FeLV antiserum and immunofluorescence

demonstrated that the antigens of FeLV were frequently found in the glomeruli of cats with underlying lymphosarcoma [488, 489]. About one-third (29 of 79) of cats from a single household had a histologic diagnosis of GN in another study; most of these cats had persistent FeLV viremia [488]. The overall incidence of ICGN was low in the general population of cats with CKD [96, 97], but ICGN was documented in about one-third of cats with hematopoietic neoplasms linked with FeLV in one study [487]. IgG was demonstrated in these complexes, but the antigen was not definitely identified as FeLV. Subepithelial, subendothelial, and mesangial dense deposits were observed on EM [487]. Immune complexes within glomeruli of cats with FeLV and GN have been reported with antibodies toward group specific viral antigens in some cats [488, 489]. Infection with FeLV or feline immunodeficiency virus (FIV) was more frequent in cats with ICGN than in cats without ICGN in one study of cats with CKD; the magnitude of proteinuria was not separated out by retroviral status [97]. Details about the magnitude of proteinuria in cats with FeLV were not provided in early pathology-oriented reports, but proteinuria based on increases in UPC is expected in cats with substantial glomerular lesions.

Feline Immunodeficiency Virus

Renal involvement with FIV is common and often associated with glomerular, tubular, and interstitial lesions that are similar to those seen with HIV nephropathy. Selective and nonselective glomerular proteinuria has been reported [490]. Proteinuria (UPC > 0.4) was more common in cats with FIV than in cats without infection, but there was no difference in the degree of azotemia in one study [491]. In another study, median UPC was 0.21 (0.07–0.87) in 30 cats with natural FIV compared to median UPC 0.18 (0.22–0.37) in healthy cats [430]. Infection with FIV was three times more common (10 of 36) than infection with FeLV (3 of 37) in one study of CKD in cats [97].

The median UPC was 1.17 (0.18–14.00) in 21 cats with natural FIV infection in one study [492]. Glomerular changes were documented in 18 of these 21 cats with the thickening of mesangial matrix and occasional segmental glomerulosclerosis in 9 of 21 cats. Membranoproliferative GN occurred in 3 of 21 cats with granular deposition of IgG, IgM, and C3 immune complexes. Glomerular amyloid deposition was found in 8 of 21 and interstitial amyloid was identified in 7 of 21 cats. Intraluminal PAS positive proteinaceous casts were common [492]. Amyloid deposits were found in kidneys examined from 12 of 34 cats with naturally acquired FIV in another study; 10 of 12 cats had amyloid that was focally distributed, whereas 2 had diffuse distribution. Amyloid deposits were identified in both the medullary interstitium and glomeruli. All amyloid deposits were potassium permanganate-sensitive indicating secondary amyloidosis. Twelve of 16 cats with CKD as the presenting clinical problem had renal amyloid deposits in this study [493].

Feline Infectious Peritonitis (FIP)

Sixty of 85 cats with naturally occurring fatal FIP were diagnosed with membranous, membranoproliferative, or mesangioproliferative GN in one study. In those with GN, 53 cats had the effusive form of FIP and 7 had the noneffusive form. Findings of electron dense deposits (22 of 31) and granular immunofluorescence for IgG (4 of 10) and complement (4 of 10) supported a diagnosis of ICGN. Direct immunofluorescence did not detect the coronavirus causing FIP in renal tissue. Interference by blocking antibodies or complement was suggested as a possibility for the failure to detect the FIP virus, but elution studies were not performed [494]. Deposits of C3 and IgG were shown in the mesangium for 12 of 14 cats with experimental (six of six kittens) and naturally occurring (six of eight) FIP of another study [495]. High titers of anticoronavirus antibodies and low levels of complement in the circulation added support for the development of immune-complex-mediated glomerular disease [495]. Urinalysis has almost never been included in FIP reports, so details of renal proteinuria and FIP are not generally available [496–504]. In one report, proteinuria was reported to be "common" in those with renal involvement, but details were not provided [505]. However, increased glomerular proteinuria and increased UPC are expected due to the nature and severity of the glomerular lesions that develop in some clinical cats with advanced FIP. Renal proteinuria could also be attributed to nonglomerular origin from pyogranulomatous inflammation that can occur in the kidneys of some cats [496, 501, 505]. Rarely, pyogranulomas have been noted in the urinary bladder [496] that could add a component of postrenal proteinuria.

Feline Morbillivirus (FeMV)

FeMV infection may have some role in the development of tubulointerstitial lesions of CKD in cats, but this has not been proven. FeMV positive cats in one study had significantly lower USG than in healthy cats. The median UPC was significantly higher in FeMV cats (0.20; 0.08–1.03) compared to healthy cats (0.1; 0.04–0.25), but was not different from that in CKD cats (0.23; 0.20–0.80). UPC in FeMV cats was 0.2–0.4 in 5 of 13 and >0.4 in 1 of 13 cats. This mild increase in proteinuria in the FeMV cats was characterized as tubular in origin due to the appearance of an increased number and intensity of LMW proteins and decreased uromodulin [62].

NEPHROTIC SYNDROME

NS is one manifestation of PLN usually characterized by concurrent severe glomerular proteinuria, hypoalbuminemia, varying amounts of peripheral edema and body cavity effusion (third-spacing), and hyperlipidemia (high cholesterol and or triglycerides). Thromboembolic events associated with a hypercoagulable state may or may not be present. Excretory renal function is variably decreased as some are azotemic and some are not. Systemic hypertension commonly accompanies NS, possibly more so than in those with non-nephrotic glomerular diseases. The documentation of minimal body cavity effusions

may require ultrasonography [20, 102, 217, 304, 506, 507]. NS is considered to occur rarely or uncommonly in dogs and cats with glomerular disease, but has the potential to occur in association with any of the reported glomerulopathies in dogs or cats An accurate incidence for the occurrence of NS compared to non-nephrotic glomerular disease in dogs and cats is not known, as those with NS are more likely to undergo diagnostic evaluation than those with clinically silent proteinuria [506, 507]. Most cases of NS have been described at initial presentation when severe glomerular barrier dysfunction was diagnosed, though NS occurs at times in those with known glomerular disease when other factors such as increasing magnitude of proteinuria or more severe hypoalbuminemia develop later.

Not all patients with very high UPC and low serum albumin develop ascites and peripheral edema, so the pathophysiology of NS is not simply a consequence of severe glomerular proteinuria and development of low oncotic pressure associated with hypoalbuminemia. Intrinsic increases in renal tubular avidity for sodium and subsequent increase in vascular volume and hydrostatic pressure is one possibility that may exist in patients that develop NS. An activated renin–angiotensin–aldosterone system (RAAS), ADH, and sympathetic nervous system may also play a role in the development of edema following the perception of hypovolemia [102, 136, 506, 507]. It should also be noted that some patients with marginally increased glomerular proteinuria and minimal hypoalbuminemia develop NS, though uncommonly [506].

The documentation of NS does not align with any particular histopathological glomerular disease [217, 506], though NS appears to be more common in cats with membranous nephropathy at the time of their evaluation. Minimal change glomerular disease is rarely described in association with NS in dogs [79, 508] or cats [80], though it is a common diagnosis in human pediatric patients with NS [20, 73, 74, 506]. Ascites and peripheral edema in combination with hypoalbuminemia and proteinuria are typical findings in dogs and cats with NS. Liver and GI disease must be excluded as the primary causes for hypoalbuminemia in cases suspected to have NS. The documentation of NS is a negative prognostic indicator for survival in both dogs and cats [506, 507]. In dogs that were not azotemic in one study, NS dogs survived significantly less than dogs with non-nephrotic glomerular disease for reasons that were not apparent. There was no difference in survival when each group was azotemic, though survival for both groups was far less when azotemic (≥1.5 serum creatinine) [217].

The treatment of NS usually entails the use of antiproteinuria treatments using ACE-I, ARB, mineralocorticoid receptor blocker (MRB), or some combination of these drugs as discussed below, as well as the use of diuretics to lessen effusions and peripheral edema. Furosemide has been recommended for dogs with pulmonary edema or hyperkalemia and spironolactone for dogs with abdominal or thoracic effusion [136, 509]. Anticoagulants to oppose the accelerated clotting potential with NS include the use of aspirin, unfractionated heparin, and clopidogrel. Antihypertensive treatments will often be needed to treat systemic hypertension that is common in NS patients [7, 304, 506, 507, 509]. Standard of care for azotemic patients with NS should also be employed.

TREATMENT OF RENAL PROTEINURIA

INTRODUCTION AND GOALS

Therapeutic plans designed to normalize or at least reduce the degree of renal proteinuria in patients with CKD are usually undertaken with the goal to reduce the risk for progressive nephron loss [7, 20, 93, 136, 509]. The removal of an inciting cause (e.g. HW disease, pyometra, hyperthyroidism, systemic infectious diseases) of renal proteinuria should always be sought and treated if possible, but often a precise cause for the glomerular injury and proteinuria cannot be identified with certainty. It may not be possible to effectively remove the cause for glomerular injury (e.g. FeLV, FIV, neoplasia, and SLE) even when it is identified. The effective treatment of isolated renal proteinuria is more readily provided than that in patients that have renal proteinuria in addition to various combinations of azotemia, systemic hypertension, and hypoalbuminemia in severe cases.

The treatment of persistent renal proteinuria often involves some combination of nutritional modification, omega-3 polyunsaturated fatty acid (PUFA) supplementation, control of hypertension, and the administration of drugs to inhibit RAAS (ACE-I, ARB, and or MRB) (Figure 7.16). Antithrombotic drugs that inhibit platelet function are sometimes prescribed. Successful treatment should stabilize CKD or slow the progression (based on serum biochemistry for surrogates of GFR), ideally maintain the UPC at less than 0.5, and should stabilize body weight and BCS. An in-depth review for the treatment of renal proteinuria is beyond the scope of this book, so the interested reader is referred to a number of resources that are likely to be useful in providing more details [7, 14, 136, 212–215, 326, 372, 509–512]. Referral to an internist with special expertise in nephrology should be considered when renal proteinuria does not respond to standard therapy employed in general practice. Patients with some combination of severe renal proteinuria, moderate-to-severe renal azotemia, rapid escalation in the degree of renal azotemia, progressive decreases in serum albumin and any associated effusions, severe systemic hypertension, and thromboembolic events are also likely to benefit from referral to a specialty center with access to emergency and critical care services.

In general, the presence of renal proteinuria is a negative prognostic indicator in dogs and cats with azotemic CKD, and the prognosis is worse for those with a greater magnitude of proteinuria [7, 167, 207]. The effect of treatment with diet or drugs given to achieve a specific targeted level of reduced proteinuria has not been reported in prospective studies of dogs or cats with CKD. Treatment has been recommended to reduce the magnitude of proteinuria in patients with azotemic CKD and UPC > 0.4 (cats) and >0.5 (dogs) (Figure 7.8b). The magnitude of renal proteinuria during CKD usually decreases during successful treatment of systemic hypertension, though there may be residual proteinuria not amenable to antihypertensive drug treatment. A reduction in the magnitude of renal proteinuria that is induced or exacerbated by systemic hypertension is an initial goal for treatment. In patients without azotemic CKD, the treatment of renal proteinuria has been recommended when the UPC exceeds 2.0 [14]. The antiproteinuric goal is to achieve a UPC < 0.5 or at least a 50% reduction in UPC over baseline following treatment [136, 372].

It has not yet been determined if treatments for IRIS CKD Stage 1 that are designed to lower MA with diets or drugs should be prescribed to improve outcome in survival or stability of renal function. The long-term effects of stable MA or borderline increased UPC levels on renal function or survival during primary glomerular disease or systemic disease in dogs or cats are not known [15]. It is common in human medicine to try to limit the level of MA in patients with DM and systemic hypertension as one way to prevent or slow the development of progressive chronic nephropathy [513–515].

DIETARY THERAPY

Dietary recommendations will vary as to whether the animal with renal proteinuria has azotemia or not, the magnitude of the renal proteinuria (marginally versus greatly increased), and the current level of dietary protein intake. The amount of dietary protein content recommended is given more priority in patients with a high level of renal proteinuria that do not have azotemia, a scenario that usually involves dogs with glomerular disease and not cats. In azotemic patients, dietary phosphorus intake usually assumes the most importance in addition to some degree of dietary protein restriction. The nuances of prescribing a particular renal diet are beyond the scope of this chapter; consultation with a veterinary nutritionist is valuable in these instances.

In nonazotemic patients with a high level of renal proteinuria, an important first step in decision making is to collect a detailed dietary history so that the current amount of protein intake (g/100 kcal) is determined. This history needs to account for the sometimes-substantial impact of treats, rawhides, and dental chews on daily protein intake in addition to that from the main diet. Dietary protein intake should then be reduced accordingly if protein intake is determined to be high. One common approach for use in dogs is to reduce the protein intake by 25–50% from the current intake to see if the feeding of the new lower protein diet lessens the magnitude of the renal proteinuria. A reduction in phosphorus content (mg/100 kcal) of the diet is of less concern in the nonazotemic patient with glomerular proteinuria compared to those with azotemic CKD, but excess phosphorus intake should be avoided [512]. More severe restriction of dietary protein intake by feeding a renal diet may be indicated if the chosen lower protein maintenance diet does not sufficiently reduce the renal proteinuria [511, 512]. The mechanism for how

(a)

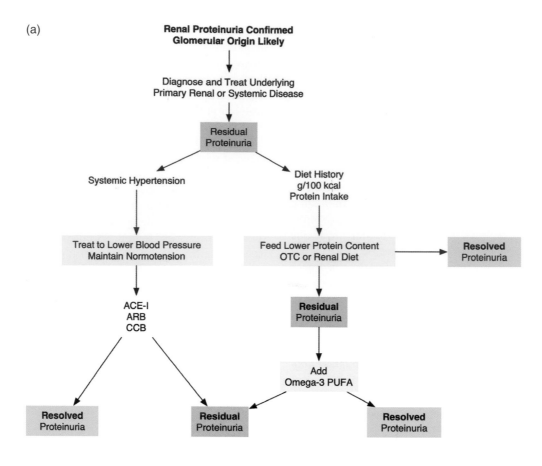

(b)

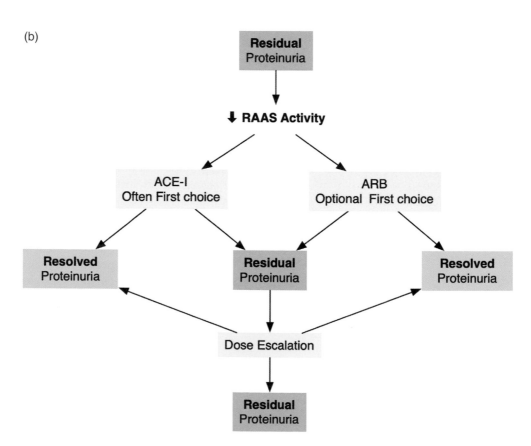

FIGURE 7.16 (Continued)

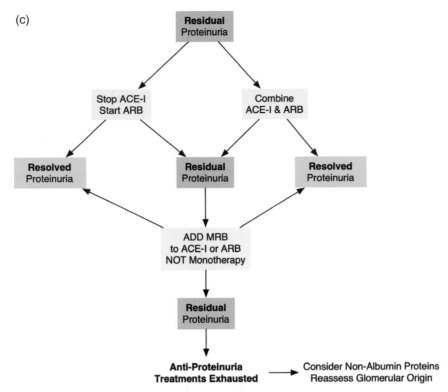

FIGURE 7.16   (a) An initial management approach to persistent renal proteinuria in those without hypoalbuminemia. Control of systemic hypertension often lessens glomerular proteinuria. The feeding of a lower protein content diet can result in decreased renal proteinuria and the addition of omega-3 PUFA mitigates glomerular proteinuria in some in some dogs and cats. Resolved proteinuria refers to a UPC that ideally has ideally decreased to <0.2, or from 0.2 to ≤0.4 in the cat and 0.2 to ≤0.5 in the dog. Alternatively, resolved proteinuria can refer to a decrease in UPC by at least 50% from the previously elevated baseline. See Figure 7.16b for treatment options in those that fail to substantially decrease proteinuria at this point. ACE-I — angiotensin converting enzyme inhibitor; ARB = angiotensin receptor blocker; CCB = calcium channel blocker; OTC = over the counter. (b) Possible treatment options for patients that have residual proteinuria after control of systemic hypertension, and after treatment with dietary modification and omega-3 PUFA. Dose escalation with either an ACE-I or an ARB frequently mitigates glomerular proteinuria. See Figure 7.16c for treatment options in patients that have residual proteinuria despite maximal doses of either an ACE-I or an ARB as monotherapy. RAAS = renin angiotensin aldosterone system; ACE-I = angiotensin converting enzyme inhibitor; ARB = angiotensin receptor blocker. (c) Possible scheme for treatment of residual proteinuria that persists following ACE-I or ARB as monotherapy. Switching treatment from an ACE-I to an ARB has more powerful effects to reduce glomerular proteinuria in some patients. Combining an ACE-I with an ARB can exert more proteinuria reduction than with either drug alone in some patients. When residual proteinuria exists at this point, consider adding in an MRB. It is important to follow the patient closely during combination therapy to ensure that dangerous hyperkalemia does not develop. If residual proteinuria is still apparent after various combinations of treatment with an ACE-I, ARB, and MRB, traditional antiproteinuric treatments have been exhausted. In these instances, it is possible that the renal proteinuria is comprised of mostly nonalbumin proteins. Sometimes it is not possible to adequately reduce the magnitude of renal proteinuria despite aggressive treatment designed to do so. Not shown in this figure is the potential anti-proteinuric effects of vitamin D metabolite treatment and those from SGLT inhibitor treatment (see text). ACE-I = angiotensin converting enzyme inhibitor; ARB = angiotensin receptor blocker; MRB = mineralocorticoid receptor blocker.

reduction in dietary protein can result in less glomerular proteinuria is discussed below.

The feeding of a renal diet is often the first treatment prescribed for those with IRIS stage 2, 3, and 4 CKD. This is usually prescribed for reasons other than targeted reduction in glomerular proteinuria, though this is one benefit that happens in some CKD patients often attributed to lower dietary protein intake [512, 516–519]. Standard "renal diets" for dogs typically provide approximately 3.0–4.0 g/100 kcal of dietary protein. Some early renal diets increase the dietary protein content to near 6.0 g/100 kcal, whereas maintenance diets can provide >14 g/100 kcal of protein content.

It is important to recognize that the definition of what comprises a "renal diet" is not standardized or accepted by all experts in this area. First-generation renal diets were usually defined on the degree of their protein restriction. There continues to be a trend to increase the amount of protein that can be safely fed to CKD patients while still maintaining a reduced intake of phosphorus. Commercially available renal diets continue to emerge with nutrient profiles that are not monolithic, particularly regarding higher protein content diet options that still provide reduced dietary phosphate intake. Additionally, some newer diets provide phosphorus restriction but with a less pronounced increase in the Ca:P ratio that is potentially important to lessen the emergence of hypercalcemia in some CKD patients, especially cats.

Renal diets are generally modified to a varying degree to be lower in content compared to maintenance diets based on a per 100 kcal basis of protein, phosphorus, and salt as well as increased in content of dietary omega-3 fatty acids, antioxidants, and bicarbonate precursors such as salts of citrate. However, since there are multiple nutrient changes in renal diets, it is not possible to know with certainty which change(s) in the nutrient profile is primarily responsible for any beneficial or harmful effects that occur in CKD patients due to the potential for multiple interactions between the nutrients that have been altered. Changes in nutrients other than dietary protein may be as important, or more so, in limiting the progression of CKD, as has been shown for the restriction of dietary phosphorus intake and supplementation with omega-3 dietary oils [86, 520].

There appears to be a link between high dietary phosphorus intake, an inverse Ca:P ratio <1.0 in the diet, the level of circulating phosphorus, phosphorus retention within the body, urinary phosphate levels, and glomerular proteinuria in those with and without CKD. High dietary phosphorus intake can lead to loss of glomerular barrier integrity and proteinuria following endothelial and vascular damage in association with decreased nitric oxide production. Proteinuria has been significantly related to the level of circulating phosphorus in humans and in experimental rodents in some studies [86, 521–523]. Higher serum and urinary phosphate levels lessened the antiproteinuric effect during low dietary protein intake in one study of human CKD [524]. High phosphorus intake resulted in a proximal tubulopathy associated with glucosuria and MA as well as decreased GFR in experimental cats of one study, presumably secondary to toxic effects of high tubular fluid phosphorus concentrations [84]. MA and the UAC significantly increased in addition to the detection of renal mineralization and increased PTH and FGF23 in cats consuming a high content of inorganic phosphate in the diet of another study. A potential contribution from increased PTH or FGF23 to the development of renal proteinuria in CKD could exist from the phosphaturic effects of these molecules that increase toxic concentrations of tubular fluid phosphorus [85]. A safe upper limit for dietary intake of the different phosphate salts in commercial foods has not been established for dogs and cats. Though no commercial pet food has yet been proven to create renal injury or CKD in dogs or cats, limiting the amount of highly soluble or highly biologically available phosphate salts in the diet seems to be a prudent consideration [86].

The feeding of higher dietary protein to normal animals and to those with various levels of reduction in nephron mass is generally associated with higher GFR, higher BUN despite higher GFR, and minor decreases or no change in serum creatinine. Adaptations within surviving nephrons contribute to increased transglomerular passage of plasma proteins, proteinuria, and progressive renal injury [103, 199, 327, 328, 356,

525–528]. Feeding of dietary protein in the form of meat may increase the serum creatinine concentration slightly independent of excretory renal function. The magnitude of these changes depends on the quantity, type, and digestibility of protein that was fed, the timing for the collection of blood samples following feeding, and the level of underlying renal function. An increased BUN following higher dietary protein intake occurs in healthy animals, but a greater magnitude of this increase appears to occur more frequently in animals with underlying renal disease and decreased GFR. See Chapter 1 for more details about the effects of diet on BUN and serum creatinine.

The feeding of a renal diet to animals with CKD has a variable effect on UPC and the progression of CKD. A reduction in dietary protein intake can improve glomerular hemodynamics that potentially slows the rate of CKD progression. The mechanism for this salutary dietary effect is not known with certainty, but it may involve less afferent arteriolar renal vasodilation following decreased dietary protein intake. The magnitude of glomerular proteinuria decreases by a variable degree following reduction of dietary protein intake with clinical or experimental CKD [328, 528]. It is important to note that findings from dietary treatment studies in dogs or cats with experimentally created CKD may not be directly applicable to those with spontaneous CKD, but conclusions from studies of experimental CKD provided the basis for development of renal diets to be prescribed for those with clinical CKD.

Experimental CKD in Dogs

Increased BUN without a change in serum creatinine was found following the feeding of higher dietary protein to CKD dogs with 75% reduction of nephron mass. Dogs with higher dietary protein intake had greater GFR at baseline that persisted after reduction in nephron mass for up to four years in these dogs. Proteinuria based on 24-hour excretion did not progressively increase over time and was not significantly related to amount of dietary protein [355, 356, 527]. The frequency and severity of glomerular lesions were highest in dogs consuming higher dietary protein, but overall, the lesions were graded as minimal by light microscopy. Ultrastructural evaluation revealed relatively minor renal lesions that were not related to the level of dietary protein intake or the level of renal function based on GFR. An increase in the number of mesangial cells and mesangial matrix along with GBM splitting and folding were the most commonly described ultrastructural lesions. There was no apparent relationship between renal lesions on light and ultrastructural microscopy with proteinuria or renal functional changes [356].

In dogs with surgically induced loss of nephron mass of another study [529], the feeding of a maintenance diet for 40 weeks resulted in higher mortality than in dogs fed diets with lower protein content. BUN was significantly higher in dogs consuming the maintenance diet compared to those eating protein-restricted diets. The ratio of BUN to serum creatinine was closely correlated with dietary protein intake and was highest in dogs consuming the maintenance diet. GFR did not progressively decrease over time in dogs of any dietary group in this study, but GFR was lower in dogs fed protein-restricted diets. Urinary protein excretion increased following nephron mass reduction and further increased over time in dogs consuming the maintenance diet but not for dogs consuming diets lower in protein content. Urinary protein excretion was lower in dogs consuming protein-restricted diets. It was concluded that the feeding of protein-restricted diets to CKD dogs mitigated renal proteinuria in this study [529].

Dogs with 11/12 nephrectomy were fed either a high-protein or moderate-protein diet for eight weeks [359]. GFR did not further decline over time in this study. GFR and the magnitude of proteinuria were increased in dogs consuming higher dietary protein. Proteinuria was generally higher in dogs with lower GFR. Renal lesions (glomerulosclerosis and interstitial inflammation) were observed in all dogs regardless of diet. Renal lesions were more severe in dogs consuming higher dietary protein, but the feeding of low dietary protein did not prevent the development of renal lesions [359].

The effect of feeding diets that varied by combinations of high or low protein with high or low phosphorus content was studied in dogs with 15/16 nephrectomy. Greater survival and longer periods of stability for GFR were found in dogs with lower intake of phosphorus, whereas dietary intake of protein had no effect. UPC increased over the 24 months of this study from about 1.0 at baseline to between 2.0 and 3.0, but there was no significant effect of dietary protein or phosphorus intake on the UPC. Numerically greater mean proteinuria was found in dogs fed higher dietary protein content, but this did not achieve statistical significance [200].

In another group of dogs with the remnant model of CKD, the feeding of a protein replete diet that was restricted in calcium and phosphorus was compared to the feeding of a diet replete in protein, calcium, and phosphorus for 24 months. GFR and survival were lower in dogs fed the fully replete diet. UPC was increased before dietary treatment was started and increased over time, but there was no effect of diet on urinary protein excretion [530].

GFR, renal plasma flow (RPF), and urinary protein excretion were studied in dogs with normal renal mass and those with 15/16 nephrectomy before and after the feeding of casein as a protein meal [525]. Increased GFR and RPF occurred in both groups of dogs 1.5–8 hours after the ingestion of the meal, with maximal increases documented at 4–5 hours. The magnitude of percentage increase in GFR and RPF over baseline was less in dogs with nephron mass loss, supporting the concept that dogs with loss of nephron mass have less renal reserve. A casein meal increased urinary protein excretion in dogs with severe reduction in nephron mass, but not in dogs with normal mass in this study [525]. In another study of dogs with 3/4 nephrectomy, dietary protein intake had no effect on the magnitude of proteinuria determined in 24 hour urine collection over 48 months [356].

Experimental CKD in Cats

Young female cats with 5/6 nephrectomy were compared to control cats and followed for one year in one study. Following renal mass reduction, GFR was reduced by two-third, whereas significant increases in systemic BP and proteinuria were found. GFR remained stable in all cats during the year of observation. GFR and proteinuria were significantly higher in all cats fed the higher protein/calorie diet, but no pattern for increasing proteinuria was found in any group of cats. Cats fed the higher protein diet consumed more calories than cats consuming the lower protein content from palatability differences in these formulations. GFR did not progressively decrease in cats with 5/6 nephrectomy regardless of diet fed. A significant increase in renal lesions (glomerulosclerosis and glomerular tuft adhesions) on light and electron microscopic evaluation was found in CKD cats eating the higher protein/calorie diet, similar to those described for rats and some studies of dogs with reduced renal mass. The feeding of diets restricted in protein/calories resulted in decreased proteinuria and less glomerular lesions. This model of reduced renal mass in cats did not show progression based on the reduction of GFR as has been reported in rats with severe reduction in renal mass [360]. Cats with induced azotemic CKD that were fed a low-protein diet had reduced serum urea nitrogen concentrations, despite lower GFRs, compared with cats with CKD fed a high-protein diet [531].

A similar lack of progression of CKD has been shown in some studies of dogs with remnant kidneys, as discussed previously, but progression with decrement in GFR has been shown in other studies of dogs [347, 357]. It is possible that reduction in GFR due to progressive CKD would be demonstrated if cats had been studied longer or if the degree of renal mass reduction were more severe [360].

Various combinations of high and low protein with high- and low-calorie diets were fed for one year to cats with CKD created by 11/12 nephrectomy in another study [361]. Glomerular lesions that developed were considered to be mild and were not affected by intake of protein, calories, or an interaction between the two. GFR was decreased following nephrectomy but did not further decrease over time in any diet treatment group. UPC significantly increased from baseline following the reduction of renal mass but did not increase further over time; all UPC remained in the reference range up to 0.3. Diets replete in protein had no effect on GFR, glomerular lesions, or nonglomerular lesions. Diets replete in calories were associated with a mild increase in nonglomerular lesions. Findings from this study challenged the conventional wisdom of feeding diets lower in protein content in an attempt to prevent the progression of CKD in cats [361].

Clinical CKD in Humans

The feeding of lower protein content diets to humans with CKD resulted in the reduction of proteinuria regardless of the baseline level of proteinuria in one study. The degree of proteinuria reduction at three months was similar to that obtained in CKD patients treated with ACE-I, achieving a mean maximal reduction of $47 \pm 27\%$ over baseline. Dietary protein restriction exerted beneficial effects to lower proteinuria regardless of whether ACE-I had been prescribed or not. It appeared that dietary modification was able to potentiate reduction in proteinuria when added to pharmacological intervention [532]. One meta-analysis of human CKD indicated that lower protein intake delayed progression and reduced mortality when compared to unrestricted dietary protein intake [533]. A later meta-analysis of human CKD compared dietary protein intake that was categorized as low, very low, or normal. Very low dietary protein intake decreased progression in those with advanced CKD so that there was less need for dialysis, whereas low dietary protein intake compared to normal intake had little effect on progression based on need for dialysis [534].

Clinical CKD in Dogs and Cats

A reduction in dietary protein intake is often successful in the reduction of proteinuria in nonazotemic dogs with PLN. It is important to avoid too much dietary protein restriction, as this can contribute to loss of lean muscle mass [516, 535], decreased body weight, and decreased serum albumin [519]. A detailed diet history that includes all food intake (commercial pet food, human food, and treats) is essential in determining the magnitude of dietary protein intake (g/100 kcal). If the dietary intake is high (g/100 kcal), reducing the protein intake by the elimination of treats or feeding of another nonrenal food with lower protein content may be effective in reducing the proteinuria. If the protein intake is already moderate or low, the feeding of a renal diet with further restriction of dietary protein may be needed to effect a decrease in proteinuria [516]. Renal proteinuria may undergo little or no reduction following the feeding of a renal diet or a lower protein content maintenance diet in some instances.

In one study of dogs with naturally occurring CKD and mean UPC > 1.0 at baseline, the feeding of a renal diet for 24 months did not result in a significant decline in UPC when compared to the feeding of a maintenance diet [336]. In a similar study of cats with CKD, there was no difference in the feeding of a renal diet compared to the feeding of a maintenance diet on UPC; cats in this study had mean UPC < 0.3 at all time points [337]. It is controversial as to the degree of protein restriction that should be prescribed for cats with CKD, if any, especially early in the disease process [536, 537].

The UPC decreased in 42 of 44 proteinuric CKD dogs after the feeding a renal diet for 30 days in another study. Median UPC significantly decreased from 2.9 at baseline to 2.2 at 30 days. Further reduction in UPC occurred 30 days after enalapril treatment was added to the feeding of a renal diet; this effect was not seen during the addition of benazepril treatment. Median BUN and serum creatinine also significantly decreased at 30 days of feeding a renal diet in this study [517].

Nonazotemic dogs with a UPC > 1.0 that presented to a teaching hospital were fed either a renal diet and benazepril or a maintenance diet and benazepril for 60 days. Proteinuria (measured by log UPC) significantly decreased in the group consuming the renal diet but not in dogs consuming the maintenance diet. The attribution of this effect to the diet could not be confirmed with analysis of variance, possibly due to few time points and small number of dogs evaluated. No evidence for malnutrition was documented during the feeding of the renal diet to this population of proteinuric dogs [518].

Diet greatly affected the magnitude of proteinuria in one study of X-linked HN in female carrier colony dogs with stable CKD. An approximate 2.5–3.0-fold increase in mean proteinuria was attributed largely to the consumption of high-protein-content diets (8.0 g/100 kcal protein) compared to the consumption of low content protein diets (3.3 g/100 kcal protein). Mean UPC was 2.5 at baseline while consuming a maintenance diet, mean UPC increased to 4.7 during consumption of higher protein intake, and mean UPC decreased to 1.8 during the consumption of the lower protein diet. Though lower protein content diets reduced the magnitude of proteinuria, some dogs were not able to maintain their body weight or serum albumin concentrations [519].

In another study of HN, the feeding of a renal diet resulted in less splitting of GBM in both affected males and carrier female Samoyeds when compared to the feeding of a maintenance diet. The feeding of the renal diet also delayed the progression of CKD in the affected males. Salutary effects may have been from more favorable glomerular hemodynamics during the feeding of renal diet, presumably from lower protein and phosphate intake. GFR was reduced in controls and carrier females during the feeding of this renal diet. Details about proteinuria were not provided, but it is expected that proteinuria would be greatest in those with the most glomerular splitting and less proteinuria would exist in dogs with less glomerular splitting [528].

Treatment with Dietary Polyunsaturated Fatty Acids

Omega-3 PUFA treatment for dogs with clinical glomerular disease is commonly recommended, either as that provided in renal diets or prescribed as dietary supplements for potential renoprotection, reduction in renal proteinuria, and antithrombic effects. However, there is little evidence in dogs with clinical glomerular disease as to the benefits of this treatment as a single treatment [136]. Studies in CKD dogs with subtotal nephrectomy showed dramatic differences in outcomes when dietary intake of fatty acids was fed as omega-3 PUFA (menhaden fish oil), omega-6 PUFA (safflower oil), or saturated fatty acids (beef tallow) for 20 months. Supplementation with omega-6 PUFA enhanced renal injury while supplementation with omega-3 provided renoprotection. CKD dogs fed fish oil had higher GFR, less proteinuria and lower serum creatinine, cholesterol, and triglycerides than those fed safflower oil or beef tallow. Histopathology revealed less mesangial expansion, glomerulosclerosis, and interstitial inflammation in CKD dogs fed fish oil. UPC was mildly increased in all dog groups following reduction in renal mass (mean: 0.24–0.31) prior to fatty acid supplementation. At 20 months, the mean UPC was 0.60 in dogs eating fish oil, which was significantly less than dogs eating safflower oil (mean UPC of 2.55) and dogs eating beef tallow (mean UPC of 1.76). This study provided a proof of concept that specific dietary oil supplementation could exert salutary effects in CKD dogs [520]. It should be noted that the intake of fish oil in this study was quite high at approximately 760 mg of eicosapentaenoic acid (EPA) and docosahexaenoic acid (DHA)/kg of $BW^{0.75}$, which is more than two times the National Research Council (NRC) safe upper limit [538]. In the same model of CKD dogs, early effects of dietary fatty acids were studied for two months following the reduction of renal mass [539]. Low-content PUFA in the diet was compared to that supplemented with omega-3 (fish oil) or omega-6 (safflower oil). Greater damaging effects seen during omega-6 supplementation were related to an increased degree of glomerular hypertension, glomerular hypertrophy, and excretion of urinary eicosanoids. Decreased cholesterol and triglycerides during the feeding of fish oil were seen early in this study as previously shown in the 20-month study. Mean UPC following nephron mass reduction was 0.23–0.35 among groups prior to dietary change. Mean UPC increased by the end of the feeding study (0.68–0.77 by group), but there was no significant effect of different dietary fatty acid intake on UPC at this early time point.

Current recommendations for the treatment of glomerular disease and renal proteinuria are to feed a diet with an n-6 to n-3 PUFA ratio of approximately 5:1, as is often provided in commercially manufactured renal diets [136]. It has not yet been determined whether the ratio or the total absolute dose of dietary PUFA delivered is more important in determining outcomes [540]. An expert panel recommended supplementation with n-3 PUFA given at a dosage of 250–500 mg/kg of animal of body weight to maintenance diets by owners. Supplementation to renal diets has not been studied. DHA and EPA are the forms of n-3 PUFA specifically recommended to supplement the diet for dogs with glomerular disease. When PUFA has been supplemented to the diet, it is also recommended to add vitamin E at a dose of 1.1 IU/g of fish oil as an antioxidant [136].

General dose recommendations of EPA and DHA for dogs are 50–75 mg (EPA + DHA)/kg body weight, up to 140 mg EPA + DHA per $kg(BW)^{0.75}$ [512]. A general dose has been made at 30–50 mg/kg for cats [541]. This general dose is lower than the dosage recommended for patients with renal disease. One author recommends starting at 140 mg per $kg(BW)^{0.75}$ for dogs with renal disease, followed by dose escalation as needed up to the NRC safe upper limit for dogs of 370 mg per $kg(BW)^{0.75}$ depending on the severity of the condition [538]. The safe upper limit can also be expressed as 2.8 g/1000 kcal of DHA + EPA for dogs [541]. Over-the-counter fish oils vary widely in the concentrations of DHA and EPA [516] and can have other oils that are not beneficial. Fish oil is recommended over flax seed oil as dogs do not reliably convert plant-based

fatty acids to EPA and DHA. The dose for the supplementation of omega-3 should be adjusted based on the amount of omega-3 already in the diet [512, 516].

Role of Vitamin D

Hypovitaminosis D based on the assessment of various vitamin D metabolites has been associated with CKD in dogs, but the mechanisms as to how this develops are not clear. Greater decreases in vitamin D metabolite status have been reported in dogs as renal disease becomes more severe based on increasing IRIS stage [349, 542, 543]. One mechanism that could account for low circulating vitamin D metabolite status is increased urinary loss of vitamin D metabolites bound to VDBP or albumin that occur following failed tubular reabsorption in patients with CKD and proteinuria. Hypovitaminosis D also has the potential to influence the development and magnitude of renal proteinuria during CKD. This may be accounted for in some part by decreased activation of various VDR within renal tissue that is required for normal function, including that for normal podocytes to limit proteinuria [544]. In an early study of azotemic CKD dogs, serum 25(OH) vitamin D concentrations were negatively associated with UPC [542]. In another study, dogs with serum creatinine <1.4 mg/dL and UPC > 0.5 were associated with significantly lower concentrations of vitamin D metabolites (25(OH)-vitamin D, 24,25(OH)$_2$-vitamin D, and 1,25(OH)$_2$-vitamin D) compared to normal control dogs. The median UPC was 4.8 (1.7–27.5) in the proteinuric dogs compared to the normal control group with median UPC 0.1 (0.1–0.1). The urinary 25(OH)-vitamin D-to-urinary-creatinine ratio was positively correlated with the UPC and negatively correlated with serum albumin. Serum 24,25(OH)$_2$ vitamin D was negatively correlated with the UPC. Though serum 25(OH)-vitamin D declined as UPC increased, this did not achieve statistical significance (P = 0.06). There was an estimated 2.6% decrease in 25(OH)-vitamin D, 2.0% decrease in 1,25(OH)2-vitamin D, and a 4.3% decrease in 24,25(OH)2-vitamin D for each increase of 10% in UPC in this study [544]. It appears that renal proteinuria of higher levels is associated with a greater reduction in vitamin D metabolites during CKD, as concentrations of vitamin D metabolites were not significantly associated with UPC in azotemic and nonazotemic CKD dogs with a median UPC of 0.6 in another study. Significantly decreased concentrations of vitamin D metabolites developed only for IRIS CKD stages 3 and 4 in this study [543]. Studies of vitamin D metabolite repletion regarding possible mitigation of renal proteinuria, CKD progression, or mortality have yet to be reported [544].

PHARMACEUTICAL THERAPY

Overview

The classic view of the RAAS system emphasizes the generation of the octapeptide AG-II as the single biologically active molecule following a series of proteolytic enzyme reactions, starting with angiotensinogen (Figure 7.17). AG-II is generated

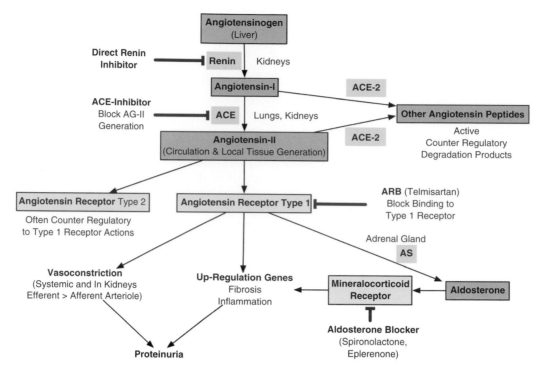

FIGURE 7.17 Classic pathways for activation of the renin–angiotensin–aldosterone system (RAAS) are emphasized in this figure (angiotensinogen to angiotensin-I to angiotensin-II). Damage to tissues is mediated following binding of excess angiotensin-II to the angiotensin type 1 receptor. Aldosterone also contributes to inflammation and fibrosis following binding to the mineralocorticoid receptor. Thick red lines show where drugs interact to decrease or block the degree of RAAS activation. These pathways are most widely recognized as a systemic response, but the same machinery and cascade happens within the kidneys (and other tissues). Newer components of the RAAS system including ANG (1–7) and alamandine which have important actions on kidney function and disease have been reviewed, but not detailed here. Source: Ames et al. [545]; Adin et al. [546]; Simoes and Teixeira [367]; Spencer et al. [547]; Santos et al. [548]; Malinowski and St Jean [549]; Goodfriend et al. [550]; Lefebvre et al. [551]; Polzin and Cowgill [509]; Vaden and Elliott [7]; Patel et al. [552]. Note: ACE – angiotensin converting enzyme; ACE-2 – angiotensin converting enzyme 2; AG-II – angiotensin-II; ARB – angiotensin receptor blocker; MR – mineralocorticoid receptor; AS – aldosterone synthase.

following the action of angiotensin-converting enzyme (ACE) on angiotensin-I [553]. AG-II can also be generated by ACE-independent chymase pathways [550]. AG-II causes preferential vasoconstriction of the efferent arteriole and enhances proximal tubular reabsorption of sodium as two major effects in the kidney; an additional effect is to inhibit renin release from the JGA [549]. It has become increasingly apparent that several other molecules are generated along this pathway that exert biologically important activity. The most important among these appears to be angiotensin 1–7 that is generated from angiotensin-I or AG-II following angiotensin II converting enzyme 2 (ACE2) activity. Angiotensin 1–7 interacts with its own receptor (Mas receptor) to provide important counter-regulatory actions that lessen the potentially deleterious effects of AG-II during RAAS activation. Decreased activity of ACE2 results in disease progression due to unopposed activity of AG-II leading to vasoconstriction, cell proliferation and hypertrophy, and fibrosis [548, 552].

Renin–angiotensin–aldosterone system inhibition (RAAS-I) is added as treatment when dietary change has not sufficiently decreased the magnitude of the proteinuria based on UPC (Figure 7.18). RAAS inhibition is the cornerstone

treatment designed to mitigate glomerular proteinuria in human medicine [23]. Decreased efferent arteriolar tone following RAAS inhibition using ACE-I or ARB reduces single-nephron GFR and transglomerular pressure as a renoprotective measure that counters glomerular hyperfiltration and proteinuria. Hyperfiltration in remnant nephrons (compensatory adaptation) occurs as the consequence of modulating the vascular tone of both the afferent and efferent arterioles. Efferent arteriolar constriction follows effects from increased AG-II and afferent arteriolar dilatation occurs from unknown mediators in remnant nephrons. Both of these changes increase single-nephron GFR and transglomerular capillary pressure, which are helpful to increase excretory renal function, but are chronically maladaptive as this contributes to further nephron loss and enhanced glomerular proteinuria [23].

RAAS-I for CKD patients without renal proteinuria has not been routinely recommended despite other mechanisms for renal damage from AG-II and aldosterone not directly related to proteinuria (Figure 7.19) [545]. The RAAS cascade has been reviewed in detail by others for the interested reader [326, 367, 545, 546, 551, 552, 555].

ACE-I Treatment Glomerular Proteinuria

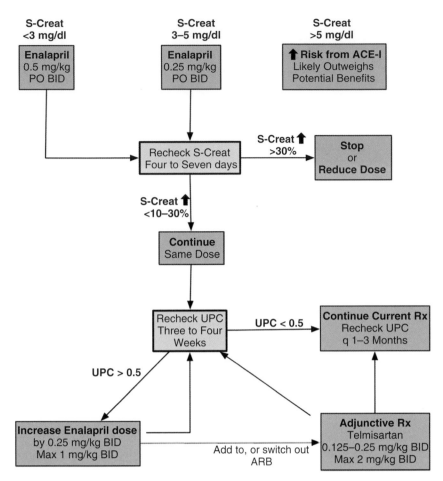

FIGURE 7.18   Potential treatment plan designed to reduce glomerular proteinuria using enalapril as an ACE-I to inhibit the RAAS in patients with CKD. In this algorithm, the initial dose of ACE-I is based on the baseline serum creatinine. Lower initial doses are suggested for patients with more severe azotemia on the premise that these patients are more likely to have adverse effects following reduction of intraglomerular pressures and reduction in GFR that then cause increases in serum creatinine. Patients that have a dramatic decrease in transglomerular pressure will have more severe increases in serum creatinine. RAAS – renin angiotensin aldosterone system; ACE-I – angiotensin converting enzyme inhibitor; ARB – angiotensin receptor blocker. Source: Adapted from Pressler [326], #669.

High concentrations of AG-II and aldosterone exert harmful effects in the heart, vessels, and kidneys during sustained RAAS activity. Harmful effects can occur from AG-II or aldosterone from the circulation or from that locally generated within tissues. The kidneys contain the complete apparatus for local generation of AG-II and aldosterone, and enhanced RAAS activity within the kidney is known to occur in the dog and cat with CKD [7, 325, 363, 510, 545, 547]. Enhanced intrarenal RAAS signals and activity within the kidneys is a characteristic of CKD and is important in the progression of CKD [550, 556]. AG-II exerts many effects beyond its well-known hemodynamic effects as it functions as a cytokine that promotes renal growth, fibrosis, and inflammation. High levels of AG-II are generated within renal tissue independent of systemic RAAS activity that contributes to these adverse effects of advancing CKD [41, 554].

Reduction in RAAS activity confers benefits to the kidneys of dogs and cats with CKD following some combination of reduction in systemic and intraglomerular BP that translates into a decrease in the magnitude of glomerular proteinuria. These desired outcomes with effective treatment help to preserve renal tissue and renal functions. Nonhemodynamic effects of RAAS-I may also contribute to reduction in glomerular proteinuria by reducing angiotensin II-induced mesangial cell proliferation, reducing production of proinflammatory and profibrotic cytokines, in addition to increasing renal vasodilation with preferential effect on the efferent arterioles [41, 322, 325, 545, 551, 557–559].

The preferential dilation of the efferent arteriole decreases glomerular capillary pressure and glomerular proteinuria [41, 545]. In a model of rats with glomerular proteinuria treated with lisinopril, tight junction proteins in the

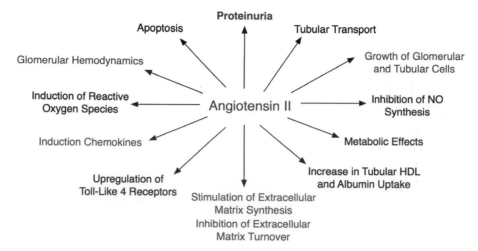

FIGURE 7.19 Effects of Angiotensin-II in renal disease. Angiotensin-II is a cytokine with many damaging effects on the kidney, beyond its classically known function as a hemodynamic mediator. Not shown are the damaging renal effects of the mineralocorticoid aldosterone during RAAS activation in CKD, many of which are difficult to separate out from those created by Angiotensin-II. NO = nitric oxide; HDL = high density lipoprotein; RAAS = renin angiotensin aldosterone system; CKD = chronic kidney disease; SNFGR – single nephron GFR. Source: Adapted from Ruster and Wolf [554] and Spencer et al. [547].

podocyte slit pore membranes were stabilized [560]. In another study, lisinopril conferred renal functional and structural benefits by preventing further loss of podocytes and promotion of the podocyte repopulation [561].

The suppression of RAAS activity is targeted during treatment with ACE-I (such as enalapril, benazepril, lisinopril, and ramipril), ARBs (such as telmisartan), and mineralocorticoid receptor antagonists (MRAs) (such as spironolactone or eplerenone) as single agents or in some combination (Table 7.6) [545]. Hemodynamic changes (decreased glomerular pressure, decreased single-nephron GFR, and decreased transglomerular driving pressure) are thought to largely account for the reduction in glomerular proteinuria [2, 7, 105, 106, 325, 326]. The suppression of RAAS activity (ACE-I most commonly, ARB occasionally, and MRA rarely) is considered standard of care for dogs with glomerular disease to reduce the magnitude of proteinuria as a therapeutic target [7, 326, 509, 545]. A decline of UPC to <0.5 is an optimal target, but if that is not readily achieved, a reduction of UPC to less than 50% of baseline is an alternative target [136, 509].

ACE-I and ARB Treatment

Escalating doses of ACE-I are generally prescribed to effect as the first line of pharmacological treatment to reduce glomerular proteinuria. ARBs are sometimes added to ACE-I treatment when the degree of proteinuria reduction has been inadequate on ACE-I alone if systemic BP is currently well controlled. The effectiveness and safety of combination therapy with ACE-I and ARB for the control of proteinuria in veterinary patients with or without CKD is starting to emerge (see later) [509, 545]. Alternatively, ARB can be used to replace ACE-I to gain control of glomerular proteinuria, as was described in one dog with

persistent high UPC despite normal systemic BP and high doses of ACE-I [565]. The addition of MRA (spironolactone, eplerenone) to ACE-I or ARB can be considered to lessen residual proteinuria, but this has not been reported in clinical dogs or cats [509].

The use of ACE-I for control of systemic hypertension in cats was not recommended by an expert panel. The small decrease in systemic BP that is achieved during the use of ACE-I in cats with systemic hypertension is not likely to be adequate for most cats [557]. When the UPC does not adequately decrease following calcium channel blocker (CCB) treatment for hypertension in cats, treating the residual proteinuria with the addition of ACE-I may be effective to further reduce the UPC and is well tolerated [372].

Enalapril

Enalapril (an ACE-I) suppresses the classical RAAS pathway while enhancing the alternative RAAS pathway in dogs [545, 546]. Aldosterone breakthrough was common during enalapril treatment, especially in dogs that were positive for the ACE gene polymorphism of one study [546].

Enalapril treatment conferred benefits over placebo to CKD dogs with biopsy proven idiopathic GN, UPC > 3.0, and serum creatinine <3.0 mg/dL in one study. At six months, UPC had significantly declined compared to baseline in dogs treated with enalapril, whereas the UPC increased in dogs treated with placebo. Dogs treated with enalapril were more often categorized as improved or stable compared to those that progressively worsened based on some combination of serum creatinine and UPC over time [325].

The effect of enalapril treatment compared to placebo was studied in a small number of Samoyed male puppies affected with X linked HN. Enalapril treated dogs lived

Table 7.6 Management of glomerular proteinuria using oral drugs to inhibit RAAS activity.

Class	Drug	Initial dose[a]	Escalating dose[b]
ACE-I[c]	Benazepril	0.25–0.50 mg/kg PO q24h Dog and Cat	Increase by 0.5 mg/kg per day to a maximum daily dose of 2.0 mg/kg divided q12h
	Enalapril	0.25–0.50 mg/kg PO q24h Dog and Cat	Increase by 0.5 mg/kg per day to a maximum daily dose of 2.0 mg/kg divided q12h
	Lisinopril	0.25–0.5 mg/kg PO q24 hr. Dog and Cat	Increase by 0.25–0.5 mg/kg/day to a maximum daily dose of 2 mg/kg divided q12h
	Ramipril	0.125 mg/kg PO q24h Dog	Increase by 0.125 mg/kg to a maximum daily dose of 0.5 mg/kg q24h; usually given q24h
	Imidapril	0.25 mg/kg PO q 24 hr. Dog	Increase by 0.25 mg/kg q24h to a maximal daily dose of 5 mg/kg; usually given q24h
ARB[c,d] (Blocks AT-1 Receptor)	Telmisartan[e,f]	1–3 mg/kg if nonazotemic; maximum of 5 mg/kg 0.5 mg/kg if azotemic PO q24h Dog and Cat	Increase by 0.25–0.5 mg/kg to a maximal daily dose of 3 mg/kg usually given q24h
MRB[g]	Spironolactone	0.5–2 mg/kg PO q12–24h Dog	None
	Eplerenone – second generation	No clinical protocol	No clinical protocol
	Finerenone – third generation	No clinical protocol	No clinical protocol

Note: RAAS = renin angiotensin aldosterone system; ACE-I = angiotensin converting enzyme inhibitor; ARB = angiotensin receptor blocker; AT-1 = angiotensin-1 subtype for angiotensin-II receptor; MRB = mineralocorticoid blocker (aldosterone blocker).

[a] These drugs should not be used in patients that are dehydrated or with systemic hypotension; they are usually prescribed when the CKD patient is considered stable. Generally, the lower dose is chosen during the initial treatment of patients with IRIS CKD stages 3 and 4 in order to see how well the patient tolerates the drug and if excretory renal function remains stable based on serum creatinine, BUN, and or SDMA. The initial dose may need to be reduced or terminated if the animal or their kidney function does not tolerate the drug.

[b] Dose escalation is titrated to an endpoint for the reduction of UPC to a level that is normal or has decreased from overtly proteinuric to borderline proteinuric. Otherwise, a minimal goal is at least a 50% reduction from the initial baseline UPC. Dose escalation may need to be terminated if a decrease in excretory renal function (increased BUN, serum creatinine, and SDMA) is severe following these treatments. Not all patients undergo successful resolution of renal proteinuria. See text for more details.

[c] ACE-I and ARB are generally considered to exert weak antihypertensive effects as single agents, so higher doses may be needed in those with renal proteinuria and systemic hypertension. Alternatively, standard doses may be successfully used when more a powerful antihypertensive treatment is given concurrently, such as with the calcium channel blocker (CCB) amlodipine.

[d] ARB can be used as a single agent, or in combination with an ACE-I.

[e] The dose of telmisartan is different for treatment of hypertension in cats than during its use for proteinuria control. The FDA licensed dosing for treatment of hypertension in cats is listed at 1.5 mg/kg BID for two weeks and then 2 mg/kg q 24 hours.

[f] The ARB losartan was often administered as an addition to an ACE-I, historically. It is no longer recommended due to inadequate clinical effect in dogs. It exhibits low bioavailability PO, and low tissue distribution due to high protein binding [562].

[g] MRB can be considered in those that have not tolerated or failed to have a protein-lowering effect from an ACE-I or ARB. MRB are usually used as an add-on rather than as a single agent.Source: Polzin and Cowgill [509]; Lefebvre et al. [551]; Dibartola and Westropp [59]; Brown et al. [136]; Vaden and Elliott [7], Christ et al. [562]; Baek et al. [563]; Caro-Vadillo et al. [564]; Bugbee et al. [565]; Glaus et al. [566]; Coleman et al. [567]; Sent et al. [568],. See Figure 7.16, algorithms showing sequential pathways for the treatment of renal proteinuria.

1.36 longer than untreated dogs, had a slower increase in serum creatinine, slower decline in GFR, slower rate of increase in UPC, and less GBM splitting early in the disease process during evaluation from 4 to 40 weeks of age [236].

Benazepril

In a study of dogs with spontaneous CKD, benazepril was associated with a decreased UPC, decreased systemic BP, and increased GFR after 180 days of treatment [339]. Benazepril decreased UPC in cats with CKD, but an increased survival benefit was not demonstrated in one study [344]. In another study of CKD cats, UPC was 0.4 ± 0.8 at baseline and was not different by IRIS CKD stage [206]. Benazepril treatment significantly decreased UPC compared to placebo over time, but this treatment was not associated with increased survival time regardless of baseline proteinuria. A renal diet was fed to most cats in both groups. This decrease in UPC occurred at all levels of proteinuria during treatment with benazepril even in cats with a UPC < 0.2, but the greatest reduction in UPC occurred in those with higher UPC [344]. An increased UPC at baseline in untreated CKD cats was a significant and independent risk factor for shorter renal survival time. CKD cats with a baseline UPC < 0.2 lived the longest and those with a UPC > 1.0 or > 0.4 had the shortest survival time [167, 206]. Increased UPC, increased plasma phosphate, and anemia predicted which azotemic CKD cats would increase their serum creatinine by ≥25% over baseline within the next year in another study. Progression occurred in 47% of these cats. The median UPC in those that were stable was 0.14 and 0.27 in CKD cats that progressed [340].

Cats with CKD treated with placebo developed an increased UPC over time, whereas the UPC did not increase in those treated with benazepril [343]. The UPC was significantly lower at days 120 and 180 of benazepril treatment compared to placebo. Cats in IRIS CKD stage 2 or 3 progressed less frequently to CKD stage 4 when treated with benazepril. There were no differences in survival time detected during the six months of this study [343].

Telmisartan

Selective AT-1 ARBs are potentially superior to ACE-Is since alternate pathways exist that can allow escape from ACE-I to continue the generation of AG-II and aldosterone.

Dogs with azotemic CKD and a UPC > 0.5 or those that were nonazotemic with a UPC ≥ 1.0 were prospectively treated with either telmisartan (1.0 mg/kg SID) or enalapril (0.5 mg/kg BID) up to 120 days in an attempt to mitigate renal proteinuria. Dose escalation occurred at days 30 and 60 if the UPC were still > 0.5. The decrease in UPC at 30 days was significantly greater for telmisartan (−65%) compared to enalapril (−35%). More dogs had a ≥50% reduction from baseline UPC when treated with telmisartan (80% of dogs) compared to enalapril (35.3% of dogs) at 30 days. A greater antiproteinuria effect was seen during dose escalation with telmisartan than with enalapril. Telmisartan had significantly greater antiproteinuric effects

than enalapril at days 60 and 90 in dogs that were still proteinuric (UPC > 0.5) at day 30. Nearly all dogs treated with telmisartan experienced a decrease in UPC, whereas 24% of dogs treated with enalapril had increases in UPC. Combination therapy (dual-RAAS blockade) further lowered proteinuria at day 120 in those that had a UPC > 0.5 at day 90. UPC was reduced in all of these instances and UPC converted to ≤0.5 in 44% of the dogs that tolerated this treatment. However, clinically relevant azotemia developed in 31% of these dogs during the first seven days of dual-RAAS blockade, raising concerns for AKI. It was suggested that lower dose regimens for dual-RAAS blockade could still mitigate renal proteinuria without creating azotemia, but this was not studied. The greater magnitude of proteinuria reduction during the use of telmisartan is likely attributed to greater RAAS inhibition with an ARB compared to an ACE-I. A significantly greater reduction in systolic BP was seen in dogs treated with telmisartan than with enalapril, which can also lessen glomerular proteinuria. There was no difference in the safety profile (escalation in serum creatinine or potassium or decreases in serum sodium) between single treatment with telmisartan or enalapril in this study but clinically relevant azotemia requiring hospitalization occurred in 31% of dog undergoing dual treatment. It was concluded that telmisartan could be a first line choice in the control of renal proteinuria in dogs [569, 570].

The use of an ACE-I (enalapril or benazepril) alone, telmisartan alone, or an ACE-I in combination with telmisartan was compared for efficacy in the control of system hypertension and renal proteinuria in dogs with PLN in a retrospective study. Dual-RAAS blockade resulted in significantly lower systolic BP compared to monotherapy with an ACE-I (mean marginal systolic BP was 13 mmHg lower). There was no difference in the magnitude of UPC reduction between telmisartan and ACE-I used as single therapy in this study, but UPC reduction was significantly greater during dual-RAAS blockade than during telmisartan or ACE-I alone. Mean marginal UPC decreased by 2.5 during dual therapy compared to that during ACE-I alone and by 3.8 compared to telmisartan alone. An increase in serum potassium was found in 46.3% of dogs treated with ACE-I alone, in 51.2% of dogs treated with dual-RAAS blockade, and in 28% of dogs with telmisartan alone, but these increases were typically of small magnitude. Treatment was stopped due to the development of hyperkalemia in only one dog with a mild increase in serum potassium at 6.2 mEq/L during dual-RAAS blockade [571].

The combination of telmisartan with amlodipine was successful in control of systemic BP after the combination of benazepril and amlodipine had failed to control BP in a small series of dogs. UPC did not decrease in any of these dogs despite control of systemic BP [564]. Telmisartan treatment was given to 28 dogs with IRIS stage 1 and 2 CKD and proteinuria (>0.5 UPC) at baseline in an open-label study with no placebo control group. The median UPC was 4.4 (1.3–12.8) at baseline. UPC, UAC, and systolic BP significantly decreased at days 45 and 120 while on treatment. UPC decreased by 50% or more from baseline in 36% of the dogs at day 45 and in 61% of dogs at day 120. At day 120, 10 of 28 dogs had a UPC < 1.0 and a UPC < 0.5 was achieved in six of these dogs. Return to normal BP was achieved at day 120 in 10 of 17 dogs with systemic hypertension at baseline [572].

Nonazotemic dogs with UPC ≥ 2.0 and azotemic dogs with UPC ≥ 0.5 were treated with either telmisartan alone (44), telmisartan plus benazepril (5), or telmisartan with mycophenolate (7) in a retrospective study. UPC declined to < 0.5 or by ≥ 50% from baseline in those treated with telmisartan in 70% of dogs at 1 month, 68% at 3 months, 80% at 6 months, and 60% at 12 months of follow-up. A partial response with a decreased in UPC ≥ 50% was more common than a complete response to a UPC ≤ 0.5. Adverse effects of treatment were minor except in two dogs that developed clinically important azotemia (> 30% increase over baseline serum creatinine) that necessitated discontinuation of treatment. Telmisartan alone or in combination was considered effective in control of renal proteinuria in this study [573].

Telmisartan is also effective for the treatment of systemic hypertension and glomerular proteinuria in cats [326, 566, 567]. Telmisartan is licensed to reduce proteinuria associated with CKD in cats in Europe [372], and for cats with systemic hypertension in the USA (many of whom also have CKD and proteinuria). Telmisartan was found to be noninferior for the mitigation of proteinuria in CKD cats when compared to benazepril. Telmisartan decreased proteinuria at all times points in these cats, whereas benazepril did not [568]. Telmisartan can be effective in lowering systemic BP, but its effect in cats with severe increases in BP has not been determined. Extra caution and monitoring should be used if ACE-I and ARB are concurrently administered, as there can be an acute increase in serum creatinine due to greater decreases in GFR [372].

Mineralocorticoid Receptor Blockers

The mineralocorticoid receptor (MR) is expressed in a variety of tissues including the kidneys. The MR is a cytosolic receptor that moves to the cell nucleus once activated. MRs are expressed in nearly all parts of the kidneys, including podocytes and mesangial cells that can be important in the generation of glomerular proteinuria. An increased expression of MR is common in many types of CKD and increased aldosterone binding to this receptor promotes proinflammatory and profibrotic pathways, similar to that following AG-II binding to its receptor AT1. Proteinuria is enhanced during MR activation from increased levels of aldosterone. MR activation contributes to podocyte injury and proteinuria following less expression of nephrin and podocin. MRBs have the ability to reduce proteinuria, fibrosis, and inflammation in rodents and patients with differing forms of CKD, often after they are added to ACE-I or ARB treatments [545, 547, 555, 574].

The activation of the MR following aldosterone binding exerts classical physiological effects that enhance renal sodium reabsorption and potassium excretion by the renal collecting tubule. Enhanced renal reabsorption of sodium can contribute to hypertension and renal damage, but chronic MR activation promotes progressive CKD in studies of experimental animals and in humans by other mechanisms that are likely to be more important. AG-II upregulates the genes for aldosterone synthesis (Figure 7.17). Many of the processes and mechanisms creating renal damage appear to be similar to those induced by AG-II making it difficult to know for sure how much of the renal injury is from excess aldosterone or AG-II. The intrarenal generation of aldosterone can be independent from circulating aldosterone, similar to that observed for intrarenal generation and effects of AG-II. MR activation on blood vessels alters the structure and function of endothelial cells and vascular smooth muscle, leading to impaired vasodilatation, vasoconstriction, and renal injury from renal hypoxia [547].

MR activation by excess aldosterone is important in the pathogenesis and progression of CKD via increased inflammation, fibrosis, mesangial hyperplasia with increased mesangial matrix, and oxidative stress in the kidney [553, 555, 575]. MR activation in endothelium, smooth muscle, podocytes, inflammatory cells, and podocytes within renal tissue can cause structural renal damage, decreased renal functions, and proteinuria. The progression of CKD was attributed to nontumorous hyperaldosteronism in one study of cats [576]. Six of 11 elderly cats had hypokalemia at initial diagnosis and 2 others had hypokalemia later, which could have also have contributed to the CKD progression.

MRBs lessen the degree of renal injury and fibrosis during CKD, reduce the degree of proteinuria in CKD, lessen glomerular hemodynamic adaptations (decreased vasoconstrictors and increased vasodilators), reduce altered glomerular hemodynamics, and reduce the magnitude of systemic hypertension [577]. Increased aldosterone activity is inversely proportional to GFR during CKD [574]. RAAS inhibition with ACE-I or ARB that decrease generation or the effect of AG-II may not adequately lessen aldosterone generation at the same time [555, 578].

To more fully suppress the RAAS, treatment with MRB (aldosterone antagonists or mineralocorticoid antagonists MRA) is usually added to ACE-I or ARB treatment, rather than being used as a single agent [509, 545, 546]. It should be noted that the treatment role for MRA alone or in combination with ACE-I or ARB for control of systemic hypertension or renal proteinuria in dogs and cats with naturally occurring CKD has not been established [545]. It is clear that MRB limit the progression of CKD in humans [555, 577] but these effects have not been specifically studied in dogs or cats with CKD.

Spironolactone is a first-generation MRB that also binds to androgen and progesterone receptors. Eplerenone is a more selective but less potent second-generation MRB and finerenone is a third-generation nonsteroidal MRB that is highly selective, potent, and exerts the most renoprotective effects. Third-generation nonsteroidal MRB (esaxerenone, apararenone, and finerenone) appear to provide optimal benefits to human patients with CKD with lower chances of creating hyperkalemia compared to earlier generation MRBs (spironolactone and eplerenone) [555, 574].

Finerenone exhibited greater anti-inflammatory and antifibrotic effects during the treatment of CKD in preclinical studies in humans than that by earlier generation steroidal MRBs such as spironolactone or eplerenone. Finerenone further decreased albuminuria in human diabetic patients already on treatment with an ACE-I or ARB [575, 579]. MRBs have shown benefits in diabetic and nondiabetic CKD as well as during nephrotoxic AKI [555, 574]. The addition of steroidal MRB to ACE-I or ARB reduced proteinuria or albuminuria by a weighted mean of 38.7% in one meta-analysis of humans with CKD [580]. Finenerone reduced proteinuria by 31% compared to placebo in a study of humans with diabetes and CKD on maximal doses of ACE-I or ARB [575]. Some of the reduction in renal proteinuria may be conferred by decreased BP while on MRB [580].

Aldosterone breakthrough refers to the escalation of aldosterone levels following initial suppression during treatment with ACE-I or ARB. It has been estimated that aldosterone breakthrough occurs in as many as one-third of dogs with renal proteinuria treated with ACE-I or ARB [547]. Consequently, additional treatment with MRB should be considered in some cases to maintain adequate RAAS-I.

RAAS-I Treatment Contraindications and Side Effects

The use of ACE-I in CKD dogs and cats is infrequently associated with adverse effects such as systemic hypotension, sudden and sustained increases in serum creatinine, and hyperkalemia. Treatment with ACE-I or ARB predictably decreases intraglomerular pressure following the dilatation of the efferent arteriole [331, 372]. This is due to a combination of less AG-II generated to interact with the AT receptor and AG-II having less ability to interact with its receptor. An increase in serum creatinine following treatment with antihypertensive drugs can occur in animals with CKD due to some combination of decreased systemic and intraglomerular BP. A small and nonprogressive increase in serum creatinine sometimes occurs, but this is usually well tolerated by the dog or cat. ACE-I or ARB should not be administered to hypertensive dogs or cats or those with CKD that have proteinuria and normotension if they are currently dehydrated. Otherwise, there is increased risk for an acute increase in serum creatinine from decreased GFR [331, 372].

Regardless of the antihypertensive agent or class, decreases in systemic BP can result in the generation of less glomerular BP and filtration during CKD (prerenal effects). Similarly, greater intraglomerular BP and a lower serum creatinine can develop during the presence of systemic hypertension during CKD. This allows a greater fraction of high systemic BP to be transmitted to the glomerular vessels due to failed autoregulation, resulting in a higher single-nephron GFR [332, 369, 581]. Decreased single-nephron GFR does not always accompany decreased intraglomerular pressure during RAAS-I due to mesangial relaxation and an increase in glomerular surface area that helps maintain GFR [105, 106]. Consequently, the offsetting effect of reduced intraglomerular pressure and increased glomerular surface area on GFR minimizes increases in serum creatinine during treatment with ACE-I or ARB. Serum creatinine increases are usually <0.5 mg/dL and tolerated by the animal when ACE-I agents are administered to stable hydrated patients that are not in heart failure [331]. The impact of ACE-I on serum creatinine in dogs with heart disease or heart failure was considered to be minimal in one review, unless hypotension was evident from the use of some combination of diuretics, sodium restriction, and vasodilators [545]. The safety of short-term treatment with a combination of benazepril and spironolactone was demonstrated in normal dogs before and during a furosemide continuous rate infusion. Increased creatinine at 24 hours following furosemide infusion was attributed to dehydration and reduced renal perfusion pressure [582].

General guidelines in human cardiology and nephrology have suggested that increases in serum creatinine of ≤30% over baseline are generally acceptable and provide some indication that the desired end point of decreased glomerular driving pressures has been achieved [369]. Adverse cardiac and renal outcomes were reported in one study of humans when serum creatinine increased following RAAS-I with ACE-I or ARB, even when the increase was <30% over baseline. It was suggested that this increase in serum creatinine identified a high-risk population that should be more closely monitored [583].

Benazepril as monotherapy in cats with and without CKD had low risk for the development of hyperkalemia or clinically relevant increases in serum creatinine of one study in primary care private practice [584]. Combination therapy with ACE-I and spironolactone (MRB) was considered to be safe in nonazotemic dogs with mitral valve disease or DCM [545]. There was no significant difference in the mean plasma potassium concentration or in the frequency of hypokalemia or hyperkalemia in CKD cats treated with renal diet and benazepril compared to those with renal diet and placebo in one study [344]. In another series of cats with CKD, no episodes of hypotension were observed during treatment with benazepril and the occurrence of hyperkalemia (>6.0 mEq/L) was uncommon and usually of clinically insignificant magnitude (3.7% of cats at 60 days). An increase in serum creatinine of greater than 30% over baseline occurred in 11% of cats during the first 30 days and in 13.7% of cats after one to two months of benazepril treatment, but this did not adversely affect survival [584].

Combination therapy with ACE-I, ARB, and/or MRB increases the risk for the development of hyperkalemia [545]. The magnitude of this risk during treatment with these combinations has not been published in dogs or cats but this risk appears to be uncommon. Routine surveillance with serum biochemistry is warranted to ensure that clinically relevant hyperkalemia and hyponatremia do not develop during these treatments, as well as to monitor for changes in renal function based on serum creatinine, BUN, SDMA, and phosphorus.

Calcium Channel Blockers

CCBs are less effective than other hypertensives in slowing progression of CKD in humans unless normal BP is achieved. Autoregulation that should protect the glomerular capillaries against damaging effects from systemic hypertension is impaired since CCBs cause afferent arteriolar vasodilation. Afferent arteriolar dilatation allows a greater fraction of systemic BP to be delivered to the glomerular capillaries; consequently, it is important to ensure systemic BP is low enough so that further pressure injury to the glomerulus does not occur in those with underlying CKD during this treatment [585].

The use of CCBs as a single treatment for hypertension in dogs with CKD is not recommended. CCBs preferentially dilate the afferent arteriole, which can then allow more pressure to be transmitted to the glomerulus and the development of increased glomerular capillary pressure and damage. For the same reason, there is concern that combination therapy of CCB with ACE-I or ARB will blunt their expected effect of to lower glomerular pressures. ACE-I or ARB are, therefore, recommended as the first choice for the treatment of systemic hypertension in dogs with CKD [372].

CCBs often have been the first choice antihypertensive for cats due to their reliable and safe reduction in systemic BP, but increased survival time in cats with systemic hypertension has not been conclusively demonstrated following effective BP control with CCB. A decrease in systolic BP of 40–55 mmHg often results during CCB treatment in cats with >160 mmHg BP initially. Amlodipine is a CCB that has been used for safe and effective control of systemic hypertension in cats that often results in reduction of UPC [377, 586, 587]. Increased activity of the systemic or intrarenal RAAS during the use of CCB is of some concern as a negative aspect for use of CCB [588]. The ability of amlodipine to decrease renal proteinuria has not been directly compared to ACE-I or ARB in the same clinical study.

Though reduced systemic BP by itself may not predict increased survival in dogs or cats with systemic hypertension following treatment, decreased renal proteinuria in association with reduced systemic BP is considered to be renoprotective [331]. In a model of dogs with reduced renal mass and systemic hypertension, renal proteinuria was reduced to the same degree during treatment with either an ACE-I or CCB given alone, but the effect was greater when given in combination. Reduction in systemic BP was similar during treatment with either drug. Reduction in glomerular capillary pressure was shown in dogs treated with ACE-I alone, but glomerular capillary pressure was increased in dogs treated with CCB alone [589]. The reduction of proteinuria could not be accounted for solely on the basis of reduction in glomerular capillary pressure in this study [589].

Sodium-Glucose Cotransporter 2 (SGLT2) Inhibitors

SGLT2 inhibitors (e.g. empagliflozin, dapagliflozin, and canagliflozin) are a new standard of care for the treatment of human patients with progressive CKD and proteinuria in those with and without DM [23, 590]. It should be noted that salutary benefits (less albuminuria, less decrease in eGFR, less kidney failure, and less death) have been reported in human CKD patients with and without DM during SGLT2 inhibitor treatment. Antialbuminuric effects during the use of SGLT2 inhibitors occurs in humans whether or not RAAS inhibition is concurrently prescribed [591] and is independent of any lowering of circulating glucose effect [590].

The rate for decline in eGFR was significantly decreased in those with CKD compared to placebo; this renoprotective effect was greater in those with diabetes. Dapagliflozin reduced albuminuria in CKD patients (more so in those with diabetes), increased the likelihood of conversion to microproteinuria from overt proteinuria, and decreased progression to nephrotic range proteinuria. Early reduction in albuminuria was associated with less decrease in eGFR over time. The greatest benefits during SGLT2 inhibitor treatment were seen in those with more rapid progression of their CKD. Observed benefits during SGLT2 inhibitor treatment could be attributed only in part to reduction in albuminuria, as other renoprotective pathways also appeared to be operative [590, 592–594].

Additional renoprotection in CKD is provided when SGLT2 inhibitors are added to RAAS inhibition. This benefit appears to occur as glomerular hyperfiltration and glomerular capillary pressure are further reduced as a consequence of afferent arteriolar vasoconstriction, though several other mechanisms are also likely to contribute. It appears that the blockade of glucose and sodium reabsorption in the proximal tubule delivers more sodium and chloride to the macula densa, which then results in the vasoconstriction of the afferent arteriole through glomerulotubular feedback [23, 591, 595]. It is likely that this further reduction in glomerular hypertension will benefit diseased podocytes that have lost their buttressing function to effectively oppose the increased glomerular capillary pressure within compensated nephrons during CKD [23]. A generalized reduction in glomerular barotrauma may also provide benefits [591]. SGLT2 inhibitor treatment in humans with CKD lowers the risk for progressive loss of eGFR, end-stage kidney disease, or death from renal or cardiovascular factors, and extends survival time compared to placebo [590]. The use of SGLT2 inhibitors for renoprotection in veterinary CKD patients with or without proteinuria has not yet been reported.

Calcimimetics

In the kidney, the CaR is expressed on renal tubules and to a lesser extent on glomerular podocytes. The CaR may play a novel role in glomerular disease, as intracellular calcium regulation is important in the maintenance and function of the actin cytoskeleton and adhesion of podocytes. CaR expression in glomeruli is upregulated in some types of glomerular disease. The activation of the CaR on podocytes by the calcimimetic cinacalcet reduced the magnitude of proteinuria in mouse models of glomerular injury and in a small number of children with idiopathic NS in one report [596].

Residual Proteinuria

Residual proteinuria has traditionally referred to the magnitude of renal proteinuria remaining after optimal or maximal dosing of ACE-I or ARB [597]. More recently, residual proteinuria in human medicine can also refer to renal proteinuria remaining after varying single agent or combinations of treatment with ACE-I, ARB, SGLT2 inhibitors, and MRB. The degree of residual proteinuria predicted the rate of further progression of CKD and loss of excretory function (GFR) in humans in several studies [597–601]. An absent or minimal decrease in the magnitude of renal proteinuria following treatment with RAAS blockage is a strong predictor of CKD progression in humans. Higher magnitudes of residual proteinuria following standard RAAS-I treatment were associated with the development of end-stage renal disease in human patients with both diabetic and nondiabetic CKD in one study [602].

Residual proteinuria following single- or dual-RAAS inhibition was further reduced when a low-salt diet was added as treatment for humans with nondiabetic CKD in one review. The addition of a lower salt diet to ACE-I resulted in lower proteinuria than following dual therapy of ACE-I and an ARB. It was suggested that dual blockade treatment to reduce proteinuria should not be prescribed before a lower salt diet had been added onto ACE-I that failed to adequately suppress renal proteinuria [603]. The effect of a lower salt diet on renal proteinuria in dogs or cats with naturally occurring CKD has not been separated from the overall effects of a renal diet in which many components of the nutrient profile including salt have been altered.

The maximal dosing of RAAS blockers is limited by the development of hyperkalemia as an adverse effect in some patients. Treatment with vitamin D analogues in animal models can reduce proteinuria and renal fibrosis as a single treatment or in combination with ACE-I or ARB, but this effect has not been consistently reported. A meta-analysis of treatment with calcitriol or the vitamin D analogue paracalcitol during CKD in humans revealed significant reduction in residual proteinuria for most patients already on standard RAAS-I treatment [601].

Treatment with the active vitamin D analogue paracalcitol for six months significantly reduced renal proteinuria to a modest degree based on UPC in one study of humans with CKD that were compared to placebo [604]. In an eight-week short-term crossover study of human nondiabetic CKD subjects with residual proteinuria following treatment with a single RAAS-I, paricalcitol did not significantly reduce albuminuria, whereas moderate dietary sodium restriction strongly and significantly reduced residual proteinuria [605].

Though most studies have focused on the ability of calcitriol or potent vitamin D metabolite analogues for their ability to mitigate glomerular proteinuria, daily cholecalciferol treatment significantly reduced albuminuria by 53.2% compared to an increase of 7.1% with placebo in one prospective randomized open label study of human CKD at six months. Patients with low 25-hydroxyvitamin D (25D) and high PTH were treated with cholecalciferol whereas those with normal PTH irrespective of 25D status received placebo. Increased 25D status at six months was inversely related to the degree of albuminuria. Mean PTH significantly decreased in those treated with cholecalciferol but not with placebo; reductions in PTH were less than during the use of paracalcitol [606]. Unfortunately, the effects on proteinuria were not measured in a study of dogs with clinical CKD that were treated with a modified release formulation of calcifediol in a short-term pilot study (84 days) [535].

VDR activation by vitamin D metabolites exerts anti-inflammatory and anti-RAAS effects in the kidney. Relative or absolute deficits of calcitriol and calcidiol could be associated with a RAAS system that is overactivated or inadequately suppressed, which can contribute to CKD progression and glomerular proteinuria. Treatment providing VDR activation was recommended as an add-on option to reduce residual proteinuria after RAAS-I failed to adequately reduce proteinuria in one study in human medicine [607].

Treatment of Complicated Cases

The previous discussion has focused on the treatment of patients with proteinuria in the absence of other complicating factors such as hypoalbuminemia and azotemia. The presence of hypoalbuminemia and azotemia along with persistent renal proteinuria complicates treatment, requiring more aggressive therapy and monitoring (Figure 7.20). In these cases, it is useful to classify patients into "tiers" [213]. Tier 1 patients do not have azotemia or hypoalbuminemia, and this classification is used for those in which renal proteinuria is the only abnormal finding (Tier 1A) or in those where systemic hypertension is also present (Tier 1B). Tier 2 patients have hypoalbuminemia but do not have azotemia; the presence of systemic hypertension (Tier 2B) or the absence of systemic hypertension (Tier 2A) further categorizes these patients. The primary criterion for Tier 3 is the documentation of renal azotemia along with the persistence of renal proteinuria. Those in Tier 3A do not have systemic hypertension or hypoalbuminemia, while those in Tier 3B have systemic hypertension but do not have hypoalbuminemia. Tier 3C patients frequently, but not always, have systemic hypertension and also hypoalbuminemia. Patients with azotemia, systemic hypertension, and hypoalbuminemia are often the sickest, and attaining a successful outcome can be especially challenging. Such patients in primary care often benefit from referral to practices for treatment and management by those with special expertise in nephrology (experts in emergency and critical care, nephrologists, and internists).

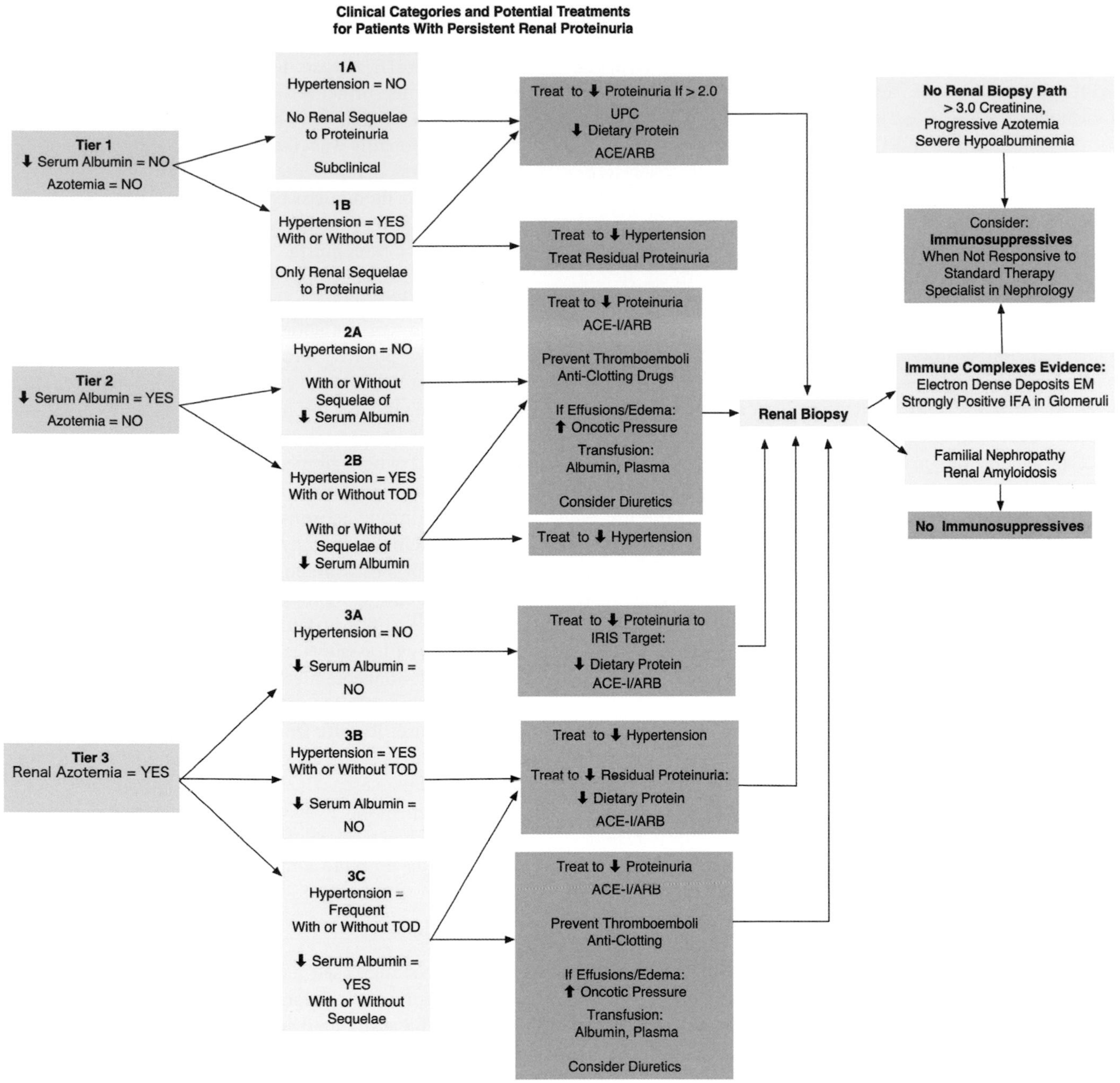

**Clinical Categories and Potential Treatments
for Patients With Persistent Renal Proteinuria**

FIGURE 7.20 Potential categorization scheme and treatment plan for clinical patients with persistent renal (glomerular) proteinuria. This is designed to be used after initial stabilization including correction of dehydration if that were present. The criteria that define what tier and sub-tier will be assigned are based on some combination for the presence or absence of systemic hypertension, hypoalbuminemia, or azotemia. TOD = target organ damage to the eyes, brain, heart, and kidneys. Sequelae from hypoalbuminemia include accelerated clotting and thromboembolic events, as well as peripheral edema and body cavity effusions associated with low oncotic pressure. Residual proteinuria refers to proteinuria that remains after intervention with diet, treatment with antihypertensives, and/or after RAAS-I with ACE-I or ARB. Source: Adapted from Littman et al. [213].

Immunosuppressive Therapy

Immunosuppressive therapy should be considered after standard treatments have failed to mitigate proteinuria and progression of CKD. Details about the use of immunosuppressive drugs or therapeutic plasma exchange for the mitigation of glomerular proteinuria and progression of CKD or AKI is beyond the scope of this chapter. It should be noted that published evidence is largely lacking that shows the benefits and limitations for the use of these various drugs alone or in combination. Treatment protocols directed toward specific glomerular diseases based on comprehensive renal biopsy results (light microscopy, IFA, and EM) have yet to be developed. A series of consensus recommendations and papers written by experts is available to those seeking more information [7, 136, 212, 214, 215, 509].

Renal biopsy is most often performed in patients with proteinuria that is trending upward, those with severe proteinuria, those with absolute hypoalbuminemia or hypoalbuminemia that is trending downward, and those with serum creatinine that is trending upward. Results from renal biopsy are most clinically informative when performed before increased serum creatinine is severe. Though sometimes results from renal biopsy are helpful when serum creatinine is >4.0 mg/dL, often times the degree of scarring and tubulointerstitial inflammation precludes a definitive glomerular diagnosis. Renal biopsy with results from light microscopy, immunofluorescent microscopy, and EM are usually needed together to make the proper diagnosis. The finding of positive glomerular immunofluorescence and electron dense deposits within glomeruli provide support for ICGN and the use of immunosuppressive drugs in select cases.

A stronger recommendation for the use of these treatments can be made for the approximately 50% of dogs with renal proteinuria that are shown on comprehensive renal biopsy to have an immune pathogenesis (electron dense deposits and unequivocal IFA positive staining within the glomeruli). Other considerations will include how active the current glomerular disease is, the magnitude of proteinuria and trending for increases, and any associations with systemic hypertension, hypoalbuminemia, effusions, and thromboembolic events.

For dogs with comprehensive renal biopsy results, immunosuppressive and anti-inflammatory treatment is recommended for those showing active glomerular disease that is severe and persistent or progressive in the absence of any identified contraindication. Rapidly acting immunosuppressive drugs (single or in combination) are recommended for dogs with a rapid rate of progression based on azotemia, severe and increasing proteinuria, and any associated hypoalbuminemia. Mycophenolate was recommended in a consensus recommendation as the first choice among immunosuppressives in dogs with rapidly progressive glomerular disease or those with evidence for immune-mediated glomerular disease. There was no consensus provided for the use of glucocorticosteroids in this population. Various combinations of mycophenolate, chlorambucil, azathioprine, cyclophosphamide, cyclosporine, and glucocorticosteroids were recommended for dogs with stable or slowly progressive glomerular disease [212].

For dogs without comprehensive renal biopsy results, immunosuppressive and anti-inflammatory treatment was recommended by a consensus panel for the treatment consideration of dogs insufficiently treated with standard therapy, when the serum creatinine was >3.0 mg/dL or azotemia was progressive, and or hypoalbuminemia was severe

(<2.0 g/dL). As noted above, there is about an equal chance to have an immunologic or nonimmunologic basis for biopsy-proven glomerular disease. This type of therapy was not recommended when proteinuria had not been confirmed to be glomerular in origin, when the age and breed suggested a familial nephropathy was likely, or when a diagnosis of renal amyloidosis was likely as determined by evaluation of renal tissue with only light microscopy [215].

Some dogs may have positive infectious disease serology and glomerular proteinuria. The evaluation of results from comprehensive renal biopsy in dogs with positive serologic status can provide evidence favoring the use of immunosuppressive therapy or not. One consensus study reinforced the concept that a positive serology for an infectious agent by itself does not confirm this agent as a cause for glomerular proteinuria. Standard treatment is initially recommended when the UPC is ≥0.5. Specific anti-infective treatment was recommended when glomerular proteinuria was found in dogs with positive infectious agent serology, despite not knowing causality in one consensus report. Treatment with standard antiproteinuria therapy and an anti-infective is recommended for dogs that are clinically stable, nonazotemic, and do not have trending increases in creatinine and UPC. It was recommended to use immunosuppressive treatment in proteinuric dogs with positive serology that have azotemic CKD, azotemic AKI, nonazotemic AKI with progressive increases in serum creatinine, or have evidence for rapidly progressive glomerular disease. Results from renal biopsy that indicate an active immunological component add support for the use of immunosuppressives, as the glomerular injury is not from the infectious agent alone. Even without results from renal biopsy, an argument has been made to use immunosuppressives to control possible immune components in this population [214].

CONCLUSION

The finding of increased amounts of proteins in the urine provides important diagnostic clues to the nature of underlying kidney and systemic diseases. It is important to initially categorize the proteinuria as prerenal, primary renal, or postrenal in origin. The anatomical and functional components of the normal glomerulus work intricately together to provide a barrier that drastically limits the transglomerular passage of plasma proteins. Renal proteinuria is often associated with less survival and increased progression of CKD, so its presence is more than just a marker of renal disease. It is also important to evaluate for the presence of systemic diseases that secondarily damage glomeruli and alter normal glomerular barrier function. Though chemistry dipstrips are the most often used method in practice, they may not be sensitive or specific for the early detection of renal proteinuria. The measurement of urine protein by UPC and MA is recommended to know with more certainty the nature and quantity of urinary proteins. The mitigation of chronic renal proteinuria is an overarching goal of treatment designed to preserve renal function and extend the life of the patient. High BP should always be treated first to see if return to normotension will also lessen renal proteinuria. In some instances, the reduction of dietary protein intake can successfully reduce renal proteinuria. Supplementation of the diet with omega-3 PUFA can be considered for its potential to further reduce renal proteinuria. In patients with residual proteinuria despite reduction in systemic BP and dietary change, reduction of RAAS activity using ACE-I or ARB alone or in combination often reduces renal proteinuria. The addition of an MRB may be considered when renal proteinuria persists despite the escalation of the doses of ACE-I or ARB. This sequential approach is often successful in lowering the level of renal proteinuria to a targeted level, but it is not possible to mitigate renal proteinuria in all cases. The long-term outcome of treatment designed to target a specified level of reduced renal proteinuria in CKD has yet to be reported for dogs and cats in prospective studies.

REFERENCES

1 Yalcin, A. and Cetin, M. (2004). Electrophoretic separation of urine proteins of healthy dogs and dogs with nephropathy and detection of some urine proteins of dogs using immunoblotting. *Revue de Médecine Vétérinaire* 155: 104–112.

2 Grauer, G.F. (2011). Proteinuria: measurement and interpretation. *Top. Companion Anim. Med.* 26: 121–127.

3 Chacar, F., Kogika, M., Sanches, T.R. et al. (2017). Urinary Tamm-Horsfall protein, albumin, vitamin D-binding protein, and retinol-binding protein as early biomarkers of chronic kidney disease in dogs. *Physiol. Rep.* 5 (11): e13262.

4 Hokamp, J.A. and Nabity, M.B. (2016). Renal biomarkers in domestic species. *Vet. Clin. Pathol.* 45: 28–56.

5 J.A., S.A., I. et al. (2018). Correlation of electrophoretic urine protein banding patterns with severity of renal damage in dogs with proteinuric chronic kidney disease. *Vet. Clin. Pathol.* 47: 425–434.

6 D'Amico, G. and Bazzi, C. (2003). Pathophysiology of proteinuria. *Kidney Int.* 63: 809–825.

7 Vaden, S.L. and Elliott, J. (2016). Management of Proteinuria in dogs and cats with chronic kidney disease. *Vet. Clin. North Am.* 46: 1115–1130.

8 Grauer, G.F. (2016). Proteinuria: Measurement and interpretation of proteinuria and albuminuria, http://www.iris-kidney.com/education/proteinuria.html.

9 DiBartola, S.P., Chew, D.J., and Jacobs, G. (1980). Quantitative urinalysis including 24-hour protein excretion in the dog. *J. Am. Anim. Hosp. Assoc.* 16: 537–546.

10 Grauer, G.F. (2007). Measurement, interpretation, and implications of proteinuria and albuminuria. *Vet. Clin. North Am.* 37 (283–295): vi–vii.

11 Harley, L. and Langston, C. (2012). Proteinuria in dogs and cats. *Can. Vet. J.* 53: 631–638.

12 Whittemore, J.C., Gill, V.L., Jensen, W.A. et al. (2006). Evaluation of the association between microalbuminuria and the urine albumin-creatinine ratio and systemic disease in dogs. *J. Am. Vet. Med. Assoc.* 229: 958–963.

13 Whittemore, J.C., Miyoshi, Z., Jensen, W.A. et al. (2007). Association of microalbuminuria and the urine albumin-to-creatinine ratio with systemic disease in cats. *J. Am. Vet. Med. Assoc.* 230: 1165–1169.

14 Lees, G.E., Brown, S.A., Elliott, J. et al. (2005). Assessment and management of proteinuria in dogs and cats: 2004 ACVIM forum consensus statement (small animal). *J. Vet. Internal Med.* 19: 377–385.

15 Langston, C. (2004). Microalbuminuria in cats. *J. Am. Anim. Hosp. Assoc.* 40: 251–254.

16 Lamb, E.J. and Jones, G.R.D. (2018). Kidney function tests. In: *Tietz Textbook of Clinical Chemistry and Molecular Diagnostics*, 6e (ed. N. Rifai, A.R. Horvath and C.T. Witter), 479–516. St. Louis, MO: Elsevier.

17 Harrison, J.F., Parker, R.W., and De Silva, K.L. (1973). Lysozymuria and acute disorders of renal function. *J. Clin. Pathol.* 26: 278–284.

18 Aguado, M.J., Garcia de Bustos, J., Ojeda, E. et al. (2000). Proteinuria caused by lysozymuria mimics nephrotic syndrome. *Nephron* 86: 183.

19 Osserman, E.F. and Lawlor, D.P. (1966). Serum and urinary lysozyme (muramidase) in monocytic and monomyelocytic leukemia. *J. Exp. Med.* 124: 921–952.

20 Delaney, M.P. and Lamb, E.J. (2018). Kidney disease. In: *Tietz Textbook of Clinical Chemistry and Molecular Diagnostics*, 6e (ed. N. Rifai, A.R. Horvath and C.T. Witter), 1256–1323. St. Louis, MO: Elsevier.

21 Summers, S.C. (2020). Feline Renal Proteinuria. *Vet. Focus.* https://vetfocus.royalcanin.com/en/https://vetfocus.royalcanin.com/en/doc-430.html: Royal Canin.

22 Hedgespeth, B. and Harrell, K. (2021). Differential diagnosis: proteinuria in dogs. *Clinicians Brief.* https://www.cliniciansbrief.com/article/differential-diagnosis-proteinuria-dogs.

23 Benzing, T. and Salant, D. (2021). Insights into glomerular filtration and albuminuria. *N. Engl. J. Med.* 384: 1437–1446.

24 Albright, R., Brensilver, J., and Cortell, S. (1983). Proteinuria in congestive heart failure. *Am. J. Nephrol.* 3: 272–275.

25 Norden, A.G., Lapsley, M., Lee, P.J. et al. (2001). Glomerular protein sieving and implications for renal failure in Fanconi syndrome. *Kidney Int.* 60: 1885–1892.

26 Vaden, S.L. (2011). Glomerular disease. *Top. Companion Anim. Med.* 26: 128–134.

27 Cianciolo, R.E., Mohr, F.C., Aresu, L. et al. (2016). World small animal veterinary association renal pathology initiative: classification of glomerular diseases in dogs. *Vet. Pathol.* 53: 113–135.

28 Naylor, R.W., Morais, M., and Lennon, R. (2021). Complexities of the glomerular basement membrane. *Nat. Rev. Nephrol.* 17: 112–127.

29 Kashtan, C.E. and Segal, Y. (2011). Genetic disorders of glomerular basement membranes. *Nephron Clin. Pract.* 118: c9–c18.

30 Littman, M.P. (2015). Emerging perspectives on hereditary glomerulopathies in canines. *Adv. Genomics Genet.* 5 (1): 179–188.

31 Tryggvason, K., Patrakka, J., and Wartiovaara, J. (2006). Hereditary proteinuria syndromes and mechanisms of proteinuria. *N. Engl. J. Med.* 354: 1387–1401.

32 Porter, P. (1964). Comparative study of the macromolecular components excreted in the urine of dog and man. *J. Comp. Pathol.* 74: 108–118.

33 Osborne, C.A. and Stevens, J.B. (1999). Biochemical analysis of urine: indications, methods, interpretation. In: *Urinalysis: A Clinical Guide to Compassionate Patient Care* (ed. C.A. Osborne and J.B. Stevens), 86–124. Shawnee Mission, KS: Bayer.

34 Pesce, A.J. (1974). Methods used for the analysis of proteins in the urine. *Nephron* 13: 93–104.

35 Welsh, G.I. and Saleem, M.A. (2011). The podocyte cytoskeleton-key to a functioning glomerulus in health and disease. *Nat. Rev. Nephrol.* 8: 14–21.

36 Kopp, J.B., Anders, H.J., Susztak, K. et al. (2020). Podocytopathies. *Nat. Rev. Dis. Primers.* 6: 68.

37 Welsh, G.I. and Saleem, M.A. (2010). Nephrin-signature molecule of the glomerular podocyte? *J. Pathol.* 220: 328–337.

38 Haraldsson, B., Nystrom, J., and Deen, W.M. (2008). Properties of the glomerular barrier and mechanisms of proteinuria. *Physiol. Rev.* 88: 451–487.

39 Deen, W.M. (2004). What determines glomerular capillary permeability? *J. Clin. Invest.* 114: 1412–1414.

40 Gaudette, S., Hughes, D., and Boller, M. (2020). The endothelial glycocalyx: structure and function in health and critical illness. *J. Vet. Emerg. Crit. Care (San Antonio)* 30 (2): 117–134.

41 de Brito Galvao, J.F., Nagode, L.A., Schenck, P.A. et al. (2013). Calcitriol, calcidiol, parathyroid hormone, and fibroblast growth factor-23 interactions in chronic kidney disease. *J. Vet. Emerg. Crit. Care (San Antonio)* 23: 134–162.

42 Thrailkill, K.M., Jo, C.H., Cockrell, G.E. et al. (2011). Enhanced excretion of vitamin D binding protein in type 1 diabetes: a role in vitamin D deficiency? *J. Clin. Endocrinol. Metab.* 96: 142–149.

43 Chesney, R.W. (2016). Interactions of vitamin D and the proximal tubule. *Pediatr. Nephrol. (Berlin, Germany)* 31: 7–14.

44 Zoja, C., Morigi, M., and Remuzzi, G. (2003). Proteinuria and phenotypic change of proximal tubular cells. *J. Am. Soc. Nephrol.* 14 (Suppl 1): S36–S41.

45 Christensen, E.I. and Nielsen, R. (2007). Role of megalin and cubilin in renal physiology and pathophysiology. *Rev. Physiol. Biochem. Pharmacol.* 158: 1–22.

46 Amsellem, S., Gburek, J., Hamard, G. et al. (2010). Cubilin is essential for albumin reabsorption in the renal proximal tubule. *J. Am. Soc. Nephrol.* 21: 1859–1867.

47 Haraldsson, B. (2010). Tubular reabsorption of albumin: it's all about cubilin. *J. Am. Soc. Nephrol.* 21: 1810–1812.

48 Schweigert, F.J., Raila, J., and Haebel, S. (2002). Vitamin a excreted in the urine of canines is associated with a Tamm-Horsfall like protein. *Vet. Res.* 33: 299–311.

49 Raila, J., Schweigert, F.J., and Kohn, B. (2014). Relationship between urinary Tamm-Horsfall protein excretion and renal function in dogs with naturally occurring renal disease. *Vet. Clin. Pathol.* 43: 261–265.

50 Bleyer, A.J. and Kmoch, S. (2016). Tamm Horsfall glycoprotein and uromodulin: it is all about the tubules! *Clin. J. Am. Soc. Nephrol.* 11: 6–8.

51 Raila, J., Forterre, S., Kohn, B. et al. (2003). Effects of chronic renal disease on the transport of vitamin a in plasma and urine of dogs. *Am. J. Vet. Res.* 64: 874–879.

52 Kohn, C.W. and Chew, D.J. (1987). Laboratory diagnosis and characterization of renal disease in horses. *Vet. Clin. North Am. Equine Pract.* 3: 585–615.

53 Putnam, F.W., Easley, C.W., Lynn, L.T. et al. (1959). The heat precipitation of Bence-Jones proteins. I. Optimum conditions. *Arch. Biochem. Biophys.* 83: 115–130.

54 Roura, X., Elliott, J., and Grauer, G.F. (2017). Proteinuria. In: *BSAVA Manual of Canine and Feline Nephrology and Urology*, 3e (ed. J. Elliott, G.F. Grauer and J.L. Westropp), 50–59. Gloucester: England British Small Animal Veterinary Association.

55 Syme, H. and Elliott, J. (2011). Proteinuria and microalbuminuria. In: *Nephrology and Urology of Small Animals* (ed. J. Bartges and D. Polzin), 410–414. West Sussex, UK: Wiley Blackwell.

56 Vaden, S.L. and Grauer, G.F. (2011). Glomerular disease. In: *Nephrology and Urology of Small Animals* (ed. J. Bartges and D. Polzin), 538–546. West Sussex, UK: Wiley Blackwell.

57 Vaden, S.L. (2017). Glomerular Diseases. In: *Textbook of Veterinary Internal Medicine*, 8e (ed. S. Ettinger, E.C. Feldman and E. Cote), 1959–1971. St. Louis Missouri: Elsevier.

58 DiBartola, S.P., Chew, D.J., and Schenck, P.A. (2010). Diseases of the glomerulus. In: *Canine and Feline Nephrology and Urology*, 2e (ed. D.J. Chew, S.P. DiBartola and P.A. Schenck), 218–239. St. Louis, Missouri: Elsevier.

59 Dibartola, S.P. and Westropp, J.L. (2020). Glomerular disease. In: *Small Animal Internal Medicine*, 6e (ed. R. Nelson and G. Cotuto), 675–685. St. Louis, MO: Elsevier.

60 Schneider, S.M., Cianciolo, R.E., Nabity, M.B. et al. (2013). Prevalence of immune-complex glomerulonephritides in dogs biopsied for suspected glomerular disease: 501 cases (2007–2012). *J. Vet. Internal Med.* 27 (Suppl 1): S67–S75.

61 Cianciolo, R.E., Brown, C.A., Mohr, F.C. et al. (2013). Pathologic evaluation of canine renal biopsies: methods for identifying features that differentiate immune-mediated glomerulonephritides from other categories of glomerular diseases. *J. Vet. Internal Med.* 27 (Suppl 1): S10–S18.

62 Crisi, P.E., Dondi, F., De Luca, E. et al. (2020). Early renal involvement in cats with natural feline morbillivirus infection. *Animals (Basel)* 10 (5): 828.

63 Wright, N.G. and Cornwell, H.J. (1983). Experimental canine adenovirus glomerulonephritis: histological, immunofluorescence and ultrastructural features of the early glomerular changes. *Br. J. Exp. Pathol.* 64: 312–319.

64 Crowell, W.A. and Barsanti, J.A. (1983). Membranous glomerulopathy in two feline siblings. *J. Am. Vet. Med. Assoc.* 182: 1244–1245.

65 Nash, A.S. and Wright, N.G. (1983). Membranous nephropathy in sibling cats. *Vet. Rec.* 113: 180–182.

66 Zeugswetter, F., Hittmair, K.M., de Arespacochaga, A.G. et al. (2007). Erosive polyarthritis associated with *Mycoplasma gateae* in a cat. *J. Feline Med. Surg.* 9: 226–231.

67   Bennett, D. and Nash, A.S. (1988). Feline immune-based polyarthritis: a study of thirty-one cases. *J. Small Anim. Pract.* 29: 501–523.

68   Johnson, K.C. and Mackin, A. (2012). Canine immune-mediated polyarthritis: part 2: diagnosis and treatment. *J. Am. Anim. Hosp. Assoc.* 48: 71–82.

69   Johnson, K.C. and Mackin, A. (2012). Canine immune-mediated polyarthritis: part 1: pathophysiology. *J. Am. Anim. Hosp. Assoc.* 48: 12–17.

70   Furrow, E., Jaeger, J.Q., Parker, V.J. et al. (2016). Proteinuria and lipoprotein lipase activity in Miniature Schnauzer dogs with and without hypertriglyceridemia. *Vet. J.* 212: 83–89.

71   Smith, R.E., Granick, J.L., Stauthammer, C.D. et al. (2017). Clinical consequences of hypertriglyceridemia-associated proteinuria in miniature schnauzers. *J. Vet. Internal Med.* 31: 1740–1748.

72   Crowell, W.A. and Leininger, J.R. (1976). Feline glomeruli: morphologic comparisons in normal, autolytic, and diseased kidneys. *Am. J. Vet. Res.* 37: 1075–1079.

73   Vilafranca, M., Wohlsein, P., Leopold-Temmler, B. et al. (1993). A canine nephropathy resembling minimal change nephrotic syndrome in man. *J. Comp. Pathol.* 109: 271–280.

74   Aresu, L., Martini, V., Benali, S.L. et al. (2017). European veterinary renal pathology service: a survey over a 7-year period (2008–2015). *J. Vet. Internal Med.* 31: 1459–1468.

75   Gori, E., Pierini, A., Lippi, I. et al. (2019). Urinalysis and urinary GGT-to-urinary creatinine ratio in dogs with acute pancreatitis. *Vet. Sci.* 6 (1): 27.

76   Paltrinieri, S., Mangiagalli, G., and Ibba, F. (2018). Use of urinary gamma-glutamyl transferase (GGT) to monitor the pattern of proteinuria in dogs with leishmaniasis treated with N-methylglucamine antimoniate. *Res. Vet. Sci.* 119: 52–55.

77   Ibba, F., Mangiagalli, G., and Paltrinieri, S. (2016). Urinary gamma-glutamyl transferase (GGT) as a marker of tubular proteinuria in dogs with canine leishmaniasis, using sodium dodecylsulphate (SDS) electrophoresis as a reference method. *Vet. J.* 210: 89–91.

78   Winiarczyk, D., Michalak, K., Adaszek, L. et al. (2019). Urinary proteome of dogs with kidney injury during babesiosis. *BMC Vet. Res.* 15: 439.

79   Brown, M.R., Cianciolo, R.E., Nabity, M.B. et al. (2013). Masitinib-associated minimal change disease with acute tubular necrosis resulting in acute kidney injury in a dog. *J. Vet. Internal Med.* 27: 1622–1626.

80   Backlund, B., Cianciolo, R.E., Cook, A.K. et al. (2011). Minimal change glomerulopathy in a cat. *J. Feline Med. Surg.* 13: 291–295.

81   Grauer, G.F., Oberhauser, E.B., Basaraba, R.J. et al. (2002). Development of microalbuminuria in dogs with heartworm disease [abstract 103]. *J. Vet. Internal Med.* 16: 352.

82   Grauer, G.F., Culham, C.A., Cooley, A.J. et al. (1987). Clinicopathologic and histologic evaluation of *Dirofilaria immitis*-induced nephropathy in dogs. *Am. J. Trop. Med. Hyg.* 37: 588–596.

83   Page, R.L., Stiff, M.E., McEntee, M.C. et al. (1990). Transient glomerulonephropathy associated with primary erythrocytosis in a dog. *J. Am. Vet. Med. Assoc.* 196: 620–622.

84   Dobenecker, B., Webel, A., Reese, S. et al. (2018). Effect of a high phosphorus diet on indicators of renal health in cats. *J. Feline Med. Surg.* 20: 339–343.

85   Alexander, J., Stockman, J., Atwal, J. et al. (2018). Effects of the long-term feeding of diets enriched with inorganic phosphorus on the adult feline kidney and phosphorus metabolism. *Br. J. Nutr.* 12 (3): 249–269.

86   Laflamme, D., Backus, R., Brown, S. et al. (2020). A review of phosphorus homeostasis and the impact of different types and amounts of dietary phosphate on metabolism and renal health in cats. *J. Vet. Internal Med. Am. College Vet. Internal Med.* 34: 2187–2196.

87   Grauer, G.F., Culham, C.A., Dubielzig, R.R. et al. (1989). Experimental *Dirofilaria immitis*-associated glomerulonephritis induced in part by in situ formation of immune complexes in the glomerular capillary wall. *J. Parasitol.* 75: 585–593.

88   Clinkenbeard, K.D., Cowell, R.L., and Tyler, R.D. (1988). Disseminated histoplasmosis in dogs: 12 cases (1981–1986). *J. Am. Vet. Med. Assoc.* 193: 1443–1447.

89   Yang, T.J. (1987). Pathobiology of canine cyclic hematopoiesis (review). *in vivo* 1: 297–302.

90   Bovee, K.C., Joyce, T., Blazer-Yost, B. et al. (1979). Characterization of renal defects in dogs with a syndrome similar to the Fanconi syndrome in man. *J. Am. Vet. Med. Assoc.* 174: 1094–1099.

91   Yearley, J.H., Hancock, D.D., and Mealey, K.L. (2004). Survival time, lifespan, and quality of life in dogs with idiopathic Fanconi syndrome. *J. Am. Vet. Med. Assoc.* 225: 377–383.

92   Levtchenko, E., Blom, H., Wilmer, M. et al. (2003). ACE inhibitor enalapril diminishes albuminuria in patients with cystinosis. *Clin. Nephrol.* 60: 386–389.

93   Vaden, S.L., Pressler, B.M., Lappin, M.R. et al. (2004). Effects of urinary tract inflammation and sample blood contamination on urine albumin and total protein concentrations in canine urine samples. *Vet. Clin. Pathol.* 33: 14–19.

94   Meindl, A.G., Lourenco, B.N., Coleman, A.E. et al. (2019). Relationships among urinary protein-to-creatinine ratio, urine specific gravity, and bacteriuria in canine urine samples. *J. Vet. Internal Med.* 33: 192–199.

95   Brown, C.A., Elliott, J., Schmiedt, C.W. et al. (2016). Chronic kidney disease in aged cats: clinical features, morphology, and proposed pathogeneses. *Vet. Pathol.* 53: 309–326.

96   Rayhel, L.H., Quimby, J.M., Cianciolo, R.E. et al. (2020). Clinicopathologic and pathologic characteristics of feline proteinuric kidney disease. *J. Feline Med. Surg.* 22 (12): 1219–1229.

97   Rossi, F., Aresu, L., Martini, V. et al. (2019). Immune-complex glomerulonephritis in cats: a retrospective study based on clinicopathological data, histopathology and ultrastructural features. *BMC Vet. Res.* 15: 303.

98   Vessieres, F., Cianciolo, R.E., Gkoka, Z.G. et al. (2019). Occurrence, management and outcome of immune-complex glomerulonephritis in dogs with suspected glomerulopathy in the UK. *J. Small Anim. Pract.* 60: 683–690.

99   Braun, N., Grone, H.J., and Schena, F.P. (2009). Immunological and non-immunological mechanisms of proteinuria. *Minerva Urol. Nefrol.* 61: 385–396.

100   Nabity, M.B., Lees, G.E., Cianciolo, R. et al. (2012). Urinary biomarkers of renal disease in dogs with X-linked hereditary nephropathy. *J. Vet. Internal Med.* 26: 282–293.

101 Toblli, J.E., Bevione, P., Di Gennaro, F. et al. (2012). Understanding the mechanisms of proteinuria: therapeutic implications. *Int. J. Nephrol.* 2012: 546039.

102 Perico, N., Remuzzi, A., and Remuzzi, G. (2016). Mechanisms and consequences of proteinuria. In: *Brenner and Rector's the Kidney 10th Edition*, 10e (ed. K. Skorecki, G.M. Chertow, P.A. Marsden, et al.), 1780–1806. Philadelphia, PA: Elsevier e1788.

103 Remuzzi, G. and Bertani, T. (1998). Pathophysiology of progressive nephropathies. *N. Engl. J. Med.* 339: 1448–1456.

104 Remuzzi, G. (1999). Nephropathic nature of proteinuria. *Curr. Opin. Nephrol. Hypertens.* 8: 655–663.

105 Brown, S.A. and Brown, C.A. (1995). Single-nephron adaptations to partial renal ablation in cats. *Am. J. Physiol.* 269: R1002–R1008.

106 Brown, S.A., Finco, D.R., Crowell, W.A. et al. (1990). Single-nephron adaptations to partial renal ablation in the dog. *Am. J. Physiol.* 258: F495–F503.

107 Baron, D.N. and Newman, F. (1958). Assessment of a new simple colorimetric test for proteinuria. *Br. Med. J.* 1: 980–981.

108 Roche D. (2015). Chemstrip Package Insert.

109 Free, A.H., Rupe, C.O., and Metzler, I. (1957). Studies with a new colorimetric test for proteinuria. *Clin. Chem.* 3: 716–727.

110 Bertholf, R.L. (2014). Proteins and albumin. *Lab. Med.* 45: e25–e41.

111 Pugia, M.J., Lott, J.A., Profitt, J.A. et al. (1999). High-sensitivity dye binding assay for albumin in urine. *J. Clin. Lab. Anal.* 13: 180–187.

112 James, G.P., Bee, D.E., and Fuller, J.B. (1978). Proteinuria: accuracy and precision of laboratory diagnosis by dip-stick analysis. *Clin. Chem.* 24: 1934–1939.

113 Bowie, L., Smith, S., and Gochman, N. (1977). Characteristics of binding between reagent-strip indicators and urinary proteins. *Clin. Chem.* 23: 128–130.

114 Gyure, W.L. (1977). Comparison of several methods for semiquantitative determination of urinary protein. *Clin. Chem.* 23: 876–879.

115 Hinberg, I.H., Katz, L., and Waddell, L. (1978). Sensitivity of in vitro diagnostic dipstick tests to urinary protein. *Clin. Biochem.* 11: 62–64.

116 Siemens, H.D. (2010). Multi Stix package insert.

117 ABaxis (2017). VetScan UA10 Urine Test Strips Package Insert.

118 Kragh-Hansen, U. (1981). Molecular aspects of ligand binding to serum albumin. *Pharmacol. Rev.* 33: 17–53.

119 Lind, K.E., Kragh-Hansen, U., and Moller, J.V. (1974). Protein binding of small molecules. V. Binding of bromphenol blue by chemical modifications of human serum albumin. *Biochim. Biophys. Acta* 371: 451–461.

120 Flores, R. (1978). A rapid and reproducible assay for quantitative estimation of proteins using bromophenol blue. *Anal. Biochem.* 88: 605–611.

121 Strasinger, S.K. and Di Lorenzo, M.S. (2014). Chemical examination of urine. In: *Urinalysis and Body Fluids*, 71–97. Philadelphia: F.A. Davis Company.

122 Sink, C.A. and Weinstein, N.M. (2012). Proteinuria. In: *Practical Veterinary Urinalysis*, 113–132. Ames, IA: Wiley.

123 Sink, C.A. and Weinstein, N.M. (2012). Routine urinalysis:chemical analysis. In: *Practical Veterinary Urinalysis*, 29–53. Ames, IA: Wiley.

124 Rizzi, T.E., Valenciano, A., Bowles, M. et al. (2017). Urine chemistry. In: *Atlas of Canine and Feline Urinalysis*, 53–65. Hoboken, NJ: Wiley.

125 Tripathi, N.K., Gregory, C.R., and Latimer, K.S. (2011). Urinary system. In: *Duncan and Prasse's Veterinary Laboratory Medicine: Clinical Pathology*, 5e (ed. K.S. Latimer), 253–294. Ames, Iowa: Wiley Blackwell, Wiley.

126 Miyazaki, M., Kamiie, K., Soeta, S. et al. (2003). Molecular cloning and characterization of a novel carboxylesterase-like protein that is physiologically present at high concentrations in the urine of domestic cats (*Felis catus*). *Biochem. J.* 370: 101–110.

127 Miyazaki, M., Yamashita, T., Hosokawa, M. et al. (2006). Species-, sex-, and age-dependent urinary excretion of cauxin, a mammalian carboxylesterase. *Comp. Biochem. Physiol.* 145: 270–277.

128 Miyazaki, M., Fujiwara, K., Suzuta, Y. et al. (2011). Screening for proteinuria in cats using a conventional dipstick test after removal of cauxin from urine with a Lens culinaris agglutinin lectin tip. *Vet. J.* 189: 312–317.

129 Stockham, S.L. and Scott, M.A. (2008). Urinary system. In: *Fundamentals of Veterinary Clinical Pathology*, 708–840. Ames, IA: Blackwell Publishing.

130 Moore, F.M., Brum, S.L., and Brown, L. (1991). Urine protein determination in dogs and cats: comparison of dipstick and sulfasalicylic acid procedures. *Vet. Clin. Pathol.* 20: 95–97.

131 Elliott, J. and Sargent, H.J. (2020). Detection of early chronic kidney disases in cats. *Vet. Focus.* http://vetfocus.royalcanin.com/en/doc420.html?utm_medium=newsletter&utm_source=en&utm_campaign=doc-420&utm_content=1632 422-fM1nG6T4Jt2B466: Royal Canin.

132 Jansen, B.S. and Lumsden, J.H. (1985). Sensitivity of routine tests for urine protein to hemoglobin. *Can. Vet. J.* 26: 221–223.

133 Alleman, R. and Wamsley, H.L. (2017). Complete urinalysis. In: *BSAVA Manual of Canine and Felne Nephrology and Urology*, 2e (ed. J. Elliott, G.F. Grauer and J.L. Westropp), 60–83. UK: Waterwells.

134 Vientos-Plotts, A.I., Behrend, E.N., Welles, E.G. et al. (2018). Effect of blood contamination on results of dipstick evaluation and urine protein-to-urine creatinine ratio for urine samples from dogs and cats. *Am. J. Vet. Res.* 79: 525–531.

135 Nabity, M.B. (2011). Urine protein and microalbuminuria. In: *Nephrology and Urology of Small Animals* (ed. J. Bartges and D. Polzin), 58–61. West Sussex, UK: Wiley Blackwell.

136 Brown, S., Elliott, J., Francey, T. et al. (2013). Consensus recommendations for standard therapy of glomerular disease in dogs. *J. Vet. Internal Med.* 27 (Suppl 1): S27–S43.

137 Grimes, M., Heseltine, J.C., Nabity, M.B. et al. (2020). Characteristics associated with bacterial growth in urine in 451 proteinuric dogs (2008-2018). *J. Vet. Internal Med.* 34: 770–776.

138 Dooley, M.P., Pineda, M.H., Hopper, J.G. et al. (1990). Retrograde flow of spermatozoa into the urinary bladder of dogs during ejaculation or after sedation with xylazine. *Am. J. Vet. Res.* 51: 1574–1579.

139 Dooley, M.P., Pineda, M.H., Hopper, J.G. et al. (1991). Retrograde flow of spermatozoa into the urinary bladder of cats during electroejaculation, collection of semen with an artificial vagina, and mating. *Am. J. Vet. Res.* 52: 687–691.

140 Ferguson, J.M. and Renton, J.P. (1988). Observation on the presence of spermatozoa in canine urine. *J. Small Anim. Pract.* 29: 691–694.

141   Hubbert, W.T. (1972). Bacteria and spermatozoa in the canine urinary bladder. *Cornell Vet.* 62: 13–20.

142   Prober, L.G., Johnson, C.A., Olivier, N.B. et al. (2010). Effect of semen in urine specimens on urine protein concentration determined by means of dipstick analysis. *Am. J. Vet. Res.* 71: 288–292.

143   Tvedten, H. (2016). Urine total protein concentration in clinically normal dogs. *Vet. Clin. Pathol.* 45: 395–396.

144   Fry, M.M. (2011). Urinalysis. In: *Nephrology and Urology of Small Animals* (ed. J. Bartges and D. Polzin), 46–57. Chichester: Wiley.

145   Lyon, S.D., Sanderson, M.W., Vaden, S.L. et al. (2010). Comparison of urine dipstick, sulfosalicylic acid, urine protein-to-creatinine ratio, and species-specific ELISA methods for detection of albumin in urine samples of cats and dogs. *J. Am. Vet. Med. Assoc.* 236: 874–879.

146   Brobst, D. (1989). Urinalysis and associated laboratory procedures. *Vet. Clin. North Am.* 19: 929–949.

147   Cabarkapa, V., Deric, M., Ilincic, B. et al. (2016). The laboratory aspects of proteinuria. *Med. Pregl.* 69: 197–202.

148   Hanzlicek, A.S., Roof, C.J., Sanderson, M.W. et al. (2012). Comparison of urine dipstick, sulfosalicylic acid, urine protein-to-creatinine ratio and a feline-specific immunoassay for detection of albuminuria in cats with chronic kidney disease. *J. Feline Med. Surg.* 14: 882–888.

149   Welles, E.G., Whatley, E.M., Hall, A.S. et al. (2006). Comparison of Multistix PRO dipsticks with other biochemical assays for determining urine protein (UP), urine creatinine (UC) and UP:UC ratio in dogs and cats. *Vet. Clin. Pathol.* 35: 31–36.

150   Rovin, B.H. (2019). Assessment of urinary protein excretion and evaluation of isolated non-nephrotic proteinuria in adults. https://www.uptodate-com.proxy.lib.ohio-state.edu/contents/assessment-of-urinary-protein-excretion-and-evaluation-of-isolated-non-nephrotic-proteinuria-in-adults?search=Assessment%20of%20urinary%20protein%20excretion%20and%20evaluation%20of%20isolated%20 (accessed September 27, 2019).

151   Rossi, G., Bertazzolo, W., Binnella, M. et al. (2016). Measurement of proteinuria in dogs: analytic and diagnostic differences using 2 laboratory methods. *Vet. Clin. Pathol.* 45: 450–458.

152   Giraldi, M., Rossi, G., Bertazzolo, W. et al. (2018). Evaluation of the analytical variability of urine protein-to-creatinine ratio in cats. *Vet. Clin. Pathol.* 47: 448–457.

153   Trumel, C., Diquelou, A., Lefebvre, H. et al. (2004). Inaccuracy of routine creatinine measurement in canine urine. *Vet. Clin. Pathol.* 33: 128–132.

154   Rossi, G., Giori, L., Campagnola, S. et al. (2012). Evaluation of factors that affect analytic variability of urine protein-to-creatinine ratio determination in dogs. *Am. J. Vet. Res.* 73: 779–788.

155   Scarpa, P. (2019). Urinalysis: What can go wrong? *Vet. Focus* 29.2 https://vetfocus.royalcanin.com/en/doc-224.html: Royal Canin.

156   Spierto, F.W., Hannon, W.H., Gunter, E.W. et al. (1997). Stability of urine creatinine. *Clin. Chim. Acta* 264: 227–232.

157   Giraldi, M., Paltrinieri, S., Rossi, G. et al. (2021). Influence of preanalytical factors on feline proteinuria. *Vet. Clin. Pathol.* 50 (3): 369–375.

158   Tefft, K.M., Shaw, D.H., Ihle, S.L. et al. (2014). Association between excess body weight and urine protein concentration in healthy dogs. *Vet. Clin. Pathol.* 43: 255–260.

159   Yoshimoto, M., Tsukahara, H., Saito, M. et al. (1990). Evaluation of variability of proteinuria indices. *Pediatr. Nephrol. (Berlin, Germany)* 4: 136–139.

160   Hoskins, J.D., Turnwald, G.H., Kearney, M.T. et al. (1991). Quantitative urinalysis in kittens from four to thirty weeks after birth. *Am. J. Vet. Res.* 52: 1295–1299.

161   Russo, E.A., Lees, G.E., and Hightower, D. (1986). Evaluation of renal function in cats, using quantitative urinalysis. *Am. J. Vet. Res.* 47: 1308–1312.

162   Monroe, W.E., Davenport, D.J., and Saunders, G.K. (1989). Twenty-four hour urinary protein loss in healthy cats and the urinary protein-creatinine ratio as an estimate. *Am. J. Vet. Res.* 50: 1906–1909.

163   Bertieri, M.B., Lapointe, C., Conversy, B. et al. (2015). Effect of castration on the urinary protein-to-creatinine ratio of male dogs. *Am. J. Vet. Res.* 76: 1085–1088.

164   Faulks, R.D. and Lane, I.F. (2003). Qualitative urinalyses in puppies 0 to 24 weeks of age. *J. Am. Anim. Hosp. Assoc.* 39: 369–378.

165   Lane, I.F., Shaw, D.H., Burton, S.A. et al. (2000). Quantitative urinalysis in healthy beagle puppies from 9 to 27 weeks of age. *Am. J. Vet. Res.* 61: 577–581.

166   Laroute, V., Chetboul, V., Roche, L. et al. (2005). Quantitative evaluation of renal function in healthy beagle puppies and mature dogs. *Res. Vet. Sci.* 79: 161–167.

167   Syme, H.M., Markwell, P.J., Pfeiffer, D. et al. (2006). Survival of cats with naturally occurring chronic renal failure is related to severity of proteinuria. *J. Vet. Internal Med.* 20: 528–535.

168   Marynissen, S.J., Willems, A.L., Paepe, D. et al. (2017). Proteinuria in apparently healthy elderly dogs: persistency and comparison between free catch and cystocentesis urine. *J. Vet. Internal Med.* 31: 93–101.

169   Willems, A., Paepe, D., Marynissen, S. et al. (2017). Results of screening of apparently healthy senior and geriatric dogs. *J. Vet. Internal Med.* 31: 81–92.

170   Paepe, D., Verjans, G., Duchateau, L. et al. (2013). Routine health screening: findings in apparently healthy middle-aged and old cats. *J. Feline Med. Surg.* 15: 8–19.

171   Nabity, M.B., Boggess, M.M., Kashtan, C.E. et al. (2007). Day-to-Day variation of the urine protein: creatinine ratio in female dogs with stable glomerular proteinuria caused by X-linked hereditary nephropathy. *J. Vet. Internal Med.* 21: 425–430.

172   LeVine, D.N., Zhang, D., Harris, T. et al. (2010). The use of pooled vs serial urine samples to measure urine protein:creatinine ratios. *Vet. Clin. Pathol.* 39: 53–56.

173   Shropshire, S., Quimby, J., and Cerda, R. (2018). Comparison of single, averaged, and pooled urine protein:creatinine ratios in proteinuric dogs undergoing medical treatment. *J. Vet. Internal Med.* 32: 288–294.

174   IRIS (2017). IRIS Staging of CKD - Modified 2017. http://www.iris-kidney.com/pdf/IRIS_2017_Staging_of_CKD_09May18.pdf.

175   Lamb, E.J. and Jones, G.R.D. (2018). Kidney function tests. In: *Tietz Textbook of Clinical Chemistry and Molecular Diagnostics*, 5e (ed. N. Rifai, A.R. Horvath and C.T. Witter), 479–516. St. Louis, MO: Elsevier.

176   Rizzi, T.E., Valenciano, A., Bowles, M. et al. (2017). *Urine Chemistry Atlas of Canine and Feline Urinalysis*, 53–65. Hoboken, N.J.: Wiley.

177 Bertholf, R.L. (2014). Proteins and Albumin. *Lab. Med.* 45 (1): e25–e41.

178 Miyazaki, M., Kamiie, K., Soeta, S. et al. (2003). Molecular cloning and characterization of a novel carboxylesterase-like protein that is physiologically present at high concentrations in the urine of domestic cats (Felis catus). *Biochem. J.* 370 (Pt 1): 101–110.

179 Miyazaki, M., Yamashita, T., Hosokawa, M. et al. (2006). Species-, sex-, and age-dependent urinary excretion of cauxin, a mammalian carboxylesterase. *Comp. Biochem. Physiol. B Biochem. Mol. Biol.* 145 (3-4): 270–277.

180 Miyazaki, M., Fujiwara, K., Suzuta, Y. et al. (2011). Screening for proteinuria in cats using a conventional dipstick test after removal of cauxin from urine with a Lens culinaris agglutinin lectin tip. *Vet. J.* 189 (3): 312–317.

181 Moore, F.M., Brum, S.L., and Brown, L. (1991). Urine protein determination in dogs and cats: comparison of dipstick and sulfasalicylic acid procedures. *Vet. Clin. Pathol.* 20 (4): 95–97.

182 Elliott, J. and Sargent, H.J. (2020). Detection of early chronic kidney disases in cats. *Vet. Focus* (30.1) https://vetfocus.royalcanin.com/en/scientific/detection-of-early-chronic-kidney-disease-in-cats.

183 Bagley, R.S., Center, S.A., Lewis, R.M. et al. (1991). The effect of experimental cystitis and iatrogenic blood contamination on the urine protein/creatine ratio in the dog. *J. Vet. Internal Med.* 5: 66–70.

184 Jessen, L.R. (2019). Proteinuria in dogs. *Clin. Brief* 43 (October): https://www.cliniciansbrief.com/article/proteinuria-dogs-2019.

185 Wilde, H.M., Banks, D., Larsen, C.L. et al. (2008). Evaluation of the Bayer microalbumin/creatinine urinalysis dipstick. *Clin. Chim. Acta* 393: 110–113.

186 Mardell, E.J. and Sparkes, A.H. (2006). Evaluation of a commercial in-house test kit for the semi-quantitative assessment of microalbuminuria in cats. *J. Feline Med. Surg.* 8: 269–278.

187 Pressler, B.M., Vaden, S.L., Jensen, W.A. et al. (2002). Detection of canine microalbuminuria using semiquantitative test strips designed for use with human urine. *Vet. Clin. Pathol.* 31: 56–60.

188 Radecki, S.V., R.E. D, and Jensen, W.A. (2003). Effect of age and breed on the prevalence of microalbuminuria in dogs [abstract 110]. *J. Vet. Internal Med.* 17: 406.

189 Pressler, B.M. (2015). Clinical approach to advanced renal function testing in dogs and cats. *Clin. Lab. Med.* 35: 487–502.

190 Bacic, A., Kogika, M.M., Barbaro, K.C. et al. (2010). Evaluation of albuminuria and its relationship with blood pressure in dogs with chronic kidney disease. *Vet. Clin. Pathol.* 39: 203–209.

191 Lees, G.E., Jensen, W.A., Simpson, D.F. et al. (2002). Persistent albuminuria precedes onset of overt proteinuria in male dogs with X-linked hereditary nephropathy. *J. Vet. Internal Med.* 16: A 108.

192 Hsieh, O.F., Lees, G.E., Clark, S.E. et al. (2005). Development of albuminuria and overt proteinuria in heterozygous (carrier) female dogs with X-linked hereditary nephropathy (XLHN) [abstract 118]. *J. Vet. Internal Med.* 19: 432.

193 Vaden, S.L., Jensen, W.A., Longhofer, S. et al. (2001). Longitudinal study of microalbuminuria in soft-coated wheaten terriers [abstract 115]. *J. Vet. Internal Med.* 15: 300.

194 Schaefer, H., Kohn, B., Schweigert, F.J. et al. (2011). Quantitative and qualitative urine protein excretion in dogs with severe inflammatory response syndrome. *J. Vet. Internal Med.* 25: 1292–1297.

195 Crivellenti, L.Z., Silva, G.E., Borin-Crivellenti, S. et al. (2016). Prevalence of glomerulopathies in canine mammary carcinoma. *PLoS One* 11: e0164479.

196 Lien, Y.H., Hsiang, T.Y., and Huang, H.P. (2010). Associations among systemic blood pressure, microalbuminuria and albuminuria in dogs affected with pituitary- and adrenal-dependent hyperadrenocorticism. *Acta Vet. Scand.* 52: 61.

197 Giori, L., Tricomi, F.M., Zatelli, A. et al. (2011). High-resolution gel electrophoresis and sodium dodecyl sulphate-agarose gel electrophoresis on urine samples for qualitative analysis of proteinuria in dogs. *J. Vet. Diagn. Invest.* 23: 682–690.

198 Zini, E., Bonfanti, U., and Zatelli, A. (2004). Diagnostic relevance of qualitative proteinuria evaluated by use of sodium dodecyl sulfate-agarose gel electrophoresis and comparison with renal histologic findings in dogs. *Am. J. Vet. Res.* 65: 964–971.

199 Zandi-Nejad, K., Eddy, A.A., Glassock, R.J. et al. (2004). Why is proteinuria an ominous biomarker of progressive kidney disease? *Kidney Int. Suppl.* 66 (82): S76–S89.

200 Finco, D.R., Brown, S.A., Crowell, W.A. et al. (1992). Effects of dietary phosphorus and protein in dogs with chronic renal failure. *Am. J. Vet. Res.* 53: 2264–2271.

201 Cravedi, P. and Remuzzi, G. (2013). Pathophysiology of proteinuria and its value as an outcome measure in chronic kidney disease. *Br. J. Clin. Pharmacol.* 76: 516–523.

202 Cravedi, P., Ruggenenti, P., and Remuzzi, G. (2012). Proteinuria should be used as a surrogate in CKD. *Nat. Rev. Nephrol.* 8: 301–306.

203 Center, S.A., Smith, C.A., Wilkinson, E. et al. (1987). Clinicopathologic, renal immunofluorescent, and light microscopic features of glomerulonephritis in the dog: 41 cases (1975–1985). *J. Am. Vet. Med. Assoc.* 190: 81–90.

204 Center, S.A., Wilkinson, E., Smith, C.A. et al. (1985). 24-Hour urine protein/creatinine ratio in dogs with protein-losing nephropathies. *J. Am. Vet. Med. Assoc.* 187: 820–824.

205 DiBartola, S.P., Spaulding, G.L., Chew, D.J. et al. (1980). Urinary protein excretion and immunopathologic findings in dogs with glomerular disease. *J. Am. Vet. Med. Assoc.* 177: 73–77.

206 King, J.N., Tasker, S., Gunn-Moore, D.A. et al. (2007). Prognostic factors in cats with chronic kidney disease. *J. Vet. Internal Med.* 21: 906–916.

207 Jacob, F., Polzin, D.J., Osborne, C.A. et al. (2005). Evaluation of the association between initial proteinuria and morbidity rate or death in dogs with naturally occurring chronic renal failure. *J. Am. Vet. Med. Assoc.* 226: 393–400.

208 Cavalcante, C.Z., Kogika, M.M., Simões, D.M.N. et al. (2007). Microalbuminuria in dogs with hyperadrenocorticism and relationship to blood pressure. *J. Vet. Intern. Med.* 21: 647–647.

209 Citron, L.E., Weinstein, N.M., Littman, M.P. et al. (2020). Urine cortisol-creatinine and protein-creatinine ratios in urine samples from healthy dogs collected at home and in hospital. *J. Vet. Internal Med. Am. College Vet. Internal Med.* 34: 777–782.

210 Duffy, M.E., Specht, A., and Hill, R.C. (2015). Comparison between urine protein: creatinine ratios of samples obtained from dogs in home and hospital settings. *J. Vet. Internal Med. Am. College Vet. Internal Med.* 29: 1029–1035.

211 Walker, D., Syme, H.M., Markwell, P., and Elliot, J. (2004). Predictors of survival in healthy, non-azotaemic cats (abstr). *J. Vet. Intern. Med.* 18: 123.

212 Segev, G., Cowgill, L.D., Heiene, R. et al. (2013). Consensus recommendations for immunosuppressive treatment of dogs with glomerular disease based on established pathology. *J. Vet. Internal Med.* 27 (Suppl 1): S44–S54.

213 Littman, M.P., Daminet, S., Grauer, G.F. et al. (2013). Consensus recommendations for the diagnostic investigation of dogs with suspected glomerular disease. *J. Vet. Internal Med.* 27: S19–S26.

214 Goldstein, R.E., Brovida, C., Fernandez-Del Palacio, M.J. et al. (2013). Consensus recommendations for treatment for dogs with serology positive glomerular disease. *J. Vet. Internal Med.* 27 (Suppl 1): S60–S66.

215 Pressler, B., Vaden, S., Gerber, B. et al. (2013). Consensus guidelines for immunosuppressive treatment of dogs with glomerular disease absent a pathologic diagnosis. *J. Vet. Internal Med.* 27 (Suppl 1): S55–S59.

216 Cowgill, L.D. and Polzin, D.J. (2013). Vision of the WSAVA renal standardization project. *J. Vet. Internal Med.* 27 (Suppl 1): S5–S9.

217 Klosterman, E.S., Moore, G.E., de Brito Galvao, J.F. et al. (2011). Comparison of signalment, clinicopathologic findings, histologic diagnosis, and prognosis in dogs with glomerular disease with or without nephrotic syndrome. *J. Vet. Internal Med.* 25: 206–214.

218 Dambach, D.M., Smith, C.A., Lewis, R.M. et al. (1997). Morphologic, immunohistochemical, and ultrastructural characterization of a distinctive renal lesion in dogs putatively associated with Borrelia burgdorferi infection: 49 cases (1987–1992). *Vet. Pathol.* 34: 85–96.

219 Vaden, S.L., Littman, M.P., and Cianciolo, R.E. (2013). Familial renal disease in soft-coated wheaten terriers. *J. Vet. Emerg. Crit. Care (San Antonio)* 23: 174–183.

220 Picut, C.A. and Lewis, R.M. (1987). Comparative pathology of canine hereditary nephropathies: an interpretive review. *Vet. Res. Commun.* 11: 561–581.

221 Lees, G.E. (2013). Kidney diseases caused by glomerular basement membrane type IV collagen defects in dogs. *J. Vet. Emerg. Crit. Care (San Antonio)* 23: 184–193.

222 Finco, D.R., Duncan, J.D., Crowell, W.A. et al. (1977). Familial renal disease in Norwegian Elkhound dogs: morphologic examinations. *Am. J. Vet. Res.* 38: 941–947.

223 Littman, M.P. (2011). Protein-losing nephropathy in small animals. *Vet. Clin. North Am.* 41: 31–62.

224 Littman, M.P. (2017). Genetic basis for urinary tract diseases. In: *BSAVA Manual of Canine and Feline Nephrology and Urology Gloucester* (ed. J. Elliott, G.F. Grauer and J.L. Westropp), 172–184. England British Small Animal Veterinary Association.

225 Harvey, S.J., Zheng, K., Sado, Y. et al. (1998). Role of distinct type IV collagen networks in glomerular development and function. *Kidney Int.* 54: 1857–1866.

226 Zheng, K., Thorner, P.S., Marrano, P. et al. (1994). Canine X chromosome-linked hereditary nephritis: a genetic model for human X-linked hereditary nephritis resulting from a single base mutation in the gene encoding the alpha 5 chain of collagen type IV. *Proc. Natl. Acad. Sci. U. S. A.* 91: 3989–3993.

227 Benali, S.L., Lees, G.E., Nabity, M.B. et al. (2016). X-linked hereditary nephropathy in Navasota dogs: clinical pathology, morphology, and gene expression during disease progression. *Vet. Pathol.* 53: 803–812.

228 Davidson, A.G., Bell, R.J., Lees, G.E. et al. (2007). Genetic cause of autosomal recessive hereditary nephropathy in the English Cocker Spaniel. *J. Vet. Internal Med.* 21: 394–401.

229 Nowend, K.L., Starr-Moss, A.N., Lees, G.E. et al. (2012). Characterization of the genetic basis for autosomal recessive hereditary nephropathy in the English Springer Spaniel. *J. Vet. Internal Med.* 26: 294–301.

230 Freudiger, U. (1965). Die kongenitale Nierenrindenhypoplasie beim bunten Cocker-Spaniel. *Schweizer Archiv für Tierheilkunde SAT* 107: 547–566.

231 Krook, L. (1957). The pathology of renal cortical hypoplasia tn the dog. *Nord. Vet. Med.* 9: 161–176.

232 Persson, F., Persson, S., and Asheim, J. (1961). Renal cortical hypoplasia in dogs a clinical study on uraemia and secondary hyperparathyreoidism. *Acta Vet. Scand.* 2: 68–84.

233 Finco, D.R., Kurtz, H.J., Low, D.G. et al. (1970). Familial renal disease in Norwegian Elkhound dogs. *J. Am. Vet. Med. Assoc.* 156: 747–760.

234 Robinson, W.F., Huxtable, C.R., and Gooding, J.P. (1985). Familial nephropathy in Cocker Spaniels. *Aust. Vet. J.* 62: 109–112.

235 Koeman, J.P., Ezilius, J.W., Biewenga, W.J. et al. (1989). Familial nephropathy in cocker spaniels. *Dtw* 96: 174–179.

236 Grodecki, K.M., Gains, M.J., Baumal, R. et al. (1997). Treatment of X-linked hereditary nephritis in Samoyed dogs with angiotensin converting enzyme (ACE) inhibitor. *J. Comp. Pathol.* 117: 209–225.

237 Jansen, B., Thorner, P., Baumal, R. et al. (1986). Samoyed hereditary glomerulopathy (SHG). Evolution of splitting of glomerular capillary basement membranes. *Am. J. Pathol.* 125: 536–545.

238 Thorner, P., Baumal, R., Valli, V.E. et al. (1989). Abnormalities in the NC1 domain of collagen type IV in GBM in canine hereditary nephritis. *Kidney Int.* 35: 843–850.

239 Littman, M.P., Wiley, C.A., Raducha, M.G. et al. (2013). Glomerulopathy and mutations in NPHS1 and KIRREL2 in soft-coated Wheaten Terrier dogs. *Mamm. Genome* 24: 119–126.

240 Littman, M.P., Dambach, D.M., Vaden, S.L. et al. (2000). Familial protein-losing enteropathy and protein-losing nephropathy in Soft Coated Wheaten Terriers: 222 cases (1983–1997). *J. Vet. Internal Med.* 14: 68–80.

241 Nash, A.S., Kelly, D.F., and Gaskell, C.J. (1984). Progressive renal disease in Soft-coated Wheaten Terriers: possible familial nephropathy. *J. Small Anim. Pract.* 25: 479–487.

242 Littman, M. and Raducha, M.G. (2014). P. H. prevalence of variant alleles associated with protein-losing nephropathy in Airedale Terriers. *J. Vet. Intern. Med.* 28: 1366.

243 Yau, W., Mausbach, L., Littman, M.P. et al. (2018). Focal segmental glomerulosclerosis in related miniature schnauzer dogs. *Vet. Pathol.* 55: 277–285.

244 Lorbach, S.K., Hokamp, J.A., Quimby, J.M. et al. (2020). Clinicopathologic characteristics, pathology, and prognosis of 77 dogs with focal segmental glomerulosclerosis. *J. Vet. Intern. Med.* 34 (5): 1948–1956.

245 Leung, N., Drosou, M.E., and Nasr, S.H. (2018). Dysproteinemias and glomerular disease. *Clin. J. Am. Soc. Nephrol.* 13: 128–139.

246 Mao, S. and Zhang, J. (2016). Role of complement in glomerular diseases. *J. Recept. Signal Transduct. Res.* 36: 319–325.

247 Dixon, F.J., Feldman, J.D., and Vazquez, J.J. (1961). Experimental glomerulonephritis. The pathogenesis of a laboratory model resembling the spectrum of human glomerulonephritis. *J. Exp. Med.* 113: 899–920.

248 Wright, N.G. and Nash, A.S. (1983). Glomerulonephritis in the dog and cat. *Irish Vet. J.* 37: 4–8.

249 Nash, A.S. and Wright, N.G. (1988). Glomerulonephritis in the dog. In: *Renal Disease in Dogs and Cats Comparative and Clinical Aspects* (ed. A.R. Michell), 105–117. Blackwell Scientific Publications.

250 Purswell, E.K., Lashnits, E.W., Breitschwerdt, E.B. et al. (2020). A retrospective study of vector-borne disease prevalence in dogs with proteinuria: southeastern United States. *J. Vet. Internal Med.* 34: 742–753.

251 Wright, N.G., Nash, A.S., Thompson, H. et al. (1981). Membranous nephropathy in the cat and dog. A renal biopsy and follow-up study of sixteen cases. *Lab. Invest.* 45: 269–277.

252 Cole, L.P., Jepson, R., Dawson, C. et al. (2020). Hypertension, retinopathy, and acute kidney injury in dogs: a prospective study. *J. Vet. Internal Med. Am. College Vet. Internal Med.* 34: 1940–1947.

253 Troia, R., Gruarin, M., Grisetti, C. et al. (2018). Fractional excretion of electrolytes in volume-responsive and intrinsic acute kidney injury in dogs: diagnostic and prognostic implications. *J. Vet. Internal Med.* 32: 1372–1382.

254 Zamagni, S., Troia, R., Zaccheroni, F. et al. (2020). Comparison of clinicopathological patterns of renal tubular damage in dogs with acute kidney injury caused by leptospirosis and other aetiologies. *Vet. J.* 266: 105573.

255 Knopfler, S., Mayer-Scholl, A., Luge, E. et al. (2017). Evaluation of clinical, laboratory, imaging findings and outcome in 99 dogs with leptospirosis. *J. Small Anim. Pract.* 58: 582–588.

256 Zaragoza, C., Barrera, R., Centeno, F. et al. (2003). Characterization of renal damage in canine leptospirosis by sodium dodecyl sulphate-polyacrylamide gel electrophoresis (SDS-PAGE) and Western blotting of the urinary proteins. *J. Comp. Pathol.* 129: 169–178.

257 Grauer, G.F., Burgess, E.C., Cooley, A.J. et al. (1988). Renal lesions associated with Borrelia burgdorferi infection in a dog. *J. Am. Vet. Med. Assoc.* 193: 237–239.

258 Littman, M.P. (2013). Lyme nephritis. *J. Vet. Emerg. Crit. Care (San Antonio)* 23: 163–173.

259 Littman, M.P., Gerber, B., Goldstein, R.E. et al. (2018). ACVIM consensus update on Lyme borreliosis in dogs and cats. *J. Vet. Internal Med.* 32: 887–903.

260 Hutton, T.A., Goldstein, R.E., Njaa, B.L. et al. (2008). Search for Borrelia burgdorferi in kidneys of dogs with suspected "Lyme nephritis". *J. Vet. Internal Med.* 22: 860–865.

261 Levy, S.A., Dambach, D.M., Barthold, S.W. et al. (1993). Canine Lyme borreliosis. *Compend. Contin. Educ. Pract. Vet.* 15: 833–846.

262 Cork, L.C., Morris, J.M., Olson, J.L. et al. (1991). Membranoproliferative glomerulonephritis in dogs with a genetically determined deficiency of the third component of complement. *Clin. Immunol. Immunopathol.* 60: 455–470.

263 Carpenter, J.L., Andelman, N.C., Moore, F.M. et al. (1988). Idiopathic cutaneous and renal glomerular vasculopathy of greyhounds. *Vet. Pathol.* 25: 401–407.

264 Jepson, R.E., Cardwell, J.M., Cortellini, S. et al. (2019). Cutaneous and renal glomerular vasculopathy: what do we know so far? *Vet. Clin. North Am.* 49: 745–762.

265 Holm, L.P., Hawkins, I., Robin, C. et al. (2015). Cutaneous and renal glomerular vasculopathy as a cause of acute kidney injury in dogs in the UK. *Vet. Rec.* 176: 384.

266 Cowan, L.A., Hertzke, D.M., Fenwick, B.W. et al. (1997). Clinical and clinicopathologic abnormalities in greyhounds with cutaneous and renal glomerular vasculopathy: 18 cases (1992–1994). *J. Am. Vet. Med. Assoc.* 210: 789–793.

267 Holm, L. and Walker, D. (2018). Dealing with cutaneous and renal glomerular vasculopathy in dogs. *In Pract.* 10: 426–438.

268 Hertzke, D.M., Cowan, L.A., Schoning, P. et al. (1995). Glomerular ultrastructural lesions of idiopathic cutaneous and renal glomerular vasculopathy of greyhounds. *Vet. Pathol.* 32: 451–459.

269 Stevens, K.B., O'Neill, D., Jepson, R. et al. (2018). Signalment risk factors for cutaneous and renal glomerular vasculopathy (Alabama rot) in dogs in the UK. *Vet. Rec.* 183: 448.

270 Holloway, S., Senior, D., Roth, L. et al. (1993). Hemolytic uremic syndrome in dogs. *J. Vet. Internal Med.* 7: 220–227.

271 Dell'Orco, M., Bertazzolo, W., Pagliaro, L. et al. (2005). Hemolytic-uremic syndrome in a dog. *Vet. Clin. Pathol.* 34: 264–269.

272 Chantrey, J., Chapman, P.S., and Patterson-Kan, J.C. (2002). Haemolytic-uraemic syndrome in a dog. *J. Vet. Med.* 49: 470–472.

273 Noris, M. and Remuzzi, G. (2015). Glomerular diseases dependent on complement activation, including atypical hemolytic uremic syndrome, membranoproliferative glomerulonephritis, and C3 glomerulopathy: core curriculum 2015. *Am. J. Kidney Dis.* 66: 359–375.

274 Noris, M., Mescia, F., and Remuzzi, G. (2012). STEC-HUS, atypical HUS and TTP are all diseases of complement activation. *Nat. Rev. Nephrol.* 8: 622–633.

275 Barbour, T., Johnson, S., Cohney, S. et al. (2012). Thrombotic microangiopathy and associated renal disorders. *Nephrol. Dial. Transplant.* 27: 2673–2685.

276 Rortveit, R., Lingaas, F., Bonsdorff, T. et al. (2012). A canine autosomal recessive model of collagen type III glomerulopathy. *Lab. Investig. J. Tech. Methods Pathol.* 92: 1483–1491.

277 Rortveit, R., Eggertsdottir, A.V., Thomassen, R. et al. (2013). A clinical study of canine collagen type III glomerulopathy. *BMC Vet. Res.* 9: 218.

278 Rortveit, R., Reiten, M.R., Lingaas, F. et al. (2015). Glomerular collagen V codeposition and hepatic perisinusoidal collagen III accumulation in canine collagen type III glomerulopathy. *Vet. Pathol.* 52: 1134–1141.

279 Koeman, J.P., Biewenga, W.J., and Gruys, E. (1994). Proteinuria associated with glomerulosclerosis and glomerular collagen formation in three Newfoundland dog littermates. *Vet. Pathol.* 31: 188–193.

280 Hood, J.C., Robinson, W.F., Huxtable, C.R. et al. (1990). Hereditary nephritis in the bull terrier: evidence for inheritance by an autosomal dominant gene. *Vet. Rec.* 126: 456–459.

281 Hood, J.C., Savige, J., Hendtlass, A. et al. (1995). Bull terrier hereditary nephritis: a model for autosomal dominant Alport syndrome. *Kidney Int.* 47: 758–765.

282 Hood, J.C., Huxtable, C., Naito, I. et al. (2002). A novel model of autosomal dominant Alport syndrome in Dalmatian dogs. *Nephrol. Dial. Transplant.* 17: 2094–2098.

283 Picut, C.A. and Lewis, R.M. (1987). Juvenile renal disease in the Doberman Pinscher: ultrastructural changes of the glomerular basement membrane. *J. Comp. Pathol.* 97: 587–596.

284 Chew, D.J., DiBartola, S.P., Boyce, J.T. et al. (1983). Juvenile renal disease in Doberman Pinscher dogs. *J. Am. Vet. Med. Assoc.* 182: 481–485.

285 Wilcock, B.P. and Patterson, J.M. (1979). Familial glomerulonephritis in Doberman Pinscher dogs. *Can. Vet. J.* 20: 244–249.

286 Rha, J.Y., Labato, M.A., Ross, L.A. et al. (2000). Familial glomerulonephropathy in a litter of beagles. *J. Am. Vet. Med. Assoc.* 216 (46–50): 32.

287 Wakamatsu, N., Surdyk, K., Carmichael, K.P. et al. (2007). Histologic and ultrastructural studies of juvenile onset renal disease in four Rottweiler dogs. *Vet. Pathol.* 44: 96–100.

288 Lavoue, R., van der Lugt, J.J., Day, M.J. et al. (2010). Progressive juvenile glomerulonephropathy in 16 related French Mastiff (Bordeaux) dogs. *J. Vet. Internal Med.* 24: 314–322.

289 Lavoue, R., Trumel, C., Smets, P.M. et al. (2015). Characterization of proteinuria in Dogue de Bordeaux dogs, a breed predisposed to a familial glomerulonephropathy: a retrospective study. *PLoS One* 10: e0133311.

290 Casal, M.L., Dambach, D.M., Meister, T. et al. (2004). Familial glomerulonephropathy in the Bullmastiff. *Vet. Pathol.* 41: 319–325.

291 Oksanen, A. and Sittnikow, K. (1972). Familial nephropathy with secondary hyperparathyroidism in three young dogs. *Nord. Vet. Med.* 24: 278–280.

292 Reusch, C., Hoerauf, A., Lechner, J. et al. (1994). A new familial glomerulonephropathy in Bernese mountain dogs. *Vet. Rec.* 134: 411–415.

293 Minkus, G., Breuer, W., Wanke, R. et al. (1994). Familial nephropathy in Bernese mountain dogs. *Vet. Pathol.* 31: 421–428.

294 de Morais, H.S., DiBartola, S.P., and Chew, D.J. (1996). Juvenile renal disease in golden retrievers: 12 cases (1984–1994). *J. Am. Vet. Med. Assoc.* 209: 792–797.

295 Kerlin, R.L. and Van Winkle, T.J. (1995). Renal dysplasia in Golden Retrievers. *Vet. Pathol.* 32: 327–329.

296 Finco, D.R. (1976). Familial renal disease in Norwegian Elkhound dogs: physiologic and biochemical examinations. *Am. J. Vet. Res.* 37: 87–91.

297 Wiersma, A.C., Millon, L.V., van Dongen, A.M. et al. (2005). Evaluation of canine COL4A3 and COL4A4 as candidates for familial renal disease in the Norwegian elkhound. *J. Hered.* 96: 739–744.

298 Picut, C.A. and Lewis, R.M. (1987). Microscopic features of canine renal dysplasia. *Vet. Pathol.* 24: 156–163.

299 Hoppe, A., Swenson, L., Jönsson, L. et al. (1990). Progressive nephropathy due to renal dysplasia in shih tzu dogs in Sweden: a clinical pathological and genetic study. *J. Small Anim. Pract.* 31: 83–91.

300 O'Brien, T.D., Osborne, C.A., Yano, B.L. et al. (1982). Clinicopathologic manifestations of progressive renal disease in Lhasa Apso and Shih Tzu dogs. *J. Am. Vet. Med. Assoc.* 180: 658–664.

301 DiBartola, S.P., Chew, D.J., and Boyce, J.T. (1983). Juvenile renal disease in related Standard Poodles. *J. Am. Vet. Med. Assoc.* 183: 693–696.

302 Kaufman, C.F., Soirez, R.F., and Tasker, J.P. (1969). Renal cortical hypoplasia with secondary hyperparathyroidism in the dog. *J. Am. Vet. Med. Assoc.* 155: 1679–1685.

303 Klopfer, U., Neumann, F., and Trainin, R. (1975). Renalcortical hypoplasia in a keeshond litter. *Vet. Med. Small Anim. Clin.* 70: 1081–1083.

304 Cook, A.K. and Cowgill, L.D. (1996). Clinical and pathological features of protein-losing glomerular disease in the dog: a review of 137 cases (1985–1992). *J. Am. Anim. Hosp. Assoc.* 32: 313–322.

305 DiBartola, S.P., Tarr, M.J., Parker, A.T. et al. (1989). Clinicopathologic findings in dogs with renal amyloidosis: 59 cases (1976–1986). *J. Am. Vet. Med. Assoc.* 195: 358–364.

306 Benson, M.D., DiBartola, S.P., and Dwulet, F.E. (1989). A unique insertion in the primary structure of bovine amyloid AA protein. *J. Lab. Clin. Med.* 113: 67–72.

307 Benson, M.D., Dwulet, F.E., and DiBartola, S.P. (1985). Identification and characterization of amyloid protein AA in spontaneous canine amyloidosis. *Lab. Investig. J. Tech. Methods Pathol.* 52: 448–452.

308 DiBartola, S.P., Benson, M.D., Dwulet, F.E. et al. (1985). Isolation and characterization of amyloid protein AA in the Abyssinian cat. *Lab. Investig. J. Tech. Methods Pathol.* 52: 485–489.

309 DiBartola, S.P., Reiter, J.A., Cornacoff, J.B. et al. (1989). Serum amyloid A protein concentration measured by radial immunodiffusion in Abyssinian and non-Abyssinian cats. *Am. J. Vet. Res.* 50: 1414–1417.

310 DiBartola, S.P., Tarr, M.J., and Benson, M.D. (1986). Tissue distribution of amyloid deposits in Abyssinian cats with familial amyloidosis. *J. Comp. Pathol.* 96: 387–398.

311 Kluve-Beckerman, B., Dwulet, F.E., DiBartola, S.P. et al. (1989). Primary structures of dog and cat amyloid A proteins: comparison to human AA. *Comp. Biochem. Physiol. B* 94: 175–183.

312 Mason, N.J. and Day, M.J. (1996). Renal amyloidosis in related English foxhounds. *J. Small Anim. Pract.* 37: 255–260.

313 Boyce, J.T., DiBartola, S.P., Chew, D.J. et al. (1984). Familial renal amyloidosis in Abyssinian cats. *Vet. Pathol.* 21: 33–38.

314 Bowles, M.H. and Mosier, D.A. (1992). Renal amyloidosis in a family of beagles. *J. Am. Vet. Med. Assoc.* 201: 569–574.

315 DiBartola, S.P., Tarr, M.J., Webb, D.M. et al. (1990). Familial renal amyloidosis in Chinese Shar Pei dogs. *J. Am. Vet. Med. Assoc.* 197: 483–487.

316 Rivas, A.L., Tintle, L., Meyers-Wallen, V. et al. (1993). Inheritance of renal amyloidosis in Chinese Shar-pei dogs. *J. Hered.* 84: 438–442.

317 Inman, A.L., Allen-Durrance, A.E., Cianciolo, R.E. et al. (2021). Familial nephropathy in Bracchi Italiani: 8 cases (2012–2019). *J. Am. Vet. Med. Assoc.* 259: 1422–1427.

318 Chew, D.J., DiBartola, S.P., Boyce, J.T. et al. (1982). Renal amyloidosis in related Abyssinian cats. *J. Am. Vet. Med. Assoc.* 181: 139–142.

319 Kramer, H. (2017). Kidney disease and the westernization and industrialization of food. *Am. J. Kidney Dis.* 70: 111–121.

320 Perico, N., Remuzzi, A., and Remuzzi, G. (2020). Pathophysiology of proteinuria. In: *Brenner and Rector's the Kidney*, 11e (ed. Y. ISL, G.M. Chertow, V. Luyckx, et al.), 978–1006.e1009. Philadelphia, PA: Elsevier.

321 Shankland, S.J. and Mathieson, P.W. (2016). The podocyte. In: *Brenner and Rector's the Kidney 10th Edition*, 10e (ed. K. Skorecki, G.M. Chertow, P.A. Marsden, et al.), 112–121.e113. Philadelphia, PA: Elsevier.

322 Taal, M.W. (2020). Mechanisms of progression of chronic kidney disease. In: *Brenner and Rector's the Kidney*, 11e (ed. Y. ISL, G.M. Chertow, V. Luyckx, et al.), 1742–1789. Philadelphia, PA: Elsevier.

323 de Seigneux, S., Courbebaisse, M., Rutkowski, J.M. et al. (2015). Proteinuria increases plasma phosphate by altering its tubular handling. *J. Am. Soc. Nephrol.* 26: 1608–1618.

324 de Seigneux, S., Wilhelm-Bals, A., and Courbebaisse, M. (2017). On the relationship between proteinuria and plasma phosphate. *Swiss Med. Wkly.* 147: w14509.

325 Grauer, G.F., Greco, D.S., Getzy, D.M. et al. (2000). Effects of enalapril versus placebo as a treatment for canine idiopathic glomerulonephritis. *J. Vet. Internal Med.* 14: 526–533.

326 Pressler, B. (2013). A practical guide to antiproteinuric drugs in dogs. *Vet. Med.* 108: 392–397.

327 Brenner, B.M., Hostetter, T.H., and Humes, H.D. (1978). Molecular basis of proteinuria of glomerular origin. *N. Engl. J. Med.* 298: 826–833.

328 Brenner, B.M., Meyer, T.W., and Hostetter, T.H. (1982). Dietary protein intake and the progressive nature of kidney disease: the role of hemodynamically mediated glomerular injury in the pathogenesis of progressive glomerular sclerosis in aging, renal ablation, and intrinsic renal disease. *N. Engl. J. Med.* 307: 652–659.

329 Brenner, B.M. and Humes, H.D. (1977). Mechanics of glomerular ultrafiltration. *N. Engl. J. Med.* 297: 148–154.

330 Kalantar-Zadeh, K., Jafar, T.H., Nitsch, D. et al. (2021). Chronic kidney disease. *Lancet* 398: 786–802.

331 Brown, S., Atkins, C., Bagley, R. et al. (2007). Guidelines for the identification, evaluation, and management of systemic hypertension in dogs and cats. *J. Vet. Internal Med.* 21: 542–558.

332 Palmer, B.F. and Clegg, D.J. (2018). Renal considerations in the treatment of hypertension. *Am. J. Hypertens.* 31: 394–401.

333 Lewko, B., Welsh, G.I., and Jankowski, M. (2015). Editorial: podocyte pathology and nephropathy. *Front. Endocrinol. (Lausanne)* 6: 145.

334 Delitsikou, V., Jarad, G., Rajaram, R.D. et al. (2020). Klotho regulation by albuminuria is dependent on ATF3 and endoplasmic reticulum stress. *FASEB J.* 34: 2087–2104.

335 Jacob, F., Polzin, D.J., Osborne, C.A. et al. (2003). Association between initial systolic blood pressure and risk of developing a uremic crisis or of dying in dogs with chronic renal failure. *J. Am. Vet. Med. Assoc.* 222: 322–329.

336 Jacob, F., Polzin, D.J., Osborne, C.A. et al. (2002). Clinical evaluation of dietary modification for treatment of spontaneous chronic renal failure in dogs. *J. Am. Vet. Med. Assoc.* 220: 1163–1170.

337 Ross, S.J., Osborne, C.A., Kirk, C.A. et al. (2006). Clinical evaluation of dietary modification for treatment of spontaneous chronic kidney disease in cats. *J. Am. Vet. Med. Assoc.* 229: 949–957.

338 Wehner, A., Hartmann, K., and Hirschberger, J. (2008). Associations between proteinuria, systemic hypertension and glomerular filtration rate in dogs with renal and non-renal diseases. *Vet. Rec.* 162: 141–147.

339 Tenhundfeld, J., Wefstaedt, P., and Nolte, I.J. (2009). A randomized controlled clinical trial of the use of benazepril and heparin for the treatment of chronic kidney disease in dogs. *J. Am. Vet. Med. Assoc.* 234: 1031–1037.

340 Chakrabarti, S., Syme, H.M., and Elliott, J. (2012). Clinicopathological variables predicting progression of azotemia in cats with chronic kidney disease. *J. Vet. Internal Med.* 26: 275–281.

341 Jepson, R.E., Brodbelt, D., Vallance, C. et al. (2009). Evaluation of predictors of the development of azotemia in cats. *J. Vet. Internal Med. Am. College Vet. Internal Med.* 23: 806–813.

342 Geddes, R.F., Elliott, J., and Syme, H.M. (2015). Relationship between plasma fibroblast growth Factor-23 concentration and survival time in cats with chronic kidney disease. *J. Vet. Internal Med.* 29: 1494–1501.

343 Mizutani, H., Koyama, H., Watanabe, T. et al. (2006). Evaluation of the clinical efficacy of benazepril in the treatment of chronic renal insufficiency in cats. *J. Vet. Internal Med.* 20: 1074–1079.

344 King, J.N., Gunn-Moore, D.A., Tasker, S. et al. (2006). Tolerability and efficacy of benazepril in cats with chronic kidney disease. *J. Vet. Internal Med.* 20: 1054–1064.

345 O'Neill, D.G., Church, D.B., McGreevy, P.D. et al. (2015). Longevity and mortality of cats attending primary care veterinary practices in England. *J. Feline Med. Surg.* 17: 125–133.

346 O'Neill, D.G., Church, D.B., McGreevy, P.D. et al. (2014). Prevalence of disorders recorded in dogs attending primary-care veterinary practices in England. *PLoS One* 9: e90501.

347 Finco, D.R., Brown, S.A., Brown, C.A. et al. (1999). Progression of chronic renal disease in the dog. *J. Vet. Internal Med.* 13: 516–528.

348 Lippi, I., Guidi, G., Marchetti, V. et al. (2014). Prognostic role of the product of serum calcium and phosphorus concentrations in dogs with chronic kidney disease: 31 cases (2008–2010). *J. Am. Vet. Med. Assoc.* 245: 1135–1140.

349 Cortadellas, O., Fernandez del Palacio, M.J., Talavera, J. et al. (2010). Calcium and phosphorus homeostasis in dogs with spontaneous chronic kidney disease at different stages of severity. *J. Vet. Internal Med.* 24: 73–79.

350 Rudinsky, A.J., Harjes, L.M., Byron, J. et al. (2018). Factors associated with survival in dogs with chronic kidney disease. *J. Vet. Internal Med.* 32: 1977–1982.

351 Liao, Y.L., Chou, C.C., and Lee, Y.J. (2019). The association of indoxyl sulfate with fibroblast growth factor-23 in cats with chronic kidney disease. *J. Vet. Internal Med.* 33 (2): 686–693.

352 Chen, C.N., Chou, C.C., Tsai, P.S.J. et al. (2018). Plasma indoxyl sulfate concentration predicts progression of chronic kidney disease in dogs and cats. *Vet. J.* 232: 33–39.

353 Bradley, R., Tagkopoulos, I., Kim, M. et al. (2019). Predicting early risk of chronic kidney disease in cats using routine clinical laboratory tests and machine learning. *J. Vet. Internal Med.* 33: 2644–2656.

354 Finco, D.R., Brown, S.A., Crowell, W.A. et al. (1994). Effects of aging and dietary protein intake on uninephrectomized geriatric dogs. *Am. J. Vet. Res.* 55: 1282–1290.

355 Bovee, K.C., Kronfeld, D.S., Ramberg, C. et al. (1979). Long-term measurement of renal function in partially nephrectomized dogs fed 56, 27, or 19% protein. *Invest. Urol.* 16: 378–384.

356 Robertson, J.L., Goldschmidt, M., Kronfeld, D.S. et al. (1986). Long-term renal responses to high dietary protein in dogs with 75% nephrectomy. *Kidney Int.* 29: 511–519.

357 Bourgoignie, J.J., Gavellas, G., Martinez, E. et al. (1987). Glomerular function and morphology after renal mass reduction in dogs. *J. Lab. Clin. Med.* 109: 380–388.

358 Polzin, D.J., Osborne, C.A., and Adams, L.G. (1991). Effect of modified protein diets in dogs and cats with chronic renal failure: current status. *J. Nutr.* 121: S140–S144.

359 Polzin, D.J., Leininger, J.R., Osborne, C.A. et al. (1988). Development of renal lesions in dogs after 11/12 reduction of renal mass. Influences of dietary protein intake. *Lab. Investig. J. Techn. Methods Pathol.* 58: 172–183.

360 Adams, L.G., Polzin, D.J., Osborne, C.A. et al. (1994). Influence of dietary protein/calorie intake on renal morphology and function in cats with 5/6 nephrectomy. *Lab. Investig. J. Techn. Methods Pathol.* 70: 347–357.

361 Finco, D.R., Brown, S.A., Brown, C.A. et al. (1998). Protein and calorie effects on progression of induced chronic renal failure in cats. *Am. J. Vet. Res.* 59: 575–582.

362 Dizin, E., Hasler, U., Nlandu-Khodo, S. et al. (2013). Albuminuria induces a proinflammatory and profibrotic response in cortical collecting ducts via the 24p3 receptor. *Am. J. Physiol.* 305: F1053–F1063.

363 Lawson, J., Elliott, J., Wheeler-Jones, C. et al. (2015). Renal fibrosis in feline chronic kidney disease: known mediators and mechanisms of injury. *Vet. J.* 203: 18–26.

364 Rockey, D.C., Bell, P.D., and Hill, J.A. (2015). Fibrosis--a common pathway to organ injury and failure. *N. Engl. J. Med.* 372: 1138–1149.

365 van Beusekom, C.D. and Zimmering, T.M. (2018). Profibrotic effects of angiotensin II and transforming growth factor beta on feline kidney epithelial cells. *J. Feline Med. Surg.* 21: 780–787.

366 Benali, S.L., Lees, G.E., Castagnaro, M. et al. (2014). Epithelial mesenchymal transition in the progression of renal disease in dogs. *Histol. Histopathol.* 29: 1409–1414.

367 Simoes, E.S.A.C. and Teixeira, M.M. (2016). ACE inhibition, ACE2 and angiotensin-(1-7) axis in kidney and cardiac inflammation and fibrosis. *Pharmacol. Res.* 107: 154–162.

368 Clark, S.D., Song, W., Cianciolo, R. et al. (2019). Abnormal expression of miR-21 in kidney tissue of dogs with X-linked hereditary nephropathy: a canine model of chronic kidney disease. *Vet. Pathol.* 56: 93–105.

369 Palmer, B.F. (2002). Renal dysfunction complicating the treatment of hypertension. *N. Engl. J. Med.* 347: 1256–1261.

370 Taylor, S.S., Sparkes, A.H., Briscoe, K. et al. (2017). ISFM consensus guidelines on the diagnosis and management of hypertension in cats. *J. Feline Med. Surg.* 19: 288–303.

371 Syme, H. (2011). Hypertension in small animal kidney disease. *Vet. Clin. North Am.* 41: 63–89.

372 Acierno, M.J., Brown, S., Coleman, A.E. et al. (2018). ACVIM consensus statement: guidelines for the identification, evaluation, and management of systemic hypertension in dogs and cats. *J. Vet. Internal Med.* 32: 1803–1822.

373 Schellenberg, S., Mettler, M., Gentilini, F. et al. (2008). The effects of hydrocortisone on systemic arterial blood pressure and urinary protein excretion in dogs. *J. Vet. Intern. Med.* 22: 273–281.

374 Mathur, S., Syme, H., Brown, C.A. et al. (2002). Effects of the calcium channel antagonist amlodipine in cats with surgically induced hypertensive renal insufficiency. *Am. J. Vet. Res.* 63: 833–839.

375 Finco, D.R. (2004). Association of systemic hypertension with renal injury in dogs with induced renal failure. *J. Vet. Internal Med.* 18: 289–294.

376 Cortadellas, O., del Palacio, M.J., Bayon, A. et al. (2006). Systemic hypertension in dogs with leishmaniasis: prevalence and clinical consequences. *J. Vet. Internal Med.* 20: 941–947.

377 Jepson, R.E., Elliott, J., Brodbelt, D. et al. (2007). Effect of control of systolic blood pressure on survival in cats with systemic hypertension. *J. Vet. Internal Med.* 21: 402–409.

378 Race, G.A., Edwards, J.E., and Scheifley, C.H. (1956). Albuminuria in congestive heart failure. *Circulation* 13: 329–333.

379 Jackson, C.E., Solomon, S.D., Gerstein, H.C. et al. (2009). Albuminuria in chronic heart failure: prevalence and prognostic importance. *Lancet* 374: 543–550.

380 Currie, G. and Delles, C. (2013). Proteinuria and its relation to cardiovascular disease. *Int. J. Nephrol. Renovasc. Dis.* 7: 13–24.

381 Pouchelon, J.L., Atkins, C.E., Bussadori, C. et al. (2015). Cardiovascular-renal axis disorders in the domestic dog and cat: a veterinary consensus statement. *J. Small Anim. Pract.* 56: 537–552.

382 Wegria, R., Capeci, N.E., Blumenthal, M.R. et al. (1955). The pathogenesis of proteinuria in the acutely congested kidney. *J. Clin. Invest.* 34: 737–743.

383 Brewer, R., Wang, M., Zhang, K. et al. (2012). A canine model of chronic heart failure and renal insufficney (caridoreanl syndrome). *J. Am. Coll. Cardiol.* S59: E969.

384 Vaden, S.L., Turman, C.A., Harris, T.L. et al. (2010). The prevalence of albuminuria in dogs and cats in an ICU or recovering from anesthesia. *J. Vet. Emerg. Crit. Care (San Antonio)* 20: 479–487.

385 Whittemore, J.C., Marcum, B.A., Mawby, D.I. et al. (2011). Associations among albuminuria, C-reactive protein concentrations, survival predictor index scores, and survival in 78 critically ill dogs. *J. Vet. Internal Med.* 25: 818–824.

386 Prudic, R.A., Saba, C.F., Lourenco, B.N. et al. (2018). Prevalence of proteinuria in a canine oncology population. *J. Small Anim. Pract.* 59: 496–500.

387 Di Bella, A., Maurella, C., Cauvin, A. et al. (2013). Proteinuria in canine patients with lymphoma. *J. Small Anim. Pract.* 54: 28–32.

388 Pressler, B.M., Proulx, D.R., Williams, L.E. et al. (2003). Urine albumin concentration is increased in dogs with lymphoma or osteosarcoma [abstract 101]. *J. Vet. Internal Med.* 17: 404.

389 Saam, D.E., Liptak, J.M., Stalker, M.J. et al. (2011). Predictors of outcome in dogs treated with adjuvant carboplatin for appendicular osteosarcoma: 65 cases (1996–2006). *J. Am. Vet. Med. Assoc.* 238: 195–206.

390 Shephard, R.J. (1985). Adaptation to exercise in the cold. *Sports Med. (Auckland NZ)* 2: 59–71.

391 Epstein, J.B. and Zambraski, E.J. (1979). Proteinuria in the exercising dog. *Med. Sci. Sports* 11: 348–350.

392 Joles, J.A., Sanders, M., Velthuizen, J. et al. (1984). Proteinuria in intact and splenectomized dogs after running and swimming. *Int. J. Sports Med.* 5: 311–316.

393 Gary, A.T., Cohn, L.A., Kerl, M.E. et al. (2004). The effects of exercise on urinary albumin excretion in dogs. *J. Vet. Internal Med.* 18: 52–55.

394 Durocher, L., Hinchcliff, K., Williamson, K. et al. (2006). Lack of microalbuminuria in sled dogs following exercise. *Equine Comp. Exercise Physiol.* 3: 1–2.

395 Boesken, W.H., Mamier, A., Neumann, H. et al. (1983). Does febrile proteinuria exist? *Klin. Wochenschr.* 61: 917–922.

396 Bruchim, Y., Horowitz, M., and Aroch, I. (2017). Pathophysiology of heatstroke in dogs – revisited. *Temperature (Austin)* 4: 356–370.

397 Hall, E.J., Carter, A.J., and O'Neill, D.G. (2020). Dogs don't die just in hot cars-exertional heat-related illness (heatstroke) is a greater threat to UK dogs. *Animals (Basel)* 10: 8–1324.

398 Hall, E.J., Carter, A.J., and O'Neill, D.G. (2020). Incidence and risk factors for heat-related illness (heatstroke) in UK dogs under primary veterinary care in 2016. *Sci. Rep.* 10: 9128.

399 Segev, G., Bruchim, Y., Berl, N. et al. (2018). Effects of fenoldopam on kidney function parameters and its therapeutic efficacy in the management of acute kidney injury in dogs with heatstroke. *J. Vet. Internal Med.* 32: 1109–1115.

400 Romanucci, M. and Salda, L.D. (2013). Pathophysiology and pathological findings of heatstroke in dogs. *Vet. Med. (Auckland NZ)* 4: 1–9.

401 Segev, G., Daminet, S., Meyer, E. et al. (2015). Characterization of kidney damage using several renal biomarkers in dogs with naturally occurring heatstroke. *Vet. J.* 206: 231–235.

402 Drobatz, K.J. and Macintire, D.K. (1996). Heat-induced illness in dogs: 42 cases (1976–1993). *J. Am. Vet. Med. Assoc.* 209: 1894–1899.

403 Krum, S.H. and Osborne, C.A. (1977). Heatstroke in the dog: a polysystemic disorder. *J. Am. Vet. Med. Assoc.* 170: 531–535.

404 Shapiro, Y., Rosenthal, T., and Sohar, E. (1973). Experimental heatstroke. A model in dogs. *Arch. Intern. Med.* 131: 688–692.

405 Matz, R. (1986). Hypothermia: mechanisms and countermeasures. *Hosp. Pract. (Off. Ed)* 21: 45–48. 54–48, 63–71.

406 Fitzgerald, F.T. and Jessop, C. (1982). Accidental hypothermia: a report of 22 cases and review of the literature. *Adv. Intern. Med.* 27: 128–150.

407 Caragelasco, D.S., Kogika, M.M., Martorelli, C.R. et al. (2017). Urine protein electrophoresis study in dogs with pituitary dependent hyperadrenocorticism during therapy with trilostane. *Pesq. Vet. Bras.* 37: 734–740.

408 Smets, P.M., Lefebvre, H.P., Meij, B.P. et al. (2012). Long-term follow-up of renal function in dogs after treatment for ACTH-dependent hyperadrenocorticism. *J. Vet. Internal Med.* 26: 565–574.

409 Smets, P.M., Lefebvre, H.P., Kooistra, H.S. et al. (2012). Hypercortisolism affects glomerular and tubular function in dogs. *Vet. J.* 192: 532–534.

410 Smets, P.M., Lefebvre, H.P., Aresu, L. et al. (2012). Renal function and morphology in aged beagle dogs before and after hydrocortisone administration. *PLoS One* 7: e31702.

411 Smets, P., Meyer, E., Maddens, B. et al. (2010). Cushing's syndrome, glucocorticoids and the kidney. *Gen. Comp. Endocrinol.* 169: 1–10.

412 Waters, C.B., Adams, L.G., Scott-Moncrieff, J.C. et al. (1997). Effects of glucocorticoid therapy on urine protein-to-creatinine ratios and renal morphology in dogs. *J. Vet. Internal Med.* 11: 172–177.

413 Lees, G.E., Willard, M.D., and Dziezyc, J. (2002). Glomerular proteinuria is rapidly but reversibly increased by short-term prednisone administration in heterozygous (carrier) female dogs with X-linked hereditary nephropathy [abstract 102]. *J. Vet. Internal Med.* 16: 352.

414 Cavalcante, C.Z., Kogika, M.M., Bacic, A. et al. (2013). Avaliação da albuminúria e da eletroforese de pro¬teínas urinárias de cães com hiperadrenocorticismo e a relação com a pressão arterial sistêmica. *Pesq. Vet. Bras.* 33: 1364–1370.

415 Ortega, T.M., Feldman, E.C., Nelson, R.W. et al. (1996). Systemic arterial blood pressure and urine protein/creatinine ratio in dogs with hyperadrenocorticism. *J. Am. Vet. Med. Assoc.* 209: 1724–1729.

416 Hurley, K.J. and Vaden, S.L. (1998). Evaluation of urine protein content in dogs with pituitary-dependent hyperadrenocorticism. *J. Am. Vet. Med. Assoc.* 212: 369–373.

417 Herring, I.P., Panciera, D.L., and Werre, S.R. (2014). Longitudinal prevalence of hypertension, proteinuria, and retinopathy in dogs with spontaneous diabetes mellitus. *J. Vet. Internal Med.* 28: 488–495.

418 Kogika, M.M., Cavalcante, C.Z., Simoes, D.M.N. et al. (2007). Microalbuminuria in dogs with diabetes mellitus. *J. Vet. Intern. Med.* 21: 647–647.

419 Struble, A.L., Feldman, E.C., Nelson, R.W. et al. (1998). Systemic hypertension and proteinuria in dogs with diabetes mellitus. *J. Am. Vet. Med. Assoc.* 213: 822–825.

420 Mazzi, A., Fracassi, F., Dondi, F. et al. (2008). Ratio of urinary protein to creatinine and albumin to creatinine in dogs with diabetes mellitus and hyperadrenocorticism. *Vet. Res. Commun.* 32 (Suppl 1): S299–S301.

421 Al-Ghazlat, S.A., Langston, C.E., Greco, D.S. et al. (2011). The prevalence of microalbuminuria and proteinuria in cats with diabetes mellitus. *Top. Companion Anim. Med.* 26: 154–157.

422 Paepe, D., Ghys, L.F., Smets, P. et al. (2015). Routine kidney variables, glomerular filtration rate and urinary cystatin C in cats with diabetes mellitus, cats with chronic kidney disease and healthy cats. *J. Feline Med. Surg.* 17: 880–888.

423 DiBartola, S.P. and Brown, S.A. (2000). The kidney and hyperthyroidism. In: *Kirk's Current Veterinary Therapy XIII* (ed. J.D. Bonagura), 337–339. Philadelphia WB: Saunders.

424 Langston, C.E. and Reine, N.J. (2006). Hyperthyroidism and the kidney. *Clin. Tech. Small Anim. Pract.* 21: 17–21.

425 Williams, T.L., Peak, K.J., Brodbelt, D. et al. (2010). Survival and the7 development of azotemia after treatment of hyperthyroid cats. *J. Vet. Internal Med.* 24: 863–869.

426 Syme, H.M. and Elliott, J. (2003). The prevalence of hypertension in hyperthyroid cats at diagnosis and following treatment. *J. Vet. Internal Med.* 17: 754.

427 Vaske, H.H., Schermerhorn, T., and Grauer, G.F. (2016). Effects of feline hyperthyroidism on kidney function: a review. *J. Feline Med. Surg.* 18: 55–59.

428 van Hoek, I., Lefebvre, H.P., Peremans, K. et al. (2009). Short- and long-term follow-up of glomerular and tubular renal markers of kidney function in hyperthyroid cats after treatment with radioiodine. *Domest. Anim. Endocrinol.* 36: 45–56.

429 Syme, H.M. and Elliott, J. (2001). Evaluation of proteinuria in hyperthyroid cats. *J. Vet. Internal Med.* 15: 299.

430 Ghys, L.F., Paepe, D., Taffin, E.R. et al. (2015). Serum and urinary cystatin C in cats with feline immunodeficiency virus infection and cats with hyperthyroidism. *J. Feline Med. Surg.* 18 (8): 658–665.

431 Niessen, S.J., Church, D.B., and Forcada, Y. (2013). Hypersomatotropism, acromegaly, and hyperadrenocorticism and feline diabetes mellitus. *Vet. Clin. North Am.* 43: 319–350.

432 Peterson, M.E., Taylor, R.S., Greco, D.S. et al. (1990). Acromegaly in 14 cats. *J. Vet. Internal Med. Am. College Vet. Internal Med.* 4: 192–201.

433 Gunn-Moore, D. (2005). Feline endocrinopathies. *Vet. Clin. North Am.* 35: 171–210, vii.

434 Niessen, S.J., Petrie, G., Gaudiano, F. et al. (2007). Feline acromegaly: an underdiagnosed endocrinopathy? *J. Vet. Internal Med.* 21: 899–905.

435 Greco, D.S. (2012). Feline acromegaly. *Top. Companion Anim. Med.* 27: 31–35.

436 Furrow, E. (2020). Hypertriglyceridemia-associated proteinuria in miniature schnauzers. *Vet. Focus* 30.1, https://vetfocus.royalcanin.com/en/doc-400.html: Royal Canin.

437 Furrow, E., Lees, G.E., Brown, C.A. et al. (2017). Glomerular lesions in proteinuric miniature schnauzer dogs. *Vet. Pathol.* 54: 484–489.

438 Fournel, C., Chabanne, L., Caux, C. et al. (1992). Canine systemic lupus erythematosus. I: a study of 75 cases. *Lupus* 1: 133–139.

439 Monier, J.C., Ritter, J., Caux, C. et al. (1992). Canine systemic lupus erythematosus. II: antinuclear antibodies. *Lupus* 1: 287–293.

440 Smee, N.M., Harkin, K.R., and Wilkerson, M.J. (2007). Measurement of serum antinuclear antibody titer in dogs with and without systemic lupus erythematosus: 120 cases (1997–2005). *J. Am. Vet. Med. Assoc.* 230: 1180–1183.

441 Drazner, F.H. (1980). Systemic lupus erythematosus in the dog. *Compend. Contin. Educ.* 2: 243–254.

442 Grindem, C.B. and Johnson, K.H. (1983). Systemic lupus erythematosus: literature review and report of 42 new canine cases. *J. Am. Anim. Hosp. Assoc.* 19: 489–503.

443 Grindem, C.B. and Johnson, K.H. (1984). Amyloidosis in a case of canine systemic lupus erythematosus. *J. Comp. Pathol.* 94: 569–573.

444 Hannah, F. (2013). Case study: three cats with SLE and erosive polyarthritis. *Companion Anim.* 18 (6): 256–263.

445 Yang, T.J. (1987). Gray collie syndrome. *J. Am. Vet. Med. Assoc.* 191: 390–391.

446 Dale, D.C., Rodger, E., Cebon, J. et al. (1995). Long-term treatment of canine cyclic hematopoiesis with recombinant canine stem cell factor. *Blood* 85: 74–79.

447 Cheville, N.F., Cutlip, R.C., and Moon, H.W. (1970). Microscopic pathology of the gray collie syndrome. Cyclic neutropenia, amyloidosis, enteritis, and bone necrosis. *Pathol. Vet.* 7: 225–245.

448 DiGiacomo, R.F., Hammond, W.P., Kunz, L.L. et al. (1983). Clinical and pathologic features of cyclic hematopoiesis in grey collie dogs. *Am. J. Pathol.* 111: 224–233.

449 Maddens, B., Heiene, R., Smets, P. et al. (2011). Evaluation of kidney injury in dogs with pyometra based on proteinuria, renal histomorphology, and urinary biomarkers. *J. Vet. Internal Med.* 25: 1075–1083.

450 Sant'Anna, M.C., Martins, G.F., Flaiban, K.K.M.C. et al. (2019). Protein-to-creatinine urinary in the early diagnosis of renal injury in canine pyometra. *Pesq. Vet. Brasil.* 39: 186–191.

451 de Schepper, J., van der Stock, J., Capiau, E. et al. (1987). Renal injury in dogs with pyometra. *Tijdschr. Diergeneeskd.* 112 (Suppl 1): 124S–126S.

452 Maddens, B., Daminet, S., Smets, P. et al. (2010). Escherichia coli pyometra induces transient glomerular and tubular dysfunction in dogs. *J. Vet. Internal Med. Am. College Vet. Internal Med.* 24: 1263–1270.

453 Obel, A., Nicander, L., and Asheim, A. (1964). Light and electron microscopical studies of the renal lesions in dogs with pyometra. *Acta Vet. Scand.* 5: 146–178.

454 Whitney, J.C. (1969). Polydipsia in the dog – symposium. 2. Polydipsia and its relationship to pyometra. *J. Small Anim. Pract.* 10: 485–489.

455 Koenhemsi, L., Toydemir, S., Ucmak, M. et al. (2016). Evaluation of early renal disease in bitches with pyometra based on renal doppler measurements. *Vet. Med.* 61: 344–347.

456 Heiene, R., Kristiansen, V., Teige, J. et al. (2007). Renal histomorphology in dogs with pyometra and control dogs, and long term clinical outcome with respect to signs of kidney disease. *Acta Vet. Scand.* 49: 13.

457 Heiene, R., Moe, L., and Molmen, G. (2001). Calculation of urinary enzyme excretion, with renal structure and function in dogs with pyometra. *Res. Vet. Sci.* 70: 129–137.

458 Stone, E.A., Littman, M.P., Robertson, J.L. et al. (1988). Renal dysfunction in dogs with pyometra. *J. Am. Vet. Med. Assoc.* 193: 457–464.

459 Asheim, A. (1964). Renal function in dogs with Pyometra. 8. Uterine infection and the pathogenesis of the renal dysfunction. *Acta Pathol. Microbiol. Scand.* 60: 99–107.

460 Sandholm, M., Vasenius, H., and Kivisto, A.K. (1975). Pathogenesis of canine pyometra. *J. Am. Vet. Med. Assoc.* 167: 1006–1010.

461 Asheim, A. (1965). Pathogenesis of renal damage and polydipsia in dogs with pyometra. *J. Am. Vet. Med. Assoc.* 147: 736–745.

462 Qurollo, B.A., Buch, J., Chandrashekar, R. et al. (2019). Clinicopathological findings in 41 dogs (2008–2018) naturally infected with Ehrlichia ewingii. *J. Vet. Internal Med.* 33: 618–629.

463 Abramowsky, C.R., Powers, K.G., Aikawa, M. et al. (1981). *Dirofilaria immitis*. 5. Immunopathology of filarial nephropathy in dogs. *Am. J. Pathol.* 104: 1–12.

464 Aikawa, M., Abramowsky, C., Powers, K.G. et al. (1981). Glomerulonephropathy induced by *Dirofilaria immitis* infection. *Am. J. Trop. Med. Hyg.* 30: 84–91.

465 Buoro, I.B. and Atwell, R.B. (1983). Urinalysis in canine dirofilariasis with emphasis on proteinuria. *Vet. Rec.* 112: 252–253.

466 Ludders, J.W., Grauer, G.F., Dubielzig, R.R. et al. (1988). Renal microcirculatory and correlated histologic changes associated with dirofilariasis in dogs. *Am. J. Vet. Res.* 49: 826–830.

467 Hormaeche, M., Carreton, E., Gonzalez-Miguel, J. et al. (2014). Proteomic analysis of the urine of *Dirofilaria immitis* infected dogs. *Vet. Parasitol.* 203: 241–246.

468 Carreton, E., Falcon-Cordon, Y., Rodon, J. et al. (2020). Evaluation of serum biomarkers and proteinuria for the early detection of renal damage in dogs with heartworm (*Dirofilaria immitis*). *Vet. Parasitol.* 283: 109144.

469 Dalton, G.O. Jr., Bruce, L.A., and Huber, T.L. (1971). Effect of *Dirofilaria immitis* on renal function in the dog. *Am. J. Vet. Res.* 32: 2087–2089.

470 Simpson, C.F., Gebhardt, B.M., Bradley, R.E. et al. (1974). Glomerulosclerosis in canine heartworm infection. *Vet. Pathol.* 11: 506–514.

471 Wong, M.M. (1964). Studies on microfilaremia in dogs. Ii. Levels of microfilaremia in relation to immunologic responses of the host. *Am. J. Trop. Med. Hyg.* 13: 66–77.

472 Wong, M.M., Suter, P.F., Rhode, E.A. et al. (1973). Dirofilariasis without circulating microfilariae: a problem in diagnosis. *J. Am. Vet. Med. Assoc.* 163: 133–139.

473 Grauer, G.F., Culham, C.A., Bowman, D.D. et al. (1988). Parasite excretory-secretory antigen and antibody to excretory-secretory antigen in body fluids and kidney tissue of *Dirofilaria immitis* infected dogs. *Am. J. Trop. Med. Hyg.* 39: 380–387.

474 Grauer, G.F., Culham, C.A., Dubielzig, R.R. et al. (1988). Effects of a specific thromboxane synthetase inhibitor on development of experimental *Dirofilaria immitis* immune complex glomerulonephritis in the dog. *J. Vet. Internal Med.* 2: 192–200.

475 Atkins, C.E., DeFrancesco, T.C., Coats, J.R. et al. (2000). Heartworm infection in cats: 50 cases (1985–1997). *J. Am. Vet. Med. Assoc.* 217: 355–358.

476 Kramer, L.H., Tamarozzi, F., Morchon, R. et al. (2005). Immune response to and tissue localization of the Wolbachia surface protein (WSP) in dogs with natural heartworm (*Dirofilaria immitis*) infection. *Vet. Immunol. Immunopathol.* 106: 303–308.

477 Morchon, R., Carreton, E., Grandi, G. et al. (2012). Anti-Wolbachia surface protein antibodies are present in the urine of dogs naturally infected with *Dirofilaria immitis* with circulating microfilariae but not in dogs with occult infections. *Vector Borne Zoonotic Dis.* 12: 17–20.

478 Morchon, R., Ferreira, A.C., Martin-Pacho, J.R. et al. (2004). Specific IgG antibody response against antigens of *Dirofilaria immitis* and its Wolbachia endosymbiont bacterium in cats with natural and experimental infections. *Vet. Parasitol.* 125: 313–321.

479 Ciaramella, P., Oliva, G., Luna, R.D. et al. (1997). A retrospective clinical study of canine leishmaniasis in 150 dogs naturally infected by Leishmania infantum. *Vet. Rec.* 141: 539–543.

480 Roura, X., Fondati, A., Lubas, G. et al. (2013). Prognosis and monitoring of leishmaniasis in dogs: a working group report. *Vet. J.* 198: 43–47.

481 Poli, A., Abramo, F., Mancianti, F. et al. (1991). Renal involvement in canine leishmaniasis. A light-microscopic, immunohistochemical and electron-microscopic study. *Nephron* 57: 444–452.

482 Zatelli, A., Borgarelli, M., Santilli, R. et al. (2003). Glomerular lesions in dogs infected with Leishmania organisms. *Am. J. Vet. Res.* 64: 558–561.

483 Palacio, J., Liste, F., and Gascon, M. (1995). Urinary protein/creatinine ratio in the evaluation of renal failure in canine leishmaniasis. *Vet. Rec.* 137: 567–568.

484 Proverbio, D., Spada, E., de Giorgi, G.B. et al. (2016). Proteinuria reduction after treatment with miltefosine and allopurinol in dogs naturally infected with leishmaniasis. *Vet. World* 9: 904–908.

485 Jeraj, K.P., Hardy, R., O'Leary, T.P. et al. (1985). Immune complex glomerulonephritis in a cat with renal lymphosarcoma. *Vet. Pathol.* 22: 287–290.

486 Anderson, L.J. and Jarrett, W.F. (1971). Membranous glomerulonephritis associated with leukaemia in cats. *Res. Vet. Sci.* 12: 179–180.

487 Glick, A.D., Horn, R.G., and Holscher, M. (1978). Characterization of feline glomerulonephritis associated with viral-induced hematopoietic neoplasms. *Am. J. Pathol.* 92: 321–332.

488 Jakowski, R.M., Essec, M., Hardy, W.D. et al. (1980). Membranous glomerulonephritis in a household cluster of cats persistently viremic with feline leukemia virus. *Third Int. Feline Leukemia Virus Meeting* 1981: 141–149.

489 Hardy, W.D. Jr. (1974). Immunology of oncornaviruses. *Vet. Clin. North Am.* 4: 133–146.

490 Poli, A., Abramo, F., Taccini, E. et al. (1993). Renal involvement in feline immunodeficiency virus infection: a clinicopathological study. *Nephron* 64: 282–288.

491 Baxter, K.J., Levy, J.K., Edinboro, C.H. et al. (2012). Renal disease in cats infected with feline immunodeficiency virus. *J. Vet. Internal Med.* 26: 238–243.

492 Poli, A., Tozon, N., Guidi, G. et al. (2012). Renal alterations in feline immunodeficiency virus (FIV)-infected cats: a natural model of lentivirus-induced renal disease changes. *Viruses* 4: 1372–1389.

493 Asproni, P., Abramo, F., Millanta, F. et al. (2013). Amyloidosis in association with spontaneous feline immunodeficiency virus infection. *J. Feline Med. Surg.* 15: 300–306.

494 Hayashi, T., Ishida, T., and Fujiwara, K. (1982). Glomerulonephritis associated with feline infectious peritonitis. *Nihon Juigaku Zasshi* 44: 909–916.

495 Jacobse-Geels, H.E., Daha, M.R., and Horzinek, M.C. (1980). Isolation and characterization of feline C3 and evidence for the immune complex pathogenesis of feline infectious peritonitis. *J. Immunol.* 125: 1606–1610.

496 Pedersen, N.C. (2009). A review of feline infectious peritonitis virus infection: 1963–2008. *J. Feline Med. Surg.* 11: 225–258.

497 Pedersen, N.C. (2014). An update on feline infectious peritonitis: diagnostics and therapeutics. *Vet. J.* 201: 133–141.

498 Tasker, S. (2018). Diagnosis of feline infectious peritonitis: update on evidence supporting available tests. *J. Feline Med. Surg.* 20: 228–243.

499 Riemer, F., Kuehner, K.A., Ritz, S. et al. (2016). Clinical and laboratory features of cats with feline infectious peritonitis – a retrospective study of 231 confirmed cases (2000–2010). *J. Feline Med. Surg.* 18: 348–356.

500 Paltrinieri, S., Comazzi, S., Spagnolo, V. et al. (2002). Laboratory changes consistent with feline infectious peritonitis in cats from multicat environments. *J. Vet. Med.* 49: 503–510.

501 Norris, J.M., Bosward, K.L., White, J.D. et al. (2005). Clinicopathological findings associated with feline infectious peritonitis in Sydney, Australia: 42 cases (1990–2002). *Aust. Vet. J.* 83: 666–673.

502 Tsai, H.Y., Chueh, L.L., Lin, C.N. et al. (2011). Clinicopathological findings and disease staging of feline infectious peritonitis: 51 cases from 2003 to 2009 in Taiwan. *J. Feline Med. Surg.* 13: 74–80.

503 Sparkes, A.H., Gruffydd-Jones, T.J., and Harbour, D.A. (1994). An appraisal of the value of laboratory tests in the diagnosis of feline infectious peritonitis. *J. Am. Anim. Hosp. Assoc.* 30: 345–350.

504 Sparkes, A.H., Gruffydd-Jones, T.J., and Harbour, D.A. (1991). Feline infectious peritonitis: a review of clinicopathological changes in 65 cases, and a critical assessment of their diagnostic value. *Vet. Rec.* 129: 209–212.

505 Pedersen, N.C. (1976). Feline infectious peritonitis: something old, something new. *Feline Pract.* 6: 42–46, 48–51.

506 Pressler, B. (2011). Nephrotic syndrome. In: *Nephrology and Urology of Small Animals* (ed. J. Bartges and D. Polzin), 415–421. West Sussex, UK: Wiley Blackwell.

507 Klosterman, E.S. and Pressler, B.M. (2011). Nephrotic syndrome in dogs: clinical features and evidence-based treatment considerations. *Top. Companion Anim. Med.* 26: 135–142.

508 Sum, S.O., Hensel, P., Rios, L. et al. (2010). Drug-induced minimal change nephropathy in a dog. *J. Vet. Internal Med.* 24: 431–435.

509 Polzin, D. and Cowgill, L.D. (2017). Management of glomerulopathies. In: *BSAVA Manual of Canine and Feline Nephrology and Urology*, 3e (ed. J. Elliott, G.F. Grauer and J.L. Westropp), 278–290. Gloucester, England British: Small Animal Veterinary Association.

510 Coleman, A.E. and Elliott, J. (2019). Inhibition of the renin-angiotensin-aldosterone system in cats and dogs: The emerging role of angiotensin II receptor blockers. International Renal Interest Society (IRIS). http://www.iris-kidney.com/education/renin-angiotensin-aldosterone-system.html (accessed December 17 2019).

511 Parker, V.J. and Freeman, L.M. (2011). Association between body condition and survival in dogs with acquired chronic kidney disease. *J. Vet. Internal Med.* 25: 1306–1311.

512 Parker, V.J. (2021). Nutritional management of dogs and cats with CKD. *Vet. Clin. North Am.* 51 (3): 685–710.

513 Ruggenenti, P., Cortinovis, M., Parvanova, A. et al. (2021). Preventing microalbuminuria with benazepril, valsartan, and benazepril-valsartan combination therapy in diabetic patients with high-normal albuminuria: a prospective, randomized, open-label, blinded endpoint (PROBE) study. *PLoS Med.* 18: e1003691.

514 Marquez, D.F., Ruiz-Hurtado, G., Segura, J. et al. (2019). Microalbuminuria and cardiorenal risk: old and new evidence in different populations. *F1000Res* 8: 1659.

515 Viazzi, F., Cappadona, F., and Pontremoli, R. (2016). Microalbuminuria in primary hypertension: a guide to optimal patient management? *J. Nephrol.* 29: 747–753.

516 Parker, V.J. and Freeman, L.M. (2012). Nutritional Management of Protein-Losing Neprhopathy. Dogs *Compendium*. July E1-E5.

517 Zatelli, A., Roura, X., D'Ippolito, P. et al. (2016). The effect of renal diet in association with enalapril or benazepril on proteinuria in dogs with proteinuric chronic kidney disease. *Open Vet. J.* 6: 121–127.

518 Cortadellas, O., Talavera, J., and Fernandez del Palacio, M.J. (2014). Evaluation of the effects of a therapeutic renal diet to control proteinuria in proteinuric non-azotemic dogs treated with benazepril. *J. Vet. Internal Med.* 28: 30–37.

519 Burkholder, W.J., Lees, G.E., LeBlanc, A.K. et al. (2004). Diet modulates proteinuria in heterozygous female dogs with X-linked hereditary nephropathy. *J. Vet. Internal Med.* 18: 165–175.

520 Brown, S.A., Brown, C.A., Crowell, W.A. et al. (1998). Beneficial effects of chronic administration of dietary omega-3 polyunsaturated fatty acids in dogs with renal insufficiency. *J. Lab. Clin. Med.* 131: 447–455.

521 Chang, A.R. and Anderson, C. (2017). Dietary phosphorus intake and the kidney. *Annu. Rev. Nutr.* 37: 321–346.

522 Shuto, E., Taketani, Y., Tanaka, R. et al. (2009). Dietary phosphorus acutely impairs endothelial function. *J. Am. Soc. Nephrol.* 20: 1504–1512.

523 Stevens, K.K., Denby, L., Patel, R.K. et al. (2017). Deleterious effects of phosphate on vascular and endothelial function via disruption to the nitric oxide pathway. *Nephrol. Dial. Transplant.* 32: 1617–1627.

524 Di Iorio, B.R., Bellizzi, V., Bellasi, A. et al. (2013). Phosphate attenuates the anti-proteinuric effect of very low-protein diet in CKD patients. *Nephrol. Dial. Transplant.* 28: 632–640.

525 Brown, S.A. and Finco, D.R. (1992). Characterization of the renal response to protein ingestion in dogs with experimentally induced renal failure. *Am. J. Vet. Res.* 53: 569–573.

526 Bovee, K.C. and Kronfeld, D.S. (1981). Reduction of renal hemodynamics in uremic dogs fed reduced protein diets. *J. Am. Anim. Hosp. Assoc.* 17: 277–285.

527 Bovee, K.C. (1991). Influence of dietary protein on renal function in dogs. *J. Nutr.* 121: S128–S139.

528 Valli, V.E., Baumal, R., Thorner, P. et al. (1991). Dietary modification reduces splitting of glomerular basement membranes and delays death due to renal failure in canine X-linked hereditary nephritis. *Lab. Investig. J. Techn. Methods Pathol.* 65: 67–73.

529 Polzin, D.J., Osborne, C.A., Hayden, D.W. et al. (1984). Influence of reduced protein diets on morbidity, mortality, and renal function in dogs with induced chronic renal failure. *Am. J. Vet. Res.* 45: 506–517.

530 Finco, D.R., Brown, S.A., Crowell, W.A. et al. (1992). Effects of phosphorus/calcium-restricted and phosphorus/calcium-replete 32% protein diets in dogs with chronic renal failure. *Am. J. Vet. Res.* 53: 157–163.

531 Adams, L.G., Polzin, D.J., Osborne, C.A. et al. (1993). Effects of dietary protein and calorie restriction in clinically normal cats and in cats with surgically induced chronic renal failure. *Am. J. Vet. Res.* 54: 1653–1662.

532 Chauveau, P., Combe, C., Rigalleau, V. et al. (2007). Restricted protein diet is associated with decrease in proteinuria: consequences on the progression of renal failure. *J. Ren. Nutr.* 17: 250–257.

533 Fouque, D. and Laville, M. (2009). Low protein diets for chronic kidney disease in non diabetic adults. *Cochrane Database Syst. Rev.* CD001892.

534 Hahn, D., Hodson, E.M., and Fouque, D. (2018). Low protein diets for non-diabetic adults with chronic kidney disease. *Cochrane Database Syst. Rev.* 10: CD001892.

535 Parker, V.J., Rudinsky, A.J., Benedict, J.A. et al. (2020). Effects of calcifediol supplementation on markers of chronic kidney disease-mineral and bone disorder in dogs with chronic kidney disease. *J. Vet. Internal Med.* 34: 2497–2506.

536 Polzin, D.J. and Churchill, J.A. (2016). Controversies in veterinary nephrology: renal diets are indicated for cats with international renal interest society chronic kidney disease stages 2 to 4: the pro view. *Vet. Clin. North Am.* 46: 1049–1065.

537 Scherk, M.A. and Laflamme, D.P. (2016). Controversies in veterinary nephrology: renal diets are indicated for cats with international renal interest society chronic kidney disease stages 2 to 4: the con view. *Vet. Clin. North Am.* 46: 1067–1094.

538 Bauer, J.E. (2011). Therapeutic use of fish oils in companion animals. *J. Am. Vet. Med. Assoc.* 239: 1441–1451.

539 Brown, S.A., Brown, C.A., Crowell, W.A. et al. (2000). Effects of dietary polyunsaturated fatty acid supplementation in early renal insufficiency in dogs. *J. Lab. Clin. Med.* 135: 275–286.

540 Lenox, C.E. (2015). Timely topics in nutrition: an overview of fatty acids in companion animal medicine. *J. Am. Vet. Med. Assoc.* 246: 1198–1202.

541 Lenox, C.E. (2016). Role of dietary fatty acids in dogs & cats. *Today's Vet. Pract.* 83–88.

542 Galler, A., Tran, J.L., Krammer-Lukas, S. et al. (2012). Blood vitamin levels in dogs with chronic kidney disease. *Vet. J.* 192: 226–231.

543 Parker, V.J., Harjes, L.M., Dembek, K. et al. (2017). Association of Vitamin D metabolites with parathyroid hormone, fibroblast growth Factor-23, calcium, and phosphorus in dogs with various stages of chronic kidney disease. *J. Vet. Internal Med.* 31 (3): 791–798.

544 Miller, M.S., Rudinsky, A.J., Brett, G. et al. (2020). Association between vitamin D metabolites, vitamin D binding protein, and proteinuria in dogs. *J. Vet. Intern. Med.* 34 (6): 2468–2477.

545 Ames, M.K., Atkins, C.E., and Pitt, B. (2019). The renin-angiotensin-aldosterone system and its suppression. *J. Vet. Internal Med.* 33: 363–382.

546 Adin, D., Atkins, C., Domenig, O. et al. (2020). Renin-angiotensin aldosterone profile before and after angiotensin-converting enzyme-inhibitor administration in dogs with angiotensin-converting enzyme gene polymorphism. *J. Vet. Internal Med.* 34 (2): 600–606.

547 Spencer, S., Wheeler-Jones, C., and Elliott, J. (2020). Aldosterone and the mineralocorticoid receptor in renal injury: a potential therapeutic target in feline chronic kidney disease. *J. Vet. Pharmacol. Ther.* 43: 243–267.

548 Santos, R.A.S., Sampaio, W.O., Alzamora, A.C. et al. (2018). The ACE2/angiotensin-(1-7)/MAS Axis of the renin-angiotensin system: focus on angiotensin-(1-7). *Physiol. Rev.* 98: 505–553.

549 Malinowski, J.T. and St Jean, D.J. (2018). Next-generation small molecule therapies for heart failure: 2015 and beyond. *Bioorg. Med. Chem. Lett.* 28: 1429–1435.

550 Goodfriend, T.L., Elliott, M.E., and Catt, K.J. (1996). Angiotensin receptors and their antagonists. *N. Engl. J. Med.* 334: 1649–1654.

551 Lefebvre, H.P., Brown, S.A., Chetboul, V. et al. (2007). Angiotensin-converting enzyme inhibitors in veterinary medicine. *Curr. Pharm. Des.* 13: 1347–1361.

552 Patel, V.B., Zhong, J.C., Grant, M.B. et al. (2016). Role of the ACE2/angiotensin 1-7 Axis of the renin-angiotensin system in heart failure. *Circ. Res.* 118: 1313–1326.

553 Agarwal, R., Anker, S.D., Bakris, G. et al. (2020). Investigating new treatment opportunities for patients with chronic kidney disease in type 2 diabetes: the role of finerenone. *Nephrol. Dial. Transplant.* 37 (6): 1014–1023.

554 Ruster, C. and Wolf, G. (2006). Renin-angiotensin-aldosterone system and progression of renal disease. *J. Am. Soc. Nephrol.* 17: 2985–2991.

555 Patel, V., Joharapurkar, A., and Jain, M. (2021). Role of mineralocorticoid receptor antagonists in kidney diseases. *Drug Dev. Res.* 82: 341–363.

556 Mitani, S., Yabuki, A., Taniguchi, K. et al. (2013). Association between the intrarenal renin-angiotensin system and renal injury in chronic kidney disease of dogs and cats. *J. Vet. Med. Sci.* 75: 127–133.

557 Brown, S.A., Brown, C.A., Jacobs, G. et al. (2001). Effects of the angiotensin converting enzyme inhibitor benazepril in cats with induced renal insufficiency. *Am. J. Vet. Res.* 62: 375–383.

558 Brown, S.A., Finco, D.R., Brown, C.A. et al. (2003). Evaluation of the effects of inhibition of angiotensin converting enzyme with enalapril in dogs with induced chronic renal insufficiency. *Am. J. Vet. Res.* 64: 321–327.

559 Taal, M.W. (2020). Classification and management of chronic kidney disease. In: *Brenner and Rector's the Kidney*, 11e (ed. Y. ISL, G.M. Chertow, V. Luyckx, et al.), 1946–1976.e1947. Philadelphia, PA: Elsevier.

560 Macconi, D., Ghilardi, M., Bonassi, M.E. et al. (2000). Effect of angiotensin-converting enzyme inhibition on glomerular basement membrane permeability and distribution of zonula occludens-1 in MWF rats. *J. Am. Soc. Nephrol.* 11: 477–489.

561 Macconi, D., Sangalli, F., Bonomelli, M. et al. (2009). Podocyte repopulation contributes to regression of glomerular injury induced by ACE inhibition. *Am. J. Pathol.* 174: 797–807.

562 Christ, D.D., Wong, P.C., Wong, Y.N. et al. (1994). The pharmacokinetics and pharmacodynamics of the angiotensin II receptor antagonist losartan potassium (DuP 753/MK 954) in the dog. *J. Pharmacol. Exp. Ther.* 268: 1199–1205.

563 Baek, I.H., Lee, B.Y., Lee, E.S. et al. (2013). Pharmacokinetics of angiotensin II receptor blockers in the dog following a single oral administration. *Drug Res. (Stuttg)* 63: 357–361.

564 Caro-Vadillo, A., Daza-González, M.A., Gonzalez-Alonso-Alegre, E. et al. (2018). Effect of a combination of telmisartan and amlodipine in hypertensive dogs. *Vet. Rec. Case Rep.* 6 (2): e000471.

565 Bugbee, A.C., Coleman, A.E., Wang, A. et al. (2014). Telmisartan treatment of refractory proteinuria in a dog. *J. Vet. Internal Med.* 28: 1871–1874.

566 Glaus, T.M., Elliott, J., Herberich, E. et al. (2019). Efficacy of long-term oral telmisartan treatment in cats with hypertension: results of a prospective European clinical trial. *J. Vet. Internal Med.* 33: 413–422.

567 Coleman, A.E., Brown, S.A., Traas, A.M. et al. (2019). Safety and efficacy of orally administered telmisartan for the treatment of systemic hypertension in cats: results of a double-blind, placebo-controlled, randomized clinical trial. *J. Vet. Internal Med.* 33: 478–488.

568 Sent, U., Gossl, R., Elliott, J. et al. (2015). Comparison of efficacy of long-term oral treatment with telmisartan and benazepril in cats with chronic kidney disease. *J. Vet. Internal Med.* 29 (6): 1479–1487.

569 Lourenço, B.N., Coleman, A.E., Brown, S. et al. (2019). Efficacy of telmisartan for the treatment of persistent canine renal proteinuria. *J. Vet. Intern. Med.* 33: 2370.

570 Lourenco, B.N., Coleman, A.E., Brown, S.A. et al. (2020). Efficacy of telmisartan for the treatment of persistent renal proteinuria in dogs: a double-masked, randomized clinical trial. *J. Vet. Internal Med.* 34: 2478–2496.

571 Fowler, B.L., Stefanovski, D., Hess, R.S. et al. (2021). Effect of telmisartan, angiotensin-converting enzyme inhibition, or both, on proteinuria and blood pressure in dogs. *J. Vet. Internal Med.* 35 (3): 1231–1237.

572 Miyagawa, Y., Akabane, R., Sakatani, A. et al. (2020). Effects of telmisartan on proteinuria and systolic blood pressure in dogs with chronic kidney disease. *Res. Vet. Sci.* 133: 150–156.

573 Lecavalier, J., Fifle, L., and Javard, R. (2021). Treatment of proteinuria in dogs with telmisartan: a retrospective study. *J. Vet. Internal Med.* 35 (4): 1810–1818.

574 Ingelfinger, J.R. and Rosen, C.J. (2020). Finerenone – halting relative hyperaldosteronism in chronic kidney disease. *N. Engl. J. Med.* 383: 2285–2286.

575 Bakris, G.L., Agarwal, R., Anker, S.D. et al. (2020). Effect of Finerenone on chronic kidney disease outcomes in type 2 diabetes. *N. Engl. J. Med.* 383: 2219–2229.

576 Javadi, S., Djajadiningrat-Laanen, S.C., Kooistra, H.S. et al. (2005). Primary hyperaldosteronism, a mediator of progressive renal disease in cats. *Domest. Anim. Endocrinol.* 28: 85–104.

577 Barrera-Chimal, J., Girerd, S., and Jaisser, F. (2019). Mineralocorticoid receptor antagonists and kidney diseases: pathophysiological basis. *Kidney Int.* 96: 302–319.

578 Allison, S.J. (2021). Finerenone in chronic kidney disease. *Nat. Rev. Nephrol.* 17: 13.

579 Bakris, G.L., Agarwal, R., Chan, J.C. et al. (2015). Effect of Finerenone on albuminuria in patients with diabetic nephropathy: a randomized clinical trial. *JAMA* 314: 884–894.

580 Currie, G., Taylor, A.H., Fujita, T. et al. (2016). Effect of mineralocorticoid receptor antagonists on proteinuria and progression of chronic kidney disease: a systematic review and meta-analysis. *BMC Nephrol.* 17: 127.

581 Grauer, G.F. (2015). Feline chronic kidney disease. *Today's Vet. Pract.* 5: 36–41.

582 Adin, D., Atkins, C., Wallace, G. et al. (2021). Effect of spironolactone and benazepril on furosemide-induced diuresis and renin-angiotensin-aldosterone system activation in normal dogs. *J. Vet. Internal Med.* 35: 1245–1254.

583 Schmidt, M., Mansfield, K.E., Bhaskaran, K. et al. (2017). Serum creatinine elevation after renin-angiotensin system blockade and long term cardiorenal risks: cohort study. *BMJ* 356: j791.

584 Lavallee, J.O., Norsworthy, G.D., Huston, C.L. et al. (2017). Safety of benazepril in 400 azotemic and 110 non-azotemic client-owned cats (2001–2012). *J. Am. Anim. Hosp. Assoc.* 53: 119–127.

585 Griffin, K.A. and Bidani, A.K. (2008). Potential risks of calcium channel blockers in chronic kidney disease. *Curr. Cardiol. Rep.* 10: 448–455.

586 Henik, R.A. and Snyder, P.S. (1997). Treatment of systemic hypertension in cats with amlodipine besylate. *J. Am. Anim. Hosp. Assoc.* 33: 226–234.

587 Elliott, J., Barber, P.J., Syme, H.M. et al. (2001). Feline hypertension: clinical findings and response to antihypertensive treatment in 30 cases. *J. Small Anim. Pract.* 42: 122–129.

588 Jepson, R.E., Syme, H.M., and Elliott, J. (2014). Plasma renin activity and aldosterone concentrations in hypertensive cats with and without azotemia and in response to treatment with amlodipine besylate. *J. Vet. Internal Med.* 28: 144–153.

589 Brown, S.A., Walton, C.L., Crawford, P. et al. (1993). Long-term effects of antihypertensive regimens on renal hemodynamics and proteinuria. *Kidney Int.* 43: 1210–1218.

590 Heerspink, H.J.L., Stefansson, B.V., Correa-Rotter, R. et al. (2020). Dapagliflozin in patients with chronic kidney disease. *N. Engl. J. Med.* 383: 1436–1446.

591 Heerspink, H.J.L., Kosiborod, M., Inzucchi, S.E. et al. (2018). Renoprotective effects of sodium-glucose cotransporter-2 inhibitors. *Kidney Int.* 94: 26–39.

592 Tuttle, K.R. (2021). Forecasting therapeutic responses by albuminuria and eGFR slope during the DAPA-CKD trial. *Lancet Diabetes Endocrinol.* 9: 727–728.

593 Jongs, N., Greene, T., Chertow, G.M. et al. (2021). Effect of dapagliflozin on urinary albumin excretion in patients with chronic kidney disease with and without type 2 diabetes: a prespecified analysis from the DAPA-CKD trial. *Lancet Diabetes Endocrinol.* 9: 755–766.

594 Heerspink, H.J.L., Jongs, N., Chertow, G.M. et al. (2021). Effect of dapagliflozin on the rate of decline in kidney function in patients with chronic kidney disease with and without type 2 diabetes: a prespecified analysis from the DAPA-CKD trial. *Lancet Diabetes Endocrinol.* 9: 743–754.

595 Heerspink, H.J., Perkins, B.A., Fitchett, D.H. et al. (2016). Sodium glucose cotransporter 2 inhibitors in the treatment of diabetes mellitus: cardiovascular and kidney effects, potential mechanisms, and clinical applications. *Circulation* 134: 752–772.

596 Muhlig, A.K., Steingrover, J., Heidelbach, H.S. et al. (2022). The calcium-sensing receptor stabilizes podocyte function in proteinuric humans and mice. *Kidney Int.* 101 (6): 1186–1199.

597 Humalda, J.K., Goldsmith, D.J., Thadhani, R. et al. (2015). Vitamin D analogues to target residual proteinuria: potential impact on cardiorenal outcomes. *Nephrol. Dial. Transplant.* 30: 1988–1994.

598 Ruggenenti, P., Perna, A., Remuzzi, G. et al. (2003). Retarding progression of chronic renal disease: the neglected issue of residual proteinuria. *Kidney Int.* 63: 2254–2261.

599 Ivory, S.E., Packham, D.K., Reutens, A.T. et al. (2013). Residual proteinuria and eGFR predict progression of renal impairment within 2 years in type 2 diabetic patients with nephropathy who are receiving optimal treatment with angiotensin receptor blockers. *Nephrology (Carlton)* 18: 516–524.

600 Imai, E., Haneda, M., Chan, J.C. et al. (2013). Reduction and residual proteinuria are therapeutic targets in type 2 diabetes with overt nephropathy: a post hoc analysis (ORIENT-proteinuria). *Nephrol. Dial. Transplant.* 28: 2526–2534.

601 de Borst, M.H., Hajhosseiny, R., Tamez, H. et al. (2013). Active vitamin D treatment for reduction of residual proteinuria: a systematic review. *J. Am. Soc. Nephrol.* 24: 1863–1871.

602 Minutolo, R., Gabbai, F.B., Provenzano, M. et al. (2018). Cardiorenal prognosis by residual proteinuria level in diabetic chronic kidney disease: pooled analysis of four cohort studies. *Nephrol. Dial. Transplant.* 33: 1942–1949.

603 Slagman, M.C., Waanders, F., Hemmelder, M.H. et al. (2011). Moderate dietary sodium restriction added to angiotensin converting enzyme inhibition compared with dual blockade in lowering proteinuria and blood pressure: randomised controlled trial. *BMJ* 343: d4366.

604 Fishbane, S., Chittineni, H., Packman, M. et al. (2009). Oral paricalcitol in the treatment of patients with CKD and proteinuria: a randomized trial. *Am. J. Kidney Dis.* 54: 647–652.

605 Keyzer, C.A., van Breda, G.F., Vervloet, M.G. et al. (2017). Effects of vitamin D receptor activation and dietary sodium restriction on residual albuminuria in CKD: the ViRTUE-CKD trial. *J. Am. Soc. Nephrol.* 28: 1296–1305.

606 Molina, P., Gorriz, J.L., Molina, M.D. et al. (2014). The effect of cholecalciferol for lowering albuminuria in chronic kidney disease: a prospective controlled study. *Nephrol. Dial. Transplant.* 29: 97–109.

607 Santoro, D., Caccamo, D., Lucisano, S. et al. (2015). Interplay of vitamin D, erythropoiesis, and the renin-angiotensin system. *Biomed. Res. Int.* 2015: 145828.

Atlas

CELLULAR ELEMENTS

RED BLOOD CELLS

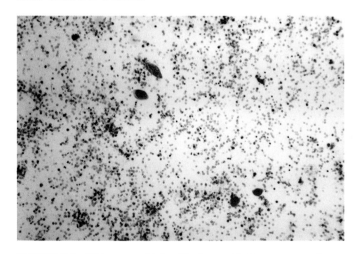

FIGURE 8.1   Urine was obtained by free catch from a young dog. TNTC RBC with a few large squamous epithelial cells. It is not possible at this power to tell if other cells types are there or not (42X).

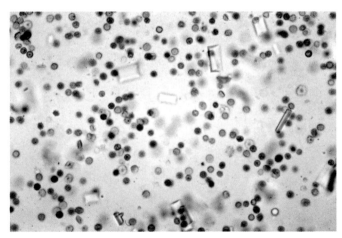

FIGURE 8.2   Note numerous intact RBC in urine sediment from a cat with idiopathic cystitis. Some RBC stain dark red and others stain light orange. There are occasional struvite crystals (relatively flat sheet appearance) and rare WBC (168X SediStain).

Urinalysis in the Dog and Cat, First Edition. Dennis J. Chew and Patricia A. Schenck.
© 2023 John Wiley & Sons, Inc. Published 2023 by John Wiley & Sons, Inc.

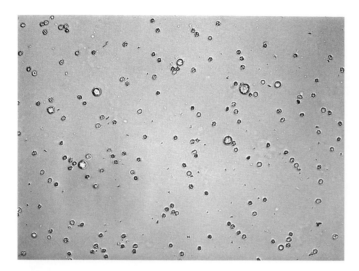

FIGURE 8.3 Urinary sediment image acquired by Sedi-Vue® automated microscopy. Most of the cells are RBC with a few WBC that are considerably larger than the RBC. Source: Courtesy of Dr. Ronald Lyman, Ft. Pierce, FL.

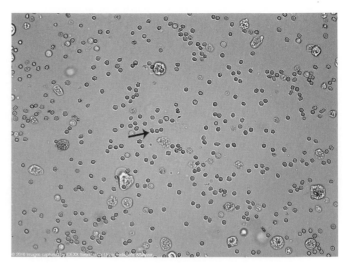

FIGURE 8.5 Urinary sediment image acquired by SediVue®. Numerous RBC are easily seen as the predominant cell type, some of which are crenated (arrow). A few easily identified neutrophils are also in this field. The WBC are at least 2.5 times the size of the RBC. The largest cells that are round to oblong are likely urothelial cells. Source: Courtesy of IDEXX Laboratories. Copyright © 2022, IDEXX Laboratories, Inc. All rights reserved. Used with permission.

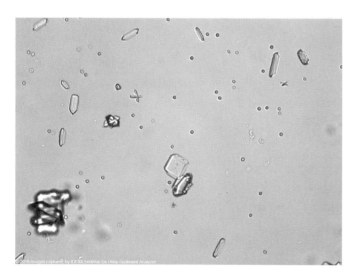

FIGURE 8.4 Urinary sediment digital image of urine sediment acquired by SediVue®. Notice the small size of the RBC compared to the much larger struvite crystals. Source: Courtesy of IDEXX Laboratories. Copyright © 2022, IDEXX Laboratories, Inc. All rights reserved. Used with permission.

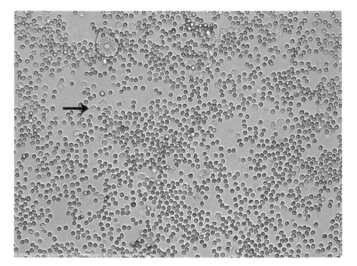

FIGURE 8.6 Urinary sediment image acquired by SediVue®. Note numerous RBC with homogenous size and dark appearance; they are the smallest cells in this field. Look more closely to identify WBC that are much lighter in color (ghost-like; arrow) and larger than RBC. Some of the WBC appear in small clumps. One very large epithelial cell assuming a tear drop shape is seen at the top left of this field; this is a squamous epithelial cell. Squamous cells often display sharp edges which are not seen in this particular cell. In a single area of this field is the appearance of what could be a few bacteria. Source: Courtesy of IDEXX Laboratories. Copyright © 2022, IDEXX Laboratories, Inc. All rights reserved. Used with permission.

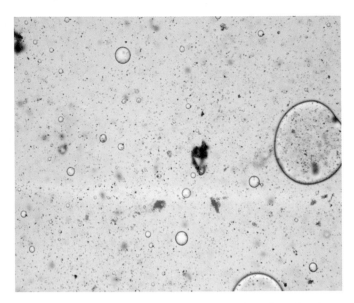

FIGURE 8.7 Note numerous round clear droplets of varying size that do not take up stain. These are typical for lipid droplets from urine sediment in cats. These should not be confused with red blood cells. The very large sphere at the far right and bottom are artifacts from an air bubble under the cover slip during preparation for microscopy.

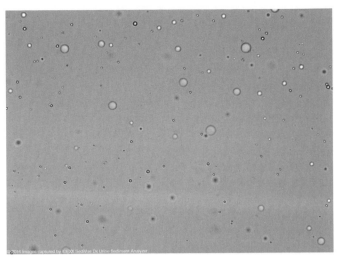

FIGURE 8.8 Multiple lipid droplets captured with SediVue®. Lipid droplets accumulate in a similar plane above the other urinary elements, so they are not counted or confused with RBC or crystals. Source: Courtesy of IDEXX Laboratories. Copyright © 2022, IDEXX Laboratories, Inc. All rights reserved. Used with permission.

WHITE BLOOD CELLS

(a)

(b)

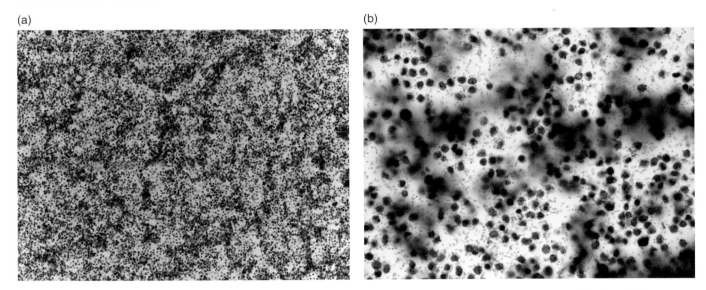

FIGURE 8.9 (a) Very cellular crowded field at low power. It is not possible to identify the cells without further magnification. (b) Upon higher magnification, nearly all the cells are neutrophils. A large number of bacteria are obvious between the WBC.

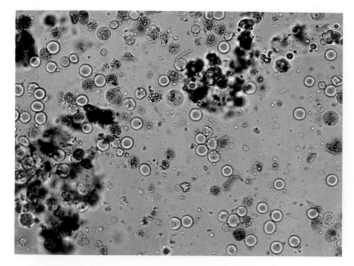

FIGURE 8.10 Urine sediment from a dog with major neurological problems that include inability to fully empty the bladder. The dog had a long history of urinary infections. Note numerous RBC and WBC and some cells that cannot be readily identified. Particulate debris of unknown origin is seen in some areas of this field. Some of the particulates appear to be cocci, which is better confirmed with urine cytology.

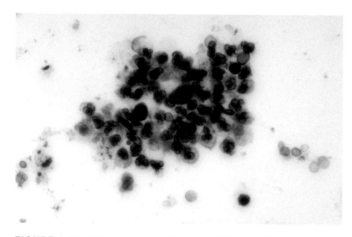

FIGURE 8.11 Urine sediment from a middle-aged female Doberman with stranguria and masses within the bladder detected on ultrasonography. A large clump of WBC is seen staining mostly with red uptake into the nuclei, with some taking up blue. A few RBC are also seen. There are rare particulate elements that could be bacteria. There are no epithelial cells in this field. Polypoid cystitis was the diagnosis.

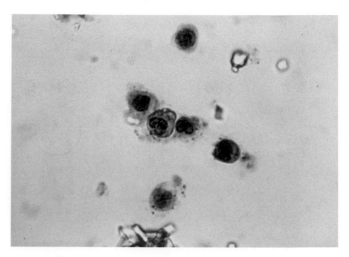

FIGURE 8.12 Clump of three neutrophils with red staining nuclei, three free-floating WBC, and clump of struvite crystals (bottom of picture).

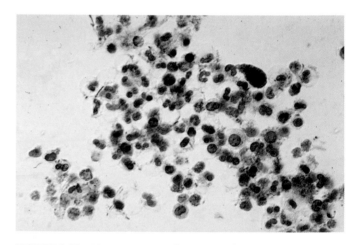

FIGURE 8.13 Numerous WBC (neutrophils) and many are in clumps. Nuclei of neutrophils stain mostly blue, but some are red. Notice fine linear structures between the neutrophils that are rods. Occasional nonsquamous epithelial cells are seen. A pure culture of *Escherichia coli* was isolated from this urine. Clumps of WBC, rather than individual cells, are more indicative of an infectious agent in the urine. There is loss of nuclear detail in some of the WBC.

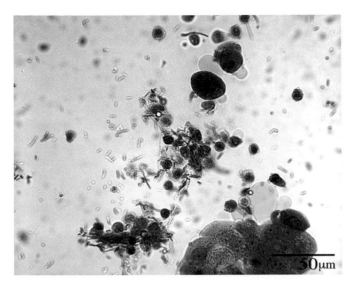

FIGURE 8.14 Note small clumps of WBC with numerous rod bacteria between the WBC. Some bacteria are free-floating. Many of the neutrophils are not so easy to identify since the cytoplasm has shrunk tightly around the nuclei. The typical lobulated nucleus is seen in a few of the neutrophils. A few large free epithelial cells are seen at the top of this field. A large clump of epithelial cells with central nuclei are seen at the bottom right of this field. It is likely that the clump of transitional cells is "reactive" in the face of the other indicators of inflammation. Source: Reproduced by permission of Dr. Michael Horton, Fairborn, OH.

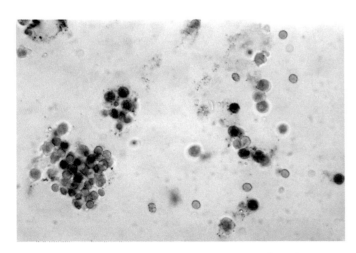

FIGURE 8.15 Urine sediment from a dog with pyelonephritis. Note the large clump of RBC and mostly blue staining WBC on the far left of this field. Nuclear detail of the red staining WBC in other parts of the field is more distinct.

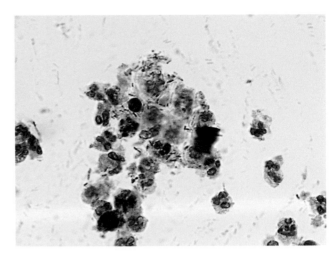

FIGURE 8.16 Oil immersion view of urine sediment from a dog with bacterial UTI. Most WBC are in clumps with obvious rod-shaped bacteria in-between the WBC. The multilobulated nature of the nucleus of the neutrophils is easy to see.

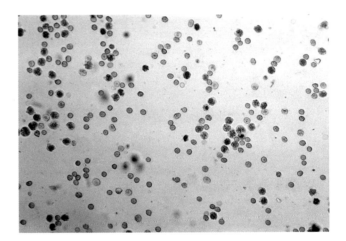

FIGURE 8.17 Numerous RBC with stain uptake predominates in this field; some RBC do not take up the stain. Increased numbers of WBC are seen among the RBC. The pattern of nuclear segmentation of the neutrophils can still be seen but nuclear detail is poor due to degeneration.

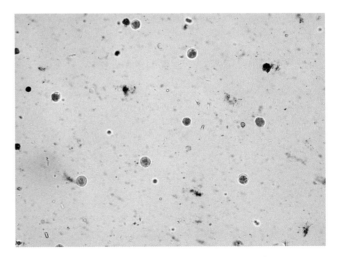

FIGURE 8.18 Mild increase in numbers of WBC with rare RBC in this stained sediment. Cytoplasm is swollen in several WBC.

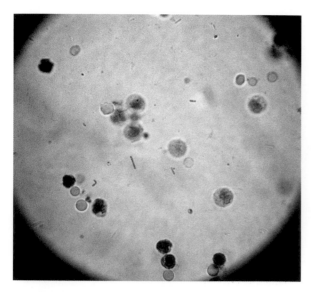

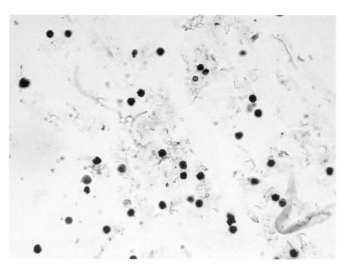

FIGURE 8.19 Image captured through the microscope eyepiece using a handheld iPhone. Note small cluster of three neutrophils in central field with pale blue staining nuclei. These neutrophils are swollen and the nuclei have undergone some degeneration. There are occasional RBC that do not take up stain. Also note free-floating rod bacteria. Other WBC have red staining nuclei and scant cytoplasm.

FIGURE 8.20 Urine sediment from a dog with a urinary tract infection. WBC that are blue staining are easier to identify than the WBC that are staining red. Many of the red staining WBC are smaller as the cytoplasm has contracted around the nucleus. A few RBC are available to compare the size of WBC as at least 2–2.5× larger than the RBC. Rod bacteria are seen in between the cells and sometimes can be seen protruding from the surface of the WBC. The lightly pink staining element at the lower right of the image could be confused for a cast, but its width varies too much and is likely mucus.

(a)

(b)

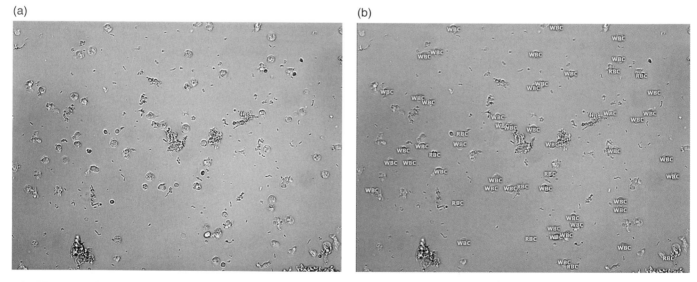

FIGURE 8.21 (a) SediVue® acquired image of urinary sediment from a cat with CKD, USG of 1.017, and a pure culture of *Escherichia coli*. Note numerous WBC (neutrophils), some RBC, and quite a few bacteria recognized as rods. The results were officially reported as 47 WBC/HPF, eight RBC/HPF, absent cocci, and present rods. (b) Screenshot of how SediVue® recognized and labeled urinary sediment findings. Notice that most but not all cells are labeled. Bacteria in this field are not labeled. Source: Reproduced with permission of Dr. Carmen Colitz, Jupiter, FL.

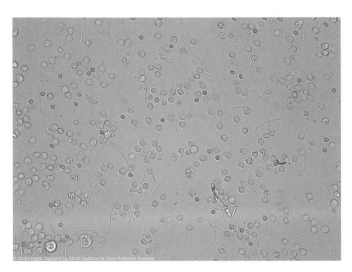

FIGURE 8.22 Many WBC, far fewer RBC, and multiple long rods. Image acquired by SediVue®. Source: Courtesy of IDEXX Laboratories. Copyright © 2022, IDEXX Laboratories, Inc. All rights reserved. Used with permission.

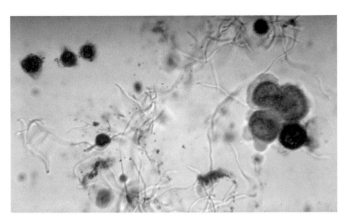

FIGURE 8.25 This is an oil-immersion view of a wet-mount urinary sediment. Three WBC with red staining nuclei are in the upper left corner. There is a three epithelial cell clump on the right of image. Many very elongated bacterial organisms show how *Escherichia coli* can grow in urine. Source: Reproduced by permission of Dr. Richard A. Scott, Animal Medical Center, NY, NY.

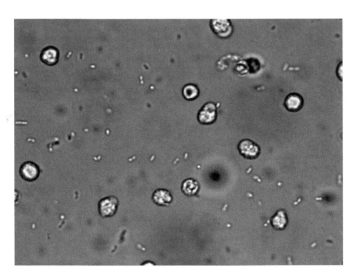

FIGURE 8.23 Numerous WBC and bacteria. The bacteria are cocci. Image acquired by Zoetis VETSCAN® UA Urine Analyzer. Reproduced with permission of Zoetis

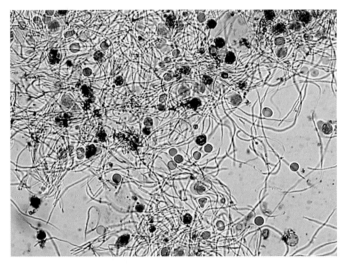

FIGURE 8.26 Stained urinary sediment from a dog with pyelonephritis. The most striking feature about this urinary sediment image is the abundance of long filamentous bacteria. Notice many WBC and RBC (pale stain) among the bacteria. Many of the WBC (most have blue nuclei) display degenerative changes likely the result of the toxic urinary environment from the urinary infection. At first glance, filamentous bacteria can be confused with fungal elements. *Escherichia coli* was isolated at >30 000 cfu/mL in pure culture from a cystocentesis sample. There is nothing pathognomonic about the findings in this urine sediment leading to the diagnosis of bacterial pyelonephritis, which requires the integration of findings from urinalysis, urine culture, clinical signs, and urinary tract imaging.

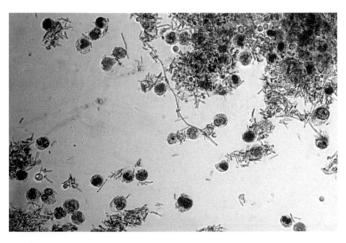

FIGURE 8.24 Large numbers of bacterial rods and moderate number of WBC. Some rods are elongated.

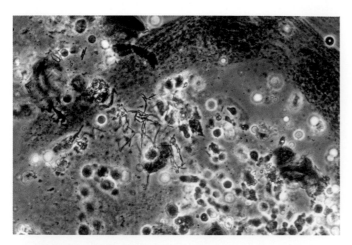

FIGURE 8.27 Phase contrast microscopy urine sediment from a dog. This method of microscopy can be used to convincingly confirm the presence of bacteria. Note the rod bacteria grouped together in the center of the image. There is a large accumulation of mucus at the top of the image. Source: Reproduced by permission of Dr. Michael Horton, Fairborn OH.

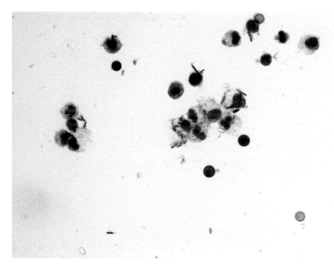

FIGURE 8.28 Dog with bacterial urinary tract infection. Note clump of WBC in the center of the image. Some bacteria are adherent to the WBC and some have been phagocytized inside the cell.

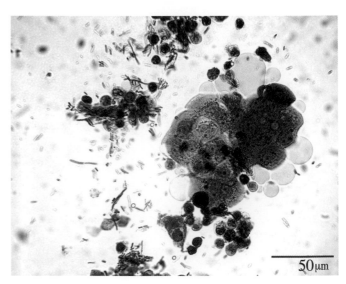

FIGURE 8.29 Note large clump of nonsquamous epithelial cells of similar size with central nuclei. There are several clumps of WBC with red-staining nuclei and numerous linear bacteria (rods) in between WBC; some bacteria are free-floating. It is possible that the large clump of urothelial cells resulted from desquamation secondary to urinary infection and inflammation. Though the clump of epithelial cells could be "reactive," this could occur in those with a urinary infection and urothelial neoplasia. Dry-mount cytology is recommended to further evaluate this patient for neoplasia. Source: Reproduced by permission of Dr. Michael Horton, Fairborn, OH.

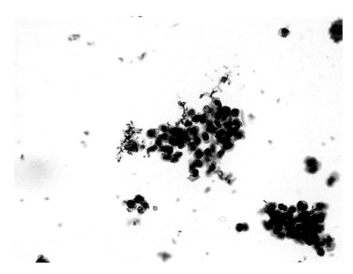

FIGURE 8.30 Clumps of deeply staining dark red and blue nuclei of neutrophils. There is scant cytoplasm around the nuclei, but their segmented nature can still be seen. Bacterial rods are seen in between the WBC and also free.

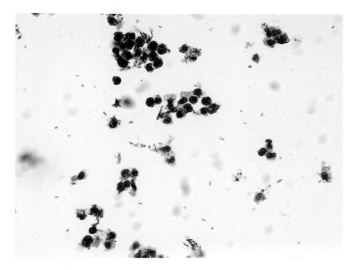

FIGURE 8.31 Several clumps of WBC with bacteria in between and around them. Nuclei stain red with little cytoplasm visible around some of the WBC.

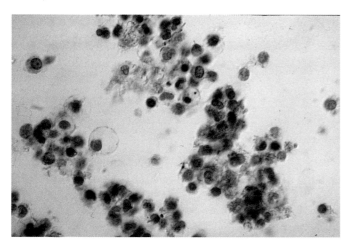

FIGURE 8.32 Clumps of WBC with bacterial rods within the clumps are obvious in this field (168×). Some of the neutrophils display swollen cytoplasm.

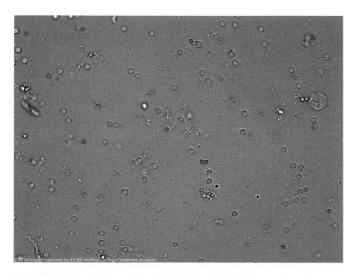

FIGURE 8.33 Image acquired by SediVue®. WBC predominate in this field with one epithelial cell (far upper right) and many rod bacteria. Source: Courtesy of IDEXX Laboratories. Copyright © 2022, IDEXX Laboratories, Inc. All rights reserved. Used with permission.

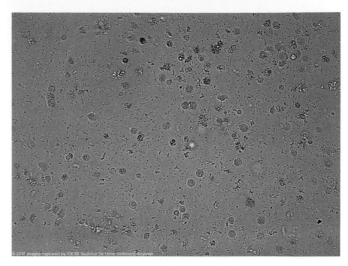

FIGURE 8.34 Moderate numbers of WBC, rare RBC, and many bacteria (some rods and possibly some cocci) are seen. SediVue® image. Source: Courtesy of IDEXX Laboratories. Copyright © 2022, IDEXX Laboratories, Inc. All rights reserved. Used with permission.

ORGANISMS (INCLUDING PARASITES)

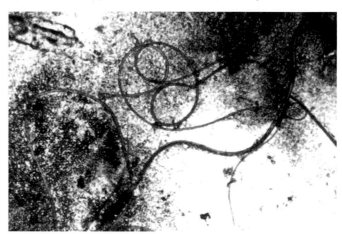

FIGURE 8.35 Mature *Capillaria spp.* worms in urine sediment from a naturally infected Whippet. Eggs seen within the worms confirm that they are adults and not larvae. Source: Reproduced by permission of Dr. David Senior.

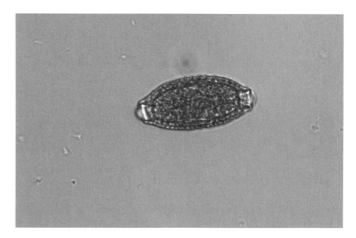

FIGURE 8.36 Image captured by SediVue®. *Pearsonema spp* (*Capillaria spp.*) ova. Adult worms live in the bladder and can cause clinical signs or be nonclinical. Source: Courtesy of IDEXX Laboratories. Copyright © 2022, IDEXX Laboratories, Inc. All rights reserved. Used with permission.

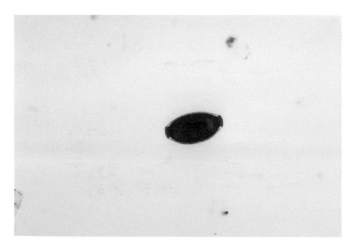

FIGURE 8.37 *Capillaria* ova in urine from a cat. This cat did not have clinical signs related to the urinary tract.

(a)

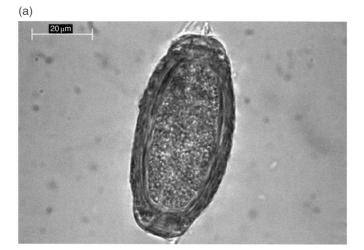

(b)

FIGURE 8.38 (a) Mature egg of *Capillaria plica*. (b) Immature egg of *Capillaria plica*. Source: From Basso et al. [1]. Used with permission.

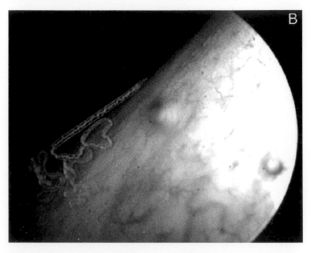

FIGURE 8.39 Adult *Capillaria plica* worms attached to the mucosa of the urinary bladder as seen during cystoscopy. Source: From Basso et al. [1]. Used with permission.

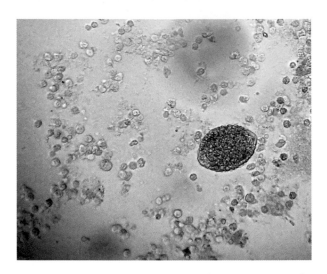

FIGURE 8.40 Unstained sediment. Ova of *Dioctophyma renale*, and degenerating WBC and RBC. Source: Courtesy of Dr. Marcia Kogika, USP, Sao Paulo, Brazil.

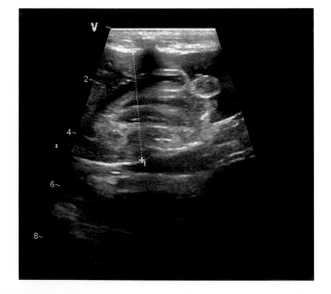

FIGURE 8.41 *Dioctophyma renale* adult worm shown during ultrasonography of the right kidney from a dog that presented for hematuria. Source: Courtesy of Dr. Marcia Kogika, USP, Sao Paulo, Brazil.

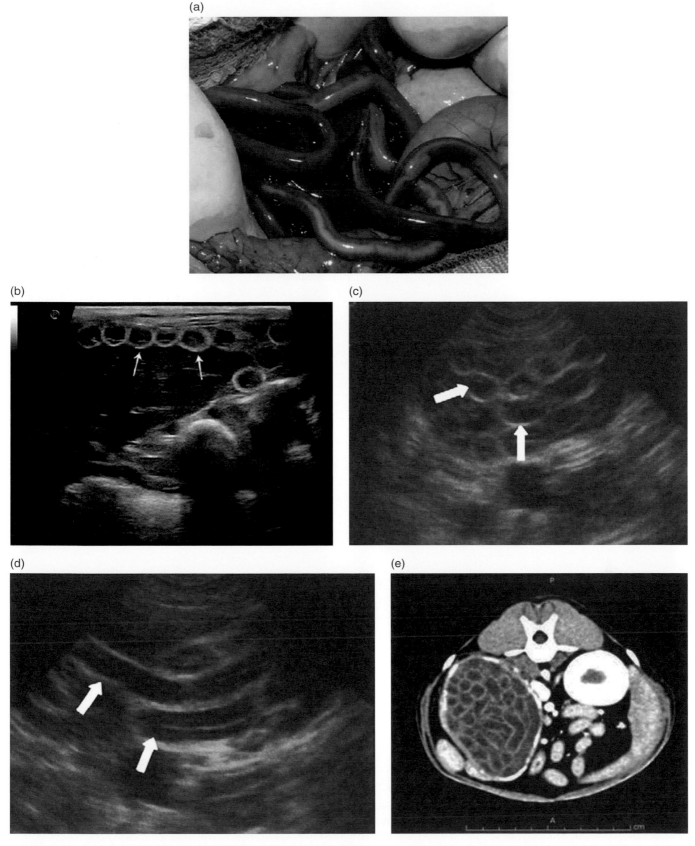

FIGURE 8.42 (a, b, c, d, e) (a) Adult *Dioctophyme renale* being removed from a kidney. (b) An ultrasound demonstrating an end-on view of segments of *Dioctophyme renale*. (c) Ultrasonogram of transverse view of kidney showing a ring-like appearance of the parasite with a highly echogenic wall and anechoic central area. (d) Ultrasonogram in longitudinal view of the same kidney showing the parasite as bands. (e) CT of the right kidney of another dog. Note uptake of contrast in the atrophic renal cortex along with a ring like and band appearance of the parasite in the enlarged right kidney. Normal size and contrast uptake in the left kidney. Source: (c and d) Ferreira et al. [2]. (a, b and e) Rahal et al. [3].

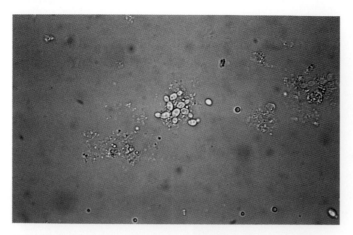

FIGURE 8.43 Clump of budding yeast in central and far right field. WBC are rare.

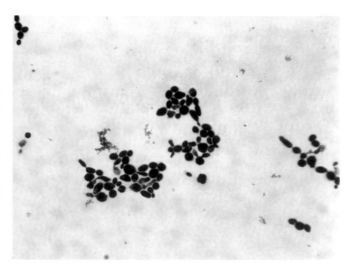

FIGURE 8.44 Cytoprep examination of urine confirming the presence of yeast.

(a)

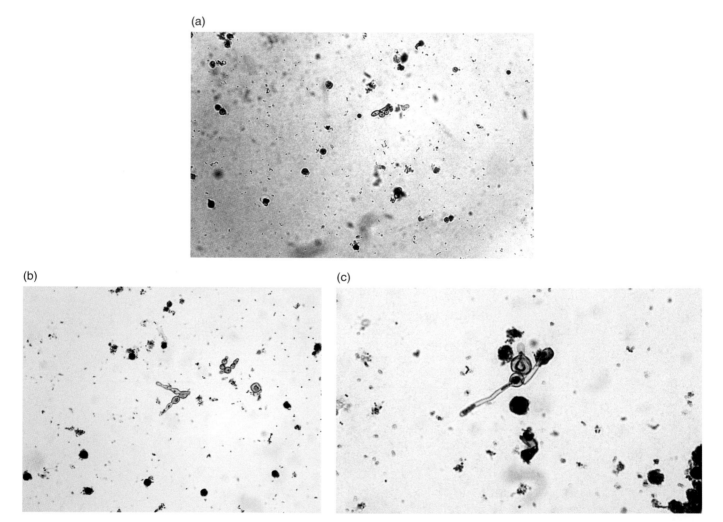

(b)

(c)

FIGURE 8.45 (a) Note the mild increase in WBC and abundant bacteria in the background of this image; most bacteria appear to be cocci. There is a small group of budding yeast (yellowish color) near the top of this image. (b) Urine sediment from same cat as in (a). Closer view of budding yeast. There are moderate numbers of neutrophils with contracted cytoplasm. Some WBC have bacteria protruding from their surface. (c) Same urine sediment as from (a) and (b). Note budding yeast that appears to be extending into a more filamentous form. A WBC with contracted cytoplasm is just above and below these organisms. Note the clump of WBC at the lower right of this image. Source: Reproduced with permission of Dr. Mary Ann Crawford, Oradell, NJ.

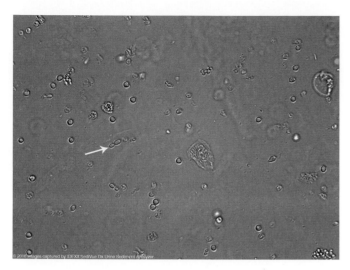

FIGURE 8.46 Image acquired by SediVue®. Budding yeast (arrow) are the most important and unusual element to note in this field. There are moderate numbers of WBC, rare RBC, a few nonsquamous epithelial cells and one squamous epithelial cell. Source: Courtesy of IDEXX Laboratories. Copyright © 2022, IDEXX Laboratories, Inc. All rights reserved. Used with permission.

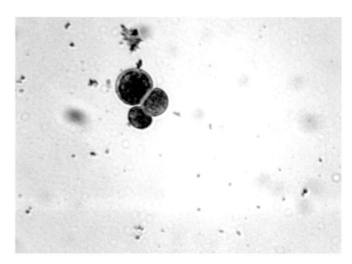

FIGURE 8.48 Cryptococcus in urine from a cat.

(a) (b)

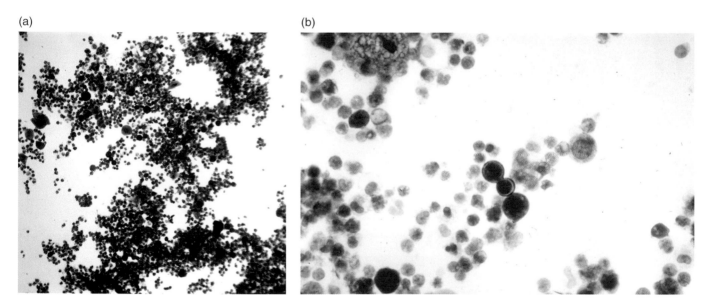

FIGURE 8.47 Urine from a 5 ½ year old male German Shepherd mix dog with disseminated Blastomycosis. (a) Highly cellular urinary sediment at lower power magnification. There are numerous WBC, occasional transitional epithelial cells and some highly round prominent elements near the top of this field that need further identification. (b) Higher power view of field showing wall structure of *Blastomyces* organisms. Many degenerate neutrophils are also in this field. Source: Reproduced with permission of Dr. James Brace, The Ohio State University.

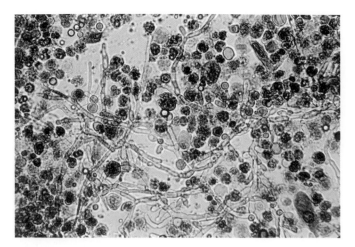

FIGURE 8.49 Many degenerate neutrophils are seen throughout this field. Occasional transitional epithelial cells and many septate hyphae of Candida are also observed.

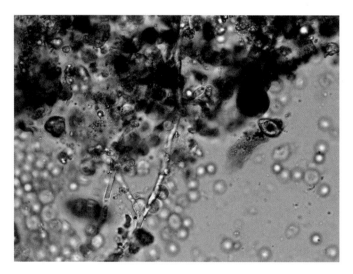

FIGURE 8.50 In this field, the RBC and WBC are out of focus in the background. In a slightly different plane of focus, branching and septate hyphae of a fungal organism can be seen. Off to the right in this field is also a single ovum of *Capillaria*. The fungal infection was a consequence of long-term antibiotic and steroid therapy in conjunction with an inability to fully empty the bladder.

EPITHELIAL CELLS

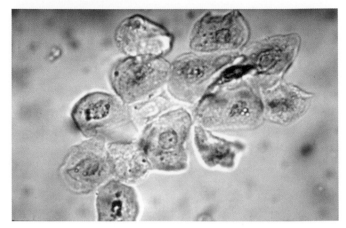

FIGURE 8.51 Unstained sediment showing a large clump of squamous epithelial cells. Voided specimen from a female dog. Notice flattened surfaces of these very large cells. Source: Reproduced with permission of Dr. Richard Scott, Animal Medical Center, New York, NY.

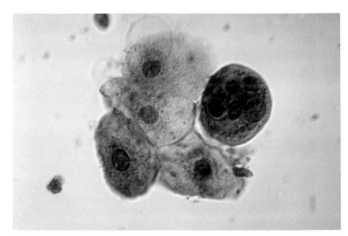

FIGURE 8.52 Clump of squamous epithelial cells. One epithelial cell appears to have phagocytized several WBC. Source: Reproduced with permission Dr. Richard Scott, Animal Medical Center, New York, NY.

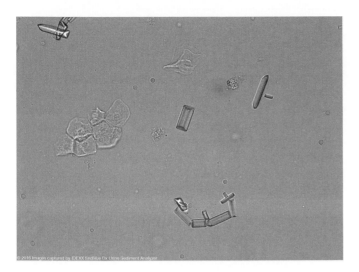

FIGURE 8.53   One clump of squamous epithelial cells at left of field and one free squamous epithelial cell at top of field. Struvite crystals are also observed. Image captured by SediVue®. Source: Courtesy of IDEXX Laboratories. Copyright © 2022, IDEXX Laboratories, Inc. All rights reserved. Used with permission.

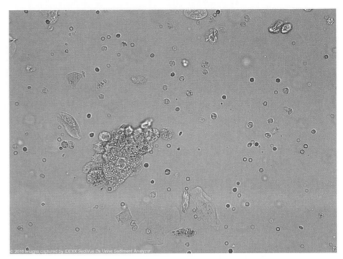

FIGURE 8.55   Image acquired by SediVue®. Large clump of nonsquamous epithelial cells to left of center. There are also a few squamous epithelial cells which are quite large; one is folded on itself (left central field). Moderate numbers of RBC and WBC accompany the epithelial cells. Source: Courtesy of IDEXX Laboratories. Copyright © 2022, IDEXX Laboratories, Inc. All rights reserved. Used with permission.

(a)   (b)

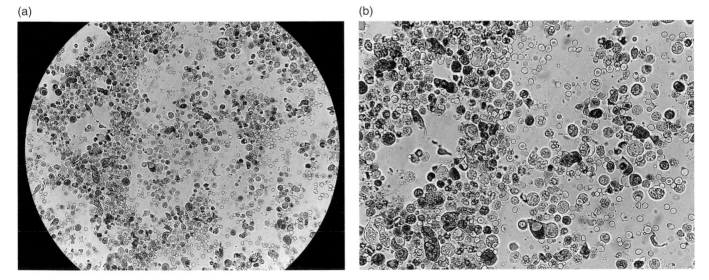

FIGURE 8.54   (a) Image captured through microscope eyepiece using a handheld digital phone camera showing an obviously cellular sediment. Higher power microscopy identified the cells as WBC, nonsquamous epithelial cells, and RBC (see b). (b) Higher power image from (a). Image captured through microscope eyepiece using a handheld digital phone camera. RBC are the smallest cells seen with pale stain; WBC are larger than the RBC and have blue staining nuclei. The largest cells are nonsquamous epithelial cells (transitional cells). Most of the epithelial cells stain red but some do not take up stain. This sediment is from a dog undergoing treatment for transitional cell carcinoma and was obtained by cystocentesis with ultrasound guidance.

(a)

(b)

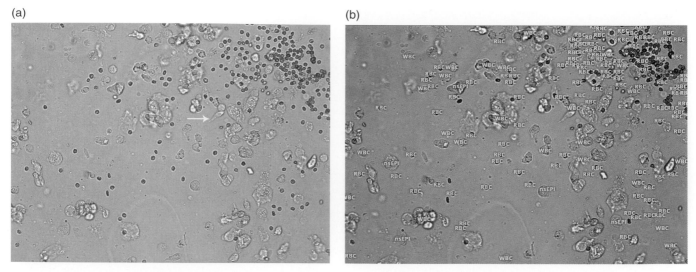

FIGURE 8.56 (a) SediVue® acquired image. There are many RBC, especially in the upper right corner of this image. Moderate WBC are seen, and some are in clumps (lower left field). The largest cells are nonsquamous epithelial cells; most are free but there is one clump at the center top field. One small epithelial cell is seen with a tail (arrow). No bacteria are observed. (b) Identification of elements in urine sediment as assigned by SediVue®. Note that not all cells are labeled. This happens with more frequency when urinary elements are crowded and when elements are clumped. It is always a good idea to check what an automated analyzer is reporting and compare that to your own visual inspection of the digital images collected by the machine. Source: Reproduced by permission of Dr. Carmen Colitz, Jupiter, FL.

(a)

(b)

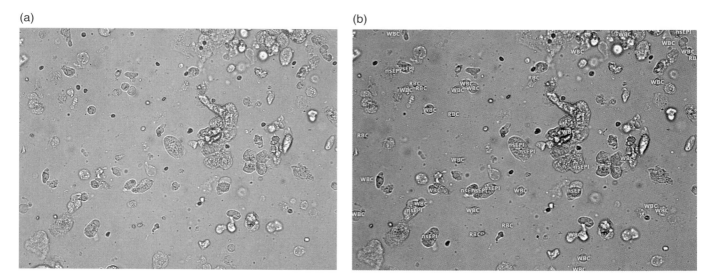

FIGURE 8.57 (a, b) Unlabeled digital image and screenshot of labels to identity elements in urine sediment as assigned by SediVue®. Many WBC, some RBC, and many nonsquamous epithelial cells are seen in this field. Not all elements are identified with a label. Source: Reproduced by permission of Dr. Carmen Colitz, Jupiter, FL.

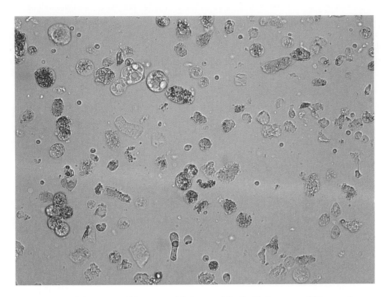

FIGURE 8.58   Image captured by SediVue® from an older cat with ketoacidotic diabetes mellitus and pancreatitis. Moderate RBC and WBC. There is a cluster of large round nonsquamous epithelial cells at top of this image. There are also occasional free nonsquamous epithelial cells. A WBC cluster of smaller round cells appears at the lower left. Though not identified by the analyzer, there are a few elements that are linear with parallel walls that are suspected to be granular casts. Source: Reproduced with permission of Dr. Ron Lyman, Ft Pierce, FL.

(a)   (b)

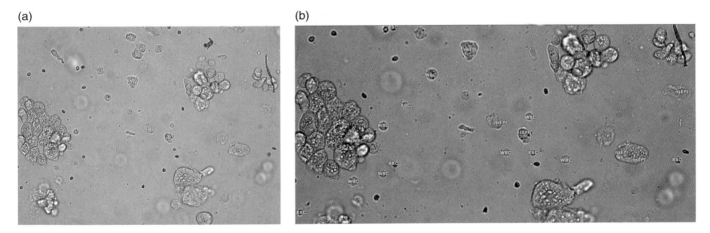

FIGURE 8.59   (a, b) Three clumps of WBC – a large clump on the left and two smaller clumps on the right. The largest cells are nonsquamous epithelial cells. Some smaller nonsquamous epithelial cells are seen at the top center field. Source: Reproduced by permission of Dr. Carmen Colitz, Jupiter, FL. Image acquired by SediVue®.

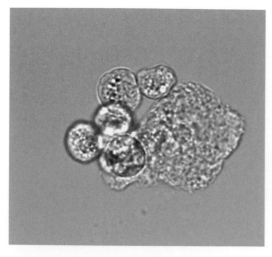

FIGURE 8.60 Image acquired by SediVue®. Small clump of nonsquamous epithelial cells. A single large squamous epithelial cell is to the right of the clump.Source: Courtesy of IDEXX Laboratories. Copyright © 2022, IDEXX Laboratories, Inc. All rights reserved. Used with permission.

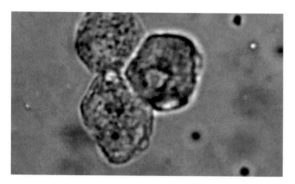

FIGURE 8.61 Clump of squamous epithelial cells. Image acquired by VETSCAN® SA Sediment Analyzer. Reproduced with permission of Zoetis.

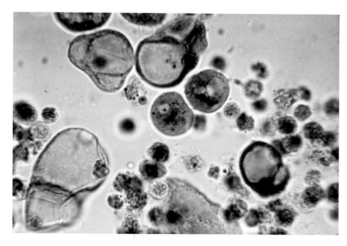

FIGURE 8.62 Epithelial cells distended with lipid accumulation. These are sometimes called "signet" cells and occur as part of cellular degeneration. Several WBC that have poorly defined cellular detail are in the background. Source: Reproduced with permission of Dr. Richard Scott, Animal Medical Center, New York, NY.

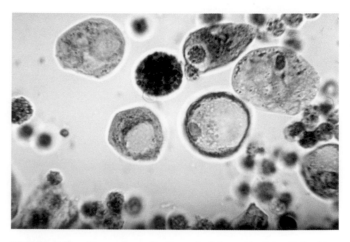

FIGURE 8.63 Signet ring cells. Several of the epithelial cells in this field display lipid degeneration. Several WBC with poor detail are seen at the lower field. Source: Reproduced with permission of Dr. Richard Scott, Animal Medical Center, New York, NY.

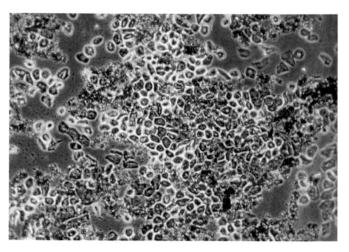

FIGURE 8.64 Sheets of renal epithelium as observed during phase microscopy. Source: Reproduced with permission Dr. Michael Horton, Fairborn, OH.

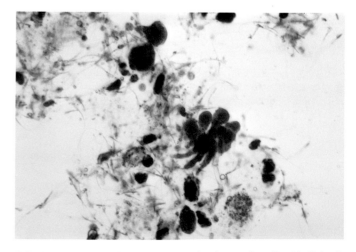

FIGURE 8.65 Urine from a dog. Note the clump of small epithelial cells with tails. Nuclear degeneration precludes definitive assessment of the position of the nucleus within these cells, but some appear to be basal. Renal origin epithelial cells. Nuclear positing and detail would be better analyzed with dry mount cytology.

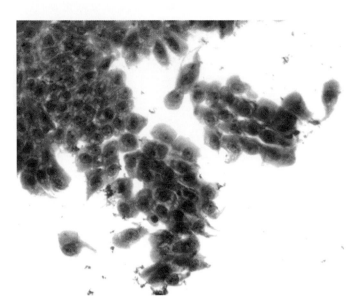

FIGURE 8.66 Large sheet of small epithelial cells, some of which have tails. The cells with more basal positioning of nuclei suggest renal origin. Dry mount cytology would provide greater cellular detail.

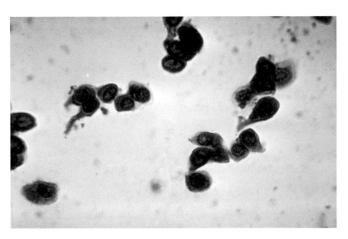

FIGURE 8.67 Small epithelial cells, some in clusters. A few of the epithelial cells have "tails" (caudate cells). Cytology is needed to provide more detail for these cells. Based on the history and the absence of other cell types, it was concluded that these cells arose from the kidney. This dog had a diagnosis of AKI. Source: Reproduced with permission Dr. Richard Scott, Animal Medical Center, New York, NY.

(a)   (b)

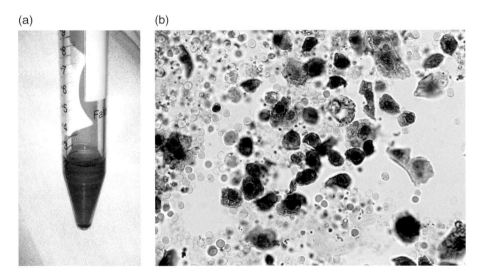

FIGURE 8.68 (a) Urine tube post centrifugation. Pedicel at the bottom was quite cellular with renal epithelial cells. (b) Urine from a cat. WBC and RBC are easy to identify. The epithelial cells are round to ovoid to cuboidal. Nuclei of the epithelia cells are noted to be basal in many of the cells supporting renal tubular origin for these epithelial cells.

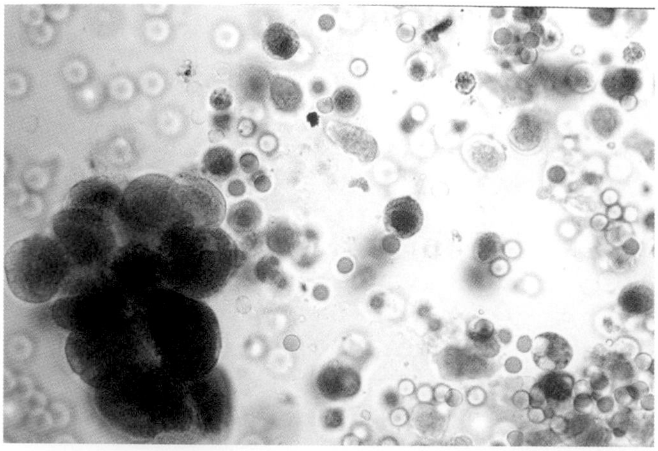

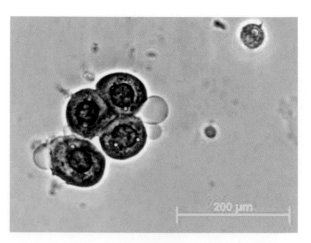

FIGURE 8.69 Large clump of nonsquamous epithelial cells left lower field. These cells stain both blue and red but cellular detail is lacking. Occasional free transitional epithelial cells and WBC are seen. It is not possible from examination of this urine sediment to tell if this is a "reactive" clump of epithelial cells or those that are neoplastic.

FIGURE 8.70 Stained urine microscopy. Note clump of four transitional epithelial cells. Clumps are usually more clinically significant than single epithelial cells. The nuclei look normal. There is one poorly stained WBC toward the upper right; note that transitional epithelial cells are usually 2–2.5 times the size of WBC. This clump does not have definitive character for neoplasia. It could still be a neoplastic condition, or it could represent desquamation in the face of urinary tract infection, trauma, or abrasion from urinary stones. Source: Reproduced with permission of Dr. Michael Horton, Fairborn, OH.

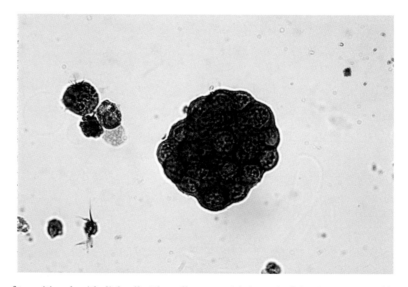

FIGURE 8.71 Large cluster of transitional epithelial cells. The cells are so tightly packed that it is not possible to describe the cellular details further. Submission of urine sediment for cytology will reveal more cellular detail. Diagnosis was transitional cell carcinoma in a dog.

(a)

(b)

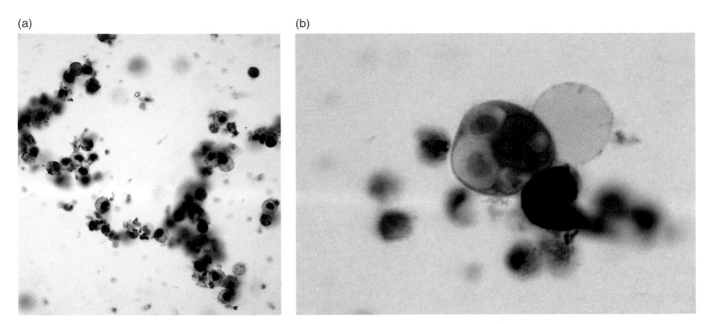

FIGURE 8.72 (a) Voided urine sample from a female dog with TCC of the urethra. This image shows several neutrophils and some bacteria, but not atypical epithelial cells. Many of the neutrophils show swollen cytoplasm.(b) Voided urine sample from a female dog with TCC of the urethra. This image shows a single raft of epithelium with some malignant character. Cells around this clump are out of focus and cannot be identified.

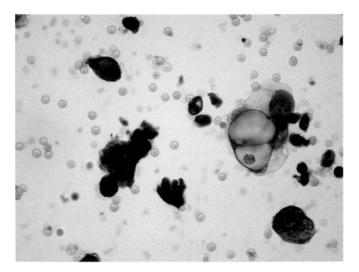

FIGURE 8.73 Clumps and free transitional epithelium. TCC of urinary bladder in a Shetland Sheepdog. Note the large blue staining clump in the right of this field. Several of the cells in this clump are lipid distended. Moderate RBC are in the background.

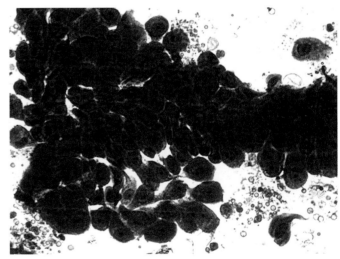

FIGURE 8.74 Large clump of epithelial cells. Voided specimen from a dog. There are several lipid droplets in this field. Transitional cell carcinoma (urothelial carcinoma) was the diagnosis.

(a) (b)

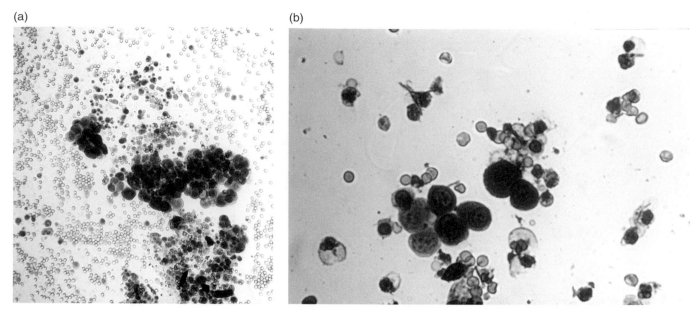

FIGURE 8.75 (a) Highly cellular sediment with numerous RBC, some WBC, and clumps of round blue- and red-staining epithelial cells. The dog was evaluated for one day of macroscopic hematuria. (b) Higher magnification of the same urine sediment as in (a). Clump of blue- and red-staining epithelial cells. The nuclei are particularly large compared to the cytoplasm. Orange staining RBC are in background as are a few WBC. These epithelial cells should be further evaluated with cytology. The diagnosis in this dog was transitional cell carcinoma of the bladder.

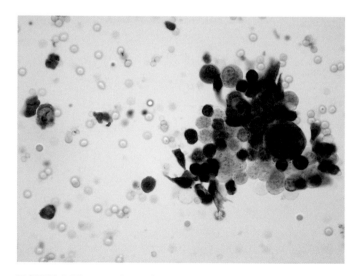

FIGURE 8.76 Note large clump of epithelial cells of widely varying size. Some take up the blue stain and others take up the red stain. Cell shape is round to ovoid to cuboidal. Some of the epithelial cells have tails. RBC are in the background. The diagnosis was TCC of the urinary bladder in a Shetland Sheepdog.

CASTS

HYALINE

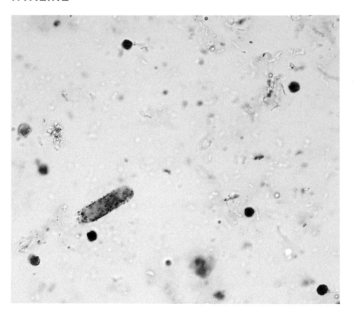

FIGURE 8.77 Hyaline cast is visible in lower left field. Note many linear bacteria in the background as well as a mild increase in WBC. Particle debris appears to adhere to the outside of the hyaline cast. Urine culture was positive for large growth of bacteria, but it is not possible to tell from this image alone if the urinary infection is confined to the lower urinary tract, or if it extends to the kidneys.

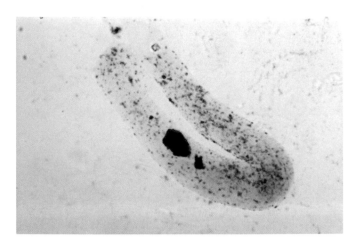

FIGURE 8.78 Hyaline cast. Note that this cast is bent on itself. There are several particles taking up stain either within or on the cast.

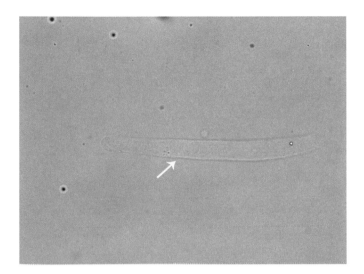

FIGURE 8.79 Pure hyaline cast (arrow). The portion of this cast is more easily seen in its middle. Outlines of the walls of this cast fade at each end of the cast. It is very easy to miss hyaline casts without proper adjustment of the microscope lighting. Source: Reproduced with permission of Dr. Heather L. Wamsley, Bradenton, FL.

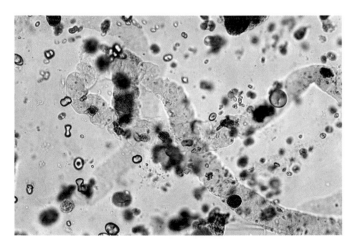

FIGURE 8.80 Long Hyaline Cast. Notice light pink staining and some convolutions of this cast. Calcium carbonate crystals in the background. Urine sample is from a horse.

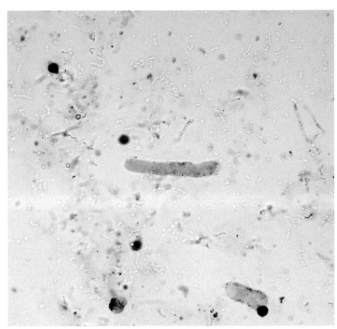

FIGURE 8.81 Two hyaline casts and numerous bacteria in the background. A few degenerate WBC are in this field but are largely out of focus.

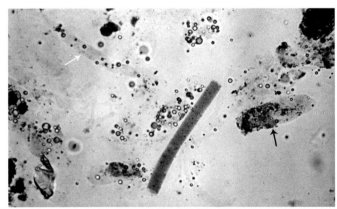

FIGURE 8.82 Hyaline casts. Hyaline cast upper left part of this field (white arrow) – note the parallel walls and transparent nature. A single waxy cast is in the central field – it is deep staining pink and has abrupt ends. Some hyaline casts are difficult to see as is often the case. One cast in the far-right field is mostly hyaline at one pole and granular at the other pole (mixed cast; black arrow).

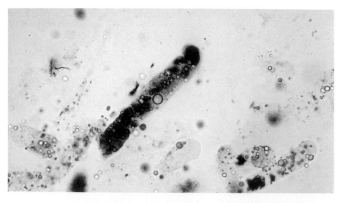

FIGURE 8.83 Several hyaline casts are seen throughout this field. All of the hyaline casts have refractile granules within them that could be lipid or could represent filtered plasma protein precipitates from abnormal glomerular permeability. The hyaline cast in the center stains more intensely than the other casts and has the most granules.

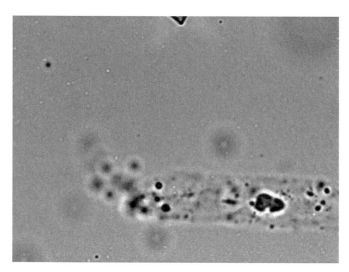

FIGURE 8.84 Hyaline cast. There are a few granules but the predominant composition of this cast is matrix protein. Source: Image acquired by VETSCAN® SA Sediment Analyzer. Reproduced with permission of Zoetis.

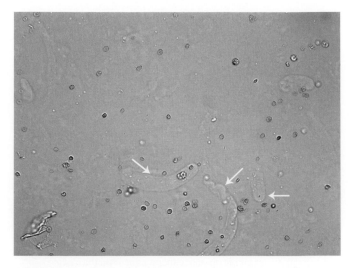

FIGURE 8.85 Notice three hyaline casts in lower half of the image (white arrows) acquired during SediVue® automated microscopy. RBC are also in the background. Several other hyaline casts are faint in this image but are routinely identified during automated microscopy. Source: Courtesy of IDEXX Laboratories. Copyright © 2022, IDEXX Laboratories, Inc. All rights reserved. Used with permission.

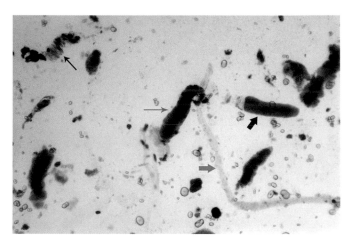

FIGURE 8.86 Cylindroid. Note the long thin pink staining cast from the middle to the right of the image (large gray arrow). This is a special type of hyaline cast in which it formed within a tubular lumen that is compressed, from intrarenal edema, hemorrhage, or inflammation. The darker staining cast in the middle of this panel would be classified as coarsely granular cast (small gray arrow) based on the appearance of the top part of this cast. The cast at the upper left would be categorized as a degenerating cellular or coarsely granular cast (small black arrow). The darker pink cast that is translucent is a waxy cast (large black arrow). Calcium carbonate crystals are in the background – this sample is from a horse.

GRANULAR CASTS – DEGENERATING CELLULAR, COARSE, FINE

(a)

(b)

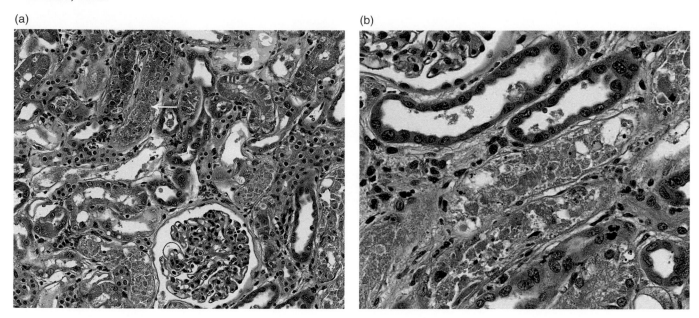

FIGURE 8.87   (a) Renal histopathology from a dog with acute tubular necrosis (ATN with severe AKI) at (20×). Note the large amount of intratubular debris and cellular remnants (arrow) that can contribute to granular cast formation according to the classic theory. Normal glomerulus is at bottom of field. (b) Higher power view from the same case above in (a) showing the coarse nature of intraluminal necrotic debris that can contribute to granular cast formation. Tubules near top left show stretching of tubular epithelium to cover damaged area over basement membrane. Source: Courtesy of Dr. Steven Weisbrode, The Ohio State University College of Veterinary Medicine.

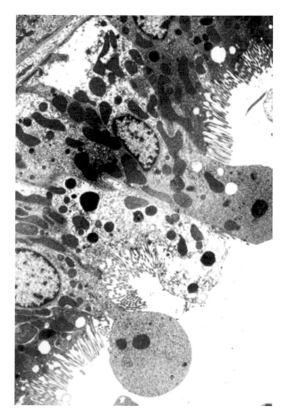

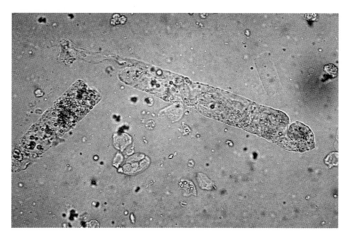

FIGURE 8.89   Two granular casts in a dog with acute nephritis. The cast to the right has abundant matrix protein without granules in some places. Unstained.

FIGURE 8.88   Electron micrograph showing proximal tubular injury 18 hours post ethylene glycol exposure in a dog. Note blebbing of proximal renal tubular cell into tubular lumen. Cells could be shed into the tubular lumen, or organelles could be released that could contribute to granular cast formation more distally. Source: From Smith et al. [4]. Used with permission.

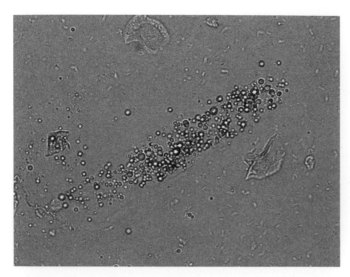

FIGURE 8.90 Granular cast. Refractile granules within this cast are also seen free in the urine. It is likely that these granules are lipid. A few squamous epithelial cells are in the background along with bacteria. Source: Reproduced with permission of Dr. Heather L. Wamsley, Bradenton, FL.

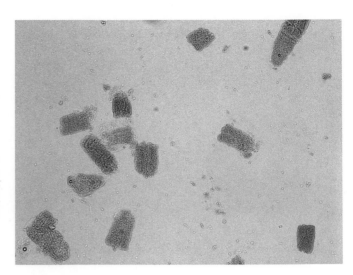

FIGURE 8.92 High powered microscopy field from the same urine sediment as in Figure 8.91. Numerous finely granular casts are identified at this power. The green stain is from bile pigments in the urine. Bilirubin associated nephropathy with accelerated granular cast formation is likely in this dog. Source: Reproduced with permission of Dr. Heather L. Wamsley, Bradenton, FL.

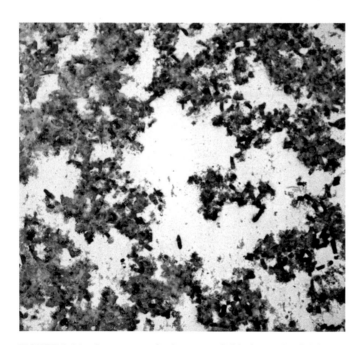

FIGURE 8.91 Low powered microscopy field of unstained urinary sediment from a dog. Note the bright green staining to unidentified elements in the background. Also note a "shower" of casts that appear dark. Characterization of these casts is not possible at this power. Urine chemistry was strongly positive for bilirubin. Source: Reproduced with permission of Dr. Heather L. Wamsley, Bradenton, FL.

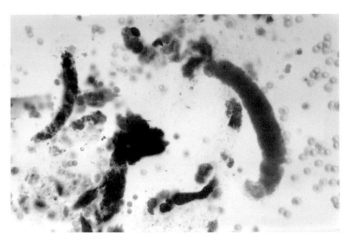

FIGURE 8.93 Two easily identified coarsely granular casts are on the left side of this image. One large waxy cast is on the right side. Many RBC and some WBC are also visible, but they are not in the same plane of focus as are the casts.

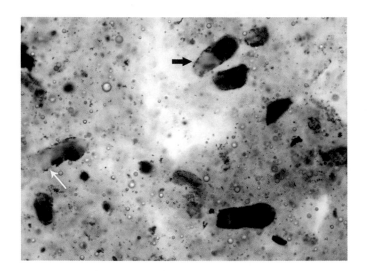

FIGURE 8.94 Hyaline and granular casts (stained sediment). An obvious hyaline cast is to the far left of this field (small white arrow). The cast at top center (large black arrow) is a mixed granular/hyaline cast but would be referred to as a granular cast since that is the more important component. Two other granular casts are seen further to the right. Many lipid droplets and particulate debris of unknown origin is in the background.

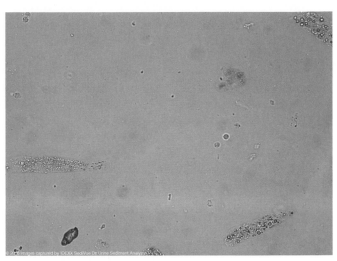

FIGURE 8.96 Image captured by SediVue®. Three granular casts; upper right corner, lower right, and far left fields. Source: Courtesy of IDEXX Laboratories. Copyright © 2022, IDEXX Laboratories, Inc. All rights reserved. Used with permission.

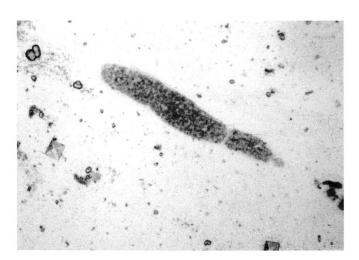

FIGURE 8.95 Granular cast in stained sediment. This cast has coarse granules that take up a pink stain. There is one obvious calcium oxalate dihydrate crystal in the left mid field.

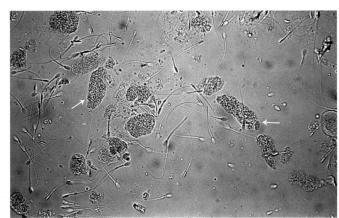

FIGURE 8.97 Two short granular casts (white arrows). Many sperm. Several unidentified round epithelial cells. Granular degeneration of nonsquamous epithelial cells can mimic the appearance of granular casts, but they are usually more rounded on the ends.

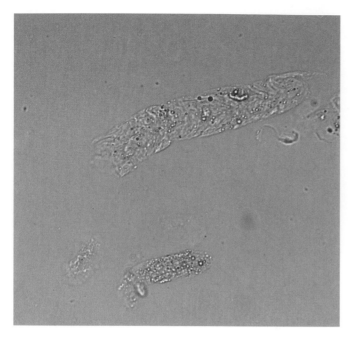

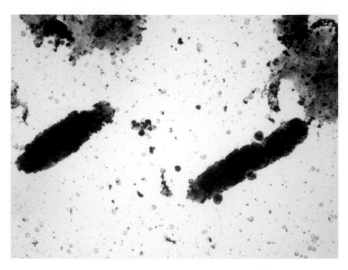

FIGURE 8.100 Two coarsely granular casts in urine sediment from a kitten. Numerous RBC and some WBC are noted in the background.

FIGURE 8.98 Image captured by SediVue®. Granular cast on bottom of field and hyaline cast at top. The hyaline cast on top does have a few granules within but it would still be classified as hyaline. Source: Courtesy of IDEXX Laboratories. Copyright © 2022, IDEXX Laboratories, Inc. All rights reserved. Used with permission.

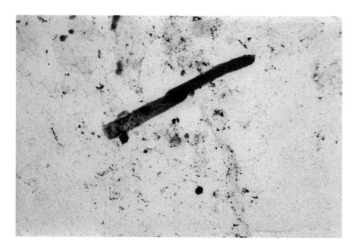

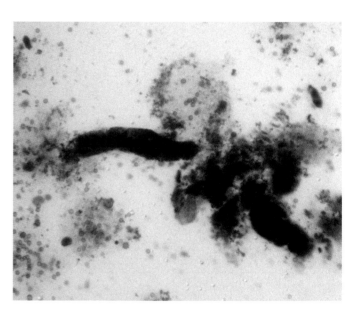

FIGURE 8.101 Coarsely granular casts. Faint staining RBC in the background. There is quite a bit of unidentifiable granular debris in between the casts.

FIGURE 8.99 Coarse granular cast. Donkey in renal failure.

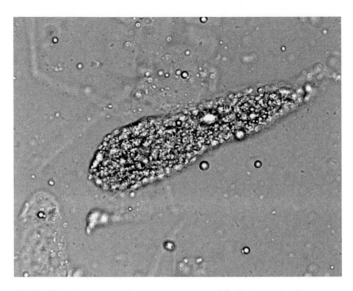

FIGURE 8.102 Granular cast in center of field. Unstained.

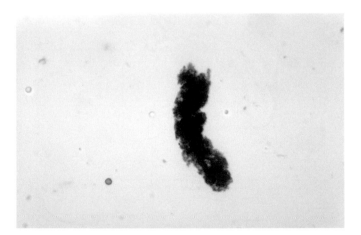

FIGURE 8.103 Coarsely granular cast.

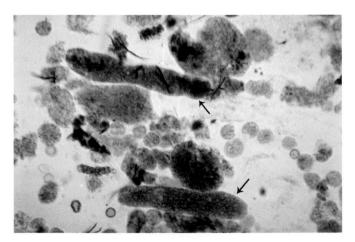

FIGURE 8.104 Two finely granular casts (black arrows). Bilirubin crystals are apparent near the granular cast at the top of this field. Several nonsquamous epithelial cells and WBC are also in this field, but some are lacking in cellular detail. The two largest cells at the top of this field are squamous epithelium.

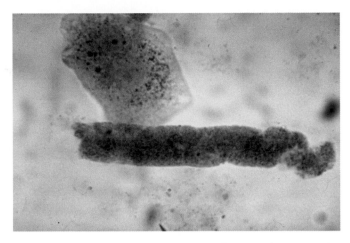

FIGURE 8.105 Finely granular cast. Very fine granules exist in this cast. Large squamous epithelial cell at the top of this field.

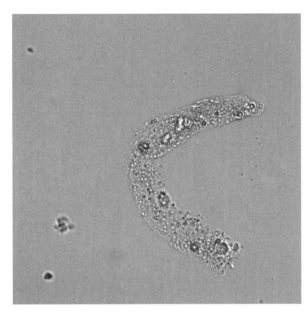

FIGURE 8.106 Image acquired by SediVue®. Finely granular cast. Source: Courtesy of IDEXX Laboratories. Copyright © 2022, IDEXX Laboratories, Inc. All rights reserved. Used with permission.

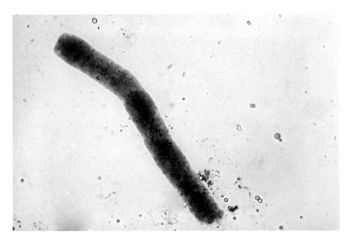

FIGURE 8.107 Finely granular cast. Note very fine stippling within this cast. Some areas of this cast appear waxy.

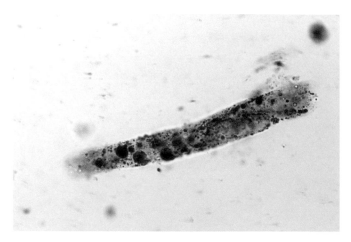

FIGURE 8.108 Granular and degenerating cellular cast. The cells within the cast cannot be definitively identified.

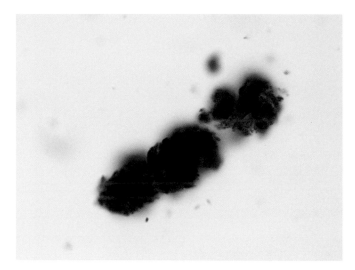

FIGURE 8.109 Granular and cellular cast. The lower portion of this cast is mostly coarsely granular and the upper portion is cellular. The cellular component appears to be RTE.

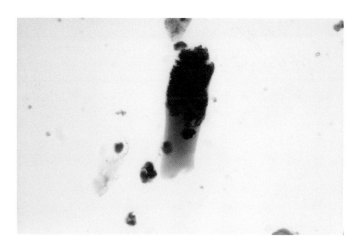

FIGURE 8.110 Coarsely granular cast. Coarse granules are located at the top portion of this cast and mostly hyaline at the other end. There are a few degenerating cells within this cast too. This cast could be classified as a degenerating cellular cast.

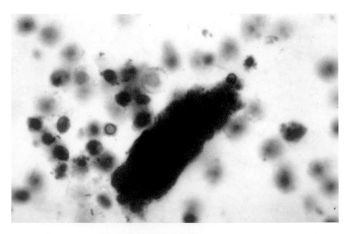

FIGURE 8.111 The single cast in this field has a fine granular pattern that can be seen at the periphery of the cast. There also appear to be much larger granules that could be degenerating cells. Numerous RBC and some WBC are in the background.

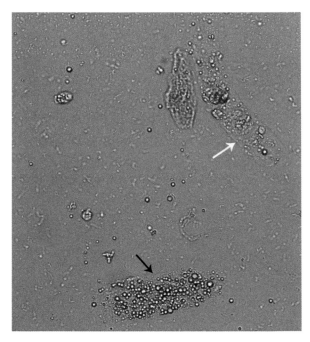

FIGURE 8.112 Granular casts. The cast at the top right of this image has a few coarse and fine granules (white arrow). There is a large squamous epithelial cell just to the left of this cast. The cast at the bottom (black arrow) has many globular granules that could be lipid, or alternatively precipitates of filtered plasma proteins. Many punctate bacteria appear in the background. Source: Reproduced with permission of Dr. Heather L. Wamsley, Bradenton, FL.

(a)

(b)

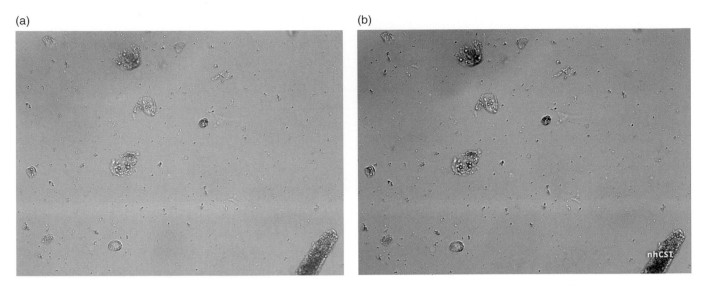

FIGURE 8.113 (a) Image captured by SediVue® automated microscopy. Note one nonhyaline (granular) cast in lower right corner. Many round punctate particles in background are likely bacteria in cocci form. (b) Same as in (a), with on screen notation of nhCST (nonhyaline cast). Round cells that are free or in a small clump were not identified by the sediment reader. Source: Courtesy of Dr. Ronald Lyman, Ft. Pierce, FL.

(a)

(b)

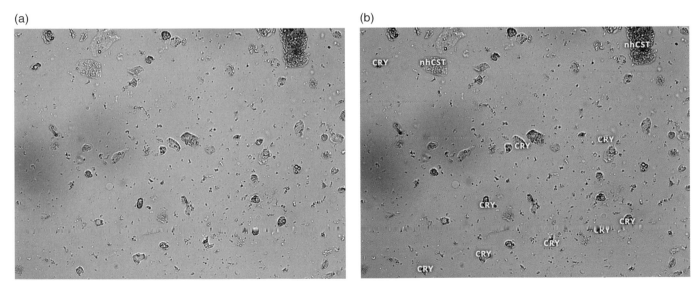

FIGURE 8.114 (a) Note two nonhyaline casts (granular) identified during SediVue® automated microscopy. (b) Same field as figure above. CRY – suspected crystalluria but not further identified. Upon review by laboratory personnel, elements labeled as CRY were not crystals. This is why it is still important to have a human confirm the reported identification of abnormal sediment. New neural networks and their associated algorithms are more likely to result in improved identification. Source: Courtesy of Dr. Ronald Lyman, Ft. Pierce, FL.

(a) (b) (c)

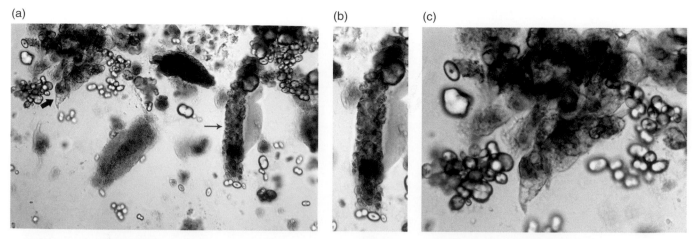

FIGURE 8.115 (a) Cellular cast and clump of renal tubular epithelial (RTE) cells. The single cast that appears with vertical orientation on the right side of this field (small black arrow) at first appears to be granular, but closer inspection reveals that the cast is largely composed of cells some of which are neutrophils. There is a large clump of RTE in the upper left corner of this field. Note tails and basal orientation of some of the nuclei in the RTE (thick black arrow). Calcium carbonate crystals in the background. One large squamous epithelial cell middle-left field. Urine sample from a horse. (b, c) Enlarged view cutouts from the lower power view in (a). (b) Cells in the cast can be seen. WBC are identified as some of the cells at the periphery of the cast. (c) Renal tubular epithelium.

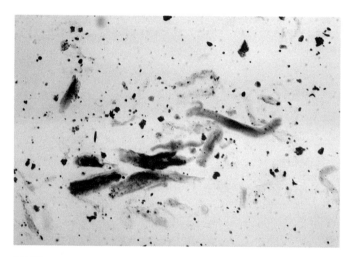

FIGURE 8.116 Shower of hyaline to finely granular (mixed) casts.

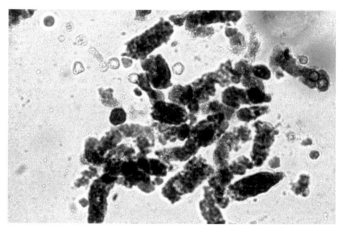

FIGURE 8.118 Shower of granular casts. Urinary sediment from a dog. New methylene blue stain. Source: Reproduced with permission of Dr. Michael Horton, Fairborn OH.

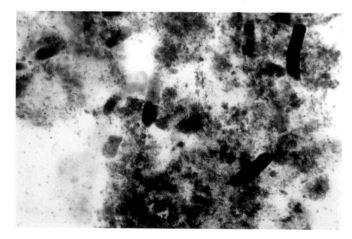

FIGURE 8.117 Several casts at high power view. Coarse granules are in several of these casts. Much particulate debris is in the background. This type of debris has been observed and described as cellular detritus in patients with severe AKI. This dog was in the midst of severe azotemic acute renal failure.

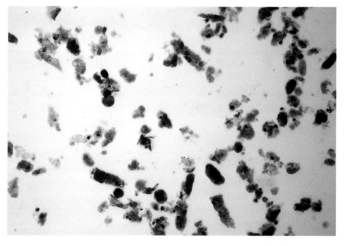

FIGURE 8.119 Several coarsely granular casts; occasional finely granular cast; free RTE. Occasional WBC. Urine sediment from a dog with leptospirosis.

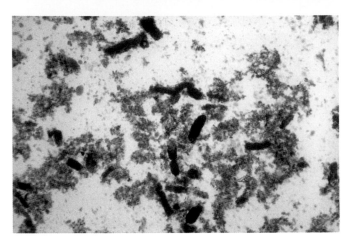

FIGURE 8.120 Shower of granular casts. Abundant course background debris that could be associated with necrosis of renal cells.

FIGURE 8.121 Numerous coarsely granular casts.

(a)

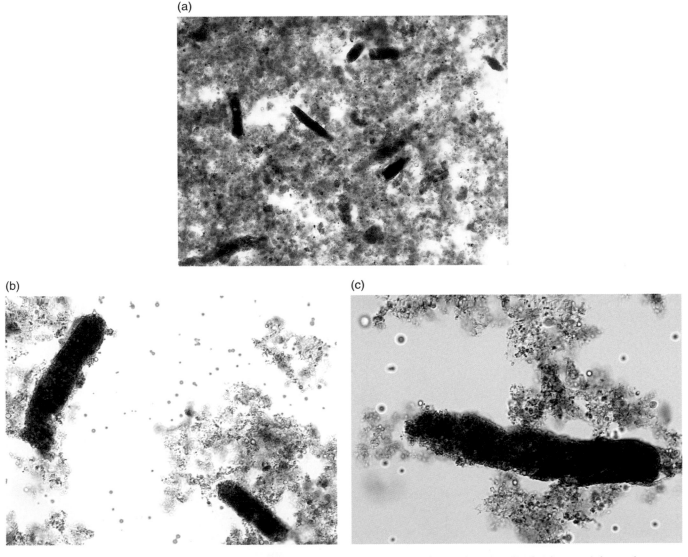

(b)

(c)

FIGURE 8.122 (a) Multiple casts in low power view. There are abundant particulate spheres of varying size that have an inherent brown color throughout the background. The urine was a muddy brown color before centrifugation. (b) Coarsely granular casts. Higher power view of casts; same sediment as shown in (a). This dog had myoglobinuria. We presume that the granular precipitates that are free and within the casts are myoglobin. (c) Coarsely granular cast – high power view. This is from a dog with myoglobinuria. Abundant amorphous material is in the background. Source: Dr. Felipe Galvao, Downers Grove, IL.

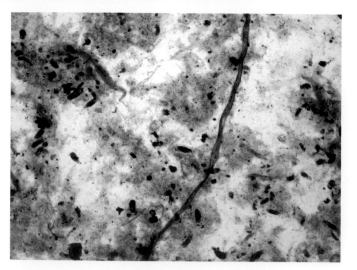

FIGURE 8.123 Numerous casts at low power view. This is sediment from a dog on a cast watch while receiving amikacin treatments. There is a large strand in the middle of this field that is an artifact from the collection of voided urine.

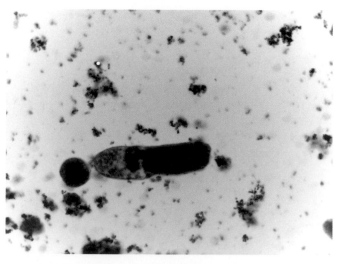

FIGURE 8.126 Granular cast. Amikacin treatment cast watch.

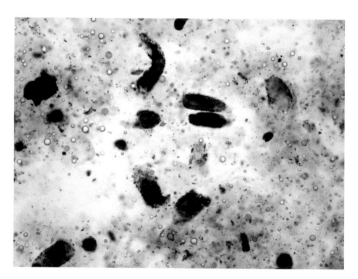

FIGURE 8.124 Granular casts in a dog on amikacin treatments (high power). Note also numerous refractile lipid droplets.

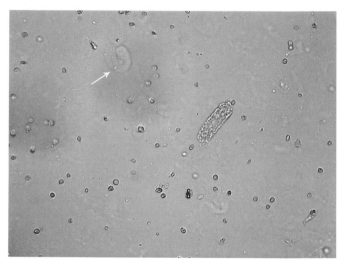

FIGURE 8.127 SediVue® acquired image. One hyaline cast in upper field (arrow). A probable granular cast in the mid right of center part of this field – not identified by the analyzer during automated microscopy. Several RBC are seen in this field but only averaged 1–5/ HPF. This dog was on a "cast watch" as part of surveillance for renal damage during treatment with the aminoglycoside antibiotic amikacin. Source: Courtesy of Dr. Ronald Lyman.

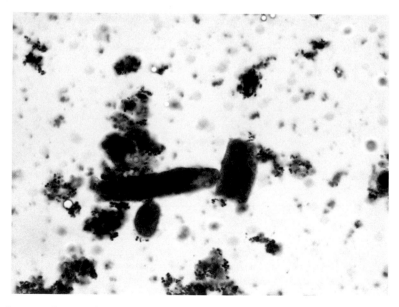

FIGURE 8.125 Several granular casts. Cast watch while on amikacin treatment.

WAXY CASTS

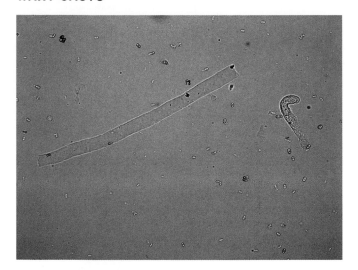

FIGURE 8.128 Waxy cast to the left and smaller granular cast to the right in this image. Source: Reproduced with permission of Dr. Heather L. Wamsley, Bradenton, FL.

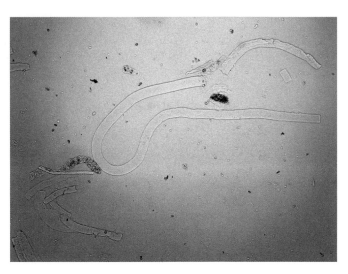

FIGURE 8.130 Several waxy casts. There is one cast in the middle left part of this image that is not waxy; it is either coarsely granular, cellular, or degenerating cellular in nature. Source: Reproduced with permission of Dr. Heather L. Wamsley, Bradenton, FL.

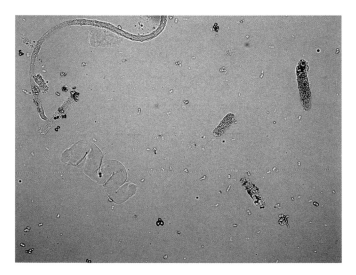

FIGURE 8.129 Waxy and granular casts. One highly convoluted waxy cast is seen in the lower left of this image. Two granular casts appear to the far right and right of middle. A long fiber artifact is seen in the upper left of this image that should not be confused with a cast (pseudocast). Source: Reproduced with permission of Dr. Heather L. Wamsley, Bradenton FL.

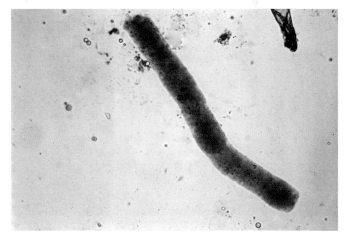

FIGURE 8.131 Mostly waxy cast. This is an example of transition from a finely granular to a waxy cast. Note that granules can still be identified in this cast at some locations and not at others.

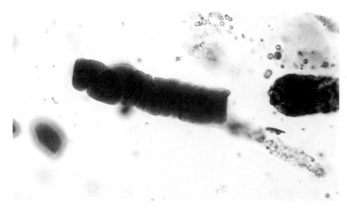

FIGURE 8.132 Waxy cast. The waxy cast in the center of this image is stained deeply pink and displays corrugations. A granular element to the far right at first looks like it could be a cast, but the very round end suggests that this is a degenerating epithelial cell.

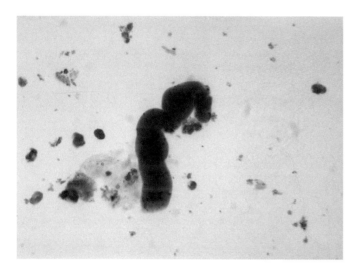

FIGURE 8.133 Waxy cast. Intense pink stain uptake is noticed along with some convolutions that represent where the cast was formed.

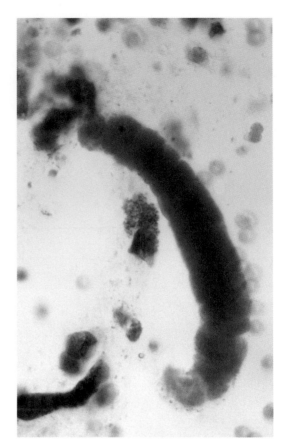

FIGURE 8.135 Waxy cast with intense uptake of pink stain. RBC and WBC are in the background.

(a)

(b)

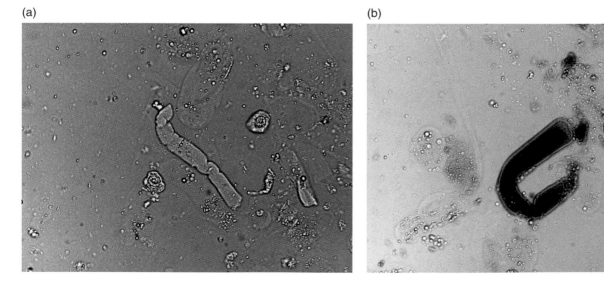

FIGURE 8.134 (a) Waxy cast (unstained). This cast is opaque, has multiple indentations, and blunt ends. There is one broad very faint hyaline cast just to the right of the waxy cast. Two nonsquamous epithelial cells are also seen in this field. (b) Waxy cast (stained). Same sediment as from Figure 8.58a. This waxy cast intensely takes up blue stain, and is bent on itself. A few calcium oxalate crystals are also in this field.

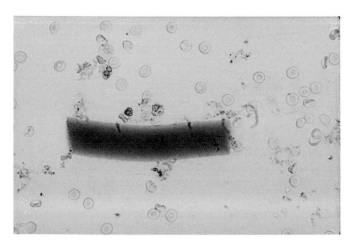

FIGURE 8.136 Waxy cast. Notice several cracks along the top border in this image. Numerous concave faint staining RBC and a few WBC are in the background.

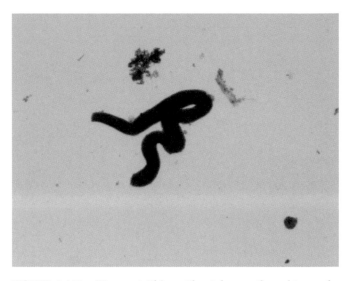

FIGURE 8.139 Waxy cast. This cast has taken up the red to purple stain intensely. A single degenerating WBC is seen at the lower right corner of this image.

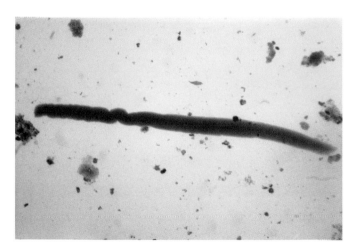

FIGURE 8.137 Waxy cast. This cast is very long and displays one convolution at the left in this field.

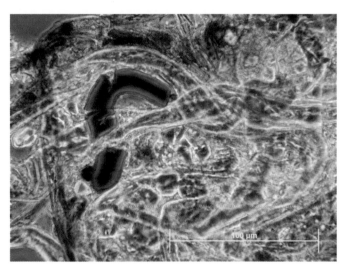

FIGURE 8.140 Waxy cast (phase microscopy). Notice the sharp lines of fracture along the exterior border of this cast. Source: Reproduced by permission of Dr. Michael Horton, Fairborn Ohio.

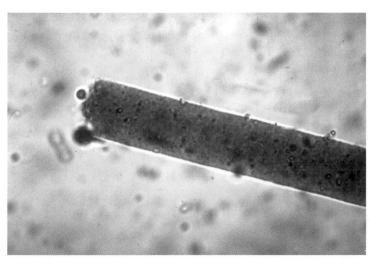

FIGURE 8.138 Waxy cast, unstained sediment.

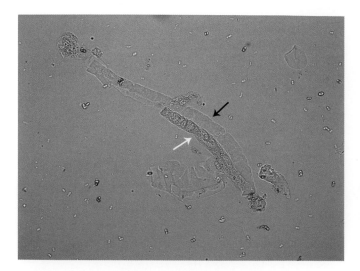

FIGURE 8.141 Waxy and cellular cast. Waxy cast is at the top of this image (black arrow). Right below the waxy cast is a cellular cast (white arrow). A second waxy cast is below the cellular cast but is not as easy to identify as it has been folded on itself. Source: Reproduced with permission of Dr. Heather L. Wamsley, Bradenton, FL.

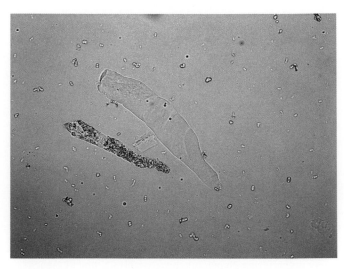

FIGURE 8.143 Waxy and granular cast. The waxy cast at the top is very wide and would be considered to be a "broad cast". The cast below the waxy cast is a coarsely granular cast. Source: Reproduced with permission of Dr. Heather L. Wamsley, Bradenton, FL.

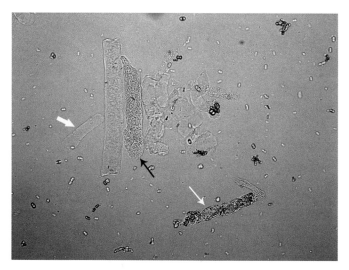

FIGURE 8.142 Waxy and granular casts. There are three casts in vertical orientation left of mid center; all three are waxy, but the one in the middle appears to have a finely granular pattern that has not made the final transition to waxy character (black arrow). It is unclear whether the cast on the far left is a waxy or hyaline cast (large white arrow). The cast with more horizontal orientation is a coarsely granular cast (small white arrow). Source: Reproduced with permission of Dr. Heather L. Wamsley, Bradenton, FL.

CELLULAR CASTS

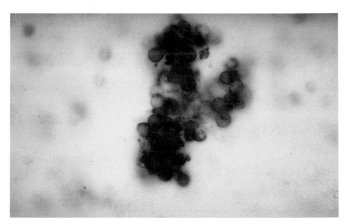

FIGURE 8.144 RBC cast. Note close association of RBC within a linear array. RBC come out of the cast quickly after entering urine and they are unusual to see unless when examining very fresh urine from patients with acute to subacute glomerular disease. Source: Reproduced by permission of Dr. Richard A. Scott, Animal Medical Center, NYC, NY.

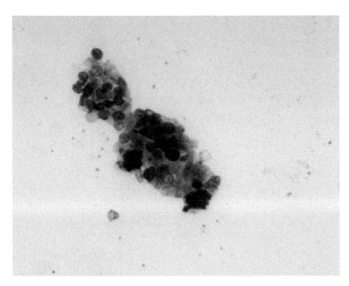

FIGURE 8.145 RBC cast. RBC are easy to identify in the portion of the cast to the upper left and middle. Urine sediment was from a patient with glomerulonephritis.

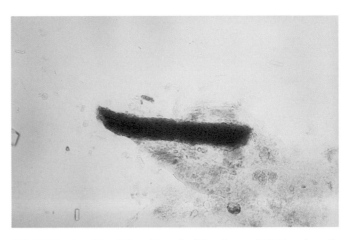

FIGURE 8.147 Blood Cast. Note the faint shape of RBC as the cell membranes and pigment are lost from the previously intact RBC in the cast. The significance for the presence of a blood cast is the same as that for an RBC cast, usually from glomerular leakage of RBC into Bowman's space due to acute glomerular inflammation. Urine sediment from critical illness foal.

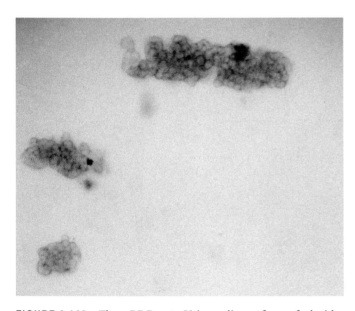

FIGURE 8.146 Three RBC casts. Urine sediment from a foal with critical illness.

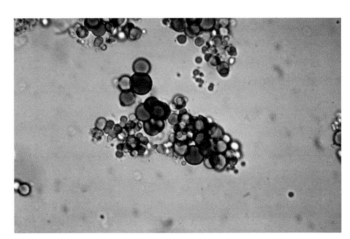

FIGURE 8.148 RBC cast. RBC are packed within parallel walls in this cast. Some RBC to the left of the cast are free. Source: Reproduced with permission of Dr. Richard A. Scott, Animal Medical Center, New York, NY.

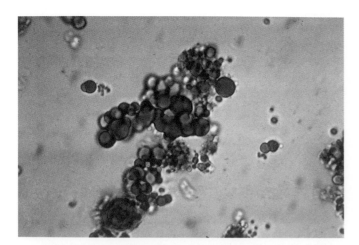

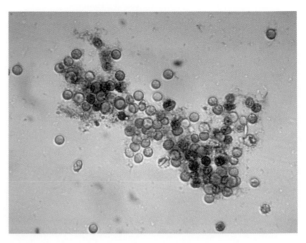

FIGURE 8.149 Possible RBC cast. RBC appear in a linear array to the left. Large round cell at bottom of the image is a nonsquamous epithelial cell. Source: Reproduced with permission of Dr. Richard A. Scott, Animal Medical Center, New York, NY.

FIGURE 8.150 Suspected RBC cast. Note linear array of RBC. Parallel walls of this suspected cast exist for a short distance. Clumping artifacts are usually more irregular unless there is a mucus or fibrin strand that allows a linear alignment. Source: Reproduced by permission of Dr. Richard A. Scott, Animal Medical Center, New York, NY.

(a) (b)

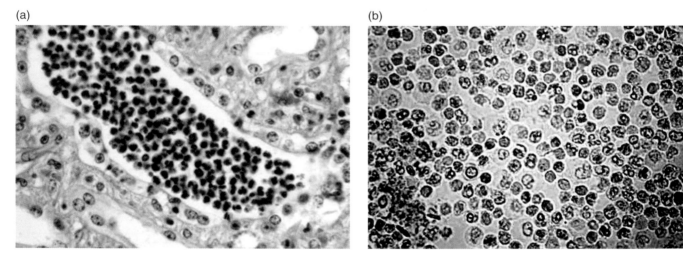

FIGURE 8.151 (a) Renal histopathology from a dog with pyelonephritis. The tubular lumen is filled with neutrophils. This is the first step in the formation of a cellular cast composed of WBC. Source: Reproduced by permission of Dr. Donald Meuten – North Carolina State University. (b) Urine sediment from dog with pyelonephritis. There are numerous WBC. Most of the neutrophils have well preserved morphology. Despite intrarenal WBC cast formation, none were observed in urine at this particular time. Shedding of WBC casts can be intermittent. If only WBC are seen in the urine, it is not possible to make the diagnosis of pyelonephritis unless the WBC are also trapped within a cast. Source: Used with permission of Dr. Donald Meuten, North Carolina State University.

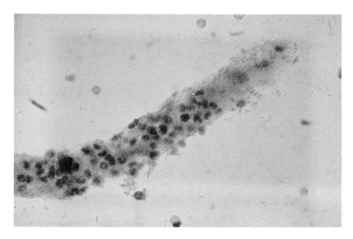

FIGURE 8.152 Cellular cast of white blood cells. High power view showing nature of cells as neutrophils. The right end of this cast has very few cells.

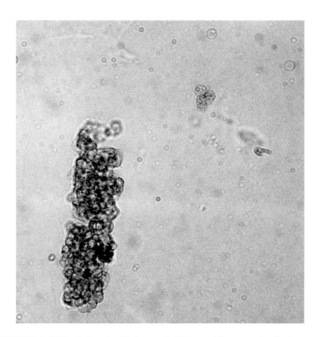

FIGURE 8.155 Mixed cellular cast. This cast is comprised of mostly neutrophils. Urine from a foal with critical illness.

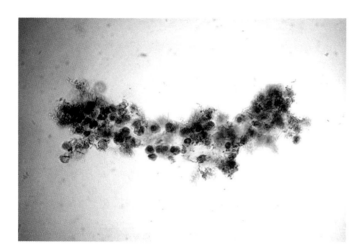

FIGURE 8.153 WBC cast with bacteria. Neutrophils predominate in this cast. This cast appears to be breaking up into two well defined pieces of what was originally a longer cast. The right end of this cast is the most convincing that it really is a cast due to the tight packing of cells and well-defined parallel walls. This cast also contains linear structures that appear to be bacterial rods.

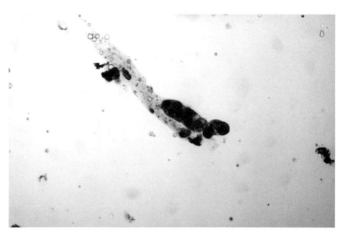

FIGURE 8.156 Hyaline and renal tubular cell casts. Note the light pink staining hyaline cast in the center of this field and the cellular cast to the right comprised of renal tubule epithelial cells. This urine sediment is from a cat following a perineal urethrostomy surgery and the development of pyelonephritis.

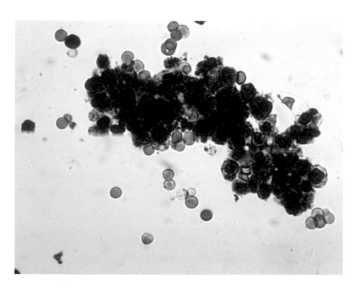

FIGURE 8.154 WBC cast. There are two areas of the cast with parallel walls. The cast appears to be fractured one-third of the way from the right. Free RBC are seen in the background.

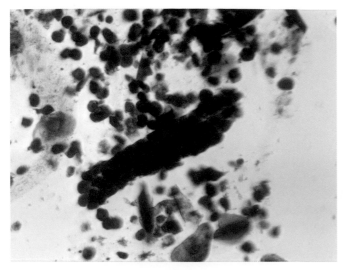

FIGURE 8.157 Cellular cast consisting of renal tubular epithelial cells (RTE). Notice the parallel rows of similar size small epithelial cells within this cast. This tight packing of epithelium in an orderly way suggests that a segment of connected epithelium was lost into the tubular lumen at the same time. Note numerous free small round epithelial cells that are the same size as those within the cast. The small free epithelial cells in the urine look very similar to the cells trapped in the cast but their nuclear detail is lacking to provide more evidence that they are RTE. Urine sediment was from a young nonazotemic Yorkshire Terrier with lead poisoning.

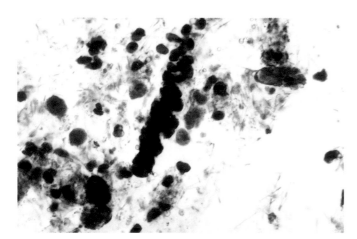

FIGURE 8.158 Cellular cast; renal tubular epithelium. Urine sediment was examined in a young male German Shepherd dog initially suspected to have ethylene glycol poisoning. This dog was examined by the emergency service and found to have azotemia and a USG of 1.018. There were no calcium oxalate crystals identified during microscopy. Note the linear cluster of small epithelial cells contained in the cast in the middle of this image. Also note the free small epithelial cells that are presumably renal tubular epithelial cells. There are numerous sperm, which can be found in urine from normal intact male dogs. Ischemic nephropathy (AKI) associated with a pericardial diaphragmatic hernia caused this cast to develop.

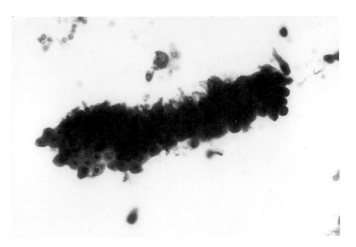

FIGURE 8.159 Cellular cast; renal tubular epithelium. This cellular cast is packed with renal tubular epithelium. There are a few free small epithelial cells and RBC in the background. Urine sediment from a dog with heartworm disease (before treatment).

(a)

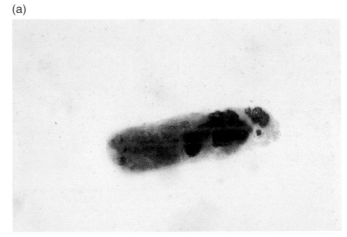

(b)

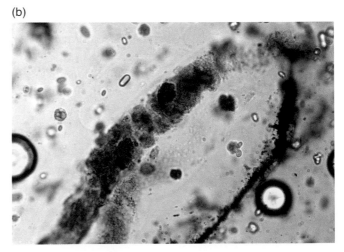

FIGURE 8.160 (a) Degenerating cellular cast. This is likely to be a renal tubular epithelial cast based on the size of the cells. Urine sediment from a horse with gentamicin toxicity. (b) Degenerating cellular cast. This is likely to be a renal tubular epithelial cast based on the size of the cells. Calcium carbonate crystals in the background. Urine sediment from a horse with gentamicin toxicity.

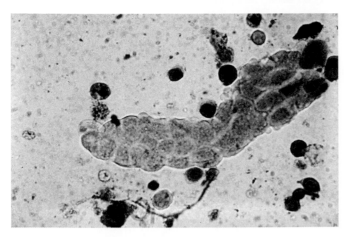

FIGURE 8.161   Cellular cast; renal tubular epithelium. The cells are larger than from WBC or RBC embedded in a cast. These cells have lost considerable detail but the cell size fits with that of RTE. A single RBC is seen for size comparison just below the cast to the left. The free cells in the background are likely RTE.

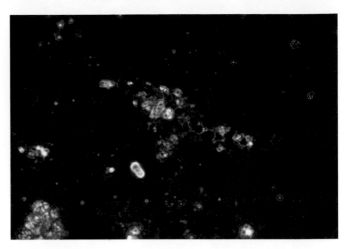

FIGURE 8.163   Cellular cast (phase microscopy). An RTE cast is in the center of this image. A few calcium oxalate crystals are also in the background. Urinary sediment from a cat with ethylene glycol intoxication. Source: Reproduced by permission of Dr. Michael Horton, Fairborn, OH.

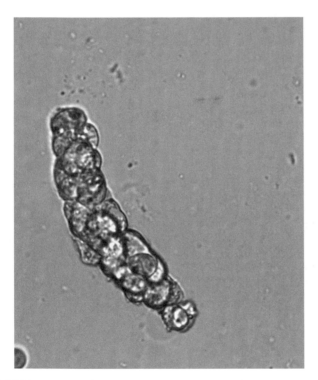

FIGURE 8.162   Cellular cast; renal tubular epithelium. Image acquired by SediVue®. Source: Courtesy of IDEXX Laboratories. Copyright © 2022, IDEXX Laboratories, Inc. All rights reserved. Used with permission.

(a)   (b)

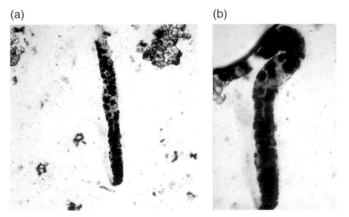

FIGURE 8.164   (a) Cellular cast; renal tubular epithelium. Low power magnification. Calcium carbonate crystals are in the background. The size of the cells is bigger than RBC and WBC, so these cells are likely to be renal tubular epithelium. Urine sediment from a horse with myoglobinuric AKI due to "tying up." (b) Cellular cast; renal tubular epithelium. Higher power magnification. The RTE have undergone some degenerative change. Urine sediment from a horse with myoglobinuric AKI due to "tying up." Calcium carbonate crystals are in the background.

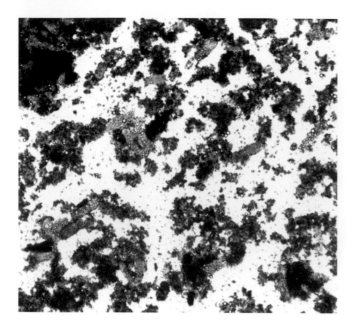

FIGURE 8.165 Shower of uric acid casts, low power (10× objective). Unstained urine sediment showing casts packed with amorphous crystals. Many small amorphous crystals are in the background along with several lipid droplets. The urine was cloudy and contained these casts one day after treatment of lymphoma with l-asparaginase. Serum uric acid concentration was high and infrared spectroscopy identified the crystals to be 100% uric acid dihydrate. Source: Figure is from figure 3 in Tvedten et al. [5]. Used with permission.

STRUVITE CRYSTALS

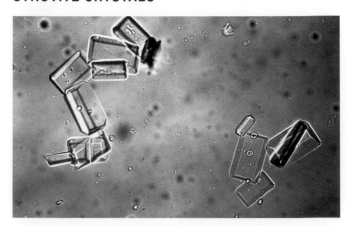

FIGURE 8.166 Clusters of struvite crystals in stained sediment. Occasional RBC in this field. Urine sediment from a cat with idiopathic cystitis.

(a)

(b)

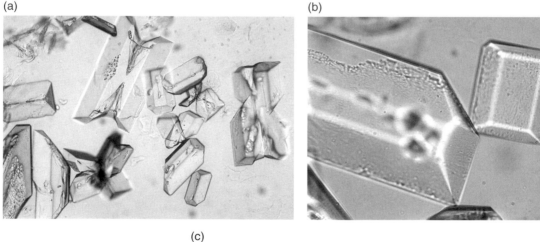

(c)

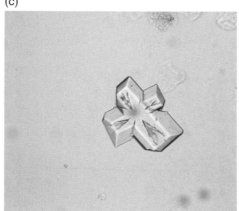

FIGURE 8.167 (a) Struvite (unstained sediment). Clusters of struvite and two large crystals growing in an X-shape. (b) Struvite crystals. High power view showing edges and three-dimensional nature of this crystal type. (c) Struvite crystals. Crystals are growing perpendicular to each other. Source: Reproduced with permission of Dr. Michael Horton, Fairborn, OH.

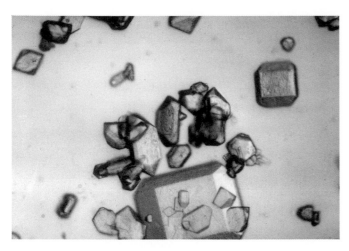

FIGURE 8.168 Struvite crystals, high power view. Source: Reproduced by permission of Dr. Richard Scott, Animal Medical Center, New York, NY.

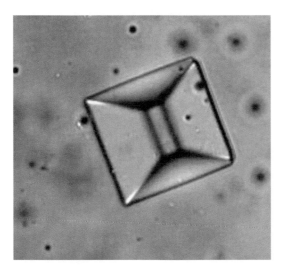

FIGURE 8.169 Struvite crystal (high magnification). Three-dimensional nature of this crystal is apparent. Image acquired by VETSCAN® SA Sediment Analyzer. Reproduced with permission of Zoetis.

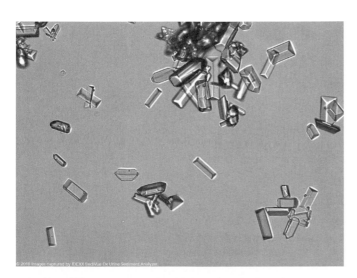

FIGURE 8.170 Struvite crystals. Image acquired by SediVue®. Source: Courtesy of IDEXX Laboratories. Copyright © 2022, IDEXX Laboratories, Inc. All rights reserved. Used with permission.

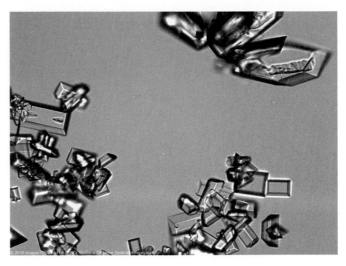

FIGURE 8.171 Struvite crystals. Most of the crystals are in clusters. Image acquired by SediVue®. Source: Courtesy of IDEXX Laboratories. Copyright © 2022, IDEXX Laboratories, Inc. All rights reserved. Used with permission.

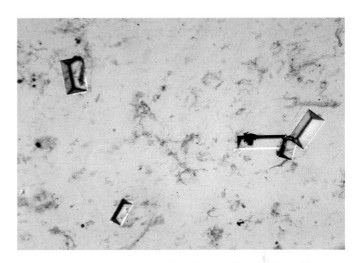

FIGURE 8.172 Struvite crystals (stained sediment). Very distinct edges show the three-dimensional nature of this crystal.

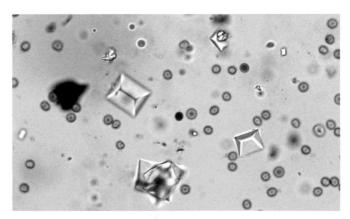

FIGURE 8.173 Struvite crystals and numerous RBC.

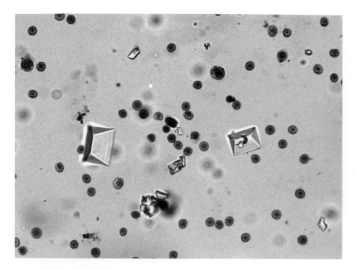

FIGURE 8.174 Struvite crystals (stained sediment). Many crenated RBC and rare WBC in the background.

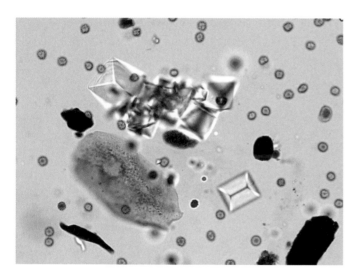

FIGURE 8.175 Struvite crystals – stained sediment. Many RBC and one large squamous epithelial cell.

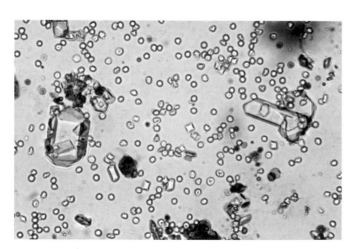

FIGURE 8.176 Struvite crystals, numerous RBC, and rare WBC (stained sediment). RBC are pale staining. Urine from cat with idiopathic cystitis. Source: Reproduced by permission of Dr. Michael Horton, Fairborn, OH.

(a)

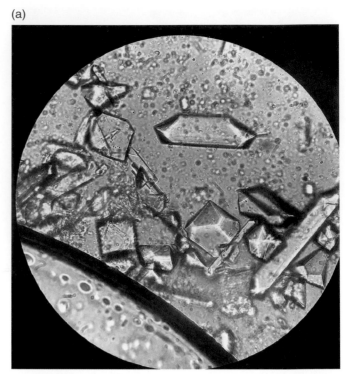

(b)

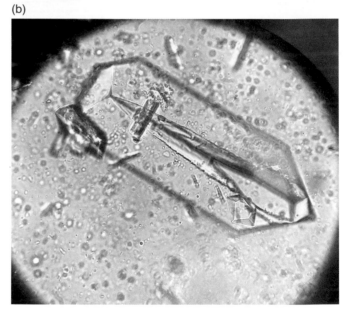

FIGURE 8.177 (a) Struvite crystals. Edge of air bubble at bottom left of image. Image acquired with a digital camera through the microscope eyepiece. (b) Struvite crystal. One large struvite crystal is seen along with other crystalline material that cannot be identified in this field. Image acquired with a digital camera through the microscope eyepiece. Source: Reproduced with permission of Dr. Felipe Galvao, Downers Grove, IL.

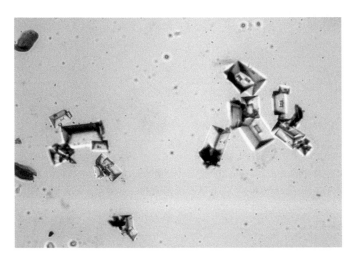

FIGURE 8.178 Struvite crystals. Classic coffin-lid appearance to small clusters of struvite crystals. Two squamous epithelial cells at far left of image.

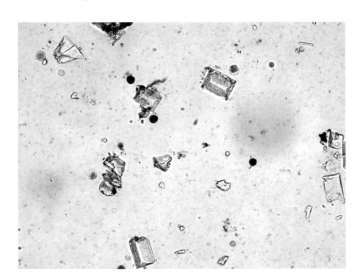

FIGURE 8.179 Struvite crystals.

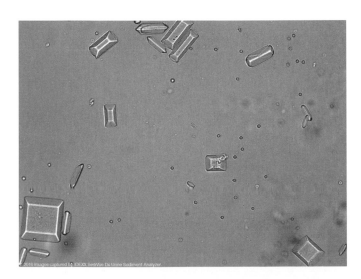

FIGURE 8.180 Struvite crystals. A moderate number of RBC are in the background. Image acquired by SediVue®. Source: Courtesy of IDEXX Laboratories. Copyright © 2022, IDEXX Laboratories, Inc. All rights reserved. Used with permission.

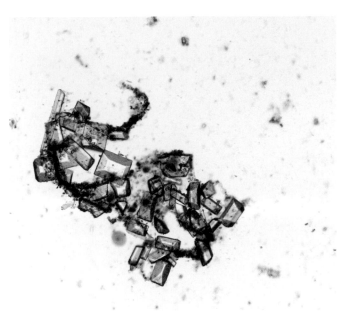

FIGURE 8.181 Struvite cluster. Crystals are aligned along a mucus thread.

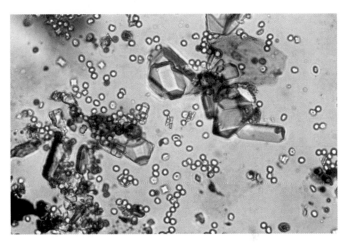

FIGURE 8.182 Struvite crystal clusters. Numerous RBC and rare WBC in the background. Urine from cat with idiopathic cystitis. Source: Reproduced with permission of Dr. Michael Horton, Fairborn, OH.

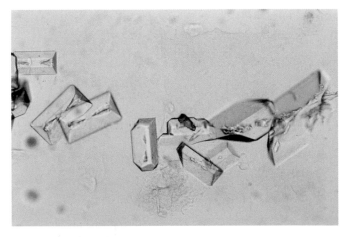

FIGURE 8.183 Struvite clusters.

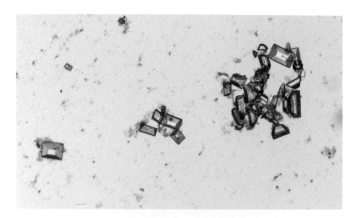

FIGURE 8.184 Struvite clusters. Single struvite crystal to the left shows deep three-dimensional nature of this crystal.

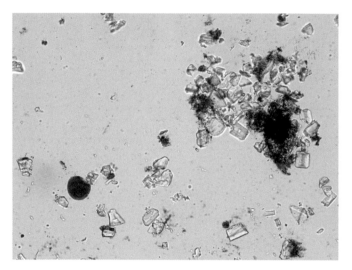

FIGURE 8.185 Struvite crystals in a dog. Most crystals are in clusters. One nonsquamous epithelial cell is on the far left of this image.

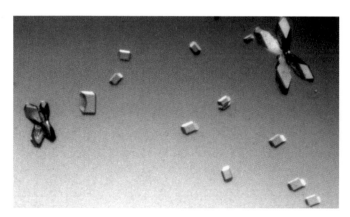

FIGURE 8.186 Struvite crystals. The large crystals at the far right and far left have a butterfly appearance.

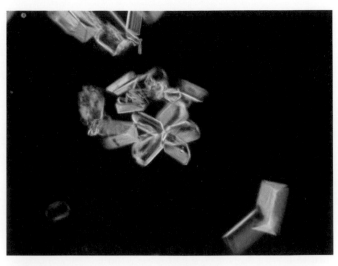

FIGURE 8.187 Struvite crystals (darkfield microscopy). Source: Reproduced by permission of Dr. Michael Horton, Fairborn, OH.

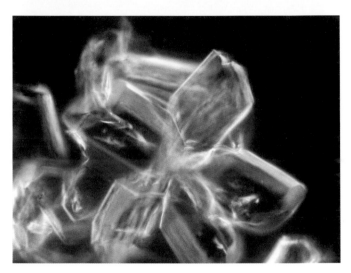

FIGURE 8.188 Struvite crystals (high power view darkfield microscopy). Source: Reproduced by permission of Dr. Michael Horton, Fairborn, OH.

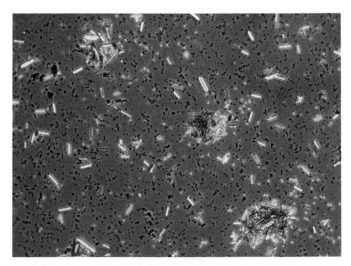

FIGURE 8.189 Struvite crystals (phase microscopy). Struvite crystals exist in clumps and those that are free. Multiple punctate structures in background appear to be cocci. Source: Reproduced by permission of Dr. Michael Horton, Fairborn, OH.

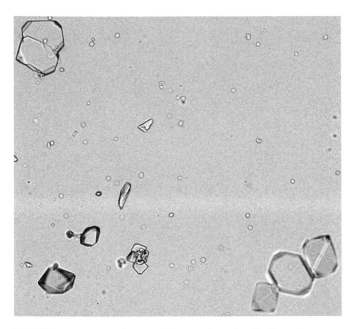

FIGURE 8.190 Struvite crystals. Note the refractile lines that are observed in some crystals as their edges line up perpendicular to the microscopic lens. Source: Reproduced with permission of Dr. Heather L. Wamsley, Bradenton, FL.

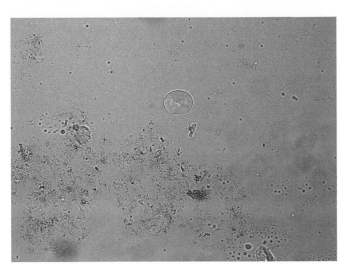

FIGURE 8.192 Amorphous phosphate crystals. The identity of the large round to oval crystal at the top of this image is unknown. Source: Reproduced with permission Dr. Heather L. Wamsley, Bradenton, FL.

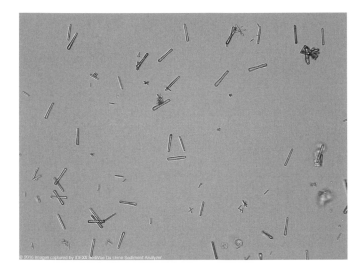

FIGURE 8.191 Phosphate crystals. Image acquired by SediVue®. The automated reader identified these crystals as nonstruvite and nonoxalate crystals. Source: Courtesy of IDEXX Laboratories. Copyright © 2022, IDEXX Laboratories, Inc. All rights reserved. Used with permission.

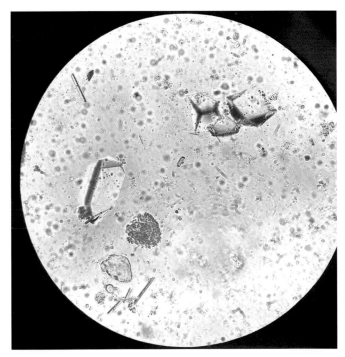

FIGURE 8.193 Struvite crystals (unstained sediment). The classic nature with three-dimensional appearance of several struvite crystals is seen. Some crystals are needle-like and many others are amorphous. Small round cells are out of focus in the background, but are likely to be RBC. Image acquired with a digital camera through the microscope eyepiece. Source: Reproduced with permission of Dr. Felipe Galvao, Downers Grove, IL.

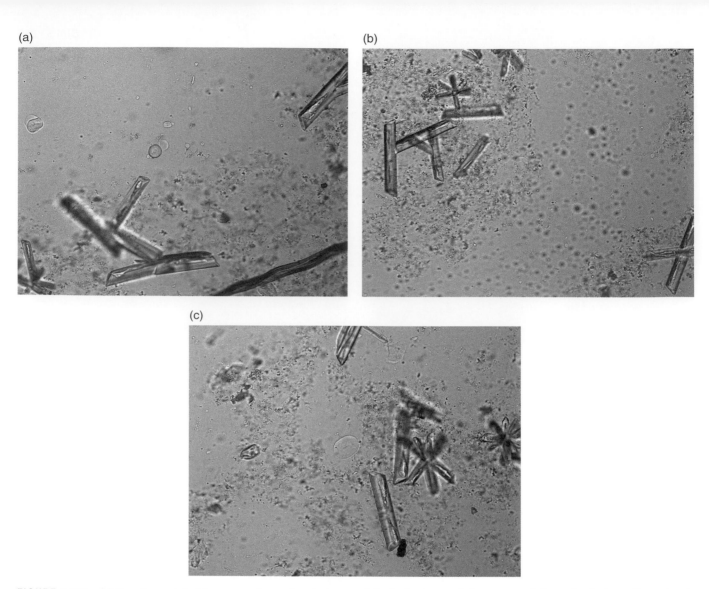

FIGURE 8.194 (a) Struvite crystals. Many amorphous phosphate crystals in the background. Larger crystals have classic three-dimensional shape of struvite. USG of 1.056 with a pH of 8.5. Some of the particulate matter was confirmed as cocci on cytology with Wright's stain. (b) Struvite crystals. Many amorphous phosphate crystals in the background. Some cocci among particulates in background. (c) Struvite crystals. Many amorphous phosphate crystals in the background. Note two starburst clusters to the right in this image. USG of 1.056 with a pH of 8.5. Source: Reproduced by permission of Dr. Heather L. Wamsley, Bradenton, FL.

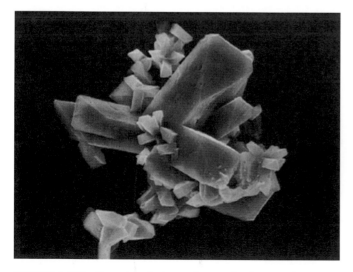

FIGURE 8.195 Scanning electron micrograph of magnesium ammonium phosphate crystals in urine sediment of a four-year-old domestic longhaired cat. (Original magnification, ×4400). Source: From Osborne et al. [6]. Used with permission.

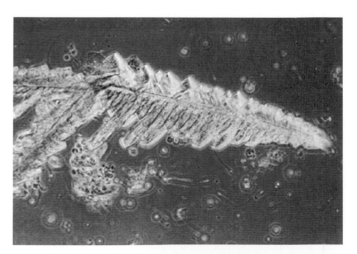

FIGURE 8.196 Photomicrograph of urine sediment containing aggregates of struvite crystals. Note the orderly arrangement of individual struvite crystals forming the aggregate. (Unstained; polarized light microscopy; original magnification, ×64.) Source: From Osborne et al. [6]. Used with permission.

CALCIUM OXALATE CRYSTALS

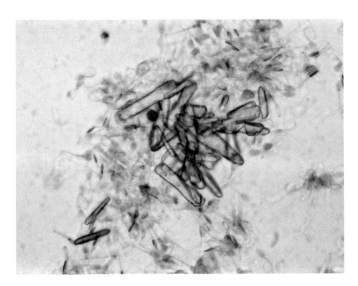

FIGURE 8.197 Calcium oxalate monohydrate crystals. Many sperm are observed in the background. Urine sediment from a dog with ethylene glycol poisoning.

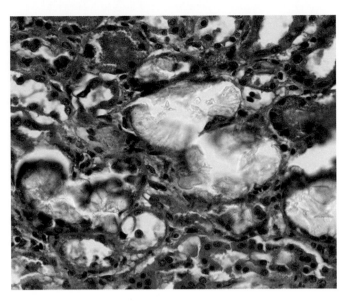

FIGURE 8.199 Renal histopathology from a dog with ethylene glycol poisoning. Note large number of intratubular calcium oxalate crystals. There appears to be some tubular necrosis in areas that are in close apposition to these crystals. Crystals are more often an indicator of ethylene glycol poisoning than a creator of severe AKI by themselves. Source: Courtesy of Dr. Steven Weisbrode, The Ohio State University College of Veterinary Medicine.

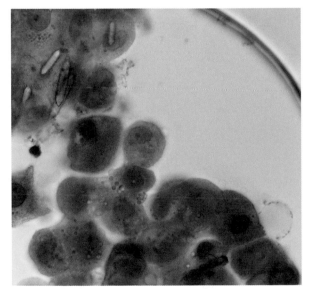

FIGURE 8.198 Calcium oxalate monohydrate crystals. Note picket fence shape crystals in the upper left of this image. The crystals are overlying RTE. Margin of an air bubble is seen in the upper right field. Ethylene glycol poisoning in a dog.

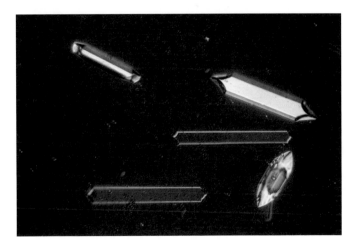

FIGURE 8.200 Calcium oxalate monohydrate crystals seen with polarizing light. The crystal at the right bottom of this field has a hemp seed appearance with a budding daughter crystal.

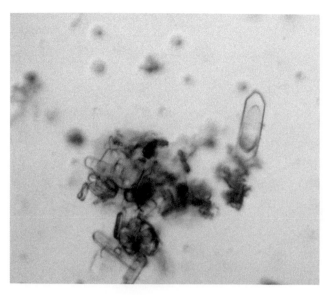

FIGURE 8.201 Calcium oxalate monohydrate crystals. Faint appearance of budding daughter crystal overlying the large crystal to the right.

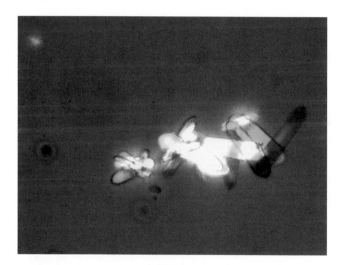

FIGURE 8.202 Calcium oxalate monohydrate crystals (polarizing light). Source: Courtesy of Dr. Gerry Thornhill, Purdue University, W. Lafayette, IN.

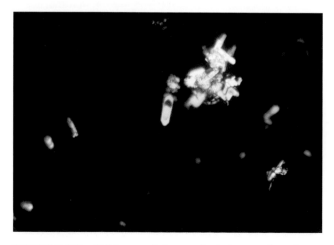

FIGURE 8.203 Calcium oxalate monohydrate crystals under polarizing light.

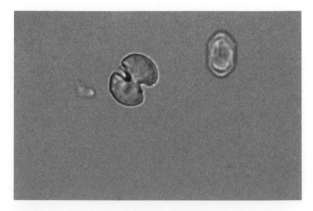

FIGURE 8.204 Calcium oxalate monohydrate crystals. Magnified view showing budding daughter crystal to the right and a sheath shape to the left (dumbbell). Source: Reproduced with permission of Dr. Heather L. Wamsley, Bradenton, FL.

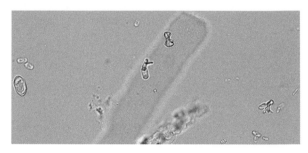

FIGURE 8.205 Calcium oxalate monohydrate crystals. The crystal to the far left appears to have a budding daughter crystal protruding. Waxy or hyaline cast in background is out of focus. Source: Reproduced with permission of Dr. Heather L. Wamsley, Bradenton, FL.

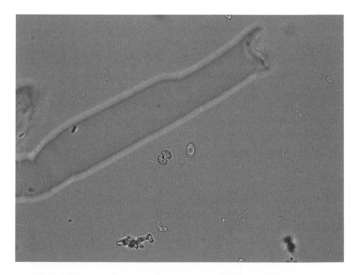

FIGURE 8.206 Calcium oxalate monohydrate crystals. These crystals are quite small. There is one budding daughter crystal to the right just below the cast. Hyaline cast in background. Source: Reproduced with permission of Dr. Heather L. Wamsley, Bradenton, FL.

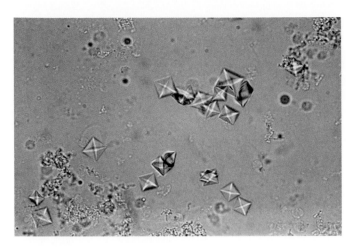

FIGURE 8.207 Calcium oxalate dihydrate crystals. Amorphous particulates are in the background that are not identified. Faint WBC and RBC are in the background.

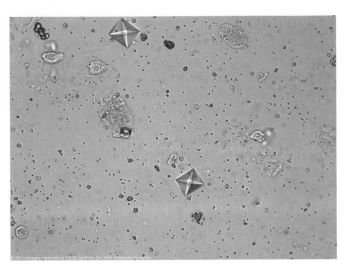

FIGURE 8.209 Calcium oxalate dihydrate crystals. Image acquired by SediVue®. Two large calcium oxalate crystals are in this field. One squamous and several nonsquamous epithelial cells are also in this field, as are occasional RBC and rare WBC. Particulate debris in background is not identified. Source: Courtesy of IDEXX Laboratories. Copyright © 2022, IDEXX Laboratories, Inc. All rights reserved. Used with permission.

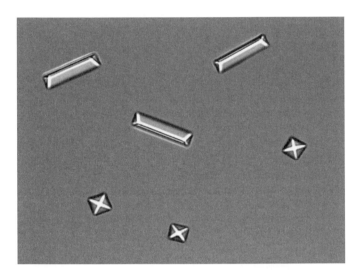

FIGURE 8.208 Calcium oxalate dihydrate and struvite crystals. The top three crystals are struvite and the lower three crystals are calcium oxalate dihydrate (Maltese cross within rhomboids). Image acquired by VETSCAN® SA Sediment Analyzer. Reproduced with permission of Zoetis.

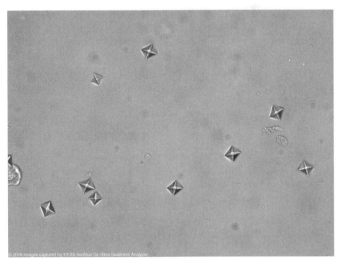

FIGURE 8.210 Calcium oxalate dihydrate crystals. Image acquired by SediVue®. Classic rhomboid shape with Maltese cross structure within the crystal. Rare RBC are faintly seen and are much smaller than the crystals. Source: Courtesy of IDEXX Laboratories. Copyright © 2022, IDEXX Laboratories, Inc. All rights reserved. Used with permission.

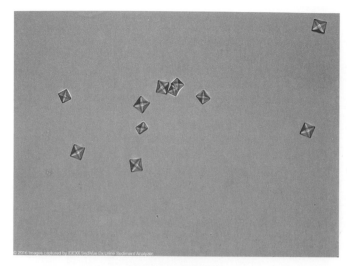

FIGURE 8.211 Calcium oxalate dihydrate crystals. Image acquired by SediVue®.Source: Courtesy of IDEXX Laboratories. Copyright © 2022, IDEXX Laboratories, Inc. All rights reserved. Used with permission.

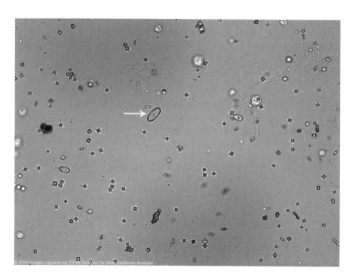

FIGURE 8.212 Calcium oxalate dihydrate and monohydrate crystals. Image acquired by SediVue®. Numerous small square crystals characteristic of calcium oxalate dihydrate dominate this field. The two largest crystals (center top and center left) are ovoid (hemp seed-like; arrow) and are calcium oxalate monohydrate. Source: Courtesy of IDEXX Laboratories. Copyright © 2022, IDEXX Laboratories, Inc. All rights reserved. Used with permission.

URATE CRYSTALS

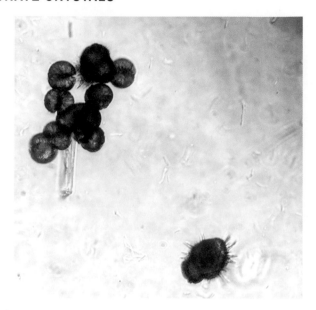

FIGURE 8.213 Urate crystals. A few of the round brownish crystals have extensions or protrusions from the crystal surface that make it easy to identify them. A single struvite crystal is seen underneath the cluster of urate crystals.

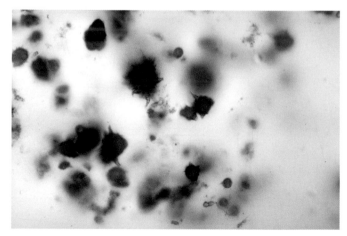

FIGURE 8.214 Ammonium biurate crystals. Note spicules that protrude as a characteristic feature of this crystal.

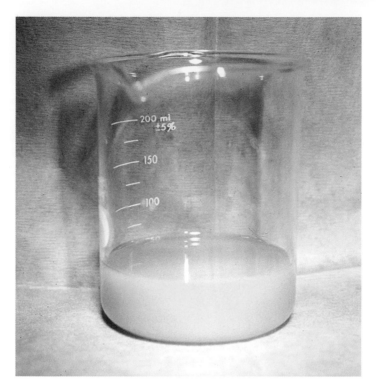

FIGURE 8.215 Opaque urine from a Dalmatian dog with urate urolithiasis. Source: Courtesy of Dr. Joe Bartges, University of Georgia, Athens, GA.

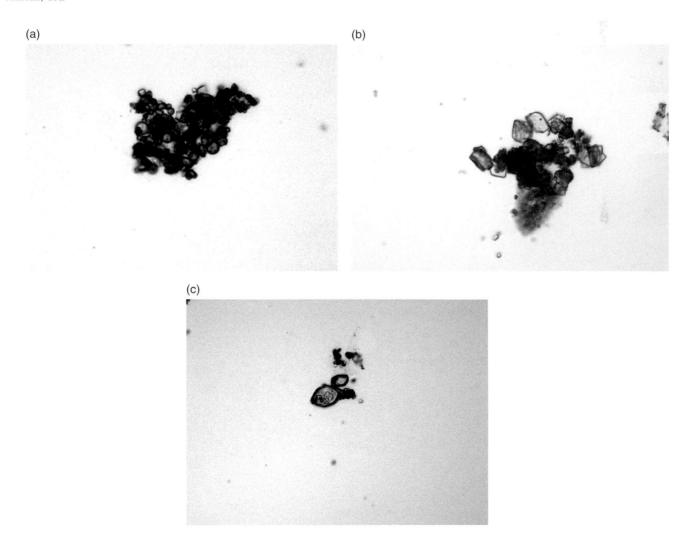

FIGURE 8.216 (a) Urates from a Dalmatian dog with urate urolithiasis. (b) Urates. Higher magnification of urate crystal cluster from a Dalmatian dog with urate urolithiasis. (c) Urates. Higher magnification of individual urate crystals from a Dalmatian dog with urate urolithiasis.

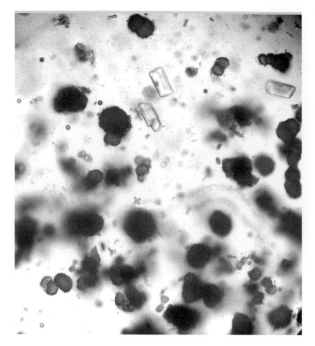

FIGURE 8.217 Ammonium biurate crystals. Urine sediment from a Yorkshire Terrier with the diagnosis of a portosystemic shunt. There are also a few struvite crystals in this field.

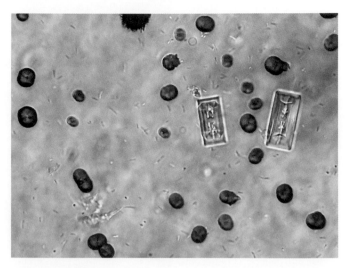

FIGURE 8.219 Urate and struvite crystals. The two clear crystals to the right are struvite The other crystals are urates most of which are round. A few of the urate crystals do have protrusions. Without protrusions from the surface, it can be difficult to accurately identify urate crystals.

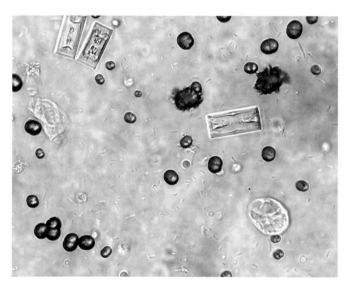

FIGURE 8.218 Urate and struvite crystals. A few of the urate crystals have characteristic protrusions. Most of the urate crystals are round and in small clumps, some appearing to be bivalve. It is difficult to identify urate crystals that do not have protrusions from their surface. There are three struvite crystals in this field as well as a few squamous epithelial cells. There are occasional RBC and WBC in the background. Moderate numbers of bacteria are visible.

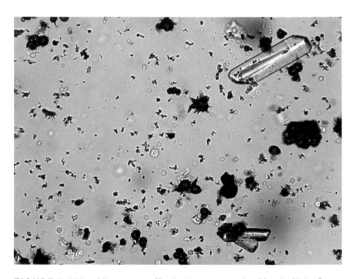

FIGURE 8.220 Urate crystalluria. Image acquired by SediVue®. Some of the urate crystals have typical protrusions. Other urate crystals are round and in clumps. There is one large struvite crystal in the upper right of this field. Source: Courtesy of IDEXX Laboratories. Copyright © 2022, IDEXX Laboratories, Inc. All rights reserved. Used with permission.

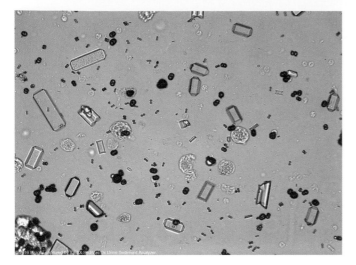

FIGURE 8.221   Ammonium urate and struvite crystals. Image acquired by SediVue®. The larger clear crystals are struvite. The darker ones either alone or in clusters are ammonium urate. Note also the presence of moderate numbers of nonsquamous epithelial cells and RBC; rare WBC. Source: Courtesy of IDEXX Laboratories. Copyright © 2022, IDEXX Laboratories, Inc. All rights reserved. Used with permission.

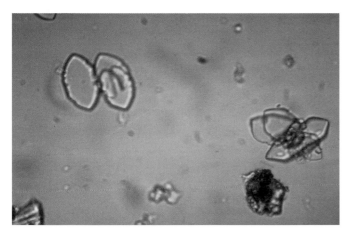

FIGURE 8.222   Urate crystals. Source: Reproduced with permission of Dr. Richard Scott, Animal Medical Center, New York, NY.

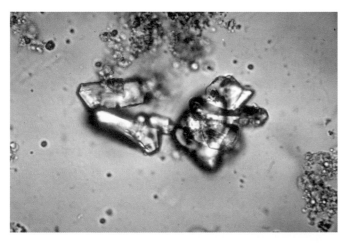

FIGURE 8.223   Urate crystals. Source: Reproduced with permission of Dr. Richard Scott, Animal Medical Center, New York, NY.

Unusual or Rare Crystals

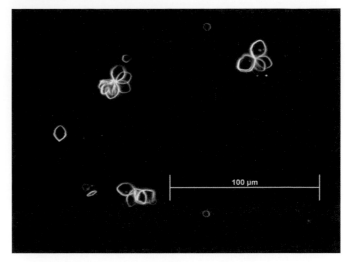

FIGURE 8.224   Uric acid or xanthine crystals. Phase microscopy. Source: Reproduced with permission of Dr. Michael Horton, Fairborn, OH.

(a)

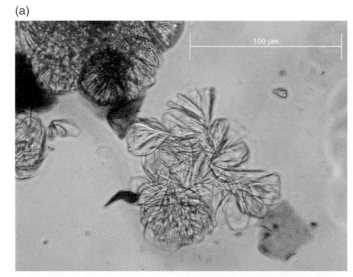

(b)

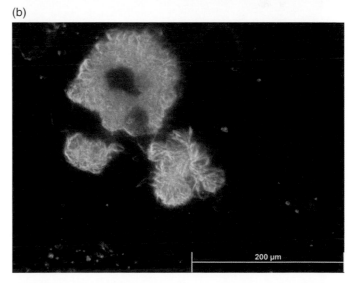

FIGURE 8.225   (a) Suspected xanthine crystals in clusters; dog on treatment with allopurinol. Squamous epithelial cell at bottom right. Source: Reproduced with permission of Dr. Michael Horton, Fairborn, OH. (b) Suspected xanthine crystals; dog on allopurinol treatment. Phase microscopy. Source: Reproduced with permission of Dr. Michael Horton, Fairborn, OH.

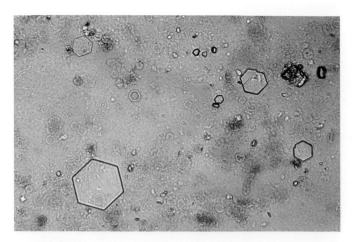

FIGURE 8.226 Cystine crystals. Six sided flat clear crystals are seen in this field. One crystal (middle right) has a small notch. Another crystal (top right) has what appears to be a notch, but closer inspection reveals what is likely to be piece of another cystine crystal on top of it. Many degenerate WBC are seen in the background. Male Bassett Hound with cystine urolithiasis. Source: Courtesy of Dr. Stephen DiBartola, The Ohio State University College of Veterinary Medicine.

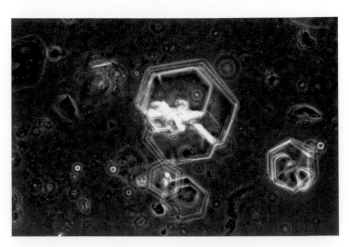

FIGURE 8.228 Cystine crystals. Phase microscopy. Urine sediment from a young Siamese female cat with cystine urolithiasis. Source: Reproduced with permission of Dr. Michael Horton, Fairborn, OH.

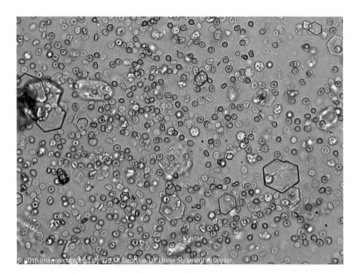

FIGURE 8.227 Cystine crystals. Image acquired by SediVue®. Many RBC, occasional WBC and rare squamous epithelial cells. Source: Courtesy of IDEXX Laboratories. Copyright © 2022, IDEXX Laboratories, Inc. All rights reserved. Used with permission.

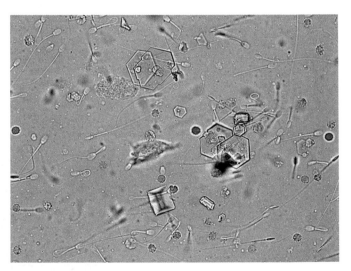

FIGURE 8.229 Cystine crystals in sheets. There is one struvite crystal at the bottom middle of this image. Numerous sperm are present. Increased numbers of RBC with rare WBC are also in this field. Source: Reproduced with permission of Dr. Heather L. Wamsley, Bradenton, FL.

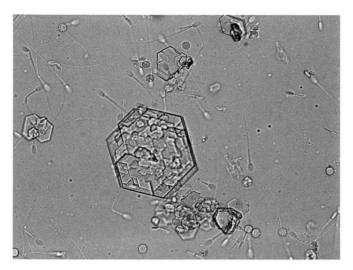

FIGURE 8.230 Cystine crystals. The central large crystal displays sheets of cystine on top of each other. Many sperm and several WBC cells in background. Source: Reproduced with permission of Dr. Heather L. Wamsley, Bradenton, FL.

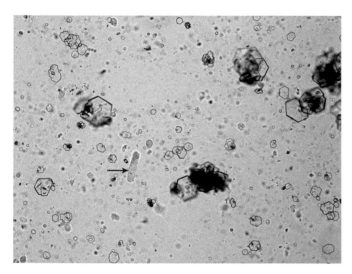

FIGURE 8.231 Cystine crystals. Numerous RBC and one granular cast (arrow center left) are visible in this field. Source: Reproduced with permission of Dr. Heather L. Wamsley, Bradenton, FL.

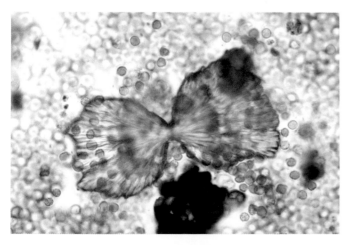

FIGURE 8.232 Sulfa crystals. Numerous RBC in background. Urine sediment from a dog on sulfa treatment.

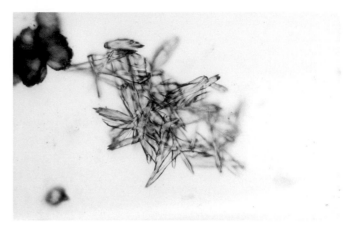

FIGURE 8.233 Sulfa crystals. Urine sediment from a dog treated with sulfisoxazole.

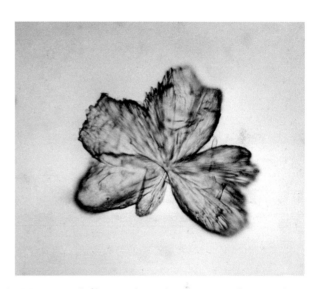

FIGURE 8.234 Sulfa crystals. High power magnification of urine sediment from a dog.

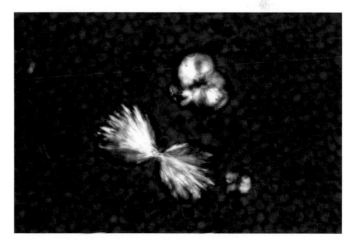

FIGURE 8.235 Sulfa crystals seen with polarizing microscopy. There are numerous RBC slightly out of focus in the background. Urine sediment from a dog on sulfa treatment.

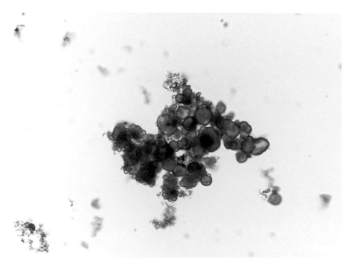

FIGURE 8.236 Melamine–cyanuric acid crystals. Urine sediment for a cat with AKI and CKD due to ingestion of food contaminated with melamine and cyanuric acid.

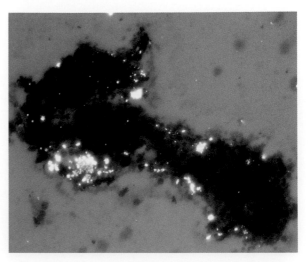

FIGURE 8.238 Melamine–cyanuric acid crystals (most likely). Cytology from a fine needle aspirate from the kidney of a cat with AKI. RTE are observed in this field, many of which are broken. Many of the crystals are associated with the RTE and some appear to be within the RTE. These crystals exhibit birefringence. Birefringence of crystals from a kidney aspirate in an animal with AKI could also be observed in those with ethylene glycol poisoning and deposition of calcium oxalate crystals within the renal tubules. It was confirmed that this cat was eating food contaminated with melamine and cyanuric acid. Source: Courtesy of Dr. Maxey Wellman The Ohio State University.

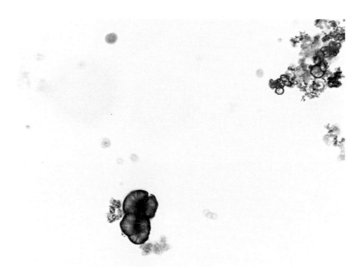

FIGURE 8.237 Melamine–cyanuric acid crystals. Notice the radial striations in this small clump of crystals at the bottom of the image. Urine sediment from cat with AKI and CKD from melamine and cyanuric acid food contamination.

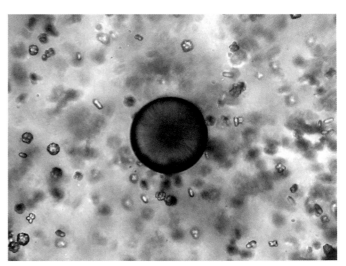

FIGURE 8.239 Calcium carbonate crystals. One large brown colored calcium carbonate crystal with central radiations. Many aggregates of much smaller crystals are present.

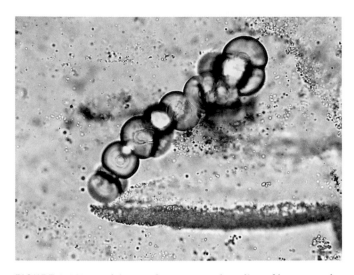

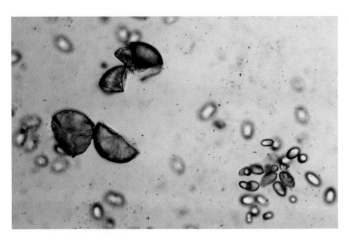

FIGURE 8.240   Calcium carbonate crystals. A line of large round calcium carbonate crystals can be seen in the middle of this image. These crystals are more yellow than is common for calcium carbonate. There are numerous amorphous calcium carbonate crystals in the background. Urine sediment from a horse and urine pH of 8.0.

FIGURE 8.241   Calcium carbonate crystals. Fan shaped crystals with central radiations are seen in the darker brown crystals. The ovoid clearer crystals are another morphology for calcium carbonate crystals. Urine sediment from a horse.

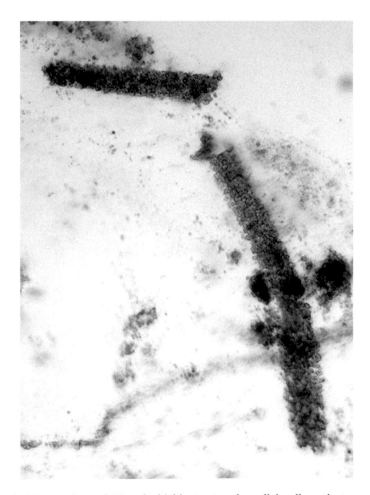

FIGURE 8.242   Two crystal casts (calcium carbonate). Note the highly structured parallel walls on the two casts (one at top and the other at right of image). The granules inside the cast look the same as the free calcium carbonate crystals. At first glance, the granules could be confused with RBC in an RBC cast, but these granules are smaller than would be seen with RBC and there was no uptake of supravital stain as would occur with RBC. Wispy mucous strands are out of focus in the background. Urine sediment from a horse.

(a)

(b)

(c)

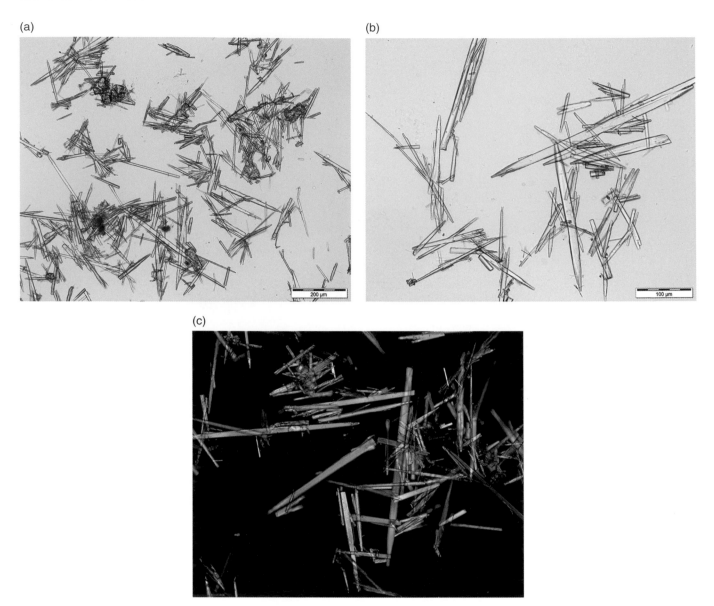

FIGURE 8.243 (a–c) Mannitol crystals. Voided urine sample from a one-month old female kitten, shortly after IV mannitol was administered (0.5 gm/kg over 20 minutes) for suspected brain edema. Note the numerous long rectangular or needle shaped crystals. A is 100× and B is 200× brightfield microscopy. C is 200× under polarizing light. Identical appearing crystals that were also birefringent on polarizing light were identified when a 25% mannitol solution was diluted in a small amount of saline. Source: Courtesy of Dr. Bin Xi Wu and Dr. Bill Vernau, UC Davis School of Veterinary Medicine 2021.

(a)

(b)

(c)

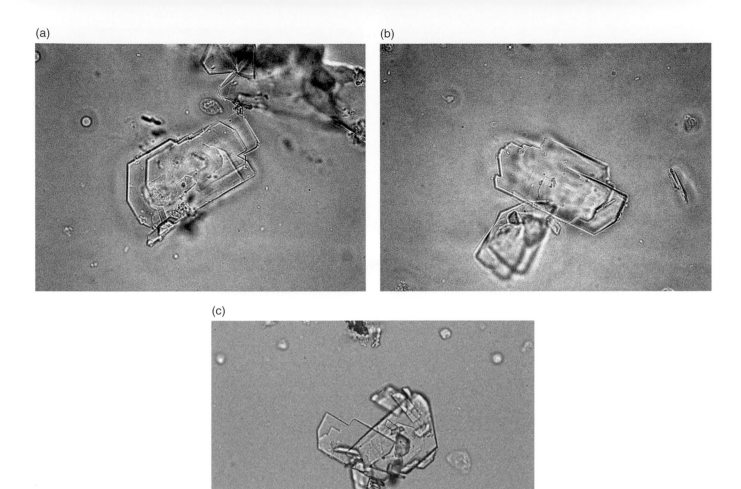

FIGURE 8.244 (a) Cholesterol crystals. Note characteristic notches. (b) Cholesterol crystals. (c) Cholesterol crystals. Note the flat clear crystal with notches. Source: Reproduced with permission of Dr. Heather L. Wamsley, Bradenton, FL.

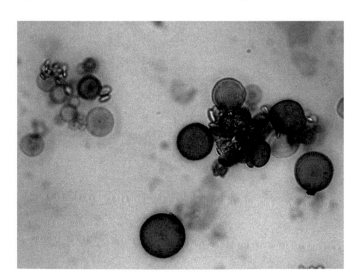

FIGURE 8.245 Leucine crystals and biliary fluid. The brown crystals with internal concentric rings are leucine crystals. There are also clusters of unidentified smaller clear crystals. Source: Reproduced with permission of Dr. Heather L. Wamsley, Bradenton, FL.

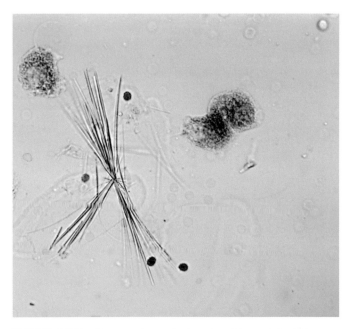

FIGURE 8.246 Presumptive cyclophosphamide crystals. Urine sediment from a dog receiving Cytoxan chemotherapy. A few RBC and nonsquamous epithelial cells are in the background.

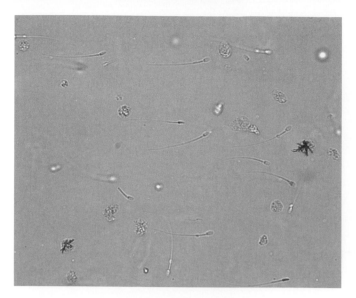

FIGURE 8.247 Bilirubin crystals. Image acquired by SediVue®. Two sets of dark bilirubin crystals are seen in this field. Multiple sperm, occasional nonsquamous epithelial cells, and rare WBC are seen in the background. Source: Courtesy of IDEXX Laboratories. Copyright © 2022, IDEXX Laboratories, Inc. All rights reserved. Used with permission.

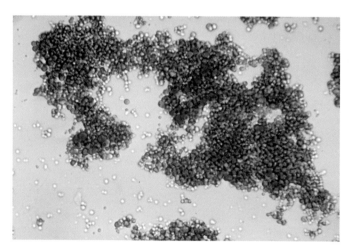

FIGURE 8.248 Hemoglobin crystals. Note varying size of the orange to brown color hemoglobin crystals. Urine sediment from a dog with systemic hemolysis. Source: Reproduced with permission of Dr. Richard Scott.

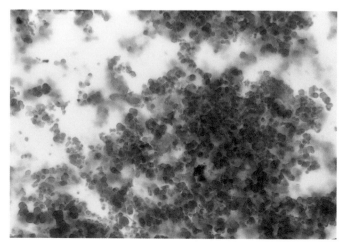

FIGURE 8.249 Precipitates of hemoglobin crystals in a dog with systemic hemolysis. Great Dane with splenic torsion. These globular crystals were originally reported as numerous RBC.

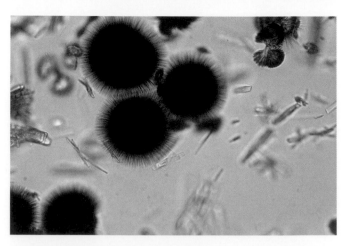

FIGURE 8.250 Unidentified crystals. Medium- and large-size spherical crystals with multiple fine linear protrusions from their surfaces. A crystal cluster exists in a sheath form (upper right of this field).

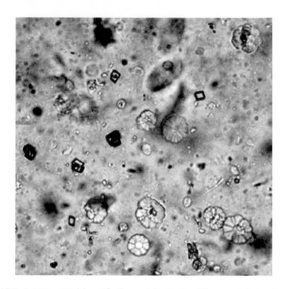

FIGURE 8.251 Unidentified crystals. Daisy-like crystals in dog urine. (Bright-field microscopy, 400×). Source: From Fogazzi et al. [7]. Used with permission.

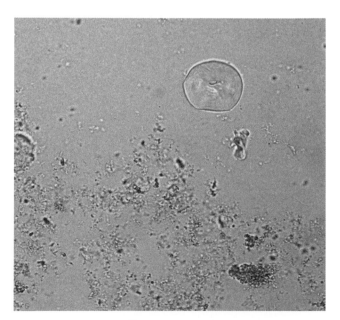

FIGURE 8.252 Unidentified round crystal among abundant amorphous phosphate crystals. Source: Reproduced with permission of Dr. Heather L. Wamsley, Bradenton, FL.

ARTIFACTS AND MISCELLANEOUS ELEMENTS

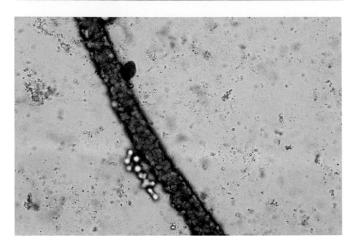

FIGURE 8.253 Pseudocast formed from crystals that have been compressed together. Amorphous crystals in the background.

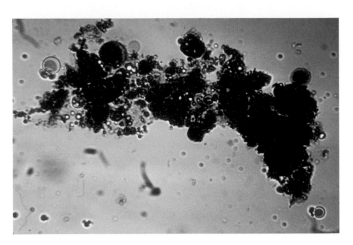

FIGURE 8.255 Pseudocast. Clumps of cells and granules appear in a disorganized way in the left part of this structure. The portion of the structure to the far right could easily be misidentified as a granular cast but it should be assessed with the clump it accompanies.

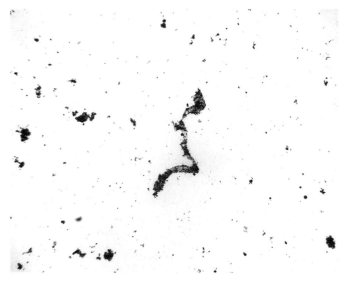

FIGURE 8.254 Pseudocast. Very low power view of what appears to be cellular cast, especially at the lower left portion of the linear structure. This structure is much larger than casts would appear at this power, however. This is a prostatic "plug" from a dog with prostatic bleeding.

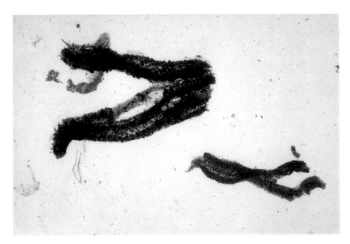

FIGURE 8.256 Pseudocasts. Large wispy structures are observed. Note that many of the particles appear to be adhering to the structure and do not look like they are embedded as would occur in a true cast. The wispy end of one linear structure in the lower right also is not typical for a cast. Mucous strands in urine can allow this to happen as is more frequently the case in horses.

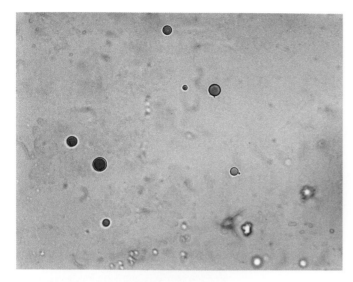

FIGURE 8.257 Urine sediment following Sudan stain. Note red uptake of spheres confirming their lipid content.

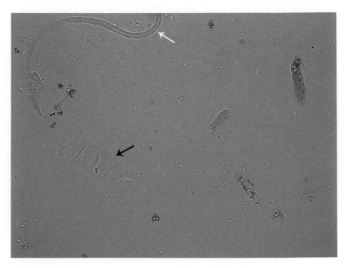

FIGURE 8.259 Fiber artifact. Note the linear structure in the upper left corner (white arrow). Three granular and one waxy cast (black arrow) are also in this field. Bacteria are also noted.

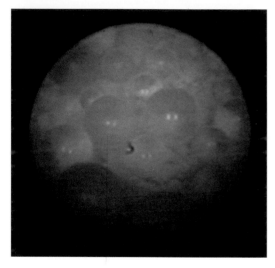

FIGURE 8.258 Lipid droplets seen on the wall of the bladder from a cat during cystoscopy. Lipids ascend from the dependent portion of the bladder, whereas crystals fall by gravity. Lipiduria is often considered normal in cat urine.

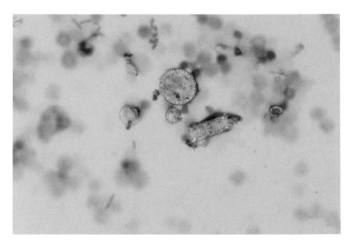

FIGURE 8.260 Contaminants from the environment observed in the center and center-right field in the urine sediment from a sample collected by the owner in a container they provided. Cells and bacteria are out of focus in another plane. Source: Reproduced with permission of Dr. Heather L. Wamsley, Bradenton, FL.

REFERENCES

1 Basso, W., Spänhauer, Z., Arnold, S., and Deplazes, P. (2014). *Capillaria plica* (syn. *Pearsonema plica*) infection in a dog with chronic pollakiuria: challenges in the diagnosis and treatment. *Parasitol. Int.* **63** (1): 140–142.

2 Ferreira, V.L., Medeiros, F.P., July, J.R., and Raso, T.F. (2010). Dioctophyma renale in a dog: clinical diagnosis and surgical treatment. *Vet. Parasitol.* 168 (1–2): 151–155.

3 Rahal, S.C., Mamprim, M.J., Oliveira, H.S. et al. (2014). Ultrasonographic, computed tomographic, and operative findings in dogs infested with giant kidney worms (Dioctophyme renale). *J. Am. Vet. Med. Assoc.* 244 (5): 555–558.

4 Smith, B.J., Anderson, B.G., Smith, S.A., and Chew, D.J. (1990). Early effects of ethylene glycol on the ultrastructure of the renal cortex in dogs. *Am. J. Vet. Res.* 51 (1): 89–96.

5 Tvedten, H., Lilliehöök, I., Rönnberg, H., and Pelander, L. (2019). Massive uric acid crystalluria and cylinduria in a dog after l-asparaginase treatment for lymphoma. *Vet. Clin. Pathol.* 48 (3): 425–428.

6 Osborne, C.A., Lulich, J.P., Ulrich, L.K., and Bird, K.A. (1996). Feline crystalluria. Detection and interpretation. *Vet. Clin. North Am. Small Anim. Pract.* 26 (2): 369–391.

7 Fogazzi, G.B., Anderlini, R., Canovi, S. et al. (2017). Daisy-like crystals: A rare and unknown type of urinary crystal. *Clin. Chim. Acta* 471: 154–157.

Frequently Asked Questions (FAQ)

CHAPTER 9

CHAPTER 1 – RENAL ANATOMY AND RENAL FUNCTIONS

FAQ-01   I usually assume that a patient with a serum creatinine and blood urea nitrogen (BUN) within the reference range does not have kidney disease. Am I safe in this assessment?

A: No. A normal BUN or serum creatinine does not necessarily indicate the presence or absence of kidney disease. It is important to remember that BUN and serum creatinine concentrations do not escalate until 50–75% or more of the original nephron mass and glomerular filtration rate (GFR) are reduced (depending on the value for creatinine used for the upper reference limit), so renal disease could still exist. The evaluation of a complete urinalysis (UA) with emphasis on urine specific gravity (USG), proteinuria, and cylindruria will help provide more information as to whether kidney disease exists or not. Renal imaging can also be helpful in determining the presence of renal disease when there are changes in size or shape, echotexture, or corticomedullary junction distinction. Some with primary renal disease do not have abnormalities on renal imaging.

FAQ-02   I understand that it is difficult in private practice to actually measure GFR using conventional research methods that are highly accurate. Is there something I can do that measure GFR with enough accuracy to be clinically useful?

A: YES. You can give an IV injection of iohexol (the same molecule used for contrast urography) followed by the collection of blood samples at timed intervals over a few hours. The rate for the disappearance of iohexol is proportional to the GFR. Only a few laboratories offer the analysis of this molecule unfortunately. The laboratory will calculate the GFR based on the body weight and timing of the blood samples.

FAQ-03   When is the measurement of GFR something that I need to consider in my patients that I suspect have renal disease?

A: The value of GFR is particularly useful in the evaluation of patients that have normal concentrations of BUN, serum creatinine, and symmetric dimethylarginine (SDMA), but yet you still have concerns about the level of renal functions. This is often the situation in those with polyuria/polydipsia (PU/PD)

and minimally concentrated urine based on USG. A low GFR in this scenario supports the presence of nonazotemic renal disease that could be associated with the low USG.

FAQ-04   A five-year-old dog with chronic renal disease has a serum phosphorus concentration of 7.1 mg/dL. This result is not cause for concern because it falls within my diagnostic laboratory's reference range for phosphorus (i.e. 3.5–8.5 mg/dL), right?

A: No. Unfortunately, many diagnostic laboratories have reference ranges for serum phosphorus concentration that go up to 8 mg/dL or higher. The reason is because young growing animals with ongoing physiological bone growth have been included in the population used to determine the reference range. A normal mature dog or cat should have a serum phosphorus concentration no greater than 5.5 mg/dL. So, there is reason for concern in this dog especially regarding renal function. The targeted goal for serum phosphorus in chronic kidney disease (CKD) patients is ideally near the middle of the reference range and less than 4.7 mg/dL when possible.

FAQ-05   Which is better in the evaluation of patients with suspected renal disease, BUN or serum creatinine concentration?

A: Neither one is better than the other. Both the BUN and serum creatinine concentrations are insensitive tests for the evaluation of renal function during the early stages of nephron loss. Depending on the upper limits used in the reference range, both the BUN and serum creatinine concentrations begin to increase when 50–75% or more of the nephrons are nonfunctional. BUN, however, is affected by more nonrenal factors than is the serum creatinine concentration, but both have pitfalls in their interpretation. Hence, it is recommended that clinicians evaluate both the BUN and serum creatinine concentrations at the same time.

FAQ-06   My clinic uses a reference laboratory that does not offer SDMA as part of routine biochemistry measurement. Am I missing out on a better way to look for diseases associated with decreased GFR?

A: Yes and No. It is true that SDMA outperforms creatinine for the earlier detection of CKD in both dogs and cats. This means that SDMA will increase above the reference range before creatinine will increase as CKD develops and progresses, especially

Urinalysis in the Dog and Cat, First Edition. Dennis J. Chew and Patricia A. Schenck.
© 2023 John Wiley & Sons, Inc. Published 2023 by John Wiley & Sons, Inc.

when the patient has had loss of lean muscle mass (muscle generates creatinine). Greater efficiency in the early diagnosis of CKD can be gained while using creatinine when the upper reference range is lowered to 1.6 for the cat and 1.4 in the dog. Also, trending increases in creatinine within the reference range are useful as are trends for decreasing USG in the earlier detection of CKD.

FAQ-07   I have a patient with a repeatable increase in SDMA, but the BUN and serum creatinine are in the mid reference range. The USG is 1.030 and higher at times. How do I handle this discordance?

A: This type of discordance is common since SDMA escalates before creatinine in many instances of developing CKD. Trending increases in creatinine and or trending decreases in USG provide support that SDMA has been providing accurate information about the presence of renal disease. The measurement of systolic blood pressure and urine protein-to-creatinine ratio (UPC) along with renal imaging by ultrasound (ULS) may provide more information about the progression of CKD.

FAQ-08   Can I trust artificial intelligence/machine learning (AI/ML) algorithms that are designed to predict a future diagnosis of CKD?

A: No currently available algorithm is perfect in the prediction of a future diagnosis of CKD using commonly measured analytes (BUN, creatinine, USG, body weight, age, species, protein on dipstrip, urinary pH, and white blood cells [WBC] count on complete blood count [CBC]). These algorithms look for small changes over time in order to make this prediction. A positive prediction for the prediction of CKD over a defined time (one year and two years) would act as an alarm system, warning the attending veterinarian to look more closely at the patient and to measure blood pressure and evaluate proteinuria by UPC or microalbumin (MA). AI/ML for the diagnosis of or prediction of a future diagnosis is in its infancy in veterinary medicine. No studies yet exist to show treatment interventions delay a future CKD diagnosis using AI/ML.

FAQ-9   On preoperative screening, a seemingly healthy dog has a BUN of 40 mg/dL (30 mg/dL upper reference limit) and a serum creatinine concentration of 1.2 mg/dL (1.6 mg/L upper reference limit). I thought both of these tests usually increased together in the presence of renal disease.

A: The most likely cause for such results is that the blood samples were taken within a few (four to eight) hours after a protein-rich meal, which can result in an increased BUN without a corresponding increase in serum creatinine concentration. A blood sample should be collected after a 12-hour fast and re-submitted to the laboratory. Dehydration can also result in an increased BUN concentration relative to serum creatinine concentration because urea can be passively reabsorbed into the blood from the renal tubules during decreased tubular flow whereas creatinine cannot. In this instance, the USG is expected to be high due to the renal conservation of water if renal function is normal. Gastrointestinal (GI) hemorrhage is

another possible reason why the BUN concentration could be increased disproportionately because the whole blood is a type of high-protein meal. Alternatively, the increased BUN concentration may accurately reflect poor renal function, while the lower serum creatinine concentration reflects reduced muscle mass in a cachectic animal.

FAQ-10   I get excited to see the BUN decline when my azotemic patients are eating a renal diet. I tell the owners that this decrease in BUN means that excretory renal function has increased due to the beneficial effects of the renal diet.

A: Actually, this decrease in BUN may have nothing to do with any increase in kidney function. When the animal is eating a diet low in protein content but adequate in calories, BUN concentration often decreases because less nitrogenous waste products are generated. In such a situation, BUN concentration is not a good indicator of renal function.

FAQ-11   I have an older cat with stable CKD over the past two years. Serum creatinine stays at nearly 2.4 mg/dL on all the samples measured every three months. My assessment of this stable serum creatinine concentration is that the CKD is not currently progressive. Am I correct in this thinking?

A: A "stable" serum creatinine concentration during CKD is better for the patient than one that is escalating in general. It is important to remember that animals with CKD often lose lean muscle mass that results in less generation of creatinine into the circulation. Loss of lean muscle mass in the absence of renal disease should result in a decreased serum creatinine concentration. Loss of lean muscle mass at a rate proportional to the decrease in GFR in those with renal disease will result in little to no change in serum creatinine. Stable serum creatinine concentration in the presence of ongoing lean muscle mass loss can mask the clinician's ability to appreciate the progression of renal disease.

FAQ-12   I have heard that SDMA can be used to replace the evaluation of serum creatinine in patients suspected to have CKD. Should I retire creatinine and instead focus on SDMA?

A: No, not entirely. Both creatinine and SDMA are surrogates for GFR. During the development of CKD, SDMA often increases quite a bit earlier, before increases in serum creatinine are recognized. Much of this early increase in SDMA likely occurs since SDMA is not influenced by body weight/condition whereas creatinine is. Creatinine is generated from within muscles, so with loss of lean muscle mass that often accompanies CKD, there is less creatinine entering the circulation and a lower serum creatinine will be measured. The usefulness for the evaluation of serum creatinine is improved when a lower upper reference range is used, instead of the larger population-based reference range (e.g. <1.6 mg/dL for cats and <1.4 for dogs). It is always better to measure and assess multiple surrogates of GFR at the same time to limit the chances for errors in interpretation. Discordance in results for surrogates of GFR happens at times.

FAQ-13   As I understand it, SDMA increases only in primary renal disease and not in prerenal or postrenal conditions. Is this true?

A: No. SDMA, like creatinine and BUN, will be influenced by anything that alters GFR. SDMA will increase during prerenal, postrenal, and primary renal conditions that decrease GFR. SDMA will decrease during hyperthyroidism as GFR increases.

FAQ-14   I usually bias my evaluation of serum biochemistry results in my CKD patients to BUN, creatinine, and SDMA. Are there other analytes to which I should also give attention?

A: YES. Circulating phosphorus is a very important molecule to follow for its potentially detrimental effects on soft tissue calcification and effects that can increase PTH and FGF-23. Calcium is also important especially during interactions with increased phosphorus that increase the $Ca \times P$ product. Potassium and TCO_2 (close approximator of HCO_3) also deserve your attention.

Close attention to circulating calcium, phosphorus, and $Ca \times P$ product is a good idea when following CKD patients that are treated with calcitriol.

FAQ-15   How important is it to monitor circulating calcium concentrations in dogs or cats with CKD?

A: Most patients with CKD have normocalcemia, but some will be observed with either hypocalcemia or hypercalcemia based on total serum calcium measurements. Unfortunately, discordance between total serum calcium and ionized calcium occurs frequently, especially during states of azotemic CKD. Many CKD dogs with high total serum calcium have normal ionized calcium concentrations likely due to increased concentrations of complexes that bind calcium during CKD; this phenomenon is far less common in cats. It is important to know if the high total calcium is also associated with high ionized calcium, since only increases in ionized calcium are toxic to the animal.

Trending increases in both total serum calcium and ionized calcium that are still within the reference range have recently been associated with the progression of CKD in the cat. Some cats with early stages of CKD develop hypercalcemia while eating a renal diet that is too restricted in phosphorus; the high Ca:P ratio appears to facilitate calcium absorption across the intestine.

FAQ-16   How important is it to monitor serum potassium levels in patients with CKD or acute kidney injury (AKI)?

A: Hypokalemia occurs in some patients with CKD, especially in cats. Hypokalemia can develop secondary to CKD, but it appears that hypokalemia can also create CKD. Hypokalemia can exert deleterious effects on excretory renal function and can be associated with less ability to concentrate urine. Hypokalemia results in functional changes that decrease kidney function initially but structural changes can occur later. Hyperkalemia is of concern in some patients with AKI, especially those that have oligo-anuria.

FAQ-17   Should I recommend renal biopsy more often in my persistently azotemic patients?

A: Renal biopsy should not be approached lightly because complications are possible (hemorrhage and renal damage). The kidney should be biopsied only if the results are likely to change how the patient is treated. ULS-guided biopsy of small kidneys in CKD should not be undertaken due to the risk of hemorrhage and the oftentimes unrewarding pathology findings due to extensive fibrosis. Examples of situations in which the information obtained from renal biopsy may change your approach to management include: differentiating acute from chronic renal failure when this is not apparent after thorough clinical evaluation, establishing a prognosis in AKI when the clinical course has been protracted, and differentiating glomerulonephritis (GN) from glomerular amyloidosis in those with CKD. Distinguishing between AKI caused by nephrosis or that caused by nephritis can be helpful, especially for patients suspected to have leptospirosis. It is less rewarding to perform renal biopsy in patients with stage 3 or 4 CKD, as primary renal lesions may not be apparent due to extensive tubular atrophy, glomerular sclerosis, and interstitial fibrosis. Renal biopsy earlier in the course of CKD may be especially helpful in patients with renal proteinuria if the biopsy can undergo full evaluation using light microscopy, electron microscopy, and immunofluorescent antibody (IFA). Treatment protocols are emerging in veterinary medicine that are designed for a specific histopathological diagnosis in those with GN. Systemic blood pressure should be normalized prior to renal biopsy, a procedure that should be performed by a highly skilled operator and experienced hospital that is able to deal with any complications.

FAQ-18   Why is the measurement of serum albumin and cholesterol concentrations important to monitor in patients with CKD?

A: Low serum albumin and high cholesterol during CKD can be associated with protein losing nephropathy in some dogs. The measurement of UPC is indicated now, if it has not already been determined, to assess the magnitude of proteinuria and its likely contribution to the hypoalbuminemia. High cholesterol concentration in cats with CKD is common and does not raise concern for PLN as it does in dogs. Animals consuming renal diets can develop hypoalbuminemia and hypercholesterolemia as a result of too little dietary protein.

FAQ-19   How can I best know if abdominal effusion following trauma is urine or not?

A: Following abdominocentesis, the abdominal fluid creatinine concentration to serum creatinine concentration ratio is usually >2.1 if the fluid is urine due to delayed uptake of creatinine in this fluid across the peritoneum. Urea nitrogen ratios are not as useful since urea is more readily reabsorbed from the peritoneal cavity. If the abdominal fluid-creatinine-concentration-to-serum-creatinine-concentration ratio is equivocal (i.e. ≤2:1), calculate the abdominal fluid potassium concentration to serum potassium concentration ratio. Patients with uroperitoneum will have a ratio of >1.4 (dogs) or >1.9 (cats). Determining the site of the urine leakage is the next step using some form of contrast urography. Uroabdomen occurs most often from ruptures in the bladder. The retrieval of urine following urethral catheterization does not exclude the possibility for a ruptured bladder.

FAQ-20 Last week, I euthanized a 17-year-old cat that was presented for the evaluation of anorexia and vomiting. Serum creatinine concentration was >20.0 mg/dL. The kidneys were slightly small on palpation and the cat was approximately 10% dehydrated based on skin turgor assessment. The cat was euthanized with a presumed diagnosis of azotemic CKD. On necropsy, there was a considerable amount of abdominal fluid and a small hole in the bladder surrounded by a large bruise. Could all of these findings be associated with urine leakage from the bladder into the abdomen?

A: Yes. The magnitude of azotemia does not differentiate among prerenal, primary renal, or postrenal causes. Many older cats have CKD and some degree of azotemia, but older cats also may experience bladder rupture following trauma, as was the case in this particular cat. The kidneys were normal at necropsy. It is always a good idea in any case with azotemia to ask the question, "Could it be prerenal, primary renal, or postrenal in origin?"

FAQ-21 I have heard that it is important to evaluate thyroid function in all cats with suspected or confirmed CKD. The term "masking" has been mentioned in this situation, but I am not sure just what that means.

A: Excess thyroid hormones in the body increase both renal blood flow and GFR such that excretory renal function is enhanced. This means that the surrogates of GFR (creatinine and SDMA) will be lower than during the euthyroid state. Restoration of T4 to the reference range following treatment (I-131, methimazole, and surgery) will decrease GFR and increase creatinine and SDMA concentrations. The increase in creatinine post-treatment is often mild but can be of high magnitude in some cats. For example, in a cat with a high T4 and a creatinine of 1.8 mg/dL, the post-treatment creatinine increased to 2.5 mg/dL at a time that T4 was in the reference range. The initial 1.8 mg/dL creatinine was this low because of the high thyroid status that had increased GFR, thus masking the degree of excretory renal failure that only became obvious after the T4 was reduced.

FAQ-22 I have a 14-year-old spayed female domestic shorthair cat presented for PU and PD along with severe weight loss and fairly normal appetite. A thyroid nodule is consistently palpable on the left side of the trachea. The kidneys are approximately 3.0–3.5 cm in length and feel smooth on palpation. USG is 1.019, serum creatinine is 2.0 mg/dL, and BUN is 38 mg/dL. The T4 is about 2× increased beyond the upper reference range. What can I expect following radioiodine treatment for the hyperthyroidism?

A: The creatinine is mildly increased in the face of hyperthyroidism and urine that is minimally concentrated. Hyperthyroidism increases GFR, which decreases the creatinine concentration.

So, we should expect to see some increase in serum creatinine when euthyroidism has been restored. The increase in serum creatinine following the restoration of euthyroidism is modest in most cats.

FAQ-23 I am treating a hyperthyroid cat with oral methimazole. The T4 concentration decreased to within the mid reference range at the same time that the serum creatinine increased from 1.7 to 2.4 mg/dL. Should I decrease the dose of the methimazole to keep the creatinine at a lower value?

A: No. It is unlikely that the cat knows that its current creatinine has escalated by 0.7 mg/dL. Lowering the dose of methimazole will allow the T4 to increase and that will increase GFR and lower the creatinine. The ongoing hyperthyroidism, however, will result in glomerular hypertension and progressive renal injury. So, it is better to become euthyroid and to tolerate the "exposed" increase in serum creatinine in general.

CHAPTER 2 – INTRODUCTION TO UA

FAQ-24 Is it best to perform the complete UA in-house or to send it out to a reference laboratory?

A: There is no set answer for all practice situations. If you currently perform few complete urinalyses in-house, sending urine to a reference laboratory offers a way to increase diagnostic information for your patients without consuming in-house personnel time. The training of technicians to perform in-house UA varies widely among practices. Sending urine to a reference laboratory makes sense if your technicians do not have the skill set and training needed to accurately and consistently perform urine microscopy, which is the biggest stumbling block to performing in-house UA.

Some practices have highly skilled technicians that efficiently, consistently, and accurately perform the complete UA. The workflow to make this happen is not linear and takes from about 18–22 minutes to complete. Performing in-house urinalyses allows more money to be generated for the practice compared to sending out the urine to a reference laboratory.

The sicker an animal is, the more important it is to perform the complete UA in-house so that abnormalities of importance are detected and reported. Fragile elements like cellular casts are unlikely to be detected in samples sent to reference laboratories. Lower numbers of cells and casts along with more crystals are likely to be reported from samples that undergo storage and shipping to a reference laboratory. There is less urgency to perform in-house UA for apparently normal animals (pre-op, wellness, and geriatric).

Performing the UA in-house gives the attending DVM the chance to have a conversation about the results while the owner is still at the practice. Sending the UA to a reference laboratory usually involves a 5–24-hour delay in obtaining the results, depending on when the sample is picked up and processed by the laboratory.

FAQ-25   I keep hearing about "automated" UA. Is this just a fad, or should I consider this for use in my practice? Is it better than the traditional manual methods?

A: Automated UA is not just a fad and is likely to become the standard for in-house UA in the near future. "Automated" refers to both the measurement of chemistry by urinary dipstrip and urine microscopy. USG still needs to be done manually in-house.

Urine chemistry is more accurate and more consistent when determined with a reader that removes the subjectivity of a human deciding on the degree of color reaction that will be reported.

Automated urine microscopy is very good at identifying red blood cells (RBC), WBC, epithelial cells, hyaline casts, and bacteria, but not yet as good as that determined by human experts. The algorithms used to identify urinary elements continue to improve over time and so the accuracy of reporting will continue to improve during automated microscopy. Clumping of WBC or epithelial cells is not yet part of automated reporting, and characterization of casts beyond nonhyaline is problematic.

Automated microscopy generates a report that enumerates urinary elements within three minutes. Results of the complete UA are generated within five to six minutes accounting for the time to measure USG by refractometry, automated urine chemistry, and automated microscopy. The technician still needs to take about another minute to make sure that the microscopy results on the report match up with that seen on the digital pictures taken by the machine. Workflow efficiency is improved using automated methods compared to the manual method that consumes from 18 to 22 minutes of nonlinear personnel time. Clients appreciate receiving the UA reports generated, while they are still on site and more readily understand their costs for this testing.

FAQ-26   How can I justify the expense of a machine to perform automated urine microscopy? The equipment is rather expensive.

A: Yes. The one-time expense to purchase the urine microscopy analyzer is high. If you are currently submitting few UA for complete analysis, then the use of the automated analyzer will allow the practice to ramp up to do a lot more UA without consuming a lot more personnel time while generating additional income that will pay for the machine. If you are sending out most of your UA currently, switching over to the automated analyzer will allow increased accuracy of results due to decreased generation of artifacts (e.g. crystal growth and bacterial growth) during cooling and transport and increased ability to identify elements in fresh urine that have not undergone degeneration or loss during transport to a laboratory. Fresh warm urine always wins.

If you are routinely doing UA by manual methods – you can continue to do so, or you can consider giving the automated methods a try to see how your practice workflow might improve that can allow you to perform even more complete UA.

FAQ-27   I am skeptical that a machine can be as accurate during urine microscopy as that recorded by my experienced technicians.

I have compared the results from the automated to the manual method and they are not always the same. Is it good enough?

A: You are correct that results between automated and manual methods of urine microscopy are not identical. Nor should they be. Differences in the methods as to how the urine is handled can account for this – volume, centrifugation force, and level of observer skill. Though there will be differences in the enumeration of elements, that difference is likely to be small. Differences in the identification of elements will also occur; automated methods are not as good in the identification of more uncommon elements.

YES, it is good enough for the identification of routine elements like RBC and WBC. Pretty good for the identification of squamous and nonsquamous epithelial cells. Really good at the identification of rod bacteria. Cocci identified by the machine should be confirmed on the visual analysis of digital images. Good for the identification of hyaline casts, but not able yet to determine other than nonhyaline casts – the technician must examine the digital images to determine if the nonhyaline casts are granular, waxy, or cellular. Digital pictures should also be examined to ensure that crystals other than struvite or calcium oxalate are not present.

In some instances, results from automated microscopy will be more accurate than elements reported by manual microscopy, depending on the level of expertise of the technician.

FAQ-28   I am not comfortable with the change in the reporting of results in urinary sediment from per high-power field (HPF) or per low-power field (LPF) to per μL. Why is it now considered better to report results as per μL rather than the time-honored method of per HPF or per LPF?

A: This is the future to which we should be moving. Enumeration per μL is more accurate than when reporting as per HPF or per LPF for several technical reasons related to the set up for urine microscopy. This type of counting is already conventional for hematology and fluid cytology results. The per HPF or per LPF method is an approximation of a volume that is examined, but this varies considerably by the dynamics of the microscope optics as to what is a "field," the thickness of the drop examined, and the size of the coverslip.

CHAPTER 3 – COLLECTION AND HANDLING

FAQ-29   I have been told that it is generally not worth examining urine collected by voiding and that only samples collected by cystocentesis should be submitted. Is that true?

A: No, not entirely. It is true that samples collected by cystocentesis avoid lower urinary and genital contamination with bacteria, cells, and protein, which lessens confusion as to what is pathological or not. Samples collected by cystocentesis often have extra RBC from the trauma of this method, regardless of operator skill in performing the cystocentesis. There is no easy way to know with certainty that RBC in samples collected by cystocentesis are there from underlying disease or trauma during bladder entry and manipulation of the cystocentesis needle.

Voided urine, preferably mid-stream, still generates value in the analysis of USG, urine chemistry, and urine microscopy showing the presence of abnormal elements. Also, actually going out with the client to watch the dog urinate can provide valuable information as to the nature and character of the act of urination. If the urinary sediment is silent – there is no need to collect another sample by cystocentesis. If the urine sediment is active, it might be a good idea to confirm these results using a sample collected by cystocentesis. Increased RBC shown on a sample collected by cystocentesis but absent on a voided urine sample suggests that trauma from the cystocentesis accounts for the RBC.

End-urination voided urine samples may prove especially fruitful in the identification of malignant epithelial cells from those with transitional cell carcinoma (TCC) of the bladder. Also, end-urination samples can yield more crystalline material that has settled out in the bladder at times. Initial-voided urine samples reflect more of what is going on in the urethra and genital tracts.

FAQ-30 Is it OK to culture urine collected during voiding for bacteria?

A: Culture of urine is best interpreted on samples collected by cystocentesis since bacterial contamination of the lower urogenital tract is avoided. Culture of voided urine that shows no growth provides useful results. Positive bacterial growth on voided samples is often problematic, as we often do not know with certainty that the isolated organisms are pathological or if they grew from lower urogenital (UG) contamination. Older literature indicated that this was particularly a problem in female dogs that could have abundant growth of organisms on culture of voided samples but not from the same dog's urine collected by cystocentesis. More recent thinking is that culture of voided urine can accurately reflect the presence of a bacterial urinary tract infection (UTI) if a single organism grows in large quantity (>100 000 cfu/mL in female dogs and >10 000 cfu/mL in male dogs and in cats). It is always best to culture urine collected by cystocentesis if there is uncertainty about culture results generated from voided urine or from catheterized urine samples.

FAQ-31 I was taught to never perform cystocentesis in a dog or cat with urethral obstruction (UO) and a large bladder – largely due to fears of rupturing the bladder and/or creating uroabdomen. I have heard from others that cystocentesis can safely be performed in this setting. Is this true?

A: Yes, in general when performed by an experienced operator. The procedure should be that of decompressive cystocentesis and not just removal of a small volume to submit for UA. Nearly complete evacuation of urine from the bladder allows time for the cystocentesis tract to seal in the absence of high pressure. Collection of urine by cystocentesis allows the analysis of a urine sample before urethral and bladder manipulation have taken place during attempts to relieve the UO. Contamination or dilution of the urine sample is avoided when cystocentesis is performed before alleviation of the UO. It is likely that decompressive cystocentesis facilitates relief of the UO during hydropulsion needed to flush obstructing material (plugs and stones) from the urethra into the bladder.

In cats with UO, some abdominal effusion often exists prior to any urethral manipulation, instrumentation, or cystocentesis. Some abdominal effusion can become apparent post cystocentesis, but this volume is small and is resorbed soon after UO is relieved (indwelling urethral catheter). Postcystocentesis leakage of bladder contents is less likely to occur when the bladder has undergone removal of as much urine as is feasible.

FAQ-32 I have heard that it is nearly meaningless to evaluate UA results from dogs or cats in which the urine was collected by catheter. Is this true?

A: No, depending on the operator's skill in atraumatic passage and placement of the urethral catheter. USG and most urinary dipstrip chemistry results will be clinically useful. Urinary sediment could potentially be active as an artifact due to the addition of RBC and epithelial cells as a consequence of trauma from this technique of urine collection. Bacteria can be added to the urine sample during the passage of the urinary catheter as another artifact. Bacterial culture from urine samples collected by urethral catheterization can yield large positive growth at times from contamination, especially in female dogs.

FAQ-33 I stopped performing cystocentesis in cats due to very scary episode I had in one cat that collapsed during the procedure. Is this a common adverse effect?

A: Collapse during cystocentesis rarely happens in some cats. And yes, it can be frightening to observe. This collapse is probably related to a vagal–vagal response during the procedure. Recovery following the collapse is usually rapid if there are no underlying cardiovascular problems that promoted the collapse. This has been observed in some cats that were highly agitated before the procedure. Mild sedation prior to cystocentesis is recommended in these instances. We have observed acute collapse in some male cats with UO in which removal of urine was very rapid during therapeutic decompressive cystocentesis.

FAQ-34 How can the number of crystals vary so drastically in samples collected by cystocentesis compared to voided urine?

A: In some instances, a high crystal burden can settle out into dependent regions of the bladder. Consequently, the cystocentesis needle can be aimed above the dependent regions of crystal accumulation and the recorded number of crystals will be low. We recommend agitating the bladder to resuspend crystals immediately before the cystocentesis in order to retrieve a more representative sample. Alternatively, an end-urination urine sample will retrieve the settled-out crystals. Similarly, more crystals can be retrieved via urethral catheter as bladder urine is fully emptied.

FAQ-35 I have noticed substantial discordance in urine microscopy results when the same urine sample was examined a second time shortly after the first examination. How is this possible?

A: This is not an uncommon phenomenon. It likely happens when one of the two urine samples was not well-mixed immediately before preparation of the urine sample for microscopy. Elements in urine can settle by gravity very quickly, so it is easy to submit a nonrepresentative portion of the urine above that which has settled. This is an example of a preanalytical error. It is essential to ALWAYS well-mix the urine sample before analysis.

CHAPTER 4 – PHYSICAL PROPERTIES

FAQ-36 If the urine is a medium to dark yellow color, I often assume that the urine is well concentrated. In these instances, in an animal that appears otherwise healthy, I do not measure the USG. Is this practice OK?

A: No. It is true that the amount of yellow color to the urine varies somewhat by how concentrated that urine sample is. Urine with very little color is often dilute and urine with deep yellow color is often concentrated. There are many instances of discordance between an estimated USG based on urine color and USG measured on a refractometer. It is often important to know the actual USG rather than some guesstimate. How dilute or how concentrate the sample is good to know. Urochromes largely contribute to the urine color, but their presence varies by each individual.

FAQ-37 I just examined a urine sample that appeared dark brown to black in color. The dog is sick but has no urinary signs. After centrifugation, the supernatant is the same color and there is no obvious sediment. Urine microscopy reveals very few of any type of elements. What is causing the dark coloration to this urine?

A: Since the color persisted after centrifugation and the urinary sediment was inactive, the color has to be from something dissolved in the urine rather from formed elements that would have gravitated into sediment. Though hemoglobinuria and myoglobinuria can both create pink urine, both can also appear black following some degree of oxidation in the urine. If the CBC shows normal RBC counts and appearance, hemolysis is unlikely to be generating enough hemoglobin to enter the urine. Myoglobinuria is a more likely cause in these instances. Increased serum CK is supportive for rhabdomyolysis that could allow enough myoglobin to enter and discolor the urine. Though not commonly performed, there are tests to definitively differentiate between myoglobin and hemoglobin in the urine.

FAQ-38 A three-month-old pure-bred dog is presented for evaluation of PU, PD, dilute urine (USG 1.012), and moderate azotemia (serum creatinine concentration 3.7 mg/dL). Proteinuria (2+) is found on urine dipstrip evaluation. The health status of the other littermates cannot be determined. What is the chance that this dog has a familial nephropathy?

A: It is very possible that the dog indeed has a familial nephropathy. It is also possible, however, that renal disease was acquired in utero or soon after birth as a result of nongenetic factors. Information from diagnostic imaging and UPC can provide support for this diagnosis, but renal histopathology using light microscopy, electron microscopy, and evaluation with IFA will be needed to make a definitive diagnosis.

FAQ-39 An 11-year-old castrated male German Shepherd Dog has been definitively diagnosed with hyperadrenocorticism (HAC) and treated with trilostane, leading to a hypoadrenal crisis in the past. Pre- and post-adrenocorticotropic hormone cortisol concentrations are currently within the normal range. Persistent and severe PU and PD developed in the last month. Serum biochemistry results, including BUN and serum creatinine concentrations, are normal. Urinalysis was normal, with the exception of a USG of 1.010. The USG was still 1.010 after gradual water restriction to 30 mL/lb/day. Results of abdominal radiographs and abdominal ULS imaging are normal. The dog was given 0.2 mg DDAVP orally twice a day which resulted in a USG of 1.040. The USG returned to 1.010 shortly after the DDAVP tablets were discontinued. Does this dog have central diabetes insipidus (CDI)?

A: Apparently so. The dramatic response to the DDAVP followed by a rapid return to much more dilute urine in the absence of DDAVP supplementation supports a diagnosis of CDI. The possibility of a mass lesion in the region of the pituitary gland and the hypothalamus should be considered.

FAQ-40 Is a USG in the hyposthenuric range (1.001–1.006) required to diagnose CDI?

A: No. Animals with complete CDI typically have hyposthenuria (USG 1.001–1.006), but some dogs with complete CDI can concentrate above this range despite complete absence of ADH if they are dehydrated (but usually not above USG 1.017). An alternate explanation is that the dog has partial CDI. Brain imaging (magnetic resonance imaging or computed tomography [CT]) can be performed to evaluate the hypothalamus and pituitary gland for diseases that could interrupt production or secretion of ADH.

FAQ-41 I have encountered a USG from a dog that was 1.000. I thought that might be an analytical error, so I repeated the measurement using the same urine sample and the same refractometer as before, and it was again 1.000. I have never seen a USG this low. The dog has mild PU, but I was not expecting to find a USG this low. Is this a "real" USG? The urine was collected free-catch by the owner.

A: Probably not. Something else is happening here. If the 1.000 USG were real, one would expect the dog to have severe PU/PD and that is not the case. It is possible that the sample is not really urine, or that it has been diluted accidentally with water. Repeat the USG on another sample to see if the USG is still the same or not. It most likely is NOT.

FAQ-42 The owners of a 13-week-old male Labrador retriever are having difficulty housebreaking the puppy. The dog seems to drink constantly and urinates while walking around the house. Urinalysis was normal except for a USG of 1.003. Could this dog have CDI?

A: CDI is possible, but psychogenic PD (PPD) is far more common in puppies. Some puppies drink water in excess of their physiological need. They usually outgrow this tendency by the time they are four to six months old. If necessary, PPD can quickly be differentiated from CDI during water deprivation testing (WDT). This dog's USG was >1.040 after approximately six hours of water deprivation, confirming normal urinary concentrating ability. If the dog had CDI, its USG would have remained low and would not have increased to more than 1.017 when dehydrated. Sometimes gradual WDT is needed to counteract MWO from severe PU/PD before urinary concentration capacity is fully restored.

FAQ-43 We anesthetized an 11-year-old spayed female mixed breed dog for dental extractions. Her history indicated no problems, and she was normal on physical examination before the dental procedure. CBC and serum biochemistry results also were normal before the procedure, but no UA was performed. Anesthesia and the dental procedure lasted approximately one hour, and she received some intravenous fluids during this time. The nonsteroidal anti-inflammatory drug (NSAID) carprofen and the antibiotic enrofloxacin were prescribed for one week after the procedure. A few days after release from the hospital, the owners reported that the dog was drinking quite a bit of water and urinating large volumes. Urinalysis at this time was normal except for a USG of 1.010 and trace proteinuria, and urine culture showed no growth. Serum biochemistry results at this time were still normal. A low dose dexamethasone test to evaluate for HAC was normal. What can I tell the owner?

A: More information is needed. It would have been helpful to have UA results (especially USG) before anesthesia. In dogs with underlying renal disease, UA results are likely to be abnormal long before changes in serum biochemistry become apparent. Some dogs with chronic nonazotemic renal disease decompensate after anesthesia. NSAID administration could have transiently affected urine concentration. Some dogs develop renal medullary washout (which can persist for several weeks) after anesthesia and IV fluid administration. The determination of iohexol clearance would identify if GFR is decreased despite normal BUN and serum creatinine concentrations. If GFR is decreased, the dog likely has nonazotemic chronic renal disease that has been pushed over the edge somewhat. If GFR is normal, gradual water deprivation could be performed to determine if renal medullary washout has occurred. This procedure also will help to correct renal medullary washout if it is present.

FAQ-44 Is there any benefit to perform WDT in dogs or cats suspected to have underlying CKD?

A: WDT should not be performed in an animal is known to have underlying renal disease. Dehydration that arises during this testing can pose a risk to develop AKI in the remnant nephrons if enough renal ischemia develops. The risk of ischemic renal damage during WDT is far greater in patients with diseased kidneys than in those with normal kidneys, especially if they are overtly azotemic. The reason(s) for the inability to adequately concentrate urine are readily explained by the primary renal disease and no extra benefit is gained by WDT.

In some instances, it is not clear in the nonazotemic patient if the cause of impaired ability to elaborate concentrated urine (low USG) is created by chronic renal disease or some other underlying disease associated with PU/PD. In such instances, careful monitoring during water deprivation is crucial to ensure that those with underlying kidney disease are not further injured by the WDT. The use of gradual water deprivation at home can be useful in these instances.

Desmopressin testing and/or GFR measured by iohexol clearance are often better choices to further evaluate renal function and ability to concentrate urine in fragile patients.

FAQ-45 In what diseases is WDT most likely to help me determine the definitive diagnosis?

A: WDT is used primarily as a tool to distinguish among CDI, nephrogenic diabetes insipidus (NDI), and PPD. WDT usually substantially increases in those with PPD and fails to increase the USG in those with CDI and NDI. After failed WDT, a large increase in USG following the administration of desmopressin supports the diagnosis of CDI. Failure to increase the USG after administration of desmopressin supports the diagnosis of NDI (including those with MWO).

FAQ-46 Is it better to perform a 12-hour or a 24-hour abrupt water deprivation test?

A: NEITHER. There should be no such thing as a predetermined 12-hour or 24-hour period for the abrupt WDT. WDT should be tailored to each patient individually; following USG or Uosm sequentially hourly until a steady state has been reached, or when body weight loss approaches 5%. In some instances, WDT will be over in a few hours if maximal urine concentration is achieved (as in PPD). WDT will also be terminated within a few hours if obligatory PU continues (CDI, NDI) and dehydration develops. It is essential to closely monitor all patients during WDT to ensure that they are not injured by dehydration during this testing (e.g. AKI). Some have referred to WDT as "barbaric," which it can be if the patient is not carefully monitored. Desmopressin testing usually is the next diagnostic step for those that fail WDT. Alternatively, desmopressin testing could be used instead of WDT as it is easier and safer for fragile patients, though a positive response can happen in those with CDI or those with MWO from any other cause.

FAQ-47 Can a bacterial UTI account for PU/PD in a dog? I have an older female spayed mix-breed dog that has had PU/PD and a mild increase in urgency to urinate for about three weeks. Physical examination is normal. Routine hemogram and serum biochemistry results are all normal. The USG ranges between 1.006 and 1.010. Urine dipstrip was 2+ protein and 1+ positive for blood; other urine chemistry pads were normal. Urine microscopy revealed 10–20 WBC/HPF, 5–10 RBC/HPF, 0 epi, and numerous rod bacteria. Urine culture grew >100 000 cfu/mL of *Escherichia coli*. Dexamethasone suppression testing to check for HAC was negative. Ultrasonography showed normal kidney architecture and echogenicity without pyelectasia. The ureters and bladder were also normal.

A: The conventional interpretation of this data is that bacterial UTI exists but without definitive evidence that the infection is in the kidneys. The low USG could develop from the local absorption of *E. coli* endotoxin from the lower urinary tract (LUT) that would then interfere with normal urine concentrating capacity by the kidneys. Alternatively, the UTI exists within the renal parenchyma which would also disrupt the ability to normally concentrate urine. There is no easy way to know for sure how much of a UTI exists in the LUT compared to that in the upper urinary tract with certainty.

After two weeks of urinary antibacterial treatment, urinary sediment was silent, PU/PD abated, and the USG at this time was 1.027.

FAQ-48 I have been working up a dog that has had PU/PD for the last four weeks. The UA is normal with the exception of the USG that has ranged from 1.003 to 1.010. Urine culture was negative for bacterial growth. All serum biochemistry results were normal with the exception of an ALP of 400 IU/L (<120 is normal). Circulating cortisol was suppressed following dexamethasone suppression testing to evaluate for the possibility of HAC. The owner casually mentioned that they were giving an old prescription for skin "allergies" over the past few months. This treatment was a combination pill of antihistamine and 2.5 mg of prednisolone. Is it possible that the treatment created the PU/PD and failure to concentrate urine?

A: YES. Some dogs are exquisitely sensitive to small doses of glucocorticosteroids that result in large volume PU/PD as a form of NDI. The moderate increase in ALP is likely from steroid effects on the liver.

FAQ-49 I have a 12-year-old dog with PU/PD and low USG (1.006–1.015) that has hypercalcemia as an obvious abnormality. Physical examination did not reveal any masses or lymphadenopathy. The total serum calcium is 15.2 mg/dL (upper reference is 11.8 mg/dL). Serum phosphorus was 3.0 mg/dL (3.5–5.5 mg/L reference range). Other serum biochemistry results were normal. Ionized calcium was 6.2 mg/dL (upper reference limit is 5.8 mg/dL). Is this a good time to perform WDT to see if this patient is capable of making more concentrated urine?

A: No. WDT could be hazardous for a hypercalcemic patient. Patients with ionized hypercalcemia usually cannot elaborate highly concentrated urine with this form of NDI. WDT is likely to increase the magnitude of the hypercalcemia as dehydration develops during this testing. Testing to exclude malignancy associated hypercalcemia (body cavity imaging, rectal palpation biased to the anal sac, and cytology from FNA) and measurement of PTH in relationship to ionized calcium are likely to yield valuable diagnostic information when previous testing did not yield a diagnosis. If normocalcemia can be restored, normal urinary concentrating capacity can return if there has not been permanent kidney damage from the hypercalcemia.

FAQ-50 A six-month-old intact female Labrador had a sudden onset of PU/PD and nocturia. She has yet to experience her first heat cycle. She has had intense thirst and was urinating on herself in her crate at night after she had previously been completely toilet trained.

Her creatinine was 1.3 mg/dL, P of 6.7 mg/dL, BUN of 44 mg/dL; there are no previous laboratory examinations for comparison. The USG on three separate occasions over 48 hours was 1.010 each time. Urine chemistry dipstrip was negative to trace on 2 UA and UPC was 0.22. Urine microscopy showed an inactive sediment on a sample obtained by cystocentesis. An initial POC rapid screening test (IgM toward various serovars) for Leptospirosis was negative. Her kidneys were normal size and of normal echo-architecture on ultrasonography. She is 32 lbs, which is bit low for weight at six months in a female Labrador. She appears well hydrated. Is it a good idea to perform WDT in this puppy? Could she have PPD?

A: No for WDT. Though her creatinine is at the upper part of the reference range for adult dogs, the serum creatinine is too high to be normal for a puppy (often between 0.4 and 0.8 mg/dL). She has impaired excretory renal function based on this creatinine and the BUN. Thus, it is not safe to take water away from this patient as it could create more renal injury. It is not clear how much of the renal disease is related to acute or chronic injury.

WDT would have been indicated to see if PPD were the cause of her PD/PU *if* her serum biochemical analysis revealed no other condition that could impair urinary concentrating capacity. The finding of decreased renal function identifies one category of conditions that impair the capacity to elaborate concentrated urine.

Further history revealed a one-time possible exposure to Advil tablets at a very low dose, far less than that reported to create AKI. She had no GI signs which are expected in those with NSAID toxicity.

Sequential monitoring of renal function is indicated over the next several months to see if there is further decline or improvement in excretory renal function, and if the impaired urinary concentration can improve. Normal ULS of the kidneys does not exclude the possibility for AKI or CKD (including renal dysplasia in this puppy). A UPC of 0.22 is very close to the <0.2 generally accepted as normal. When the UPC is at the tipping point for "normal," the variability in the performance of the analyzer must be considered; the actual values may really be higher or lower than those reported. Some normal dogs can have a UPC of 0.2–0.5. Also, the UPC should be sequentially monitored to see if it escalates or not. Most dogs with familial nephropathy have renal proteinuria from altered glomerular dynamics of a greater magnitude than that encountered in this dog. Polymerase chain reaction (PCR) on blood and urine that were sent to the state laboratory returned negative for leptospirosis.

If the decreased excretory function does not improve, a comprehensive renal biopsy analysis is the next step to establish a definitive diagnosis following microscopy by light (with special stains), electron microscopy, and IFA. Amoxicillin TID was started pending the final results for the Leptospirosis PCR on urine and blood.

In this dog 10 days later, PU/PD suddenly stopped. At this time, she had a 1.037 USG and a decrease in her BUN to 17 mg/dL and serum creatinine of 0.9 mg/dL. UPC was 0.17 at this recheck clinical visit. It appears that she has made a full recovery from her AKI, but it should be noted that those with an episode of AKI can be at risk for a future diagnosis of CKD.

FAQ-51 Is it a good idea to exclude HAC in most dogs prior to WDT?

A: YES, in many instances. The classic clinical signs associated with HAC are not always obvious and yet HAC could still account for the PU/PD and low USG. Screening for HAC with cortisol suppression testing makes sense in those with mostly normal serum biochemistry and inactive urinary sediment. HAC is frequently associated with renal proteinuria, but so is nonazotemic CKD. If the diagnosis of idiopathic PPD is likely, screening for HAC is not necessary. However, PPD secondary to HAC can occur at times.

FAQ-52 Can a dog or cat with CKD have PU/PD and impaired urinary concentration without an obvious increase in BUN, serum creatinine, or SDMA?

A: YES. There is a window in which enough nephron mass has been lost to impair urinary concentration, but not enough lost to cause azotemia. In dogs, impaired urinary concentration happens with some regularity when there has been between 50% and 67% loss of nephron mass. The nonazotemic window for reduced urinary concentration is far less predictable in cats with CKD.

CHAPTER 5 – CHEMICAL PROPERTIES

FAQ-53 I have on occasion observed that the urine dipstick reaction in cats is positive for WBC, but urine sediment does not show excess WBC and urine culture is negative. What causes this discordance?

A: The dipstrip reaction for WBC was designed to detect the presence of leukocyte esterase in human white cells. Pyuria in cats and dogs needs to be identified based on microscopic evaluation of fresh urinary sediment. This test is frequently negative in dogs despite the presence of WBC and positive in cats despite the absence of WBC. It is best to ignore or not report results for WBC based on chemistry dipstrip due to this level of inaccuracy.

FAQ-54 I have tentatively diagnosed Fanconi syndrome in a Basenji dog with a blood glucose concentration of 90 mg/dL, 3+ glucosuria, and 1+ proteinuria. How can I be sure the diagnosis is accurate?

A: The generalized proximal tubular transport dysfunction known as Fanconi syndrome is likely in this dog. However, remember that proteinuria and amino aciduria are not synonymous. A good screening test for amino aciduria is to send a urine sample to the University of Pennsylvania Division of Medical Genetics. The combination of glucosuria in the face of normoglycemia and aminoaciduria secures the diagnosis.

FAQ-55 Am I OK to skip measurement of USG by refractometer and instead rely on the USG measured on the chemistry dipstrip?

A: No. USG by dipstrip is far less accurate as to the actual urine concentration. USG by dipstrip does not generally line up close enough to the USG measured by refractometer to be useful. The maximal USG that can be measured and reported from the dipstrip is 1.035 based on human concentrating capacity, but this is too low a maximal point for veterinary measurement since dogs and cats can elaborate urine with USG much higher than this that is of interest. The bins for USG on the dipstrip are in increments of 0.005, which is large enough to allow the misclassification of the degree of urine concentration at the various tipping points that define adequacy of urine concentration.

FAQ-56 Is the measurement of urinary pH by dipstrip accurate enough for me to clinically manage and follow my patients with urolithiasis?

A: No. Compared to urinary pH measured by pH meter, pH determined by dipstrip is surprisingly inaccurate. Extremes in reported dipstrip pH values will be helpful in determining the effect of treatment in individual patients, but it is not possible to detect minor changes in pH by dipstrip. Bins for urinary pH on the dipstrip vary by 0.5 or 1.0 pH units depending on the brand of chemistry dipstrip. The accuracy of the dipstrip pH is considered acceptable by the manufacturer if the reported pH is within one bin above or one bin below the pH as measured by meter. For precise work when the actual urinary pH is important to know, it is best to measure urinary pH by meter.

FAQ-57 I have observed that the dipstrip pad reaction for protein is frequently trace positive or 1+ positive in patients that I can find no other abnormalities; they have an inactive urinary sediment. How much attention should I give to these low-level dipstrip pad color reactions for protein?

A: Your observation is correct; trace positive and 1+ dipstrip protein reactions are common in animals that are normal. Dry reagent pads on the urinary dipstrip detect mostly albumin and far less of nonalbumin proteins. The conventional assessment has been to presume that these low-level reactions are likely to be normal, especially when the urine is highly concentrated and the urinary sediment is inactive. Small amounts of albumin excreted into urine can measure as trace or 1+ on the dipstrip when water has been largely reabsorbed by the CT, thus increasing the concentration of albumin despite no increase in the absolute amount of albumin initially entering the urine. In cats, high concentrations of cauxin normally present in the urine are likely to activate the color reaction on the reagent pad in some cats.

FAQ-58 How much significance should I place on the finding of glucosuria (trace, 1+ or 2+ on urinary dipstrip) in cats that have either normoglycemia or mild increases in circulating glucose concentration?

A: This depends on other aspects of the clinical presentation. Diabetes mellitus is always important to exclude in the differential diagnosis as a cause for glucosuria. However, a higher magnitude of circulating glucose is expected with this diagnosis.

Cats can undergo acute epinephrine-mediated stress that results in a transient hyperglycemia that is above the renal threshold for glucose. Transporting cats to the veterinary clinic increases blood glucose concentrations high enough to allow spillover into the urine of some cats. Depending on the timing of the blood and urine sample collection, the previously high glucose concentration may have substantially declined by the time of the blood draw, but glucose spillover into urine already occurred when the circulating glucose was high.

Alternatively, a proximal tubulopathy exists that is impairing the normal capacity of the proximal renal tubules to reabsorb the usual amount of glucose that enters the tubular fluid. This can be part of the Fanconi Syndrome, but this is less common in cats than in dogs. A detailed drug and diet history should be reviewed. Some forms of AKI are associated with normoglycemic glucosuria. Recent studies have demonstrated that high dietary phosphate intake can result in glucosuria in some previously normal cats, attributed to proximal tubular dysfunction (tubular phosphatopathy), among other renal problems. Jerky treats can cause an acquired glucosuria in dogs, but I have not observed this in cats from any source of treats.

Cats that are severely ill with chronic disease have anecdotally been observed to have normoglycemic glucosuria at times. This phenomenon has not been studied or well characterized, so how often this occurs is not known. It could be an isolated glucosuria or part of an acquired Fanconi syndrome.

FAQ-59   Occasionally I detect glucosuria (urinary dipstrip positive reaction) from the urine of male cats with UO. Why does this occur in some cats?

A: Glucosuria during UO is attributed to stress hyperglycemia severe enough to allow spillover into the urine in some cats. In other cats, normoglycemia exists and the dipstrip positive reaction is attributed to "pseudo-glucosuria." Some nonglucose substance appears to be capable of activating the color reaction on the reagent pad in these instances. Glucose positive status from either mechanism returns to negative on dipstrip chemistry shortly after the UO is relieved. There are no consequences to the cat from glucosuria in this setting.

FAQ-60   How do I know for sure that trace and 1+ color reactions on the protein reagent pad are not pathological?

A: Assuming that the urinary sediment is inactive, measurement of MA should be negative or UPC should be <0.2, or at least <0.4 in the cat or <0.5 in the dog if they are normal. Otherwise, you may be finding this animal in an early stage of a disease process causing the kidney to leak mostly albumin proteins following loss of glomerular barrier function.

FAQ-61   Is it safe for me to assume that dipstrip color reactions at ≥2+ arise from extra protein added to urine from some kidney problem?

A: No. It is important to know if the urine sediment is highly active or not. Increased color reaction on the protein reagent pad is expected in some dogs and cats in which there is a large increase in the numbers of RBC or WBC in the urine from inflammation or hemorrhage, usually from the LUT. Postrenal proteinuria is common in LUT disorders that include UTI, urolithiasis, and urinary neoplasia. Prerenal proteinuria is rare and can usually be ruled out in the absence of hemoglobinemia or myoglobinemia. The hallmark of renal glomerular proteinuria is the finding of ≥2+ protein on the dipstrip in the absence of increased urine sediment findings. This should be confirmed by the measurement of UPC >0.5 in dogs and >0.4 in cats.

FAQ-62   What kind of protein does the urinary chemistry dipstrip detect?

A: This reagent pad is much more sensitive to the detection of albumin, but it can detect some nonalbumin proteins if they are in the urine in high enough concentrations. Positive reactions for protein on the dipstrip are attributed to albuminuria in most instances.

FAQ-63   How can I know if proteins from excess RBC are increasing the dipstrip reaction for protein?

A: In general, it takes a lot of RBC to cause in an increase in the color reaction of protein on the reagent pad from hemoglobin originating in the red cells. If the occult blood reaction is 1+ and the dipstrip protein reaction is 2+, the contribution of blood to the protein reaction is minimal. When the occult blood is 3+, some of the protein in that much blood could increase the color reaction on the protein reagent pad.

FAQ-64   I have encountered urine samples in which the occult blood reaction was positive despite very few RBC observed during urine microscopy. How can I reconcile these findings?

A: This type of discordance occurs with some frequency. The reagent pad for occult blood is most sensitive to the presence of free hemoglobin or myoglobin in the urine. Myoglobinuria could account for this discordance, but this is not such a common finding. Free hemoglobin from lysed RBC is a more likely explanation for this discordance. RBC that undergo lysis are often assumed to originate in the LUT, but the lysis of RBC that traverse a diseased glomerulus that become dysmorphic RBC could also account for this discrepancy.

FAQ-65   I have a middle-aged dog that has been chronically ill and has lost quite a bit of weight. On the urinary chemistry dipstrip, ketones are positive, but the glucose pad is negative. I was under the impression that ketonuria is usually associated with diabetes mellitus and the reagent pad for glucose should be positive. Blood glucose was 110 mg/dL. What am I missing here?

A: Ketonuria without glucosuria can develop during starvation and during chronic hypoglycemia. During hypoglycemia, insulin is less secreted which favors ketogenesis.

FAQ-66   2+ dipstrip glucose positive reactions have been found on sequential UA in a two-year-old dog with PU/PD for the past few months. Ketones on the dipstrip have been negative. 1+ protein was found on some of the urinalyses. Other dipstrip reactions were normal. USG varied from 1.015 to 1.025. Blood glucose was 130 mg/dL. BUN, serum creatinine, and SDMA were within the reference range. UPC or MA was not evaluated.

A: This dog has renal glucosuria and possibly acquired Fanconi syndrome. The blood glucose is well below the normal renal threshold for glucose to appear in the urine. Upon further questioning of the owners, they started feeding their dog beef jerky treats shortly before the PU/PD started. Jerky treats, often imported or made with ingredients imported from China, have been incriminated in this type of proximal tubulopathy, but a presumptive toxic molecule has not been definitively identified. Some degree of AKI is sometimes found at the same time in association with jerky treats, but not in this particular dog. PU/PD is attributed to the glucosuria from impaired proximal tubular function and resulting solute diuresis. Six weeks after stopping the jerky treats, the PU/PD resolved and glucosuria was no longer apparent. If the jerky treat history had been negative, it would be important to closely review any drugs or anesthetic exposure that could have created this tubulopathy. Azotemic AKI can be associated with glucosuria at times in other instances of glucosuria in the face of normoglycemia.

FAQ-67 I have been considering purchasing an automated reader for urine chemistry dipstrip reactions. Is this a good idea?

A: Yes. This is the future. Subjective assessment of color reaction by the human eye and brain is removed when automated readers are employed. Automated readers are capable of detecting subtle color changes on the dipstrip reagent pads that are beyond accurate detection by humans. These automated readers are cost affordable and results can be integrated into the patient's digital medical record, lessening transcription errors.

CHAPTER 6 – URINARY SEDIMENT/MICROSCOPY

FAQ-68 How important is the centrifugation speed or force of urine used prior to urine microscopy?

A: Centrifugation has traditionally been considered important in amplifying or concentrating the number of elements in urine that can be detected during microscopy. This concept of amplification has been challenged in recent times. When centrifugation is used, the centrifuge must be capable of $<400 \times G$; RPM and length of the centrifuge arm are related to the G forces generated. The centrifuge should not be set to the higher settings employed in processing serum or plasma samples; otherwise, fragile urinary elements may be destroyed (especially casts and RBC). The time that the urine is centrifuged also has an impact on any amplification and preservation of elements. In some automated microscopy analyzers, centrifugation is not used at all; instead, elements accumulate by gravity over a set time. Similarly, in some commercial laboratories analyzing multiple urine sediments sequentially, urine sits in wells on a plate for a standard time to allow settling before the sediment is examined.

FAQ-69 How important is the urine volume that undergoes centrifugation or settling prior to microscopy?

A: Not as important as we once thought. It has seemed intuitively obvious that the evaluation of a larger urine volume would allow the detection of elements not detected in smaller urine volumes as the elements become more concentrated following centrifugation, but this so-called amplification effect may be overrated. Textbooks often recommend the use of 10 mL of urine, but urine samples of this size are often not possible when collected from dogs and cats. Some veterinary laboratories routinely analyze 3 mL and others 1 mL. It is important to use the same volume each time in your practice in order to try to make semiquantitative comparisons between urinary sediment results. Recent veterinary studies have shown similar results between large and small urine volumes that underwent centrifugation prior to urine microscopy. Automated microscopy analyzers evaluate $<200\,\mu L$ that generate the enumeration of sediment results that generally match up with those by manual methods using larger volumes.

FAQ-70 Why is the need to well-mix the urine immediately before centrifugation or entry into an automated analyzer for urine microscopy emphasized so heavily?

A: Failure to well-mix a urine sample prior to centrifugation can result in a large preanalytical error in how many elements per microscopic filed or per μL will be reported. The impact of gravity on settling of urine elements is largely unappreciated for how quickly this can occur. Urine that has been standing for as little as 30–60 seconds can undergo rapid settling of elements (depending on weight and shape of the element) to the lower region of the urine tube or container. When urine to be further analyzed is aspirated from the top after some standing time, far fewer elements will be in that portion of the urine sample. If urine from the standing sample is aspirated from the bottom, far more elements will be reported from that portion. We are interested in the average number of elements in all portions of the urine, so mixing immediately before centrifugation is important in order to generate more representative results.

FAQ-71 I currently do not perform any urinalyses in house. Why should I stop sending my urine samples to a reference laboratory and perform in-house UA instead?

A: Fresh warm urine always generates more accurate results than following delay and refrigeration. The ex vivo generation of crystals or bacterial growth as artifacts can be encountered in the stored and shipped urine sample that was not there in the fresh sample. The degeneration of WBC, RBC, epithelial cells, and casts is more likely to occur in samples shipped to the reference laboratory, which can result in under-reporting of important abnormal elements. Depending on when the sample is picked up and shipped, UA results from the reference laboratory become available in about 5–24 hours. Manual in-house UA results are usually generated in less than 30 minutes. Automated in-house UA is usually completed within five minutes (USG, urine chemistry, and urine microscopy). In-house UA allows greater income to be kept within the practice rather than at the reference laboratory and also allows for a real-time conversation with the owners about the UA results, while they are still physically present.

FAQ-72   Why should I switch over from in-house manual methods of urine microscopy to in-house automated microscopy?

A: The number one reason to do this is to standardize how the urine sample is handled after it enters the analyzer; volume, centrifugation or time to settle, digital image capture, and ID of elements. Handling of urine samples often varies by the technician setting up the urine during manual microscopy. It is always very important to well-mix the urine immediately before it enters the analyzer.

The number two reason to switch over to automated microscopy is to decrease the time needed to generate the microscopy report (less than three minutes compared to 18– 22 minutes manually). This allows less consumption of technician time that can then allow you to perform more urinalyses, which is good medicine and generates more practice income.

The number three reason is to guarantee more accurate identification of common elements (RBC, WBC, epithelial cells, rod bacteria, calcium oxalate crystals, and struvite crystals) when inexperienced laboratory personnel are performing the UA.

FAQ-73   I know you are keen on automated microscopy. I understand the advantages of using this technology. What are the drawbacks associated with automated microscopy?

A: The algorithms employed by the analyzer usually accurately identify and enumerate RBC, WBC, epithelial cells, rod bacteria, hyaline casts, and calcium oxalate crystals and struvite crystals. Bilirubin, urate, and unidentified crystals are reported by some analyzers. Even so, it is a good idea for the technician to scan the digital images of the urinary sediment to ensure that the reported elements align with what is seen on the digital images. The analyzer decides which images are likely to be of most interest that are then placed at the front of the line. Many more digital images are captured, but the images with the most activity are moved to the front to allow a quick review. The technician has the ability to move other images to the front if they are deemed worthy of closer inspection.

Current algorithms for the identification and enumeration of less common elements in urine sediment are not so accurate. The technician must examine the digital images to further classify casts reported as nonhyaline to determine if they should be reported as granular, cellular, or waxy casts. Nonsquamous epithelial cells should further be classified as renal tubular epithelium (RTE) or urothelial cells. It is a good idea for the technician to determine if urothelial cells or WBC are in clumps or not. Automated reports of cocci bacteria are sometimes not accurate – so visual inspection of the digital images may be helpful to confirm the nature of "bacteria." Uncommon crystals may not be identified or they can be reported as unidentified crystals. Errors in the ID of urinary elements may be reported at an increased rate when the sediment is "crowded" with RBC or WBC. A repeat microscopy can be performed after the lysis of RBC to reduce crowding in order to more accurately identify bacteria at times or following the dilution of the sediment.

FAQ-74   Why is it so important to evaluate fresh warm urine in dogs or cats that are sick?

A: Animals that are ill are more likely to have abnormal urinary elements identified during urine microscopy that may not be there or be able to be identified when evaluated later. Cellular casts are notoriously unstable and rapidly break up within a short time (<30 minutes). RBC casts seem to be the most likely to break up (<15 minutes), such that their contribution to a cast is no longer apparent; only free RBC are then seen. The degeneration of WBC and epithelial cells that are free or within casts can quickly undergo substantial degeneration that makes their proper identification difficult or impossible. Cellular detail is preserved when microscopy is performed as soon as possible following urine collection.

FAQ-75   Should I perform urine microscopy on sediment that is unstained or stained with a supravital stain (e.g. Sternheimer-Malbin [SediStain®]; new methylene blue)?

A: My preference is to examine stained sediment during urine microscopy. Stained sediment usually makes it easier for me to identify cells when there is contrast and color difference between nuclei and cytoplasm. However, at times it is helpful to examine urine sediment without stain, especially when it is unclear if detection of bacteria is "real" or not. The best practice is to examine an unstained drop and stained drop of urine sediment on the same slide with two coverslips. Whether "to stain or not to stain" is highly debated and sometimes involves an emotional conversation; many experienced technicians prefer unstained urine microscopy. I believe that stain helps less experienced operators identify urinary elements with more certainty.

The enumeration of elements following the addition of stain adds a component of dilution; consequently, the enumeration of elements in sediment will differ slightly in those examined with stain compared to those examined without stain. It is preferable to count elements in the unstained sediment and then characterize the elements further in the stained sediment if needed.

Stain should NOT be added to urine or sediment entering an automated sediment reader. The stain ruins the ability of the algorithms to properly identify cells and crystals.

FAQ-76   Why is it recommended to examine urine sediment under low illumination?

A: Some elements in the urine sediment can have an optical density close to that of the urine around them, which means that bright light can make it more difficult to identify elements in unstained specimens. Wet field urine microscopy requires lower lighting intensity compared to microscopy of dry-mount slides. Hyaline casts are especially apt to not be seen and identified due to being "burned out" by too much light, as their optical density is so close to that of the background urine. It is a good practice to partially close the iris diaphragm and lower the substage condenser to enhance contrast and maximize one's ability to identify all the elements.

FAQ-77 Why is it that my in-house urinary sediment (manual or automated) results differ from those generated at a reference laboratory? Sometimes these results are substantial and clinically important.

A: In-house urine microscopy results are more likely to reveal elements that have been preserved (more intact casts, greater cellular detail to WBC and epithelial cells, less lysis of WBC and RBC) compared to those undergoing several hours of refrigeration and transport to a reference laboratory. Also, in-house samples are less likely to undergo substantial bacterial growth as an artifact of time. Cellular casts frequently disintegrate, and most are only identified during microscopy of fresh warm urine. It can be frustrating to see discordance in sediment results between the in-house microscopy and that reported from the reference laboratory. If you are sending in a urine because you identified something unusual or of uncertain origin, it would be good to also send in a dry mount of the urinary sediment along with the urine sample. Prepare a dry mount by spinning down the urine then taking the pellet and making smears. Not all elements that were in the wet-mount will also be in the dry mount – this is especially problematic for casts. Also, it would be helpful to the clinical pathologist at the reference laboratory to be able to examine digital images of the interesting urine sediment that you have captured, perhaps using the digital camera on your cell phone through the eyepiece of the microscope.

FAQ-78 I frequently see what appear to be "bacteria" in urine sediment that are not associated with bacterial growth on urine culture of the same sample. I am frustrated with this discordance.

A: Your frustration is understandable. Many things in urine can resemble bacteria, especially cocci. The identification of rod-like bacteria in the urine sediment much more often aligns with positive results on urine culture.

Many times, the "cocci" you have identified do look like bacteria, but they are not bacteria. Tiny crystals, cellular detritus, and small lipid droplets (cats) can look like cocci. In stained sediment, mucus staining or precipitate of stain can at times be punctate, resembling cocci. Older stain is sometimes contaminated with bacteria; examine a drop of the stain with the microscope to ensure that there are no bacteria. Old stain is also likely to have undergone some evaporation and so precipitates of crystals from chemicals in the stain can resemble cocci. Use clean and high-quality slides to minimize artifacts that could be identified as bacteria.

FAQ-79 I am concerned that the crystals reported during urine microscopy are an artifact following storage for several hours and from refrigeration. Can I rewarm and agitate a previously refrigerated urine sample in an effort to get crystals to go back in solution?

A: You are correct to be concerned about storage and refrigeration allowing crystals to come out of solution that were not there in fresh warm urine. Unfortunately, rewarming and agitating the urine does not reliably result in crystals going back into solution. If you are highly concerned about crystals in the urine sediment, it is best to examine fresh warm urine to see if they are still there.

FAQ-80 Why does our reference laboratory never report cellular casts from patients suspected to have AKI?

A: Cellular casts are very fragile and frequently degenerate during transport to a reference laboratory. They may not be seen even during in-house microscopy if there is a substantial delay between the urine collection and urine microscopy. Urine sediment should be examined within 15 minutes of collection to facilitate the identification of fragile cellular casts (RBC, WBC, and RTE).

FAQ-81 We frequently get reports of bacteria on urine microscopy with minimal pyuria and often these patients have negative urine cultures. Do these patients have UTI caused by a fastidious organism?

A: Usually not. Normal urine sediment may contain many artifacts that resemble bacteria. Most often, these reports are false positives. *Corynebacterium urealyticum* is an exception, as it is a fastidious, slow-growing organism but usually is associated with very alkaline urine pH, struvite crystalluria, and bladder encrustation with struvite along with pyuria. Bacteria without pyuria occur in some patients that are immunosuppressed, but the urine culture should be positive in those with "real" bacteria.

FAQ-82 In our practice, we believe that crystalluria is always of major concern since crystals often create disease or are at least associated with some disease. Are we correct to be so concerned?

A: The presence of crystalluria is generally overrated for any ability to predict underlying stones already formed, stones likely to form in the future, or in the pathophysiology of feline idiopathic/interstitial cystitis (FIC).

Crystalluria many times is not associated with disease or a cause of disease, depending on the specific type of crystal. Struvite and calcium oxalate crystalluria are often found in dogs and cats that have no underling disease. The presence of these crystals is not usually a risk for first-time stone growth in normal dogs and cats but could be so for recurrent of stones composed of these molecules. Urinary stones are often found without crystalluria, crystalluria often occurs without stones, and sometimes stones are found but with crystals in the urine that do not match up with the crystals in the stone.

In acutely ill animals, the identification of calcium oxalate crystals in urine sediment supports a diagnosis of ethylene glycol (EG) poisoning, especially when the urine is somewhat dilute due to the osmotic diuresis associated with the ingestion of EG early on. Calcium oxalate monohydrate crystals are more common; they are more difficult to identify than calcium oxalate monohydrate and are often reported as amorphous or unidentified crystals by less experienced laboratory personnel.

Ammonium urate crystalluria can be encountered in those with severe liver disease or more commonly in those with portosystemic shunt. They can also be encountered in those with and without urate stones and are a risk factor for recurrent urate stones especially in breeds at risk such as the Dalmatian dog. Cystine crystals are never normal as they indicate a proximal tubulopathy (congenital or acquired). Cystine crystals may or may not be associated with cystine urolithiasis.

Bilirubin crystals are often identified in urine sediment from normal dogs, especially when the urine is highly concentrated and in males. Hyperbilirubinuria from hemolysis or from primary liver disease can account for these crystals at times. Bilirubin crystals are never normal in cats, so hepatic function and disease should be further evaluated.

It is important to remember that urine storage and cooling (especially in the refrigerator) prior to microscopy can allow the ex vivo development of some crystals that were not there when the urine sample was collected. The number of crystals can also be increased over the number of baseline crystals when originally collected in these instances. If you think that these crystals and their numbers are important, it is a good idea to perform another urine microscopy on fresh warm urine.

FAQ-83   Is it possible for me to tell the site of origin from the urogenital tract when increased numbers of WBCs, RBCs, and or epithelial cells are observed in the urine sediment?

A: The morphological appearance of free WBC and RBC is not different when they arise from the upper urinary tract or LUT in general. Small epithelial cells with basal nuclei help to identify them as RTE that has entered the urine. Large squamous cells are almost always contaminants from the distal urethra, vestibule, or prepuce. It is not possible to determine the origin of urothelial cells based on size alone, but only small epithelial cells can come from the kidneys.

The finding of cellular casts – RBC, WBC, and renal tubular epithelial – indicates that at least some of these elements are arising from the kidney as they become trapped in casts. Rarely, the finding of dysmorphic RBC can indicate glomerular disease as the RBC become damaged as they traverse a diseased glomerulus.

FAQ-84   I have a three-year-old dog in my practice that was normal until two days ago. Now, the dog is moribund. It is severely dehydrated and has a 1.010 USG with several granular casts per low power microscopic field in the urinary sediment. Abnormal serum chemistry results include a serum creatinine concentration of 6.1 mg/dL, serum phosphorus concentration of 9.0 mg/dL, and serum total calcium concentration of 18.2 mg/dL. What is the prognosis for this dog?

A: The isosthenuric USG, granular cylindruria, and azotemia are likely a consequence of ionized hypercalcemia. The severe hypercalcemia and hyperphosphatemia suggest exposure to a vitamin D metabolite such as found in cholecalciferol-based rat bait or calcipotriene in antipsoriasis cream. Some of the hyperphosphatemia is likely due to excretory renal failure. How much azotemia is primary and how much is prerenal cannot be determined at the time of presentation because hypercalcemia interferes with urinary concentrating ability. Repeated measurement of serum creatinine concentration after IV fluid therapy has corrected dehydration will allow you to determine how much, if any, of the azotemia was prerenal in origin. Given the magnitude of the increased serum total calcium, the ionized calcium is likely to be also increased, if the history for acute disease is correct. If the azotemia is

chronic instead, then increased circulating calcium complexes can increase the total calcium without increasing the ionized calcium. The measurement of serum ionized calcium concentration would be useful to make this distinction. The persistence of ionized hypercalcemia in the face of azotemia increases the risk for the development of additional primary renal lesions. Rapid reversal of hypercalcemia is crucial to the successful treatment of this dog.

FAQ-85   I have a five-year-old spayed female Labrador retriever in my clinic that presented to our office with a sudden onset of anorexia, vomiting, and lethargy × two days. Her physical examination was unremarkable. There was no history of previous PU or PD. Her USG is 1.015 with 3+ dipstrip proteinuria, Urine microscopy revealed an average of four granular casts per low power microscopic field, occasional renal tubular epithelial cell casts, and rare free RTE. Her UPC is 7.2. Serum biochemistry results include a serum creatinine concentration of 9.3 mg/dL, serum phosphorus concentration of 8.5 mg/dL, and hypoalbuminemia (1.5 g/dL). Her serum creatinine concentration has not decreased following IV fluids. Her kidneys are normal sized with normal renal pelves, but they are hyperechoic with loss of corticomedullary distinction on ultrasonography. Her Lyme titer is positive. Is this azotemic AKI or CKD, and what is the prognosis?

A: Many of her laboratory findings point to at least a component of AKI, but this disease has likely been ongoing longer than the time the dog has been displaying clinical signs based on the hypoalbuminemia.

The 3+ dipstick proteinuria and the UPC of 7.2 (normal <0.2) in a urine that is isosthenuric and has an inactive sediment (except for cylindruria) is the hallmark of glomerular proteinuria. The magnitude of the proteinuria indicates a severe breakdown in glomerular barrier integrity, but this magnitude cannot be used to predict the underlying histopathology. Based on the finding of RTE and epithelial cell casts, some of the proteinuria is likely tubular in origin.

An excess number of granular casts is traditionally considered to result from tubular degeneration at an accelerated rate (nephrotoxins, renal ischemia, and renal infections). That is possible in this case, but it is also possible that plasma proteins entering urine at a high rate are precipitating in the matrix protein form the granules in the cast as a less appreciated mechanism. The finding of free RTE and epithelial cell casts supports acute renal tubular injury as these cells are shed into the urine. The finding of epithelial casts is never normal and indicates a severe renal tubular insult.

Hypoalbuminemia is not a usual feature of azotemic AKI early on, especially before treatment with IV fluids. An exception to this can be with rapidly progressive glomerulonephritis (RPGN). The severe proteinuria is most compatible with glomerular disease; this magnitude of proteinuria is not common with most causes of AKI.

Differential diagnosis at this point should include leptospirosis, RPGN (with or without *Borrelia* positive status), amyloidosis with acute medullary necrosis, or a chronic glomerulopathy with acute exacerbation. Renal biopsy will be an important tool to establish a definitive diagnosis and offer a prognosis. Unfortunately, advanced azotemia associated with renal amyloidosis or RPGN has a grave prognosis, especially when found in association with hypoalbuminemia. The positive Lyme titer is not necessarily helpful because many normal dogs in endemic regions have positive titers without obvious clinical disease. The positive titer could indicate exposure rather than active disease.

FAQ-86   Can a bacterial UTI exist without an increase in the number of WBC identified during urine microscopy?

A: Not typically. Most true UTI (based on quantitative bacterial growth cfu/mL) will have increased WBC detected. The odds of a UTI being present are higher if WBCs are seen in association with bacteria at the same time.

  The degree of pyuria can be lessened or blunted in some dogs or cats with CKD, HAC, exogenous glucocorticosteroid administration, or diabetes mellitus at times of large quantitative bacterial growth.

FAQ-87   I examined a urinary sediment that showed large numbers of rod bacteria, but no other elements. How can I account for this?

A: The most likely explanation is the contamination of the urine sample with bacteria during the collection process and then a delay in analysis or refrigeration. Remember that bacterial organisms can double their numbers every 20 minutes at room temperature.

FAQ-88   I was startled to see what appeared to be fungal organisms in the urinary sediment – long filamentous connected organisms. There were many WBC and some RBC in this sediment also. Urine culture revealed >100 000 cfu/mL of *E. coli*. No fungal elements were isolated despite the microbiology laboratory using special media to aid their growth. The culture plate was observed for seven days and still no fungal organisms grew. Why were fungal organisms not isolated?

A: They were not fungal organisms in the first place. *E. coli* can assume a filamentous morphology when growing in urine that can be confused with fungi.

FAQ-89   I have a dog with a proven bacterial UTI (*Staphylococcus spp.*), but I cannot see organisms in the urinary sediment. Why cannot I identify these bacterial organisms?

A: It takes a critical mass of bacteria to be seen in a wet-mount microscopy, estimated at >10 000 cfu/mL for rods and >100 000 cfu/mL for cocci. Thus, the bacteria could be there but not able to be seen by the human eye. A dry-mount cytology from the urine sediment allows microscopy under oil immersion that will more readily reveal bacterial organisms if they are really there.

FAQ-90   I frequently review reports of "bacteria" in urinary sediment on my urinalyses, but often the urine culture from the same sample does not grow any bacteria. What accounts for the discordance between bacteria observed during microscopy and failure of bacterial growth in the microbiology laboratory?

A: First of all, it is important to remember that not everything reported as "bacteria" in the urinary sediment really are bacteria. Many particulate artifacts occur in urine sediment and can be confused with bacteria, especially cocci. Small crystals, lipid droplets (cats), cellular detritus, punctate staining of mucus, and stain precipitate can resemble cocci. When "rods" are reported in the UA, they are more likely to be "real" bacteria compared to when cocci are reported.

  The bottle of supravital stain is rarely contaminated with bacteria, but it is still a good idea to periodically examine a drop of the stain alone to ensure that there are no bacteria in order to exclude this artifact in the reporting of bacteria.

  Sometimes the bacteria are real in the urine sediment, but they are "dead in the urine," which means that they will not grow at the microbiology laboratory. This is an uncommon occurrence and is more likely to occur with fastidious organisms. Most routine uropathogens grow readily in urine transported in a timely manner to a reference laboratory.

  If you are concerned that you are getting false-negative bacterial culture results due to storage of urine samples or that growth has been inhibited during transport to the laboratory, consider plating out the urine sample immediately after collection and send the plate to the laboratory after initial incubation if overnight growth is detected.

FAQ-91   The dipstrip for WBC is frequently positive in urine from cats, but urine microscopy usually fails to identify excess WBC. Why is there such discordance in the identification of WBC during urine microscopy with that noted on the WBC dipstrip (esterase) color reaction?

A: The WBC reagent pad is designed to detect esterase in WBC from humans. It is not accurate for use in the urine of dogs or cats and should not be reported, or ignored if it is reported. This reagent pad for WBC is frequently falsely positive for WBC as compared to visual observation during urine microscopy in cats.

FAQ-92   I spend a lot of time looking for and trying to identify crystals during urine microscopy, especially in patients with LUT signs. When I see crystals, I become concerned about the likely presence of urinary stones.

A: The presence of crystalluria in no way guarantees that urinary stones are present at the same time. Many normal animals have crystalluria and will never develop a stone. Crystalluria can be a normal physiological phenomenon especially when the urine sample is highly concentrated (high USG) and stored under refrigeration as the crystals may not have been there at the time the sample was collected (ex vivo development).

  The absence of crystalluria never excludes the presence of a urinary stone either, as most of the crystals may be within the urinary stone. Many animals with urolithiasis do not have crystalluria. When a urinary stone exists within the urinary tract, the type of crystals in the urine does not always align with the chemical composition of the urolith.

  The number and chemical type of crystalluria may be more helpful in trying to reduce a recurrent episode of urolithiasis during management with drugs, water, and diet.

FAQ-93 I pay extra attention during urine microscopy of urine from cats with FIC and get excited when I find struvite crystalluria. Someone recently told me that crystalluria during FIC is pretty much meaningless. Is that true?

A: YES, that is true in most instances. Crystalluria during FIC is usually that of struvite, but its presence is not related to the pathophysiology of this disease. The number and type of crystals matters only if the cat is forming a stone or a urethral plug. Crystalluria is a contributing, but not a primary driving, factor as urethral plugs form. Crystalluria is not known to damage the urothelium and create cystitis directly, as is commonly misunderstood by the profession. Neither struvite nor calcium oxalate crystals are known to "harpoon" the mucosa. Under rare circumstances, crystalluria could contribute to cystitis if the crystals were to adhere to the bladder wall when the GAG layer was diminished or the urothelium has been denuded.

FAQ-94 In animals with documented crystalluria and urinary stones, I do not submit the urinary stones in order to save the clients some money on the assumption that the mineral analysis of the stone will be the same as that of the crystals in the urine. Is this an acceptable practice?

A: No. Crystals in the urine may not match up with the chemical composition within the urolith. It is important to submit the stone for quantitative analysis to know with certainty the nature of the stone. It is also important to determine if the layers of the stone are all the same, or if the exterior and interior components of the stone differ in chemical composition. Sometimes the crystals currently in the urine match up with the superficial layer of the stone but not with the chemical nature of its interior. Veterinary laboratories interested in urolithiasis are available to perform quantitative analysis on submitted stones.

FAQ-95 A 10-year-old female spayed Persian cat is presented for routine geriatric evaluation. The owner reports no specific problems with the cat except for some mild weight loss. The cat has been fed a diet that has been marketed to "promote urinary health." Serum biochemistry shows a total serum calcium concentration of 12.3 mg/dL. After subcutaneous fluids overnight, the total serum calcium concentration modestly decreases to 11.9 mg/dL (upper reference range is 11.3 mg/dL). A plain abdominal radiograph shows a small radiopaque ureteral stone on the right side. The ULS examination of the kidneys shows them to be slightly small (3.0 cm in length) but otherwise normal without evidence of pyelectasia on either side. There was no evidence for masses or infiltrative lesions. Other analytes on routine biochemistry are normal. What diagnostic tests should be done, and how should the cat be managed?

A: Serum ionized calcium should be evaluated. The cat's body should be carefully examined and palpated for masses that could be associated with hypercalcemia. A panel of calciotrophic hormones (e.g. PTH, calcitriol, 25-hydroxycholcalciferol, and PTHrP) should be determined. If the PTH and PTHrP are low and the 25(OH)-vitamin D results normal, the cat likely has idiopathic hypercalcemia (IHC).

FAQ-96 I usually expect a cat with recent clinical LUT signs of irritative voiding to be positive for hematuria and proteinuria on UA. Sometimes the urine is surprisingly devoid of any abnormal elements or protein. These cats appear to have cystitis, but I cannot prove that based on results from UA. Can a cat have classic signs of cystitis and yet have a relatively normal UA?

A: YES. Although hematuria and proteinuria are often detected during an active clinical episode of FIC, this disease is characterized by a waxing and waning course. It depends on the precise timing that the urine was collected during this process. Another urine shortly after the first one may reveal hematuria and proteinuria.

FAQ-97 I am wondering about the significance of "rafts" of nonsquamous epithelial cells (urothelial cells) detected during urine microscopy of voided urine from an older female dog that has had recurrent bacterial UTI over the past six months. Is this more significant than the finding of free nonsquamous epithelial cells?

A: YES in many instances. Desquamation of urothelial cells into the urine can occur during bacterial UTI, urolithiasis, and urothelial carcinoma (UCC or TCC). The desquamation of occasional free urothelial cells into urinary sediment can be observed in any of these conditions. The finding of "rafts" – aggregated clusters of urothelial cells – is more alarming for its potential to indicate UCC. The nature of the cells within the rafts is very important to help distinguish cancer from reactive changes secondary to inflammation and or trauma. Sometimes, changes in the cells within the raft are highly suggestive for neoplasia, but the call as to neoplastic or reactive is better made on dry-mount cytology of urine sediment.

The finding of free urothelial cells or rafts of urothelial cells in the absence of many WBC and bacteria increases the chances that these cells are neoplastic. Many dogs with UCC (TCC) have increases in urothelial cells and RBC in urinary sediment as the predominant change. Since about half of dogs with UCC (TCC) have a bacterial UTI at the same time, the findings of bacteria and increased numbers of WBC along with increased RBC make it difficult to know for certain how much of the increase in urothelial cells is from a reactive or neoplastic process.

Other supportive findings on physical examination and urinary tract imaging bias the interpretation for the finding of increased numbers of urothelial cells during urine microscopy. Bladder or urethral masses identified on palpation or imaging (contrast urography or ultrasonography) increase the likelihood that an increased number of urothelial cells in the urine sediment have arisen from neoplasia.

Full histopathological evaluation of tissue samples from the bladder or urethra is the gold standard to distinguish inflammatory from neoplastic disease. If tissue biopsy is not feasible, positive Cadet BRAF and CADET BRAF PLUS test results (based on PCR to detect mutations in cells shed into urine) can be helpful. The BRAF mutation is detected in approximately 85% of dogs with UCC. CADET® *BRAF* PLUS detects DNA copy number changes and is used for dogs with clinical signs of TCC/UCC that are not associated with a *BRAF* mutation, increasing the overall sensitivity to detect a TCC/UCC to over 95% for eligible samples.

FAQ-98 When I see abnormal cells during urine microscopy, is it better to send an entire urine sample to the laboratory or should I make smears of the urine sediment for urine cytology and send those?

A: Send BOTH. Sending a dry-mount cytology slide of urinary sediment from a fresh urine sample allows cellular morphology to be preserved in case that the cells decreased in number or quality during storage and transport of the urine sample sent to the laboratory.

FAQ-99 I have identified clusters or "rafts" of highly malignant appearing urothelial cells during urine microscopy of a dog with stranguria. An increased number of RBC was the only other significant finding during urine microscopy. The urine was collected by initial, mid-stream, and end-stream voiding. The cytology of the urine sediment was highly supportive for UCC. Ultrasonography and contrast cystography failed to document any masses. Where is the UCC located?

A: It is not possible to determine the LUT origin of urothelial cell rafts based on their appearance alone. It becomes more likely that the tumor is within the urethra, as that area is difficult to image completely during ultrasonography. A rectal exam should be performed with bias toward palpation of the urethra. A thickened urethra in associated with urothelial rafts is highly supportive, but not pathognomonic, for UCC of the urethra. Proliferative urethritis is the other major differential diagnosis. Urethrocystoscopy is the imaging technique most likely to disclose the location and extent of disease in these instances.

FAQ-100 Is there any difference in the clinical interpretation of excess WBC in the urine that are free compared to clusters or clumps of WBC?

A: YES. I believe that a clinical distinction is likely despite lack of study in this area. Free WBC enter the urine during any type of inflammatory process, most commonly with bacterial UTI. The finding of an increased number of free WBC in association with bacteria in the urinary sediment usually means that a bacterial UTI is present (based on large quantitative bacterial growth in the microbiology laboratory). Clumps of WBC most often develop, in my opinion, from an infectious agent that is causing the WBC to clump, whether or not the infectious agent is easily seen in other areas during urine microscopy. Close inspection of the clump of WBC often reveals bacteria between the WBC. This finding is most helpful in suggesting UTI as the diagnosis when bacteria are not identified elsewhere during urine microscopy.

FAQ-101 Is there any clinical significance to the finding of phagocytized bacteria within WBC during urine microscopy?

A: YES. Since it takes some time for WBC to engulf bacteria in the urine, this means the bacteria in the urine were not added from contamination during the urine collection and thus occurred within the urinary tract.

FAQ-102 I have a 10-month-old female Weimaraner presented for a history of severe hematuria (identified when the dog urinated on a snowbank). Although shocking to the owner, the hematuria seems to be of no concern to the dog (no straining, no increased frequency, and no apparent pain). Routine UA shows too numerous to count RBC in the sediment but no other abnormal elements. Urine culture was negative and imaging studies with survey radiographs and ultrasonography revealed no lesions within the upper and LUT. Could this be a case of idiopathic benign hematuria?

A: Idiopathic benign hematuria is rare, and the diagnosis should always be approached with some skepticism. However, if no other cause for the hematuria can be identified, it should be considered. Painless hematuria is the hallmark of upper urinary tract bleeding. Renal neoplasia must be considered in these instances, but this diagnosis would be unusual in such a young dog. Coagulopathy would be an unusual cause for this presentation as the only site for bleeding; thrombocytopenia should be excluded from the start.

Cystoscopy should be performed to evaluate the urine emanating from the ureteral orifices in the trigone region. In most dogs with idiopathic benign hematuria, the blood comes only from one kidney, but it sometimes is observed from the other kidney at a later time.

The dog may be managed conservatively until it can be determined if the hemorrhage will be long-standing or severe enough to cause anemia. The obviously affected kidney should be preserved if possible, since bleeding can occur at another time in the contralateral kidney.

Newer knowledge suggests that this type of renal bleeding may not really be "idiopathic" since the endoscopic visualization of the renal pelvis can disclose a bleeding vascular lesion that can be cauterized in some instances. Also, the sequential occlusion of the branches of the renal artery to the affected kidney can stop the renal bleeding at other times.

FAQ-103 Should I ignore reports of hyaline casts at two to four per LPF reported from a UA as part of a wellness examination of an older dog? Her CBC and routine biochemistry were normal. Her USG was 1.047; her chemistry dipstrip showed a trace protein reaction, pH of 5.5, negative blood, negative glucose, negative ketones, and negative bilirubin.

A: No. You should not ignore the detection of hyaline cylindruria; it could be an artifact of no importance if their presence is transient, or it could represent something brewing in the kidney. Up to two hyaline casts per LPF can be considered "normal" especially in highly concentrated urine. The combination of the 1.047 USG and the 5.5 pH favor the precipitation of Tamm–Horsfall protein (THP) that comprises hyaline casts. The presence of hyaline casts at four per LPF is higher than usual, but still might be normal in this particular situation. It would be good to repeat the urine microscopy on other urine samples to see if the hyaline cylindruria persists or not. It would be useful to know if the hyaline casts persist in urine samples that are less concentrated, as is more likely to occur in urine within a few hours after eating and drinking.

Hyaline cylindruria is the least consistent cast that can indicate renal disease. This cast easily forms and easily dissolves (especially in alkaline urine). There are quite a few non-renal factors that can contribute to hyaline cast formation, including passive congestion to the kidney, fever, seizures, and "stress," but these conditions are also usually associated with proteinuria. Protein within tubular lumens favors the precipitation of the THP matrix protein.

Since renal proteinuria favors hyaline cast formation, it would be good to quantitatively measure urine protein with UPC or MA. Trace protein on the dipstrip in a urine sample with a USG is likely to be "normal."

The persistence of chronic hyaline cylindruria is not normal and could indicate an ongoing nephropathy that should be followed. Hyaline cylindruria as the single abnormal finding during urine microscopy in an otherwise normal animal is not common. Urine should be sequentially followed since changes in urine often occur long before changes in serum biochemistry are detected. Trending USG, urinary proteins, BUN, serum creatinine, and SDMA should be charted.

FAQ-104   What is going on in a dog that is seemingly well, but the UA reveals three to five finely granular casts per LPF as the only microscopic finding of concern during a routine yearly visit. USG measured by the refractometer is 1.014 and there was a 1+ protein reaction on the dipstrip. There are no previous UA results for comparison. CBC is normal. Serum creatinine is mildly increased at 1.9 mg/dL (reference range <1.5 mg/dL). The serum creatinine was repeated over the next month, and it was still increased to the same magnitude. He is a seven-year-old castrated male mixed-breed dog weighing 54 lbs (60 lbs last year); level of activity and appetite are good.

A: Up to one granular cast per LPF can be normal in concentrated urine. This urine is isosthenuric, so any reported casts are of concern. The 1+ dipstrip proteinuria is likely to be pathological and should be followed up with a UPC. The proteinuria and granular cylindruria are of concern in the face of isosthenuria and mild azotemia.

Granular casts are most often thought to arise from the intrarenal degeneration of cells that entered the tubular lumens. Accelerated renal tubular degeneration from any cause should be considered, including that from subacute leptospirosis. An alternative explanation is that the granules within the cast formed as precipitates of plasma proteins that have entered the tubular fluid. The UPC in this case was 2.7 in the face of an inactive sediment (except for the granular cylindruria), so renal proteinuria is a distinct possibility due to loss of glomerular barrier integrity.

Even though the dog appears to be normal to the owners, something is brewing at a high enough level within the kidneys to decrease the level of functional renal mass. Weight loss is often a clinical sign associated with progressive CKD. All the causes for glomerular proteinuria and development of CKD should be reviewed and investigated.

FAQ-105   Is there any clinically important difference in the finding of coarsely versus finely granular casts during urine microscopy? I have a dehydrated sick cat with both finely and coarsely granular cylindruria reported in the UA.

A: YES, though this is not often appreciated. It is likely that coarse granules in these casts are the result of renal tubular cell degeneration. Finely granular casts can arise from both cellular degeneration and plasma protein precipitates. My impression is that coarsely granular casts are associated with more aggressive acute (or acute on chronic) kidney diseases. In those with coarsely granular casts, degenerating cells within the cast can be seen at times, which supports the notion that the coarse granules arose from cells. Standard textbooks assert that there is no difference for clinical interpretation between the finding of finely or coarsely granular casts. Some laboratories report only as granular casts without description as to whether they are finely or coarsely granular, which I think is unfortunate.

FAQ-106   Why are RBC casts never reported in UA from my patients?

A: These are the most fragile of the cellular casts and breakup very quickly after the urine has been collected. If they were there in the first place, they are not going to be seen during urine microscopy performed after 15–30 minutes following collection.

Pure RBC casts are rarely found in those with various renal diseases even when examining urine sediment within minutes of urine collection. RBC casts are more likely to be found in aggressive acute diseases of the glomerulus (such as RPGN), which are not very common in veterinary medicine.

RBC mixed in with RTE and WBC are seen on occasion, but their origin may not be glomerular. The RBC in these instances enter the cast at the same place that the WBC and RTE enter.

RBC casts are very unlikely to ever be seen and reported from urine samples that have been stored and shipped to a reference laboratory. Since these casts often form in the sickest animals, urine microscopy of fresh warm urine is needed in order to know that they are there. RBC casts are most likely to be identified in animals presenting to emergency critical care services, IF the urine sample is examined immediately.

It is possible that RBC casts also occur in less severe glomerular diseases, but a concerted effort to examine fresh urine quickly is not generally performed in veterinary medicine or veterinary nephrology.

FAQ-107   What is the significance for the finding of WBC casts during microscopy? I have an azotemic CKD cat that has not been doing well. 0–1 WBC casts per LPF were found during urine microscopy. No other type of cast or abnormal element was identified in the urinary sediment.

A: The finding of even one cellular cast is important as it indicates activity within the kidney. The reporting of WBC casts is uncommon in veterinary medicine since they do not occur in many renal diseases and they break up quickly after they are formed. I suspect that you examined fresh warm urine to even know that they were there.

The finding of WBC casts identifies renal inflammation, most commonly caused by bacterial pyelonephritis. Bacteria were not identified within the cast or free in the urine; urine culture was negative. The negative urine culture does NOT exclude the possibility for active pyelonephritis from bacteria. Free WBC at <5 per HPF were considered normal.

Pure WBC casts are sometimes identified during acute interstitial nephritis, but mixed cell types (RBC, WBC, epithelial cell) are more common. Eosinophils can comprise many of the WBC in these instances when caused by drug allergy. WBC mixed in casts with RBC and RTE occurs at times in those with acute interstitial nephritis, acute tubular necrosis, and active glomerular disease. WBC within casts that have undergone extensive degeneration may be reported as granular casts and can be easily confused with RTE.

FAQ-108 How concerned should I be about the identification of one to two RTE cellular casts per HPF during urine microscopy? These casts were first identified at day 5 of treatment with amikacin. We perform a "cast watch" as part of a surveillance program while any of our patients are treated with a nephrotoxin. I am treating a dog that has severe pneumonia with a standard dose of amikacin; this dog had normal renal function and a resistant organism isolated from a tracheal wash before treatment was started. UA prior to treatment was considered normal with a USG of 1.034, negative protein on dipstrip, and an inactive urinary sediment.

A: The presence of RTE cellular casts indicates that the renal tubules are undergoing a severe insult. The nephrotoxin must be stopped immediately to stop further renal injury. Unfortunately, further renal injury may still occur, especially since aminoglycosides (AG) persist within the renal tissues for a long time. The appearance of RTE within casts or free RTE in the urine can occur before a decrease in USG, an increase in urinary protein, or an increase in serum creatinine or SDMA.

    The RTE cast most often forms following the agglutination of damaged RTE as they desquamate into the renal tubular lumen and matrix protein. Conglutination is when an area of continuous RTE sloughs into the tubular lumen and is associated with more severe renal injury. In these instances, there is no matrix protein in the cast.

FAQ-109 Is the prognosis worse in renal disease patients in which waxy casts are identified?

A: Yes. Waxy casts can form in any specific type of CKD, in which local nephron stasis is substantial. In the traditional theory, waxy casts develop as the final transformational product following degeneration of cells to granular and then to waxy in composition (translucent material). This process takes the longest time for any cast to develop within the kidney. In order for this to occur, the earlier forms of cast material must be retained within the tubules for a long enough time for this to occur, suggesting local nephron stasis of urine flow. Otherwise, granular casts would be excreted instead.

    In an alternate theory, waxy casts form following the prolonged retention of hyaline casts with the tubular lumens. In both theories, waxy cast formation requires substantial intrarenal retention time in order to allow the waxy protein to fully develop.

    Waxy casts are very stable and can be identified in the urine long after other types of casts have disintegrated.

FAQ-110 Is the prognosis always worse in patients that have "broad casts" identified during urine microscopy? A current patient has 0–2 "broad" granular casts per LPF and 1–2 "broad" hyaline casts per LPF. Urine microscopy also revealed 5–10 WBC per HPF, 3–5 RBC per HPF, 3 hyaline casts per HPF, and occasional granular casts. This urine came from a dog with stable CKD that has gradually progressed from a serum creatinine of 2.3 mg/dL to 4.1 mg/dL over the past six months. 1+ protein on chemistry dipstrip and a USG of 1.013 were also noted.

A: YES, in general. Broad casts are much wider than the usual casts indicating that they formed in the CT or in pathologically dilated portions of the tubules. They are often two to three times the width of standard sized casts. In this setting, the finding of broad casts is more ominous for the prognosis than in those without them. Sometimes following the conversion of oligo-anuria to greater urine volume production, broad casts can suddenly appear in the urine, a scenario that can have a better prognosis.

FAQ-111 What comprises the background material, sometimes particulate in nature, that I occasionally observe during urine microscopy?

A: Not all things observed during urine sediment microscopy can be identified. This material is often referred to as "debris" of unknown origin. This debris could represent cellular breakdown detritus that is normal, or breakdown from increased numbers of cellular elements in the sediment. A peculiar type of background debris is sometimes observed during urine microscopy from patients with severe forms of AKI, likely following tubular necrosis. The terms "mung" or "gradeaux" are colloquial or slang terms sometimes used to describe this debris.

CHAPTER 7 – PROTEINURIA

FAQ-112 Is there any reason to order a UPC or microalbuminuria test if the dipstick for protein is negative or only shows only a trace?

A: YES, especially in those with minimally concentrated urine. In animals with suspected renal disease, systemic hypertension, HAC, or hyperthyroidism, the UPC or microalbuminuria test may detect proteinuria indicative of early renal damage because these tests detect much lower concentrations of protein than does the dipstick methodology.

    In many instances a trace or 1+ protein dipstrip reaction in highly concentrated urine will be associated with a negative MA and an UPC <0.2.

FAQ-113 Is there any reason to order a UPC test if the dipstick for protein is 1+ or 2+ on a urine sample with a specific gravity of 1.050 and negative urine sediment examination?

A: YES. This magnitude of proteinuria on dipstick evaluation could be pathologic or could be a consequence of the concentrated nature of the urine sample. The UPC corrects for the concentrated nature of the urine since both the numerator and denominator will be similarly affected by the magnitude of urine concentration.

FAQ-114 Urinalysis on a voided urine sample from a dog with stranguria shows dark pink color, 100–150 red blood cells per high-power field (RBCs/HPF), 20–30 WBCs/HPF, and 3+ proteinuria on dipstick analysis. The urine UPC was 4.7 (normal <0.5). Is the UPC reliable in this situation?

A: No, at least not for figuring out if the proteinuria is renal in origin with certainty. There certainly are abnormal amounts of protein in the urine sample, but the origin of the proteinuria remains obscure. The urinary sediment is very active with RBC and WBC which can result in some increase in the measurement of urinary protein. Also, it is likely that plasma proteins can enter the urine at the site(s) that WBC and RBC enter the urine during bleeding or inflammation. We are clinically interested in determining if proteins in the urine came from the kidneys or not. It is likely that some, if not all, of the proteinuria is emanating from a LUT disease in this dog, based on clinical signs and the magnitude of the urinary sediment activity.

It is still possible that some of the proteinuria is renal in origin, but this is not currently possible to distinguish given the sediment activity. The repeat measurement of the UPC after the underlying LUT disease has been successfully treated and the urinary sediment has become inactive will then allow the UPC to determine if there are still relevant amounts of protein in the urine that is likely coming from the kidneys.

The conventional wisdom that the UPC cannot be used to determine renal proteinuria in those with an active sediment has been challenged in recent times. Some with an active sediment do not increase their UPC as might be anticipated. I do not recommend measurement of a UPC or MA in those with pink or red urine due to the possibility that the protein is coming from the same place where all the RBC emanate. Renal proteinuria is most readily determined when the urine sediment is inactive.

FAQ-115 When should angiotensin-converting enzyme (ACE) inhibitors or an angiotensin II receptor blocker (ARB) be administered to dogs or cats with CKD?

A: Conventional wisdom dictates that renin–angiotensin–aldosterone system (RAAS) inhibition with an angiotensin-converting enzyme inhibitor (ACE-I) or an ARB will lessen glomerular proteinuria, but that does not always translate into an increased survival benefit for dogs and cats. Greater stability of CKD (less progression) has been shown in some studies of dogs and cats with CKD that were treated with benazepril. ACE inhibitors and ARB lower high intraglomerular pressure (glomerular hypertension) by preferentially dilating the efferent arteriole which decreases GFR, transglomerular pressures, and glomerular proteinuria.

Conventional renin–angiotensin–aldosterone system inhibition (RAAS-I) is prescribed during CKD only if the patient has glomerular proteinuria that potentially can be mitigated and followed. This path of reasoning may be flawed. Assuming that most animals with naturally occurring renal disease also suffer from glomerular hypertension in remnant nephrons, it is logical to provide treatment designed to decrease the glomerular hypertension thought to be pivotal in

the progression of CKD, whether or not they have glomerular proteinuria. The main drawback of treatment in this situation is that there is no marker to follow showing that the treatment is effective or it is not, as is the case in those with proteinuria.

RAAS-I can be effective in the treatment of systemic hypertension associated with CKD, though usually not as powerful a lowering effect as that achieved with a calcium channel blocker (amlodipine). It is a good thing to lessen increased systemic blood pressure so that this increased blood pressure is not transmitted to already damaged glomerular beds in those with CKD and already existing glomerular hypertension. Reduction in systemic blood pressure is often associated with a decline in glomerular proteinuria.

FAQ-116 Should I consider treatment with an ACE-I or ARB in order to mitigate renal proteinuria in patients without azotemia?

A: YES, if there is enough renal proteinuria. The ACVIM Consensus statement from 2005 recommends treatment for this group if they have a UPC ≥2.0. This makes sense since most nephrologists think that glomerular proteinuria is a risk factor for the progression of CKD and possibly its development initially. An even stronger argument for this type of treatment can be made if hypoalbuminemia exists or serum albumin trending in that direction. The use of this treatment should not be employed, when possible, until after infectious diseases and attendant immune responses have been excluded or treated as the cause for renal proteinuria.

It is always a good idea to measure systemic blood pressure and ensure that normotension exists or is achieved post treatment with antihypertensive medications. The restoration of normotension from the hypertensive state is often associated with some decline in renal proteinuria, but it may not mitigate proteinuria to normal (UPC <0.2 or at least <0.5).

A detailed diet history needs to be collected and analyzed focusing on dietary protein intake (g/100 kcal). Some dogs with renal proteinuria are consuming high dietary protein and if so, changing to a lower protein content diet can mitigate the degree of renal proteinuria in some instances.

If the dog is already consuming a moderate to low protein in the diet, pharmacological intervention to provide RAAS inactivation is the next step using an ACE-I or an ARB.

FAQ-117 I have failed to gain adequate control of renal proteinuria in a dog with CKD despite enalapril dose escalation to 1.0 mg/kg twice daily. Systemic diseases that can create renal proteinuria were not found. The dog is also eating a renal diet. The initial UPC was 3.8 and the UPC after treatment has not substantially changed (3.2–4.3). Systolic blood pressure remains normal. Is there anything more I can do to further lower the amount of renal proteinuria?

A: Residual proteinuria is the term used to describe a higher than desired amount of proteinuria following treatment. Dietary protein reduction can lower renal proteinuria (lower UPC), but there is often residual proteinuria. ACE-I can be successful in restoration of UPC to a lower level but not always to <0.5. A decrease in UPC of at least 50% from baseline is a reasonable goal in many instances. Dose escalation with enalapril has not been successful in mitigating the renal proteinuria in this case. Adding in an ARB on top of the ACE-I or swapping out the ACE-I for an ARB (telmisartan) can be successful in gaining further reduction in the UPC. Recent evidence in both the dog and the cat shows that the ARB telmisartan exerts more anti-proteinuria effects than an ACE-I.

Adding in an MRB such as spironolactone on top of an ACE-I or an ARB can further lessen renal proteinuria in some cases. MRB are not usually chosen for monotherapy. When dual or triple therapy is employed to provide RAAS-I, it is important to ensure that sodium and potassium levels in the blood do not change much.

It is possible that all efforts to reduce renal proteinuria fail. This could happen because the glomerular disease is severe and the glomeruli remain leaky despite favorable changes in glomerular hemodynamics that usually lessen the transglomerular passage of plasma proteins. It is also possible that the proteinuria is tubular in origin, in which case the above treatments would not be expected to work.

FAQ-118 Is it true that treatment with ACE inhibitors or an ARB can create or aggravate azotemia?

A: YES in some patients, especially those with azotemic CKD. Patients with azotemic CKD have high intraglomerular pressures that maintain a high single-nephron GFR (super nephrons following nephron mass loss) as part of the compensatory response to nephron mass loss. High single-nephron GFR is maintained by some combination of afferent arteriolar dilatation and or efferent arteriolar constriction.

Intraglomerular pressure will decrease during RAAS-I (ACE-I, ARB). This causes single-nephron GFR to decline as there is now less efferent arteriolar vasoconstriction (less AG-II generated, or less AG-II effect at its receptor) to provide resistance that drives filtration. Consequently, BUN, serum creatinine, and SDMA concentrations can increase to some degree during treatment depending on the magnitude of decreased GFR that ensues. A 20–30% increase in serum creatinine concentration above baseline is generally considered acceptable and indicates that the drug has had a measurable effect to lower intraglomerular pressure. Most patients showing this magnitude of increase in serum creatinine do not show worsening of clinical signs.

In some CKD animals, there is no increase in the blood concentration for surrogates of GFR following treatment. This could happen because single-nephron GFR did not decrease enough to document impaired excretory function in blood tests. Alternatively, less AG-II effect can result in mesangial cell relaxation and increased glomerular surface area available for filtration with attendant increased GFR. It is possible to reduce intraglomerular pressure (a desired endpoint to help damaged glomeruli to survive longer in CKD), which will decrease GFR, but this effect then might be countervailed by increased glomerular surface area available for filtration resulting in a net change of close to zero in GFR.

Some CKD patients experience a spike in their serum creatinine values, but often this is within tolerable limits. These minor increases in serum creatinine often return to baseline values. In some patients, the serum creatinine continues to decrease over time suggesting an ongoing salutary effect on the excretory function within the damaged glomeruli.

FAQ-119 Is benazepril preferable to enalapril for treatment of renal proteinuria or systemic hypertension in dogs and cats with CKD?

A: There is no obvious advantage to either one over the other. Both benazepril and enalapril are prodrugs. Benazeprilat and enalaprilat are the active forms of the drug following the metabolism of the parent molecules, and both are cleared by the kidneys. Benazeprilat undergoes more clearance by the liver than enalaprilat, and less benazeprilat accumulates in the serum in patients with CKD, so this is a potential advantage. Both drugs have similar ability to inhibit ACE. It appears that there is little if any difference in the clinical effects between these drugs in their ability to decrease glomerular proteinuria or to decrease systemic hypertension.

FAQ-120 Is it safe to prescribe ACE-I or ARB to CKD patients that are in late IRIS stage 3 or stage 4 patients?

A: The notion that it is dangerous to provide RAAS-I to CKD patients with more advanced azotemia (more severe decreases in GFR) is commonly accepted in veterinary medicine, but there are known salutary effects from RAAS-I in some studies of humans with more advanced azotemia. It is true that dogs and cats with more severe azotemia are more fragile and that less AG-II effect during such treatment could further decrease GFR to such an extent that serum creatinine will increase too much for the animal to tolerate. In those with more advanced azotemia during CKD, starting at lower doses once daily and then escalating the dose gradually as needed to effect can be effectively employed in some instances without greatly increasing the level of azotemia. There will be some cases that do not tolerate even low dose protocols.

FAQ-121 Is it true that providing RAAS-I with ACE-I or ARB treatment in CKD patients is likely to mitigate renal proteinuria only when the patient also has systemic hypertension?

A: No. Successful RAAS-I can lower intraglomerular pressure, decrease proteinuria, and slow progression of CKD independent of their effects on systemic blood pressure. It is true that a return to normal systemic blood pressure often reduces glomerular proteinuria to some degree, but additional antiproteinuria effects are gained from the beneficial intraglomerular hemodynamic changes.

FAQ-122 I have been taught that renal biopsy does not change how CKD will be managed in most patients. Is renal biopsy of any value in dogs or cats with CKD, especially those with renal proteinuria?

A: YES. Renal biopsy to establish a specific diagnosis has always had value to distinguish renal amyloidosis from GN, or AKI from CKD. To refine the prognosis, it is important to know if renal proteinuria during CKD is from amyloidosis, as this is a relentless progressive disease. Some cases of GN are slowly progressive, and some can be treated if they are found to be immune-complex mediated.

YES for renal biopsy to have a precise histopathological diagnosis IF a comprehensive microscopic evaluation of the renal tissue will be conducted. This includes light microscopy with special stains, IFA, and TEM in order to really know what is going on. Evaluation by only light microscopy will allow the differentiation of amyloidosis from other glomerulopathies, but any other specific glomerulopathy will not be able to identified. Comprehensive biopsy results are needed to determine whether the disease is likely to be a familial nephropathy/glomerulopathy or if it is immune-complex mediated. Now that we perform many more comprehensive renal biopsies in proteinuric animals, we are learning the natural history of the specific glomerulopathy and what treatments are likely best for that particular disease.

Undergoing a renal biopsy is not a trivial procedure and is best performed in animals that have normal size or enlarged kidneys and those with minimal azotemia. Renal biopsy is not likely to change the treatment in those with advanced azotemia in CKD (serum creatinine >4.0 mg/dL) due to the degree of fibrosis and tubulointerstitial nephritis that often is already in place – it may not be possible to identify the initiating lesions in these instances. This rule is not etched in stone – we have on occasion biopsied the kidneys of proteinuric CKD patients with serum creatinine >4.0 mg/dL and normal sized kidneys. In this scenario, immune-complex GN can be identified in some patients, which then provides support to start immunosuppressive treatment.

FAQ-123   What is the risk to the CKD proteinuric patient that undergoes renal biopsy?

A: The benefit-to-risk ratio has been improved with the development of ULS-guided renal biopsy techniques. The quality of the biopsy and the safety for the trajectory of the biopsy needle are operator dependent. Despite a high experience and skill set of the operator, macroscopic renal hemorrhage can occur, but severe blood loss is uncommon. Microscopic RBC in urine sediment are expected for up to a week following the biopsy.

FAQ-124   A dog with weight loss has moderately concentrated urine (USG 1.026) and a UPC of 12.1. The reference laboratory indicates that amyloidosis is the likely diagnosis. Is this a reliable method to make a diagnosis of glomerular amyloidosis?

A: No. Although it is generally true that patients with glomerular amyloidosis tend to have the highest UPCs, glomerular amyloidosis cannot be reliably differentiated from GN by the magnitude of proteinuria alone. Some animals with amyloidosis have lower UPCs and patients with GN can have very high UPCs. Renal biopsy with use of appropriate stains (e.g. Congo red with polarizing light) and techniques (e.g. immunohistochemistry using peroxidase-antiperoxidase methodology) are necessary to accurately distinguish glomerular amyloidosis from GN on light microscopy.

FAQ-125   Should I worry about an adult dog with a UPC of 0.33 if all else is normal?

A: The UPC is in a gray area that could be normal, or it could indicate an early renal lesion. Normal UPC is <0.5, but most dogs are <0.2. The presence of microalbuminuria (<2.5 mg/dL is normal) would indicate some dysfunction of the glomerular barrier. The damage could have occurred in the past and be nonprogressive or the microalbuminuria could indicate an early stage of what may become progressive glomerular injury despite the absence of clinical signs. Thus, the follow-up monitoring of microalbuminuria in this asymptomatic dog is warranted. If microalbuminuria and the UPC increase over time, glomerular injury is ongoing, and its cause should be investigated because the animal potentially is at risk for the development of chronic renal disease and failure. Blood pressure also should be evaluated to see if systemic hypertension could be a factor contributing to the proteinuria.

FAQ-126   A dog with biopsy-confirmed glomerular amyloidosis has a serum creatinine concentration of 2.6 mg/dL, USG of 1.015, proteinuria of 3+ dipstrip analysis, and a UPC of 3.7. Several hyaline and waxy casts are observed on urine sediment examination. Serum albumin is normal. Given the grave prognosis for amyloidosis, should euthanasia be recommended to the owner?

A: No. Not yet in this particular patient since this dog is in late IRIS stage 2. Renal amyloidosis generally is a relentlessly progressive disease, and the presence of moderate to severe azotemia warrants a grave prognosis. The waxy and hyaline casts are related to the glomerular proteinuria in this dog. Most experience in veterinary medicine, however, has been with dogs with amyloidosis and advanced renal failure. Such patients have relatively short survival times (months). The prognosis may not be as grave when amyloidosis is discovered at an earlier stage (i.e. proteinuria with minimal azotemia). Survival time can be associated with serum amyloid A (SAA) concentrations in some species, but this has not been evaluated in dogs or cats. It is unknown whether or not treatment with ACE inhibitors is beneficial for dogs with glomerular amyloidosis, as is often the case with GN.

FAQ-127   Over the past month, a dog with CKD has had a stable serum creatinine concentration of 8.0–9.0 mg/dL. The urine sediment is inactive, the protein dipstrip reaction is 4+, and the UPC is greater than 10. The kidneys are hyperechoic and small on ULS examination. Should a renal biopsy be performed?

A: No. A renal biopsy is unlikely to be helpful in this situation and may be harmful. Technical difficulties are more likely when performing a biopsy of a small kidney. Renal bleeding may be substantial. Furthermore, the small kidneys may have extensive interstitial fibrosis, and it may not be possible to determine the underlying primary lesion (e.g. glomerular, interstitial, tubular) that led to chronic renal failure. The likelihood of obtaining useful diagnostic information is small compared with the risk of complications for the patient.

CHAPTER 10 Case Studies

| CASE EXAMPLE: | Urinalysis Case Number: 1 |

Source of Specimen:
    Cystocentesis ☐   Voided (Stream part) ☒   mid stream   Post-Void (location) ☐
    Expressed ☐   Catheterized ☐
Volume: 3 mL
Refrigeration: Yes ☐   No ☒
Elapsed Time Before Analysis: 30 minutes
Stain: Yes ☒   No ☐

Color: Brown
Appearance: Opaque
Specific Gravity: 1.039
pH: 7.0
Protein: 100 mg/dL
Occult Blood: 4+
    Hemolyzed: ☐
    Intact: ☐
Glucose: Negative
Ketones: Negative
Bilirubin: Negative

Casts per LPF:
    Hyaline 0
    Granular rare/LPF
    Cellular 0

WBC per HPF: 5–7/HPF
    Free   ☒
    Clumped   ☐
RBC per HPF: Too numerous to count
Epithelial Cells per HPF: 1–2/HPF.
    Type: Squamous: ☒   Transitional: Free ☐   Clumped ☐   Renal: ☐

Crystals per HPF: None ☒
    Type: Struvite ☐   Calcium Oxalate ☐   Urate ☐   Other ☐

Bacteria per HPF: None ☒
    Type: Rods ☐   Cocci ☐   Mixed ☐

Miscellaneous:

Urinalysis in the Dog and Cat, First Edition. Dennis J. Chew and Patricia A. Schenck.
© 2023 John Wiley & Sons, Inc. Published 2023 by John Wiley & Sons, Inc.

Signalment: Two-year-old spayed female Weimaraner dog.

History and Physical Examination: She has had pinkish-to-brown urine observed by the owners for at least six months. She is normal in every other respect, as is her physical examination. She has had no clinical urinary tract signs.

Interpretation of Urinalysis: The brown color to the urine is often due to the presence of hemoglobin oxidation products or myoglobin in the urine. Since there are TNTC RBC, the color is attributed to RBC and oxidation of hemoglobin. The urine is well concentrated at 1.039 USG. The pH of 7.0 could be in part accounted for by the amount of bleeding into the urine (plasma pH of 7.4). The 2+ protein on the dipstrip is likely from the proteins in the numerous RBC and plasma entering the urine. The rare granular cast per LPF is considered normal in the face of the 1.039 USG. The mild increase in WBC is most likely from the entry of blood into the urine; less likely it is from inflammation. The squamous epithelial cells are not of concern as they are almost always contaminants from the lower urogenital tract especially in samples collected during voiding or catheterization.

Hematuria is the most important finding in this urinalysis. There is a high amount of occult blood on dipstrip and RBC during microscopy. The origin of the RBC cannot be determined on findings from the urinalysis alone.

Further Diagnostics and Assessment: The finding of painless hematuria usually indicates upper urinary tract disease (kidneys, ureters). Differential diagnosis for painless hematuria should include renal neoplasia, nephrolithiasis, renal pelvic blood clot from trauma, and benign essential renal hematuria. Neoplasia is unlikely in a well dog with hematuria of this duration. Benign essential renal hematuria is the most likely consideration at this point.

A hemogram was normal with the exception of a mild microcytic anemia attribute to the chronic blood loss. Routine serum biochemistry was normal. Urine culture on a sample obtained by cystocentesis was negative.

Urinary tract imaging with radiographs and ultrasonography was normal. Urethrocystoscopy revealed no anatomical abnormalities, but bright red blood was seen from a urine jet emanating from the left ureteral orifice.

No treatment to interrupt the renal bleeding was provided. Iron supplementation over the next six months resulted in resolution of the microcytic anemia.

Final Diagnosis: Benign essential renal hematuria.

CASE EXAMPLE: Urinalysis Case Number: 2

Source of Specimen:
Cystocentesis ☒   Voided (Stream part) ☐   Post-Void (location) ☐
Expressed ☐   Catheterized ☐
Volume: 2   mL
Refrigeration: Yes ☐   No ☒
Elapsed Time Before Analysis: 40 mins
Stain: Yes ☐   No ☒

Color: Dark amber
Appearance: Cloudy
Specific Gravity: 1.039
pH: 6.5
Protein: 100 mg/dL
Occult Blood: 2+
   Hemolyzed: ☒
   Intact: ☒
Glucose: Negative
Ketones: Negative
Bilirubin: Negative

Casts per LPF: 0
   Hyaline
   Granular
   Cellular

WBC per HPF: 1–3
   Free   ☒
   Clumped   ☐
RBC per HPF: 15-20
Epithelial Cells per HPF: 1–3
   Type: Squamous: ☐   Transitional: Free ☒   Clumped ☐   Renal: ☐

Crystals per HPF: None ☐
   Type: Struvite ☒ Few   Calcium Oxalate ☐   Urate ☐   Other ☐

Bacteria per HPF: None ☐
   Type: Rods ☐   Cocci ☒ Moderate   Mixed ☐

Miscellaneous:

Signalment: Three-year-old spayed female Domestic Shorthair cat.

History and Physical Examination: The current owner complaint is pollakiuria, stranguria, and hematuria for the past four days. This cat does not always use the litterbox for urinations during the past year. The cat is otherwise normal. Abdominal palpation is normal with the exception of some discomfort during palpation of the bladder; no masses were detected.

Interpretation of Urinalysis: The occult blood positive reaction on the dipstrip and the increased numbers of RBC are the main abnormalities to be observed from this urinalysis. Some of the RBC may have been added by the cystocentesis method of urine collection. Sometimes during cystocentesis, the needle more readily adds RBC to the urine when there is an underlying inflammatory process in the bladder wall. There is no pyuria but there were a few extra free non squamous epithelial cells observed. Desquamation of urothelial cells can occur during urinary tract neoplasia and inflammation during cystitis or urolithiasis. A few struvite crystals were observed in urine that is well concentrated and with a pH of 6.5.

Moderate numbers of cocci that are reported are not aligned with an increase in the number of WBC, so there is suspicion that these bacteria may not be "real." Caution must be used in the interpretation of reported bacteria because many artifacts in urine can be misinterpreted as bacteria, especially in cats. Brownian motion of small particles in urine sometimes leads to the interpretation of these particles as bacteria. Small crystals, lipid droplets, cellular debris, mucus threads, and precipitated stain can all resemble bacteria.

Further Diagnostics and Assessment: Urinary tract imaging with abdominal radiographs and ultrasonography were normal, excluding the presence of urolithiasis. Urinary sediment cytology was negative for bacteria, and quantitative urine culture was negative for bacterial growth. The cocci described in the urinary sediment apparently were artifacts. Reports of bacteria on urine sediment examination that are not substantiated by bacterial culture of urine are common.

Crystalluria need not be present to diagnose idiopathic/interstitial cystitis, and most cats with this disorder have few or no crystals in their urine sediment, especially when consuming diets designed to promote urinary acidification.

Final Diagnosis: Idiopathic/interstitial cystitis.

CASE EXAMPLE: Urinalysis Case Number: 3

Source of Specimen:

Cystocentesis ☐   Voided (Stream part) ☐   Post-Void (location) ☒ Floor/table/cage

Expressed ☐   Catheterized ☐

Volume: mL

Refrigeration: Yes ☒   No ☐

Elapsed Time Before Analysis: 6 hours

Stain: Yes ☒   No ☐

Color: Brown
Appearance: Cloudy
Specific Gravity: 1.024
pH: 8.0
Protein: 100 mg/dL
Occult Blood: 3+
  Hemolyzed: ☐
  Intact: ☒
Glucose: Negative
Ketones: Negative
Bilirubin: Negative

Casts per LPF: 0
  Hyaline
  Granular
  Cellular

WBC per HPF: 20–30
  Free   ☐
  Clumped   ☒
RBC per HPF: 10-20
Epithelial Cells per HPF: 4–6
  Type: Squamous: ☒   Transitional: Free ☒   Clumped ☐   Renal: ☐

Crystals per HPF: None ☒
  Type: Struvite ☒ Few   Calcium Oxalate ☐   Urate ☐   Other ☐

Bacteria per HPF: None ☐
  Type: Rods ☐   Cocci ☒ Few   Mixed ☐

Miscellaneous:

Signalment: Nine-year-old spayed female German Shepherd Dog.

History and Physical Examination: This dog had increased frequency and straining to urinate over the past three days with occasional urinary spotting "accidents" in the house. Some red discoloration was observed by the owners in the dog's urine, and an unusually strong odor was noticed. There was no change in water consumption or daily urine volume output. This dog had normal appetite, bowel movements, and attitude. A urine sample was collected by the owner from a small puddle on thee floor.

The dog is bright, alert, and hydration assessed as normal based on skin turgor. Mild mucopurulent vaginal discharge is noted. The bladder is small and possibly thickened on abdominal palpation; the dog is very uncomfortable during the palpation of the bladder.

Interpretation of Urinalysis: Urinalysis results are from a post-voided sample; it was aspirated from a urine puddle in the house by the owner. Since she has a vulvar discharge, it is likely that some inflammatory elements will be picked up as the urine passes through the vestibule and vulva as a form of extra-urinary contamination.

Brown cloudy urine is abnormal and likely due to the inflammatory elements identified during urine microscopy. The USG of 1.024 shows at least modest urine concentrating capacity. Any consideration for a urinary concentrating defect cannot be made at this time as we do not know the time of the day and relationship to when the dog ate and drank as to when the sample was collected. Bacterial urinary infection can impair urine concentration at times.

The high urine pH (8.0) is compatible with infection by a urease-producing organism (e.g. *Staphylococcus aureus*, *Proteus* spp.). In this setting, urea is hydrolyzed to ammonium and carbonate ions. The carbonate ions bind hydrogen ions and remove them from solution resulting in more alkaline urine. Infection by cocci is suspected based on the appearance of the bacterial organisms in the urine sediment. The presumptive diagnosis is bacterial urinary tract infection, suspect for *S. aureus*.

The 2+ proteinuria on the dipstrip is attributed to postrenal contamination with proteins associated with the active urinary sediment.

The predominant element identified during urine microscopy was the WBC (20–30/HPF). Lesser numbers of RBC (10–20/HPF) accompany the WBC as part of an inflammatory process. Clumping of leukocytes in the urine often adds support for an underlying bacterial etiology. Contamination from the genital tract also must be considered because the sample was voided, and the dog had a mucopurulent vaginal discharge. The report of "few cocci" is likely to be real and not an artifact given the inflammatory response (WBC, RBC, and +2 protein). Increased numbers of squamous epithelial cells are likely from genital tract contamination from the voided sample. Increased numbers of nonsquamous epithelial cells (urothelial) are likely from desquamation association with the inflammatory process.

Further Diagnostics and Assessment: Based on the uncertainty for the origin of the elements in the active sediment on the voided urine sample, another sample was obtained by cystocentesis. All the urinalysis results were very similar, except that squamous epithelial cells were no longer identified. Culture of the sample collected by cystocentesis grew a pure culture of *S. aureus* at >30 000 cfu/mL that was susceptible to all the routine urinary antimicrobials.

Another option while awaiting urine culture results to return could have been to perform a urine cytology to confirm the presence of cocci.

Since *Staphylococcus* species are associated with initiation and growth of struvite stones in the dog, an abdominal radiograph was taken to exclude the presence of radiodense urinary calculi. None were found.

The dog's clinical signs resolved within three days of starting a 10-day course of oral amoxicillin. Given the age of the dog, if long-term response to treatment is poor, the clinician should consider additional diagnostic testing (e.g. contrast radiography, ultrasonography, and urine cytology) to rule out urinary tract neoplasia or other structural abnormality.

Final Diagnosis: Bacterial UTI due to *S. aureus*.

CASE EXAMPLE: Urinalysis Case Number: 4

Source of Specimen:
  Cystocentesis ☐   Voided (Stream part) ☐   Post-Void (location) ☐
  Expressed ☐   Catheterized ☒
Volume: mL
Refrigeration: Yes ☐   No ☒
Elapsed Time Before Analysis:
Stain: Yes ☒   No ☒

Color: Dark brown
Appearance: Turbid
Specific Gravity: 1.025
pH: 6.5
Protein: 100 mg/dL
Occult Blood: 3+
  Hemolyzed: ☒
  Intact: ☐
Glucose: Negative
Ketones: Negative
Bilirubin: Negative

Casts per LPF:
  Hyaline
  Granular 3–4
  Cellular

WBC per HPF: 3–6
  Free   ☒
  Clumped   ☐
RBC per HPF: 5-10
Epithelial Cells per HPF: 3–6
  Type: Squamous: ☐   Transitional: Free ☒   Clumped ☐   Renal: ☐

Crystals per HPF: None ☒
  Type: Struvite ☐   Calcium Oxalate ☐   Urate ☐   Other ☐

Bacteria per HPF: None ☒
  Type: Rods ☐   Cocci ☐   Mixed ☐

Miscellaneous: Many precipitates of hemoglobin with varying size globules

Signalment: Three-year-old intact male Great Dane.

History and Physical Examination: Vomiting and anorexia of one-week duration were noted. The owner reports red to dark urine over the past few days without any urinary distress (no stranguria, pollakiuria, or dysuria). Daily urine volume is about the same as usual, and there is no increased thirst. There is no history of trauma and no exposure to rodenticides.

The dog was painful on abdominal palpation and the spleen was markedly enlarged. The mucous membranes were slightly pale.

Interpretation of Urinalysis: Dark brown turbid urine is attributed to the +3-occult blood reaction that is mostly from free hemoglobin in the urine (positive for hemolyzed blood but not for intact RBC). There were only minor increases in the WBC and intact RBC during urine microscopy. Increased transitional epithelial cells are attributed to urinary catheterization used to collect the urine sample.

The urine is moderately concentrated with a USG of 1.025. The strong occult blood reaction is mostly due to the presence of free hemoglobin in the urine (very few RBC were identified in the sediment and the occult blood was negative for intact RBC). Based on later laboratory data, the positive protein reaction on the dipstrip is attributed to prerenal delivery of free hemoglobin from hemolysis into the urine.

The presence of granular cast cylindruria identified during urine microscopy is of concern for the possibility of AKI and accelerated renal tubular degeneration. Alternatively, granules within the casts could result from precipitates of hemoglobin into the cast matrix protein following systemic hemolysis.

Precipitated hemoglobin in the urine sediment can sometimes be confused with red blood cells; therefore, the sediment should be reviewed to confirm that the reported red blood cells do not represent precipitated hemoglobin (hemoglobin pigmenturia versus hematuria). In this particular case, numerous precipitates of hemoglobin were initially identified as intact RBC in error, but upon closer inspection, these globules varied widely in size, unlike for RBC.

Hemoglobinuria following systemic hemolysis can be associated with several conditions in dogs, including transfusion reaction, disseminated intravascular coagulation, postcaval dirofilariasis syndrome, heat stroke, zinc toxicity, severe hypophosphatemia, red cell enzyme deficiencies, and autoimmune hemolytic anemia. The young age of the dog and the presence of splenomegaly on physical examination led to the suspicion of splenic torsion.

The presumptive diagnosis was splenic torsion with hemoglobinuria and possible hemoglobinuric nephrosis.

Further Diagnostics and Assessment: The hemogram disclosed moderate anemia (PCV 27%) with target cells, polychromasia, and red cell fragmentation supporting the finding of a hemolytic process. The platelet count was 78 000 μlL. A biochemical profile was normal except for a mild increase in alkaline phosphatase (178 IU/L). The heartworm and Coombs' tests were negative, but fibrin degradation products were detected in serum.

Abdominal radiographs confirmed marked splenomegaly and ultrasonography showed diffuse enlargement of the spleen with uniform echogenicity. Exploratory laparotomy revealed splenic torsion and splenectomy was performed.

The mechanism of hemolysis and hemoglobinuria in splenic torsion is unknown but may be due to microangiopathy and damage to red cells by intraluminal fibrin strands. This is supported by the presence of red cell fragments on the hemogram. The presence of thrombocytopenia and fibrin degradation products support a diagnosis of concurrent disseminated intravascular coagulation. Renal damage as indicated by the presence of granular casts was subclinical, and azotemia did not develop in this dog.

Final Diagnosis: Splenic torsion with systemic hemolysis and DIC; probable hemoglobinuric nephrosis; prerenal proteinuria.

CASE EXAMPLE: Urinalysis Case Number: 5

Source of Specimen:
    Cystocentesis ☒   Voided (Stream part) ☐   Post-Void (location) ☐
    Expressed ☐   Catheterized ☐
Volume: mL
Refrigeration: Yes ☐   No ☒
Elapsed Time Before Analysis:
Stain: Yes ☐   No ☒

Color:	Straw
Appearance:	Slightly cloudy
Specific Gravity:	1.019
pH:	6.5
Protein:	100 mg/dL
Occult Blood:	1+
Hemolyzed:	☐
Intact:	☐
Glucose:	Negative
Ketones:	Negative
Bilirubin:	Negative

Casts per LPF: 0
    Hyaline
    Granular
    Cellular

WBC per HPF: 30–40
    Free   ☐
    Clumped   ☒
RBC per HPF: 10–15
Epithelial Cells per HPF: 5–7
    Type: Squamous: ☐   Transitional: Free ☒   Clumped ☐   Renal: ☐

Crystals per HPF: None ☒
    Type: Struvite ☐   Calcium Oxalate ☐   Urate ☐   Other ☐

Bacteria per HPF: None ☐
    Type: Rods ☒ Few   Cocci ☐   Mixed ☐

Miscellaneous:

Signalment: Seven-year-old spayed female Domestic Shorthair cat.

History and Physical Examination: This cat stopped eating during the past week and is less active; the owners are unsure of water consumption and urine output. They have noted an increased volume/weight of clumping litter in the litter box in recent times. The owners also suspect mild weight loss over the past several months.

The cat was thin and had reduced skin turgor. We do not have a previous weight with which to compare today's weight. The kidneys were small and irregular, and the cat resisted palpation that was interpreted to be pain. A small thyroid nodule on the left side was suspected on palpation of the neck. The bladder was moderately full. The cat had a grade II/VI right sternal border systolic murmur. Systolic blood pressure was 175 mmHg on repeated measurements.

Interpretation of Urinalysis: The slightly cloudy appearance to the urine sample is attributed to the active urine sediment findings. The 1.019 USG is far less than should occur in a cat with dehydration based on skin turgor changes and anorexia. The 2+ dipstrip proteinuria is abnormal, especially in urine that is minimally concentrated and is likely associated with the inflammatory findings in the urine sediment. The protein could be renal or postrenal in origin. The 1+ occult blood for intact RBC matches up with the 10–15 RBC per HPF seen on urine microscopy. The RBC are likely originating from the same process adding WBC to the urine, but some RBC could have been added from the trauma of cystocentesis.

The finding of 30–40 WBC per HPF, 10–15 RBC per HPF, 5–7 free transitional cells per HPF, and few rod bacteria on urine microscopy from a sample collected by cystocentesis supports the presence of an inflammatory process caused by bacterial urinary infection. The report of rods in the urine is more convincing than the finding of cocci in general. Clumping of WBC often indicates that organisms are between the WBC causing the clumping. The site of the infection as upper or lower urinary tract cannot be determined.

The presence of small and irregular kidneys with pain upon palpation suggests the possibility of pyelonephritis superimposed on CKD. The possibility for hyperthyroidism exists, but this diagnosis is difficult to make with certainty in the face of nonthyroidal illness.

Further Diagnostics and Assessment: The hemogram disclosed leukocytosis (41 000/μL) due to neutrophilia (37 000/μL) and a left shift (2000 bands/μL). The PCV (28%) and plasma proteins (7.6 g/dL) were normal. The biochemical profile disclosed azotemia (BUN 68 mg/dL, creatinine 4.1 mg/dL), hyperphosphatemia (8.5 mg/dL), decreased serum bicarbonate (10 mEq/L), and mild hypokalemia (3.2 mEq/L). Serum thyroxine concentration was 2.1 μg/dL, well within the reference range.

Abdominal ultrasonography showed that the kidneys were smaller than normal and had increased medullary echogenicity. Mild pelvic dilatation also was noted.

Bacterial culture of the urine grew a pure culture of >30 000 cfu/mL of *Escherichia coli* that was susceptible to most of the common urinary antimicrobials.

The cat was treated with intravenous fluids and intravenous sodium cephalothin. There was improvement in the cat's attitude and appetite over the next four days. The cat was treated with cephalexin for two weeks.

At re-evaluation, the cat was doing well and had a good appetite. A hemogram showed resolution of the leukocytosis, but the PCV was now mildly decreased (21%). The biochemical profile showed improvement in azotemia (BUN 43 mg/dL, creatinine 2.6 mg/dL) and resolution of hypokalemia, metabolic acidosis, and hyperphosphatemia. Urinalysis on a urine sample collected by cystocentesis showed resolution of pyuria and no bacteria were observed. Urine specific gravity was 1.017. The protein on the dipstrip had declined to trace positive at this time.

Final Diagnosis: Azotemic CKD, *E. coli* bacterial UTI, pyelonephritis; hyperthyroidism is likely.

CASE EXAMPLE: Urinalysis Case Number: 6

Source of Specimen:
 Cystocentesis ☐ Voided (Stream part) ☐ Post-Void (location) ☒ Floor/table/cage
 Expressed ☐   Catheterized ☐
Volume: mL
Refrigeration: Yes ☐ No ☒
Elapsed Time Before Analysis: 10 minutes
Stain: Yes ☒ No ☐

Color: Light yellow
Appearance: Cloudy
Specific Gravity: 1.010
pH: 6.5
Protein: 30 mg/dL
Occult Blood: Trace
 Hemolyzed: ☐
 Intact: ☐
Glucose: Negative
Ketones: Negative
Bilirubin: Negative

Casts per LPF:
 Hyaline
 Granular
 Cellular 3-5 Renal Tubular Epithelial

WBC per HPF: 0–1
 Free   ☒
 Clumped ☐
RBC per HPF: 3–5
Epithelial Cells per HPF: 5–10
 Type: Squamous: ☐ Transitional: Free ☐ Clumped ☐ Renal: ☒

Crystals per HPF: None ☒
 Type: Struvite ☐   Calcium Oxalate ☐   Urate ☐   Other ☐

Bacteria per HPF: None ☒
 Type: Rods ☐   Cocci ☐   Mixed ☐

Miscellaneous: Many sperm

Signalment: Five-year-old intact male German Shepherd Dog.

History and Physical Examination: Presented to the emergency service for the evaluation of acute onset of vomiting and severe lethargy. The owner reports rapid breathing and possible exposure to antifreeze containing ethylene glycol.

Temperature was 100.1 F, respiratory rate was 60, and heart rate was 170. Pulses were weak. The dog was lethargic and estimated to be 8% dehydrated based on skin turgor and dryness of mucous membranes. Heart sounds were muffled, and lung sounds were normal. The dog became progressively weaker and collapsed during the exam.

Interpretation of Urinalysis: The initial urine sample was collected before any treatments were started. The USG of 1.010 in the face of dehydration indicates impaired urine concentration that could be caused by a number of different disorders, including ethylene glycol ingestion. An osmotic diuresis happens shortly after the ingestion of ethylene glycol and its renal excretion before it is metabolized. AKI of any other cause is also under consideration as the cause for isosthenuria.

A biased examination of the urine sediment was performed to see if there were any calcium oxalate dihydrate or monohydrate crystals that could support the diagnosis of ethylene glycol intoxication, but none were found. However, absence of oxalate crystalluria does not exclude a diagnosis of ethylene glycol intoxication. Some animals with ethylene glycol intoxication have oxalate crystalluria within six hours of toxin ingestion; the number of crystals observed will depend on the amount consumed, the degree of metabolism, and the timing of the urine sample.

The presence of a large number of free small epithelial cells and renal tubular epithelial cell casts indicate that the kidneys are being actively damaged by some disease process (e.g. nephrotoxins, ischemia, or nephritis).

Further Diagnostics and Assessment: Thoracic radiographs disclosed an enlarged cardiac silhouette. Gas-filled bowel loops were observed in the pericardial sac resulting in a diagnosis of pericardial diaphragmatic hernia.

Serum creatinine concentration was 3.7 mg/dL and BUN was 120 mg/dL. Azotemia in combination with a 1.010 USG immediately incriminates primary renal disease. The hematocrit was 54% and total protein concentration was 8.1 g/dL. A rapid point-of-care test for Leptospirosis was negative. Abdominal ultrasonography showed kidneys of normal size and a mild increase in echogenicity.

Dehydration was rapidly corrected, and the extracellular fluid volume expanded by intravenous administration of lactated Ringer's solution to improve renal perfusion. Surgery was performed to decompress the hernia. The BUN and serum creatinine concentrations returned to normal within 72 hours after surgery and the hematocrit and total protein concentrations also returned to normal 24 hours after beginning fluid therapy.

The original identification of free renal tubular epithelial cells and epithelial cell casts in the urine sediment are attributed to ischemic AKI, secondary to reduced renal perfusion from the pericardial hernia and ECF volume contraction.

The initial azotemia is considered to be partly prerenal because it resolved with fluid therapy, but some of the azotemia is attributed to AKI since the USG was isosthenuric. Prerenal azotemia alone should result in elaboration of a USG >1.030.

Final Diagnosis: Prerenal and primary-renal azotemia; ischemic AKI; pericardial diaphragmatic hernia.

CASE EXAMPLE: Urinalysis Case Number: 7

Source of Specimen:
    Cystocentesis ☐   Voided (Stream part) ☒ Midstream   Post-Void (location) ☐
    Expressed ☐   Catheterized ☐
Volume: 2 mL
Refrigeration: Yes ☐   No ☒
Elapsed Time Before Analysis:
Stain: Yes ☒   No ☐

Color:	Amber
Appearance:	Cloudy
Specific Gravity:	1.031
pH:	7.5
Protein:	100 mg/dL
Occult Blood:	2+
Hemolyzed:	☒
Intact:	☒
Glucose:	Negative
Ketones:	Negative
Bilirubin:	Negative

Casts per LPF: 0
   Hyaline
   Granular
   Cellular

WBC per HPF: 5–10
   Free   ☒
   Clumped ☐
RBC per HPF: 20–30
Epithelial Cells per HPF: 10–15
   Type: Squamous: ☐   Transitional: Free ☒   Clumped ☒   Renal: ☐

Crystals per HPF: None ☒
   Type: Struvite ☐   Calcium Oxalate ☐   Urate ☐   Other ☐

Bacteria per HPF: None ☒
   Type: Rods ☐   Cocci ☐   Mixed ☐

Miscellaneous:

Signalment: 10-year-old spayed female mixed-breed dog.

History and Physical Examination: This dog has been taking a longer time to urinate over the past several months. Stranguria has been noted over the past few weeks, and a small amount of red color has been observed in the urine on the ground. She has been licking her vulvar area more than usual during this time. Appetite and attitude are normal.

The dog was bright and alert and in good body condition. Moderately severe dental tartar and lenticular sclerosis in both eyes were noted. No abnormalities were detected on abdominal palpation and thoracic auscultation. Rectal palpation revealed a firm irregular thickening (approximately 1.5-cm diameter) of the urethra along the pelvic floor; no pelvic lymphadenopathy was palpated.

Prominent urethral thickening can be caused by urothelial neoplasia (TCC) most commonly, or proliferative urethritis. UTI is not likely to account for this degree of urethral change by itself.

Interpretation of Urinalysis: UA results are from a mid-stream voided urine collection. Voided urine, compared to cystocentesis, can provide more diagnostic material at times when the disease is mostly within the urethra.

Cloudy urine is accounted for by the active sediment findings (RBC, WBC, epithelial cells). The 1.031 USG shows adequate concentrating ability. The 7.5 pH on dipstrip can indicate the presence of a urease positive bacterial UTI or could represent a protracted post-prandial alkaline tide (we do not know the timing of the urine collection in relationship to fasting or feeding). The 2+ protein is likely associated with the active urinary sediment findings. The 2+ occult blood aligns with the microscopic reports of RBC in the urinary sediment. The dipstrip showed both intact RBC and free hemoglobin on the dipstrip. The free hemoglobin is attributed to lysed RBC in the urine.

The predominant findings during microscopy were the increased RBC (20–30 per HPF), increased free and clumped transitional epithelial cells (10–15 per HPF), and a modest increase in WBC (5–10 per HPF). No bacteria were identified. These findings indicate the presence of inflammation, desquamation of epithelial cells, and hemorrhage. The pyuria could be the result of a bacterial UTI despite absence of identified bacteria. "Rafts" or clumps of urothelial cells are always of concern that they could arise from urinary tract neoplasia, but they sometimes arise during UTI and urolithiasis. There was no comment as to the morphology of the free or clumped epithelial cells, unfortunately.

The two differentials that need to be distinguished are TCC (UCC) of the urethra and proliferative urethritis.

Further Diagnostics and Assessment: CBC, serum biochemistry, thoracic radiographs, and abdominal radiographs were normal. Ultrasonography of the bladder was not performed since urethrocystoscopy was planned instead.

Unstained urine sediment from a voided urine collection was smeared on glass slides and submitted for standard dry mount cytology. Alternatively, urine could be submitted to the laboratory to then prepare the slides for cytology. Urine was not collected by cystocentesis since the process seemed to predominantly involve the urethra. Alternatively, aspiration biopsy of the urethra could have been performed during the passage of a urethral urinary catheter. Urine cytology from the voided urine sample revealed anaplastic transitional cells, some of which were binucleated.

A urinary catheter was passed into the urethra during the use of a handheld vaginoscope. The catheter was advanced with some resistance approximately 3–4 cm into the urethra. A sample of catheterized urine was submitted for bacterial culture and sensitivity and returned with >10 000 cfu/mL *Escherichia coli*. This level of quantitative bacterial growth of rods usually aligns with bacteria reported in the urinalysis, but that was not true in this case.

Urinary endoscopy showed a roughened and irregular distal and mid-urethral mucosa. The proximal urethra, bladder neck, and bladder appeared normal except for focal hemorrhages. Projections of tissue into the urethral lumen that are attached on both ends that are typical of proliferative urethritis were not observed. Biopsy material retrieved using forceps resulted in the histopathologic diagnosis transitional cell carcinoma (UCC).

The dog was treated with amoxicillin for the bacterial urinary tract infection and with piroxicam for its palliative effects in dogs with transitional cell carcinoma. The dog improved considerably within the first month after beginning treatment but still had some difficulty urinating. The dog did reasonably well for approximately nine months after which time she began to lose weight, had a reduced appetite, and increased difficulty urinating. At that time, the owner elected euthanasia.

Final Diagnosis: Transitional cell carcinoma (urothelial cell carcinoma) of the urethra; bacterial UTI.

CASE EXAMPLE: Urinalysis Case Number: 8

Source of Specimen:

Cystocentesis ☐   Voided (Stream part) ☒ Midstream   Post-Void (location) ☐

Expressed ☐   Catheterized ☐

Volume: 3 mL

Refrigeration: Yes ☐   No ☒

Elapsed Time Before Analysis: 60 minutes

Stain: Yes ☒   No ☐

Color: Amber
Appearance: Cloudy
Specific Gravity: 1.033
pH: 8.0
Protein: 100 mg/dL
Occult Blood: 2+
  Hemolyzed: ☐
  Intact: ☒
Glucose: Negative
Ketones: Negative
Bilirubin: Negative

Casts per LPF: 0
  Hyaline
  Granular
  Cellular

WBC per HPF: 10–15
  Free   ☒
  Clumped   ☐
RBC per HPF: 15–20
Epithelial Cells per HPF: 10-15 Nonsquamous; Rare Squamous
  Type: Squamous: ☒   Transitional: Free ☒   Clumped ☐   Renal: ☐

Crystals per HPF: None ☒
  Type: Struvite ☐   Calcium Oxalate ☐   Urate ☐   Other ☐

Bacteria per HPF: None ☐
  Type: Rods ☐   Cocci ☒ Few   Mixed ☐

Miscellaneous:

Signalment: Eight-year-old spayed female Scottish Terrier dog.

History and Physical Examination: The owner reports the recent observation of blood in the dog's urine. The dog's urine during voiding is initially yellow but blood is observed toward the end of urination. There is also an increased frequency in urination. The dog seems systemically well with a good appetite and attitude. The dog was alert and in good body condition. There was moderately severe dental tartar. The bladder was thickened on abdominal palpation but without pain. No masses were palpated within the bladder wall or within the bladder lumen. Palpation of the kidneys was normal. Rectal examination was normal.

The history and physical examination findings in this dog are compatible with bladder neoplasia, cystic calculi, or a bacterial urinary tract infection. Scottish Terriers have the greatest risk for any dog breed to develop urothelial neoplasia (TCC or UC), so it is essential to rule this diagnosis in or out.

Interpretation of Urinalysis: Cloudy urine is attributed to the active urinary sediment (RBC, WBC, and epithelial cells). A USG of 1.033 shows good concentrating capacity. A highly alkaline urinary pH of 8.0 often develops in the presence of a urease-producing bacterial UTI (*Staphylococcus*, *Proteus*, mycoplasma spp). The 2+ proteinuria on dipstrip is attributed to postrenal origin from the inflammatory/hemorrhagic increases in RBC and WBC observed during urine microscopy. The 2+ occult blood color reaction on the dipstrip was only for intact RBC, which matches up with the 15–20 RBC per HPF identified during microscopy. Pyuria at 10–15 WBC per HPF in association with some cocci in urinary sediment supports the presence of a bacterial UTI. Pyuria could also be secondary to inflammation arising from a bladder tumor or urinary stones. The finding of rare squamous epithelial cells is not clinically relevant as they sometimes enter normal urine that is collected by voiding. The 10–15 free transitional cells per HPF are clinically relevant, but no further details about their appearance was provided. Desquamation of transitional cells of this magnitude into urine is most common with urothelial neoplasia, but reactive desquamation from urolithiasis or UTI is still possible. Epithelialcyturia in a Scottish Terrier is worrisome for the diagnosis of urothelial neoplasia.

Further Diagnostics and Assessment: A hemogram and biochemical profile were within normal limits. Thoracic radiographs were normal. An end-urination voided urine sample was collected and submitted for cytology. Results of urine cytology showed increased numbers of transitional cells with some atypical cytological features. Some of these cells were binucleate but differentiating neoplastic from reactive epithelial cells was not possible.

A focal mass involving the cranioventral aspect of the bladder was identified on both contrast cystography and bladder ultrasonography. Portions of the mass projected into the bladder lumen, but not in a way typical for polypoid cystitis. A urethrogram was normal. There were no lesions at the trigone, the location where about two-third of TCC develop. No urinary stones were identified.

A sample of catheterized urine was submitted for bacterial culture and sensitivity and returned with >30000 cfu/mL *Staphylococcus aureus*. The dog was treated with cefadroxil for the bacterial urinary tract infection.

At exploratory cystotomy, a 3-cm mass was identified and was removed from the bladder by partial cranial cystectomy. Histopathology revealed the mass to be a transitional cell carcinoma. This diagnosis could have been achieved following cystoscopy, but surgery was chosen instead in order to remove what appeared to be a focal cranial bladder mass.

The dog improved considerably after surgery and did well for approximately 21 months while treated with piroxicam for its palliative effects on TCC. At 21 months, there was a recurrence of clinical signs and imaging studies disclosed multiple masses within the bladder. The owner elected euthanasia.

If the diagnosis had been in question earlier and the owners were unwilling to go further to get a tissue diagnosis, submission of a test to detect the BRAF mutation in epithelial cells shed into urine might have secured the diagnosis of TCC or UCC. The BRAF mutation exists in about 85% of dogs with this tumor.

Final Diagnosis: TCC of bladder apex. *Staphylococcus* UTI.

CASE EXAMPLE: Urinalysis Case Number: 9

Source of Specimen:
 Cystocentesis ☒ Voided (Stream part) ☐   Post-Void (location) ☐
 Expressed ☐   Catheterized ☐
Volume: 3 mL
Refrigeration: Yes ☐ No ☒
Elapsed Time Before Analysis:
Stain: Yes ☐ No ☒

Color: Straw
Appearance: Clear
Specific Gravity: 1.019
pH: 6.5
Protein: 1000 mg/dL
Occult Blood: Negative
 Hemolyzed: ☐
 Intact: ☐
Glucose: Negative
Ketones: Negative
Bilirubin: Negative

Casts per LPF: 2–4
 Hyaline 2–4
 Granular
 Cellular

WBC per HPF: 0–3
 Free ☒
 Clumped ☐
RBC per HPF: 1–3
Epithelial Cells per HPF: Occasional
 Type: Squamous: ☐ Transitional: Free ☒ Clumped ☐ Renal: ☐

Crystals per HPF: None ☒
 Type: Struvite ☐ Calcium Oxalate ☐   Urate ☐ Other ☐

Bacteria per HPF: None ☒
 Type: Rods ☐ Cocci ☐   Mixed ☐

Miscellaneous:

Signalment: Six-year-old spayed female mixed-breed dog.

History and Physical Examination: Decreased appetite, weight loss, and a bloated appearance of the abdomen were noted by the owners over the past month. The dog was thin and had a dry haircoat. The abdomen was distended, and a fluid wave was balloted. Hydration based on skin turgor was assessed as normal.

Interpretation of Urinalysis: The USG of 1.019 shows minimally concentrated urine, but it is not possible to tell if this is physiological or pathological by itself. The clear appearance to the urine aligns with a mostly inactive urinary sediment (only hyaline casts were seen during microscopy). Despite collection by cystocentesis, there was no increase in RBC in urinary sediment or occult blood dipstrip reaction. The most striking finding from the urinalysis is the 4+ dipstrip proteinuria. Remember that the urinary chemistry dipstrip for protein is most sensitive for the detection of urinary albumin. The hallmark of glomerular origin proteinuria is the finding of proteinuria associated with an inactive urinary sediment, as in this case. The observation of 2–4 hyaline casts per LPF is attributed to glomerular proteinuria, which favors the precipitation of the THP matrix protein. The presumptive diagnosis was glomerular disease (glomerulonephritis or amyloidosis). The marked proteinuria and the ballotable fluid wave in the abdomens provide suspicion for the presence of the nephrotic syndrome (NS).

Further Diagnostics and Assessment: The UPC was very high at 17.0, which confirms renal proteinuria, most of which is likely albumin. Dogs with advanced glomerular amyloidosis often have values above 10.0, but those with glomerulonephritis may have values that can range up to 40.0. GN and renal amyloidosis can have widely differing prognoses, so a renal biopsy is necessary to distinguish these two diseases. Amyloidosis is generally considered to be a relentlessly progressive disease.

A hemogram was normal except for low plasma proteins (5.0 g/dL; normal = 6.0–8.0 g/dL). On serum biochemistry, the dog was nonazotemic but had hypercholesterolemia (436 mg/dL), hypoalbuminemia (1.2 g/dL), and low serum proteins (4.5 g/dL). A sample of fluid obtained by abdominocentesis was interpreted as a pure transudate, attributed to the low oncotic pressure from the low circulating albumin.

The combination of severe glomerular proteinuria, hypoalbuminemia, hypercholesterolemia, and varying amounts of edema or body cavity effusions defines nephrotic syndrome (NS). NS can also be associated with accelerated clotting.

Ultrasound-guided renal biopsy was performed after assessment of buccal mucosal bleeding time (1 minute; normal = <2 minutes) and systolic blood pressure by Doppler technique (110 mmHg; normal = 100–140 mmHg). Results of routine histopathology and immunofluorescence microscopy resulted in a diagnosis of membranous glomerulonephritis associated with immune complexes.

When possible, an antigen hunt (HW, SLE, vector-borne titers, and leptospirosis) is undertaken in an effort to find an antigen that could be eliminated from the dog's body with treatment. Often, the offending antigen is not determined no matter how extensive the antigen search. An extensive panel of possible antigens is costly and this owner did not allow the attending DVM to submit such tests.

A sodium-restricted diet, furosemide, and the ACE-I enalapril were prescribed for this dog. Re-evaluation at four weeks showed stable laboratory results with continued proteinuria. Re-evaluation at six months showed resolution of ascites, normal serum cholesterol concentration, and improvement in serum albumin concentration. The magnitude of the proteinuria had substantially declined (UPC of 2.9) and there still was no azotemia.

GN associated with immune complexes and NS are rarely observed to spontaneously go into remission. Perhaps the antigen provoking the development and deposition of immune complexes was no longer active. In many dogs with ICGN, persistent renal proteinuria and progression of intrarenal lesions continue unless aggressive immunosuppressive treatments are provided.

Final Diagnosis: Glomerulonephritis, nephrotic syndrome.

CASE EXAMPLE: Urinalysis Case Number: 10

Source of Specimen:
    Cystocentesis ☐   Voided (Stream part) ☐   Post-Void (location) ☒ Floor/table/cage
    Expressed ☐   Catheterized ☐
Volume: 1 mL
Refrigeration: Yes ☐   No ☒
Elapsed Time Before Analysis: 10 minutes
Stain: Yes ☒   No ☐

Color: Light yellow
Appearance: Cloudy
Specific Gravity: 1.010 (on fluids)
pH: 6.5
Protein: 30 mg/dL
Occult Blood: Trace
    Hemolyzed: ☒
    Intact: ☐
Glucose: Negative
Ketones: Negative
Bilirubin: Negative

Casts per LPF:
    Hyaline
    Granular
    Cellular 5–10 renal tubular epithelial

WBC per HPF: 0–1
    Free   ☒
    Clumped   ☐
RBC per HPF: 3–5
Epithelial Cells per HPF: 10–15
    Type: Squamous: ☐   Transitional: Free ☐   Clumped ☐   Renal: ☒

Crystals per HPF: None ☒
    Type: Struvite ☐   Calcium Oxalate ☐   Urate ☐   Other ☐

Bacteria per HPF: None ☒
    Type: Rods ☐   Cocci ☐   Mixed ☐

Miscellaneous:

Signalment: Eight-month-old spayed female Yorkshire Terrier dog.

History and Physical Examination: The puppy was bumping into walls and experienced an acute onset of generalized seizures over the past 24 hours. Prior to this time the dog appeared to be normal. The dog was very quiet on physical examination, but no specific abnormalities were detected.

The differential diagnosis included concerns for toxins, hepatoencephalopathy, other metabolic disorders, and structural brain disease (encephalitis and hydrocephalus).

Interpretation of Urinalysis: The urine sample was collected as a post-void sample from the cage floor. The urine was described as cloudy, likely due to increased urinary sediment activity associated with free RTE and RTE casts. The low urine specific gravity (1.010) could have been the result of intravenous fluid therapy or due to renal tubular damage (see sediment activity). Unfortunately, there were no urinalysis results obtained before fluid therapy was initiated. 1+ protein on the chemistry dipstrip is likely indicative of renal proteinuria, especially in urine of low USG, but this was not further pursued with a UPC or MA test. The trace + reaction for occult blood occurred for free hemoglobin during the finding of 3–5 RBC per HPF; it is conceivable lysis of some RBC occurred in this instance. The occult blood reaction is more sensitive to free hemoglobin than to that in the intact RBC.

The most striking change during urine microscopy is the "shower" (5–10 per LPF) of cellular casts containing RTE. The 10–15 per HPF free epithelial cells were small. They had similar size and shape as those observed in the accompanying casts, suggesting common origin in the kidney (i.e. renal tubular epithelium). Some of the free epithelial cells had basal nuclei adding further credence to their identity as tubular in origin. Many of the RTE casts were tubular fragments, as entire contiguous tubular segments had sloughed into the urine rather than the addition of sporadic cells to a matrix protein.

Cellular casts are not found in normal urine. The finding of excessive numbers of renal tubular epithelial cells and epithelial cell casts/tubular fragments indicates marked damage to the renal tubular epithelium.

Further Diagnostics and Assessment: Examination of a blood smear on the CBC showed basophilic stippling and nucleated RBC in the absence of anemia. Based on these findings and the history, blood lead was submitted and returned with a concentration of >150 ug/dL (normal, <20 ug/dL) confirming the diagnosis of lead poisoning. Further questioning of the owners revealed that they lived in a very old house and were scraping paint from the interiors, the likely source for the puppy to ingest lead. BUN, serum creatinine, and serum phosphorus concentrations were initially normal and remained so throughout treatment. All other routine serum biochemical parameters were normal. Treatment consisted of IV calcium ethylene diamine tetraacetate (EDTA), intravenous fluids, and anticonvulsants as needed. The dog responded well to therapy.

Even though this dog remained nonazotemic, an episode of AKI can predict a future diagnosis of CKD associated with the initial nephron drop out in some animals. Consequently, routine twice yearly evaluation of serum biochemistry and urinalysis was recommended.

Final Diagnosis: Nonazotemic AKI due to nephrotoxic agents (lead and calcium EDTA).

CASE EXAMPLE: Urinalysis Case Number: 11

Source of Specimen:
    Cystocentesis ☒   Voided (Stream part) ☐   Post-Void (location) ☐
    Expressed ☐   Catheterized ☐
Volume: 5   mL
Refrigeration: Yes ☐   No ☒
Elapsed Time Before Analysis: 5 minutes
Stain: Yes ☐   No ☒

Color: Pale yellow
Appearance: Clear
Specific Gravity: 1.014
pH: 6.5
Protein: Trace
Occult Blood: 0
    Hemolyzed: ☐
    Intact: ☐
Glucose: Negative
Ketones: Negative
Bilirubin: Negative

Casts per LPF:
    Hyaline
    Granular 0–1
    Cellular 0–1 WBC

WBC per HPF: 0–2
    Free   ☒
    Clumped   ☐
RBC per HPF: 1–2
Epithelial Cells per HPF: 0
    Type: Squamous: ☐   Transitional: Free ☐   Clumped ☐   Renal: ☐

Crystals per HPF: None ☒
    Type: Struvite ☐   Calcium Oxalate ☐   Urate ☐   Other ☐

Bacteria per HPF: None ☒
    Type: Rods ☐   Cocci ☐   Mixed ☐

Miscellaneous:

Signalment: Six-year-old spayed female Doberman Pinscher dog.

History and Physical Examination: Sudden onset of severe polyuria and polydipsia that was ongoing for one week. The dog is otherwise well. There were no abnormal findings on physical examination.

Interpretation of Urinalysis: The isosthenuric USG of 1.014 supports the historical complaint of PU/PD. The trace protein reaction on the dipstrip could indicate pathological proteinuria in a urine sample that is not concentrated, but this was not pursued further with UPC or MA testing.

The observation of cellular casts in urine is always abnormal and indicates some active process in the kidneys. White blood cell casts (0–1 per LPF) are associated with renal inflammation that is most commonly caused by bacterial infection (i.e. pyelonephritis). An occasional granular cast can be normal in concentrated urine. In the presence of a low USG and cellular casts, the presence of granular casts indicates renal tubular injury. Granules can form in casts as cells degenerate. The presence of WBC casts was likely detected in this case because of how quickly urine microscopy was performed after urine was collected. WBC casts are known to break up quickly, so they are infrequently identified during microscopy at later times.

The finding of only a few free white blood cells and no bacteria observed in the urine sediment does not support the diagnosis of a bacterial UTI. However, pyuria and bacteriuria can be intermittent and are not always observed in animals with upper urinary tract infection.

The presumptive diagnosis was bacterial pyelonephritis.

Further Diagnostics and Assessment: A routine serum biochemistry profile and hemogram were performed to evaluate renal function and any potential systemic response to the suspected renal infection – results were normal. Renal function is often normal in acute pyelonephritis in animals that are well hydrated. Neutrophilia and left shift can be observed in dogs with acute pyelonephritis, but often it is an early and transient finding. Bacterial urine culture returned with no growth of bacteria.

The dog was treated with a cephalosporin antibiotic for four weeks on the suspicion of upper urinary tract infection despite the negative culture. Polyuria and polydipsia resolved within four days and the dog appeared to be normal two years later. Urine specific gravity values greater than 1.025 were observed on numerous subsequent urinalyses.

Final Diagnosis: Pyelonephritis, bacterial.

CASE EXAMPLE: Urinalysis Case Number: 12

Source of Specimen:
    Cystocentesis ☐   Voided (Stream part) ☐   Post-Void (location) ☐
    Expressed ☐   Catheterized ☒
Volume: 5   mL
Refrigeration: Yes ☐   No ☒
Elapsed Time Before Analysis: 30 minutes
Stain: Yes ☒   No ☐

Color: Pale yellow
Appearance: Hazy
Specific Gravity: 1.008
pH: 5.5
Protein: 100 mg/dL
Occult Blood: 1+
   Hemolyzed: ☒
   Intact: ☐
Glucose: Negative
Ketones: Negative
Bilirubin: Negative

Casts per LPF:
   Hyaline
   Granular 3–5, fine and coarse
   Cellular

WBC per HPF: 5–10
   Free   ☒
   Clumped   ☐
RBC per HPF: 3–5
Epithelial Cells per HPF: 0
   Type: Squamous: ☐   Transitional: Free ☐   Clumped ☐   Renal: ☐

Crystals per HPF: None ☒
   Type: Struvite ☐   Calcium Oxalate ☐   Urate ☐   Other ☐

Bacteria per HPF: None ☒
   Type: Rods ☐   Cocci ☐   Mixed ☐

Miscellaneous:

Signalment: Five-year-old castrated male Border Collie dog.

History and Physical Examination: The owner reports that the dog has urinated in the house and was observed to be lethargic while being watched by a friend when the owner was out of town; the owner believes the dog is producing a larger urine volume and drinking quite a bit more water for the past 7–10 days. He is well house-trained and has not urinated in the house since he was a puppy. The dog seems to be "off" to the owners and is not as eager to finish his meals. He has free range of their farm for a few hours each day. Normal temperature, pulse, and respiration were found at presentation. Hydration based on skin turgor was assessed as normal. The dog was alert but very quiet during physical examination. No abnormalities were detected.

Interpretation of Urinalysis: The presence of a low USG at 1.008 supports the historical concern for polyuria and polydipsia. A 2+ protein dipstrip reaction usually indicates pathological proteinuria especially in urine that is not concentrated. The 1+ positive occult blood reaction for free hemoglobin on the dipstrip reagent pad may reflect lysis of erythrocytes despite limited numbers of erythrocytes in the urinary sediment. The proteinuria and mild pyuria (5–10 free WBC per HPF) could result from a bacterial urinary tract infection or nonbacterial inflammation; no bacteria were identified in the urinary sediment. The proteinuria with a low USG and minimal sediment abnormalities warrants follow-up with a UPC and or MA. The three to five finely and coarsely granular casts per LPF in the face of 1.008 USG point to an intrarenal process with accelerated cellular degeneration in order to form these granular casts. Alternatively, some of the granular casts could represent precipitates of filtered proteins.

The presumptive diagnosis was renal disease of unknown cause to account for the dilute urine, proteinuria, and cylindruria.

Further Diagnostics and Assessment: The hemogram disclosed mild thrombocytopenia (72 000/μL) and hyperproteinemia (8.1 g/dL) with a normal leukogram. The biochemical profile disclosed azotemia (BUN 70 mg/dL and creatinine 7.1 mg/dL), hyperphosphatemia (8.4 mg/dL), hyponatremia (134 mEq/L), hypochloremia (106 mEq/L), and hypokalemia (3.0 mEq/L). A clotting profile was within normal limits except for mild thrombocytopenia.

Radiographs and abdominal ultrasonography revealed enlarged kidneys (9–9.5 cm long) with poor corticomedullary distinction on ultrasonography.

Urine culture yielded no growth and the urine protein-to-creatinine ratio was 4.0. The high UPC can indicate tubular and or glomerular origin in those with leptospirosis (see serology below).

The dog's azotemia and hyperphosphatemia became progressively worse over the next few days (serum creatinine 9.3 mg/dL, BUN 101 mg/dL, and serum phosphorus 9.5 mg/dL) and the dog became oliguric. An exploratory laparotomy was performed to place a peritoneal dialysis catheter and a renal biopsy was taken. The surgeon remarked that the kidneys were very swollen, and that the renal parenchyma bulged from the incision that was made in the renal capsule. Histopathology disclosed acute interstitial nephritis characterized by infiltration of neutrophils, lymphoplasmacytes, and severe edema. The dog was treated with ampicillin and aluminum hydroxide and underwent peritoneal dialysis for approximately two weeks.

Serology for leptospirosis was performed twice over a 10-day interval. A fourfold increase in titer was found for serovars *pomona* and *bratislava* and a twofold increase for *grippotyphosa*. At the time of release from the hospital, the dog's serum creatinine concentration was 2.4 mg/dL and BUN was 40 mg/dL. After the amoxicillin treatment, doxycycline was given to the dog in order to help clear leptospiral organisms from the kidneys. The dog eventually made a full recovery.

Final Diagnosis: Azotemic AKI due to leptospirosis.

CASE EXAMPLE: Urinalysis Case Number: 13

Source of Specimen:
Cystocentesis ☐   Voided (Stream part) ☐   Post-Void (location) ☒ Floor/table/cage
Expressed ☐   Catheterized ☐
Volume: 2 mL
Refrigeration: Yes ☐   No ☒
Elapsed Time Before Analysis: 60 minutes
Stain: Yes ☒   No ☐

Color:	Light pink
Appearance:	Cloudy
Specific Gravity:	1.008
pH:	6.5
Protein:	100 mg/dL
Occult Blood:	2+
Hemolyzed:	☐
Intact:	☒
Glucose:	Negative
Ketones:	Negative
Bilirubin:	Negative

Casts per LPF: Waxy 1-2; occasional broad cast
    Hyaline 1–2
    Granular 2–4
    Cellular

WBC per HPF: 1–3
    Free   ☒
    Clumped   ☐
RBC per HPF: 10–15
Epithelial Cells per HPF: 0-1
    Type: Squamous: ☐   Transitional: Free ☒   Clumped ☐   Renal: ☐

Crystals per HPF: None ☒
    Type: Struvite ☐   Calcium Oxalate ☐   Urate ☐   Other ☐

Bacteria per HPF: None ☐
    Type: Rods ☐   Cocci ☒ Few   Mixed ☐

Miscellaneous: Urinalysis was performed 2 days postoperative; on IV fluids and antibiotics

Signalment: Four-year-old castrated male Domestic Longhair cat.

History and Physical Examination: The cat had experienced four episodes of urethral obstruction over the past six months. During each episode, the cat was treated by use of an indwelling urinary catheter for at least 24 hours, antibiotics, and glucocorticoids. The cat has had signs of lower urinary tract irritation between episodes of urethral obstruction (e.g. stranguria and pollakiuria). Perineal urethrostomy was performed to prevent future episodes of obstruction and the surgical procedure went well. A region of urethral stricture was observed and corrected during surgery. Urine flow through the urethrostomy site was excellent. The cat had a poor appetite postoperatively and was lethargic. Body temperature was 103.0 °F; normal auscultation of heart and lungs, hydration based on skin turgor, and abdominal palpation were found on physical examination. The bladder was small and nonpainful, and the kidneys were normal to mildly enlarged, but not painful.

Interpretation of Urinalysis: This urine sample was collected from the surface of the exam table two days after surgery. It is not possible to assess urinary concentrating capacity since the USG of 1.008 was measured while the cat was on IV fluids; no presurgical or prefluids USG was determined. The cylindruria (see later on microscopy) and low USG could indicate the presence of primary renal disease. The 2+ proteinuria and the 2+ occult blood along with the 10–15 RBC per HPF are attributed to the underlying inflammation and hemorrhage from the urethral obstructions, intervening cystourethritis, and surgical trauma. Pyuria is not present, but the cat is being treated with antibiotics and this could reduce pyuria even in the presence of infection. Also, one to three WBCs per HPF in dilute urine may be more clinically relevant than a similar number in concentrated urine. Lastly, treatment with glucocorticoids may have suppressed WBC diapedesis into urine. The few cocci-like bacteria are difficult to interpret because the sample was collected from a cleaned litter pan.

Most alarming in this urinalysis is the degree and type of cylindruria. The finding of granular casts at two to four per LPF in urine that is not concentrated likely indicates renal tubular cell degeneration. The one to two hyaline casts per LPF were surprising to find as it is more difficult for these casts to form in urine that is this dilute. The presence of broad casts (hyaline and granular) suggests dilatation of some portions of the nephron. The finding of waxy casts is of concern as this implies substantial intrarenal stasis. The presence of waxy casts suggests some chronicity since waxy casts take the longest time to be formed in the kidney.

At this point, the presumptive diagnosis was chronic pyelonephritis.

Further Diagnostics and Assessment: Mild leukocytosis with a left shift was observed on the hemogram; it was not present two days before surgery. Renal function as evaluated by BUN and serum creatinine concentrations was normal before and after surgery. Ultrasound examination after surgery showed bilateral dilatation of the renal pelves and diverticulae. These findings provide support for a diagnosis of pyelonephritis. Pyelonephritis could have been caused by bacterial infection that was not documented and/or by multiple episodes of urethral obstruction affecting the kidneys.

After surgery, bacterial culture of a midstream voided sample of urine returned with no bacterial growth at a time when the cat was being treated with antibiotics. Several days after changing antibiotics, the cat's fever abated, and he began to eat. He was treated with antibiotics for six weeks. Serial urinalysis showed resolution of the cylindruria, but the USG at 1.020–1.025 remained lower than expected for normal cats (≥1.035 USG) on several urine samples. He had no further episodes of urethral obstruction or signs of lower urinary tract inflammation during the next year. Surveillance of renal function was suggested based on our suspicion for early CKD.

Final Diagnosis: Pyelonephritis.

CASE EXAMPLE: Urinalysis Case Number: 14

Source of Specimen:
  Cystocentesis ☒   Voided (Stream part) ☐   Post-Void (location) ☐
  Expressed ☐   Catheterized ☐
Volume: 4   mL
Refrigeration: Yes ☐   No ☒
Elapsed Time Before Analysis:
Stain: Yes ☐   No ☒

Color: Straw
Appearance: Clear
Specific Gravity: 1.016
pH: 6.0
Protein: 500 mg/dL
Occult Blood: Negative
  Hemolyzed: ☐
  Intact: ☐
Glucose: Negative
Ketones: Negative
Bilirubin: Negative

Casts per LPF: Waxy 0–2
  Hyaline occasional
  Granular
  Cellular

WBC per HPF: 5–7
  Free   ☒
  Clumped   ☐
RBC per HPF: 0–3
Epithelial Cells per HPF: 5–7
  Type: Squamous: ☐   Transitional: Free ☒   Clumped ☐   Renal: ☐

Crystals per HPF: None ☒
  Type: Struvite ☐   Calcium Oxalate ☐   Urate ☐   Other ☐

Bacteria per HPF: None ☒
  Type: Rods ☐   Cocci ☐   Mixed ☐

Miscellaneous:

Signalment: Eight-year-old intact male Basset Hound dog.

History and Physical Examination: Poor appetite for the past few weeks and vomiting two to three times a day for the past week have been observed. Prior to this time, the dog had no known prior health problems. On physical examination, the dog had a dry haircoat and was slightly thin. The dog's skin turgor was decreased suggesting moderate dehydration. The prostate was moderately enlarged with some loss of the median raphe, but not painful. Fundic examination revealed partial retinal detachment in the left eye and several retinal hemorrhages in the right eye. Systolic blood pressure measured by Doppler was 190 mmHg (normal = 110–140 mmHg).

Interpretation of Urinalysis: The 1.016 USG during dehydration shows impaired urinary concentrating capacity as the USG at these times should be much higher (>1.040 USG). The dog had not received any drugs (e.g. corticosteroids, furosemide) that might have interfered with concentrating ability.

The presence of heavy proteinuria (500 mg/dL) based on urinary dipstrip with low urine specific gravity and mostly inactive urinary sediment suggests the presence of underlying glomerular disease (glomerulonephritis, glomerular amyloidosis, or glomerulosclerosis).

The mild increase in leukocytes (five to seven free WBC) in the urine sediment may reflect underlying prostatic disease, a bacterial urinary tract infection, nonspecific change during inflammatory renal disease, or may be clinically insignificant. There were no bacteria identified during urine microscopy to further indicate bacterial urinary infection.

The presumptive diagnosis at this point was glomerular disease (glomerulonephritis, amyloidosis, and glomerulosclerosis).

Further Diagnostics and Assessment: A nonregenerative anemia (PCV 34%) and lymphopenia (500/μL) were noted on the CBC. A serum biochemical panel revealed increases in BUN of 145 mg/dL, creatinine of 8.4 mg/dL, phosphorus of 9.2 mg/dL, cholesterol of 402 mg/dL, and a CK of 875 IU/L. Decreased serum bicarbonate at 11 mEq/L, albumin at 1.8 g/dL, and total proteins at 5.3 g/dL were also observed.

Abdominal radiographs were performed to evaluate renal size and showed the kidneys to be at the upper limit of normal in size. Prostatomegaly and mild splenomegaly were also noted. Quantitative urine culture was negative for bacterial growth.

The dog was treated with intravenous lactated Ringer's solution, famotidine, aluminum hydroxide, and amlodipine. After two days of fluid therapy, azotemia was improved but not resolved (BUN 85 mg/dL and creatinine 6.1 mg/dL). Serum phosphorus and bicarbonate concentrations had returned to normal. The nonregenerative anemia was more severe with a PCV of 30%. These changes were attributed to rehydration and resolution of prerenal azotemia. Blood pressure gradually returned to normal during escalating doses of amlodopine.

The owner elected to have ultrasound-guided renal biopsy performed despite a guarded prognosis. On light microscopy, glomeruli were hypocellular with presence of amorphous pink material on H&E-stained sections. This material demonstrated green birefringence when stained with Congo red and examined by polarization microscopy. Moderately severe interstitial fibrosis and infiltration of lymphocytes and plasma cells also were observed. Tubular atrophy and focal tubular dilatation were also noted.

The UPC was initially 6.4 and declined to 2.8 when high systemic blood pressure was controlled. Addition of an ACE-I or ARB to further reduce glomerular proteinuria was considered but not implemented. The reason that renal amyloidosis develops is often elusive, but chronic infectious, inflammatory, and neoplastic diseases are found at times. It is possible that prostatic disease contributed to the development of renal amyloidosis in this case, but the prostate was not further evaluated.

Final Diagnosis: CKD; Glomerular amyloidosis with secondary chronic tubulointerstitial nephritis.

CASE EXAMPLE: Urinalysis Case Number: 15

Source of Specimen:
    Cystocentesis ☒   Voided (Stream part) ☐   Post-Void (location) ☐
    Expressed ☐   Catheterized ☐
Volume: 3   mL
Refrigeration: Yes ☐   No ☒
Elapsed Time Before Analysis:
Stain: Yes ☒   No ☐

Color: Yellow
Appearance: Clear
Specific Gravity: 1.017
pH: 7.5
Protein: Negative
Occult Blood: Negative
   Hemolyzed: ☐
   Intact: ☐
Glucose: Negative
Ketones: Negative
Bilirubin: Negative

Casts per LPF: 0
   Hyaline
   Granular
   Cellular

WBC per HPF: 0–3
   Free   ☒
   Clumped   ☐
RBC per HPF: 5–8
Epithelial Cells per HPF: Rare
   Type: Squamous: ☐   Transitional: Free ☒   Clumped ☐   Renal: ☐

Crystals per HPF: None ☐
   Type: Struvite ☒   Calcium Oxalate ☐   Urate ☐   Other ☒ Ammonium biurate

Bacteria per HPF: None ☒
   Type: Rods ☐   Cocci ☐   Mixed ☐

Miscellaneous: Few to moderate numbers of crystals were identified

Signalment: Three-year-old spayed female Miniature Schnauzer dog.

History and Physical Examination: Presented for the evaluation of vague signs of intermittent lethargy and anorexia, and occasional vomiting. The owner also reports a few episodes of urinating in the house overnight. This dog has always been a relatively big water drinker; large urine volumes were described by the owner. No urinary distress with dysuria, hematuria, or pollakiuria were observed. The dog was small for its age. She was quiet on physical examination and was well hydrated. She had a dry haircoat, mild scaling, and several comedones along the dorsum. No other abnormalities were noted.

Interpretation of Urinalysis: The 1.017 USG supports the contention that the dog has PU/PD. Urinary sediment was inactive except for the finding of a few struvite crystals and a moderate number of ammonium biurate crystals. The urinary pH of 7.5 could indicate a postprandial alkaline tide or that following UTI with a urease producing bacteria. There were no bacteria or excess WBC noted on urine microscopy. The slight increase in RBC (5–8 per HPF) could have been due to the trauma of cystocentesis or underlying disease of the urinary tract such as urolithiasis. Rare nonsquamous epithelial cells could be normal or from urolithiasis. The UA findings are nonspecific, but a low USG and ammonium biurate crystalluria raises the concerns about the presence of a portosystemic shunt.

Further Diagnostics and Assessment: The hemogram disclosed low plasma proteins (5.0 g/dL) and mild microcytosis (MCV 57 fl). Serum biochemistry disclosed low serum proteins (4.8 g/dL), low BUN (5 mg/dL), and mild hypoalbuminemia (2.0 g/dL). Liver enzyme concentrations were normal. Quantitative urine culture was negative for bacterial growth.

Survey abdominal radiographs showed a few mildly radiopaque cystic calculi and the liver was small based on the angle of the gastric gas shadow. Resting serum bile acids were 85 μmol/L and the postprandial serum bile acids were 325 μmol/L. These results were compatible with a portosystemic shunt, which was confirmed by rectal scintigraphy.

A mesenteric venous angiogram identified a single extrahepatic shunt that was partially ligated at surgery. Also at surgery, a cystotomy was performed and several small, smooth, tetrahedral, brownish–green cystic calculi were removed and submitted for quantitative analysis. The results of analysis indicated that the core of the calculi consisted of 100% ammonium acid urate whereas the outer covering of the calculi was 90% struvite (magnesium ammonium phosphate) and 10% hydroxyapatite (calcium phosphate). The dog recovered well from surgery and was treated with a diet restricted in protein.

Final Diagnosis: Portosystemic shunt and ammonium urate urolithiasis.

CASE EXAMPLE: Urinalysis Case Number: 16

Source of Specimen:
    Cystocentesis ☒   Voided (Stream part) ☐   Post-Void (location) ☐
    Expressed ☐   Catheterized ☐
Volume: 4 mL
Refrigeration: Yes ☒   No ☐
Elapsed Time Before Analysis: 10 hr refrigeration
Stain: Yes ☒   No ☐

Color: Yellow
Appearance: Clear
Specific Gravity: 1.025
pH: 6.5
Protein: Negative
Occult Blood: Negative
   Hemolyzed: ☐
   Intact: ☐
Glucose: Negative
Ketones: Negative
Bilirubin: Negative

Casts per LPF: 0
   Hyaline
   Granular
   Cellular

WBC per HPF: 0
   Free   ☐
   Clumped   ☐
RBC per HPF: 1–3
Epithelial Cells per HPF: 0
   Type: Squamous: ☐   Transitional: Free ☐   Clumped ☐   Renal: ☐

Crystals per HPF: None ☐
   Type: Struvite ☒ Many   Calcium Oxalate ☐   Urate ☐   Other ☐

Bacteria per HPF: None ☒
   Type: Rods ☐   Cocci ☐   Mixed ☐

Miscellaneous:

Signalment: Two-year-old castrated male Burmese cat.

History and Physical Examination: This cat had one episode of urethral obstruction three months ago. A urethral plug was retrieved at that time, and it was observed to contain struvite upon a smash preparation of the plug. The owner was instructed to feed the cat a canned food diet with moderate acidifying potential. A bacterial urine culture one month after the episode of urethral obstruction showed no bacterial growth. Three months after the initial episode of urethral obstruction, the cat was doing well with no clinical signs referable to the urinary tract. Physical examination at this time was completely normal.

Interpretation of Urinalysis: The USG of 1.025 is in the range expected for cats eating canned food. None of the dipstrip chemical test results or urine sediment findings suggest any active inflammation at the present time. The finding of marked struvite crystalluria prompts concern about the potential of recurrence of struvite plugs and urethral obstruction should another episode of cystitis or urethritis develop. Struvite crystalluria in the presence of hematuria and proteinuria, however, would be more cause for concern. The urine is moderately acidic and only moderately concentrated, which suggests that few struvite crystals should form. The fact that the urine sample was collected during the evening and was refrigerated for over 12 hours before analysis must also be considered. Refrigeration of the sample may have resulted in the artifactual precipitation of struvite crystals.

Further Diagnostics and Assessment: No crystals were observed on the examination of a fresh warm urine sample. The crystals in the previous UA were an artifact of prolonged refrigeration of the urine before analysis. Struvite crystalluria by itself is not a disease and should not be overinterpreted, especially in samples that have been refrigerated.

Final Diagnosis: Normal; artefactual crystalluria.

CASE EXAMPLE: Urinalysis Case Number: 17

Source of Specimen:
    Cystocentesis ⊠   Voided (Stream part) ☐   Post-Void (location) ☐
    Expressed ☐   Catheterized ☐
Volume: 3 mL
Refrigeration: Yes ☐   No ⊠
Elapsed Time Before Analysis: 45 minutes
Stain: Yes ⊠   No ☐

Color:	Yellow
Appearance:	Cloudy
Specific Gravity:	1.030
pH:	7.0
Protein:	100 mg/dL
Occult Blood:	2+
Hemolyzed:	⊠
Intact:	⊠
Glucose:	Negative
Ketones:	Negative
Bilirubin:	Negative

Casts per LPF:
   Hyaline
   Granular
   Cellular

WBC per HPF: 10–15
   Free   ⊠
   Clumped   ☐
RBC per HPF: 15-20
Epithelial Cells per HPF: 5–7
   Type: Squamous: ☐   Transitional: Free ⊠   Clumped ☐   Renal: ☐

Crystals per HPF: None ☐
   Type: Struvite ⊠ Few   Calcium Oxalate ⊠ Few   Urate ☐   Other ☐

Bacteria per HPF: None ⊠
   Type: Rods ☐   Cocci ☐   Mixed ☐

Miscellaneous:

Signalment: Five-year-old spayed female Bichon Frise dog.

History and Physical Examination: Dysuria and hematuria for three weeks are the current complaints. The dog has been on antimicrobial treatment during the past three weeks as prescribed by another veterinary hospital. Multiple episodes of recurrent urinary tract infection that have occurred over the past 18 months were treated with several antimicrobials (e.g. amoxicillin, cefadroxil, and trimethoprim-sulfadiazine). The dog would respond to antimicrobial therapy, and clinical signs (e.g., dysuria, hematuria, and increased frequency) stopped several days after beginning antibiotic therapy. Clinical signs returned several weeks after discontinuing antibiotics. No additional studies had been performed.

The dog was alert and friendly with a normal body temperature, pulse, and respiration. He was normally hydrated based on skin turgor. Palpation of the caudal abdomen in the region of the bladder revealed crepitation. There were no other abnormalities detected on abdominal palpation or during chest auscultation.

Interpretation of Urinalysis: Urine was collected by cystocentesis. The USG of 1.030 shows adequate urinary concentration. The pH of 7.0 could be attributed to the inflammatory process. The 2+ protein and 2+ occult blood on chemistry dipstrip are from the inflammatory reaction and or bleeding in the lower urinary tract. Urine microscopy shows an active urinary sediment with 10–15 WBC per HPF, 15–20 RBC per HPF, and 5–7 free nonsquamous epithelial cells, compatible with a UTI or urolithiasis. Urinary tract cancer would be unlikely based on the history. Some of the increased RBC might arise from the cystocentesis. Zero bacteria were seen during urine microscopy. A few struvite and a few oxalate crystals were observed in urinary sediment examined within 45 minutes post collection, so they are not likely an artifact of delayed examination.

The presence or absence of crystalluria often does not align with the presence or absence of urinary stones. Both struvite and calcium oxalate crystals may be observed in the urine of normal dogs. UTI can still exist even when bacteria are not observed during urine microscopy as it takes a high cfu/mL of bacteria to be easily identified in a wet mount.

The Bichon Frise breed has a higher relative risk for urolithiasis than many other breeds. Recurrent urinary tract infections could be the cause or consequence of urolithiasis. Bacterial urinary tract infection is known to predispose dogs to struvite urolithiasis, and bacterial urinary tract infection can occur secondarily in dogs with other types of primary metabolic urolithiasis including calcium oxalate urolithiasis.

The presumptive diagnosis at this point was bacterial urinary tract infection; possible urolithiasis (struvite or oxalate) based on bladder palpation.

Further Diagnostics and Assessment: Bacterial culture and sensitivity were performed on a sample of urine collected by cystocentesis and disclosed >30 000 cfu/mL of enterococci, which was sensitive only to tetracycline, chloramphenicol, amoxicillin-clavulanic acid, and enrofloxacin.

Plain abdominal radiographs disclosed the presence of many small (<5 mm) radiopaque cystic calculi. The dog was anesthetized, the bladder infused with saline, and voiding hydropropulsion performed. Approximately 50–60 small and smooth calculi were retrieved. A follow-up plain abdominal radiograph was negative for the presence of additional calculi. Quantitative stone analysis revealed its composition to be 90% struvite (magnesium ammonium phosphate) and 10% hydroxyapatite (calcium phosphate).

The dog was released from the hospital on a course of enrofloxacin for three weeks with instructions to return for a bacterial culture of a urine sample obtained by cystocentesis while the dog was on antimicrobial therapy and then again later after treatment had been stopped.

Six months later, routine urinalysis disclosed pyuria but there were no urinary stones on urinary tract imaging. The dog was asymptomatic, but bacterial culture of a urine sample collected by cystocentesis grew 3000 cfu/mL of *Escherichia coli*. ISCAID guidelines recommend to not treat dogs that are culture positive and without clinical signs. Based on the history of many UTI having clinical signs in this dog and its previous development of infection-related urinary stones, antimicrobial treatment was again administered to this dog. The urine was negative for bacterial growth five days after completion of this course of antimicrobial therapy.

This dog has had multiple reinfections as the type of recurrent UTI (versus relapsing or persistent UTI). Struvite stone development in dogs is often associated with bacterial UTI; more so with *Staphylococcus* and *Proteus* than with *E. coli* or enterococcus. This dog has not yet had the kind of diagnostic workup that could reveal why new bacterial UTI develop on such a frequent basis. A search for, and correction of, anatomical abnormalities that can predispose to urinary infection should be undertaken including the evaluation of vulvar conformation (hidden vulva syndrome), vestibulovaginal bands, ectopic ureters, proliferative urethritis, polypoid cystitis, and urachal diverticulum. Vestibulovaginal urethrocystoscopy is especially useful in the identification of anatomical abnormalities that can predispose to reinfection types of UTI.

Final Diagnosis: Recurrent bacterial UTI due to reinfections.

CASE EXAMPLE: Urinalysis Case Number: 18

Source of Specimen:
    Cystocentesis ☒   Voided (Stream part) ☐   Post-Void (location) ☐
    Expressed ☐   Catheterized ☐
Volume: 3 mL
Refrigeration: Yes ☐   No ☒
Elapsed Time Before Analysis:
Stain: Yes ☐   No ☒

Color:	Light yellow
Appearance:	Clear
Specific Gravity:	1.020
pH:	6.0
Protein:	100 mg/dL
Occult Blood:	1+
Hemolyzed:	☒
Intact:	☒
Glucose:	Trace
Ketones:	Negative
Bilirubin:	Negative

Casts per LPF:
   Hyaline
   Granular
   Cellular

WBC per HPF: 3–5
   Free   ☒
   Clumped   ☐
RBC per HPF: 10–15
Epithelial Cells per HPF: 0
   Type: Squamous: ☐   Transitional: Free ☐   Clumped ☐   Renal: ☐

Crystals per HPF: None ☐
   Type: Struvite ☐   Calcium Oxalate ☒ Moderate   Urate ☐   Other ☐

Bacteria per HPF: None ☒
   Type: Rods ☐   Cocci ☐   Mixed ☐

Miscellaneous: Both mono- and dihydrate present. Crystals vary greatly in shape and size; some are similar to what we used to call "hippurate-like."

Signalment: Six-year-old castrated male Domestic Shorthair cat.

History and Physical Examination: The cat had been missing for three days; it returned very lethargic and would not eat. On the morning of its return, the cat vomited four times. This cat was apparently completely healthy prior to this disappearance.

The cat had a body temperature of 98.5 °F and was estimated to be 8% dehydrated based on skin turgor. The bladder was intact but small on palpation and the kidneys feel slightly enlarged, but not painful. No other abnormalities were found on the palpation of the abdomen. The heart rate was 160 beats per minute and no murmurs were auscultated. The femoral pulses were weak. The lungs were normal on auscultation. There were no external signs of trauma.

Interpretation of Urinalysis: The USG of 1.020 indicates impaired urine concentration in the face of dehydration. A USG >1.045 is expected in a dehydrated cat with normal renal function.

The 2+ dipstrip proteinuria in a minimally concentrated urine is pathological, but its origin as to renal or post-renal is not yet clear. Protein may be entering the urine at the same place that 1+ occult blood, RBC at 10–15 per HPF, and WBC at 3–5 per HPF are entering the urine. The presence of a moderate number of "hippurate-like" crystals (calcium oxalate monohydrate) in the urine sediment in a cat with this history is supportive of a diagnosis of ethylene glycol intoxication. What have previously been called "hippurate-like" crystals have more recently been recognized to be calcium oxalate monohydrate (whewellite) crystals. These crystals can be quite small and easily missed without careful examination of the urine sediment. Calcium oxalate monohydrate crystals occur more commonly with ethylene glycol intoxication that do calcium oxalate dihydrate crystals (i.e. the familiar so-called Maltese cross crystals or weddellite). The absence of cylindruria does not rule out AKI because any casts that may have

formed may still be trapped within the renal tubules if the cat is oliguric (see later).

Calcium oxalate crystalluria in an acutely sick animal always brings the possibility for ethylene glycol intoxication to the forefront, especially when these crystals are identified in those with urine that is not maximally concentrated.

The presumptive diagnosis was ethylene glycol intoxication and nephrotoxicity.

Further Diagnostics and Assessment: The serum creatinine concentration was 6.7 mg/dL, BUN was 219 mg/dL, phosphorus was 12.0 mg/dL, total CO_2 was 10.1 mEq/L, and calcium was 5.8 mg/dL. The low total CO_2 suggests the presence of metabolic acidosis, and the low calcium concentration could reflect chelation of calcium by metabolites of ethylene glycol. The 1.020 USG in combination with increased creatinine confirms the presence of primary renal disease. Renal ultrasonography revealed marked hyperechogenicity of normal sized kidneys, findings that support a diagnosis of AKI from ethylene glycol intoxication.

The measurement of serum osmolality and the calculation of the osmolal gap may provide supportive data for a diagnosis of ethylene glycol intoxication, depending upon when ingestion occurred (i.e. the osmolal gap may be increased if ingestion occurred within the past 24 hours).

The cat deteriorated over the next three days and died during aggressive fluid therapy. No urine production was observed (anuria). BUN, creatinine, and phosphorus concentrations increased progressively, and hyperkalemia (7.2 mEq/L) was observed.

At necropsy, the cat was overhydrated, and other findings were typical of ethylene glycol-associated nephrotoxicity (e.g. intratubular calcium oxalate crystal deposition, acute tubular necrosis).

Final Diagnosis: Ethylene glycol toxicity; Azotemic Anuric AKI.

CASE EXAMPLE: Urinalysis Case Number: 19

Source of Specimen:
    Cystocentesis ☒   Voided (Stream part) ☐   Post-Void (location) ☐
    Expressed ☐   Catheterized ☐
Volume: 2 mL
Refrigeration: Yes ☐   No ☒
Elapsed Time Before Analysis: 60 minutes
Stain: Yes ☒   No ☐

Color:	Red
Appearance:	Cloudy
Specific Gravity:	1.058
pH:	5.5
Protein:	100 mg/dL
Occult Blood:	3+
Hemolyzed:	☒
Intact:	☒
Glucose:	Negative
Ketones:	Negative
Bilirubin:	Negative

Casts per LPF: 0
   Hyaline
   Granular
   Cellular

WBC per HPF: 7–10
   Free   ☒
   Clumped ☐
RBC per HPF: 60–80
Epithelial Cells per HPF: 5–7
   Type: Squamous: ☐   Transitional: Free ☒   Clumped ☐   Renal: ☐

Crystals per HPF: None ☐
   Type: Struvite ☐   Calcium Oxalate ☒ Few   Urate ☐   Other ☐

Bacteria per HPF: None ☒
   Type: Rods ☐   Cocci ☐   Mixed ☐

Miscellaneous: Occasional sperm

Signalment: Eight-year-old spayed female Domestic Shorthair cat.

History and Physical Examination: The owner reports increased frequency of attempts to urinate in the litter pan and occasional urinations outside the litter pan during the past three weeks. Blood in the urine was observed when the cat urinated on the kitchen floor one time. This cat has been eating a dry, high-protein, acidifying, magnesium-restricted diet for the past four years. This cat has been otherwise healthy.

This cat was fond to be bright, alert, and had good body condition. The finding of a small firm bladder and resistance to palpation in the caudal abdomen were the only abnormal findings from the physical examination.

Interpretation of Urinalysis: The finding of red cloudy urine is mostly attributed to RBC in the urine. The USG of 1.058 shows highly concentrated urine indicating good renal function, but this high an USG can be a risk factor for the development of urolithiasis or for FIC. The urinary pH of 5.5 is quite low, but compatible with the acidifying diet that is being fed. Highly acid urine is a risk factor for oxalate but not for struvite urolithiasis. The 2+ proteinuria and 3+ occult blood are associated with urinary tract bleeding. 3+ occult blood is high enough to increase the proteinuria level on the dipstrip reading to some degree from the hemoglobin in the RBC.

Microscopy showing 60–80 RBC per HPF matches with the 3+ occult blood dipstrip reading as the most significant finding. There are minor increases in WBC and free transitional epithelial cells compatible with inflammation (bacterial or nonbacterial), trauma, and desquamation. Free epithelial cells are not commonly identified in those with FIC but are more commonly detected in those with urolithiasis. Neoplasia of the lower urinary tract is possible in an older cat but is rare in younger cats. The presence of calcium oxalate crystals in the urine is of limited diagnostic value as these crystals may be present in normal cats and dogs and may be absent in animals with calcium oxalate urolithiasis.

The presumptive diagnosis was calcium oxalate urolithiasis based on the dietary history, the very low urinary pH, and the abnormal palpation of the bladder.

Further Diagnostics and Assessment: Survey abdominal radiographs disclosed the presence of a single radiopaque cystic calculus compatible with struvite or calcium oxalate. Given the dietary history and the very low urinary pH, calcium oxalate urolithiasis was deemed more likely.

Quantitative bacterial urinary culture revealed no growth on a sample retrieved by cystocentesis.

A cystotomy was performed and a single roughened pale-yellow calculus was removed from the bladder and submitted for quantitative analysis. The analysis of the calculus showed that it was composed of 100% calcium oxalate dihydrate.

The hematuria gradually resolved within the first week after surgery and a follow-up urinalysis one month later was normal. It was recommended that the cat's diet be changed to a canned food that was less acidifying and somewhat lower in protein. If possible, achieving a targeted USG <1.030 would be ideal to lessen the chances for recurrence of urinary stones. The litter pan was to be changed frequently and the cat was to have access to fresh water at all times. The cat was found to be normal during reevaluation at 6 and 12 months.

Final Diagnosis: Calcium oxalate urolithiasis.

CASE EXAMPLE: Urinalysis Case Number: 20

Source of Specimen:
    Cystocentesis ☐   Voided (Stream part) ☐   Post-Void (location) ☐
    Expressed ☐   Catheterized ☒
Volume: 8   mL
Refrigeration: Yes ☐   No ☒
Elapsed Time Before Analysis: 30 minutes
Stain: Yes ☒   No ☐

Color:	Amber
Appearance:	Cloudy
Specific Gravity:	1.029
pH:	5.5
Protein:	100 mg/dL
Occult Blood:	2+
Hemolyzed:	☐
Intact:	☐
Glucose:	Negative
Ketones:	Negative
Bilirubin:	Negative

Casts per LPF: 0
   Hyaline
   Granular
   Cellular

WBC per HPF: 10–15
   Free   ☒
   Clumped ☐
RBC per HPF: 20–25
Epithelial Cells per HPF: 5–10
   Type: Squamous: ☒   Transitional: Free ☒   Clumped ☐   Renal: ☐

Crystals per HPF: None ☐
   Type: Struvite ☐   Calcium Oxalate ☐   Urate ☐   Other ☒ Cystine, moderate

Bacteria per HPF: None ☒
   Type: Rods ☐   Cocci ☐   Mixed ☐

Miscellaneous:

Signalment: Three-year-old castrated male Newfoundland dog.

History and Physical Examination: This dog had three days of dysuria and pollakiuria but was otherwise well. Physical examination was normal except that the bladder was mildly enlarged. There was resistance to passage of a 9 Fr urinary catheter, but a 3.5 Fr catheter passed easily, and a urine sample was collected.

Interpretation of Urinalysis: Urine concentration at 1.029 is very close to the cutoff point of 1.030 expected from normal dogs. Based on refractometer performance, the USG may actually be a bit lower or higher than that reported. This sample was collected several hours after the dog last ate and drank water, so the reported USG is likely less concentrated than that from a first morning sample before eating and drinking.

The pH is highly acidic at 5.5 which can influence the precipitation of some types of crystals, such as cystine. The positive reaction for occult blood matches up with RBC observed in the urinary sediment at 10–15 per HPF. Urinary protein was positive at 2+. Increased WBC at 10–15 per HPF and increased numbers of squamous and free transitional epithelial cells are also reported. Cystine crystals were observed during urine microscopy.

Overall, the UA indicates that urinary tract inflammation or trauma is associated with hemorrhage and desquamation of urothelial cells in addition to pyuria. Some of the RBC and epithelial cells could be added from urinary catheterization used to collect the sample. Alternatively, RBC and epithelial cells could be added from the trauma of urolithiasis. Cystine crystalluria is never normal and results from a disorder of proximal tubular transport of cystine and possibly other AA. Cystinuria can be found in isolation or when cystine urolithiasis exists; some breeds have a predilection for this genetic abnormality.

Additional Information: Cystine calculi are usually radiolucent, so contrast urography was performed. Urethral calculi were identified following a positive contrast urethrogram. Cystic calculi were identified during double contrast urethrography right after the urethrogram was completed. Ultrasonography would have identified the radiolucent calculi in the bladder, but not in the urethra; thus contrast urography was used instead of ultrasonography.

Retropulsion under anesthesia was successful in pushing the urethral calculi into the bladder. Surgical removal of the bladder stones confirmed them to be 100% cystine.

Final Diagnosis: Cystine urolithiasis, cystic and urethral; partial urethral obstruction.

CASE EXAMPLE: Urinalysis Case Number: 21

Source of Specimen:
    Cystocentesis ☒   Voided (Stream part) ☐   Post-Void (location) ☐
    Expressed ☐   Catheterized ☐
Volume: 3 mL
Refrigeration: Yes ☐   No ☒
Elapsed Time Before Analysis: 45 minutes
Stain: Yes ☒   No ☐

Color:	Orange
Appearance:	Clear
Specific Gravity:	1.032
pH:	6.0
Protein:	30 mg/dL
Occult Blood:	Negative
Hemolyzed:	☐
Intact:	☐
Glucose:	Negative
Ketones:	Negative
Bilirubin:	3+

Casts per LPF:
  Hyaline
  Granular 2–3
  Cellular

WBC per HPF: 2–4
  Free   ☒
  Clumped   ☐
RBC per HPF: 1–3
Epithelial Cells per HPF: Occasional
    Type: Squamous: ☐   Transitional: Free ☒   Clumped ☐   Renal: ☒

Crystals per HPF: None ☐
    Type: Struvite ☐   Calcium Oxalate ☐   Urate ☐   Other ☒ Bilirubin, moderate

Bacteria per HPF: None ☒
    Type: Rods ☐   Cocci ☐   Mixed ☐

Miscellaneous: Some small epithelial cells may be RTE

Signalment: Six-year-old spayed female mixed-breed dog.

History and Physical Examination: Current complaints included anorexia, lethargy, and vomiting 48–72 hours after eating raw bacon. Body temperature was 103.2 °F, the dog was lethargic, approximately 7% dehydrated, and had icteric mucous membranes. She was uncomfortable and resisted attempts at abdominal palpation.

Interpretation of Urinalysis: Urine color that was orange was attributed to the abundant bilirubin pigment in the urine. The 1.032 USG in the face of dehydration indicates moderately concentrated urine. This degree of urine concentration is considered minimally appropriate, as young normal dogs with dehydration often have USG higher than this. 1+ protein on the dipstrip could be "normal" or it could be renal in origin, since the urinary sediment is mostly inactive. Bilirubinuria is considered marked with a 3+ reaction on the dipstrip and moderate numbers of bilirubin crystals observed during urine microscopy. A low-level bilirubin positive dipstrip reaction can be normal in dogs at times, especially in males with concentrated urine. This degree of bilirubin reactivity on the dipstrip pad is abnormal, as are the moderate numbers of bilirubin crystals. Bilirubinuria can occur following systemic hemolysis, primary liver disease, or biliary obstructive disease. The two to three granular casts per LPF are of concern in this setting as to the possibility for AKI that could be developing from volume contraction severe enough to create renal ischemia, or from biliary nephrosis.

Bilirubinuria is the pivotal problem in this urinalysis that deserves the most attention.

Further Diagnostics and Assessment: The hemogram showed a leukocytosis (41 600/µL) due to neutrophilia (37 900/µL) and a left shift (2500/µL) compatible with a severe inflammatory process. Serum direct bilirubin was 6.9 mg/dL and alkaline phosphatase was 2690 IU/L. Alanine aminotransferase was 250 IU/L, amylase was 876 IU/L, and lipase 754 IU/L. Serum canine pancreatic lipase concentration was increased, and a tentative diagnosis of acute pancreatitis was tendered. Serum creatinine and BUN were initially within the reference range. Abdominal ultrasound disclosed dilatation of the extra- and intrahepatic biliary system and the pancreas was diffusely enlarged and hyperechoic. The gall bladder also was enlarged and there was a small amount of peritoneal effusion present. Other abdominal viscera were assessed as normal.

A UPC of 1.8 was compatible with glomerular origin proteinuria that was originally suspected on the 1+ dipstrip proteinuria. Renal proteinuria is fairly common in dogs with acute pancreatitis and can have prognostic significance. Leaky glomeruli happen for reasons that are not entirely clear in those with pancreatitis and SIRS.

The bilirubinuria and bilirubin crystals are compatible with the extrahepatic biliary obstruction and increased excretion of direct-reacting bilirubin in the urine secondary to the pancreatitis.

The dog was treated medically for pancreatitis by intravenous fluid therapy, parental nutrition, and antibiotics. It responded poorly and exploratory laparotomy was performed. The pancreas was severely enlarged and inflamed and contained a moderately large organizing abscess. The dog was euthanized at the time of surgery and no necropsy was performed that could provide further details.

Final Diagnosis: Biliary obstruction secondary to pancreatitis; Ischemic AKI or biliary nephrosis; renal proteinuria.

CASE EXAMPLE: Urinalysis Case Number: 22

Source of Specimen:
    Cystocentesis ☐   Voided (Stream part) ☒ Midstream   Post-Void (location) ☐
    Expressed ☐   Catheterized ☐
Volume: 3   mL
Refrigeration: Yes ☐   No ☒
Elapsed Time Before Analysis: 15 minutes
Stain: Yes ☒   No ☐
Comments: urine was collected immediately following the expulsion of the urethral plug

Color: Red
Appearance: Cloudy
Specific Gravity: 1.060
pH: 7.0
Protein: 300 mg/dL
Occult Blood: 4+
    Hemolyzed: ☐
    Intact: ☐
Glucose: Negative
Ketones: Negative
Bilirubin: Negative

Casts per LPF: 0
    Hyaline
    Granular
    Cellular

WBC per HPF: 3–5
    Free   ☒
    Clumped   ☐
RBC per HPF: 50-60
Epithelial Cells per HPF: 1–3
    Type: Squamous: ☐   Transitional: Free ☒   Clumped ☐   Renal: ☐

Crystals per HPF: None ☐
    Type: Struvite ☒ Few   Calcium Oxalate ☐   Urate ☐   Other ☐

Bacteria per HPF: None ☒
    Type: Rods ☐   Cocci ☐   Mixed ☐

Miscellaneous: Capillaria eggs - occasional

Signalment: Three-year-old castrated male Domestic Shorthair cat.

History and Physical Examination: Straining to urinate and drops of blood in the litter pan were observed over the past week. The cat also was making more frequent trips to the litter pan and staying in the pan for much longer than usual. His appetite was normal until yesterday and is now poor. The cat had been otherwise healthy and had not been to a veterinarian since receiving its vaccinations as a kitten.

The cat was obviously uncomfortable based on its crying and posture. Abdominal palpation revealed an enlarged, turgid bladder that was very painful. The cat was slightly dehydrated based on skin turgor. The tip of the penis was reddened, and some white mucoid material was observed at the external urethral meatus. Gentle massage of the distal penis dislodged some of the white, mucoid material and was followed by the passage of a good stream of urine. A smash preparation of a part of the urethral plug did not reveal any crystalline material. This was unexpected since most urethral plugs contain struvite.

Interpretation of Urinalysis: The urine was red and cloudy due to the high numbers of RBC in the urinary sediment. The USG of 1.060 is highly concentrated and is an appropriate response to the noted dehydration. The urinary dipstrip pH of 7.0 is tending toward neutrality, which is expected in cats not eating and during episodes of urethral obstruction. The exudation of plasma into the urine as a result of the inflammation may also have contributed to the urine pH of 7.0 in this cat. The 3+ protein and 4+ occult blood on urinary dipstrip are associated with urinary bleeding as supported by the 50–60 RBC per HPF seen during urine microscopy. The high numbers of RBC can be part of an inflammatory process but can also reflect trauma to the urothelium encountered during high bladder pressure achieved during urethral obstruction. When there are maximal occult blood reactions on the dipstrip, some increase in dipstrip protein is also

expected to occur from hemoglobin in the RBC. A trivial increase in WBC at 3–5 per HPF was seen in the urinary sediment, likely from blood contamination of the urine or from mild inflammation. The mild increase in transitional cells at one to three per HPF shed into the urine could be accounted for by the effects of urethral obstruction and high-pressure trauma exerted on the urothelium, or from increased desquamation secondary to inflammation. Sometimes increased urothelial cells are shed into the urine as part of the inflammatory process leading to urethral obstruction, similar to that sometimes observed in nonobstructive FIC. The small numbers of struvite crystals likely formed from a combination of urine stasis and the urinary pH of 7.0. Struvite becomes increasingly insoluble in urine when the urinary pH is 6.8 and higher. The struvite crystals were identified during urine microscopy shortly after collection, so they are not an artifact of cooling and storage of the urine sample. The finding of *Capillaria* eggs was entirely unexpected. The adult *Capillaria* parasite can be an incidental finding or can cause hematuria due to associated cystitis in some instances. No bacteria were identified in the urinary sediment.

The working diagnosis at this point was urethral obstruction secondary to sterile cystitis, possibly as a consequence of *Capillaria* infestation of the bladder.

Further Diagnostics and Assessment: Quantitative bacterial culture of a voided mid-stream urine sample returned with no growth. Histopathology on the submitted mucoid urethral plug revealed that the plug contained numerous ova and adult parasites of *Capillaria*. In this cat, the presence of *Capillaria* was pathologic.

The cat's dehydration was corrected by administration of subcutaneous fluids. The urethra remained patent following the passage of the mucoid urethral plug, and the cat was discharged on fenbendazole to treat *Capillaria*.

Final Diagnosis: Urethral obstruction due to *Capillaria*.

CASE EXAMPLE: Urinalysis Case Number: 23

Source of Specimen:
    Cystocentesis ☐   Voided (Stream part) ☐   Post-Void (location) ☐
    Expressed ☐   Catheterized ☒
Volume: 5   mL
Refrigeration: Yes ☐   No ☒
Elapsed Time Before Analysis:
Stain: Yes ☐   No ☒

Color: Yellow
Appearance: Slightly turbid
Specific Gravity: 1.023
pH: 6.0
Protein: 100 mg/dL
Occult Blood: Negative
   Hemolyzed: ☐
   Intact: ☐
Glucose: 4+
Ketones: 2+
Bilirubin: 1+

Casts per LPF: 0
   Hyaline
   Granular
   Cellular

WBC per HPF: 10–15
   Free   ☒
   Clumped ☐
RBC per HPF: 7–10
Epithelial Cells per HPF: 5-7
   Type: Squamous: ☐   Transitional: Free ☒   Clumped ☐   Renal: ☐

Crystals per HPF: None ☒
   Type: Struvite ☐   Calcium Oxalate ☐   Urate ☐   Other ☐

Bacteria per HPF: None ☒
   Type: Rods ☐   Cocci ☐   Mixed ☐

Miscellaneous:

Signalment: Nine-year-old intact male German Shepherd Dog.

History and Physical Examination: Lethargy and anorexia of five days duration were reported prior to hospitalization. Weight loss and greatly increased water consumption were observed by the owner over the past few weeks, but urinations were not observed. This dog has been very healthy until recently. The dog was found to be lethargic, thin, and slightly dehydrated based on skin turgor. Increased inspiratory bronchovesicular sounds were heard during thoracic auscultation and an abdominal component to respirations was noted. TPR was normal and the heart auscultated normally.

Interpretation of Urinalysis: The yellow urine was slightly turbid, which is attributed to the increased number of WBC, RBC, and epithelial cells identified during urine microscopy. Urinary pH by dipstrip was 6.0; a higher urinary pH is expected in an anorectic dog. The ketone positive status on urinary dipstrip may be associated with ketoacidosis and acid urine production. The 2+ protein positive reagent pad on the dipstrip could be from proteins added from the lower urinary tract, given the 10–15 WBC per HPF, 7–10 RBC per HPF, and the 5–7 free transitional cells observed in the urinary sediment. The slight increase in RBC is not likely due to the method of urine collection since the urinary catheter passed easily. The 4+ glucosuria and the 2+ ketonuria are strikingly abnormal findings in this urinalysis that support a diagnosis of ketoacidotic diabetes mellitus. The 1+ bilirubin could be a normal finding in a male dog at times, but given the

likely diagnosis of diabetes mellitus, there is concern for liver disease acquired from the diabetes mellitus that accounts for the bilirubinuria. The combination of proteinuria, mild pyuria, and mild hematuria could signify the presence of a urinary tract infection, but no bacterial were identified (quantitative bacterial urine culture later returned with no growth). Renal proteinuria is known to occur in some dogs and cats with diabetes mellitus.

Further Diagnostics and Assessment: The blood glucose was 855 mg/dL, which far exceeds the renal threshold that allows glucose to appear in the urine (spill over). Serum total CO_2 was 8 mEq/L indicating severe metabolic acidosis. Moderate azotemia was present based on a serum creatinine concentration of 3.2 mg/dL and a BUN of 54 mg/dL. The USG of 1.023 was lower than expected in a dehydrated dog. This is partially a result of solute diuresis due to glucosuria and ketonuria, but underlying renal disease also may have contributed to the low urine specific gravity. Blood pH was 7.017 indicating severe acidosis. The dog was treated with IV fluids and insulin that resulted in a much lower blood glucose concentration at 250 mg/dL and much less glucosuria. Ketonuria resolved during these treatments. The dog's serum creatinine concentration decreased to 2.3 mg/dL and the BUN to 41 mg/dL during fluid therapy indicating a component of prerenal azotemia. One month later during successful treatment of the diabetes mellitus, the creatinine was almost normal at 1.8 mg/dL.

Final Diagnosis: Ketoacidotic diabetes mellitus.

CASE EXAMPLE: Urinalysis Case Number: 24

Source of Specimen:
    Cystocentesis ☐   Voided (Stream part) ☒ end stream   Post-Void (location) ☐
    Expressed ☐   Catheterized ☐
Volume: 2 mL
Refrigeration: Yes ☐   No ☒
Elapsed Time Before Analysis: 30 minutes
Stain: Yes ☒   No ☐

Color: Yellow
Appearance: Clear
Specific Gravity: 1.038
pH: 6.5
Protein: Negative
Occult Blood: Negative
   Hemolyzed: ☐
   Intact: ☐
Glucose: Negative
Ketones: Negative
Bilirubin: Negative

Casts per LPF: 0
   Hyaline
   Granular
   Cellular

WBC per HPF: 0–1
   Free   ☒
   Clumped ☐
RBC per HPF: 0–1
Epithelial Cells per HPF: 0
   Type: Squamous: ☐   Transitional: Free ☐   Clumped ☐   Renal: ☐

Crystals per HPF: None ☒
   Type: Struvite ☐   Calcium Oxalate ☐   Urate ☐   Other ☐

Bacteria per HPF: None ☒
   Type: Rods ☐   Cocci ☐   Mixed ☐

Miscellaneous:

Signalment: Three-month-old intact female Labrador Retriever dog.

History and Physical Examination: The owners have been having difficulty in training their puppy to not urinate in the house or in the crate during the day. She came into the veterinary clinic to see if there was anything wrong with her that could be causing her to drink so much water. She is active, growing well, eating vigorously (meal fed twice daily), and has normal bowel movements. She seems to "drink a lot of water." The owners were not sure if she was producing a larger volume of urine or not, but she takes about 15 seconds to finish voiding, quite a bit longer than the other dog in the household. Her physical examination was normal.

Interpretation of Urinalysis: This urine sample was collected by voiding in the late afternoon at the veterinary hospital. The urinalysis is normal in every aspect. The 1.038 USG is not compatible with excessive water drinking and urinations, at least not in the time proximity this sample was collected. PPD is often associated with episodic polydipsia that drives the polyuria at certain times of the day, so the finding of one USG that shows high urine concentration does not exclude samples at other times of the day that are far less concentrated.

Further Diagnostics and Assessment: Serum biochemistry and CBC were normal. The owner purchased an inexpensive refractometer online and collected urine samples at various times of the day and recorded the USG. USG first thing in the morning (before the meal and drinking) was 1.035 and 1.030 on two consecutive days. Samples later in the day showed USG of 1.004, 1.008, 1.015, 1.024, and 1.030. Following the evening meal, the USG was 1.014 and then 1.020 and 1.025 before bedtime. Such wide differences in USG demonstrate that normal concentrating ability can and did happen at some periods of the day. PPD is the only condition associated with such wide swings in the USG over one day. In this puppy, it appears that high volumes of water drinking follow the meals. She tolerated mild water restriction, which resulted in less urine volume production. She outgrew PPD by six months of age. It is not unusual for dogs with PPD presenting to a veterinary hospital to have USG >1.030 depending on the time of the day that the sample was collected. Some dogs that are hospitalized for part of the day also suddenly stop water drinking due to the shock of the visit and elaborate urine of much higher USG than before the visit.

Final Diagnosis: Primary (psychogenic) Polydipsia.

CASE EXAMPLE: Urinalysis Case Number: 25

Source of Specimen:
 Cystocentesis ☐ Voided (Stream part) ☒ beginning stream Post-Void (location) ☐
 Expressed ☐ Catheterized ☐
Volume: 3 mL
Refrigeration: Yes ☐ No ☐
Elapsed Time Before Analysis: 30 minutes
Stain: Yes ☒ No ☐

Color: Slight pink
Appearance: Cloudy
Specific Gravity: 1.030
pH: 7.0
Protein: 2+
Occult Blood: 2+
 Hemolyzed: ☐
 Intact: ☒
Glucose: Negative
Ketones: Negative
Bilirubin: Negative

Casts per LPF: 0
 Hyaline
 Granular
 Cellular

WBC per HPF: 5–8
 Free ☒
 Clumped ☐
RBC per HPF: 20–25
Epithelial Cells per HPF: 0–2
 Type: Squamous: ☐ Transitional: Free ☒ Clumped ☐ Renal: ☐

Crystals per HPF: None ☒
 Type: Struvite ☐ Calcium Oxalate ☐ Urate ☐ Other ☐

Bacteria per HPF: None ☒
 Type: Rods ☐ Cocci ☐ Mixed ☐

Miscellaneous:

Signalment: 11-year-old spayed female mixed-breed dog.

History and Physical Examination: A pink tinge has been noted in some of her urinations over the past month. She has a mild increase in the frequency of urinations and some straining to urinate at times. Her water intake is unchanged, and her overall urine volume has not increased. She is doing well systemically. Her general physical examination is normal with the exception of a mildly thickened urinary bladder. Rectal examination is normal.

Interpretation of Urinalysis: The urine sample was collected only from the beginning urine stream by accident (the goal was for a mid-stream sample). The urine is slightly pink and cloudy due to the increased numbers of RBC at 20–25 per HPF and WBC at 5–8 per HPF. The USG of 1.030 shows adequate urine concentration. Some of the 2+ protein on the dipstrip is associated with urinary tract bleeding as shown in the sediment with intact RBC and with the occult blood reaction on the dipstrip. Very few free transitional epithelial cells were observed during urine microscopy and they were of normal morphology. The predominant abnormality on this UA is the finding of increased RBC with a mild increase in WBC without identification of bacteria. Causes for this can include bacterial UTI, lower urinary tract stones, and urothelial neoplasia. In an older dog with mostly hematuria and some thickening of the bladder wall, it is essential to exclude TCC (UCC).

Further Diagnostics and Assessment: Abdominal radiographs were taken to exclude the presence of radiopaque urinary calculi; these images were normal. Abdominal ultrasonography was normal with the exception of mild thickening of the bladder wall especially prominent near the trigone. There was no hydronephrosis. CBC and routine serum biochemistry were normal.

Given our concern for the possibility of urothelial carcinoma, another urine sample was collected in the hope of having more urothelial cells to examine during microscopy of a wet mount slide and then submission of urinary sediment for cytological evaluation. This sample was specifically collected at the end of urination when she strained a bit. This end-urination sample was loaded with free and clumped urothelial cells that enabled a diagnosis of TCC (UCC) to be established. Due to the trigonal bladder thickening and the dog's age, getting the second sample for urinalysis by cystocentesis was avoided in an effort to avoid needle tracking of any neoplastic cells that might be harvested.

Final Diagnosis: TCC (UCC) urinary bladder.

CASE EXAMPLE: Urinalysis Case Number: 26

Source of Specimen:
Cystocentesis ☒   Voided (Stream part) ☐   Post-Void (location) ☐
Expressed ☐   Catheterized ☐
Volume: 3   mL
Refrigeration: Yes ☐   No ☒
Elapsed Time Before Analysis: 60 minutes
Stain: Yes ☒   No ☐

Color: Slight pink
Appearance: Cloudy
Specific Gravity: 1.028
pH: 6.5
Protein: Negative
Occult Blood: Negative
    Hemolyzed: ☐
    Intact: ☐
Glucose: Negative
Ketones: Negative
Bilirubin: Negative

Casts per LPF: 0
    Hyaline
    Granular
    Cellular

WBC per HPF: 0–1
    Free   ☐
    Clumped   ☐
RBC per HPF: 0–2
Epithelial Cells per HPF: 0
    Type: Squamous: ☐   Transitional: Free ☐   Clumped ☐   Renal: ☐

Crystals per HPF: None ☒
    Type: Struvite ☐   Calcium Oxalate ☐   Urate ☐   Other ☐

Bacteria per HPF: None ☒
    Type: Rods ☐   Cocci ☐   Mixed ☐

Miscellaneous:

Signalment: Six-year-old intact male Pit Bull dog.

History and Physical Examination: Yearly wellness examination. The owners had no complaints and the dog appears to be systemically well. Physical examination was normal. UA was submitted along with blood testing as part of the annual wellness program for dogs ≥5 years old.

Interpretation of Urinalysis: All findings on this UA are normal. The USG of 1.028 is close to the tipping point of ≥1.030 USG expected from normal dogs. That rule of expected USG depends on when the urine was collected in relationship to eating and drinking, as USG varies considerably throughout the day in normal dogs. Also, USG refractometer accuracy can vary by as much as ±0.004 depending on the specific refractometer and the operator.

Further Diagnostics and Assessment: A few days later, the USG was 1.043 on a post-voided sample collected by the owners at home (before the morning meal).

Final Diagnosis: Normal.

CASE EXAMPLE: Urinalysis Case Number: 27

Source of Specimen:
  Cystocentesis ☒   Voided (Stream part) ☐ beginning stream   Post-Void (location) ☐
  Expressed ☐   Catheterized ☐
Volume: 3   mL
Refrigeration: Yes ☐   No ☒
Elapsed Time Before Analysis: 10 minutes
Stain: Yes ☒   No ☐
Comments: ULS guided cystocentesis

Color: Colorless
Appearance: Cloudy
Specific Gravity: 1.012
pH: 6.0
Protein: 3+
Occult Blood: 1+
    Hemolyzed: ☒
    Intact: ☒
Glucose: 1+
Ketones: Negative
Bilirubin: Negative

Casts per LPF:
    Hyaline 0
    Granular 3-5 coarse and finely granular
    Cellular 1-2 RBC, 0-1 RTE

WBC per HPF: 3–5
    Free   ☒
    Clumped   ☐
RBC per HPF: 5–7
Epithelial Cells per HPF: 1–2
    Type: Squamous: ☐   Transitional: Free ☐   Clumped ☐   Renal: ☒

Crystals per HPF: None ☒
    Type: Struvite ☐   Calcium Oxalate ☐   Urate ☐   Other ☐

Bacteria per HPF: None ☒
    Type: Rods ☐   Cocci ☐   Mixed ☐

Miscellaneous:

Signalment: Six-year-old intact male Labrador Retriever dog.

History and Physical Examination: This dog has had total anorexia for the past three days preceded by progressive vomiting, lethargy, and depression over the past seven days. He has been drinking more water than usual, but there is no observed change in the volume of urine produced. 101.1 °F, 150 HR, 35 RR. Dehydration is assessed at 8% based on skin turgor. Chest auscultation is normal. The left kidney palpates of normal size; the right kidney was not identified. Bladder volume was moderate and non-painful. The rest of the abdomen palpated normally.

Interpretation of Urinalysis: The cloudy appearance of this sample is mostly attributed to the various types of cylindruria (granular, RTE, RBC). The USG of 1.012 is inappropriate for a dog with overt dehydration in which the USG should be >1.030. The low USG in conjunction with the cylindruria points to a major kidney problem. The 3+ dipstrip proteinuria along with the low USG and a urinary sediment without too many RBC or WBC usually indicates glomerular origin proteinuria. The 1+ occult blood (hemolyzed and intact) is in concordance with the five to seven RBC per HPF identified during urine microscopy. Since the suspicion for active glomerular disease is high, it is possible that some of the RBC traveled across the damaged glomerulus to appear as dysmorphic RBC. Some of dysmorphic RBC, if they were there, could have undergone lysis. Particular attention to the morphology of the RBC as to whether they could be dysmorphic or not was not given.

The central abnormal findings of importance are the high magnitude proteinuria on dipstrip and the high level cylindruria during microscopy. The three to five finely and coarsely granular casts per LPF are compatible with the proteinuria leading to precipitation of plasma proteins as granules, or as granules that appear following cellular degeneration of RBC, WBC, or RTE within the tubular lumens. The finding of 0–1 RTE cellular casts per LPF indicates an active process that promotes desquamation of renal tubular cells into the cast matrix protein. The finding of one to two free RTE per HPF is likely from the same cause as for the RTE casts. The most interesting and possibly important cast identified is that of the RBC cast at 1–2 per LPF. The finding of even one RBC cast is highly abnormal, often indicating glomerular bleeding into tubular lumens. Integrating the finding of severe proteinuria with the presence of RBC casts suggests a highly active glomerulonephritis. The finding of free RTE and RTE casts suggests a component of AKI from tubular injury. The mild increase in WBC at 3–5 per HPF in the absence of bacteria is compatible with renal inflammation, especially in the face of the cylindruria.

Further Diagnostics and Assessment: On serum biochemistry, a BUN of 120 mg/dL, creatinine of 3.2 mg/dL, phosphorus of 7.2 mg/dL, and serum albumin of 2.0 g/dL were noted abnormalities. The finding of azotemia at the same time as a 1.012 USG before any treatment indicates primary renal disease. Since the dog was known to be dehydrated, a combination of prerenal and primary renal azotemia exists.

The UPC was 8.4 (normal <0.5) and the urine culture was negative. Serologic testing was positive for Lyme's disease and negative for other vector-borne diseases.

Renal biopsy revealed a severe glomerulopathy with immune complex deposition. Focal areas of acute tubular necrosis were also evident, as were the appearance of intraluminal RBC casts.

Final Diagnosis: Borrelia associated RPGN; RBC casts; Renal proteinuria.

CASE EXAMPLE: Urinalysis Case Number: 28

Source of Specimen:
Cystocentesis ☐   Voided (Stream part) ☐   Post-Void (location) ☒ litter NoSorb
Expressed ☐   Catheterized ☐
Volume: 2 mL
Refrigeration: Yes ☒   No ☐
Elapsed Time Before Analysis: 3 hours
Stain: Yes ☒   No ☐
Comments: The owner brought in sample collected at home

Color: Amber
Appearance: Clear
Specific Gravity: 1.042
pH: 6.5
Protein: Trace
Occult Blood: 3+
    Hemolyzed: ☒
    Intact: ☐
Glucose: Negative
Ketones: Negative
Bilirubin: Negative

Casts per LPF: 0
    Hyaline 0
    Granular 0
    Cellular 0

WBC per HPF: 0
    Free   ☐
    Clumped   ☐
RBC per HPF: 0
Epithelial Cells per HPF: 0
    Type: Squamous: ☐   Transitional: Free ☐ Clumped ☐   Renal: ☐
    Frequency of Type:

Crystals per HPF: None ☐   Few ☒   Moderate ☐   Many ☐
    Type: Struvite ☒   Calcium Oxalate ☐   Urate ☐   Other ☐

Bacteria per HPF: None ☐   Few ☒   Moderate ☐   Many ☐
    Type: Rods ☐   Cocci ☒   Mixed ☐

Miscellaneous Findings/Comments:

Signalment: Six-year-old spayed female Domestic Shorthair Cat.

History and Physical Examination: One-month recheck of previous episode of idiopathic cystitis; no current clinical signs. Cat is apparently healthy in all regards. The physical examination is normal.

Interpretation of Urinalysis: Results are from a post-voided sample collected from the litterbox filled with nonabsorbent litter. The sample was collected from the litterbox and stored in the refrigerator for about two hours before driving to the veterinary clinic. The USG of 1.042 indicates good capacity to elaborate highly concentrated urine. The dipstrip reaction was strongly positive for hemolyzed blood and negative for intact RBC and there were no RBC seen during microscopy of urinary sediment. There was no evidence for systemic hemolysis or muscle damage that could have added pigments to the urine to activate the occult blood dipstrip color reaction. The trace protein reaction on the dipstrip does not often indicate pathological proteinuria in those that are well and with highly concentrated urine.

The few cocci-like bacteria reported are likely to be seen when urine is collected post voiding from a litter box. The few struvite crystals that were reported is not surprising in concentrated urine that has cooled, and is often normal. The ex vivo precipitation of crystals is more likely in samples that have been refrigerated.

Further Diagnostics and Assessment: Upon further questioning of the owner, it was determined that the litterbox is frequently washed out with water and then disinfected with bleach. It is likely that the positive occult blood reaction is from residual bleach contamination of the sample.

Another sample of post-voided urine from the litter box was collected after thorough rinsing with water and no bleach disinfectant. This was done the next week and the reaction for blood was negative.

Final Diagnosis: Falsely positive occult blood due to bleach contamination.

CASE EXAMPLE: Urinalysis Case Number: 29

Source of Specimen:
    Cystocentesis ☐   Voided (Stream part) ☒ Midstream   Post-Void (location) ☐
    Expressed ☐   Catheterized ☐
Volume: 8   mL
Refrigeration: Yes ☐   No ☒
Elapsed Time Before Analysis: 20 minutes
Stain: Yes ☒   No ☐

Color: Yellow
Appearance: Slightly cloudy
Specific Gravity: 1.035
pH: 7.0
Protein: 2+
Occult Blood: Trace
   Hemolyzed: ☐
   Intact: ☒
Glucose: Negative
Ketones: Negative
Bilirubin: Negative

Casts per LPF:0
   Hyaline
   Granular
   Cellular

WBC per HPF: 30–40
   Free   ☒
   Clumped ☐
RBC per HPF: 5–10
Epithelial Cells per HPF: 3–5
   Type: Squamous: ☒   Transitional: Free ☒   Clumped ☐   Renal: ☐

Crystals per HPF: None ☒
   Type: Struvite ☐   Calcium Oxalate ☐   Urate ☐   Other ☐

Bacteria per HPF: None ☐
   Type: Rods ☐   Cocci ☒ Few   Mixed ☐

Miscellaneous:

Signalment: Six-month-old intact female Great Dane dog.

History and Physical Examination: Pollakiuria for seven days and increased licking of the vulva were the primary concerns of the owner. The dog was otherwise doing well, growing normally, and she had a high level of activity. There was no PU/PD and nor was blood noted in the urinations. A small volume of yellow discharge was noted coming from her vulva along with signs of perivulvar irritation. Her vulvar conformation was normal and there was no "hooding." The rest of the physical examination was normal.

Interpretation of Urinalysis: This urine was a midstream voided sample reported to be slightly cloudy and yellow, with a USG that was well concentrated at 1.035. The 2+ protein and the trace occult blood for intact RBC were attributed to the active urine sediment with 30–40 WBC per HPF, 5–10 RBC per HPF, and the 3–5 epithelial cells per HPF (squamous and free transitional cells). A few cocci were also identified.

The active sediment indicates inflammation, but the location of the inflammation as to the bladder, urethra, or genital (vestibular or vulvar) is not clear. Puppy "vaginitis" could account for this, but the bladder could be involved. Cocci in this voided specimen could easily have been added from the genital tract.

Further Diagnostics and Assessment: A follow-up UA by cystocentesis was obtained later the same day and revealed no pyuria or bacteriuria. The active sediment on the voided sample compared to absence of abnormal elements from the cystocentesis sample localizes the inflammatory process distal to the bladder. Urine culture on this sample collected by cystocentesis was negative. An anoscope was used to visualize the vestibule, which showed extensive follicular change consistent with puppy vaginitis. Vestibular douching with a dilute iodine solution was administered once daily for seven days. Clinical signs resolved without the use of antibiotics over the next month. The term "vaginitis" is misleading as the inflammatory process is mostly within the vestibule and not the vagina as viewed during cystoscopy.

Final Diagnosis: Puppy "vaginitis."

CASE EXAMPLE: Urinalysis Case Number: 30

Source of Specimen:
    Cystocentesis ☐   Voided (Stream part) ☐   Post-Void (location) ☒ cage pads
    Expressed ☐   Catheterized ☐
Volume: 2 mL
Refrigeration: Yes ☐   No ☒
Elapsed Time Before Analysis: 30 minutes
Stain: Yes ☒   No ☐

Color:	very pale
Appearance:	clear
Specific Gravity:	1.008
pH:	6.5
Protein:	Negative
Occult Blood:	Negative
Hemolyzed:	☐
Intact:	☐
Glucose:	Negative
Ketones:	Negative
Bilirubin:	Negative

Casts per LPF: 0
  Hyaline
  Granular
  Cellular

WBC per HPF: 0-1
  Free   ☒
  Clumped   ☐
RBC per HPF: 0
Epithelial Cells per HPF: 0
  Type: Squamous: ☐   Transitional: Free ☐   Clumped ☐   Renal: ☐

Crystals per HPF: None ☒
  Type: Struvite ☐   Calcium Oxalate ☐   Urate ☐   Other ☐

Bacteria per HPF: None ☐
  Type: Rods ☐   Cocci ☐   Mixed ☒ few

Miscellaneous: ICU patient on IV fluids. Foreign material and fiber seen in sediment

Signalment: Three-year-old spayed female mixed-breed dog.

History and Physical Examination: Acute watery diarrhea ongoing for over one day is the presenting complaint. The dog is well vaccinated and has been healthy to this point. The dog was an estimated 7–8% dehydrated based on skin turgor and had some fluid filled bowl loops noted on abdominal palpation. The rest of the physical examination was unremarkable. IV fluids are being administered to correct dehydration.

Interpretation of Urinalysis: A post-voided urine sample was obtained from the cage pads. About 2 mL of urine was aspirated from the wet pads. The urine was very pale and clear with a USG of 1.008. Dipstrip pad color reactions were all normal. Urine sediment was inactive for RBC, WBC, and epithelial cells. The few rods and cocci bacteria along with foreign material and fibers in the sediment are attributed to contamination of urine in the cage pads.

Further Diagnostics and Assessment: Routine biochemistry showed a normal BUN and serum creatinine. Other biochemistry results were also normal with the exception of mild hypokalemia (3.5 mEq/L). Isosthenuria is common and expected in patients on IV fluids. The dog quickly recovered with a diagnosis of nonspecific enteritis. Two weeks later the owners dropped off a voided urine specimen that had a USG of 1.042.

Final Diagnosis: Isosthenuria during IV fluid administration.

CASE EXAMPLE: Urinalysis Case Number: 31

Source of Specimen:
    Cystocentesis ☐   Voided (Stream part) ☒ Midstream   Post-Void (location) ☐
    Expressed ☐   Catheterized ☐
Volume: 6 mL
Refrigeration: Yes ☐   No ☒
Elapsed Time Before Analysis: 40 minutes
Stain: Yes ☒   No ☐

Color: Light yellow
Appearance: Clear
Specific Gravity: 1.016
pH: 6.5
Protein: 1+
Occult Blood: Negative
   Hemolyzed: ☐
   Intact: ☐
Glucose: 2+
Ketones: Negative
Bilirubin: Negative

Casts per LPF: 0
   Hyaline
   Granular
   Cellular

WBC per HPF: 0–1
   Free   ☒
   Clumped   ☐
RBC per HPF: 0–1
Epithelial Cells per HPF: 0
   Type: Squamous: ☐   Transitional: Free ☐   Clumped ☐   Renal: ☐

Crystals per HPF: None ☒
   Type: Struvite ☐   Calcium Oxalate ☐   Urate ☐   Other ☐

Bacteria per HPF: None ☒
   Type: Rods ☐   Cocci ☐   Mixed ☐

Miscellaneous:

Signalment: Four-year-old castrated male Golden Retriever dog.

History and Physical Examination: The owners complain that their dog has had increased water drinking for the past four to five weeks. He also has an increased need to void outside and with larger than normal urine volume. The dog is otherwise systemically normal. Physical examination is unremarkable. The dog is not receiving any medication other than monthly heartworm prevention.

Interpretation of Urinalysis: The USG of 1.016 is lower than expected for urine produced over the day for normal dogs. This USG supports the accuracy of the history for PUPD. If the low USG were the only abnormal finding, it would be good to repeat the USG before the dog ate or drank in the morning in order to get a better appreciation for urine concentrating capacity. The 2+ glucosuria adds credence to the low USG being representative of diminished urine concentrating ability, possibly due to osmotic diuresis associate with glucosuria. The 1+ dipstrip protein reaction in urine with this low a USG indicates that proteinuria could be a problem. Glucosuria is the pivotal finding on this urinalysis with diabetes mellitus and renal glucosuria being the differential considerations. Findings from urine microscopy were inactive.

Further Diagnostics and Assessment: CBC, routine serum biochemistry, and a UPC were sent to the laboratory. Blood glucose was 110 mg/dL thus excluding diabetes mellitus as the cause for the glucosuria. Glucosuria plus normal blood glucose concentrations define some type of renal glucosuria due to a proximal tubulopathy. All other analytes on the serum biochemistry were normal including BUN, serum creatinine, and SDMA. UPC was 1.1, supporting the presence of renal proteinuria in the face of an inactive urinary sediment. Acquired Fanconi syndrome appears to be likely. Further questioning about exposure to medications that could cause this were negative, but the dietary history was positive for the feeding of both beef and chicken jerky treats over the past three to four months. Jerky treats with ingredients from China have been implicated in this type of acquired renal glucosuria, but the specific compound creating this has not been identified. Fanconi syndrome requires the finding of aminoaciduria, but urinary testing for this was not done.

After discontinuing the feeding of any jerky treats, the severity of the PU/PD abated over the next two months. At that time the USG was 1.025 and the dipstrip was negative for glucose and for protein.

Final Diagnosis: Acquired renal glucosuria (possibly Fanconi syndrome) due to the feeding of jerky treats.

CASE EXAMPLE: Urinalysis Case Number: 32

Source of Specimen:
　Cystocentesis ☐　　Voided (Stream part) ☒ Endstream　　　Post-Void (location) ☐
　Expressed ☐　　　　Catheterized ☐
Volume: 5　mL
Refrigeration: Yes ☒　　No ☐
Elapsed Time Before Analysis: 2 hours
Stain:　　　Yes ☒　　No ☐

Color:　　　　　　　Yellow
Appearance:　　　　Clear
Specific Gravity:　　1.012
pH:　　　　　　　　6.0
Protein:　　　　　　Neg
Occult Blood:　　　 Neg
　Hemolyzed:　　　☐
　Intact:　　　　　☐
Glucose:　　　　　　Neg
Ketones:　　　　　　Neg
Bilirubin:　　　　　Trace

Casts per LPF: 0
　Hyaline
　Granular
　Cellular

WBC per HPF: 1–2
　Free　　　☒
　Clumped　☐
RBC per HPF: 2–3
Epithelial Cells per HPF: 0–1
　Type: Squamous: ☒　　Transitional: Free ☐　　Clumped ☐　　Renal: ☐

Crystals per HPF: None ☒
　Type: Struvite ☐　　　Calcium Oxalate ☐　　　Urate ☐　　Other ☐

Bacteria per HPF: None ☐
　Type: Rods ☐　　　Cocci ☒ few　　　Mixed ☐

Miscellaneous:

Signalment: Nine-year-old spayed female Pit Bull dog.

History and Physical Examination: Episodic extreme thirst over the past six weeks. Polydipsia was associated with larger than normal urine volume at times when she has been drinking a lot.

Interpretation of Urinalysis: The 1.012 USG supports the history of PU/PD. The rest of the UA is completely normal; a few squamous epithelial cells can be seen in voided urine.

Further Diagnostics and Assessment: The history of episodic large volume water drinking is compatible with psychogenic water drinking, so the measurement of several other USG would be informative to know if the urine can be concentrated above the original USG of 1.012. CBC and routine serum biochemistry values were within the reference ranges.

The owners collected urine samples first thing in the morning before eating and drinking and at other random times of the day. USG on several of these samples was >1.030; the USG was between 1.010 and 1.020 on some samples. USG that vacillates over a short time period from isosthenuria to well-concentrated occurs in those with psychogenic polydipsia. Further history revealed that pig's ears were being used as the favorite treat for this dog over the past two months. Some treats like pig's ears and rawhide may be high in salt content. Further bouts of excess water drinking ceased as soon as the pig's ear treats were stopped. History that enquires about ingestion of treats that could be salty, including chips, is helpful at times in obscure cases of polydipsia.

Final Diagnosis: Physiological polydipsia due to ingestion of salty treats.

CASE EXAMPLE: Urinalysis Case Number: 33

Source of Specimen:
    Cystocentesis ☒   Voided (Stream part) ☐   Post-Void (location) ☐
    Expressed ☐   Catheterized ☐
Volume: 4   mL
Refrigeration: Yes ☐   No ☒
Elapsed Time Before Analysis: 60 minutes
Stain: Yes ☒   No ☐

Color: Colorless
Appearance: Clear
Specific Gravity: 1.002
pH: 6.0
Protein: Neg
Occult Blood: Neg
    Hemolyzed: ☐
    Intact: ☐
Glucose: Neg
Ketones: Neg
Bilirubin: Neg

Casts per LPF: 0
    Hyaline
    Granular
    Cellular

WBC per HPF: 0–1
    Free   ☒
    Clumped   ☐
RBC per HPF: 0–2
Epithelial Cells per HPF: 0
    Type: Squamous: ☐   Transitional: Free ☐   Clumped ☐   Renal: ☐

Crystals per HPF: None ☒
    Type: Struvite ☐   Calcium Oxalate ☐   Urate ☐   Other ☐

Bacteria per HPF: None ☒
    Type: Rods ☐   Cocci ☐   Mixed ☐

Miscellaneous: Urine sample collected before the morning meal and drinking

Signalment: 10-year-old female spayed Gordon Setter dog.

History and Physical Examination: PU/PD ongoing for at least six weeks; dog is always thirsty and needing to go outside to urinate a lot more than usual. She is still eating well with normal constitutional signs and activity. Physical examination is not remarkable, including palpation of normal kidneys. Neurological examination is also normal.

Interpretation of Urinalysis: The 1.002 USG is very dilute and is classified as hyposthenuric. There is nothing else on the UA results that helps us figure out why the USG is so low.

Further Diagnostics and Assessment: CBC is normal. Serum biochemistry is mostly normal; serum sodium was 158 mEq/L which is slightly above the reference range. The finding of hypernatremia suggests that there is obligatory polyuria resulting in loss of free water and the ensuing hypernatremia. PPD is very unlikely, as serum sodium is usually normal to low. CDI and NDI are still under consideration as the cause. There is no apparent cause for NDI to this point.

Several random USG ranged from 1.002 to 1.010 when collected over the next few days. Serum osmolality was 336 and urine osmolality was 80 mOsm/L more precisely documenting hyposthenuria with a U/S osmolality ratio of 0.24. A ratio of 1.0 would define isosthenuria. Water deprivation testing is contraindicated in the presence of hypernatremia. Instead, desmopressin testing was performed using eye drops. Within hours there was a marked decrease in water intake and volume of urine produced. USG later this day was 1.018. Desmopressin was continued as daily treatment and USG further increased to 1.025 and 1.027 over the next several days. Serum sodium decreased to 144 mEq/L during desmopressin treatment, demonstrating an adequate reabsorption of free water from renal tubular fluid under the influence of exogenous ADH (desmopressin). The dramatic increase in USG following exogenous ADH treatment supports the diagnosis of CDI. Such an increase in USG would not happen in those with NDI.

MRI of the brain showed a mass in the pituitary gland. This mass underwent radiation treatment and the dog lived another 18 months.

Final Diagnosis: CDI – complete; pituitary tumor.

CASE EXAMPLE: Urinalysis Case Number: 34

Source of Specimen:
    Cystocentesis ☒   Voided (Stream part) ☐   Post-Void (location) ☐
    Expressed ☐   Catheterized ☐
Volume: 6   mL
Refrigeration: Yes ☐   No ☒
Elapsed Time Before Analysis: 45 minutes
Stain: Yes ☒   No ☐

Color:	Dark yellow
Appearance:	Slightly cloudy
Specific Gravity:	1.068
pH:	6.0
Protein:	Trace
Occult Blood:	Neg
Hemolyzed:	☐
Intact:	☐
Glucose:	Neg
Ketones:	Neg
Bilirubin:	Neg

Casts per LPF: 0
    Hyaline
    Granular
    Cellular

WBC per HPF: 1–2
    Free   ☒
    Clumped   ☐
RBC per HPF: 1–3
Epithelial Cells per HPF: 0
    Type: Squamous: ☐   Transitional: Free ☐   Clumped ☐   Renal: ☐

Crystals per HPF: None ☐
    Type: Struvite ☒ Rare   Calcium Oxalate ☐   Urate ☐   Other ☐

Bacteria per HPF: None ☒
    Type: Rods ☐   Cocci ☐   Mixed ☐

Miscellaneous:

Signalment: Two-year-old castrated male Domestic Shorthair cat.

History and Physical Examination: Acute onset of vomiting and anorexia ongoing for two days. Vomitus was noted to contain plant material in foamy fluid. This cat had been well in all aspects prior to this episode. Temperature was 101.1°F, heart rate was 100, and respiratory rate was 20. The cat was depressed and an estimated 8% dehydrated based on skin turgor. Heart and lung sounds were normal. There was no resistance or pain during abdominal palpation. Abdominal organs were normal on palpation. The working diagnosis was acute gastritis due to ingestion of irritating plants.

Interpretation of Urinalysis: The slightly cloudy urine in this case cannot be attributed to an active urinary sediment – sometimes cloudy urine is encountered in normal animals. The 1.068 USG shows highly concentrated urine that is appropriate in the face of dehydration. The response of the body with normal kidneys is to reclaim as much water as possible from the collecting tubules under the influence of high circulating ADH levels. The hypothalamic–pituitary-renal axis for urine concentration is intact. The trace protein reaction on the urine chemistry dipstrip is likely attributed to normal amounts of protein in the urine that had its concentration increased by extensive reabsorption of water around that protein within the collecting tubules. Alternatively, dehydration could have impaired normal glomerular barrier function (loss of glomerular polyanion) to allow some plasma proteins to enter the tubular fluid. Without blood gas parameters to evaluate, we do not know how appropriate or not the urinary pH of 6.0 is. The rare struvite crystals are expected in urine that is this highly concentrated.

Further Diagnostics and Assessment: Abdominal radiographs did not support the presence of a GI obstruction or linear foreign body. The PCV and TP were mildly increased supporting the presence of dehydration. Serum biochemistry results were within the reference ranges, though BUN, creatinine, sodium and albumin were near the top of the reference ranges, attributed to the dehydration.

The cat did well with SQ fluids and NPO over the next two days. The vomiting abated and the cat started eating its usual foods. At re-evaluation the cat's hydration was now assessed as normal, a USG was 1.031 (just finishing SQ fluids), and protein on urinary chemistry dipstrip was negative.

Final Diagnosis: Normal urinalysis with highly concentrated urine during dehydration.

CASE EXAMPLE: Urinalysis Case Number: 35

Source of Specimen:
    Cystocentesis ☐   Voided (Stream part) ☐   Post-Void (location) ☐
    Expressed ☒   Catheterized ☐
Volume: 3   mL
Refrigeration: Yes ☐   No ☒
Elapsed Time Before Analysis: 60 minutes
Stain: Yes ☒   No ☐

Color: Light pink
Appearance: Slightly cloudy
Specific Gravity: 1.042
pH: 6.5
Protein: 2+
Occult Blood: 4+
    Hemolyzed: ☐
    Intact: ☒
Glucose: Neg
Ketones: Neg
Bilirubin: Neg

Casts per LPF: 0
    Hyaline
    Granular
    Cellular

WBC per HPF: 1–3
    Free   ☒
    Clumped   ☐
RBC per HPF: 60 to 80
Epithelial Cells per HPF: 0
    Type: Squamous: ☐   Transitional: Free ☐   Clumped ☐   Renal: ☐

Crystals per HPF: None ☒
    Type: Struvite ☐   Calcium Oxalate ☐   Urate ☐   Other ☐

Bacteria per HPF: None ☒
    Type: Rods ☐   Cocci ☐   Mixed ☐

Miscellaneous:

Signalment: Six-year-old castrated male Orange Tabby cat.

History and Physical Examination: Yearly wellness evaluation. The owners have no concerns about this cat as he is doing very well. He has never had any urinary issues and uses the litter box all the time. Physical examination is normal. Urine was collected during palpation to express urine; it took quite a bit of force to expel the sample as is often the case in male cats.

Interpretation of Urinalysis: The slightly pink and cloudy urine is attribute to the high numbers of RBC identified during urine microscopy. The 1.042 USG is compatible with healthy kidneys in most instances. The 4+ occult blood reaction on urine chemistry dipstrip was positive for only intact RBC. During urine microscopy, the finding of intact RBC at 60–80 per HPF aligns with the dipstrip findings of occult blood. The 2+ protein reaction on the chemistry dipstrip is likely emanating from the large amount of blood in the urine; hemoglobin in RBC can activate the protein pad if present in high quantity.

Further Diagnostics and Assessment: The owners were sent home with a nonresorbable kitty litter to collect a urine sample at home. On this post-voided sample one week later, the occult blood reaction was negative and there were only two to four RBC per HPF seen during urine microscopy.

It is not recommended to collect urine samples by expression if there is any resistance to its expulsion. The force required to expel the urine will be enough at times to traumatize the bladder and add blood and protein to the sample that was not there before this maneuver. Forceful expulsion of urine may also push infected urine up the ureteral openings in the bladder as another possible adverse effect that can create an upper UTI when only a lower UTI initially existed. Sometimes gentle palpation of the bladder results in a voiding response that allows a voided or post-voided sample to be collected with minimal trauma.

Final Diagnosis: Iatrogenic hematuria from bladder expression.

CASE EXAMPLE: Urinalysis Case Number: 36

Source of Specimen:
    Cystocentesis ☐   Voided (Stream part) ☐   Post-Void (location) ☐
    Expressed ☐   Catheterized ☒
Volume: 5 mL
Refrigeration: Yes ☒   No ☐
Elapsed Time Before Analysis: 12 hours
Stain: Yes ☒   No ☐

Color:	Pink to red
Appearance:	Cloudy
Specific Gravity:	1.031
pH:	7.0
Protein:	1+
Occult Blood:	4+
Hemolyzed:	☒
Intact:	☒
Glucose:	Neg
Ketones:	Neg
Bilirubin:	Neg

Casts per LPF: 0
   Hyaline
   Granular
   Cellular

WBC per HPF: 3–6
   Free   ☒
   Clumped   ☐
RBC per HPF: 100-120
Epithelial Cells per HPF: Occasional
   Type: Squamous: ☐   Transitional: Free ☒   Clumped ☐   Renal: ☐

Crystals per HPF: None ☐
   Type: Struvite ☒ Moderate   Calcium Oxalate ☐   Urate ☐   Other ☐

Bacteria per HPF: None ☒
   Type: Rods ☐   Cocci ☐   Mixed ☐

Miscellaneous:

Signalment: Four-year-old castrated male Domestic Shorthair cat.

History and Physical Examination: Straining to urinate for three days; some bloody spots were observed in the litter pan. The cat is not eating at all today. There had been no previous urinary history. He was apparently healthy prior to what is going on now. A biased physical examination toward the abdomen revealed a turgid and painful bladder. The cat is mildly dehydrated based on skin turgor and has a normal TPR. The cat is slightly depressed. Heart and lung sounds are normal. The cat is treated as an emergency with urethral obstruction. Retrograde flushing of the urethra allowed passage of an indwelling urinary catheter.

Interpretation of Urinalysis: Urine was gently aspirated from the urinary catheter, the first 3 mL discarded and then the next 5 ml submitted to the laboratory. Since it was in the mid-evening, the UA was performed the next morning.

The pink to red cloudy urine is attributed to RBC in the sample. The 1.031 USG in a dehydrated cat could indicate impaired renal function, BUT this sample was adulterated with flush solution needed to unblock the urethra and pass the urinary catheter. So, the sample is diluted to some extent from this procedure. The USG could also be lower than expected from healthy cats if the cat is in postrenal failure from the urethral obstruction. Determining the cause of the lower than expected USG would be better served on a sample collected by cystocentesis prior to unblocking procedures, thus avoiding dilution from flush solution. The 7.0 pH is attributed to anorexia, contamination with plasma proteins, and urinary stasis. The 4+ occult blood reaction occurred due to the presence of intact and hemolyzed RBC. Increased lysis of RBC that were originally intact in the sample could have occurred during the over 12 hours of storage in the refrigerator prior to analysis. Urine microscopy confirms the presence of an abundance of RBC (100–120 per HPF) and very few WBC; these findings are typical for cats with obstruction related to idiopathic cystitis/urethritis, but could also be observed following urinary bladder bleeding that occurs during complete urethral obstruction and bladder overdistension. Occasional free transitional epithelial cells could enter urine secondary to desquamation of epithelial cells during the obstructing process, but they could also potentially have been acquired from passage of the urinary catheter. The moderate numbers of struvite crystals are expected in a urine sample with a pH of 7.0 (struvite is far less soluble at a urinary pH of ≥6.7) especially during urinary stasis. Urine storage under refrigeration also could easily have contributed to increased numbers of these crystals as an artifact. Crystalluria is not a primary creator of urethral obstruction, but they do contribute to urethral plug formation. No bacteria were observed in this sample, which is not surprising since the vast majority of cats with urethral obstruction have sterile urine at presentation.

Further Diagnostics and Assessment: Serum biochemistry at the time of presentation showed a minimal increase in BUN and serum creatinine that was most likely postrenal in origin, though some could have been prerenal. The cat did well in the hospital and was released urinating on its own by day 3 after presentation. Ten days after release from the hospital, a repeated UA collected by cystocentesis showed trace occult blood, neg protein, three to five RBC per HPF, 0 crystals, and 0 bacteria. USG at that time was 1.047.

Final Diagnosis: Hematuria and struvite crystalluria associated with urethral obstruction. Dilution of urine with flush solution suspected. Postrenal and prerenal azotemia.

CASE EXAMPLE: Urinalysis Case Number: 37

Source of Specimen:
    Cystocentesis ☒   Voided (Stream part) ☐   Post-Void (location) ☐
    Expressed ☐   Catheterized ☐
Volume: 3 mL
Refrigeration: Yes ☐   No ☒
Elapsed Time Before Analysis: 45 minutes
Stain: Yes ☒   No ☐

Color:	Light yellow
Appearance:	Clear
Specific Gravity:	1.025
pH:	6.0
Protein:	Neg
Occult Blood:	Neg
Hemolyzed:	☐
Intact:	☐
Glucose:	Neg
Ketones:	Neg
Bilirubin:	2+

Casts per LPF: 0
  Hyaline
  Granular
  Cellular

WBC per HPF: 1–3
  Free   ☒
  Clumped ☐
RBC per HPF: 0–1
Epithelial Cells per HPF: 0
  Type: Squamous: ☐   Transitional: Free ☐   Clumped ☐   Renal: ☐

Crystals per HPF: None ☐
  Type: Struvite ☐   Calcium Oxalate ☐   Urate ☐   Other ☒ Bilirubin

Bacteria per HPF: None ☒
  Type: Rods ☐   Cocci ☐   Mixed ☐

Miscellaneous:

Signalment: Two-year-old spayed female Siamese cat.

History and Physical Examination: She has been a healthy cat until the last two months. She is no longer as playful or active as she used to be. She is still eating but has always been on the thin side and now weighs 6 lbs. TPR and skin turgor are normal. Abdominal palpation is normal as are heart and lung sounds.

Interpretation of Urinalysis: A 1.025 USG is less than that expected from healthy cats; cats with <1.035 USG often have diseases affecting urine concentration. The 2+ dipstrip pad reaction for bilirubin and the bilirubin crystals identified during urine microscopy are highly abnormal in cats, especially a sick cat. The less than expected USG in this cat could be related to the same process causing the bilirubinuria. Bilirubinuria and bilirubin crystals can be normal findings in dogs, especially male dogs.

Further Diagnostics and Assessment: Further testing toward liver disease and liver function are indicated. The sclera and mucous membranes were re-examined to see if icterus might have been overlooked during the initial physical examination; no icterus was found. CBC showed a mild nonregenerative anemia with no evidence for hemolysis. Serum biochemistry revealed increased values for ALT and ALP. Total bilirubin was very slightly increased above the reference range. Pre-prandial serum bile acids were mildly increased. Ultrasonography showed a slightly small liver with no evidence for portosystemic shunting

Final Diagnosis: Primary liver disease; a precise cause will need liver biopsy results.

CASE EXAMPLE: Urinalysis Case Number: 38

Source of Specimen:
    Cystocentesis ☐   Voided (Stream part) ☒ midstream   Post-Void (location) ☐
    Expressed ☐   Catheterized ☐
Volume: 6   mL
Refrigeration: Yes ☒   No ☐
Elapsed Time Before Analysis: 2 hours
Stain: Yes ☐   No ☐

Color:	Pale yellow
Appearance:	Clear
Specific Gravity:	1.013
pH:	6.0
Protein:	Neg
Occult Blood:	+2
Hemolyzed:	☐
Intact:	☒
Glucose:	Neg
Ketones:	Neg
Bilirubin:	Neg

Casts per LPF:
    Hyaline
    Granular 1–2
    Cellular

WBC per HPF: 0–1
    Free   ☐
    Clumped   ☐
RBC per HPF: 10–15
Epithelial Cells per HPF: 0
    Type: Squamous: ☐   Transitional: Free ☐   Clumped ☐   Renal: ☐

Crystals per HPF: None ☒
    Type: Struvite ☐   Calcium Oxalate ☐   Urate ☐   Other ☐

Bacteria per HPF: None ☐
    Type: Rods ☐   Cocci ☒ Rare   Mixed ☐

Miscellaneous: The owners collected the urine sample at home as requested by the veterinary clinic.

Signalment: Nine-year-old spayed female Golden Retriever dog.

History and Physical Examination: Three months of PU/PD is the primary complaint. Otherwise, the dog appears to be healthy, active, eating well, and maintaining its weight. Physical examination reveals an overweight dog (90 lbs on a medium frame). There is no abdominal organomegaly, heart and lung sounds are good, hydration is normal, and mucous membranes are pink.

Interpretation of Urinalysis: The pale clear urine aligns with the finding of a 1.013 USG. Urine microscopy reveals 1–2 granular casts per LPF and 10–15 RBC as the abnormal findings. The increased number of RBC seen during urine microscopy aligns with the positive occult blood dipstrip reaction. Rare cocci that were reported are likely contaminants that entered the urine during the collection process, especially in the absence of increased WBC. The finding of casts in isosthenuric urine is of interest, as it is more difficult for casts to form in urine that is dilute. The RBC are not an artifact following trauma from the method of collection since this was a voided sample.

Many disorders could result in the finding of isosthenuria including kidney disease given the increased number of granular casts. Since the protein on the dipstrip is negative, the granules in the casts are not likely precipitates of plasma proteins crossing the glomerular barrier. Granules traditionally are thought to arise as cells undergo accelerated degradation.

Further Diagnostics and Assessment: Three other random USG were measured at 1.004, 1.006, and 1.010 indicating hyposthenuria to isosthenuria. The CBC showed a mild neutrophilia without left shift and lymphopenia compatible with a stress response. The pivotal abnormal serum biochemistry results included a calcium of 15.2 mg/dL (high), phosphorus of 3.1 mg/dL (low), and a creatinine of 2.1 mg/dL (minor increase). The combination of high calcium and low phosphorus suggests the activation of the PTH/PTHrP receptor. Ionized calcium was high at 6.7 mg/dL, PTH was high at 10 pmol/L, and PTHrP was zero. Ultrasound of the neck revealed a single enlarged parathyroid gland (6 mm diameter) on the left side; other parathyroid glands could not be found. Chest radiographs were normal. Abdominal radiographs revealed multiple small radiodense cystic calculi. Abdominal ultrasound showed that both kidneys were normal in size, but increased echogenicity of the renal cortex was seen in both kidneys. Rectal exam with particular emphasis on the anal sac to rule out anal gland adenocarcinoma as the cause for hypercalcemia was negative.

The abnormal renal sonography in association with the increased number of granular casts indicates primary renal disease. The low USG could arise from CKD secondary to chronic hypercalcemia or could have directly arisen as a form of NDI from the hypercalcemia. The increased RBC in urine sediment are attributed to trauma from the presumed-to-be calcium-containing cystic calculi.

The dog underwent parathyroidectomy of one gland. Histopathology confirmed the presence of a parathyroid adenoma. Hypercalcemia resolved soon after surgery and the PU/PD ceased at the same time. Cystotomy was performed under the same anesthesia to remove the cystic calculi; they returned as 100% calcium oxalate.

At the one-month re-evaluation, serum calcium and phosphorus were normal as was the creatinine. UA at this time revealed a USG of 1.033 and urine sediment was negative for RBC and no casts were identified.

Final Diagnosis: NDI due to hypercalcemia. Hypercalcemia caused by primary hyperparathyroidism. Cystic calculi secondary to hypercalcemia.

CASE EXAMPLE: Urinalysis Case Number: 39

Source of Specimen:
  Cystocentesis ☒   Voided (Stream part) ☐   Post-Void (location) ☐
  Expressed ☐   Catheterized ☐
Volume: 6   mL
Refrigeration: Yes ☐   No ☒
Elapsed Time Before Analysis: 60 minutes
Stain: Yes ☒   No ☐

Color: Very pale yellow
Appearance: Clear
Specific Gravity: 1.005
pH: 6.5
Protein: 1+
Occult Blood: Neg
  Hemolyzed: ☐
  Intact: ☐
Glucose: Neg
Ketones: Neg
Bilirubin: Neg

Casts per LPF: 0
  Hyaline
  Granular
  Cellular

WBC per HPF: 0–2
  Free   ☒
  Clumped   ☐
RBC per HPF: 0–1
Epithelial Cells per HPF: 0
  Type: Squamous: ☐   Transitional: Free ☐   Clumped ☐   Renal: ☐

Crystals per HPF: None ☒
  Type: Struvite ☐   Calcium Oxalate ☐   Urate ☐   Other ☐

Bacteria per HPF: None ☒
  Type: Rods ☐   Cocci ☐   Mixed ☐

Miscellaneous:

Signalment: Four-year-old intact male Basset Hound dog.

History and Physical Examination: This dog has had chronic otitis problems over the past two years. He has been treated with many different types of ear drops with various antibiotics and anti-inflammatory medications. Over the past month, he developed a big increase in water consumption and in the volume of urine that he voids. His general overall health is good. He is not neutered because he is used as breeding stock, though he has only bred one bitch a year ago. His physical examination is normal with the exception of moderate amounts of dental tartar and a slight cranial displacement of the prostate appreciated during rectal examination.

Interpretation of Urinalysis: Pale colorless urine aligns with the USG of 1.005. A 1+ protein urine chemistry dipstrip reaction could be clinically significant in the face of such a low USG and inactive urinary sediment.

Further Diagnostics and Assessment: Two additional random USG returned at 1.004 and 1.007. UPC was 1.4 (normal <0.5).

Brucella canis testing was negative; this test was submitted since he is a breeding dog and *B. canis* can result in GN with proteinuria. CBC and routine serum biochemistry were within the reference ranges. Review of the drug history indicated that the ears have been treated for at least the past four weeks with betamethasone drops. Antibiotics have been given locally in the ears in the past, but none recently.

Glucocorticosteroids can be absorbed into the circulation following topical application to inflamed ears and eyes. Some dogs are exquisitely sensitive to small amounts of glucocorticosteroids that impair urine concentration. Chronic steroid administration can also result in glomerular proteinuria.

All ear drops containing steroids were stopped. PU/PD abated over the next two to three weeks. Recheck of the UA showed a USG of 1.023 and negative protein on the dipstrip.

Final Diagnosis: NDI due to systemic absorption of glucocorticoids from the ears.

CASE EXAMPLE: Urinalysis Case Number: 40

Source of Specimen:
    Cystocentesis ☐   Voided (Stream part) ☒ Midstream   Post-Void (location) ☐
    Expressed ☐   Catheterized ☐
Volume: 5   mL
Refrigeration: Yes ☐   No ☒
Elapsed Time Before Analysis: 60 minutes
Stain: Yes ☒   No ☐
Comments: Cephalosporin oral treatment for pyoderma for 3 weeks

Color:	Light yellow
Appearance:	Slightly cloudy
Specific Gravity:	1.015
pH:	6.0
Protein:	2+
Occult Blood:	1+
Hemolyzed:	☒
Intact:	☒
Glucose:	Neg
Ketones:	Neg
Bilirubin:	Neg

Casts per LPF:
    Hyaline
    Granular 0–1
    Cellular 0–1 WBC

WBC per HPF: 10–12
    Free   ☒
    Clumped   ☐
RBC per HPF: 5 to 10
Epithelial Cells per HPF: 0–1
    Type: Squamous: ☐   Transitional: Free ☐   Clumped ☐   Renal: ☒

Crystals per HPF: None ☒
    Type: Struvite ☐   Calcium Oxalate ☐   Urate ☐   Other ☐

Bacteria per HPF: None ☒
    Type: Rods ☐   Cocci ☐   Mixed ☐

Miscellaneous:

Signalment: Six-year-old spayed female black Labrador Retriever dog.

History and Physical Examination: She has had multiple episodes of pyoderma over the past two years that are often difficult to clear. She has been treated for the past three weeks with oral cephalexin and the skin lesions have mostly cleared. She has not been herself for the past three days as she is lethargic and not eating as much. Her water intake has increased along with an increase in her urine volume. Aside from her residual pyoderma, her physical examination is not remarkable.

Interpretation of Urinalysis: Since pyoderma dogs may have concurrent bacterial UTI, a UA was performed prior to the start of the cephalosporin. The UA was considered normal with a USG of 1.039, negative protein, negative occult blood, and an inactive urinary sediment. CBC and routine serum biochemistry were also normal.

The lightly colored urine in the current sample is attributed to how dilute the urine is with a USG of 1.015. The 1.015 USG supports the accuracy in the history for PU/PD. The slightly cloudy urine is attributed to proteinuria, intact and lysed RBC, pyuria, cylindruria, and epitheliuria. Free epithelial cells were characterized as renal tubular epithelial cells. The identification of occasional WBC cellular casts and granular casts are important findings, as is the identification of RTE. WBC casts occur most commonly in those with bacterial pyelonephritis but can occur in any renal inflammatory condition at times. No bacteria were identified during urine microscopy.

Cephalosporins are generally safe and not likely to be directly nephrotoxic. Rarely, cephalosporins can create renal damage following an allergic reaction and AIN.

Further Diagnostics and Assessment: Quantitative urine culture returned with no growth (cystocentesis sample). CBC was normal except for the finding of a mild eosinophilia. Serum biochemistry was normal except for mild increases in serum creatinine (2.2 mg/dL) and BUN (39 mg/dL). UPC was 1.6.

Urine cytology was performed to better identify the nature of the WBC and the suspected renal tubular epithelial cells. 60% of the WBC were found to be eosinophils that would have escaped detection relying on wet-mount urine microscopy. One cellular cast was available to examine, and it revealed that the WBC were mostly eosinophils. Eosinophils may easily escape identification during wet-mount urine microscopy. The basal positioning of the small epithelial cells further support that these are RTE and not urothelial cells.

The eosinophiliuria, free and in casts, is compatible with an allergic reaction within the kidneys. Though rare, acute interstitial nephritis (AIN) following treatment with cephalosporins can occur, as with many other antibiotics. The presence of free renal tubular epithelial cells is compatible with this type of AIN and resulting tubular damage. The finding of decreased excretory renal function (increased creatinine and BUN) is expected if the AIN is severe enough.

The proteinuria is assessed as renal in origin, with protein additions to the urine from the interstitial nephritis. Some tubular proteinuria (lack of reabsorption) is a possibility depending on the degree of renal tubular impairment.

Cephalosporin treatments were stopped and a decision to not use them again in the future was made as it seemed likely that AIN was secondary to this drug. A renal biopsy would be necessary to confirm this diagnosis, but that procedure was not chosen.

Six weeks later, excretory renal function values had returned to their original baseline pre-treatment numbers and the magnitude of water drinking and urine production were markedly reduced. USG was 1.028, dipstrip reactions were negative for protein and occult blood, and the urinary sediment was silent.

Final Diagnosis: NDI and AIN secondary to cephalosporin allergic reaction; AKI.

CASE EXAMPLE: Urinalysis Case Number: 41

Source of Specimen:
    Cystocentesis ☐   Voided (Stream part) ☒ Mid-stream   Post-Void (location) ☐
    Expressed ☐   Catheterized ☐
Volume: 10   mL
Refrigeration: Yes ☒   No ☐
Elapsed Time Before Analysis: 120 minutes
Stain: Yes ☒   No ☐

Color: Pale
Appearance: Clear
Specific Gravity: 1.004
pH: 6.0
Protein: Neg
Occult Blood: Neg
   Hemolyzed: ☐
   Intact: ☐
Glucose: Neg
Ketones: Neg
Bilirubin: Neg

Casts per LPF: 0
   Hyaline
   Granular
   Cellular

WBC per HPF: 1–3
   Free   ☒
   Clumped ☐
RBC per HPF: 0–1
Epithelial Cells per HPF: 2–3
   Type: Squamous: ☒   Transitional: Free ☐   Clumped ☐   Renal: ☐

Crystals per HPF: None ☒
   Type: Struvite ☐   Calcium Oxalate ☐   Urate ☐   Other ☐

Bacteria per HPF: None ☐
   Type: Rods ☐   Cocci ☒ Rare   Mixed ☐

Miscellaneous:

Signalment: Four-year-old intact female Gordon Setter dog.

History and Physical Examination: This dog is a breeding bitch and is currently six weeks pregnant. One week ago, she suddenly started drinking lots of water. The dog's urine volume was not well observed by the owners as she is housed in a kennel. She has had two previous litters without any problems and no association with polydipsia. She whelped four puppies in each of her previous litters. Ultrasound shows that there are eight puppies in utero at six weeks for this pregnancy. She is eating well and acting normally other than the increased water intake. Physical examination shows a moderately distended abdomen as expected with her pregnancy. There is no vulvar discharge. Her nipples are enlarged probably from previous nursing of litters. TPR, hydration, and heart and lung sounds are normal. The dog belongs to a veterinarian.

Interpretation of Urinalysis: The most striking finding is the hyposthenuria with a USG of 1.004. Everything else on the UA is normal. The few cocci reported are attributed to contamination during passage of urine along the vestibule and vulva during collection of a voided sample. CDI, NDI, and PPD are the usual differentials for hyposthenuria. There was some concern about the possibility of an upper bacterial UTI causing the dilute urine and polydipsia, but this is less likely in the absence of proteinuria and pyuria.

Further Diagnostics and Assessment: The owner collected several random USG from voided urine over three days. USG varied from 1.002 to 1.006. CBC and serum biochemical profile showed no abnormal findings. PPD is not likely since there is usually more vacillation in USG between high and lower values when urine concentration is analyzed sequentially multiple times. There were no conditions associated with NDI that were disclosed on routine serum biochemistry. Water deprivation testing could be dangerous to the fetuses and pregnant mother, so this was not considered.

In the absence of more common diagnoses, gestational diabetes was considered possible or probable. Gestational DI has not been reported in the veterinary literature, to my knowledge, but this diagnosis has been suspected based on anecdotal evidence. This condition occurs rarely in pregnant humans in the last trimester, likely caused by the elaboration of vasopressinase by the uterus in those with multiple fetuses and a large placental weight. Normal amounts of ADH are released into the circulation. This form of DI occurs due to the enhanced degradation of ADH. The PU/PD in pregnant woman can be controlled with the administration of desmopressin which is not easily degraded by vasopressinase. In this dog, no treatment was given.

After whelping, there was a dramatic decrease in water drinking and the USG one week later was 1.033. All eight puppies were normal upon delivery, and until they were weaned from the bitch when they were eight weeks of age. Gestational DI could occur with more frequency than appreciated in veterinary medicine since this form of PU/PD and hyposthenuria is reversible following whelping. It would have been interesting to see the response to desmopressin. A dramatic increase in USG would add further support to the diagnosis of gestational DI. In this case, the polydipsia and hyposthenuria were mostly a nuisance for the dog and owner. It is interesting that GDI did not develop in earlier pregnancies, possibly because of the smaller number of fetuses and lower placental weight.

Final Diagnosis: Gestational diabetes insipidus.

CASE EXAMPLE: Urinalysis Case Number: 42

Source of Specimen:
    Cystocentesis ☒   Voided (Stream part) ☐   Post-Void (location) ☐
    Expressed ☐   Catheterized ☐
Volume: 3   mL
Refrigeration: Yes ☐   No ☒
Elapsed Time Before Analysis: 30 minutes
Stain: Yes ☒   No ☐

Color:	Pale
Appearance:	Clear
Specific Gravity:	1.012
pH:	5.5
Protein:	1+
Occult Blood:	Neg
Hemolyzed:	☐
Intact:	☐
Glucose:	Neg
Ketones:	Neg
Bilirubin:	Neg

Casts per LPF:
  Hyaline
  Granular 0–1
  Cellular

WBC per HPF: 0–1
  Free   ☒
  Clumped ☐
RBC per HPF: 1–3
Epithelial Cells per HPF: 0
  Type: Squamous: ☐   Transitional: Free ☐   Clumped ☐   Renal: ☐

Crystals per HPF: None ☒
  Type: Struvite ☐   Calcium Oxalate ☐   Urate ☐   Other ☐

Bacteria per HPF: None ☒
  Type: Rods ☐   Cocci ☐   Mixed ☐

Miscellaneous:

Signalment: Three-year-old spayed female Domestic Shorthair cat.

History and Physical Examination: This cat presented to an ER in a moderate state of collapse. She was not able to pick up her head and had a "hanging head" posture. She had been unwell for at least the last week when her food intake markedly decreased. Her litter pan had markedly increased size and number of the clumping litter spots. She was also observed to be drinking water, something that the owners never noticed before. Her general health and activity were thought to be normal until the past few weeks. She was thin and weighed 7 lbs with loss of some muscle mass. Based on skin turgor, she was assessed as mildly dehydrated. Her mucous membranes were light pink. There was a two of six systolic murmur with normal heart rhythm. Both kidneys were smaller and harder than normal during abdominal palpation. The bladder was moderately full. Systolic blood pressure by Doppler was 185 mmHg (normal is less than 165 mmHg).

Interpretation of Urinalysis: The pale clear urine aligns with the 1.012 USG. 1+ protein on the chemistry dipstrip in urine with an inactive urine sediment could be pathological. The 0–1 granular casts per LPF technically could be normal, but in urine that is this dilute, it is likely more important for some intrarenal process. The 1.012 USG in the face of dehydration indicates impaired urine concentration due to reasons yet to be disclosed.

Further Diagnostics and Assessment: CBC showed a mild nonregenerative anemia with a PCV of 24%. Abnormalities on serum biochemistry included a creatinine of 2.9 mg/dL, BUN of 43 mg/dL, sodium of 162 mEQ/L, and potassium of 2.2 mEq/L. UPC was 0.9. T4 was normal. Abdominal radiographs confirmed that the kidneys were small, and without renal mineralization or urinary tract stones.

This cat has azotemic CKD, but IRIS staging based on creatinine should not be done until the cat is rehydrated. The high serum sodium is attributed to loss of free water (NDI). The low potassium at 2.2 mEq/L is the most striking biochemical abnormality and could result in the cat's demise if not treated properly. The administration of IV fluids, even with substantial amounts of potassium supplementation, can further lower potassium and threaten the cat's life. Oral potassium supplementation and SQ fluids were given for the next 24 hours before IV fluids were started.

The 1.012 USG could arise from the CKD alone, or in conjunction with the low potassium. Hypokalemia can result in NDI and can also create primary renal lesions that result in CKD. Hypokalemia at the time of CKD diagnosis is common in cats, but not usually to this severe degree. Hypokalemia can result in NDI without structural lesions or CKD with structural lesions; CKD can result in hypokalemia. NDI without structural lesions during hypokalemia is reversible when normokalemia is restored. Hypokalemia also exerts negative effects on GFR as a functional phenomenon.

The cat was released to the owner after three days of hospitalization. At that time, the creatinine had declined to 2.2 mg/dL and the potassium increased to 3.9 mEq/L. Systolic blood pressure on amlodipine treatment declined to 165 mmHg. Some of the initial azotemia was responsive to volume repletion, restoration of normokalemia, or both.

At the one-month evaluation, serum creatinine was 1.7 mg/dL, serum potassium was 4.4 mEq/L and the cat was feeling much better. USG increased to 1.022 at this visit. UPC at 0.8 was about the same as it was at the initial presentation. The high UPC (<0.4 normal) is likely from the underlying CKD with some contribution from systemic hypertension. UPC declined to 0.5 when systolic blood pressure was 145 mmHg another month later. USG at this time increased further to 1.029 possibly due to better control of systemic hypertension and less effect from pressure diuresis. Antiproteinuria treatment with benazepril did not further lower the UPC at subsequent visits.

The increase in USG from 1.012 to 1.022 and then to 1.029 over time suggests that some of the initially low USG was from the effects of hypokalemia (NDI). Some of the initially low USG could also have developed from "pressure diuresis" from the severe systolic hypertension. Urine concentration does not generally increase during CKD of other types.

Final Diagnosis: NDI from CKD, hypokalemic nephropathy, systemic hypertension.

CASE EXAMPLE: Urinalysis Case Number: 43

Source of Specimen:
    Cystocentesis ☐   Voided (Stream part) ☒ Unknown   Post-Void (location) ☐
    Expressed ☐   Catheterized ☐
Volume: 6   mL
Refrigeration: Yes ☒   No ☐
Elapsed Time Before Analysis: 180 minutes
Stain: Yes ☐   No ☒
Comments: Urine sample collected at home by owners after requested to do so by their veterinarian

Color:	Colorless
Appearance:	Clear
Specific Gravity:	1.037
pH:	6.5
Protein:	Neg
Occult Blood:	Neg
Hemolyzed:	☐
Intact:	☐
Glucose:	Neg
Ketones:	Neg
Bilirubin:	Neg

Casts per LPF: 0
  Hyaline
  Granular
  Cellular

WBC per HPF: 0–2
  Free   ☒
  Clumped   ☐
RBC per HPF: 2–4
Epithelial Cells per HPF: 2–3
    Type: Squamous: ☒   Transitional: Free ☐   Clumped ☐   Renal: ☐

Crystals per HPF: None ☒
    Type: Struvite ☐   Calcium Oxalate ☐   Urate ☐   Other ☐

Bacteria per HPF: None ☒
    Type: Rods ☐   Cocci ☐   Mixed ☐

Miscellaneous:

Signalment: Two-year-old mixed-breed intact female dog.

History and Physical Examination: This bitch whelped her first litter of seven puppies three days ago. The pregnancy and delivery of the pups went well. Shortly after whelping, she had a large increase in the volume of her water drinking; she is now drinking at least two to three times the volume of water that she did previously. The owners noted that there has been no change in the volume of urine produced; they are very observant owners. The bitch has no previous abnormal medical history. The pups are vigorously nursing many times a day. The bitch is normally hydrated, and her physical examination is normal in the face of her recent pregnancy and delivery. There is no vulvar discharge, and her mammary glands are enlarged due to engorgement with milk. The owners were frightened by the sudden increase in water drinking.

Interpretation of Urinalysis: Results from the urinalysis are almost entirely normal. The increased number of squamous epithelial cells reported are attributed to the recent whelping and changes along the birth canal. The USG of 1.037 indicates adequate urinary concentrating capacity. PD is almost always linked with PU in pathological conditions in order to maintain hydration as a compensatory mechanism, but not in this case. The high USG is not compatible with PU/PD at this time. PPD is not likely since the history indicates high volume of water intake at all times of drinking; PPD usually has bursts of high and normal volume of water intake over time in association. Much lower USG is expected in those with active drinking due to PPD. Lactation requires an increased caloric and water intake to make milk for the puppies. Polydipsia is attributed to the need to for the bitch to keep up with the fluid volume lost during milk production, which can be extensive from the seven puppies that are nursing. It is likely that the bitch is a little "dry" in the circulation which favors the release of ADH and resulting high USG.

Further Diagnostics and Assessment: Out of an abundance of caution, USG was measured from urine samples collected at home randomly over the next several days. The USG was >1.035 in all samples. No further diagnostics were performed since the bitch and pups were doing so well. Within several days after weaning, her water intake dramatically decreased adding further support to the conclusion that she had physiological PD to keep up with her milk production.

Final Diagnosis: Physiological polydipsia without polyuria during lactation.

CASE EXAMPLE: Urinalysis Case Number: 44

Source of Specimen:
  Cystocentesis ☐   Voided (Stream part) ☒ midstream   Post-Void (location) ☐
  Expressed ☐   Catheterized ☐
Volume: 5   mL
Refrigeration: Yes ☐   No ☒
Elapsed Time Before Analysis: 45 minutes
Stain: Yes ☒   No ☐
Comments: Mild vulvar discharge

Color: Light yellow
Appearance: Cloudy
Specific Gravity: 1.018
pH: 6.0
Protein: 2+
Occult Blood: 1+
  Hemolyzed: ☐
  Intact: ☒
Glucose: Neg
Ketones: Neg
Bilirubin: Neg

Casts per LPF: 0
  Hyaline
  Granular
  Cellular

WBC per HPF: 10–15
  Free   ☒
  Clumped   ☒
RBC per HPF: 5–10
Epithelial Cells per HPF: 2–3
  Type: Squamous: ☒   Transitional: Free ☐   Clumped ☐   Renal: ☐

Crystals per HPF: None ☒
  Type: Struvite ☐   Calcium Oxalate ☐   Urate ☐   Other ☐

Bacteria per HPF: None ☐
  Type: Rods ☒   Cocci ☒   Mixed ☐

Miscellaneous:

Signalment: Nine-year-old intact female German Shepherd Dog.

History and Physical Examination: This dog has had a nonremarkable past medical history. She was in heat about eight weeks ago. She has been very healthy until just this past week in which she started to drink more and urinate a larger urine volume. She is still eating but not as much as before. She has had regular heat cycles twice a year without any problems. She has never had puppies. Temperature is slightly increased at 102.8 °F and she is slightly depressed with a heart rate of 160 and respiratory rate of 15 with normal heart and lung sounds. Her skin turgor is normal. Mucous membranes are pink with normal refill time. Abdominal palpation suggests a fullness to the abdomen but specific organomegaly could not be defined. A slight purulent vulvar discharge is present.

Interpretation of Urinalysis: The cloudy urine is attributed to the increased numbers of cellular elements identified during urine microscopy (RBC, WBC, and squamous epithelial cells). The occult blood on the dipstrip at 1+ is supported by the 5–10 RBC per HPF seen on microscopy. Both free and clumped WBC are seen in excess numbers in the urinary sediment (10–15 WBC per HPF) along with both rods and cocci. Since there is a vulvar purulent discharge, some of the increased number of WBC and bacteria could be added from the genital tract especially from a voided specimen. Some of the 2+ dipstrip positive reaction for protein is attributed to the same process that is adding extra WBC to the urine, but renal proteinuria cannot be excluded at this time. The 2+ proteinuria in the face of the low USG at 1.018 supports that the proteinuria is "real" but not its origin. PU/PD and a low USG in a dog that is slightly ill eight weeks after the last heat cycle mandates that pyometra be at the top of the differential list.

Further Diagnostics and Assessment: CBC showed an obvious leukocytosis (60,000 WBC) with a left shift and some toxic changes in the white cells. Serum biochemistry was normal. UPC was 2.8 in the face of an active sediment. Abdominal radiographs revealed an obvious soft tissue enlargement that was determined to be the uterus.

After a few hours of IV fluids, the dog underwent an OHE without complications. Cystocentesis for urine culture was obtained just after the celiotomy. She was sent home on antibiotics for a presumed bacterial UTI. Urine culture later returned with >10 000 cfu/mL of a pure growth of *Escherichia coli* that was susceptible to all common urinary antibacterials.

One month after her OHE, the leukocytosis with left shift had resolved. UA at this time revealed an inactive urinary sediment, negative protein and occult blood on dipstrip. USG was 1.030. UPC at this visit was 0.3, suggesting the original UPC of 2.8 was from inflammatory contamination and not glomerular disease that is sometimes encountered in dogs with pyometra. Dogs with pyometra often have a bacterial UTI with the same organism that is within the pyometra. This UTI is often presumed to be in the lower urinary tract, but some studies suggest that the infection can be in the kidneys.

Impaired urinary concentration during pyometra represents a form of NDI that can occur from the effects of endotoxin on the concentrating mechanism in the collecting tubules. Some dogs with pyometra have pre-existing CKD that can account for impaired urine concentration too, but that was not likely in this dog since much greater urine concentration emerged following OHE.

Pyometra should always be the first rule-out in an intact bitch with a history of PU/PD and a recent heat cycle. Multiple previous heat cycles without pregnancy predispose to the development of pyometra.

Final Diagnosis: Pyometra; NDI from UTI endotoxin.

CASE EXAMPLE: Urinalysis Case Number: 45

Source of Specimen:
Cystocentesis ☐   Voided (Stream part) ☐   Post-Void (location) ☒ Table top
Expressed ☐   Catheterized ☐
Volume: 3   mL
Refrigeration: Yes ☐   No ☒
Elapsed Time Before Analysis: 40 minutes
Stain: Yes ☒   No ☐

Color: Yellow
Appearance: Clear
Specific Gravity: 1.024
pH: 6.5
Protein: 1+
Occult Blood: Neg
  Hemolyzed: ☐
  Intact: ☐
Glucose: Neg
Ketones: Neg
Bilirubin: Neg

Casts per LPF: 0
  Hyaline
  Granular
  Cellular

WBC per HPF: 1–2
  Free   ☒
  Clumped   ☐
RBC per HPF: 0–1
Epithelial Cells per HPF: 0
  Type: Squamous: ☐   Transitional: Free ☐   Clumped ☐   Renal: ☐

Crystals per HPF: None ☒
  Type: Struvite ☐   Calcium Oxalate ☐   Urate ☐   Other ☐

Bacteria per HPF: None ☐
  Type: Rods ☐   Cocci ☒ Few   Mixed ☐

Miscellaneous:

Signalment: 12-year-old castrated male Domestic Shorthair cat.

History and Physical Examination: This cat is presented for evaluation of weight loss and wanting to eat all the time for the past two months. She looks much thinner to the owners but is still quite active. Her litter box contains much more fecal material and the urine clumps of litter are larger than before. This year she weighs 8 lbs; she was 10 lbs one year ago. She is thin with a BCS of 2/5. Her skin turgor is reduced but this could be due to her weight loss. Body temperature is normal. Her heart rate is 170, respiratory rate of 20, normal lung sounds, and a two of six systolic murmur during auscultation. Both kidneys are easily palpated and assessed to be small. The bladder is medium in size. There is a questionable thyroid slip. Systolic blood pressure was increased at 178 mmHg.

Interpretation of Urinalysis: Since this sample was a post-voided one taken from a metal tabletop, it is not surprising that a few bacteria were identified during urine microscopy. The 1.024 USG is the most important finding on this UA. Most healthy cats have a USG ≥1.035. The combination of increased appetite accompanied by weight loss, a possible thyroid slip, and systemic hypertension heavily suggests hyperthyroidism as the diagnosis. The lower than expected USG is not often encountered in cats with hyperthyroidism as the singular diagnosis but is common in those with concomitant CKD. The increased volume of the clumping litter aligns with the USG. The 1+ protein on the chemistry dip-strip could indicate renal proteinuria in the face of an inactive urinary sediment, a finding that can occur in CKD, hyperthyroidism, and during systemic hypertension.

Further Diagnostics and Assessment: CBC was normal with a HCT of 42%. Abnormal serum biochemistry revealed a creatinine of 2.3 mg/dL, BUN of 42 mg/dL, phosphorus of 6.6 mg/dL, and SDMA of 24 µg/dL. ALT was increased at 320 IU/L. T4 was 6.8 µg/dL (upper ref. limit is 3.5 µg/dL). UPC was 0.7.

There is concern that a return to euthyroidism will result in an increase in creatinine after the enhancing effects of thyroxine on GFR are removed. A methimazole challenge could be performed to see what the renal function looks like at a time of normal T4. That was not done and the cat was treated with I-131. Eight weeks after I-131 treatment, the T4 decreased to 2.5 µg/dL and the creatinine escalated to 2.6 mg/dL but the cat was acting great. The return to euthyroidism unmasks the level of renal function that exists without enhancing effects of thyroid hormones on GFR. Some of the increase in creatinine might be attributed to an increase in lean muscle mass as the cat had gained 1 lb by this time. Systolic blood pressure decreased to 160 mmHg and the UPC decreased to 0.3 when a normal T4 had been achieved.

Final Diagnosis: Hyperthyroidism; CKD; Systolic hypertension.

CASE EXAMPLE: Urinalysis Case Number: 46

Source of Specimen:

Cystocentesis ☒ Voided (Stream part) ☐ Post-Void (location) ☐
Expressed ☐ Catheterized ☐
Volume: 5 mL
Refrigeration: Yes ☐ No ☒
Elapsed Time Before Analysis: 20 minutes
Stain: Yes ☐ No ☒

Color:	Pale yellow
Appearance:	Slightly cloudy
Specific Gravity:	1.010
pH:	6.0
Protein:	2+
Occult Blood:	1+
Hemolyzed:	☒
Intact:	☐
Glucose:	Neg
Ketones:	Neg
Bilirubin:	Neg

Casts per LPF: Nonhyaline "suspected"
   Hyaline
   Granular
   Cellular

WBC per HPF: 4
   Free ☒
   Clumped ☐
RBC per HPF: 10
Epithelial Cells per HPF: 1–2 Nonsquamous
   Type: Squamous: ☐ Transitional: Free ☒ Clumped ☐ Renal: ☐

Crystals per HPF: None ☒
   Type: Struvite ☐ Calcium Oxalate ☐ Urate ☐ Other ☐

Bacteria per HPF: None ☐
   Type: Rods ☐ Cocci ☒ "suspected" Mixed ☐

Miscellaneous: Manual review of captured digital images in-house did not confirm presence of any casts; parasite eggs that were discovered during manual review of images were considered to be Capillaria or Dioctophyma by house staff.

Signalment: Five-year-old castrated male Domestic Shorthair cat.

History and Physical Examination: This cat has been progressively going downhill for the past three weeks. He has not been eating much, and vomiting has been increasing in severity. Owners have not observed any stools or urinations in the litter box for the past several days. Compared to last year, he has lost 1.5 lbs and now weighs 9 lbs. He is moderately dehydrated based on skin turgor. There is some abdominal resentment during palpation, but not near the bladder. The bladder is small and soft. The cat was hospitalized for further diagnostic evaluation.

Interpretation of Urinalysis: This urine report follows that from automated microscopy. The 1.010 USG in the face of dehydration shows impaired urinary concentration. The pale urine aligns with the 1.010 USG. The cloudy urine is attributed to the increased number of RBC and WBC identified during urine microscopy. 2+ protein on the dipstrip with a minimally active urine sediment could be renal in origin, but it could also be from the lower urinary tract – more information is needed to confirm this possibility. The 10 RBC per HPF could be increased slightly in number following trauma from cystocentesis or could be from underlying urinary tract pathology. The four WBC per HPF in a urine with a low USG is likely to indicate urinary tract inflammation. "Suspect" cocci were noted by the analyzer – they were still suspect during manual review of digital images captured by the analyzer. "Suspect" nonhyaline casts were noted by the autoanalyzer. Manual review of digital images did not confirm the presence of any casts. It is likely that what the analyzer thought were nonhyaline casts were the parasite eggs, as they have a granular appearance and are somewhat linear. In-house staff were not certain if the parasitic eggs were those from *Capillaria* or from *Dioctophyma*.

Further Diagnostics and Assessment: Chest radiographs were normal. Abdominal radiographs showed both kidneys to be on the upper limit of what would be normal to slightly enlarged. These kidneys looked a bit "plump." There were several minimally radiopaque small cystic calculi in the dependent part of the bladder and two such densities in the trigone. Ultrasonography revealed bilateral hydronephrosis (dilated renal pelves and diverticulae) and proximal hydroureter. No stones were identified on ULS, but detailed description of the bladder, trigone, or distal ureters were not provided.

Because of the hydronephrosis and the parasite eggs in the urine sediment, there was concern from house staff that *Dioctophyma* was more likely to be the parasite rather than *Capillaria*. However, *Dioctophyma* is almost always a disease of dogs and not cats and this process usually destroys one kidney, often the right kidney. *Dioctophyma* would not likely cause hydroureter. The eggs of *Dioctophyma* and *Capillaria* (*Pearsonema*) are very different in morphological appearance. Consultation with a clinical pathologist confirmed that the eggs were those of *Capillaria*. The finding of *Capillaria* is often an incidental finding in cats that are free of lower urinary tract signs. In cats with lower urinary tract signs, *Capillaria* can be associated with pollakiuria, dysuria, and hematuria that respond to antiparasitic treatment.

The cat's PCV was 26% in association with a total protein of 8.0 at a time of dehydration. The PCV is likely lower when rehydrated. BUN was 198 mg/dL, creatinine 18 mg/dL, SDMA >100 μg/dL, phosphorus >15 mg/dL, calcium 6.7 mg/dL, glucose 138 mg/dL, triglycerides 117 mg/dL, sodium 146 mEq/L, potassium 9.7 mEq/L, chloride 104 mEq/L. The high magnitude azotemia indicates severe loss of GFR due to some combination of prerenal, primary renal, and postrenal factors. The 9.7 mEq/L for potassium is at life-threatening levels. Due to financial constraints and a guarded to grave prognosis, treatment was not pursued; the cat died within hours at home with the owners.

The obstructive process is likely related to current or past calcium oxalate urolithiasis.

Final Diagnosis: Incidental *Capillaria* eggs; Obstructive nephropathy, severe azotemia, hydronephrosis, hydroureter.

CASE EXAMPLE: Urinalysis Case Number: 47

Source of Specimen:
Cystocentesis ☒   Voided (Stream part) ☐   Post-Void (location) ☐
Expressed ☐   Catheterized ☐
Volume: 4   mL
Refrigeration: Yes ☐   No ☒
Elapsed Time Before Analysis: 5 minutes
Stain: Yes ☐   No ☒

Color: Pale yellow
Appearance: Slightly cloudy
Specific Gravity: 1.057
pH: 5.0
Protein: 1+ (30 mg/dL)
Occult Blood: 1+ (250 /uL)
   Hemolyzed: ☐
   Intact: ☒
Glucose: 4+ (1000 mg/dL)
Ketones: Neg
Bilirubin: Neg

Casts per LPF: Rare
   Hyaline "suspected"
   Granular "suspected"
   Cellular

WBC per HPF: 1
   Free   ☒
   Clumped   ☐
RBC per HPF: < 1
Epithelial Cells per HPF: < 1 /HPF
   Type: Squamous: ☒ Transitional: Free ☒   Clumped ☐   Renal: ☐

Crystals per HPF: None ☒
   Type: Struvite ☐   Calcium Oxalate ☐   Urate ☐   Other ☐

Bacteria per HPF: None ☒
   Type: Rods ☐   Cocci ☐   Mixed ☐

Miscellaneous: Results were generated by an automated urine chemistry strip reader and automated urine microscopy. Manual review of captured digital images in-house confirmed the presence of rare hyaline and granular casts. Some "hyaline" casts were observed to have granules or droplets within.

Signalment: Five-year-old spayed female Domestic Shorthair cat

History and Physical Examination: This cat was relinquished to a shelter with the history that the cat had been skinny but had been "fattened" up with tasty food. At initial presentation, the cat was thought to be lethargic and mildly dehydrated (skin turgor). TPR was normal and the cat was noted to have some muscle wasting with a BCS 3 of 9. A CBC and routine chemistry panel blood work were submitted in addition to a screening UA.

Interpretation of Urinalysis: This urine report was generated by an automated urine chemistry and automated microscopy analyzer. The 1.057 USG shows an ability to elaborate highly concentrated urine. Urinary protein was 1+ (30 mg/dL) and the urinary glucose was 4+ (1000 mg/dL) on two separate automated readings a few hours apart. Urinary sediment activity associated with WBC or RBC was absent. 1+ protein could easily occur in urine with such a high USG and so might not be clinically important (this did not turn out to be the case – see further below).

4+ glucose (1000 mg/dL) is considered "heavy" glucosuria, something most often caused by diabetes mellitus and hyperglycemia. Diabetes mellitus was removed from differential considerations since the blood glucose on a glucometer was 108 mg/dL, leaving renal glucosuria as the cause (failure of proximal tubules to properly reabsorb the small amounts of glucose filtered across the glomerulus from plasma into tubular fluid).

The main question from the referring DVM was if the high USG could be attributed to the large amount of glucose in the urine. No. USG is increased somewhat by the presence of this much glucose in the urine, but glucose in the urine minimally increases the USG.

A small amount of occult blood was detected, but only one RBC per HPF. Some of the occult blood reaction might be attributed to lysed RBC that were previously intact.

Small numbers of hyaline and nonhyaline casts were "suspected" by the automated sediment analyzer. Manual review of the nonhyaline casts revealed them to be granular casts. Hyaline casts were confirmed also during the manual review. Some of the "hyaline" casts had granules or droplets within. The pH of 5.0 is very acidic, which favors the precipitation of THP (Tamm–Horsfall mucoprotein) that is the matrix protein within hyaline casts. The USG of 1.057 also favors hyaline cast formation due to concentration of THP within tubular fluid and presumably a slow tubular flow rate. Some of the droplets within the hyaline casts were noted on review of digital images to be refractile, indicating that they could be lipid droplets. Alternatively, these "droplets"

are precipitates of plasma proteins abnormally leaking across the glomerulus into tubular fluid. Granules in casts can arise from cellular degeneration or from precipitates of plasma proteins.

Further Diagnostics and Assessment: In-house biochemistry revealed a creatinine of 1.8 mg/dL, BUN of 42 mg/dL, an amylase 1660 IU/L, and a total protein of 8.5 g/dL as the abnormalities noted. A fPL (feline-specific pancreatic lipase) SNAP test was normal as was the CBC. Creatinine was 1.6 mg/dL, BUN 43 mg/dL, and SDMA was 12 μg/L on a renal panel sent to a reference laboratory.

The urinalysis was also run manually in-house later the same day. The USG was 1.056 with a pH of 6.5, 3+ (500 mg/dL) protein, glucose of 500 mg/dL, and 2+ occult blood. This amount of occult blood is not enough to increase the urinary protein reading. Urine microscopy revealed only granular casts this time. The blood glucose was again well within normal limits at 103 mg/dL on the glucometer.

Notice that the amount of protein varied from 1+ to 3+ on dipstrip urine chemistry between the three samples analyzed. Some of this variability is attributed to the semiquantitative nature of this method. The "bin" assigned for how positive the color reaction was can actually be one bin below or one bin higher than that which was reported when measured a second time. If a second urine sample were analyzed hours to days later, biological variability for the excretion of protein could also account for some of this variation in the reported magnitude of proteinuria.

A UPC returned at 1.0 indicating that the 1+ protein was pathological and not just an artifact of the highly concentrated urine. This amount of proteinuria could reflect tubular origin proteinuria and could also include small amounts of filtered albumin that would normally otherwise be reabsorbed following filtration. A bias attributing the renal proteinuria to tubular origin may be assessed due to the proximal tubular disorder leading to the renal glucosuria. Proteinuria could not be attributed to systemic hypertension as systolic blood pressure was 125 mmHg on several serial measurements.

This cat is up for adoption, but clearly something is brewing in this cat's body that is allowing the development of renal glucosuria and cylindruria. Adoptive owners should be warned of this unknown, and urinary parameters should be periodically followed.

Final Diagnosis: Granular and hyaline cylindruria; renal proteinuria; renal glucosuria; IRIS stage 1 or early stage 2 CKD.

Glossary

Acetonuria: presence of acetone (a ketone body) in the urine (see Ketonuria). Acetone accounts for the sweet smell of breath in some ketoacidotic patients.

Acidic: refers to urinary pH of <7.0 (urine pH of 7.0 is considered neutral). Dipstrip measurement in urine is highly inaccurate for precise pH.

Acute kidney injury (AKI): a general term that describes a variety of acute onset renal diseases that can be either azotemic or nonazotemic, and oliguric or nonoliguric depending on the degree and cause of the injury. Nephrotoxins, renal ischemia, and infectious agents (e.g. leptospirosis) are common causes of AKI characterized by varying amounts of acute tubular necrosis (ATN) or degeneration.

Acute-on-chronic kidney disease: superimposition of an acute process/injury on preexisting azotemic or nonazotemic chronic kidney disease (CKD). This process usually results in a sudden decrease in glomerular filtration rate (GFR) and increase in serum creatinine. Examples include dehydration with prerenal effects on renal perfusion, primary renal effects following renal ischemia, exposure to nephrotoxins, and renal infections, or postrenal obstruction (e.g. ureteral stones causing obstruction).

Adaptive nephron hypothesis: theory that all surviving nephrons in azotemic CKD undergo some adaptive compensatory change that contributes to an increase in single-nephron function. The remaining renal functions reflect the heterogeneous contribution by all surviving nephrons. See Intact nephron hypothesis.

Afferent arteriole: arteriole delivering blood to the glomerulus. The afferent arteriole responds with vasoconstriction or vasodilatation to a number of stimuli and is an important determinant of glomerular filtration.

Albuminuria: presence of excessive amounts of plasma albumin in the urine. Albumin can enter urine as a result of renal or postrenal diseases.

Aldosterone: mineralocorticoid steroid hormone secreted by the zona glomerulosa of the adrenal gland; important in regulation of sodium and potassium balance by effects in the distal tubule; excess levels can promote the progression of CKD.

Alkaline: refers to urinary pH of >7.0 (urine pH of 7.0 is considered neutral). Dipstrip measurement in urine is highly inaccurate for precise pH.

Amyloidosis, renal: extracellular deposition of fibrillar proteins with a beta-pleated sheet conformation within glomeruli or the renal interstitium. Reactive systemic amyloidosis is associated with a variety of infectious, inflammatory, and neoplastic diseases; no underlying cause may be found. A familial predisposition for renal amyloidosis exists in some breeds. Renal proteinuria is encountered in those in which the glomerular deposition of amyloid predominates. Prognosis is generally poor due to the relentless progression of azotemic CKD.

Angiotensin: a general term for several molecules following the initial generation of angiotensin-I from angiotensinogen facilitated by renin. Angiotensin-II is generated during exposure of angiotensin-I to angiotensin converting enzyme (ACE) in a variety of tissues. Angiotensin-II exerts potent vasoconstriction and also is involved in proinflammatory and profibrotic pathways after binding with its receptor (angiotensin receptor type 1).

Angiotension-converting enzyme inhibitor or inhibition (ACE-I): a class of drugs designed to reduce renin–angiotensin–aldosterone system (RAAS) activity. Blocks conversion of angiotensin-I to angiotensin-II and is used to reduce systemic and glomerular hypertension.

Angiotensin receptor blocker (ARB): pharmacological molecules capable of selectively blocking access of angiotensin-II to its AT-type 1 receptor. Used as one method to reduce RAAS activity; may have greater reduction in RAAS activity than ACE-I (aldosterone escape and alternate pathways for AG-II generation). Reduced AG-II activity results in the vasodilation of systemic and renal vessels which lowers systemic and glomerular blood pressure. Appears to have more antiproteinuria effect in dogs compared to ACE-I. Telmisartan is the ARB currently of most interest in the treatment of hypertension and glomerular proteinuria in dogs and cats. Treatment with losartan has been supplanted by telmisartan. Could be a first choice for proteinuria reduction or chosen when ACE-I fail.

Antidiuretic hormone (ADH): also referred to as vasopressin for its ability to increase blood pressure. Peptide hormone synthesized in the hypothalamus and secreted by the posterior pituitary in response to plasma osmolality or perception of blood pressure. ADH is a pivotal signal needed to elaborate

Urinalysis in the Dog and Cat, First Edition. Dennis J. Chew and Patricia Schenck.
© 2023 John Wiley & Sons Ltd. Published 2023 by John Wiley & Sons Ltd.

highly concentrated urine after binding to its V-2 receptors on basolateral membranes of the collecting tubules. Arginine-vasopressin is the form secreted by most mammals.

Anuria: total cessation of urine production or extremely low urine volume (< 0.1 mL/kg/hr), as can occur with very severe decreases in GFR from some forms of AKI and during total urethral or bilateral ureteral obstruction.

Aquaporins: small membrane proteins that act as semipermeable channels that facilitate water transport and have a major impact on the ability to concentrate urine.

Atypia: term to denote cells that look abnormal in shape, color, size, and nuclear to cytoplasmic character compared to normal cells from the same location. Can occur in the face of urinary infection, inflammation, precancerous conditions, and during malignancy. Can also be described as "reactive" during inflammation or infection. Atypia is NOT a specific diagnosis. Usually used to describe urothelial cells during dry-mount cytological microscopy.

Azotemia: an increase in the concentration of nitrogenous solutes in the blood, classically urea or creatinine. Azotemia indicates decreased GFR from any cause – prerenal, primary renal, postrenal, or combinations. Azotemia can also result following uroabdomen and nonrenal causes without decreased GFR.

Azotemia, prerenal: results from the lack of adequate renal perfusion needed to excrete waste products. This form of azotemia is reversible if perfusion is corrected early enough; otherwise, progression to AKI can occur. Some component often exists on top of primary and postrenal azotemia. Most often occurs in association with highly concentrated urine if the condition is pure prerenal.

Azotemia, postrenal: results following obstruction to urine outflow (acute complete urethral or bilateral ureteral process; chronic partial obstruction). Can also develop following the absorption of small molecules from urine in the peritoneal cavity following the rupture of the urinary bladder or urethra, or rarely from the accumulation of subcutaneous urine following urethral rupture. Urine concentration (urine specific gravity [USG]) varies widely and is not predictable.

Azotemia, renal or primary: results when GFR is decreased enough to cause waste product retention (creatinine, blood urea nitrogen [BUN], symmetrical dimethyl arginine [SDMA], and others) from renal lesions acquired from the many possible underlying causes of CKD or AKI. USG is usually less than 1.030 in dogs and less than 1.035 in cats. Primary renal azotemia exists in some cats with preserved ability to highly concentrate urine, but that is not common in dogs.

Bacteriuria: presence of bacteria in the urine, regardless of quantity observed during urine microscopy or urine culture.

Bacteriuria, significant: refers to a clinically relevant quantitative growth of bacteria following proper collection and handling of a urine sample. This is commonly reported in colony-forming units per mL (cfu/mL) as no growth, <1000 cfu/mL, 1000–10 000 cfu/mL, >10 000 cfu/mL, and >100 000 cfu/mL.

Baruria: very old term to describe the elaboration of urine with an unusually high USG in humans at >1.025 or >1.030. Not often used in veterinary literature, as it is too general a denotation of urine concentration; refers to a USG > 1.035 when used.

Benazepril: a commonly used ACE-I, especially for use in cats; see ACE-I.

Bence Jones proteinuria: presence of immunoglobulin light chains in the urine in patients with multiple myeloma. These proteins are heat sensitive, coagulating at 45–55 °C, but urinary electrophoresis with immunofixation is considered definitive.

Bilirubinuria: presence of bilirubin in the urine. The form of bilirubin appearing in the urine is the conjugated or direct-reacting form. Can be normal in dogs, especially males; never normal in cats.

Bowman's capsule: the combination of parietal and visceral epithelium that surrounds the glomerular capillaries, and the space between them (Bowman's space). Glomerular filtrate accumulates in this space as it heads toward the proximal tubule to become tubular fluid.

Bowman's space: see Bowman's capsule

BRAF testing: use of PCR for the detection of the BRAF mutation in cells shed into urine of dogs with urothelial or prostatic carcinoma. The BRAF gene is important in control of cell growth.

Blood urea nitrogen (BUN): commonly measured analyte to evaluate renal function. Urea nitrogen is generated by the urea cycle in the liver. Serum urea nitrogen (SUN) is the preferred term by some, as the measurement is made in serum or plasma. BUN or SUN is NOT the same as measurement of urea. Urea is measured first, converted to urea nitrogen and then reported as mg/dL or mmol/L. An increased BUN often indicates decreased GFR during prerenal and postrenal conditions as well as in various primary renal diseases. A high-protein diet, gastrointestinal hemorrhage, or absorption of urine across the peritoneal membrane during uroabdomen can also increase BUN without a decrease in GFR.

BUN-to-creatinine ratio: most helpful in those with an increased ratio during early dehydration, uroabdomen, and early upper urinary tract obstruction due to preferential reabsorption of BUN compared to creatinine. A decreasing ratio can be found during the feeding of lower protein content renal diets (RDs) during CKD.

Calcitriol: the most biologically active vitamin D metabolite, 1,25(OH)$_2$-vitamin D, following conversion from 25(OH)-vitamin D. This metabolite has the greatest affinity for the vitamin D receptor. Absolute or relatively low levels of calcitriol are part of CKD-MBD.

Calcium channel blocker (CCB): prevents or reduces the opening of calcium channels which limits the entry of calcium into cells from the extracellular space. Most classes of these blockers affect the L-type voltage gated calcium channel. The mechanism for reduction in systemic blood pressure follows arteriolar vasodilatation, reduced myocardial contractility, heart rate reduction, and a direct effect on the adrenal gland to reduce aldosterone synthesis and secretion. Amlodopine is the CCB most commonly used in veterinary medicine to treat high blood pressure, especially in cats. CCB does not lower intraglomerular pressure as much as that with ACE-I, which preferentially cause efferent arteriolar dilatation.

Calculus: general term referring to a solid concretion (stone) occurring in a hollow organ or duct. See Urolith.

Capillaria plica: parasitic worm that can inhabit the bladder; can be incidental finding or at times associated with pathology.

Cast: a cylindrical mass of material formed in the loop of Henle and distal portion of the nephron and passed in the urine; casts may be cellular, granular (coarse and fine), waxy, or hyaline. Casts consist of varying proportions of matrix protein, cells, and granules from cellular degeneration or protein precipitation.

Cast, agglutination: cellular casts that form within precipitates of matrix protein (Tamm–Horsfall protein [THP]), which holds the cells within.

Cast, conglutination: cellular cast composed of renal tubular epithelium (RTE) that sloughed into the tubular lumen with intact side-by-side cells without matrix protein participation. These casts are sometimes called renal fragments and represent a more severe intrarenal injury that the finding of agglutinated RTE.

Cast, broad: a cast that has a much wider dimension that develops in either the collecting ducts or in a pathologically dilated part of the distal nephron. Patients with broad casts may have a poorer prognosis since their presence indicates formation of casts in some dilated location of the nephron.

Cast, cellular: cast comprised of RBC, WBC, RTE, or combinations indicating some type of active renal process detected during urine microscopy.

Cast, cellular RBC: cast that contains predominantly intact RBC. The detection of this cast is associated with renal bleeding into the tubular lumens, usually from active glomerular inflammation. Can be mixed with WBC or RTE at times.

Cast, cellular WBC: cast that is predominantly composed of WBC, usually neutrophils. The detection of this cast indicates intrarenal inflammation, often that associated with pyelonephritis but can be encountered at times in those with interstitial nephritis from other causes and glomerulonephritis (GN).

Cast, cellular RTE: cast that is predominantly composed of RTE following shedding of RTE into the tubular lumens.

Cast, cylindroid: A long narrow cast, most often hyaline in nature. Interstitial infiltrates or edema are thought to compress the renal tubules in these instances.

Cast, hyaline: cast that is mostly pure precipitation of THP matrix protein. This cast forms easily and dissolves quickly especially in alkaline urine. The persistent detection of hyaline casts can indicate glomerular disease with albuminuria that favors the precipitation of THP.

Cast, granular: includes the detection of either or both fine and coarse types during urine microscopy. Granules in casts can develop during the degeneration of cells (RBC, WBC, and RTE) and include organelles. Alternatively, granules can form in casts following the precipitation of plasma proteins that leak into tubular fluid across a glomerulus that has lost its integrity to thwart passage of proteins.

Cast, shower: numerous casts that can consist of any type (hyaline, cellular, granular, and waxy).

Cast, waxy: translucent cast that represents the final degradation product from granular or cellular casts. One theory also states that waxy casts can arise from hyaline cast protein transformation. Waxy casts take the longest time of all casts to form, and so represent clinically relevant intrarenal stasis.

Central diabetes insipidus (CDI): refers to conditions in which ADH synthesis in the hypothalamus or its secretion from the pituitary gland is impaired resulting in in low circulating ADH. Impaired urinary concentration then follows as there is minimal to no ADH interaction with its V-2 receptor on the collecting ducts. Hyposthenuria is characteristic of those with complete CDI. Partial CDI can result in some urine concentration (isosthenuria to minimally concentrated).

Chemical properties of urine: A variety of analytes measured on a urinary dipstrip including pH, protein, occult blood, glucose, ketones, and bilirubin as part of the complete urinalysis.

Chromagen: a color generating molecule as part of the urinary dipstrip reagent pad designed to measure a specific analyte (e.g., glucose, protein, and occult blood); greater color reaction is related to higher concentrations of the analyte in question.

Chronic interstitial nephritis (CIN): histopathologic lesions often described in advanced stages of azotemic CKD. These lesions are considered to be nonspecific endstage lesions that develop after an initial injury to glomeruli, tubules, and or the interstitium that can no longer be identified. Lesions consist of nephron drop-out, interstitial fibrosis, interstitial infiltrates with lymphoplasmacytes, and glomerular obsolescence. CIN is more commonly confirmed in cats than in dogs.

Chronic kidney disease: Azotemic or nonazotemic disease within the kidney accounted for by various combinations of glomerular, vascular, tubular, and interstitial, lesions that have been present for one to three months. Azotemic CKD is usually progressive, but the rate of progression is variable by individual patients.

Chronic kidney disease and mineral bone disorder (CKD-MBD): term used to reflect the complex effects and interactions that follow some combination of increased PTH, parathyroid gland hyperplasia, increased phosphorus, decreased and increased ionized calcium concentration, decreased vitamin D metabolites, decreased Klotho, and increased FGF23 that occur during CKD. Renal osteodystrophy, accelerated progression of CKD, and increased mortality are among the multiple clinical syndromes associated with CKD-MBD. This term is preferred rather than the use of renal secondary hyperparathyroidism that encompasses a much narrower focus.

Clearance: the renal clearance of a substance is that volume of plasma that would have to be filtered by the kidneys per minute to account for the amount of that substance appearing in the urine per minute. Often reported in mL/min or mL/min/kg. Depending on the compound that is cleared by the kidneys, this can be an estimate of GFR or renal blood flow (RBF).

Collecting ducts (tubules): part of the nephron between the distal/connecting tubule and the renal pelvis. Under the influence of ADH, the cortical collecting tubule is permeable to water but not to urea. The medullary collecting tubule is permeable to urea and ADH further enhances both urea and water reabsorption into the interstitium. The response of the V-2 receptor on the collecting tubules to ADH is pivotally important in the capacity to elaborate concentrated or dilute urine.

Complete urinalysis: measurement and reporting of physical properties, chemical properties, and elements found during urine microscopy.

Counter-current multiplication system: concept of the counter-current multiplier and exchanger working in concert to allow maximal concentration of urine when needed.

Counter-current multiplication: an explanation as to how urine that undergoes isosmotic tubular fluid reabsorption to the end of the proximal tubule can progressively increase its tubular fluid concentration (osmolality) manyfold in the descending loop of Henle, achieve its maximal concentration at hair pin turn of Henle's loop, and then become progressively more dilute during the ascent of Henle's loop.

Counter-current exchanger: the concept of vasa recta that parallel Henle's loop deep into the medulla that allows the preservation of local areas of renal interstitial osmolality that is important in maintaining the ability to maximally concentrate urine.

Creatinine clearance: the volume of plasma that is cleared of creatinine per unit time and can be used to estimate GFR. Can be measured using exogenous or endogenous creatinine methods. Decreases before BUN or serum creatinine increase above the reference range.

Creatinine: is commonly measured in serum (and sometimes urine) to evaluate renal function. It is often preferred to the measurement and evaluation of BUN, since creatinine has less nonrenal factors to consider. Creatinine enters the circulation as a muscle breakdown product; thus, its concentration varies somewhat by lean muscle mass. Increased creatinine can develop during prerenal, primary renal, and postrenal disorders. The magnitude of increased creatinine does not align with its cause. Traditionally, serum creatinine is thought to increase above the reference range following loss of enough nephron mass to decrease the GFR by 75%. If the upper limit of the reference range is lowered to around 1.5 mg/dL, serum creatinine increases following the loss of about 50% of GFR.

Crystalluria: refers to crystals observed during urine microscopy. Oftentimes struvite and calcium oxalate crystals in urine are not pathological. Their presence can be an artifact of storage and cooling of the urine sample. In warm urine, their presence is of concern in the consideration of factors favoring recurrent urolithiasis. Cystine crystals are always pathological, urates sometimes are associated with PSS, and oxalates can be an early indicator of ethylene glycol exposure.

Culture urine, qualitative: the isolation and reporting of any quantity of organisms that grow, sometimes with the modifiers small, medium, or heavy growth.

Culture urine, quantitative: isolated bacteria are reported in colony-forming units/mL (cfu/mL). See Bacteriuria, significant.

Cylindruria: presence of casts in the urine. A very small number of hyaline and granular casts are considered "normal" in concentrated urine. The detection of casts in minimally concentrated urine likely indicates pathology.

Cystatin C: A molecule that can be used as a surrogate for GFR. Trending in human medicine to improve eGFR calculations. Not commercially available from veterinary laboratories. A clear-cut advantage over serum creatinine has not yet been demonstrated in veterinary medicine.

Cystitis: inflammation of the urinary bladder secondary to bacterial UTI, urolithiasis, neoplasia, idiopathic, chemical, or parasitic causes.

Cystocentesis: sometimes referred to as vesicopuncture. Collection of urine by transabdominal percutaneous needle puncture of the bladder. Preferred method for urine culture. Main advantage is that this method bypasses lower urogenital tract contamination of the sample. Iatrogenic hematuria is its major disadvantage.

Cytology: microscopy of specimens obtained from urine (or effusions, other body fluids) or from a fine needle aspirate

(FNA) of masses. Dry-mount examination is usually performed after centrifugation has been employed to concentrate the number of cells. Routine Wright's Giemsa or Diff Quick is used for the initial evaluation; special stains can be used if needed. Mostly used in urine to further characterize urothelial cells during concern for neoplasia, but can also be useful to evaluate for the presence of RTE, dysmorphic RBC, and to more definitively determine WBC type compared to findings from wet-mount urine microscopy.

Desmopressin (dDAVP: 1-deamino-8-D-arginine vasopressin): synthetic analogue of the naturally occurring 8-arginine vasopressin molecule, but with increased antidiuretic activity and decreased pressor activity. See Vasopressin testing.

Diabetes insipidus (DI): general term that includes central DI (complete or partial) and nephrogenic DI. Often associated with polyuria/polydipsia (PU/PD) and hyposthenuria.

Dialysis: removal of wastes and excess water that have accumulated in the circulation during azotemic AKI or CKD following osmotic or hydraulic forces in the artificial kidney during hemodialysis or across the peritoneal membrane during peritoneal dialysis.

***Dioctophyma renale* (giant kidney worm):** parasitic infection in dogs that occupy the renal pelvis or live free in the peritoneum. This worm tends to mostly involve the right kidney and can create severe hydronephrosis. Identification of characteristic worm eggs shed into urine help to establish this diagnosis.

***Dirofilaria immitis*:** the filarial worm known as heartworm; dogs are the definitive host. Microfilaria are injected into the host following mosquito bites and then pass through several larval stages. Adult worms live in the right heart and pulmonary outflow tracts. Adult worms in the caudal vena cava can be associated with caval syndrome. Can be associated with the development of GN and glomerular proteinuria in nonazotemic or azotemic CKD.

Distal tubule: short segment of the nephron immediately downstream from the macula densa, between the terminal ascending loop of Henle and the connecting tubule; fine tuning of some electrolyte reabsorption or secretion occurs in this region.

Diuresis: urine excretion in excess of the usual volume produced as a result of diseases that impair urinary concentration or following drugs that impair tubular fluid and solute reabsorption.

Dysuria: discomfort or pain upon urination; a burning sensation is present in humans able to describe this feeling. Sometimes accompanied by difficulty in starting the urinary stream.

Enalapril: a commonly used ACE-I, especially in dogs; see ACE-I.

Ethylene glycol (EG): an industrial compound found in some consumer products. It is most often found in radiator fluid, though some products are propylene glycol based (nontoxic). It can also be found in some hydraulic brake fluids, stamp pad inks, ballpoint pens, solvents, paints, plastics, films, and cosmetics. EG is clear, colorless, viscid, and sweet. Fluorescein is often added to radiator fluid to provide a yellowish–green sheen to this fluid. Consumption of EG often leads to severe toxicity and death in dogs and cats following biotransformation to toxic intermediary metabolites. EG toxicity sequentially affects the CNS, cardiopulmonary systems, and then the kidneys. EG without biotransformation is far less toxic, manifesting mostly CNS depression. EG ingestion leads to early excretion of calcium oxalate crystals seen in urinary sediment from dogs and cats. Prognosis for survival is grave (in the absence of hemodialysis) if the patient is found to be azotemic and oligoanuric.

Extracellular fluid volume (ECFV): fluid volume distributed in both the interstitial and vascular spaces; about half of total body water exists in the extracellular fluid (ECF); estimated at $0.3 \times$ weight of patient in kg as liters in adults. The regulation of ECFV is important in maintaining blood pressure and renal perfusion.

Familial glomerulopathy: A form of CKD in which the lesion mostly affects the glomerulus from some type of genetic abnormality. Mostly in dogs of certain breeds or lines. The underlying molecular lesion may or not be known depending on the specific glomerulopathy. Proteinuria is characteristic with variable rates for the progression of CKD.

Fanconi Syndrome: an acquired or congenital proximal tubular dysfunction characterized by glucosuria and generalized aminoaciduria, with varying amounts of bicarbonaturia, phosphaturia, and proteinuria.

Fatty cast: cast that contains globules of lipid within; can occur secondary to cellular degeneration within the cast or during conditions with renal proteinuria. Fat globules can be confused with the granules of precipitated plasma proteins.

Feline urologic syndrome (FUS): A term coined in the 1960s to describe cats with a constellation of lower urinary tract signs (including urethral obstruction) without reference to a specific cause. The use of this term is discouraged in favor of more specific diagnostic terms (e.g. UTI, urolithiasis, FIC/IC, and neoplasia).

Fibroblast growth factor 23 (FGF23): a specific peptide hormone (phosphatonin) that is one member of the fibroblast growth factor family. FGF23 is secreted by osteocytes and is important in phosphate and vitamin D metabolism. FGF23 promotes phosphaturia by reducing expression of the Na-P cotransporter in the proximal tubules and decreases levels of circulating calcitriol through inhibition of 1-alpha hydroxylase and stimulation of 24,25-hydroxylase systems in the kidney. FGF23 also reduces PTH synthesis early in CKD. Circulating FGF23 increases in CKD to help maintain phosphate balance and serves as a biomarker, but also may exert maladaptive effects. High affinity binding of FGF23 to its receptor requires interaction with its coreceptor alpha-Klotho.

Fish oil: a general term to describe a dietary supplement containing various amounts and types of lipids. Over-the-counter preparations can vary widely in their content of eicosapentaenoic acid (EPA), docosahexaenoic acid (DHA), other fish oils, and the ratio of omega-3 to omega-6 polyunsaturated fatty acid (PUFA).

Focal: lesions restricted to one region of the kidney without affecting other regions, (e.g. glomerular, tubular or renal interstitial). Often used to refer to a focal lesion within the glomerulus (e.g. mesangium, glomerular basement membrane [GBM], and podocytes).

Fractional clearance of electrolytes (FC(x)): the clearance of the electrolyte in question compared to the clearance of creatinine, expressed as a percentage. Since the rate of urine production (V) in the clearance equation cancels out, this can be used without measuring urine volume over time. Ux/Sx divided by Ucr/Scr X 100, where x is the electrolyte and cr is creatinine. The FC for sodium, chloride, and calcium are <1% in health. FC for phosphorus can be used as a surrogate for activity of PTH and FGF23 on proximal renal tubular function. FC for most electrolytes increase during CKD.

Functional proteinuria: transient and mild proteinuria consisting mainly of albumin, which occurs in certain situations associated with increased sympathetic nervous system activity (e.g. fever, stress, and seizures).

Glitter cells: polymorphonuclear leukocytes in urine with granules in their cytoplasm that exhibit Brownian motion; suggestive of pyelonephritis if present in urine with specific gravity >1.015.

Global: a pathologic term referring to the glomerulus and descriptive of a lesion which involves all of the glomerulus. Also called panglomerular.

Glomerular basement membrane: part of the glomerular capillary wall consisting of the combined basal lamina maintained by the endothelial cells and the podocytes; consists of three layers – lamina rara interna (endothelial side), lamina densa, and the lamina rara externa (visceral epithelial side). Various laminins, type IV collagen, nidogens, and proteoglycans comprise the GBM. The healthy GBM is freely permeable to plasma water but importantly retards passage of some plasma molecules based on size and charge selectivity.

Glomerular filtration rate: the volume of plasma filtered across the glomerular capillaries into Bowman's space per unit of time. The gold standard for the determination of GFR involves infusion of inulin and inulin measurement in urine and blood over time. Exogenous or endogenous creatinine clearance can be used for the clinical estimation of GFR. Iohexol clearance following a single IV injection also provides acceptable estimates for measurement of GFR. A GFR of 3–6 mL/min/kg is normal for dogs and 2–4 mL/min/kg is considered normal in cats, depending on the methods used. A decrease in GFR can occur due to prerenal, renal, or postrenal causes. The determination of GFR is considered the best single test of excretory renal function.

Glomerular proteinuria: proteinuria of glomerular origin due to increased filtration of plasma proteins usually through an abnormally permeable glomerular filter; albumin usually predominates in glomerular proteinuria.

Glomerulitis: inflammation of the renal glomeruli.

Glomerulonephritis: a variety of nephritis characterized primarily by an inflammatory process in the glomeruli; most cases of glomerulonephritis involve immune-mediated injury.

Glomerulonephropathy (glomerulopathy): any disease of the renal glomeruli, including glomerulonephritis, familial nephropathy, glomerular amyloidosis, and glomerulosclerosis.

Glomerulosclerosis: general term to describe an advanced lesion of CKD, in which the glomerulus has accumulated extracellular matrix produced by mesangial cells (scar). The lesion can be focal, segmental, global, or diffuse. Its presence indicates a severe glomerular injury but not its cause and often is found in association with glomerular proteinuria.

Glomerulus: the renal filtering apparatus across which plasma traverses into Bowman's space to form an ultrafiltrate. This includes the afferent and efferent arterioles as well as the glomerular capillaries (endothelium, basement membrane, podocytes, podocyte foot processes, and slit-pore membranes). In health, the glomerulus minimizes passage of plasma proteins into Bowman's space. Glomerular capillaries are uniquely situated between two arterioles.

Glucosuria: presence of detectable glucose in the urine, either due to overflow from high plasma concentrations or from decreased proximal tubular reabsorption.

Glucosuria, renal: occurs following defective proximal tubular reabsorption of filtered glucose as a single abnormality or as part of Fanconi syndrome. Blood sugar is normal.

Glycosuria: often used interchangeably with the term glucosuria.

Hematuria: presence of erythrocytes in the urine; may be detected by the naked eye (gross) or only during urine microscopy. See Occult blood.

Hemoglobinuria: presence of free hemoglobin in the urine.

Hereditary nephropathy: progressive CKD due to a genetic defect in type 4 collagen of the GBM. Can be X-Linked or autosomal recessive in certain dog breeds. Renal proteinuria occurs early in this condition.

Hippurate crystalluria: Hippurate or hippurate-like crystals were described in early reports of ethylene glycol poisoning in dogs, but these crystals were later definitively identified as calcium oxalate monohydrate.

Hydronephrosis: distension of the renal pelvis with urine due to chronic obstruction of the urinary conduit with accompanying atrophy of the renal parenchyma.

Hydropenia: deficiency of water in the body; dehydration.

Hydrostatic pressure: pressure (mm Hg) exerted by blood on the walls of blood vessels; progressively declines from the afferent arteriole along the glomerulus to the efferent arteriole; an important determinant of GFR as part of Starling's forces.

Hyperparathyroidism, renal secondary: high circulating PTH concentrations and parathyroid gland hyperplasia that result from some combination of high serum phosphorus, low ionized calcium, low 25(OH)-vitamin D, low 1,25(OH)$_2$-vitamin D, and decreased expression of CaR that enhance the synthesis and secretion of PTH during CKD (especially azotemic CKD). A component of CKD-MBD.

Hyposthenuria: elaboration of urine with an osmolality less than that of circulating plasma. The urine to plasma (serum) osmolality is less than 1.0. 50 mOsm/kg is the lowest osmolality possible in most instances. The USG is expected to be 1.001–1.007. Often found in disorders with low circulating ADH or lessened effect of ADH.

Idiopathic cystitis: no known cause for cystitis can be found. Diagnosis is made by exclusion, common in cats, rare in dogs. Has many similarities to interstitial cystitis (painful bladder syndrome) in humans with overactivation of the sympathetic nervous system.

Idiopathic hypertriglyceridemia (IHTG): the finding of increased concentrations of triglycerides during fasting without an underlying predisposing condition. This is characterized by accumulation of very-low-density lipoproteins (VLDL) or a combination of VLDL and chylomicrons. Encountered in specific breeds but especially in miniature Schnauzers. IHTG can be a risk factor for development of pancreatitis. It can also be associated with glomerular proteinuria and a specific glomerular lesion at times during CKD.

Immune complex glomerulonephritis: deposition or formation of antigen–antibody complexes within the various layers of the GBM and the mesangium. These deposits and reaction to them decrease glomerular barrier integrity so that plasma proteins, particularly albumin, now more readily cross over into tubular fluid. Often associated with progressive CKD.

Incontinence: loss of voluntary control of urination.

Intact Nephron Hypothesis: the theory of Bricker stating that in progressive CKD, damaged nephrons drop out of the functional population and no longer contribute to renal function, while the remaining functioning nephrons undergo compensatory changes and become "super nephrons." Surviving nephrons maintain renal function at low, normal, or increased levels depending on the specific single nephron. Glomerular hypertrophy, glomerular hypertension, increased single-nephron GFR, and tubular hypertrophy contribute to this "adaptation" in surviving nephrons.

International Renal Interest Society (IRIS): a panel of veterinary experts that develop an ongoing set of recommendations for diagnosis, staging or grading, and treatment of AKI and CKD.

Interstitial nephritis: nephritis due to inflammation of the interstitial tissues of the kidney; CIN refers to interstitial fibrosis and mononuclear inflammatory cell infiltrate; etiology is not specified.

Iohexol: an iodinated radiocontrast agent given IV to perform excretory urography. It allows more detailed study of renal and ureteral anatomy and can also be injected through a urinary catheter for positive contrast cystography and urethrography. GFR can be estimated following IV injection and periodic blood sampling over time. The rate for the disappearance of iohexol from the circulation is proportional to the GFR; results in mL/min/kg are provided by the reference laboratory.

Isosthenuria: elaboration of urine with nearly the same osmolality as plasma initially filtered across the glomerulus (approximately 300 mOsm/kg). The urine to plasma (serum) osmolality is close to 1.0. Classically associated with a USG of 1.008–1.012 in humans, but the range is likely higher in dogs and cats since their plasma osmolality is often higher than in humans.

Juvenile renal disease: detection of azotemic or nonazotemic renal disease in young patients, mostly identified in purebred dogs. An underlying familial genetic condition is often suspected, but this can also include a nongenetic *in utero* developmental abnormality.

Kaliopenic Nephropathy: the constellation of renal findings that can occur during potassium depletion with or without hypokalemia. This includes the development and/or accelerated progression of CKD associated with advancing tubulointerstitial lesions, mainly documented in the cat. Potassium depletion can impair urinary concentrating capacity early on in addition to reversible decrements in GFR. Characteristic ventroflexion of the neck often occurs in cats with severe hypokalemia.

Ketone Bodies: see Ketonuria.

Ketonuria: presence of acetoacetate, beta-hydroxybutyric acid, and acetone (collectively known as ketone bodies) in the urine. Ketone bodies are normally produced at low levels by the liver and undergo peripheral tissue uptake. Starvation and altered carbohydrate metabolism encountered in diabetes mellitus can increase the production of ketone bodies so that they enter urine at higher levels. The urinary dipstrip measures mostly acetoacetate.

Leptospirosis: an acute or subacute systemic infectious disease caused by pathogenic spirochetes of the genus Leptospira. Exposure to these organisms usually occurs from urine or standing water. This is diagnosed most frequently in dogs. Acute interstitial nephritis and ATN can lead to the development of azotemic AKI. PU/PD can develop as the primary sign in dogs with subacute nonazotemic AKI from leptospirosis. Some dogs have inapparent infections, and some can shed organisms into urine for a long time. Can also be associated with liver disease in concert with kidney involvement, or as the only organ identified.

Loop of Henle: parallel renal tubular array that includes the thin descending limb, thin ascending limb, and the medullary thick ascending limb of Henle's loop; in between the proximal tubule and the distal tubule. Critical for the maintenance of a hypertonic interstitium and maximal ability to concentrate urine as part of the countercurrent system with countercurrent multiplication.

Leukocyte esterase: a specific protein found in WBC that can be detected by reagent pads on some urinary dipstrips. This pad has the ability to detect intact or lysed WBC in human urine, often associated with bacterial infection or other sterile inflammatory conditions. Color reactions on dipstrips should not be reported in dogs and cats since there are many false positive and false negative reactions.

Lipiduria: the observation of refractile lipid droplets during urine microscopy; can be confirmed with Sudan staining. Frequently observed in cats as a normal finding. Can be associated with increased cellular degeneration.

Lower urinary tract: bladder and urethra

Low-molecular-weight proteinuria: excretion of proteins in urine with a molecular weight < 69 kD. Typically encountered in patients with failed tubular reabsorption of nonalbumin proteins from tubular fluid during some forms of CKD and AKI. Includes proteins from prerenal origin too.

LUTD: lower urinary tract disease(s); term was coined as an alternative to feline urologic syndrome (FUS) to try to shift focus away from FUS as a specific disease.

Macula densa (MD): specialized cells of the first portion of the distal tubule; they lie in close apposition to juxtaglomerular cells of the afferent arteriole as part of the juxtaglomerular apparatus. Cells of the MD are important in sensing tubular fluid solute flow in this region and impact afferent arteriolar tone, GFR, RBF, and renin release.

Medullary thick ascending limb (mTAL): the terminal portion of Henle's loop. The mTAL is impermeable to water but undergoes reabsorption of sodium, potassium, and chloride following entry in the cells via the Na-K-2Cl cotransporter. The thin ascending loop of Henle together with the mTAL are sometimes called the diluting segment since solute but not water is reabsorbed in this region. Delivers hypotonic urine to the distal and collecting tubule for further processing.

Medullary washout (MWO): a condition that develops following loss of renal medullary interstitial hypertonicity. Reduction of urea and sodium concentrations in this region impair elaboration of urine with maximal concentration. Longstanding PU/PD from any cause can create MWO as can conditions that increase medullary blood flow. Low circulating ADH, less expression or activity of aquaporins and urea transporters in the colleting tubules contribute to less generation of medullary hypertonicity.

Membranous nephropathy: the glomerular lesion characterized by thickening of the GBM with or without deposits of immune complexes. Often considered to be idiopathic.

Mesangioproliferative glomerulonephritis: the glomerular lesion in which mesangial cell proliferation and expansion of mesangial cell matrix predominates in this inflammatory condition.

Mesangium: the space in between the glomerular capillary loops that is not covered by basement membrane. Contains mesangial cells and mesangial matrix that provide a scaffold that help maintain normal glomerular capillary architecture. Mesangial cells contain contractile elements that can regulate the available surface area for GFR. May be predisposed to accumulation of immune complexes. Proliferation of mesangial cells and mesangial matrix contribute to the development of glomerulosclerosis, reduced GFR, and glomerular proteinuria. Mesangial cells can perform phagocytosis.

Methemoglobin: an oxidized state of hemoglobin that has changed from ferrous (Fe^{2+}) to the ferric (Fe^{3+}) state. Methemoglobinuria can account for the observation of very dark brown to black colored urine. Oxidation of hemoglobin in urine can occur during storage of urine in the bladder or in the laboratory.

Microalbuminuria (MA): detection of albumin in urine below the limit of detection for proteins measured by reagent pads on dipstrips, defined as 1–29 mg/dL. "Overt albuminuria" is defined as ≥30 mg/dL. Persistent MA develops earlier than proteinuria detected by urinary protein-to-creatinine ratio (UPC) in most instances, and indicates loss of glomerular barrier integrity. MA occurs early in CKD, systemic diseases affecting the kidneys, and in the critical care arena.

Micturition: involves the filling and storage of urine in the bladder, evacuation (voiding) of urine from the bladder, and the termination of voiding. This requires coordination between the bladder, urethra, and the autonomic and somatic nervous systems. It is not simply the passage of urine.

Midstream catch: collection of a urine sample during voiding after the initial stream has passed. This timing for collection is desirable in most instances in order to reduce the magnitude of potential contamination from the urethra, genitalia, or skin in the region. Less commonly, collection of a urine sample from the initial stream or the endstream is indicated.

Mineralocorticoid receptor blocker (MRB): pharmacological molecules (e.g. spironolactone, eplerenone, and finerenone) designed to block access of circulating aldosterone access to its mineralocorticoid receptor. Aldosterone escape happens during the use of ACE-I or ARB treatment in some settings. Suppression of aldosterone activity can be helpful in limiting glomerular proteinuria, usually after an ACE-I or an ARB has failed to sufficiently reduce renal proteinuria. Can be associated with reduced progression of CKD in humans, but this effect has not been reported in dogs or cats.

Mixed cast: Cast with more than one characteristic without a clear preponderance. Can contain more than one cell type (WBC, RBC, RTE, degenerating cellular), granules (fine or coarse; lipid or fatty), or class of cast (such as hyaline and granular).

Myoglobinuria: the presence of the muscle pigment myoglobin in the urine. The occult blood reagent pad on the urinary dipstrip turns positive in the presence of myoglobin. Definitive identification requires urinary protein electrophoresis or immunochemical methods.

Nephrectomy: removal of a kidney, complete or partial. Historically used to create experimental models of CKD in dogs and cats.

Nephritis: inflammation of the kidney; does not specify which area of the kidney is mainly involved (i.e. tubules, glomeruli, vessels, interstitium).

Nephrocalcinosis: a condition characterized by the precipitation of calcium phosphate in renal tissues, often detected in association with renal insufficiency. Sometimes detected on radiographs or sonography of the kidneys. Definitively detected on histopathology.

Nephrogenic DI (NDI): inability to concentrate urine despite normal or increased circulating ADH. Can be attributed to a number of molecular mechanisms depending on the specific underlying cause (e.g. hypercalcemia, hypokalemia, or endotoxemia). Nonazotemic CKD is a condition associated with NDI due to an insufficient number of fully functioning nephrons needed to elaborate concentrated urine. Individuals with severe forms of NDI can exhibit hyposthenuria. Minimally concentrated urine is elaborated at times in others.

Nephron: the functional anatomic unit of the kidney consisting of the renal corpuscle (Bowman's capsule and glomeruli within), proximal convoluted tubule, loop of Henle, distal convoluted tubule, and collecting tubule.

Nephritogenic: potential for giving rise to inflammation of the kidney.

Nephropathy: any disease of the kidney.

Nephropathy, familial: genetically mediated causes of CKD. This is a common cause of azotemic and nonazotemic CKD in young dogs that preferentially affects certain purebred lines. Many dogs with familial nephropathy have renal lesions that center within the glomerulus initially, and so, renal proteinuria is common.

Nephrotic syndrome: follows some type of severe chronic glomerular disease (e.g. amyloidosis and glomerulonephritis). It is characterized by varying degrees of glomerular proteinuria, hypoalbuminemia, hypercholesterolemia, ascites, and edema. There may or may not be azotemia.

Nephrotomy: incision into the kidney, often to expose the renal pelvis for stone removal.

Nocturia: passage of urine at night. This can occur in those with urinary incontinence (e.g. PSMI) or secondary to any polyuric condition in which the bladder fills up more quickly than normal. Dogs with PU/PD often wake the owners up at night to let them out to urinate.

Occult blood: detection of intact or lysed RBC in urine by chemistry dipstrip. Reagent pad color reactions are very sensitive for the detection of small quantities of hemoglobin.

This reagent pad also will detect myoglobin in the urine. Some reagent pads detect intact RBC versus free hemoglobin.

Oligoanuria: very little to no urine production as can occur in some severe forms of azotemic AKI and during complete obstructive uropathy.

Oliguria: excretion of a reduced urine volume in animals (<12–24 mL/lb/day; 0.5–1.0 mL/kg/hr) not on IV fluids. Absolute oliguria is defined as <1 mL/kg/hr while on IV fluids. Relative oliguria can exist when urine volume produced is <2–5 mL/kg/hr while on IV fluids.

Omega-3 fatty acid: a specific type of PUFA categorized by the position of the first double bond. The most common omega-3 (n-3) fatty acids are alpha-linolenic acid, EPA, and DHA. Omega-3 fatty acids appear to exert beneficial anti-inflammatory, antifibrotic, antiproteinuric, and GFR stabilizing effects in the CKD kidney. The actual dose of omega-3 fatty acids and the ratio between dietary omega-3 and omega-6 PUFA are important considerations for these salutary effects. Not synonymous with "fish oil."

Oncotic pressure (π): the osmotic pressure generated by large molecules (especially proteins) in plasma. Important in maintaining circulating blood volume. Reduced oncotic pressure can result in edema and body cavity effusions. π is an important determinant of GFR as it opposes hydrostatic pressure within the glomerulus as part of Starling's forces.

Osmolality: the concentration of osmotically active solutes per kilogram of solvent.

Osmolarity: the concentration of osmotically active solutes per liter of solution.

Osmotic pressure: the pressure generated as molecules and water move down their concentration gradient into another compartment across a semipermeable membrane. This is related to effective osmolality (tonicity).

per µL: the volume of urine in which elements in urine are counted during microscopy. This is an emerging standard for reporting of results in urinalysis that is more accurate than enumeration using per high-power field (HPF) or per low-power field (LPF).

per HPF: standard 400× total magnification is used to further identify and enumerate elements during urine microscopy. The average number of RBC, WBC, epithelial cells, and bacteria are reported after examination of at least 10 microscopic fields.

per LPF: standard 100× total magnification is used in the initial detection of elements during urine microscopy. The average number of casts and crystals are reported after examining at least 10 microscopic low-powered fields. Further identification of casts and crystals is made during HPF microscopy.

Panglomerular: same as global.

Paradoxical aciduria: the finding of acid urine during metabolic alkalosis (e.g. duodenal foreign body obstruction with vomiting), usually in association with severe hypochloremia, hyponatremia and ECFV contraction.

Pars recta (S$_3$): the distal segment of the proximal tubule that extends into the outer medulla.

Physical properties of urine: one of the three components of the complete urinalysis. Color, clarity, and odor of the urine specimen are physically evaluated, but urine concentration (USG by refractometer) is the most important physical parameter in assessment of renal function.

Podocytopathy: direct or indirect podocyte injury that results in glomerular origin proteinuria; can be associated with progression of CKD. This often occurs following alteration of molecules within the slit-pore membrane (nephrin, podocin) or loss of podocytes. Podocyte dysfunction or injury can be genetically mediated, or follow immune, infection, hemodynamic, or toxin related environmental factors. Healthy podocytes are important in the maintenance of normal glomerular architecture.

Pollakiuria: frequent passage of urine usually indicating urgency or pain from some lower urinary tract process (inflammation or partial obstruction). The volume of urine passed is usually small during these instances. Sometimes polyuric conditions will have increased frequency of voiding, but with large volumes.

Polycystic kidney disease (PKD): a form of CKD in which the number and size of cortical and medullary cysts progressively increases over time. It is an autosomal dominant disorder observed more frequently in Persian cats.

Polydipsia: an increase in the volume of water consumed by drinking. Daily water intake is >90 mL/kg/day for dogs and >45 mL/kg/day in cats in these instances. Polydipsia is usually a compensatory response in those with obligatory polyuria. Increased water intake occurs first followed by polyuria as the compensatory response in those with PPD.

Polyunsaturated fatty acids: fatty acids that contain more than one double bond in their backbone. Essential fatty acids are all PUFA, and are classified as either omega-3 (n-3) or omega-6 (n-6) depending on the placement of double bonds. The final carbon in the fatty acid chain is termed the omega carbon; omega-3 and omega-6 fatty acids have their first double bond on either the third or sixth carbon from the chain terminus, respectively. The most common omega-3 fatty acids are linolenic acid (18:3), EPA (20:5), and DHA (22:6). The most common omega-6 fatty acids are linoleic acid (18:2), and arachidonic acid (20:4). Depending on the total amount or ratio of omega-3 to omega-6 PUFA, inflammation can be either minimized or exaggerated in a variety of organs, including the kidneys.

Polyuria: passage of a larger volume of urine than normal, >20–40 mL/kg/day in dogs and >10–20 mL/kg/day in cats.

Postrenal proteinuria: addition of proteins to urine from bleeding or inflammation at anatomic sites below the kidneys, including the lower urinary and genital tracts; glomerular barrier integrity is normal.

Postvoid catch: collection of a urine sample after voiding of urine, often collected from a clean table top. Can also be less desirably collected from cage papers or pads.

Prerenal proteinuria: overload or overflow of low molecular weight proteins not normally present in plasma that are freely filtered across the normal glomerulus. These proteins enter tubular fluid in an amount that exceeds the ability of tubules to reabsorb the particular protein (e.g. myoglobin, hemoglobin, and light chains).

Progression of CKD: Refers to the inherent nature of patients with azotemic CKD to inexorably increase the number of intrarenal lesions and to further decrease excretory renal function based on GFR, serum creatinine, and SDMA. The rate for progression varies by the individual, with cats with CKD usually progressing more slowly than that in dogs.

Protein-losing nephropathy (PLN): usually refers to a clinically relevant glomerular disease, glomerular origin proteinuria, and a UPC ≥ 2.0. PLN may or may not be associated with azotemic CKD. Can be associated with varying degrees of hypoalbuminemia and edema in those with advanced disease.

Proteinuria: is a general term that refers to the detection of an abnormal amount of protein in the urine, but not the definitive nature of that protein(s). Proteinuria can be detected by urine chemistry dipstrip, UPC, MA, or urinary electrophoresis. Proteinuria can be classified as prerenal, renal, or postrenal.

Proximal tubule (PT): in between Bowman's capsule and the descending loop of Henle; includes the convoluted PT and the more distal straight portion (S3); about 2/3 of tubular fluid water and electrolytes are reabsorbed by the end of the proximal tubule.

Proximal convoluted tubule: the first portion of the proximal tubule, between Bowman's capsule and the pars recta (S$_3$).

Psychogenic polydipsia (PPD): sometimes called apparent PPD or primary polydipsia. Excess water drinking occurs in the absence of normal stimuli for thirst (dry mucous membranes, high circulating osmolality, and low blood pressure). In this instance, PD occurs first, followed by compensatory PU. Most other causes of PU/PD have obligatory PU followed by compensatory PD. USG often hyposthenuric at times but this depends on the magnitude of the water intake. Vacillation between very low and high USG supports this diagnosis.

Pseudocasts: elements observed during urine microscopy that resemble casts such as fibers, fibrin, or mucous strands and cells that accumulate along these linear structures.

Pyelitis: inflammation of the renal pelvis.

Pyelonephritis: inflammation of the renal pelvis and renal parenchyma beginning in the interstitium and extending to the tubules, glomeruli, and blood vessels; usually bacterial in nature.

Pyonephrosis: suppurative destruction of the parenchyma of the kidney with total or almost complete loss of renal function in that kidney.

Pyuria: the presence of excessive numbers of white blood cells in the urine (the presence of "pus" in the urine) indicating inflammation, but it does not by itself reveal the origin of the WBC. Often associated with bacterial infection, but can be encountered in sterile urine and inflammation from other causes (e.g. sterile urolithiasis, transitional cell carcinoma [TCC] of the bladder, acute interstitial nephritis, or acute glomerulonephritis).

Rapidly progressive glomerulonephritis: rare disease in dogs with severe acute to subacute glomerular injury. Immune complex deposition, glomerular proteinuria, RBC cast formation, and varying degrees of ATN are often part of this syndrome. Prognosis is usually poor without aggressive early immunosuppression.

Reactive cells: usually referring to the presence of urothelial cells identified during urine microscopy that are shed or desquamated into the urine secondary to inflammation associated with infection, urolithiasis, or trauma.

Red blood cell (RBC) cast: cast that contains predominantly intact RBC. Can be identified in those with active glomerular bleeding. These casts rapidly break up, so it is necessary to perform urine microscopy on fresh warm urine.

Refractometer: a device that compares the transmission of light through a urine sample to that of distilled water as an estimate of USG. Measures the bending of light as the refractive index (nD) which is then converted to a USG value. Manual methods use a shadow line to report the USG; digital devices report the USG value directly.

Renal biopsy: collection of renal tissue for histopathological evaluation. The most complete evaluation of renal tissue involves light microscopy with special stains, electron microscopy, and immunofluorescent microscopy. Needle biopsy can be obtained using ultrasound or laparoscopic guidance. Wedge biopsy from a surgical approach can also be used. Retrieved renal tissue consists mostly of cortical tissue as this path ensures enough glomeruli to allow a proper evaluation.

Renal blood flow: volume of blood delivered to the kidneys per unit time reported in mL/min or mL/min/kg. Most of the blood is delivered to the cortex with far less to the medulla. Glomerular filtration is derived from RBF. RBF is maintained at a steady level over a wide range of systemic blood pressures by autoregulation.

Renal clearance: see Clearance

Renal cortex: the outer portion of the kidney that has the highest oxygen concentration and contains most of the glomeruli, GFR, and RBF.

Renal diet: consists of a commercially available or homemade diet designed to help support renal functions and reduce progression during CKD. These diets are usually restricted to a varying degree in content (on an energy density basis) of protein, phosphorus, and salt; may also be restricted in calcium content. RDs often are supplemented with omega-3 PUFA, potassium salts, an alkalinizing source (e.g. citrate), and sometimes antioxidants. Phosphorus restriction during azotemic CKD is likely the most important dietary modification in these diets. Salutary effects during the feeding of an RD cannot be attributed to any one alteration in the nutrient profile. Not the same as a "low-protein diet", which in itself can have deleterious effects at times during CKD.

Renal disease: refers to detection of any structural and/or functional lesion(s) within the kidneys and not their extent. Renal lesions can be progressive or nonprogressive; loss of renal functions is expected when renal lesions continue to accrue. Renal disease can be focal without clinical signs or detectable adverse effect on renal functions, or these lesions can progressively increase as a continuum that results in renal insufficiency first and then azotemic renal failure.

Renal dysplasia: a particular type of familial nephropathy characterized by embryonic glomeruli, tubules, and interstitium. Renal dysplasia can be a form of azotemic or nonazotemic CKD at the time of diagnosis and tends to progressively worsen over time.

Renal failure, primary azotemic CKD: refers to an extensive loss of renal functions in association with loss of functional nephron mass. Azotemic CKD has been traditionally defined based on the finding of an increased serum creatinine concentration that has persisted for one to three months, often in association with impaired urinary concentrating capacity and some degree of renal proteinuria. Clinical signs may not be apparent with mild to moderate increases in serum creatinine.

Renal failure, primary azotemic AKI: sudden loss of functional renal mass severe enough to cause serum creatinine to escalate above the reference range, often in association with decreased ability to elaborate concentrated urine, and some combination of cylindruria, ±glucosuria, ±renal proteinuria. This renal injury may or may not be reversible following exposure to nephrotoxins, renal ischemia, or infections such as leptospirosis depending on the extent of the renal damage.

Renal fibrosis: the final common pathway that develops during progressive CKD. Characterized by the accumulation of extracellular matrix in the renal interstitium (scar) in association with nephron dropout, tubular atrophy, tubular dilatation, glomerulosclerosis, and various amounts of lymphoplasmacytic infiltration. Molecular mechanisms leading to fibrosis are not fully characterized but include enhanced RAAS activity (Angiotensin-II and aldosterone), NF-kappa Beta and TGF-B1.

Renal insufficiency, CKD: refers to the stage of CKD before overt azotemia has been detected, often in association with an impaired ability to elaborate concentrated urine. Decreased GFR is substantial but not yet advanced enough to result in azotemia. Renal insufficiency often progresses to azotemic CKD.

Renal proteinuria: exists when plasma proteins excessively cross the glomerulus, the proximal renal tubules fail to reabsorb filtered proteins, or protein is added to the urine as a result of tubulointerstitial bleeding and inflammation.

Renal medulla: the inner portion of the kidney that exists in a relatively low oxygen environment and low RBF. This area has the highest interstitial osmolality that is important for the elaboration of concentrated urine.

Renomegaly: the finding of an enlarged kidney(s) during abdominal palpation or imaging. Can be identified in those with complete or partial obstruction to one kidney, partial obstruction to both kidneys, during PKD, acromegaly, renal neoplasia, and compensatory hypertrophy. Sometimes confused with perinephric pseudocyst.

Residual proteinuria: an excessive amount of protein remaining after standard antiproteinuria treatment, usually that following the feeding of an RD and treatment with an ACE-I or ARB.

Residual urine: the volume of urine remaining in the bladder after urination. In health, the bladder evacuates nearly all its contents during voiding; <0.4 mL/kg postvoiding urine volume is considered normal

Sedi-Stain°: brand name of supravital stain developed for use in urine sediment manufactured by Becton Dickinson, Sparks, MA. The use of this stain enhances cellular detail with varying colors.

Segmental: a pathologic term referring to the glomerulus that indicates a partial involvement of that structure in the pathologic process described.

Single-nephron glomerular filtration rate (SNG-FR): GFR in nL/minute from a particular nephron. Average SNGFR is evaluated but there is considerable splay in SNGFR by nephron population. Global GFR (mL/min) follows that contributed by all the single nephrons.

Sodium-glucose cotransporter 2 (SGLT2) inhibitors: SGLT inhibitors (e.g. empagliflozin, dapagliflozin, and canagliflozin) are typically used in human medicine for better glycemic control during diabetes mellitus. They also importantly provide renoprotection during progressive CKD and proteinuria in patients with and without diabetes mellitus. Whether these salutary effects occur in dogs or cats with progressive CKD and proteinuria has not been determined.

Specific gravity, urine: the weight of urine divided by the weight of an equal volume of distilled water at the same temperature. Estimated clinically by refractometry.

Spermaturia: observation of sperm during urine microscopy.

Stranguria (strangury): passage of urine with pain and straining. Only drops of urine are expelled at times. Continued straining can occur even when the bladder contains very little volume or is completely empty.

Sulfosalicylic acid (SSA): compound added to clear urine in equal volumes that results in precipitation of urinary proteins. Albumin, globulins and Bence Jones proteins can be detected at low concentrations, so this method can be used for screening purposes or for follow-up of urinary protein dipstrip reactions. The turbidity that results following SSA is usually quantitated subjectively by visual inspection in veterinary medicine, but it can also be objectively quantitated using photometry.

Symmetrical dimethyl arginine: is a molecule that is a surrogate for estimation of GFR in dogs and cats. SDMA increases from prerenal, primary renal, and postrenal causes. SDMA increases earlier than serum creatinine in many dogs and cats with CKD, likely due to the loss of lean muscle mass that frequently develops during CKD which generates less creatinine. SDMA appears to increase on average when the GFR has decreased by 40%, compared to a decrease in GFR of 50–75% needed before serum creatinine increases in CKD.

Systemic hypertension: blood pressure that measures above the reference range in mm Hg for systolic, diastolic, and/or mean blood pressure. The measurement of systolic pressure by Doppler is considered the most reproducible and accurate in animals that are not under anesthesia. Sustained increased blood pressure increases risk for target organ damage (brain, retina, heart, kidneys). Can magnify glomerular proteinuria and progression of CKD.

Systemic inflammatory response syndrome: a dysregulated cytokine storm associated with release of acute phase reactants as a response to noxious stressors that include infection, surgery, trauma, ischemic reperfusion, and malignancy. Can lead to reversible or irreversible end organ damage. Sometimes associated with MA or increased UPC.

Tamm-Horsfall mucoprotein (uromucoid): an alpha globulin derived from the ascending loop of Henle, distal tubule, and collecting ducts; normally present in canine and feline urine at very low concentrations (0.5–1.0 mg/dL). THP is the matrix protein for urinary casts. Its concentration in urine declines in dogs with progressive CKD.

Telmisartan: an emerging ARB for treatment of systemic hypertension and glomerular proteinuria in dogs and cats; losartan is no longer recommended; see ARB.

Tonicity: the ability of a solution to cause water to move between body fluid compartments based on the concentration of impermeant solutes, largely determined by sodium and glucose. Effective osmolality is a synonym.

Tonicity, hypertonic: describes a solution, which when bathing body cells causes a net movement of water across the semipermeable cell membranes out of cells; denotes a higher osmotic activity than the solution being used for comparison.

Tonicity, hypotonic: describes a solution, which when bathing body cells causes a net movement of water across the semipermeable cell membranes into cells; denotes a lower osmotic activity than the solution being used for comparison.

Tonicity, isotonic: describes a solution in which body cells are bathed by a solution without a net flow of water across the semipermeable cell membranes; used to describe solutions which are of equal osmotic activity.

Trade-off hypothesis: theory of Bricker that the "trade-off" for maintaining external solute balance for a given solute as renal disease advances is the induction of one or more of the abnormalities of the uremic state.

Transitional cell carcinoma: a highly malignant tumor of transitional epithelium and is the most common tumor of the urinary bladder. The emerging preferred term is urothelial cell carcinoma (UCC).

Tubular proteinuria: proteinuria associated with tubular dysfunction (reduced reabsorption of protein in tubular fluid, secretion of protein or tubular necrosis); in tubular proteinuria, globulins predominate.

Upper urinary tract: kidneys and ureters.

Urea: a nitrogenous waste product synthesized in the liver that is freely filtered by GFR that undergoes varying amounts of tubular reabsorption depending on ECF volume and ADH status. Urea molecules importantly contribute to medullary hypertonicity needed for urine concentration. See also BUN.

Urea nitrogen: see BUN (SUN). Not the same as BUN.

Uremia: the constellation of clinical and biochemical abnormalities associated with a loss of a critical mass of functioning nephrons in azotemic CKD or azotemic AKI. Uremia includes the extrarenal manifestations of renal failure and is due to a critical loss of the conservation, excretory, and endocrine functions of the kidneys. Anorexia, weight loss, depression, stupor, vomiting, oral ulcers, anemia, mineralization, electrolyte and fluid imbalances, hormone deficits, and hormone increases can occur as manifestations of uremia. Uremic toxins contribute to the development of these clinical signs, but uremic toxins are incompletely understood and many have not been identified or measured.

Urethritis: inflammation of the urethra related to infection, obstruction, urethral catheterization, neoplasia, or exposure to irritating flushing solutions.

Urinalysis, complete: the systematic examination of a urine specimen which includes physical, chemical, and sediment findings.

Urinary sediment elements: leukocytes, erythrocytes, epithelial cells, casts, bacteria, fungi, parasites, sperm, crystals, and contaminants identified during urine microscopy.

Urinary sediment, active: increased numbers of WBC, RBC, nonsquamous epithelial cells, bacteria, and casts

Turbidity: an optical characteristic of urine that depends on how much scattering of light occurs when a light is beamed through the sample. Often used interchangeably with clarity and transparency. Turbidity is usually assessed manually by the naked eye during inspection of well-mixed urine in a clear container against a white backdrop. Normal urine is usually clear to slightly cloudy. Turbidity is usually reported as clear, slightly cloudy, cloudy, opaque, or flocculent. The presence of mucous, fibrin, crystalluria, WBC, RBC, epithelial cells, and bacteria contributes to increased turbidity. Some automated systems quantitatively measure light scatter as a more objective method to report turbidity.

Urinary protein-to-creatinine ratio: the ratio of total urinary protein (mg/dL) divided by urinary creatinine (mg/dL) measured by benchtop chemistry methods. A unitless number is generated that provides quantitative information about the magnitude of the proteinuria. UPC provides a correction for urine that is highly concentrated or minimally concentrated, as the urinary creatinine will correspondingly increase or decrease. A UPC <0.5 in dogs and <0.4 in cats is considered normal.

Urine concentration: assessed by USG or urine osmolality. The degree of urine concentration is compared to plasma osmolality and characterized as isosthenuric, hyposthenuric, minimally concentrated, or highly concentrated.

Urine concentration expected: random USG from healthy dogs often varies from 1.020 to 1.045 over the day. Dogs don't always drink to fulfill their physiological needs; consequently, a higher USG in dogs may be apparent in urine samples collected first thing in the AM before eating and drinking. USG for cats varies less than that in dogs over the day. An adequate USG is considered to be >1.030 in the dog and >1.035 in cat, though these tipping points should not be considered absolute. Hydration status impacts the expected USG; animals with dehydration should elaborate maximally concentrated urine if the kidneys are normal. USG is adequately concentrated in those with prerenal azotemia and minimally or nonconcentrated in those with primary renal azotemia.

Urine concentration, hypersthenuria or baruria: very old terminology rarely used today to describe urine that is concentrated greater than that of isosthenuria. Some definitions note that the USG is "unusually" high due to water loss. These terms provide little value, for it is important to know the magnitude of increase in USG above that for isosthenuria.

Urine concentration, hyposthenuria: elaboration of urine with an osmolality less than that of plasma and initial glomerular filtrate (300 mOsm/L). Urine osmolality during hyposthenuria is 50–290 mOsm/L. A USG of 1.001–1.007 is considered to be hyposthenuric. Hyposthenuria is a classic finding in those with complete CDI and can be encountered at times in those with NDI and PPD. Hyposthenuria describes urine that is truly dilute, as this degree of urine concentration is less concentrated than that of the plasma that was filtered by the glomerulus. The detection of hyposthenuria indicates that kidneys are able to actively dilute urine. The kidneys lose their ability to concentrate urine before they lose the ability to dilute urine during CKD.

Urine concentration, inappropriate: Refers to a USG that is lower than expected for healthy animals. Common finding in those with AKI and CKD, NDI, and endocrinopathies (e.g. Cushing's disease, diabetes mellitus, and diabetes insipidus).

Urine concentration, isosthenuria: describes the elaboration of urine with an osmolality similar to plasma and that of initial glomerular filtrate (approximately, 300 mOsm/L for dogs and cats). A USG in the range of 1.008–1.012 is classically considered to be isosthenuric in humans. Dogs and cats often have higher plasma osmolality than humans, so the definition of isosthenuria should have a higher range (1.008–1.017) to account for this. Persistent isosthenuria is common in azotemic AKI and CKD since those with severe disease have lost their ability to concentrate or dilute the urine.

Urine microscopy: examination of urine using brightfield microscopy at 100× (low power) and 400× (high power) to identify and enumerate elements in urine, usually following centrifugation or settling by gravity. Urine microscopy is an important part of the complete urinalysis, in addition to evaluation of physical and chemical properties.

Urinometry: a now rarely used method to estimate urine specific gravity using a flotation ball in a chamber with the urine sample.

Uroabdomen (uroperitoneum): the presence of urine in the peritoneal cavity following rupture anywhere from the kidney to the urethra. Rupture of the bladder is the most common cause following trauma or urethral obstruction. Hypernatremia, hypochloremia, and hyperkalemia develop as constituents of urine are absorbed across the peritoneum. The finding of an increase in the ratio of abdominal fluid to serum concentration for creatinine and or potassium confirms that the suspect abdominal fluid is urine.

Urolith: a crystalline concretion, which forms in the urinary tract; also known as a calculus or a stone.

Urolith, cystolith: stone in the bladder.

Urolith, nephrolith: stone in the kidney.

Urolith, urethrolith: stone in the urethra.

Urolithiasis: the disease condition associated with the formation of calculi in the urinary tract.

Uropathy: any disease of the urinary tract.

Urothelial cell carcinoma: suggested terminology to replace TCC; see Transitional cell carcinoma.

UTI: urinary tract infection, usually associated with bacterial organisms.

Vasa recta: parallel array of descending arterioles and ascending venules that arise from the efferent arterioles of juxtamedullary nephrons. This low blood flow system is responsible for preserving the local regions of interstitial hyperosmolality generated by countercurrent multiplication. Too much blood flow in this system can create MWO.

Vasopressin testing: administration of ADH (vasopressin) by injection, eye drops, or pills to determine the ability of the patient's kidneys to respond to ADH and elaborate concentrated urine. Moderate to large increases in USG occur in those with complete or partial CDI; variable responses can occur in those with MWO. Desmopressin is the form of synthetic ADH usually given.

Void: to urinate, as in the evacuation of urine from the bladder; part of micturition.

Water deprivation test (WDT): a test used to assess kidney function; it is conducted by withholding water from a patient, then observing and measuring urine output to determine the release of vasopressin and response of the kidneys (elaboration of concentrated urine). It is essential that the patient be carefully observed during the WDT so that harmful dehydration does not develop.

Index